CLINICAL MASSAGE *in the* HEALTHCARE SETTING

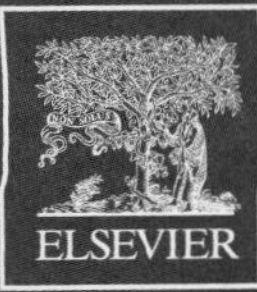

evolve

To access your Instructor Resources, visit:

http://evolve.elsevier.com/fritz/clinical

Evolve® Student Resources for ***Fritz: Clinical Massage in the Healthcare Setting,* 1st Edition** offers the following features:

Designed to work in conjunction with *Clinical Massage in the Healthcare Setting*, **Evolve Learning Resources** provides you with online, interactive resources that reinforce and expand on the concepts presented in the classroom.

Student Resources

- **Interactive Glossary!**
  Alll key terms in the book are defined and explained in this online glossary.
- **Chapter Evolve Activities.**
  Each chapter is supplemented with online content, such as further explanation of topics, a mini-image collection, matching exercises, and more!
- **Massage-related research has already been done for you!**
  Each chapter contains a list of terms related to massage research on which you can click to find the research already compiled from PubMed.

CLINICAL MASSAGE *in the* HEALTHCARE SETTING

Sandy Fritz, MS, NCTMB
Founder, Owner, Director, and Head Instructor
Health Enrichment Center
School of Therapeutic Massage and Bodywork
Lapeer, Michigan

Leon Chaitow, ND, DO
Registered Osteopathic Practitioner and Honorary Fellow
University of Westminster, London
United Kingdom

Glenn M. Hymel, EdD, LMT
Professor and Chair
Department of Psychology
Loyola University
New Orleans, Louisiana

With special contributions by

W. Randy Snyder, DC, MS, NCTMB, CHCQM
Owner/Director, College of Integrative Healthcare
Oceanside, California

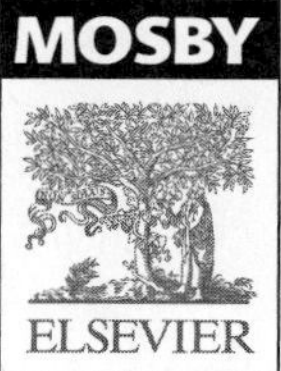

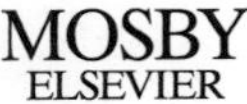

11830 Westline Industrial Drive
St. Louis, Missouri 63146

CLINICAL MASSAGE IN THE HEALTHCARE SETTING, FIRST EDITION ISBN: 978-0-323-03996-3
0-323-03996-0

Notice

Neither the Publisher nor the Authors assume any responsibility for any loss or injury and/or damage to persons or property arising out of or related to any use of the material contained in this book. It is the responsibility of the treating practitioner, relying on independent expertise and knowledge of the patient, to determine the best treatment and method of application for the patient.

The Publisher

ISBN 13: 978-0-323-03996-3
ISBN 10: 0-323-03996-0

Vice President and Publisher: Linda Duncan
Senior Editor: Kellie White
Senior Developmental Editor: Jennifer Watrous
Publishing Services Manager: Julie Eddy
Project Manager: Rich Barber
Designer: Kimberly Denando

Printed in Canada

Last digit is the print number: 9 8 7 6 5 4 3 2 1

DEDICATION

This textbook is dedicated to healthcare professionals who strive to provide competent and compassionate care. During the writing of this text, I underwent triple bypass surgery. My primary care physician, Dr. Sheila, identified vague symptoms that I would have ignored, even though I knew better. She called the emergency room at the hospital where I would go and got a recommendation from the nurses for a cardiologist. Nurses are the ones who know, by the way. Then she made the cardiologist appointment for me just in case I put it off, and she called me to make sure I went. The cardiologist worked with me to try medication for my symptoms, which were confusing and resembled acid reflux. The cardiologist was patient with me when I kept postponing the heart catheterization (the only definitive test for coronary artery disease) because some of the professional football players I worked with were playing in the Super Bowl that year. After the procedure was performed, he told me I would need bypass surgery. I then asked if it could wait a couple of weeks because I had an upcoming photo shoot for this book. He very firmly told me NO. He made sure that the best and most experienced surgeon performed my bypass. All of the nursing and support staff were great. The physicians' assistants were a little abrupt and acted impatient when I asked a bunch of questions and got after them. The doctor was glad I did.

About a year later, when I was working on the final drafts for this book, my oldest son, Greg, was hit by a car and critically injured. The police that informed us and the first responders and the paramedics on the scene went above and beyond the call of duty. The hospital chaplains, the emergency room nurses, and the trauma surgeon spent hours with us on the phone while the family made the 6-hour drive to where Greg was. They held the phone to my son's ear as we talked to him in case we did not get there in time. At the hospital, under these tragic circumstances, the staff—from the doctors to housekeeping personnel—were very caring and let their tears show. They hugged us and counseled us and helped us make the decisions about removing life support and organ and tissue donation. They stood aside as a group and wept with us while the family circled my son as he died. My daughter-in-law was pregnant, and they were especially gentle and nurturing to her.

Four months later my granddaughter was born at a different hospital. The staff knew our story and broke many rules for us so we could all be together. The nurses again were wonderful, and the doctor who delivered baby Calee was experienced. Because of this, he was able to manage some unusual circumstances that might have otherwise resulted in an emergency cesarean section. The head nurse saw me crying at the back of the birthing room-tears of joy and sorrow—and came and got me and put an ink print of baby Calee's foot on my arm that I can still see as I write this dedication.

So when I say that I dedicate this book to all these people who cared for me and my family, I hope you understand that I am speaking from all of my experiences during the writing of this book. I thank the many doctors, three different hospitals, and countless healthcare professionals. Bless their hearts, they deserve a massage.

—Sandy Fritz

For Debra Ann Hymel DiLeo and Angela Rose Hymel Songy, the two most loving & wonderful sisters any guy could ever hope to have!

—Glenn M. Hymel

FOREWORD

Massage has been referenced as the first form of medicine. However, as medicine evolved throughout the centuries and across varied societies and cultures, massage lost some of its footing in the medical field. Today, massage therapists can once again have a prominent role in the medical field. However, they have to be well trained and well versed in many aspects of modern medicine. *Clinical Massage in the Healthcare Setting* serves as a comprehensive and practical instructional textbook for massage therapists interested in pursuing medical-related work. Fritz, Chaitow & Hymel's work comprises a four-unit, well-organized volume that describes the varying facets of the modern medical field and the massage therapist's role within the hierarchical group of medical professionals.

Unit One emphasizes the rigors in maintaining professional standards and practices consistent with the medical model, and because today's medical field is a scientific field, the medical massage therapist is urged to develop an evidence-based knowledge of massage benefits. With this aim, a meticulous and authoritative chapter by Glenn Hymel reviews research methods terminology and includes a point-by-point section on how to read, evaluate, and interpret evidence-based scientific papers. A subsequent chapter is dedicated to the fundamentals of delivery and management of healthcare services, from the patient's rights and expectations, to descriptions of various medical settings (e.g, hospitals, assisted care living facilities, private medical practices), governmental healthcare systems, health insurance, record keeping, communication, legal and ethical constructs, to a brief section on getting a job as a massage therapist in the healthcare system. An entire, and necessary, chapter is devoted to the concept of preventive medicine and wellness of mind, body, and spirit and massage therapy's contributing role towards promoting a healthy lifestyle.

As opposed to the usual list of contraindications, Unit Two begins with a refreshing common sense approach that encourages therapists to consider how best to adapt massage for specific medical conditions or for regional or general body areas of concern. Chapter 6 undertakes an impressive major review of anatomical and physiological structures and systems, with particular foci on massage effects on neuroendocrine functioning, bodily fluid dynamics, the cardiovascular and respiratory systems, myofascial form, and joint and muscle structures and functions. Unit Two even contains a chapter on sanitation, including correct handwashing techniques and glove removal and disposal. The last chapters of Unit Two are dedicated to massage therapy terminology, techniques, current assessments, protocols, and applications.

Unit Three targets massage application to achieve specific outcomes in healthcare. Chapters in this unit present effective massage strategies to support the recovery process during the acute, subacute, and remodeling phases of healing and develop realistic expectations for working with people who have a chronic illness. Various factors are considered such as age, activity, type of health concern, and medical intervention as clinical reasoning becomes the method of providing appropriate massage care. The design of the unit helps the reader integrate and apply the content to be able to use massage effectively in each individual interaction between the patient and the massage therapist.

Finally, Unit Four presents case studies carefully designed to target common conditions presented to the massage therapist in the healthcare setting. In addition, each case describes related concerns, conditions, and complicating factors, so that the reader will understand that each situation is unique and requires an individualized treatment plan. The cases also reflect a category of care effectively addressed with massage, such as pain management, stress management, breathing normalization, increased mobility, and enhanced physical function. By studying each case, the student can use the model presented to help develop care plans for many different healthcare conditions.

Leon Chaitow's medical contributions are obvious throughout the book, and Sandy Fritz's clear and organized writing style and her "Just Between You and Me" boxes are insightful and humanistic. Colorful figures, illustrations, photos, and clear tables enhance the content of the material in each chapter.

A textbook of this depth serves as a one-volume primary reference source for the clinical massage therapist who desires a place in the medical profession. In particular, it is a "must have" textbook for massage therapists pursuing a career in the medical or healthcare world or for therapists who are already practicing. Massage therapy instructors, and any serious student of massage therapy, will also greatly benefit from investing in this scholarly and resourceful textbook.

Maria Hernandez-Reif, PhD
Professor
University of Alabama
Human Development and Family Studies
Tuscaloosa, Alabama

PREFACE

This text provides information for massage professionals to continue their education by preparing them to work successfully in the healthcare environment. It is a collaborative effort, which is important for reliable content. Sandy Fritz is the main author. Dr. Leon Chaitow, a trained and licensed osteopath and author, has provided content and editorial review throughout the text. Glenn M. Hymel, a psychology professor and author, has written a chapter on research, generated the Evolve site's research matrix as well as the PubMed hyperlinks for each chapter, and provided editorial review for the text. This is a great team. See the Evolve site that accompanies this book for resumes of the three authors. Our intent is to provide further educational structure for those who have successfully completed an entry level massage education. In the United States, this typically means a minimum of 500 contact hours with supervised instruction in a curriculum that covers medical terminology, anatomy, physiology, basic pathology, therapeutic massage theory and practice, ethics and professionalism, and record keeping. This content level is described in *Mosby's Fundamentals of Therapeutic Massage* and *Mosby's Essential Sciences for Therapeutic Massage: Anatomy, Physiology, Biomechanics, and Pathology*. Readers should have these textbooks as references.

MASSAGE IN HEALTHCARE

The terminology currently used to describe massage in the healthcare environment is inconsistent, so finding an appropriate name for this textbook was a challenge. Various terms are used to describe therapeutic massage in the healthcare environment, with *clinical massage* and *medical massage* being the most common. The premise of this text is that all massage is therapeutic and that the terms *clinical massage* and *medical massage* can be used interchangeably. Both tend to describe massage offered within the healthcare environment, serving people who are seeking preventive care or who have diagnosed medical conditions and are being treated at some level by a medical professional. *Clinical Massage in the Healthcare Setting* became the logical name for this textbook. There is an increasing trend for massage, as well as other complementary therapies, to be offered and integrated into the medical world.*

This textbook is specifically written to teach the massage professional how to build a successful career within traditional healthcare systems.

PURPOSE OF THIS BOOK

This Text is Not:

- **A pathology book,** although Unit Three does describe categories of illness and injury and recommendations for beneficial and safe massage treatment. You will need a good comprehensive pathology book, such as these:
  Salvo SG, Anderson SK: *Mosby's pathology for massage therapists* St. Louis, 2004, Mosby.
  Lee-Ellen C: *Pathophysiology*, ed. 3, St. Louis, 2005, Elsevier.
  Price SA, Wilson LM: *Pathophysiology: clinical concepts of disease processes*, ed. 6, St. Louis, 2002, Mosby.
- **A medications book,** although Unit Three does describe healthcare and general treatment strategies, including surgery and medication, and the Evolve site gives recommendations for the massage therapist to consider when problem-solving about the effect of massage combined with medication use. You will need a comprehensive medications book, such as these:
  Mosby's Drug Consult for Health Professions, St. Louis, Mosby, 2005.

*For specific information on how this is being done, obtain the book *Integrating Complementary Therapies in Primary Care: a Practical Guide for Health Professionals* by David Peters, Leon Chaitow, Gerry Harris, and Sue Morrison (Churchill Livingstone, 2002).

Winter H et al: *Complete guide to prescription & nonprescription drugs:* New York, 2005, Perigee Books; (revised and updated edition, October 30, 2004).

Ellsworth AJ: *Medical drug reference 2005 Textbook* (with CD-ROM PDA software), St. Louis, 2005, Mosby.

Tatro D: *Drug interaction facts 2004*, St. Louis, 2004, Facts and Comparisons.

- **A medical terminology book:** This is a must-have, along with a good medical dictionary. These medical terminology texts are recommended:

  Birmingham JJ: *Medical terminology: a self-learning text,* ed. 2, St. Louis, 1990, Mosby.

  Leonard P: *Building a medical vocabulary*, ed. 6, St. Louis, 2005, Mosby.

  Brooks ML, Brooks DL: *Basic medical language*, ed. 2, St. Louis, 2004, Mosby.

  These medical dictionaries are recommended:

  Mosby's Medical Dictionary, ed. 7, St. Louis, 2006, Mosby.

  Venes D: *Taber's Cyclopedic Medical Dictionary (Indexed) and Taber's Electronic Medical Dictionary* (CD-ROM V 3.0), ed. 20, 2005, FA Davis Co.

  Merriam-Webster's Medical Dictionary: Springfield, Massachusetts, 1995, Merriam-Webster.

  The Evolve site also has common medical terms, definitions, and abbreviations.

  All massage therapists should build a good reference library and keep it updated. The internet also provides up-to-date reference information.

This Text Does:

- Prepare you to make appropriate decisions about how to use massage to help people with pathology (disease and ailments) and various recurring types of medical care.
- Describe therapeutic massage applications and benefits in a manner acceptable for scientific communication.
- Prepare you to think and act professionally in the healthcare setting.
- Prepare you to be a contributing member of a multidisciplinary healthcare team.

FOCUS

The target populations served by the content described in this text are people who are ill or injured. There is also emphasis on preventive and wellness care. The text *Sports & Exercise Massage: Comprehensive Care in Athletics, Fitness, & Rehabilitation* (also part of the Mosby's Massage Career Development Series) targets the sport, fitness, and physical rehabilitation and orthopedic injury population. There is a significant overlap in methods and knowledge in the sports and exercise and healthcare career tracks, which all depend on the solid foundation of the theory and practice of therapeutic massage as presented in *Mosby's Fundamentals of Therapeutic Massage* and *Mosby's Essential Sciences for Therapeutic Massage*. This text has more focus on illness, acute and chronic, while the sports and exercise textbook has more focus on soft tissue injury. The target population discussed in this text has more systemic dysfunction, while those targeted in the sports and exercise massage text have physical performance-based issues that include soft tissue, joint, and osseous injury. Cardiovascular disease is discussed more in this text, while the aspects of cardiovascular rehabilitation involving exercise are discussed in the sports and exercise massage text.

Because of the focus of this text on systemic illnesses such as cancer, multiple sclerosis, diabetes, and others, and those soft tissue dysfunctions that affect the general population, much of the massage application in these chapters will be general in nature, targeting restorative mechanisms, maintenance of homeostasis, and palliative care. Soft tissue-related dysfunction targets common conditions such as headache, neck and shoulder pain, low back pain, tendinitis, bursitis, and arthritis. Pain and pain management are also important areas to consider. The relevance of the inflammatory response to seemingly unrelated diseases needs to be understood.

Various medical tests and treatments are covered, so that the massage therapist can make safe and beneficial decisions on how to use massage to complement those medical treatments being provided to the patient. Various medical environments and professionals are described (e.g., hospitals, physical therapy, private-practice physicians, mental health, chiropractic, long-term care, hospice). Unique conditions and requirements of the healthcare environment are discussed such as infection control, sanitation, HIPPA requirements, record keeping, third party insurance reimbursement, and supervision.

KEY FEATURES

The text is divided into four units.

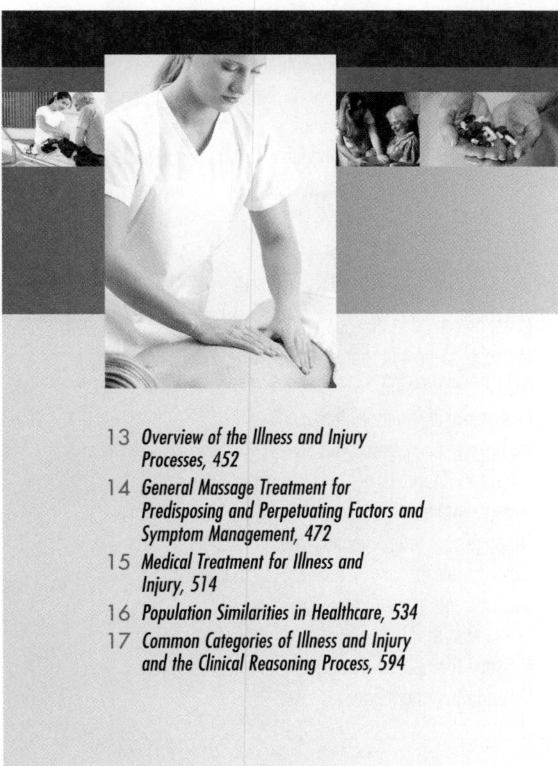
13 Overview of the Illness and Injury Processes, 452
14 General Massage Treatment for Predisposing and Perpetuating Factors and Symptom Management, 472
15 Medical Treatment for Illness and Injury, 514
16 Population Similarities in Healthcare, 534
17 Common Categories of Illness and Injury and the Clinical Reasoning Process, 594

- Unit One concentrates on information needed to work successfully in the healthcare world.
- Unit Two covers therapeutic massage application.
- Unit Three covers massage and specific treatment protocols for various medical conditions.
- Unit Four consists of a series of case studies to integrate the textbook content.

The entire textbook supports a clinical reasoning model and massage application focusing on outcomes.

The workbook section for each chapter challenges readers to expand their clinical reasoning skills.

246 UNIT TWO MASSAGE APPLICATION FOR HEALTHCARE BENEFIT

WORKBOOK

1. Choose a current bodywork method with which you are familiar (e.g., Swedish massage, reflexology, shiatsu, deep tissue massage) and describe it in terms of stimulus and forces.

   Example: Deep tissue massage (my personal pet peeve; there is no such modality, really)

   Depth of pressure—Moderate to deep
   Drag—Moderate to intense
   Duration—Intermediate (60 seconds)
   Frequency—Two or three repetitions
   Speed—Slow
   Rhythm—Even
   Consists of mechanical force application to affect connective tissue structures.
   Stimulus to deep muscles by inhibition of pressure, either to belly or attachment.
   Muscle energy methods are appropriate with primary application of localized tissue lengthening and cross-fiber stretching.

2. Watch someone give a massage (can be a video or DVD) and describe the application in terms of stimulus and force.

   Example: The massage began with superficial glide to assess skin temperature, texture, and bind. The glide assessment identified an area of bind in the midscapular region. Compressive force was increased to moderate and the direction was changed, which moved tissue into the ease position. The tissue was held for 30 seconds and then moved into the bind direction. At bind, drag was increased and sustained for 30 seconds. The tissue then was kneaded.

Found throughout the text are "Just Between You and Me" boxes, which help the reader consider the text information in relationship to the real world.

JUST BETWEEN YOU AND ME

Please don't confuse these specific treatment methods with the concept of medical massage. Most of the time, these methods are too intense and too aggressive to be used on sick or injured people. Clinical/medical massage is not a collection of methods, but rather an appropriate action in the setting of healthcare delivery.

These boxes are written by the lead au-thor, Sandy Fritz, and reflect her experiences and opinions about ma-ssage therapy practice.

Research is validating massage, making its inclusion into healthcare possible.

evolve

The following terms and expressions specific to Chapter 6 have already been used to search PubMed for the latest research literature available. The *Click Here for Massage* feature associated with this chapter on your textbook's Evolve website allows you to hyperlink to a continually updated PubMed search of research literature that corresponds to this subject.

Hyperlink Search Terms

Massage autonomic nervous system
Massage cardiovascular system
Massage central nervous system
Massage emotion neuroendocrine
Massage energy systems
Massage fluid dynamics
Massage gate control theory
Massage myofascial
Massage neuroendocrine
Massage parasympathetic nervous system
Massage respiratory system
Massage sensitization neuroendocrine function
Massage somatic nervous system
Massage sympathetic nervous system

Each chapter in the book contains a list of pertinent search terms on PubMed, which are supported with research links on the Evolve site.

The healthcare environment is a unique place requiring a specific skill set and professional set of behaviors to be successful. Recent development in mental health and general wellness and preventative care support the current trends for a more holistic approach to healthcare.

ELECTRONIC SUPPORT

Electronic ancillaries are key features of this title. The Evolve site that supports this text is extensive and includes a research matrix as well as links to research sites; access to support material such as insurance, pharmacology, and nutrition; and information expansion for most chapters. Information expansion is most heavily emphasized in the anatomy and physiology chapter, with additional material on neurotransmitters, fluid dynamics, body systems, and much more. The Evolve site also includes a comprehensive collection of PubMed hyperlinks that support best practices and justification for massage application. Each hyperlink is immediately and continuasly updated in real time wherever a user activates the link by clicking on the designated search term. A comprehensive glossary featuring key terms from all chapters is included on the Evolve site and provides audio pronunciations for some words. The Evolve content is highlighted in the book within special boxes bearing an Evolve icon.

evolve

The following terms and expressions specific to Chapter 5 have already been used to search PubMed for the latest research literature available. The *Click Here for Massage* feature associated with this chapter on your textbook's Evolve website allows you to hyperlink to a continually updated PubMed search of research literature that corresponds to this subject.

Hyperlink Search Terms

Massage anxiety
Massage cautions
Massage condition management
Massage contraindications cautions
Massage depression
Massage healing rehabilitation
Massage impingement syndromes
Massage indications
Massage mood
Massage pain fatigue management
Massage relaxation
Massage soft tissue dysfunction
Massage stress
Massage therapeutic change
Massage treatment goals

The book is also supported by an extensive DVD, playable on both set-top DVD players and in computers. It includes more than 90 minutes of technique video showing the specific applications described in the book, as well as the entire general and palliative protocol (found on the Evolve site), and several ARCHIE animations that feature biological functions and medical procedures for enhanced student learning. Each video clip and animation on the DVD is referenced in the textbook through double-numbered icons, directing the students to where they can find particular clips on the DVD.

The text can be used as a self-study tool or in a formal classroom setting. Comprehensive instructional support materials are available for the educators using this textbook. The authors are confident that achieving competency in the information covered will prepare the reader for a rewarding career in therapeutic massage in the healthcare world. The massage therapist pursuing a career in healthcare will benefit from an understanding of all these aspects of clinical massage as part of an integrated medical practice.

ACKNOWLEDGMENTS

THANK YOU TO THE FOLLOWING INDIVIDUALS

Production team: Rich Barber, Julie Eddy, Kim Denando

Editorial team: Kellie White, Jennifer Watrous, April Falast

Multimedia team: Cindy Ahlheim, Tom Pohlman, Bruce Siebert

Photographer: Jim Visser

Video team: Chuck Le Roi, Chris Roider, Christie Henry, Kelly Stallman

The models: our friends and family.

Amy Husted: Sandy's assistant, for keeping the three authors coordinated and the manuscript organized.

CONTENTS

Unit One The World of Healthcare, 1

1 Massage and Healthcare: A Professional Perspective, 2
2 Research Essentials for Massage in the Healthcare Setting, 20
3 Medical and Health-Related Professions, 54
4 Preventive Medicine, Wellness, and Lifestyle, 86

Unit Two Massage Application for Healthcare Benefit, 114

5 Indications and Contraindications to Massage, 116
6 Pertinent Anatomy and Review of Physiology, 140
7 Sanitation, 196
8 Review and Application of Massage, 208
9 Massage Application Assessment for Physical Healing and Rehabilitation, 248
10 Focused Massage Application, 314
11 General Massage Protocol and Palliative Variation, 380
12 Unique Circumstances and Adjunct Therapies, 432

Unit Three Massage Application for Specific Healthcare Outcomes, 450

13 Overview of the Illness and Injury Processes, 452
14 General Massage Treatment for Predisposing and Perpetuating Factors and Symptom Management, 472
15 Medical Treatment for Illness and Injury, 514
16 Population Similarities in Healthcare, 534
17 Common Categories of Illness and Injury and the Clinical Reasoning Process, 594

Unit Four Case Studies, 676

18 Case Studies, 678

Appendix: Massage Protocols, 759

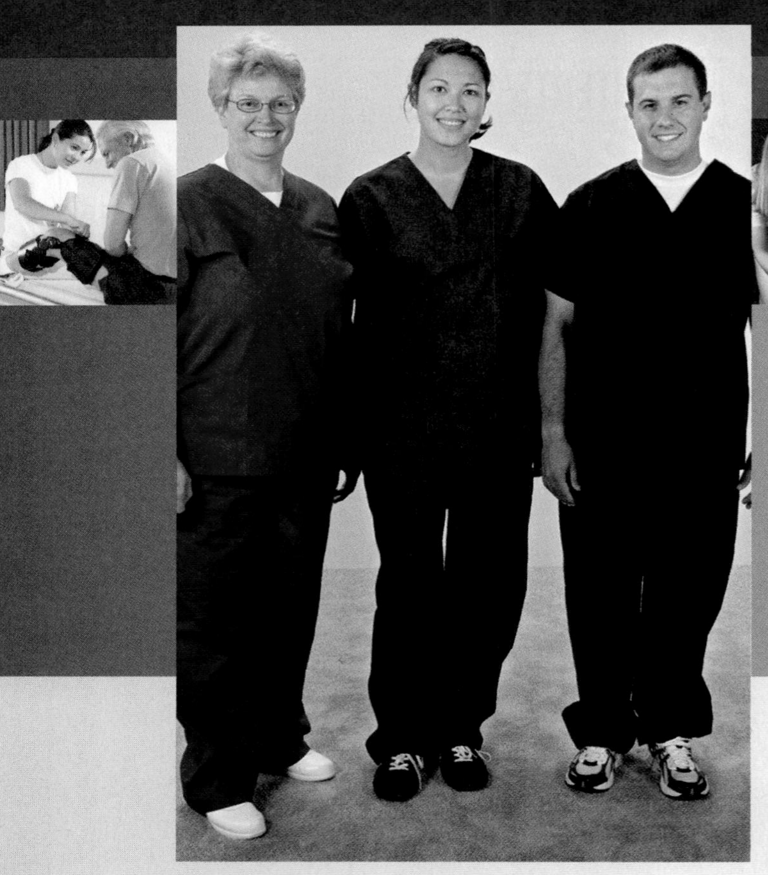

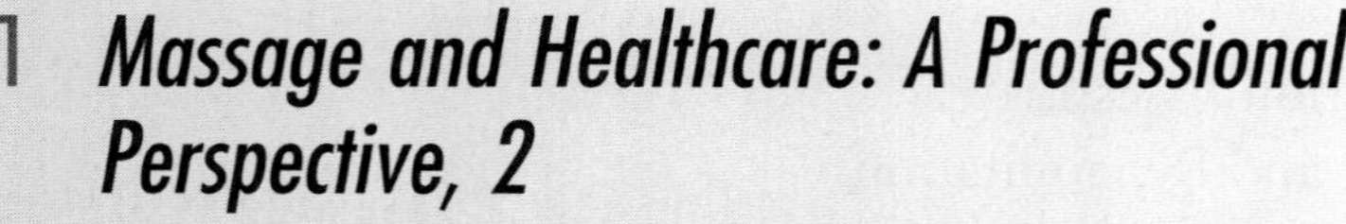

1 *Massage and Healthcare: A Professional Perspective, 2*

2 *Research Essentials for Massage in the Healthcare Setting, 20*

3 *Medical and Health-Related Professions, 54*

4 *Preventive Medicine, Wellness, and Lifestyle, 86*

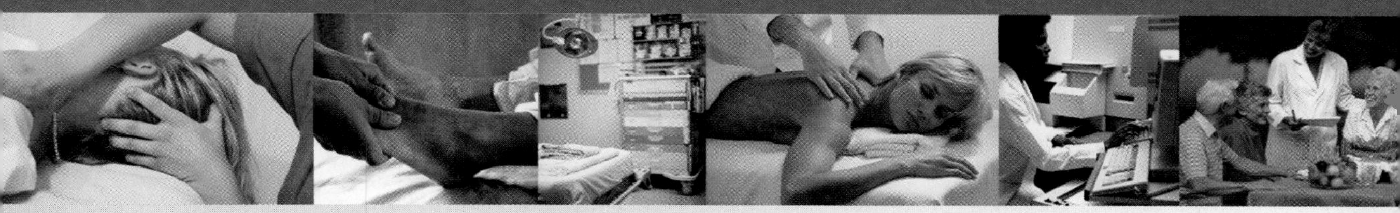

UNIT ONE

THE WORLD OF HEALTHCARE

This unit describes the integration of massage therapy into the healthcare setting. Chapter 1 provides an overview of what it is like to work with patients in the medical setting from the perspective of the main author, Sandy Fritz. It is important to have a sense of the big picture before you examine the details. It also is helpful to gain an appreciation of the personal side of a career focus from someone who has already experienced the challenges and rewards of a career in healthcare. Throughout the text you will find boxes titled Just Between You and Me. The information in these boxes will help you consider the text information in relation to the real world. The boxes are written by Sandy Fritz and reflect her experiences and opinions about massage therapy practice. Research is in the process of validating massage, making its inclusion in healthcare possible. The healthcare environment is a unique setting that requires specific sets of skills and professional behaviors for success. Recent developments in mental health, general wellness, and preventive care support the current trend toward a more holistic approach to healthcare. The massage therapist who intends to pursue a career in healthcare will benefit from an understanding of all these aspects of clinical massage as part of an integrated medical practice.

Chapter 1 Concept Map

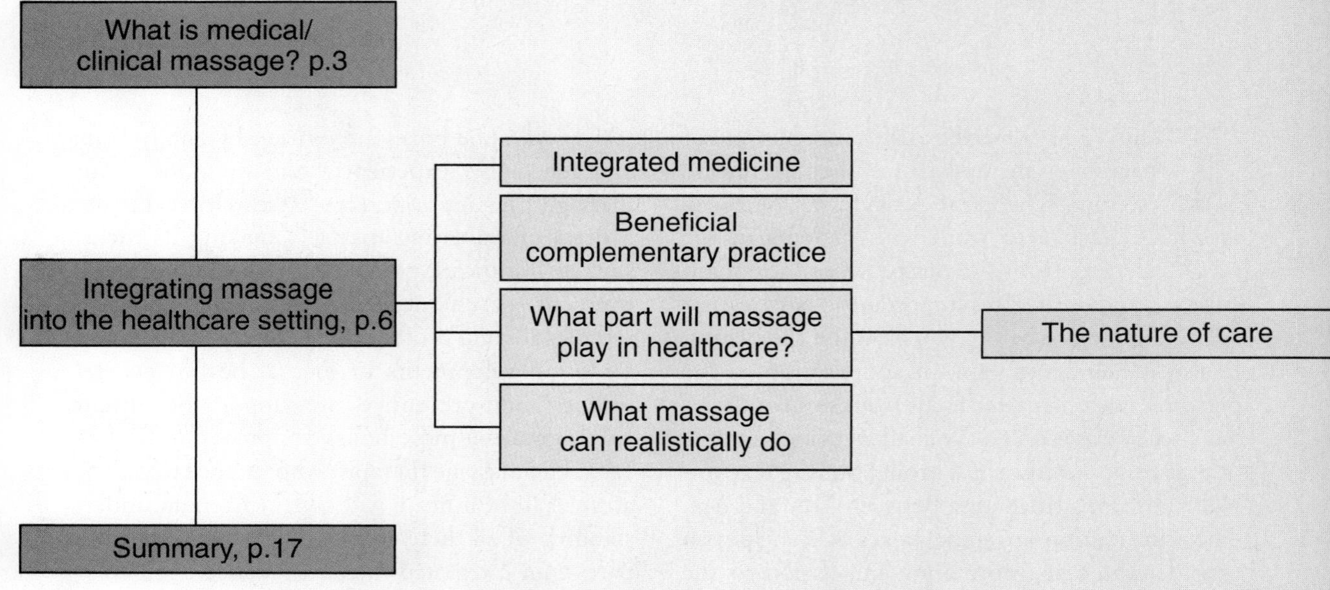

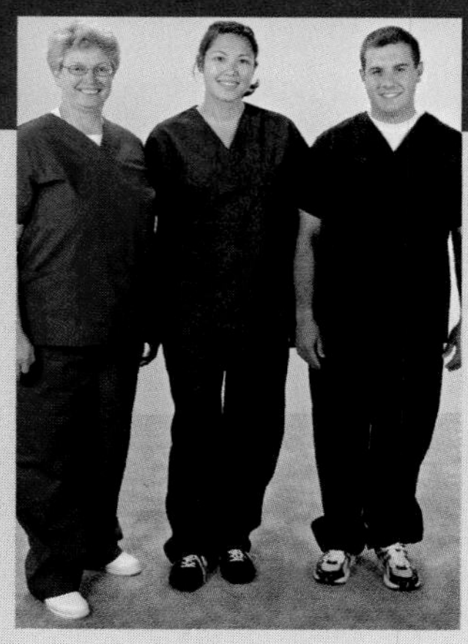

CHAPTER 1

MASSAGE AND HEALTHCARE: A PROFESSIONAL PERSPECTIVE

Key Terms

Alternative
Biomedical model
Complementary
Complementary and alternative medicine (CAM)
Ethical dilemma
Ethical distress
Ethics
Etiquette
Hierarchy
Integrated medicine
Medical/clinical massage
Medically fragile

For definitions of key terms, refer to the Evolve website.

OBJECTIVES

Upon completion of this chapter, the reader will have the information necessary to:

1 Identify the practice parameters of therapeutic massage in the healthcare setting.
2 Evaluate personal motivation for a career in the medical setting.

This chapter provides a personal* and realistic overview of massage integrated into the healthcare world. The dialog is casual, the experiences are real, and the advice is valid. This chapter represents what I would present as an instructor during orientation for a course for advanced students who want to develop the knowledge and skills to be successful in the healthcare environment. Because a textbook is a teacher, let this chapter speak to you as a caring instructor who is setting the stage for comprehensive study in a specialty career for therapeutic massage.

*Sandy Fritz is the primary author of this textbook.

WHAT IS MEDICAL/CLINICAL MASSAGE?

Definitions are difficult. As was pointed out in the introduction to this textbook, no agreement has been reached in the massage community on what constitutes the knowledge base and scope of practice for a career in therapeutic massage. Nevertheless, for this text to make sense, a definition is necessary. For the purposes of this textbook, **medical/clinical massage** (simply *massage* in the remainder of the text) is an outcome-based

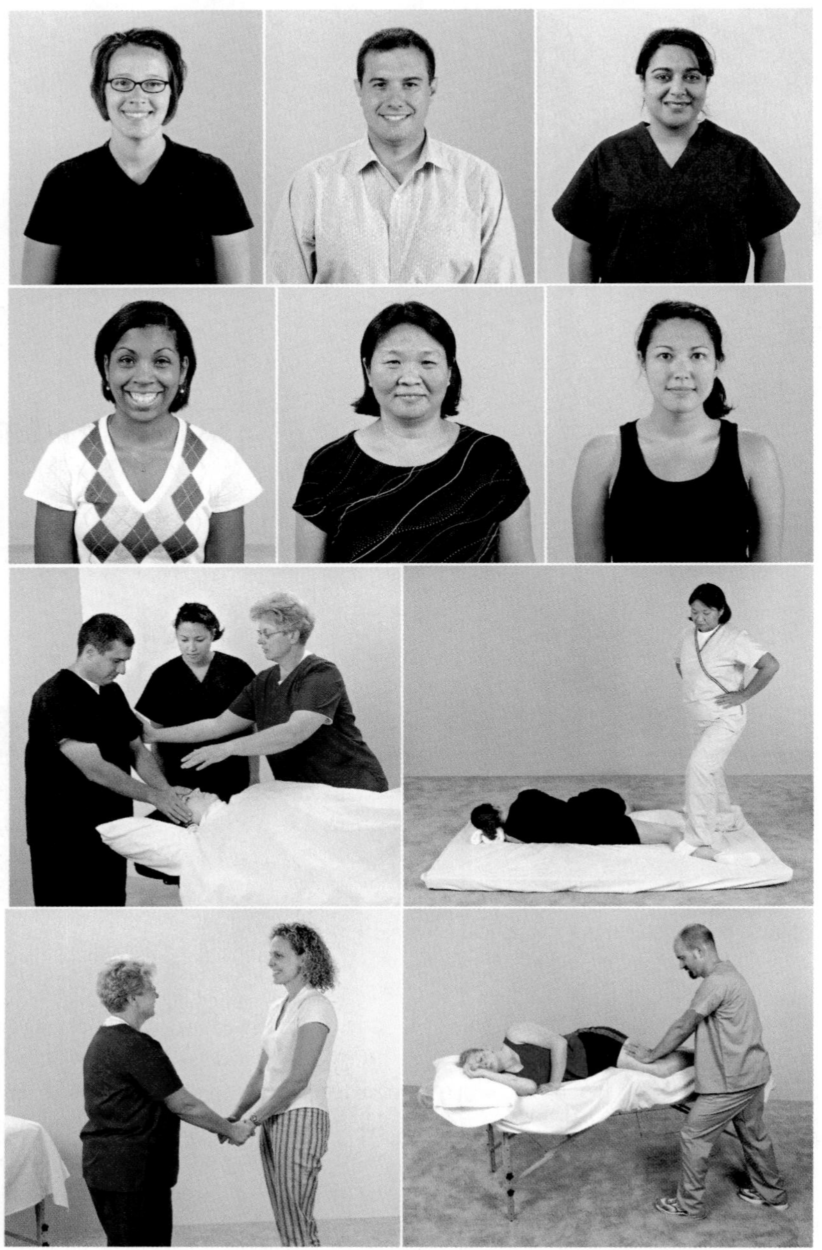

Massage therapists and patients of both genders and many different sizes, shapes, colors, cultures, and ages are working and learning how to help others in the world of healthcare.

treatment specifically targeted to address conditions that have been diagnosed by an appropriate healthcare professional. Massage is used as an aspect of a total treatment program. The focus is not on what kind of massage procedures are used, but rather on massage therapy as it relates to the diagnosis, treatment prescriptions, and determined outcomes for the patient.

Massage professionals typically call the people they work with *clients;* however, in the healthcare

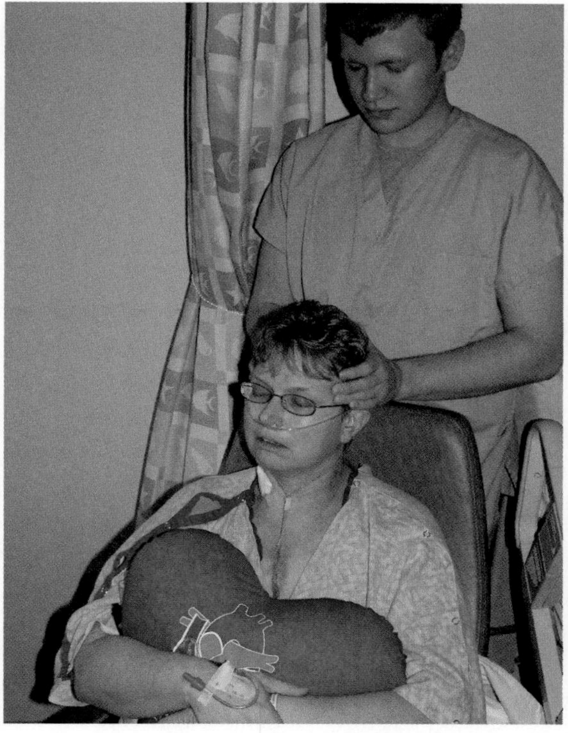

FIGURE 1-1 ■ Postsurgical massage. (Photograph courtesy Laura Cochran.)

setting, the massage therapist is working with the *patients* of the supervising healthcare providers (Figure 1-1).

Massage therapists do not diagnose. Instead, they typically work from a "prescription," following treatment orders. This is the nature of the healthcare environment. Healthcare settings are not the arena for independent practice by the massage professional or for nonproductive conflicts that may arise among the members of a multidisciplinary team. Working in the healthcare environment requires a collaborative spirit and the ability to follow orders, to relay accurate information (both written and verbal), and to contribute intelligently to the care of patients. Massage therapists who want to develop a career in this area must have a "team player" attitude and must be willing to accept supervision and instruction from medical professionals. Deference to the supervising physician, nurse, or other healthcare professional is required. Face it; they have a more comprehensive education than the typical massage therapist. They also shoulder responsibility for serious and even life-and-death decisions made during healthcare service. Healthcare professionals may not know as much about massage as you, but in general they do know more about healthcare. In choosing a career in the healthcare environment, massage therapists must understand the responsibility of providing service to people with healthcare challenges. This is not a decision that should be taken lightly (Figure 1-2).

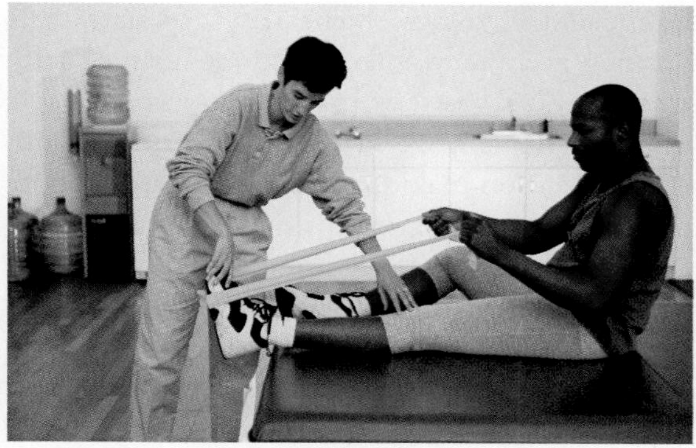

FIGURE 1-2 ■ An example of physical medicine.

Another common denominator in healthcare is the value and constraints of various types of health insurance. In some situations, such as private practice, a massage therapist may receive insurance reimbursement outside the traditional healthcare setting. Other cases require a physician referral and preauthorization. Access to health insurance–reimbursed massage care may be available if it is included as part of a person's healthcare coverage. However, in many (if not most) healthcare environments, the norm is a process of billing and reimbursement, as dictated by all the regulations governing payment for care. Massage therapists need to be able to maintain compliance with health insurance billing and reimbursement requirements. Even in private massage therapy practice, the components of team care, effective communication, and respect are essential.

Highly trained massage therapists are able to discuss the treatment plan intelligently with various medical professionals, to provide valid input, and, if disagreement arises, to state their position accurately and professionally and justify recommendations they make to supervising personnel. This is a world of ethical behavior and ethical decision making. Maintaining appropriate professional boundaries is important. The more complex a patient's condition and life circumstances are, the more balance is required of the massage therapist between dedication in service and the ability to remain somewhat neutral and objective in professional practice. Supervision and sharing the responsibility of patient care help maintain this delicate balance.

The term **medically fragile** is sometimes used to describe patients with serious and complex medical conditions. *Fragile* is a good word. Those who choose to serve people with illness and injury need to handle them like delicate glass globes. One of the biggest mistakes massage therapists make is to do too much too soon, requiring the patient to strain adaptive mechanisms even more. Because of these patients' already fragile nature, the healthcare team continually must make decisions on whether a patient can benefit from treatment or will be excessively stressed by it.

In this text, massage application is presented as an outcome-based process that is necessary to develop and/or follow treatment plans. It is assumed that the reader has completed a comprehensive entry level course of study and is proficient in the fundamentals of massage application. Those fundamentals are reviewed but not taught in this text. Some additional assumptions are made as well:

- Typically the target population is ill or injured; however, preventive healthcare is increasing, as reflected in the growing popularity of wellness programs and medical spas.
- The more injured or ill the patient, the more basic the massage application.
- Massage should support, not interfere with, medical treatment.
- Healing is a process of the body, mind, and spirit that requires a multidisciplinary approach.
- "Healing" does not necessarily mean "curing." Successful coping is a healing process.
- Living well with hope and compassion, regardless of circumstances, is an important goal of healing.
- In the healthcare setting, massage targets the body, and maintaining an appropriate scope of practice is necessary. Therefore massage therapists respect and honor the mind and spirit aspects of treatment, but they refer to appropriate professionals for patient care.
- Respect for the patient and the healthcare team is paramount.
- Dying is an important part of living and should be treated with compassion and dignity.

INTEGRATING MASSAGE INTO THE HEALTHCARE SETTING

The emerging trend in healthcare generally can be labeled the *biopsychosocial model* of medicine. The concept of health has become a metaphor for wholeness. By definition, the term **complementary** refers to approaches or therapies that are used in addition to conventional medicine treatments, such as the use of acupuncture or massage with physical therapy and medications in patients with chronic pain syndromes. The term **alternative** refers to approaches or therapies that are used instead of or in place of conventional medicine, such as the use of homeopathy and homeopathic remedies instead of pharmaceutical medications. In everyday practice, this clear distinction is lost. This text is based on the concept of massage as a complementary method, not an alternate approach to care.

The term **complementary and alternative medicine (CAM)** refers to the use of approaches, therapies, and treatments that are not considered part of the current biomedical model of medicine (Figure 1-3). The **biomedical model** is based on clearly defined philosophies and approaches to health and illness or injury that are based on the beliefs and values of Western scientific culture. CAM encompasses a broad range of philosophies and beliefs about the nature of health, healing, illness, and disease that are different from those on which the Western healthcare system is based.

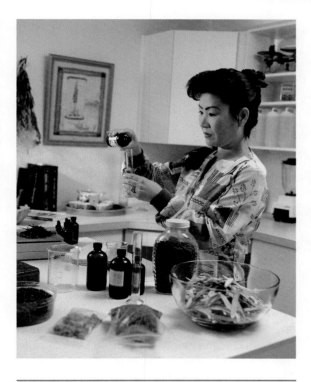

FIGURE 1-3 ■ A CAM practitioner at work.

Many complementary and alternative approaches are derived from healthcare systems from other cultures and other countries, such as the use of the meridian system and the concept of *qi* in the diagnosis and treatment of illness in traditional Chinese medicine (TCM). Other CAM approaches have emerged from visionary ideas developed by individuals such as Milton Trager or Ida Rolf.

Complementary therapies are considered whole medical systems (e.g., TCM, Ayurveda, therapeutic massage). The various systems differ somewhat in their philosophical approaches to the prevention and treatment of disease, but they have a number of common elements. These systems are based on the beliefs that:

- The body has the power to heal itself.
- Most health problems can be seen to derive from a failure of the tissues or of the individual to adapt to the biochemical, biomechanical, and/or psychosocial stressors of life.
- Healing often involves the use of multiple techniques, involving the mind, body, and spirit, to enhance the individual's adaptive capacity (self-healing), to reduce the adaptive load, or to minimize excessive symptomatic responses.
- Treatment often is individualized and depends on the presenting symptoms, as well as on the context from which they emerged and the processes involved.

Unfortunately, at this point, research conducted by the National Center for Complementary and Alternative Medicine (NCCAM) focuses on "individual therapies with an adequate experimental rationale, rather than on evaluating whole systems of medicine as they are commonly practiced."* The "whole system" approach to healthcare likely is more effective because the pieces of those systems exert synergistic influences. However, even with this research limitation, complementary modalities have been shown to be beneficial in some instances. For the sake of clarity in this text, medical practices currently derived from a biomedical, Western scientific model are called *conventional healthcare.*

Many conventional healthcare professionals express frustration and concern at the inability to effectively treat lifestyle-related illnesses, particularly those that are chronic, with standard approaches using medication, surgery, and other such methods. Nonconventional approaches to treatment of these conditions (e.g., massage) have become more accepted because the intent is to emphasize both care in a wider context of mind-body-spirit interconnectedness and the importance of supporting wellness in addition to treating the pathologic condition. The healthcare professions would be thankful if complementary methods could provide effective (and less potentially harmful) treatments for difficult-to-treat conditions by stimulating and supporting the body's self-regulatory processes.

Growing ethnic diversity makes it important to be sensitive to and respectful of cultural influences that affect a patient's behavior and beliefs (Figure 1-4). This respect extends to the historical and cultural bases of many complementary or alternative therapies. In the past, many of these vast, intricate systems have been exploited and

*Modified from National Center for Complementary and Alternative Medicine (NCCAM) Publication No. D236, October, 2004. http://nccam.nih.gov

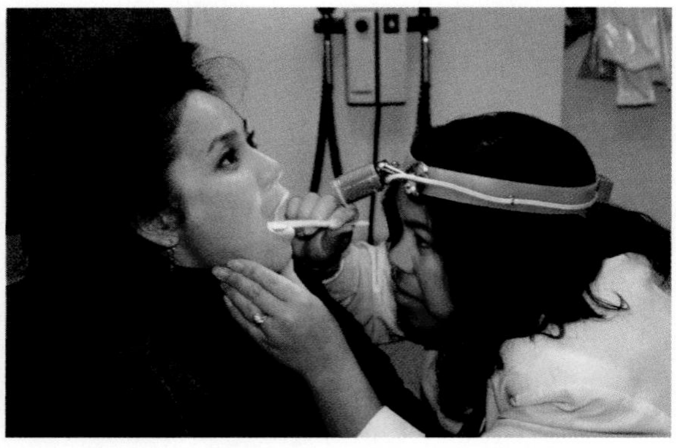

FIGURE 1-4 ■ Diversity in the clinical setting.

misused by people with insufficient training or appreciation of the depth and complexity of the system. Weekend classes in all sorts of methods have become available, leading those who attend to feel as if they can competently practice the system. This insults the extensive training and dedication of practitioners who have committed years of education and experience to becoming proficient in a specific health practice. The most common example of this is separating acupuncture from the vastness of the entire traditional Chinese medical system.

JUST BETWEEN YOU AND ME

This text describes therapeutic massage. It is a system in and of itself. It truly takes years of study and practice to become excellent at this form of therapy. It is not possible or necessary to know all the modalities or systems of healing encompassed by complementary and alternative medicine; however, some with massage training take a short-term workshop in another subject and then present qualifications as if they practice the system. You can't learn a system in 2 days. You can't really learn a system in 2 years. Typically, a practitioner needs 5 to 10 years of education and experience to really own any sort of skill, including massage. Be ethical and support interdisciplinary practice. You have decided to be a massage therapist; therefore, be the very best. Don't try to be an herbalist or a practitioner of Ayurveda, for example. Instead, learn enough about the various complementary and alternative systems so that you can refer clients when appropriate, and support and respect the professionals who have dedicated themselves to comprehensive study.

The popularity of complementary and alternative medicine is not a new phenomenon. In the past, because of the harsh approaches and unsuccessful outcomes offered by Western, or "scientifically" educated physicians, more and more people chose "alternative" healers. These treatments, which were gentler and more natural, involved the use of herbs, lifestyle changes, nutrition, and an approach that incorporated the whole person. With the increasing popularity of alternative practices, and as Western-educated physicians began to use some of those practices themselves, conventional medical practice became more interested in alternative modalities.

In 1900, many of the practitioners of medicine were "alternative" physicians.[1] In the early 1900s, the American Medical Association (AMA), which had been formed in 1847, issued a statement to its members saying that it was unethical for physicians and members of the AMA to consult, confer, or interact with "alternative" practitioners. This was the start of the exclusion of any medical approaches or treatments that were not considered within the mainstream of medicine. Other factors also contributed to the near disappearance of alternative health approaches, such as the cell theory of Rudolf Virchow (1855) and the germ theory of Louis Pasteur (1862) in the mid-1800s, followed by the discovery of x-rays in the early 1895 and then by the discovery of penicillin in 1929.

The discovery of antibiotics was a pivotal point for the emergence of conventional medicine. The use of alternative medicine reverted to more of a folk medicine practice and planted the seeds in the United States from 1920 to 1960. However, it remained an important aspect of healthcare in other parts of the world, where doctors of chiropractic (DCs), doctors of naturopathy (NDs), and doctors of osteopathy (DOs) remained active.* About 1970, alternative approaches to health and healing began to resurface in the United States.

The social upheaval of the 1960s changed the healthcare culture. Throughout the next three decades, the cost of healthcare was becoming prohibitive. The emergence of the field of psychology

*Dr. Leon Chaitow, one of the authors of this text, qualified as an ND and a DO in 1960 in the United Kingdom and joined a thriving profession.

and the study of the role of the mind in illness and disease were significant influences, as was recognition of the debilitating and sometimes fatal side effects of medications previously thought safe. The emergence of resistant strains of bacteria, the epidemic created by the spread of the human immunodeficiency virus (HIV) and acquired immunodeficiency syndrome (AIDS), and the increasing inability to medically treat "lifestyle" diseases successfully fueled a demand for change. We now are beginning to embrace and refine the concepts of multidisciplinary and interdisciplinary healthcare.

JUST BETWEEN YOU AND ME

I was a teenager in the 1960s. By the late 1970s and early 1980s, the push for alternative medicine was really taking hold. Guess who was there: the old hippies from the 1960s. Thought you might find that interesting.

People are looking for a kinder, gentler, more natural approach to health and healing. They are also looking for more choices and greater control in their health decisions, and they are less likely to accept the adverse effects of many biomedical treatments. The conventional medical system is becoming more open to integrating other systems, philosophies, approaches, and treatments into the care provided to a growing diversity of patients. These changes are the basis for the transition of many alternative practices into the contemporary healthcare category and support a more integrated care system.

In 1991 Congress established the Office of Alternative Medicine (OAM) as an agency of the National Institutes of Health (NIH), which became the National Center for Complementary and Alternative Medcine (NCCAM) in 1998. The purpose was to facilitate the evaluation of alternative medical treatments and their effectiveness through research and other initiatives. The initial budget for this undertaking was $2 million. However, before it could begin the process of evaluation, the OAM needed a classification system to better identify the alternative modalities. Initially, seven groups were created, but the classification since has been revised to five major domains[2]:

- *Alternative health systems:* Traditional, Oriental medicine, Ayurvedic (Indian) medicine, Tibetan medicine, Native American medicine, homeopathy, naturopathy.
- *Mind-body interventions:* Meditation, imagery, hypnosis, biofeedback, yoga, tai chi, qigong, prayer, spiritual healings, soul retrieval, intuitive diagnosis.
- *Biologically based therapies:* Herbal medicine, special diets (Ornish, Pritikin, Weil, South Beach, Atkins, and macrobiotic orthomolecular medicine), iridology.
- *Manipulative and body-based methods:* Chiropractic, osteopathy, craniosacral therapy, massage, reflexology, Pilates, rolfing, structural integration, Trager body work, Alexander technique.
- *Energy therapies:* Qigong, reiki, polarity therapy, therapeutic touch, electromagnetic therapies.

The NCCAM is dedicated to exploring complementary and alternative healing practices in the context of rigorous science, training CAM researchers, and disseminating authoritative information to the public and professionals.[3] The agency has recommended that CAM education be included for those studying conventional medicine and that CAM practitioners include studies in conventional medicine. The intended result is conventional providers who can discuss CAM with their patients, provide guidance on the use of CAM, and collaborate with CAM practitioners; likewise, CAM practitioners can communicate and collaborate with conventional providers, supporting collaborative care.

Some common complementary modalities that have moved into mainstream biomedical medicine are massage, acupuncture, relaxation/stress management, and herbology (Box 1-1). Massage has been incorporated into conventional healthcare practice for three main reasons: low risk, low cost, and high satisfaction. Research into the physiologic mechanisms underpinning the benefits of massage has demonstrated the *efficacy* (ability to produce a desired effect) of massage.

INTEGRATED MEDICINE

The term **integrated medicine** is used to describe a system in which mainstream, conventional medical care and complementary therapies are integrated within a practice or institution, each

Box 1-1 Complementary Medicine Treatment Approaches

Treatment approaches that commonly fall under the heading of complementary medicine include the following healthcare practices:

Acupressure	Meditation
Acupuncture	Naturopathy
Alexander technique	Nutritional therapy
Applied kinesiology	Osteopathy
Aromatherapy	Qigong
Autogenic training	Reflexology
Ayurveda	Relaxation and visualization techniques
Chiropractic	
Cranial osteopathy	Shiatsu
Environmental medicine	Tai chi
Homeopathy	Therapeutic touch
Hypnosis	Yoga
Massage	

From Peters D, Chaitow L, Harris G, Morrison S: *Integrating complementary therapies in primary care,* Edinburgh, 2002, Churchill Livingstone.

complementing the other. As a result of the growing incidence of lifestyle illnesses caused by stress, fatigue, detrimental nutritional choices, obesity, and other poor health habits, many people now recognize the overwhelming need to change their lifestyles. Often they choose integrated medicine as a means to bring about that change. The medical spa is a model of an integrated approach. The medical spa concept embraces relaxation, pleasure, and pampering combined with treatment of medical conditions. A medical spa is an ideal environment for addressing healthcare conditions that require major lifestyle changes such as weight management, chronic fatigue, some types of physical rehabilitation, and physical conditioning. Some medical spas also offer nutritional help to assist patients in making dietary lifestyle changes; this in turn can help them with managing their weight and with coping with disease and some illnesses. An example of a growing aspect of integrated healthcare is the increase in cosmetic surgery coupled with antiaging modalities that primarily target control of inappropriate inflammation and support both physical fitness and mental health.

BENEFICIAL COMPLEMENTARY PRACTICE

People usually consult complementary practitioners about mild to moderate long-term, painful, functional, and stress-related conditions and disorders, which take up a great deal of the general medical practitioner's time. Conditions that often are managed successfully with complementary therapies include undifferentiated illnesses and chronic structural, dysfunctional, and relapsing functional disorders. The results of good clinical trials suggest that complementary therapies are the treatment of choice for certain conditions. Well-designed studies have been conducted on the effectiveness of complementary methods for a range of common problems, including anxiety, fibromyalgia, asthma, irritable bowel syndrome (IBS), eczema, and migraine (see the Evolve website). Microbiologists are studying the effects of nutrition and stress on the human body, and the results of these studies probably will create a whole new realm of knowledge and understanding for treatment.

The growing acceptance of complementary therapies coincides with an increased interest in lifestyle change, health promotion, and low-technology treatments. These approaches, integrated with conventional medical care, might provide inexpensive, safe ways to address conditions that currently do not respond well to conventional care.

Conventional medicine most often is the best treatment for trauma and acute care. It provides effective treatment for many common conditions, such as acute bacterial infection, congestive heart failure, and glaucoma. Alternative or adjunctive treatments support this care. For example, pneumonia patients who receive osteopathic care (mainly soft tissue treatments) as well as medication have shorter hospital stays and better recoveries.* However, many common health problems are not easily "fixed," such as recurring mechanical back pain, headache, asthma, irritable bowel syndromes, rheumatoid arthritis, and osteoarthritis. The continuing management of these conditions is a daily challenge for the healthcare system, and the cost in both human and financial terms is high.

The accepted modalities currently available in healthcare (e.g., nursing, physiotherapy, specialist referral, counseling, and use of medications) do not necessarily meet the needs of patients whose problems are not "fixable." Other patients have

*Noll D, Shores J, Gamber R et al: Benefits of osteopathic manipulative treatment for hospitalized elderly patients with pneumonia, *J Am Osteopath Assoc* 100:776-782, 2000.

long-term relapsing structural or functional disorders, for which medical treatment often is less than satisfactory. Conceivably, people with conditions that do not respond to conventional medical care alone may have better outcomes with a combined approach that involves multiprofessional/multidisciplinary integrated healthcare. For this healthcare approach to succeed, practitioners of complementary therapies must comply with various requirements to integrate their specialties into the current healthcare system.

Practitioners of conventional healthcare have concerns about complementary and alternative practitioners, and most of these concerns are valid. If people are seen by unqualified practitioners, the risk of a missed or delayed diagnosis arises. This can have tragic results. People may waste money on ineffective treatments and discontinue or neglect effective conventional treatment. The mechanisms of benefit claimed for some complementary treatments are implausible, and many complementary therapies are scientifically unproven. Healthcare insurers need to establish whether and how complementary therapies support healthcare before authorizing routine insurance coverage. Public demand that complementary therapies be made available is growing; therefore it must be demonstrated that patients are being treated not only with a safe, effective therapy provided by a qualified practitioner, but also that the therapy is more acceptable and cost-effective for the patient's condition than the conventional medical alternatives.

The main focus of this text is therapeutic massage, which is being integrated into conventional healthcare. Massage therapists are working to meet the recommendations for a professional model of practice (Box 1-2), and it is important that they continue to press forward in these areas.

Massage has come a long way, especially in the past 5 years. Evidence-based research indicates the effectiveness of massage (Box 1-3). Avenues for appropriate education, licensure or certification, and insurance have been created. The two biggest obstacles for integrating massage into conventional healthcare are finding appropriately trained massage therapists (this textbook is intended to correct that problem) and identifying sources of funds to pay for massage. Currently, health insurance does not routinely cover therapeutic massage. Further research must be done to show that massage treatment is more cost-effective than conventional medical treatment for various conditions and that it has the same or better benefits without increased risk to the patient. Research can also document whether better outcomes are achieved when conventional medical treatment is combined with complementary methods. When this has been proved (and the massage community is confident that it will be), a major hurdle to full integration of massage into conventional healthcare will be overcome. Because most healthcare professionals in the medical setting have more education than a massage therapist does (Box 1-4), massage most likely will be incorporated into healthcare as a support service. Unfortunately, this will be at the lower end of the pay scale (discussed in more depth later).

JUST BETWEEN YOU AND ME

It seems logical that an integrated approach that combines traditional medicine and complementary medicine would best serve people seeking healthcare. The best of both disciplines makes sense because neither has all the answers. The medical community's concerns are valid. I have seen many cases (and probably been guilty of some myself) of less than desirable outcomes that are a direct result of failure to comply with the recommendations for complementary practitioners presented in Box 1-2. Everything in that model is reasonable and logical. It used to be that the support systems for compliance with this type of professionalism, including education, were not wholly in place for massage therapists. However, that is not true now. Massage therapists can be in compliance with all recommendations—no more excuses. It is time to get up to speed and be part of the team. A very spiritual and inspirational speaker once said, "A good attitude gets you to a great altitude [success]."

One more thing: Just as important, doctors and nurses have to learn about us, too.

WHAT PART WILL MASSAGE PLAY IN HEALTHCARE?

As the integration of massage into conventional healthcare proceeds, massage therapists probably will fall into the category of technical specialist/paraprofessional, with an education that is equivalent to a minimum of 1 year of college but that can be received in a vocational training

Box 1-2 Key Constituents of a Professional Practice Model for Complementary Medicine Practitioners

- **Qualifications:** Practitioners should have recognized qualification from a training establishment that is accredited by a suitable regulatory body.
- **Registration/license:** Practitioners must be registered with or licensed by a recognized professional body that requires its members to abide by codes of conduct, **ethics,** and discipline.
- **Insurance:** Practitioners must have adequate professional liability insurance coverage that applies to the period of their employment.
- **Consent to treatment:** Patients must be fully informed about the nature of the therapy and its effects, including any side effects, and have realistic expectations of its benefits. The informed consent of the patient or, in the case of young children, of the parent or guardian must be obtained and documented.
- **Medical responsibility:** Practitioners should be aware that patients referred to them for treatment remain the overall responsibility of the referring clinician. CAM practitioners should not advise discontinuation of existing treatments without the agreement of the referring clinician.
- **Documentation:** Practitioners should keep a written record of the consultation and each episode of treatment. All written and oral information should be treated as confidential, in compliance with the requirements of the Health Insurance Portability and Accountability Act (HIPAA).
- **Refusal to treat:** Practitioners have a duty not to treat a patient if they consider the treatment unsafe or unsuitable.
- **Education and training:** Practitioners should take responsibility for keeping up-to-date on developments in the practice of their therapy.
- **Quality standards:** In conjunction with other healthcare professionals, practitioners should assist with the development of local standards and guidelines for practice.
- **Audit:** Practitioners should undertake a clinical audit and report the results to the employing or commissioning practice. They should be responsible for monitoring the outcome of therapy, and the opinions of patients should be actively sought and included in any evaluation.
- **Research:** Practitioners should be expected to agree to take part in research trials to support the evaluation and development of treatment programs.
- **Health and safety:** Practitioners should comply with the requirements of health and safety legislation and should adhere to good practice in the protection of staff, patients, and the public.
- **Control of infection:** Practitioners should adhere to regulations governing infection control and follow the procedure for reporting outbreaks of infection.

Practitioners of complementary therapies, including massage, must be in compliance with these logical and attainable recommendations before a unified move can be made toward integrated medicine.

Adapted from the Scottish Department of Health 1996 Complementary Medicine and the National Health Service: Complementary medicine information pack for primary care groups, June, 2000.

Box 1-3 Research-Derived Evidence on the Effectiveness of Massage*

- Massage reduces anxiety and improves the perceived quality of life of patients with cancer.
- Massage therapy (30 minutes twice weekly for 1 month) significantly decreased anxiety and depression in women who had been sexually abused.
- Adult patients with multiple sclerosis who had massage twice weekly for 45 minutes for 5 weeks reported improved function and self-image, reduced anxiety and depression.
- Circulatory benefits include the ability to enhance lymphatic drainage as well as improved tissue oxygenation.
- Asthmatics receiving massage therapy report improved respiratory function.
- Massage can reduce pain and stiffness, even in chronic inflammatory conditions such as rheumatoid arthritis.

*Chapter 2 presents an in-depth discussion of research on the effects of massage, and the text's Evolve site provides an extensive matrix on this topic.

From Peters D, Chaitow L, Harris G, Morrison S: *Integrating complementary therapies in primary care,* Edinburgh, 2002, Churchill Livingstone.

BOX 1-4 Occupational Definitions and the Scope of Practice

The following are typical regulations governing the scope of practice for various medical professionals. Most of these regulations have been taken from the administrative rules of the Michigan Occupational Regulations Department of Licensing and Regulation and the Occupational Regulations section of the Michigan Public Health Code. Each state has its own regulations, but they are consistent enough to provide a sense of uniformity across the United States. More specific information on occupational regulations and health codes can be obtained from the department responsible for licensing and regulation in your jurisdiction.

Acupuncture

Acupuncture is a form of primary healthcare, based on traditional Chinese medical concepts, that uses acupuncture diagnosis and treatment, as well as adjunctive therapies and diagnostic techniques, to promote, maintain, and restore health, and prevent disease. Acupuncture includes but is not limited to the insertion of acupuncture needles and the application of moxibustion to specific areas of the human body.

Education/certification requirements: Licensure and certification vary by state.

Athletic Training

Athletic training is the study of athletic performance, injury prevention, and rehabilitation. It includes evaluation and assessment of injury, treatment, rehabilitation, and reconditioning of the athlete, therapeutic exercise, and use of therapeutic modalities.

Education/certification requirements: Typically a bachelor's degree or higher is required. Licensure and certification vary by state. See the National Athletic Trainers Association Board of Certification (NATABOC) for information about the requirements of a specific state.

Chiropractic

Chiropractic is the discipline within the healing arts that deals with the nervous system, its relationship to the spinal column, and its interrelationship with the other body systems. Chiropractic uses radiography to detect spinal subluxation and misalignment and adjusts related bones and tissues to establish neural integrity through techniques that use the inherent recuperative powers of the body to restore and maintain health. Examples of these techniques include the use of analytic instruments, the provision of nutritional advice, and the prescribing of rehabilitative exercise. Chiropractic does not include the performance of incisive surgical procedures or any invasive procedure that requires instrumentation, or the dispensing or prescription of drugs or medicine.

Education/certification requirements: Doctorate training/education, licensing credential, licensure.

Dentistry

Dentistry is the discipline of diagnosis, treatment, prescription, and surgery for disease, pain, deformity, deficiency, and injury of human teeth, alveolar processes, gums, jaws, and dependent tissues. Dentistry is also concerned with preventive care and the maintenance of good oral health.

Education/certification requirements: Doctorate education, licensure.

Medicine

Medicine is the diagnosis, treatment, prevention, cure, or relief of human disease, ailment, defect, complaint, or other physical or mental condition by attendance, advice, device, diagnostic test, or other means.

Education/certification requirements: Doctorate degree, licensure.

Naturopathy

Naturopathy is the combination of clinical nutrition, herbology, homeopathy, acupuncture, manipulation, hydrotherapy, massage, exercise, and psychological methods, including hypnotherapy and biofeedback, to maintain health. Naturopathic physicians use radiography, ultrasound, and other forms of diagnostic testing but do not perform major surgery or prescribe synthetic drugs.

Education/certification requirements: Typically a bachelor's degree or higher is required. Doctorate licensure and certification requirements vary by state.

Nursing

Nursing is the systematic application of substantial specialized knowledge and skill derived from the biologic, physical, and behavioral sciences to the care, treatment, counsel, and health education of individuals who are experiencing changes in the normal health process or who require assistance in the maintenance of health and the prevention or management of illness, injury, and disability.

Education/certification requirements: Associate's degree or higher, licensure.

Osteopathic Medicine

Osteopathic medicine is an independent school of medicine and surgery that uses full methods of diagnosis and treatment for physical and mental health and disease, including the prescription and administration of drugs and vitamins, surgery, obstetrics, and radiologic and electromagnetic diagnostics. Osteopathy emphasizes the interrelationship of the musculoskeletal system with other body systems.

Education/certification requirements: Doctorate, licensure.

Physical Therapy

Physical therapy is the evaluation or treatment of an individual by the use of effective physical measures, therapeutic exercise, and rehabilitative procedures, with or without devices, to prevent, correct, or alleviate a physical or mental disability. A physical therapist's duties include treatment planning, performance of tests and measurements, interpretation of referrals, instruction, consultative services, and supervision of personnel. Physical measures include massage, mobilization, and application of heat, cold, air, light, water, electricity, and sound.

Continued

BOX 1-4 **Occupational Definitions and the Scope of Practice—cont'd**

Education/certification requirements: Master's degree or higher, licensure.

Podiatry

Podiatry is the examination, diagnosis, and treatment of abnormal nails and superficial excrescences (abnormal outgrowths or enlargements) on the human hands and feet, including corns, warts, callosities, bunions, and arch troubles. It includes the medical, surgical, or mechanical treatment and physiotherapy of ailments that affect the condition of the feet. It does not include amputation of the feet or the use or administration of general anesthetics.

Education/certification requirements: Postdoctoral residency required by most states, licensure.

Psychology

Psychology is the rendering to individuals, groups, organizations, or the public, service involving the application of principles, methods, and procedures of understanding, predicting, and influencing behavior for the purpose of diagnosis, assessment, prevention, amelioration, or treatment of mental or emotional disorders, disabilities, and behavioral adjustment problems. A psychologist performs treatment by means of psychotherapy, counseling, behavior modification, hypnosis, biofeedback techniques, psychological tests, and other verbal or behavioral methods. Psychology does not include the prescription of drugs, the performance of surgery, or the administration of electroconvulsive therapy.

Education/certification requirements: Master's degree, licensure.

Modified from the Michigan Bureau of Health Professions, Lansing, Michigan, michigan.gov

setting. The model for this exists with medical assistants, respiratory therapy assistants, and physical therapy aides. The required education would translate into about 36 credits, or 1200 contact hours, which fits the current educational trend in massage. The entry level education requirement for massage presently is 500 to 750 contact hours (approximately 20 credits). This prepares the student for a career in wellness massage. To acquire the knowledge necessary to work in a medical setting (a specialty), the student would need an additional 15 or 16 credits, or 300 to 500 contact hours. The educational requirements may rise as high as an associate's degree (64 credits), and if this happens, massage therapists would be ranked with other healthcare technical specialists, such as physical therapy assistants.

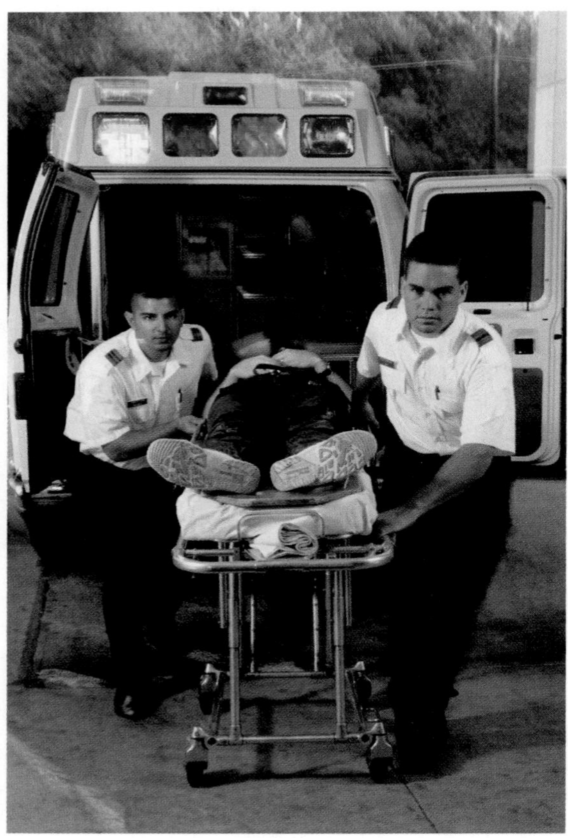

FIGURE 1-5 ■ Acute care.

The Nature of Care

Some diseases and injures are cured with medical intervention. This is especially true of acute care conditions, the area in which the science and practice of medicine shine (Figure 1-5). However, for most people, conventional healthcare interventions (e.g., medication or surgery) do not provide a cure; rather, the patient's condition is *managed,* and this situation has put a major strain on the healthcare delivery system. Because most health conditions are managed, requiring long-term care, treatment is expensive. Massage offers benefits for the management of many chronic health conditions in a potentially cost-effective manner.

The doctor and highly trained support staff are best suited to handle acute situations. This is an important distinction in the healthcare environment. Massage therapists work most effectively with patients who have chronic conditions or those whose conditions are terminal because no cure is available. The students in my advanced programs have a hard time with this. They want to *fix* it; however, if "it" can be fixed, a medical treatment of some sort (e.g., medication, surgery) most likely will be responsible for the cure. The contraindications to medical treatment in conditions that can't be cured are also important. Patients must consider the possible side effects of medication to make sure that the drug's purpose outweighs any side effects. Sometimes the treatment is worse than the disease. The difficult health problems are the ones that medical science does not know how to fix and those that develop because of poor lifestyle choices, requiring people to change their behavior (e.g., nutrition, exercise, diet modification) (Figure 1-6).

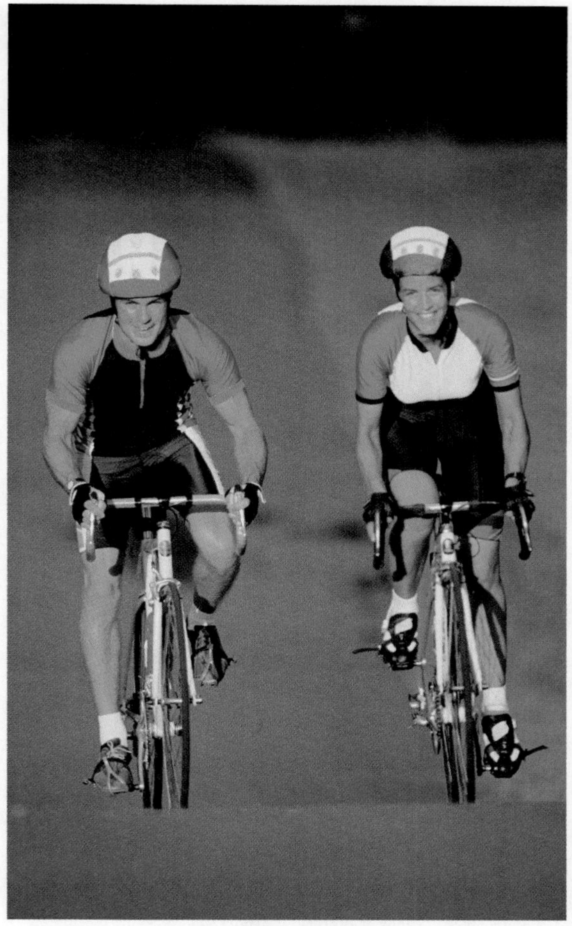

FIGURE 1-6 ■ Healthy behavior.

WHAT MASSAGE CAN REALISTICALLY DO

Massage care is supportive, not curative, for patients who are ill or hurt (Figure 1-7). Massage effectively supports various forms of medical intervention (including mental health) as well as the body's innate ability to heal itself.

The following list presents the primary uses of massage in the healthcare environment. Some of these benefits have been validated by research (see Chapter 2 and the Evolve site), and others are based on clinical experience or have been historically supported over many cultures and centuries.

- Breathing effectiveness
- Circulation (blood and lymph) support
- Comfort and pleasure
- Edema and fluid imbalance management
- Enhanced parasympathetic dominance
- Pain management
- Reduced sympathetic dominance
- Sleep support and reduced fatigue
- Soft tissue normalization (neuromuscular and myofascial)

These outcomes interface and overlap. For example, reducing sympathetic dominance could reasonably be expected to improve breathing, support sleep, and increase pain tolerance. Reducing edema can ease pain and increase circulation to an area. Neuromuscular balance allows for effective movement, and myofascial balance supports mobility and stability; together they support effective and efficient movement that encourages circulation, increases comfort, and supports productivity.

REFERENCES

1. Kligler B, Lee RA: *Integrative medicine,* McGraw Hill Professional, 2004.
2. NCCAM Publication No. D347: "What is CAM?"
3. www.nih.gov/about/almanac/organization/NCCAM.htm

JUST BETWEEN YOU AND ME

My students always want to learn how to do some sort of massage treatment that will specifically address a condition and produce a fantastic result. In close to 30 years of massage practice, this has not been my experience. Massage does not "fix it." Massage aids in the healing process; that has to be enough. If I did not somehow come to grips with this, I would have burned out professionally and quit.

Massage therapists must respect the commitment to education and service of the various healthcare professionals. I have worked for and with chiropractors, osteopathic physicians (DOs), medical doctors (MDs), physical therapists, psychologists, and athletic trainers. I have participated in these professional relationships as an employee, an independent contractor, and with mutual referral. Some health conditions with which I have worked include the following:

ADD/ADHD
Aging conditions (general)
AIDS and HIV
Allergies
Alzheimer's disease and other forms of dementia
Amputation
Anxiety
Arthritis and other types of degenerative joint disease
Athletic injury
Autism
Auto accidents
Breast reconstruction and other forms of plastic surgery
Burns
Cancer
Cardiovascular and respiratory diseases
Chronic fatigue
Closed head injury
Death and dying (hospice)
Depression
Developmental disorders
Diabetes
Eating disorders
Endocrine disorders
Epilepsy and other seizure disorders
Fibromyalgia
Headaches
Hepatitis
Irritable bowel disorders and other similar conditions
Joint replacement
Kidney disease
Low back pain
Lupus
Multiple sclerosis
Neck and shoulder pain
Organ replacement
Pain
Physical and emotional abuse
Physical rehabilitation
Post-traumatic stress disorder
Prenatal and postnatal treatments
Schizophrenia
Scleroderma
Spinal cord injury
Substance abuse
Surgery in general

And I'm sure there are others I can't remember right now. Each time a client or patient showed up with some disease, injury, or condition, I would have to look it up; ask questions; learn about the nature of the illness or injury and the various treatments, including medication, surgery, physical therapy, counseling, and so forth; and then figure out how to give a massage that would help and not harm.

Through years of practice, I have found that, regardless of the type of illness or injury, a particular summation of the symptoms helps me figure out what to do: that is, people either hurt, are tired, or both. Based on this summation, the general treatment plan typically ends up being some sort of pain management and sleep support delivered with empathy and compassion.

Over the years I have become able to identify my own burnout periods, times when I am less able to provide empathy and compassion. If you do not have heartfelt empathy and compassion, you have no business serving these clients.

I have learned the hard way about the importance of empathy and compassion, as a result of my own health issues: thyroid dysfunction, chronic joint pain, inner ear disturbances, neurochemical imbalance (tendency for anxiety and obsessive compulsive disorder), and dyslexia. I am somewhere in the menopausal realm, have glaucoma, cardiovascular disease that has been treated with triple bypass surgery, and age-related vision issues, on top of lifelong severe nearsightedness (now that's a pain!). Like so many, I struggle with weight management. I take medication for some of these conditions, use ice for a lot of others, and cope with the rest. I have undergone mental health therapy, physical therapy, and chiropractic care. I had two easy births and one horrendous one that resulted in reconstructive surgery. I underwent a yearlong course of treatment in traditional Chinese medicine and, as mentioned previously, have had major heart surgery. I have experienced the tragic death of my eldest son. I regularly use massage therapy, exercise, and other treatments. They all help, but no one thing is the total answer. I really am doing very well, and I have great kids and grandkids (who can drive me crazy, too!), coworkers, close friends, and pets. I love what I do and feel as if I have value. I hurt, but I ignore it (most of the time), because it won't harm me; I'm tired, but not all the time. I am truly thankful for the miracle of medication every morning when I take it to keep me alive and relatively sane. I might have died at one time from an illness, but I chose to live instead (which is much harder), and I could have literally dropped dead if not for the heart surgery. I grieve and cry. I am glad to be alive, and I laugh a lot at life these days. It is important that you realize that a human being is writing this textbook and as objective as I want to be, my life will influence the tone of this book and that's okay. Without all of this personal experience I doubt that I would be as tolerant and understanding of others in similar situations.

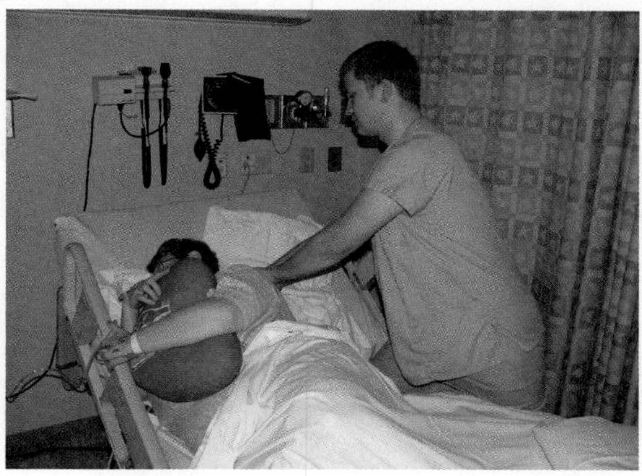

FIGURE 1-7 ■ Massage for medical purposes. (Photograph courtesy Laura Cochran.)

evolve 1-1

An additional research-based feature of this book at strategic points is the identification of key search terms/expressions used to search the expansive literature contained in PubMed. Each chapter specifies those relevant search terms/expressions that are also contained on this book's Evolve website under the heading "Evolve Links to PubMed." These web site entries are in the form of "Click Here" links to the search results within PubMed that have already been generated and that are continually updated each time the link is activated. The intent is to provide the reader with a means of continually being able to access the most current research literature of interest via the abstracts and full-text documents contained in PubMed. Because the research matrix introduced in this chapter via the Evolve website is representative rather than exhaustive, this "Evolve Links to PubMed" feature obviously allows the existing collection of studies in the matrix to be continually augmented and updated. From a practical standpoint, the proliferation of accessible research literature is best accommodated by way of this electronic option rather than an exclusive reliance on printed text.

The following terms and expressions specific to Chapter 1 have already been used to search PubMed for the latest research literature available.

Hyperlink Search Terms

Massage care
Massage clinical medical
Massage healthcare
Massage integrated medicine

SUMMARY

So there you have it, the bottom line on clinical/medical massage. Understand and appreciate that it takes a comprehensive knowledge base and effective use of clinical reasoning to pursue a career in clinical/medical massage. A textbook (such as this one), support texts as described previously, and a comprehensive course of study are all prerequisites. Congratulations on committing to continuing education. The motivation to be successful in any educational and career endeavor requires self-exploration. It is important to consider the questions in the workbook section at the end of this chapter.

What happens between the patient and the massage therapist is difficult to describe and often a unique interaction. Whatever it is, the interaction must be based on empathy, compassion, and empowerment. Massage is both a science and an art, and the two aspects are equally important. Much of this book is technical because it has to be. Look for the *Just Between You and Me* comments, written by Sandy Fritz, that are placed strategically throughout the text. They present learning tricks, little insights, dabs of humor, and snippets of experience to keep the reading from getting dull. Make sure to use the Evolve site. As is discussed in Chapter 2, research has emerged that describes and validates some of the benefits of massage in healthcare. Probably, we will never really understand it all. That's the faith part, and it's okay, as long as we commit to "do no harm." Welcome to the journey!

WORKBOOK

Respond to each of the questions. Be specific with your responses.

1. What do I want to give?

2. What do I want to get?

3. How much of this process is about serving others?

4. How much of this process is about serving me?

5. What is my main motivating force (e.g., job security, money, personal growth, status, helping others)?

6. What sacrifices will I need to make?

7. Am I willing to make the necessary sacrifices?

8. Am I willing to receive the rewards?

9. For what responsibilities will I be accountable?

10. Can I accept the responsibility?

11. Can I share the responsibility?

12. What are my limitations?

13. What can I do about my limitations?

____

____

____

14. How can I remain hopeful regardless of circumstances?

____

____

____

15. Why do I consider learning a lifelong experience?

____

____

____

16. How will I contribute to the growth of massage therapy in health care?

____

____

Chapter 2 Concept Map

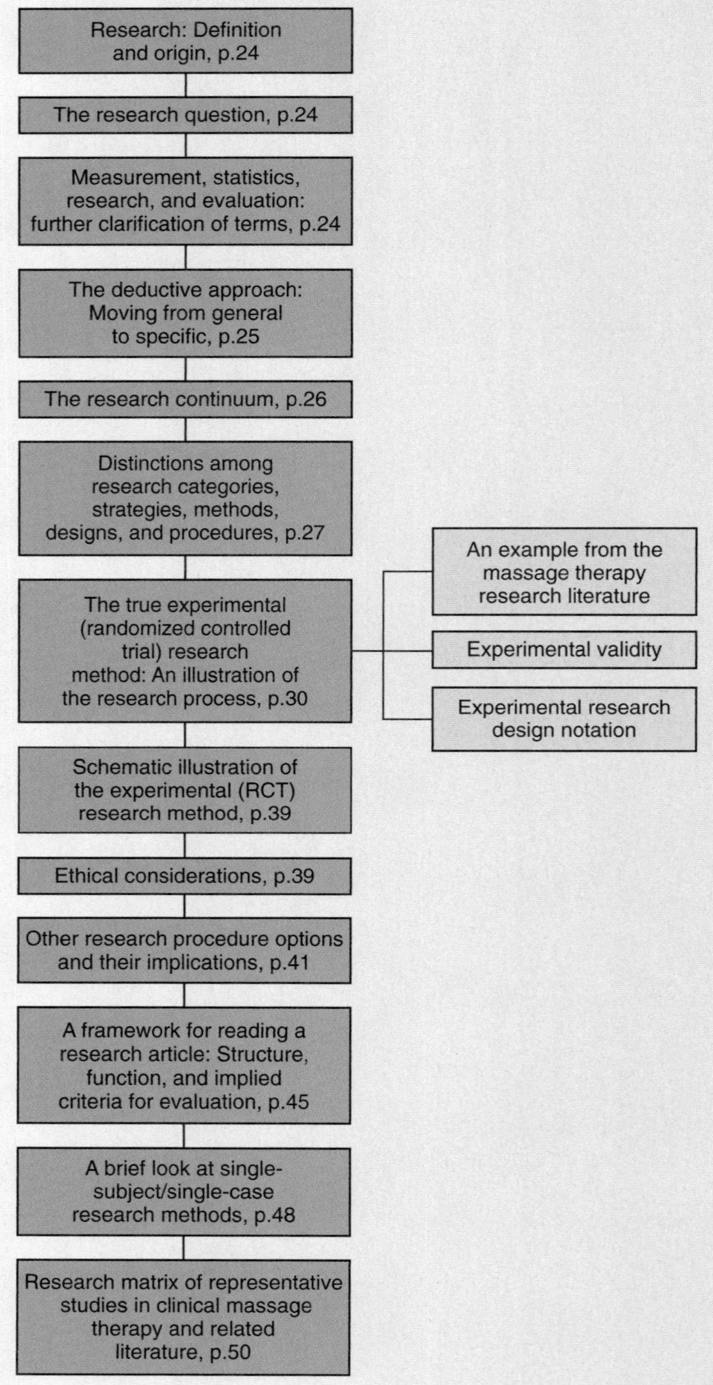

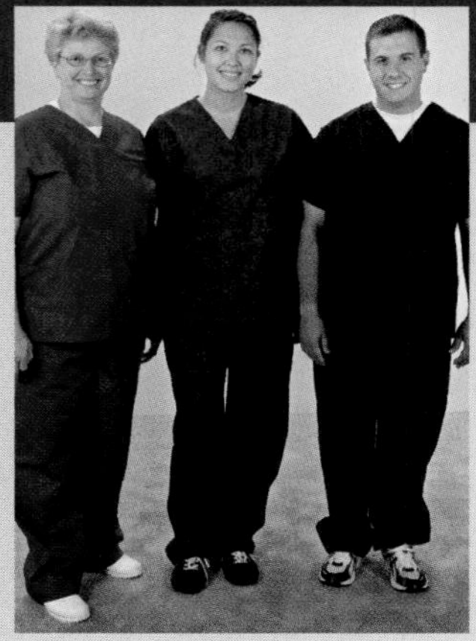

Chapter 2

RESEARCH ESSENTIALS FOR MASSAGE IN THE HEALTHCARE SETTING

Glenn M. Hymel

Key Terms

Abstract
Accessible population
Alpha (α) level
Alternative hypothesis
Between-subjects independent variable
Blinded (masked) study
Case report method
Case study method
Comparison treatment control group
Concluding section
Confidence interval (CI)
Confounding variable
Control group
Control variable
Deductive approach
Dependent variable (DV)
Discussion section
Double-blind research procedure
Effect size
Evaluation
Experimental validity
External validity
Extraneous variable
Group-specific focus
Hypothesis
Independent variable (IV)
Intact groups
Internal validity
Intervening variable
Introductory section
Manipulated independent variable
Measurement
Method section
No treatment control group
Nonmanipulated independent variable
Null (statistical) hypothesis
Open study
P value (level of significance)
Parameter
Placebo-attention control group
Placebo—sham treatment control group
Posttest
Preliminary section
Pretest
PubMed
Random assignment
Random selection
Randomized clinical trial
Randomized controlled trial (RCT)
Research
Research category
Research continuum
Research design
Research design notation
Research ethics
Research hypothesis
Research method
Research procedures
Research question
Research strategy
Results section
Sample
Single-blind research procedure
Single-case experimental method
Single-case focus
Single-case quantitative analysis method
Single-subject/single-case research methods
Standard treatment control group
Statistic
Statistical power (power analysis)
Statistics
Type I error
Variable
Waiting-list control group
Within-subjects independent variable (repeated measures)

For definitions of key terms, refer to the Evolve website.

OBJECTIVES

Upon completion of this chapter, the reader will have the information necessary to:

1 Define research.
2 Identify and explain the point of origin of any research endeavor.
3 Distinguish among the terms *measurement, statistics, research,* and *evaluation.*
4 Discuss the research process as a deductive approach.
5 Prepare a flowchart of the research continuum, displaying the progression from research category to research procedures, with an emphasis on labeling its starting and ending points as well as its three intermediate points.
6 Identify and explain each of the three research categories and discuss the one or more research strategies that define it.
7 Identify and explain the distinguishing features of a particular research strategy and discuss the two or more research methods that define it.
8 Identify and explain the distinguishing features of a particular research method and, if applicable, discuss the two or more research designs that define it.
9 Identify and explain the distinguishing features of a particular research design and, if applicable, discuss the two or more research procedures that define it.
10 Identify and explain the distinguishing features of a particular research procedure.
11 Working from the model provided by the research study presented in the chapter (Chang et al., 2002), discuss the following features of that study in the context of a true experimental, or randomized controlled trial, research method:
   - Research question and professional literature review
   - Population and sample
   - Random selection and random assignment as manifestations of randomization
   - Variables, from a research design perspective, including independent, dependent, extraneous, control, confounding, and intervening variables
   - Research hypothesis, null (statistical) hypothesis, and alternative hypothesis
   - Parameter and statistic
   - Statistical analyses, including such concepts as statistical testing and inference, alpha level (probability of a Type I error), P value (level of significance), statistical power (power analysis), confidence interval, and effect size
   - Internal validity and external validity
   - Experimental research design notation
12 Working from the example study (Chang et al., 2002), interpret and discuss a schematic illustration, in the form of an annotated flowchart, that reflects only select features of and a slight modification in that study.
13 Discuss at least three of the major ethical considerations prevalent in health science research.
14 Distinguish between comparative groups formed by random assignment or as a result of already being in place (i.e., intact).
15 Distinguish between manipulated and nonmanipulated independent variables.
16 Explain the possible options with regard to comparative groups or levels of an independent variable.
17 Distinguish among the five types of control groups: no treatment ("do nothing") control group, standard treatment control group, waiting-list control group, placebo-attention control group, and placebo–sham treatment control group.
18 Explain the distinction regarding a between-subjects independent variable and a within-subjects (repeated measures) independent variable.
19 Recognize the use of either a pretest–posttest or posttest–only set of measurement procedures in a hypothetical or actual research study and explain the rationale for each approach.
20 With regard to research methods used in the difference-oriented research strategy, distinguish between a group-specific focus and a single-case focus.
21 Explain the subtle distinction between the expressions *randomized controlled trial* and *randomized clinical trial.*
22 Distinguish between a blinded (masked) study and an open study.
23 Explain how a research article's structure and function are analogous to the concepts of anatomy and physiology.
24 Identify and discuss the six sections (and their subsections) that define the structure of a research article.
25 For each of the six sections of a research article (and their subsections), identify and explain the function served by each.
26 Provided with a list of the criteria for critiquing the six sections of a research article, explain why each criterion or

standard represents a basis for analyzing the associated section of the article.

27 Identify and characterize the four types of research methods that focus on a single subject or case of interest.

28 Explain in detail the nature and purpose of the case report research method.

29 Using the figure/matrix that identifies representative studies in the clinical massage therapy and related literature, select, read, and discuss at least three articles pertinent to the categories of patient systems, conditions, and populations.

30 Based on the figure/matrix that identifies representative studies in the clinical massage therapy and related literature, select, read, and discuss at least three articles pertinent to each of the remaining chapters in this book.

31 Access and use the *Evolve Links to PubMed* section of the book's website to identify the most current research literature available on a subject of interest.

To function well in the healthcare setting, the massage therapist must be able to justify the benefits of massage as part of a total treatment program. The medical community is a scientific community. Best practices in healthcare depend on research to ensure that medical treatments are safe, to assess the inherent risks of a treatment, and to determine whether a treatment has greater potential for benefit than risk. Massage therapy professionals have undertaken focused, massage-related research to support the efficacy, cost-effectiveness, and safe and best practice of clinical/medical massage. Massage therapists who work in the healthcare environment must be able to read critically and apply research findings appropriately. Glenn M. Hymel, author of *Research Methods for Massage and Holistic Therapies* (St Louis, 2006, Mosby), has also identified, organized, and integrated throughout the various chapters important research that supports the massage recommendations made in this text and on the Evolve website. This chapter lays the foundation for educating the reader in the correct use of research.

INTRODUCTION

This chapter provides an overview of the research process, which is essential to a better understanding of the topics covered in subsequent chapters. The current emphasis on evidence-based healthcare demands that the massage therapist have a knowledge of certain concepts, principles, and procedures that constitute the foundations of scientific investigation. With this knowledge base, the student should develop at least three capabilities at a more informed level: (1) critical reading of currently available research on massage with regard to healthcare and related topics; (2) participation as a member of a research team; and (3) collaborative communication with other healthcare professionals on issues of mutual interest.

A single chapter devoted to the research process obviously does not allow the type of exhaustive coverage that is possible in a full-length book focused entirely on the topic. Such comprehensive works are available (e.g., Gehlbach, 2002; Hulley et al., 2001; Hymel, 2006; Portney and Watkins, 2000; and Stommel and Wills, 2004), and the student is encouraged to use them as resources that certainly can build on and extend the introduction provided in this chapter. Our intent here is to provide a brief survey of the research landscape that acknowledges the three principal categories of research and their several affiliated research strategies and methods. In this process, considerably more attention is given to the true experimental (or randomized controlled trial [RCT]) research method. This emphasis reflects two realities: (1) the prevalence of research studies in massage that reflect either this specific research methodology or slight variations or modifications of it; and (2) the inclusion of research procedures in this method that ensure the degree of control and validity required for the type of research evidence appropriately demanded of healthcare professionals.

The principal sections of this chapter cover clarification of terms, such as *research, measurement, statistics,* and *evaluation;* a deductive approach to identifying various research categories, strategies, methods, designs, and procedures; specific consideration of the true experimental (randomized controlled trial) research method;

issues in research ethics; the structure and function of a research report; possible variations in research procedures; and representative studies in therapeutic massage and related literature. The representative studies section provides a matrix that crosses authors and researchers with various patient systems, conditions, and populations. The intent is not to provide exhaustive coverage and interpretation of the pertinent research literature, but rather to acknowledge representative studies of probable interest to the reader as the subsequent chapters of this book unfold.

RESEARCH: DEFINITION AND ORIGIN

Our journey through the research process starts at a rather logical point, namely, an attempt at defining exactly what we mean by the term *research.* At its most basic level, **research** can be defined as a process that explores one or more areas of interest (called *factors* or *variables*) by analyzing numeric or verbal data (or both) to advance understanding. More specifically, research is an activity that allows one or more of the following tasks to be accomplished:

- The researcher may want to characterize a variable of interest by an appeal to numeric and/or verbal data. For example, the researcher might undertake the task of characterizing the percentage of adults surveyed nationwide who have used therapeutic massage as a form of complementary and alternative healthcare. Or, the researcher might document, by means of a detailed interview, a client's individual experience and perception of therapeutic massage over a designated period as an intervention for chronic low back pain.
- The researcher may want to investigate a possible relationship between two or more variables. For instance, a research team might explore the nature of the relationship, if any, between aquatic therapy and increased range of motion for clients recovering from bilateral hip replacement surgery.
- The researcher may need to integrate or synthesize data concerning one or more variables of interest from already published sources. For example, a massage therapist might complete an exhaustive, state-of-the-art review and synthesis of what the professional literature has to say about therapeutic massage as a viable intervention for clients suffering from fibromyalgia.

THE RESEARCH QUESTION

Across all three possible tasks that define the research process is a point of origin that gives direction and meaning to the entire research effort; that critical point is the **research question** posed. For example, if one were to ask about the relationship between trigger point therapy and the alleviation of migraine headaches, a possible research effort might be to investigate whether a meaningful difference exists between trigger point therapy and a conventional, drug-specific intervention with regard to the alleviation of migraines. The origin in the research process, then, is always the research question, on which all the research activities are based.

MEASUREMENT, STATISTICS, RESEARCH, AND EVALUATION: FURTHER CLARIFICATION OF TERMS

Measurement and statistics are critical tools in both the research and evaluation processes. The term **measurement** refers to the procedure by which numeric and/or verbal data are collected to portray, in as valid and reliable a manner as possible, a factor or **variable** of interest to an investigator. For example, any testing effort of an outcome of interest (e.g., range of motion) is considered an instance of measurement. Once the measurement data have been collected, the researcher uses the applied area of mathematics known as **statistics** to analyze and better understand what the data set demonstrates. This is accomplished through the use of one or more mathematical techniques from descriptive statistics and/or inferential statistics. An example of descriptive statistics, calculating the arithmetic average, or mean, of a numeric data set, could be used to describe the central tendency of the scores in the data set. As an example of inferential statistics, a technique could be used that tells us whether the outcome measures of participants in a study's two comparison groups are indeed different in a mathematically meaningful way.

Any evaluative effort may follow immediately on the heels of measurement and statistical analysis or as a sequel to a research effort. In either case, **evaluation** is the process of making a value judgment or an assessment of merit about one or more variables of interest that have been measured and analyzed. An example might be a corporate policy decision being made to include in a company's health coverage package reimbursement for employees who use therapeutic massage for chronic pain management. Such a decision might stem at least partly from the fact that the human resource office had become aware of research demonstrating massage therapy as a viable intervention for managing chronic pain (see Cherkin et al., 2001).

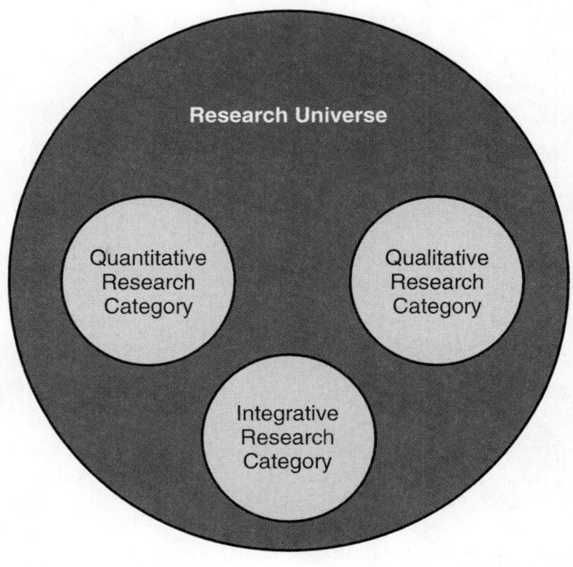

FIGURE 2-1 ■ Three subsets of the research universe: quantitative research category, qualitative research category, and integrative research category. (Modified from Hymel GM: *Research methods for massage and holistic therapies,* St Louis, 2006, Mosby.)

THE DEDUCTIVE APPROACH: MOVING FROM GENERAL TO SPECIFIC

At the most general level, the research universe comprises three subsets of research categories: the quantitative research category, the qualitative research category, and the integrative research category (Figure 2-1). The distinction among these three categories is examined shortly.

Figure 2-2 shows in a generic way the progression that occurs when a **deductive approach** is used to discuss a complex issue. As shown, the starting point is the general, or global, or panoramic view level (GL), followed by increasingly detailed levels of specificity. For our purposes, four specific levels (SLs) are shown beyond the general level.

A general level of thinking about research is the **research category.** This level is followed, in progressively increasing degrees of detail and specificity, by considering various research strategies, methods, designs, and procedures. The research process has five levels. Figures 2-3 and 2-4 provide a view of these five levels and the terminology used in the progression from the general to the most specific.

To elaborate on Figures 2-3 and 2-4, an example of the most general level (GL) could be the quantitative research category. A possible research strategy included under the quantitative research category is the difference-oriented research strategy, which matches up with specific level 1 (SL1). A simple example here might be a study investigating whether a difference exists between the presence and absence of chair massage with regard to reducing stress levels among clerical workers in a corporate setting. A viable research method affiliated with this strategy is the true experimental (RCT) research method, which represents the second specific level (SL2). A prevalent research design associated with this method is the randomized, control group, pretest–posttest design, or specific level 3 (SL3). The fourth specific level (SL4), or research procedures, ideally includes such procedures as random selection, random assignment, pretesting on relevant variables, a manipulated independent variable (in our example, the presence or absence of chair massage intervention), and posttesting on the dependent or outcome variable or variables.

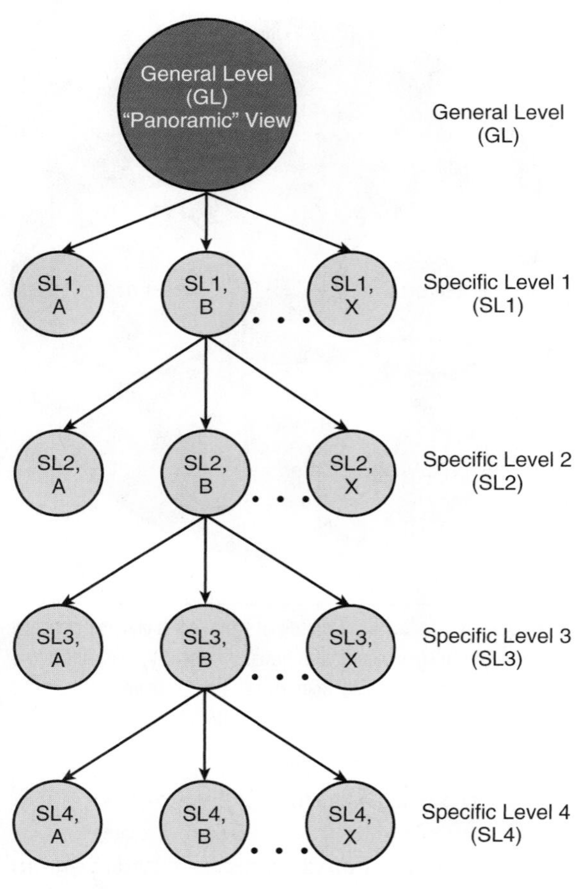

FIGURE 2-2 ■ Generic display of the progression from general to specific in the deductive approach. (Modified from Hymel GM: *Research methods for massage and holistic therapies,* St Louis, 2006, Mosby.)

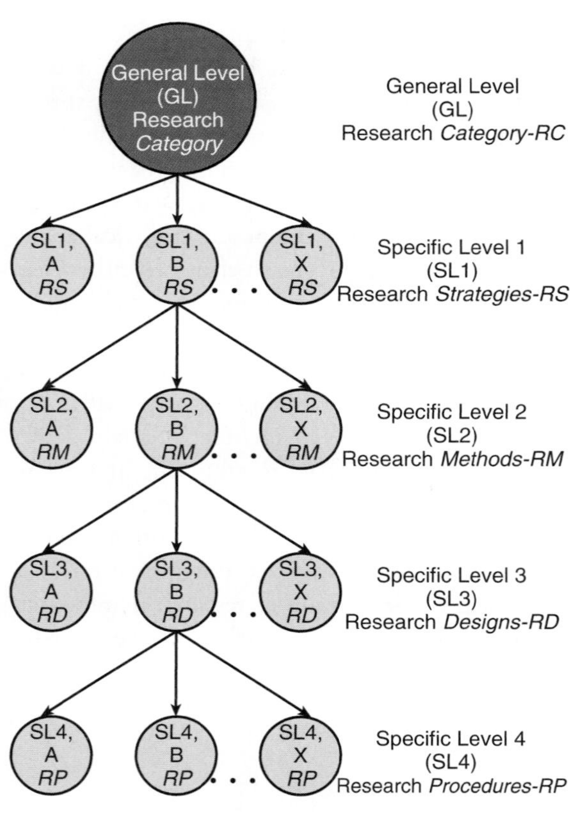

FIGURE 2-3 ■ Deductive view of the progression from the general level of research category to the specific levels of research strategies, methods, designs, and procedures. (Modified from Hymel GM: *Research methods for massage and holistic therapies,* St Louis, 2006, Mosby.)

- Research Category
  - • Research Strategies
    - • • Research Methods
      - • • • Research Designs
        - • • • • Research Procedures

FIGURE 2-4 ■ Another view of the progression from research category to research procedures. (Modified from Hymel GM: *Research methods for massage and holistic therapies,* St Louis, 2006, Mosby.)

THE RESEARCH CONTINUUM

As we have just seen, the starting point in our discussion of the research process is the research category, from which everything else flows. The endpoint, in terms of detail, is the specific set of research procedures that would have to be carried out to complete the research effort. Sandwiched in between are the so-called intermediate points that progress from research strategies to methods to designs. Figure 2-5 shows these various points in the **research continuum** and sets the stage so

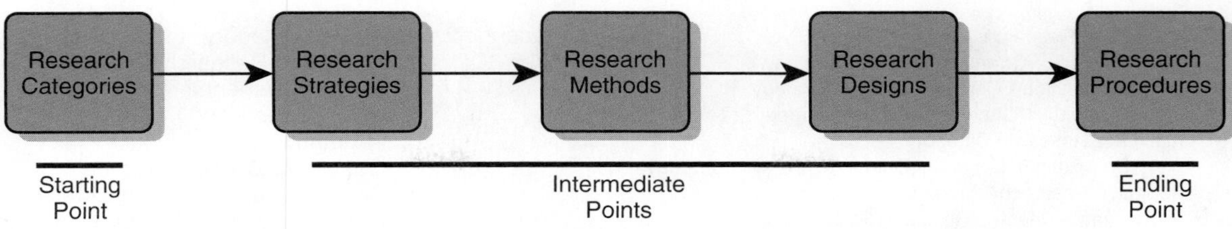

FIGURE 2-5 ■ The continuum from research categories to research procedures. (Modified from Hymel GM: *Research methods for massage and holistic therapies,* St Louis, 2006, Mosby.)

- Research Categories: Philosophically Driven
  - Quantitative: Objective Analysis, Primarily Numerical Data
  - Qualitative: Subjective and Contextual Interpretation, Primarily Verbal Data
  - Integrative: Synthesizing Effort Valued, Objective and/or Subjective Orientation, Numerical and/or Verbal Data

FIGURE 2-6 ■ Research categories and their philosophical orientations. (Modified from Hymel GM: *Research methods for massage and holistic therapies,* St Louis, 2006, Mosby.)

that we can specify what we mean by each of the options.

DISTINCTIONS AMONG RESEARCH CATEGORIES, STRATEGIES, METHODS, DESIGNS, AND PROCEDURES

RESEARCH CATEGORIES: THE MOST GENERAL LEVEL

As shown in Figure 2-1, the most general level comprises three possible research categories: the quantitative research category, the qualitative research category, and the integrative research category. The distinguishing feature of these three categories is the philosophical orientation that is basic to each (Figure 2-6).

Quantitative research is philosophically driven by a view of reality and truth that emphasizes the objective and unbiased approach to scientific investigation. This orientation is rooted primarily in numeric data that are statistically analyzed once the measurements have been demonstrated to be valid and reliable. The research that has historically dominated the basic and health sciences falls into this category (see Peat, Mellis, Williams, & Xuan, 2002). Somewhat in contrast is the qualitative research approach, which is philosophically driven by a perspective on reality and truth that relies on subjective, contextual, and highly individualistic perceptions of all that is observed and experienced. This mind set is based primarily on verbal data, which by their nature lend themselves to alternative interpretations by both the observer and the observed. Historically, the qualitative approach has been emphasized in disciplines such as anthropology and sociology; however, it has enjoyed a somewhat recent emergence in psychology and various health science professions (see Creswell, 1998).

Something of a hybrid perspective on reality and truth philosophically drives the integrative category of research. This view recognizes the equally valuable possibilities that exist in both objective analysis and subjective interpretation of the experiences under investigation. The focal point may encompass both numeric and verbal data, but a concerted effort is made to synthesize research that has already been generated in the quantitative and/or qualitative realms. In a sense, this category highlights two themes: the whole

- Quantitative Research Category
  - • • Difference-Oriented Research Strategy
  - • • Association-Oriented Research Strategy
  - • • Descriptive-Oriented Research Strategy
- Qualitative Research Category
  - • • Contextual/Interpretive-Oriented Research Strategy
- Integrative Research Category
  - • • Synthesis-Oriented Research Strategy

FIGURE 2-7 ■ Research categories and their research question–driven strategies. (Modified from Hymel GM: *Research methods for massage and holistic therapies,* St Louis, 2006, Mosby.)

may indeed be greater than simply the sum of its parts, and patterns of meaning may unfold in an area of research if a synthesizing approach is taken. Marks and Sykes (2004), Mulrow and Cook (1998), and Patterson, Thorne, Canam, & Jillings (2001) provide guidelines for the integrative approach to research.

RESEARCH STRATEGIES

Any of the three research categories is made operational, or brought to life, so to speak, by one or more of its defining research strategies (Figure 2-7). The **research strategy** is the first level of specificity or detail beyond the general research category to which it belongs; it is driven by the research question that the strategy will be investigating.

The quantitative research category has three possible research strategies, each of which reflects the type of research question that gives it direction and meaning. These three strategies are (1) the difference-oriented research strategy, (2) the association-oriented research strategy, and (3) the descriptive-oriented research strategy. The qualitative research category has only one specific research strategy, the contextual/interpretive-oriented strategy. The integrative research category likewise has one research strategy, the synthesis-oriented strategy.

RESEARCH METHODS

The **research method** is the next level of specificity in the research continuum. A research strategy is actually implemented by means of one or more research methods. Any research method is variable control driven; this simply means that the investigator's degree of control over the study's several variables (aspects or features subject to change) is what defines the research method.

- Quantitative Research Category
  - • • Difference-Oriented Research Strategy
    - • • • True Experimental (or Randomized Controlled Trial) Method
    - • • • Quasi-Experimental Method
    - • • • Single-Case Experimental Method
    - • • • Nonexperimental Comparative Groups Method
  - • • Association-Oriented Research Strategy
    - • • • Correlational Method
    - • • • Predictive Method
  - • • Descriptive-Oriented Research Strategy
    - • • • Single-Case Quantitative Analysis Method
    - • • • Survey Method
    - • • • Naturalistic/Structured Observational Method
    - • • • Case Report Method

FIGURE 2-8 ■ The quantitative research category: its affiliated research strategies and their variable control-driven methods. (Modified from Hymel GM: *Research methods for massage and holistic therapies,* St Louis, 2006, Mosby.)

Methods Used in the Quantitative Research Category

Each of the three strategies of the quantitative research category has two or more related methods (Figure 2-8):

- The difference-oriented strategy has four possible research methods: the true experimental (RCT) method, the quasi-experimental method, the single-case experimental method, and the nonexperimental comparison groups method.
- The association-oriented strategy has two research methods: the correlational method and the predictive method.
- The descriptive-oriented strategy has four possible methods: the single-case quantitative analysis method, the survey method, the naturalistic/structured observational method, and the case report method.

Methods Used in the Qualitative Research Category

As mentioned earlier, the qualitative category has only one specific strategy, the contextual/

interpretive-oriented strategy (Figure 2-9). This strategy has four methods: the case study method, the phenomenological method, the grounded theory method, and the ethnographic method.

Methods Used in the Integrative Research Category

The integrative category also has one strategy, the synthesis-oriented strategy, which has five associated research methods (Figure 2-10):

- Traditional narrative review method
- Critical systematic review method
- Meta-analytic systematic review method
- Best-evidence synthesis method
- Qualitative systematic review methods, which include meta-syntheses and meta-summaries

At this point, you may be wondering how to make sense of the many research terms just thrown at you. It is very important for you to keep in mind that our primary interest now is simply to provide a framework for, or a way of thinking about and organizing, the research process. The spectrum of various research categories, strategies, and methods is summarized in Figure 2-11.

- Qualitative Research Category
  - Contextual/Interpretive-Oriented Research Strategy
    - Case Study Method
    - Phenomenological Method
    - Grounded Theory Method
    - Ethnographic Method

FIGURE 2-9 ■ The qualitative research category: its affiliated research strategy and variable control-driven methods. (Modified from Hymel GM: *Research methods for massage and holistic therapies,* St Louis, 2006, Mosby.)

RESEARCH DESIGNS

Continuing with our deductive approach, which moves from the general to the specific, many research methods, although not all, can be further subdivided into research designs. A **research design** might be considered to be components driven. This means that in implementing a particular research method, the researcher at times faces various available options, or research designs, that involve including or excluding certain parts (components) of a study. The components the investigator chooses are precisely what defines the research design. In one design, for example, one of the components may be a measure of shoulder pain before the introduction of massage therapy; in another design, this premeasure might be omitted. That single component, the presence or absence of a premeasure, can distinguish one design from another.

Listing all the possible design subdivisions for each of the research methods already discussed is far beyond the scope of this chapter. The reader is referred to any of the research methodology textbooks cited at the outset of this chapter.

RESEARCH PROCEDURES

As with research designs, a detailed discussion of research procedures is beyond the intent of this chapter. Certain research procedures are considered on a rather limited basis as we continue to work our way through the remainder of the chapter. At this stage, it is sufficient simply to

- Integrative Research Category
  - Synthesis-Oriented Research Strategy
    - Traditional Narrative Review Method
    - Critical Systematic Review Method
    - Meta-Analytic Systematic Review Method
    - Best-Evidence Synthesis Method
    - Qualitative Systematic Review Methods
      - Qualitative Meta-Synthesis Method
      - Qualitative Meta-Summary Method

FIGURE 2-10 ■ The integrative research category: its affiliated research strategy and variable control-driven methods. (Modified from Hymel GM: *Research methods for massage and holistic therapies,* St Louis, 2006, Mosby.)

- Quantitative Research Category
  - Difference-Oriented Research Strategy
    - True Experimental (or Randomized Controlled Trial) Method
    - Quasi-Experimental Method
    - Single-Case Experimental Method
    - Nonexperimental Comparative Groups Method
  - Association-Oriented Research Strategy
    - Correlational Method
    - Predictive Method
  - Descriptive-Oriented Research Strategy
    - Single-Case Quantitative Analysis Method
    - Survey Method
    - Naturalistic/Structured Observational Method
    - Case Report Method
- Qualitative Research Category
  - Contextual/Interpretive-Oriented Research Strategy
    - Case Study Method
    - Phenomenological Method
    - Grounded Theory Method
    - Ethnographic Method
- Integrative Research Category
  - Synthesis-Oriented Research Strategy
    - Traditional Narrative Review Method
    - Critical Systematic Review Method
    - Meta-Analytic Systematic Review Method
    - Best-Evidence Synthesis Method
    - Qualitative Systematic Review Methods
      - Qualitative Meta-Synthesis Method
      - Qualitative Meta-Summary Method

FIGURE 2-11 ■ The spectrum of research categories, research strategies, and research methods.

acknowledge that a **research design** involves the implementation of several specific research procedures, which in turn involve certain activities. Research procedures are activities driven. For example, a particular design we will address shortly involves the research procedure of randomization. This randomization procedure can include both the activities of random selection and random assignment of participants in a study, or simply random assignment.

THE TRUE EXPERIMENTAL (RANDOMIZED CONTROLLED TRIAL) RESEARCH METHOD: AN ILLUSTRATION OF THE RESEARCH PROCESS

As mentioned previously, a comprehensive discussion of research methods is beyond the scope of this chapter. However, we present a fairly detailed illustration of a prevalent research method, the true experimental (RCT) research method, as exemplified by a study published in the massage therapy literature. Furthermore, this research method represents a type of scientific investigation frequently encountered specifically in the medical massage literature.

AN EXAMPLE FROM THE MASSAGE THERAPY RESEARCH LITERATURE

A study by Chang, Wang, and Chen (2002) provides an example of a true experimental (RCT) research method (Box 2-1). Certain aspects and procedures define this study as a difference-oriented research strategy in the quantitative research category.

BOX 2-1 Abstract Excerpt from a Study on the Effects of Massage on Pain and Anxiety During Childbirth

Aims. To investigate the effects of massage on pain reaction and anxiety during labor.

Background. Labor pain is a challenging issue for nurses designing intervention protocols. Massage is an ancient technique that has been widely used during labor; however, relatively little study has been undertaken to examine the effects of massage on women in labor.

Methods. A randomized controlled study was conducted between September 1999 and January 2000. Sixty primiparous women expected to have a normal childbirth at a regional hospital in southern Taiwan were randomly assigned to either the experimental ($n = 30$) or the control ($n = 30$) group. The experimental group received massage intervention, whereas the control group did not. The nurse-rated present behavioral intensity (PBI) was used as a measure of labor pain. Anxiety was measured with the visual analog scale for anxiety (VASA). The intensity of pain and anxiety between the two groups was compared in the latent phase (cervical dilation of 3 to 4 cm), active phase (dilation of 5 to 7 cm) and transitional phase (dilation of 8 to 10 cm).

Results. In both groups, a relatively steady increase was noted in pain intensity and anxiety level as labor progressed. An *t-test* demonstrated that the experimental group had significantly lower pain reactions in the latent, active, and transitional phases. Anxiety levels were significantly different between the two groups only in the latent phase. Of the 30 experimental group subjects, 26 (87%) reported that massage was helpful, providing pain relief and psychological support during labor.

Conclusions. The findings suggest that massage is a cost-effective nursing intervention that can reduce pain and anxiety during labor and that partners' participation in massage can positively influence the quality of women's birth experiences.

Modified from Chang MY, Wang SY, Chen CH: Effects of massage on pain and anxiety during labour: a randomized controlled trial in Taiwan, *J Adv Nurs* 38:68-73, 2002.

Research Question and Professional Literature Review

As stated previously, the starting point in any research study is the research question posed by the investigator at the very outset. Closely affiliated with the research question is completion of a comprehensive review of the professional literature relevant to the research question. Formulation of the research question and review of the relevant professional literature actually occur concurrently, in a sense, for several reasons. To state the research question in a specific and operational way, the researcher must already be somewhat familiar with earlier studies in a particular problem area. Likewise, an investigator must have at least the beginnings of a research question in mind to know exactly where in the vast professional literature to search in order to locate studies relevant to the problem area.

In the study by Chang et al. (2002), the implied research question is: What are the effects of massage on the degree of pain and anxiety experienced during childbirth? More specifically, is there a statistically significant difference between an experimental group receiving massage and a control group not receiving massage with regard to the degree of pain and anxiety experienced during childbirth? For the literature review, the 24 citations that are included in the body of the research report and also listed in the references section at the end identify the efforts of other investigators who have addressed a similar research interest.

Another important aspect of the research question in this study is the fact that it is a difference-oriented research question. This terminology is used because the research question basically asks whether a difference exists between the two comparison groups (i.e., the experimental group receiving the massage intervention and the control group not receiving massage) with regard to the outcome measures of degrees of pain and anxiety. Because this research question is difference oriented, the researchers must use a difference-oriented research strategy, and one of the research methods that falls under that strategy is the true experimental (RCT) method. (The details of why the research method in this study is considered a true experimental [RCT] method are addressed later in the chapter.)

Population and Sample

The report of the study by Chang et al. identifies a total of 60 women who participated in the research. However, neither the abstract nor the body of the report give the size of the original group from which the participants were recruited. That information would have allowed us to identify the number of potential study participants in the so-called **accessible population** (also known as the *set, universe,* or *macrocosm of potential participants*). From the study report, though, we can easily recognize that the **sample** (also known as the *subset* or *microcosm of actual participants*) included a total of 60 women who were members of the two comparison groups, each having 30 participants.

Randomization: Random Selection and Random Assignment

The Chang et al. study recruited the 60 participants from a regional hospital in a sequential manner; that is, as they became available through admission to the hospital to give birth. As an alternative sampling method, the researchers could have identified a set number of maternity patient admissions anticipated over a designated period; this would have allowed identification of a set number of potential study participants, or the study's accessible population. With that feature of the study in place, the researchers would have had the option of randomly selecting the 60 participants from the larger set (or universe or macrocosm) of patients who made up the accessible population. (The ramifications of **random selection** become apparent later in the chapter, in the discussion of external validity.)

As conducted, the study involved a total of 60 available participants who represented the sample. Random assignment was used to allocate 30 participants to the experimental group that received massage and 30 to the control group that did not receive massage. **Random assignment** of the participants simply means that each of the 60 subjects had an equal chance of being assigned to either comparison group. (The ramifications of random assignment are addressed later in the chapter, in the discussion of internal validity.)

Variables from a Research Design Perspective

The aspects or features of interest in a study that have the potential to vary, or change, are the study's **variables.** Several types of variables can be identified from a research design perspective. This clarification is important, because variables may also be considered from other perspectives, such as a measurement perspective or a conceptual/theoretical perspective, both of which are beyond the scope of this chapter.

Independent Variable. The **independent variable (IV)** in the study by Chang et al. is the extent to which massage therapy is provided to each of the 60 participants. Because the study has two comparison groups (i.e., one receiving massage and the other not receiving massage), the IV has two levels, or is manifested in two ways, namely, the presence and the absence of the massage therapy intervention. Level one of the IV is the presence of the massage intervention, which defines the experimental group (EG); level two of the IV is the absence of the massage intervention, which defines the control group (CG). To recap, the study has only one IV, which has two levels that represent the two comparison groups.

We can also say that the researchers are manipulating the study's one IV in that they govern (or determine) the two ways in which the IV is manifested. A **manipulated independent variable** exists when any type of treatment or intervention is used in a research study, be it a massage modality, an instructional method, a drug dosage, a medical procedure, or a psychotherapeutic intervention. Other terms for the independent variable are *stimulus variable, input variable, treatment variable,* and *causal variable.*

Dependent Variable. In a true experimental (RCT) method, the manipulated IV is considered a potential cause of some outcome or effect that is being measured among the participants. The study's outcome is viewed as a potential effect of the impact of the manipulated IV. This particular variable, then, is the study's **dependent variable (DV),** because it represents an outcome or effect that presumably is dependent on (i.e., is caused by) the manipulated IV. The DV may also be called the *response variable, output variable, outcome variable, consequent variable,* or *effect variable.* In the study by Chang et al., the researchers investigated two dependent variables, pain and the intensity of anxiety during labor.

Extraneous Variable. In studies similar to the one done by Chang et al., the researchers are principally, although not exclusively, interested in whether a meaningful relationship exists between the IV and the DV. However, many other variables are present in a study besides the manipulated IV and the DV. For example, these other variables may relate to characteristics of the study's participants or characteristics of the setting or circumstance in which the study is conducted. They are present in the study, but they are not the principal or primary focus of the researchers' interest and are considered extraneous to the study's major emphasis. Any one of these variables is referred to as an **extraneous variable** simply because it is extraneous to the study's main interest.

Extraneous variables that pertain to characteristics of the study's participants (also known as *personological* or *organismic variables*) include individual differences in traits and features that distinguish one person from another. Some examples of the vast array of such person-specific features are health status, lifestyle and work habits, intelligence, socioeconomic status, race, gender, ethnicity, motivational and compliance tendencies, behavioral habits that affect health, genetic inclinations, aptitudes, avocational interests, occupation, family of origin, self-esteem, and academic background.

Similarly, characteristics of the setting or circumstance in which a study is conducted may be extraneous to the primary concern. These may include situation-specific features such as the time of day, climatic conditions, unanticipated noise or lighting fluctuations, personal interaction dynamics of participants and others, study personnel's unintentional influence on the participants, and ergonomic features of furniture and surroundings.

In the results section of the study report by Chang et al., the researchers acknowledged several demographic and obstetric characteristics among the 60 participants, such as maternal age, maternal weight, gestational age, newborn weight, and duration of labor. Each of these is an extraneous variable in this particular study.

Control Variable. If ignored, any extraneous variable in a study has the potential to confuse the manner in which the completed study eventually is interpreted. Because of this, researchers must address these extraneous variables in such a way as to ensure that the comparison groups are equivalent at the outset of a study on as many of the extraneous variables as possible. A number of procedures can be used to achieve this equivalence of comparison groups; however, an approach that is essential to any true experimental (RCT) method is random assignment of participants to the comparison groups. This procedure was used in the study by Chang et al., resulting in the assignment of 30 participants to the experimental group and 30 to the control group. This feature of randomization allows the researcher a certain degree of latitude in assuming (although it is not guaranteed) that the two comparison groups are essentially equal on extraneous variables particularly relevant to the study. In other words, random assignment allows the researcher to view the potentially problematic extraneous variables as having been "controlled," in that the assumption (again, not a guarantee) is that the comparison groups are basically similar on any given extraneous variable. Accordingly, a variable that is so controlled is called a **control variable.**

Confounding Variable. If an extraneous variable is not appropriately controlled, it may be unequally present in the comparison groups. As a result, the variable becomes a **confounding variable.** In such cases, any differences between the two groups on a DV might very well be the result of the uncontrolled extraneous variable (i.e., confounding variable), because that variable has the effect of confusing, or confounding, proper interpretation of the study. The end result is that the true relationship between the IV and DV is somewhat disguised because of the possibility that another variable (the confounding variable) has influenced the outcome of the study in an unanticipated way. In the study by Chang et al., any one or more of the several demographic and obstetric features (e.g., maternal age, maternal weight, gestational age, newborn weight, and duration of labor) could function as a confounding variable if not adequately controlled.

Intervening Variable. An **intervening variable** is a factor that is proposed or theorized as a plausible explanation for the results obtained in a study. In more common parlance, it is the variable that explains "why we got what we got." Because this variable (sometimes called the *explanatory variable*) "intervened" at some point between the onset of the IV and eventual measurement of the DV, it now represents a viable explanation of the particular impact of the IV on the DV. In massage therapy research in general, the appeal to so-called underlying mechanisms typically captures the idea of intervening variables in that a proposed underlying mechanism represents a possible explanation of what factor came into play and why the results of the study were what they were (see Field, 2000).

In the report by Chang et al., several intervening variables were acknowledged as possible explanations for the study's findings. One of several possible explanations considered in the discussion section of the report was the effect of psychosocial factors on the nurses and midwives involved, the study participants, and the study participants' spouses. Physiological factors related to the gate control theory of pain management, increased endorphin levels, and increased vagal activity also were considered.

Hypotheses

The formulation of hypotheses is a research procedure that is critical to any scientific investigation. Just as a study's research question is informed by the investigators' familiarity with the relevant professional literature, the study's hypotheses likewise reflect the pertinent literature and are specific to the research question being investigated.

In its most basic form, a **hypothesis** is a statement that (1) is justified by or founded on some conceptual, theoretical, experiential, and/or research basis reflected in the professional literature and (2) predicts a research outcome with regard to the study's sample and/or population. Although not always stated explicitly, a study's hypotheses typically assume three different forms that are critical to the research process: the research hypothesis, the null (statistical) hypothesis, and the alternative hypothesis.

Research Hypothesis. At the very outset of a study, specifically when the research question is being formulated in the context of the relevant professional literature in the problem area, the researchers formulate the research hypothesis. The **research hypothesis** is simply a well-justified prediction of the study's anticipated outcome in the context of the study's sample. In a sense, it is the researchers' predicted answer to the study's research question in the context of the sample. In a difference-oriented research strategy, for example, the research question addressed is difference oriented, in the manner described earlier. Therefore the research hypothesis likewise is difference oriented.

The abstract presented in Box 2-1 implies a research hypothesis that could be stated as follows:

> A statistically significant difference will be found between participants in an experimental group receiving massage and those in a control group not receiving massage relative to the degrees of pain and anxiety intensity experienced during childbirth. The participants in the experimental group receiving massage will demonstrate significantly lesser degrees of pain and anxiety intensity during childbirth than will the participants in the control group not receiving massage.

This research hypothesis (1) provides a predicted answer to the study's research question, (2) is justified by or founded on some conceptual, theoretical, experiential, and/or research basis reflected in the professional literature, and (3) speaks to one or more characteristics or properties of the sample used in the study. Contrary to the fear some students of the research process have about a research hypothesis, this prediction at the outset of a study neither compromises the objectivity of the study nor suggests any type of bias on the part of the researchers. Students must keep in mind that typical studies are not conducted in some intellectual vacuum. A study is planned and implemented against the backdrop of an intellectual history and in the context of current intellectual thought. Therefore some attempt at predicting a well-founded outcome is to be expected, and the researchers must report on it at the study's conclusion, even if the actual results are contrary to the predicted outcome. Intellectual honesty and professional ethics demand no less of researchers; they must acknowledge objectively the actual results of a study, regardless of how contrary they might be to the researchers' initial predictions.

A decision to confirm or not confirm a research hypothesis is not based on direct testing of the research hypothesis; rather, the so-called null hypothesis is tested statistically to allow researchers to infer a decision on the research hypothesis.

Null (Statistical) Hypothesis. The **null (statistical) hypothesis** is a prediction of a study's outcome that (1) asserts the absence of a statistically significant relationship between or among the study's variables; (2) speaks to one or more characteristics or properties of the study's population; (3) serves as the focal point in a study's statistical analysis; and (4) provides the basis for a decision on the study's research hypothesis and alternative hypothesis (the alternative hypothesis is discussed in the following section).

For example, the study by Chang et al. implies a null hypothesis that could be stated as follows:

> No statistically significant difference will be found between participants in that segment of the population represented by the experimental group receiving massage and participants in that segment of the population represented by the control group not receiving massage relative to the degrees of pain and anxiety intensity experienced during childbirth.

This formal statement of the null hypothesis says that in the population represented by the sample, no statistically significant relationship exists between the IV (i.e., the extent of massage therapy intervention) and the DVs (i.e., the degrees of pain and anxiety intensity experienced during childbirth). This prediction takes the operational form of stating that in the population represented by the sample, no statistically significant difference exists between the two levels of the IV relative to the two DVs under investigation. Again, it is this null statement that is subjected to a study's statistical analysis, and the decision thus made about the null hypothesis becomes the basis for inferring a decision on both the research hypothesis and the alternative hypothesis. If the statistical test of a study's null hypothesis results in its rejection, the researchers may infer a confirmation of the research and alternative hypotheses.

Alternative Hypothesis. The alternative hypothesis might be viewed as something of an intermediary between the research hypothesis and the null hypothesis. More to the point, the **alternative hypothesis** is a prediction of a study's anticipated outcome in the context of the population. In a sense, it is the researchers' predicted answer to the study's research question in the context of the population (as opposed to the study's sample).

For example, the implied alternative hypothesis in the study by Chang et al. could be stated as follows:

> A statistically significant difference will be found between participants in that segment of the population represented by the experimental group receiving massage and participants in that segment of the population represented by the control group not receiving massage relative to the degrees of pain and anxiety intensity experienced during childbirth. More specifically, participants in that segment of the population represented by the experimental group receiving massage will demonstrate significantly lesser degrees of pain and anxiety intensity during childbirth than will participants in that segment of the population represented by the control group not receiving massage.

The research hypothesis and the alternative hypothesis, therefore, make identical predictions of a statistically significant difference between the levels of the IV relative to the study's two DVs in favor of the experimental group. Precisely in this sense, the alternative hypothesis is considered quite literally an alternative to the prediction of the null hypothesis.

The research hypothesis and the alternative hypothesis differ in that the research hypothesis predicts an outcome in terms of the study's sample, whereas the alternative hypothesis predicts an outcome in the context of the study's population. Thus the alternative hypothesis and the null hypothesis have in common the fact that each predicts an outcome regarding the study's population.

Parameter and Statistic

The terms *parameter* and *statistic* have very specific meanings in any discussion of the research process. **Parameter** refers to any characteristic, property, or feature of a population, whereas **statistic** pertains to any characteristic, property, or feature of a sample.

For example, part of the study by Chang et al. focuses on the average, or mean, degree of pain intensity experienced by the participants during childbirth. The mean degree of pain during childbirth can be considered a feature or property of the population from which the sample was derived. In the context of the study's population, the mean degree of pain is considered a parameter.

In a somewhat comparable way, the mean degree of pain during childbirth can be viewed as a feature or property of the sample derived from the study's population. In the context of the study's sample, the mean degree of pain is considered a statistic.

A verbal analogy may be helpful for remembering the distinction between parameter and statistic: parameter is to population as statistic is to sample. Expressed in another form, the analogy might look like this:

parameter : population :: statistic : sample

In the context of hypotheses, the research hypothesis is always a prediction specific to a sample statistic; the null and alternative hypotheses are always predictions specific to a population parameter.

Statistical Analysis

Statistical Testing and Inference. In the research process, both measurement procedures and statistical analyses are vital tools for collecting data on variables of interest and for analyzing the data to clarify understanding of the variables. For example, the study by Chang et al. established the measurement of pain and anxiety intensity levels as the two DVs and then proceeded to analyze the data sets statistically to test the study's null hypothesis.

Appropriate use of measurement and statistical testing are critical research procedures that allow investigators to make two important inferences:

- Statistical analysis of data collected on a given DV enables researchers to test the null hypothesis. The decision made regarding the null hypothesis (i.e., to reject or fail to reject the null) permits an inferential decision on both the alternative and research hypotheses.
- If a study used random selection of participants from an accessible population for the purpose of forming the sample, statistical analysis of the study's hypotheses allows an inference of what is learned about the sample back to the accessible population.

Alpha (α) Level (Probability of a Type I Error). A very important feature of scientific inquiry involving the statistical analysis of data to test hypotheses must be stated: The statistical conclusion arrived at is never absolute and is always presented in probability terms. When a null hypothesis is tested, for example, a decision to reject the null is always accompanied by an admission that a certain probability exists that this decision may be an error. That probability level, also known as the **alpha level** (sometime written as *α level*), is established before the actual analysis is completed. If the decision is to reject the null, alpha indicates the probability or likelihood that the researchers are committing a so-called **Type I error;** that is, that they are rejecting the null when in reality it should not be rejected. In the behavioral sciences, an alpha level of .05 is customary; however; in many of the basic and health science areas of research, a lower (i.e., more demanding) alpha is set, such as .01.

P Value (Level of Significance). In addition to the alpha level, another type of probability context affects any decision about the null. The **p value,** also known as the *level of significance,* indicates the likelihood or probability of obtaining the results of the statistical analysis by chance if the null hypothesis is actually valid. In a sense, the researchers are searching for statistical results that have such a low likelihood or probability of having occurred by chance, it becomes more reasonable to conclude that the results were driven by some nonchance reality, namely, an authentic relationship between or among the variables investigated.

For example, in the study by Chang et al., the statistical analysis indicates that the experimental group receiving massage had significantly lower pain reactions across all three phases of labor than did the control group. This means that the results of the statistical analysis of the data collected on the pain intensity DV have such a very low likelihood or probability of occurring by chance (if the null hypothesis is true), it is more reasonable to conclude that some nonchance reality is responsible for the findings. The nonchance reality in this case is the strong and convincing likelihood that a significant relationship exists between the IV and this DV, allowing the conclusion that the massage intervention—as contrasted with its absence—is responsible for lowering the participants' level of pain in the experimental group.

Statistical Power (power analysis). Still another type of probability context in which a null hypothesis is tested is the statistical power present when the analysis is done. The **statistical power** that exists when the data on a given DV are statistically analyzed refers to the probability or mathematical odds that the analysis will result in rejection of the null hypothesis when in fact the null is false and therefore should be rejected. Unfortunately, not all research reports provide for this type of calculation. However, a power analysis is critical, because it relates in part to the number of participants needed to establish the existence of an appropriate probability (usually at least .80) for rejecting the null if indeed it should be rejected.

Confidence Interval. Researchers in the basic, behavioral, and health sciences typically supplement or augment hypothesis testing by calculating a *confidence interval.* Various types of confidence intervals may be included in the results section of a research report, but in its most basic form, a **confidence interval (CI)** is a range of numeric values that has a certain probability of "capturing" the true population parameter under investigation in a study. For example, a 95% CI identifies both the lower and upper limits of the range of numeric values that the researchers are 95% confident actually contains or "captures" the true population parameter under investigation in a study (e.g., in the study by Chang et al., the population mean of the pain intensity level).

Effect Size. Researchers across various scientific disciplines should also report an *effect size* for their studies. As with the CI, this particular statistical concept can have several variations. In its basic form, the **effect size** is the degree or extent of influence, or "effect," of the IV on the DV. The effect size may be quantified as (1) the proportion of variation on the DV measures that can be explained or accounted for by the IV and/or (2) the size of the difference between the means of two comparison groups, as indicated in standard deviation units.

EXPERIMENTAL VALIDITY

The **experimental validity** of a difference-oriented study is the degree of control researchers are positioned to exercise over the several variables present in the investigation. In the true experimental (RCT) research method, two types of experimental validity are of paramount importance: internal validity and external validity. The internal validity issue in these studies typically is more important than the external validity issue, although the integrity of both types of validity should be ensured if possible.

Internal Validity

The issue of **internal validity** in a difference-oriented study involves the extent to which the DV measures can be traced back exclusively to the influence of the IV. The greater the degree of internal validity, the greater the researchers' ability to relate the IV to the DV in some cause-and-effect fashion. The higher level of internal validity is precisely what defines the true experimental (RCT) method as such a highly valued approach to research. The two critical research procedures that increase a study's internal validity are the use of random assignment and a manipulated IV.

Random assignment of participants to the comparison groups in a study helps control the extraneous variables that otherwise pose the risk of functioning as confounding variables. As mentioned earlier, random assignment of participants to the comparison groups or levels of the IV allows the researchers to assume (although it is not guaranteed) that the comparison groups are essentially equivalent on the major extraneous variables pertinent to the study. Once the manipulated IV has been introduced, the comparison groups can be thought of as differing only on that one single variable (i.e., the manipulated IV). The experimental group now is defined as the group receiving the experimental or treatment level of the manipulated IV being studied, and the control group is the group that is not. If a difference between the two comparison groups eventually emerges relative to the DV, the researchers can reasonably infer that this effect can be traced back to the manipulated IV; that is, to the only variable on which the participants differed. This sequence and line of reasoning become the basis for possibly inferring a causal relationship between the manipulated IV and the DV.

It should be apparent that the study by Chang et al. includes these two essential research procedures for elevating the study's internal validity. The 60 participants in the sample were randomly assigned to the experimental and control groups, and the IV was manipulated to establish, by intent and design, a planned distinction or difference between the two groups on that one single variable. Thus any difference between the two groups on either the pain intensity DV or the anxiety level DV could be traced back to the manipulated IV (i.e., the presence versus the absence of massage intervention).

External Validity

The issue of **external validity** in a study considers the extent to which the conclusions reached can be generalized from the sample to the accessible population from which the sample was derived. A study is implemented in the contexts of the participants who constitute the sample and the setting or circumstances that operationally define the research procedures used. Researchers are interested in generalizing as extensively as possible from the comparatively limited sample to the original accessible population.

Random selection of participants from the accessible population is the research procedure most critical to elevating a study's external validity. This is the case largely because random selection allows the researchers to assume that the resulting sample is an unbiased, representative subset (microcosm) of the larger population (set or macrocosm). This assumption is based on the role of random selection in ensuring that every member of the accessible population has an equal and nonzero chance of being included in the sample. Properly performed, random selection allows chance factors alone to operate in determining which participants in the accessible population become members of the sample, thereby protecting against any systematically biased influence on the selection process.

The study by Chang et al. did not use random selection; rather, participants were recruited sequentially as they entered the maternity ward in a regional hospital. Consequently, the researchers' ability to generalize their findings with confidence to an accessible population is greatly compromised. This is because the accessible population was not thoroughly defined as a known set of potential participants in terms of the size and characteristics of the group, therefore there was no way to ensure mathematically that each member of the sample had the same probability of being selected as other members.

Again, a verbal analogy may prove useful for remembering the relationship between random assignment and internal validity and the connection between random selection and external validity: random assignment is to internal validity as random selection is to external validity. Expressed in another form, the analogy would look like this:

random assignment : internal validity ::
random selection : external validity

EXPERIMENTAL RESEARCH DESIGN NOTATION

This chapter's discussion of the true experimental (RCT) type of study obviously involves quite an accumulation of concepts, principles, procedures, and terminology, which might come across as somewhat intimidating. At this point, you are strongly encouraged to keep in mind the broad context within which the discussion occurs.

Relying only on narrative descriptive labels, we could say that the study by Chang et al. is (1) a randomized, control group, posttest–only research design, which is (2) one of several possible designs affiliated with the true experimental (RCT) research method, which is (3) included in the difference-oriented research strategy, which is (4) recognized as belonging to the quantitative research category.

You undoubtedly will be relieved to learn that a certain type of **research design notation,** which takes the following form, can economically display the specifics of the preceding paragraph:

$$\begin{array}{cccc} RA & EG & X & O_{Post} \\ RA & CG & \cdot & O_{Post} \end{array}$$

The display is interpreted as follows: *RA* indicates the random assignment of participants to both the experimental group *(EG)* and the control group *(CG),* as in the study by Chang et al. *X* designates the experimental level of the manipulated IV (in the study by Chang et al., the presence of massage for the 30 participants in the experimental group). The bullet *(·)* represents the nonexperimental level of the manipulated IV (in Chang et al., the absence of massage for the 30 participants in the control group). O_{Post} indicates that both the experimental group and the control group were post-observed, or post-tested, on each of the DVs.

This simple display allows us to "read" the design of the study as being a randomized, control group, posttest–only research design. That should prompt recognition that such a research design logically belongs to the true experimental (RCT) research method because of the use of random assignment and a manipulated IV. This recognition should lead us to recall that any research method that examines the relationship between an IV and a DV must belong to the difference-oriented research strategy family, because the relationship between an IV and a DV is explored by investigating whether a difference exists between or among the two or more levels of the IV relative to the DV. If all of this is still going well for you and making sense, we should recognize that this particular research strategy is one of three possible research strategies constituting the quantitative research category.

SCHEMATIC ILLUSTRATION OF THE EXPERIMENTAL (RCT) RESEARCH METHOD

(Reflecting only select features of, and a slight modification in, the study by Chang et al, 2002)

The holistic view of the true experimental (RCT) research method, which provides a context for our discussion throughout most of this chapter, is displayed succinctly by the schematic in Figure 2-12. The schematic presents select features and a slight modification of the study by Chang et al. to allow a panoramic view of the research process as examined thus far. The very sequential and linear progression of the concepts, principles, and procedures covered up to this point should be easily recognized.

Specifically, the progression reflected in this schematic begins with the interplay between formulation of the research question and review of the professional literature. This interplay becomes the basis for initiation of the sequence of research procedures that begins with the accessible population (the slight modification in the actual study) and continues to the eventual decision to reject the null hypothesis regarding the DV of pain intensity. The interplay between the research question and the literature review also serves as the basis for the formulation of the research hypothesis at the very outset of the study and for the implied null and alternative hypotheses that follow.

ETHICAL CONSIDERATIONS

Our brief consideration of the study by Chang et al. should have caused you to reflect on some of the ethical considerations that undoubtedly arose before, during, and after the study. These include the following:

- What kind of collegial input and supervision were the researchers provided both before and during the study with respect

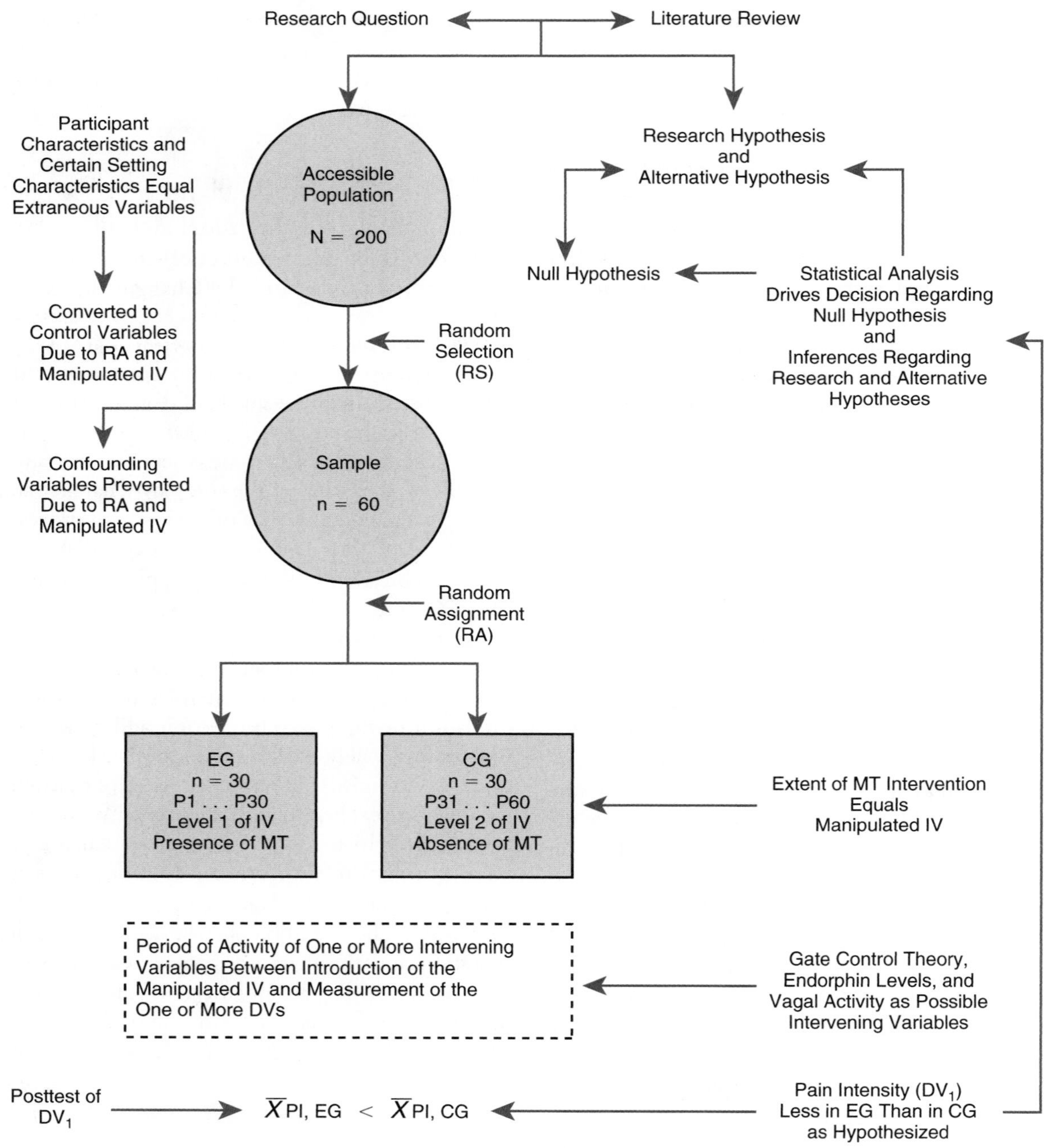

FIGURE 2-12 ■ Schematic of a true experimental (RCT) research method. The diagram reflects select features of the study by Chang et al. (2002) with a slight modification. (Modified from Hymel GM: *Research methods for massage and holistic therapies,* St Louis, 2006, Mosby.)

to the study's design and the measures taken to protect the participants during the conduct of the study?

- Was any type of institutional review of the study's proposal done before the study was implemented?
- What types of information about the study were provided to the participants before they became involved in the investigation?
- What type of consent was received from the participants before their admission to the study?

- Did the participants have the option of discontinuing their involvement at any time and without prejudice?
- Did any questions arise regarding the confidentiality of the data collected on the several variables for each participant?
- What might be the thoughts and feelings of those assigned to the control group, who did not receive the massage intervention?
- Were the study's results shared with the participants afterward?

These are just a few of several very important concerns that relate to **research ethics.** Issues pertaining to the role of an Institutional Review Board (IRB) in granting approval for the study would certainly have encompassed most if not all of these concerns. Informed consent, confidentiality, the latitude to exit the study at any time without prejudice, the entitlement of the control group participants to the experimental level of the IV, and debriefing are among an array of ethical issues that researchers must face. Scrupulously ethical conduct of research is essential, for the obvious reason that the advancement of science must not occur at the expense of the safety and well-being of research participants. A comprehensive discussion of the requirements of research ethics is beyond the scope of this chapter, but it can be found in any of the textbooks cited earlier.

OTHER RESEARCH PROCEDURE OPTIONS AND THEIR IMPLICATIONS

Our discussion of the research process thus far has focused primarily on the true experimental (RCT) method, as exemplified by the study by Chang et al. However, many other options are available, and several are relevant to difference-oriented studies in the quantitative research category.

RANDOM ASSIGNMENT OR INTACT GROUPS

The essential distinction between the true experimental (RCT) research method and the quasi-experimental research method is the random assignment of participants to the two or more levels of the IV. In the former method, participants are randomly assigned to the comparative groups. In the latter method, the comparative groups are formed not by random assignment, but rather as a function of the groups' already being in place (i.e., **intact groups**).

The presence of random assignment in the true experimental/randomized control trial method is one of two critical procedures necessary for the possibility of cause-and-effect conclusions being derived. The other critical procedure is that of the independent variable being manipulated or governed by the researcher. And it is precisely this issue that brings us to the next option requiring a decision on the part of researchers.

MANIPULATED INDEPENDENT VARIABLE OR NONMANIPULATED INDEPENDENT VARIABLE

As mentioned earlier, the IV in a difference-oriented study is also known as a *stimulus variable,* an *input variable,* or possibly a *causal variable.* With certain research questions, the researcher must manipulate or govern the dynamics associated with the IV. This is certainly the case in any study involving a treatment or intervention delivered in the present to the study's participants. This type of IV also is the focal point in research studies that are perhaps of most interest to massage therapists and other health science professionals curious about various treatment modalities and their impact on certain client outcomes.

Equally important among the research procedure options for the IV are circumstances in which the research question does not address a treatment or intervention in the present, but rather is concerned with traits, characteristics, or conditions that do not (or should not) lend themselves to being manipulated by the researcher. This is the so-called **nonmanipulated independent variable.** Our earlier acknowledgment of the nonexperimental comparative groups method and its affiliated research designs provided several examples of this type of IV.

In the context of a difference-oriented research strategy, the IV being addressed is always manifested in two or more ways regardless of whether or not it is being manipulated. This tissue leads us to yet another option that must be addressed by researchers.

POSSIBLE COMPARATIVE GROUPS OR LEVELS OF THE INDEPENDENT VARIABLE

Any independent variable in a difference-oriented study, whether manipulated or not, always is manifested in two or more ways. As mentioned previously, the ways an IV presents itself are also called the *levels* of the IV. For example, in its simplest form a true experimental design may investigate the difference between an experimental group and a control group with regard to the study's dependent variable. In a somewhat more extended manner, the same type of design may investigate the differences among three groups—two experimental groups and a control group—regarding a DV.

The nature of a study's research question leads eventually to the determination of how many comparative groups or levels of the IV will be explored for differences regarding the DV. Any researcher involved in a difference-oriented study has basically two decisions to make with regard to the research question prompting the study: (1) whether the IV is manipulated or nonmanipu lated and (2) whether the IV entails two or more comparative groups or levels that reflect how the IV is manifested.

TYPES OF CONTROL GROUPS

As we have seen, a **control group** is one of the possible comparative groups or levels of an IV investigated in a difference-oriented research strategy. Several types of control groups may appear in a study, each serving a particular purpose. They may include the following: (1) a no treatment or "do nothing" control group, (2) a standard treatment control group, (3) a waiting-list control group, (4) a placebo-attention control group, and (5) a placebo-sham treatment control group.

The **no treatment control group** (or "do nothing" control group) entails precisely what its name describes. Although this type of control group is appearing considerably less frequently in research studies, researchers use it when they want to compare one or more treatment groups to a comparable group of participants for whom no treatment or involvement is planned.

The **standard treatment control group** includes study participants who receive the healthcare treatment or intervention recognized as standard or typical for their presenting condition. This standard treatment is contrasted with one or more experimental versions or levels of the IV to determine whether any differences exist between or among the interventions with regard to one or more outcome measures of interest (i.e., the DVs). In the study by Chang et al., the control group of 30 participants undergoing childbirth obviously received standard medical treatment, but without the massage intervention that was provided to the experimental group.

The **waiting-list control group** is a group of participants who do not receive the investigative treatment or intervention during the conduct of the study, but rather are put on a waiting list and are scheduled to receive the treatment once the study is completed. This approach to forming a control group for comparison to an experimental or treatment group is one way to ensure participant welfare under two circumstances: (1) when those initially in the control group have a noncritical or nonemergency condition that might benefit from the treatment and (2) when the duration of the investigative treatment is relatively brief, such that the waiting period is not too long.

With a **placebo-attention control group,** a group of study participants who are not receiving the experimental treatment is exposed to a stimulus experience that is inert with respect to any direct anticipated impact on the outcome being investigated. Although inert as just described, the stimulus experience typically takes the form of interpersonal contact and support that provide these participants with a sense of being attended to and involved. As a result, the placebo-attention control group and the experimental group have the common experience of being "engaged." This allows any outcome differences between the groups to be attributed to the one uncommon feature across the two groups, namely, the presumed dynamic nature of the experimental treatment. For example, a childbirth labor study reported by Field, Hernandez-Reif, Taylor, Quintino, and

Burman (1997) compared the effect of having partners massage women in labor with that of having partners simply be present and react spontaneously during labor, usually in terms of the breathing coaching learned in prenatal classes.

With a **placebo-sham treatment control group,** the group of study participants being contrasted with the experimental group is exposed to a simulated treatment that feigns the intervention of a viable treatment. The presumed dynamic or viable treatment provided to the control group actually is a "pretended" or impostor-type intervention with no dynamic potential to influence the outcome measure or measures. A study by Preyde (2000) included among the four levels of the manipulated IV a sham laser (infrared) therapy intervention in which the laser was made to appear to be functioning, when in fact it was not operative.

BETWEEN-SUBJECTS INDEPENDENT VARIABLE OR WITHIN-SUBJECTS (REPEATED MEASURES) INDEPENDENT VARIABLE

The distinction involving a between-subjects IV and a within-subjects (repeated measures) IV has not been made thus far. However, this distinction is critical to two important considerations: (1) the way the study's participants become affiliated with the comparative groups of the IV and (2) the type of statistical technique eventually used to analyze the data acquired on the DV.

With regard to the way study participants become affiliated with the two or more comparative groups, a **between-subjects independent variable** (also known as a *between-subjects design*) simply means that a separate group of individuals is affiliated with each level of the IV. For example, if the IV has three levels that are being contrasted regarding the DV, then three separate groups constitute those three levels.

The advantage to using a between-subjects IV is that the experiences of a given group in a given level of the IV remain there and entail no participation with any of the other levels of the IV. An important consequence of this is that the participants' measures on the DV are specific to what they experienced within that one particular group or IV level.

The disadvantage to employing a between-subjects IV is that even with random assignment of a distinct group of participants to a specific level of the IV, no guarantee exists that the two or more comparative groups will be equivalent in terms of, for example, the individual differences the researchers are trying to control. In this circumstance researchers often act on the assumption that the comparative groups are equivalent on the extraneous variables that take the form of individual differences; however, this is nonetheless an assumption.

With a **within-subjects independent variable** (also known as a *within-subjects design*), a specific group of participants experiences each level of the IV. For example, if the IV has three levels that are being compared with regard to the DV, then the same group of participants will experience what each of the three levels of the IV has to offer.

The advantage to using the within-subjects IV is that it is an optimal way to control extraneous variables that are rooted in individual differences across participants. This is the case simply because the very same participants, and obviously the very same individual differences they represent, are present within each level of the IV. By implication, this same group of participants is measured repeatedly on the DV within each level of the IV. For this reason, the within-subjects IV is also called a *repeated measures IV.*

The disadvantage to using a within-subjects (repeated measures) IV is the risk that the participants' experience of a particular level of the IV will carry over to their experience of the other level or levels. Also, because the participants are measured repeatedly on the DV for each level, their responses to the DV under the conditions of one level may be influenced by their experience of a preceding level. This problem of *carryover effect* should be countered by a procedure known as *counterbalancing.* With counterbalancing, the participants experience each level of the IV in each and every sequential position in which the IVs' two or more levels can be placed. The participants' repeated measures on the DV then are aggregated for analysis purposes across all the possible sequential positions in which any given level might have appeared. The ultimate intent, therefore, is to have counterbalancing counteract the carryover effects.

As mentioned, a second important consideration that depends on the use of a between-subjects or a within-subjects IV is the statistical technique selected to analyze the data collected on the DV. It is sufficient to acknowledge at this point that the distinction involving between-subjects and within-subjects IVs is one of several criteria researchers must use in difference-oriented studies to ensure the selection of the most appropriate statistical technique. For example, the so-called independent groups t-test is a *possible* selection for data analysis in a difference-oriented study involving a between-subjects IV with only two levels. In a similar circumstance involving a between-subjects IV with three or more levels, the so-called one-way between-subjects analysis of variance is a *possible* selection. The word *possible* is emphasized in both examples because more criteria must come into play before a final selection of either statistical technique could be justified.

PRETEST-POSTTEST OR POSTTEST ONLY

Some of the designs mentioned earlier in the chapter specified a **pretest** or preobservation procedure relatively early in the design's sequence and specifically before introduction of the IV. In some cases the pretest is done to establish a baseline record of the participants' reactions to the DV before any type of intervention is introduced. In other cases the pretest may be done to collect data, which become the basis for identifying the two or more levels of the IV.

Almost all the designs examined thus far involved a **posttest** of the participants on the DV. In some studies this is done to examine the contrast between pretest and posttest performances. When only a posttest is administered, the intent is to rely exclusively on the contrast between or among the two or more levels of the IV with regard to just the posttest measures.

Although this discussion speaks in terms of a single measure of a DV, studies more typically examine two or more DVs. Furthermore, pretesting in a study often focuses on the accumulation of demographic data and other types of participant characterizing data that inform the researcher of the broader context in which the study is being undertaken.

GROUP-SPECIFIC OR SINGLE-CASE FOCUS

As you have seen, three of the four research methods affiliated with the difference-oriented research strategy involve manipulated and nonmanipulated IVs, which have levels that take the form of groups of participants, which are contrasted on the study's DV. These three methods are the true experimental (RCT) method, the quasi-experimental method, and the nonexperimental comparative groups method. Because each of these methods involves the comparison of groups, the issue of between-subjects or within-subjects IVs is always an important consideration.

The fourth research method affiliated with the difference-oriented research strategy relies on the use of individual participants rather than groups of participants; this is the so-called single-case experimental method. This method focuses on a single participant, who may be exposed to baseline measures, treatment variations, and post-measures somewhat comparable to those experienced in the group-specific methods. The single-case experimental method holds a great deal of potential for therapeutic massage practitioners who are interested in research that may be integrated into their individual practice. Massage therapists see many different types of clients with varying signs and symptoms that call for informed use of appropriate interventions and modalities; this situation offers practitioners the opportunity to contribute to the scientific advancement of their profession. Of course, it is critical to emphasize that standard prerequisites must be in place regarding such issues as the practitioner's research literacy and capacity, membership on a viable research team, mentor-collegial supervision, client/participant protection, and the overall ethical integrity of the entire research effort.

RANDOMIZED CONTROLLED TRIAL OR RANDOMIZED CLINICAL TRIAL

Earlier in the chapter we discussed the true experimental (RCT) method, an element of the difference-oriented research strategy. The explanation of this method involved a comparison between an experimental or treatment group and a control group; this is the context in which the term **randomized controlled trial** is used; that is, when the group compared to the experimental group is a no treatment ("do nothing") control group or possibly a waiting-list control group. However, as pointed out by Hagino (2003), the term **randomized clinical trial** is preferred when the comparison to the experimental group involves a **comparison treatment control group.** In this case three other options for control groups are possible: the standard treatment control group, the placebo-attention control group, and the placebo-sham treatment control group.

BLINDED (MASKED) OR OPEN STUDIES

The term **blinded (masked) study** refers to a study involving a research procedure in which one or more of the parties are unaware of the level of the IV to which a participant belongs. In a **single-blind research procedure,** the investigator is unaware of a participant's group membership. In a **double-blind research procedure,** neither the investigator nor the participant is aware of the participant's affiliated IV level. As noted by Ernst (2002, p.17), "Blinding patients in trials of massage therapy is probably not achievable. The same obviously applies to the therapist. In essence, this means that in clinical massage research only the evaluator-blinded trials are feasible." The complete absence of any form of blinding or masking defines a so-called **open study.**

A FRAMEWORK FOR READING A RESEARCH ARTICLE: STRUCTURE, FUNCTION, AND IMPLIED CRITERIA FOR EVALUATION

Against the backdrop of our chapter content coverage thusfar, this is perhaps the appropriate point at which to introduce what admittedly has already been implied regarding the basic format for an empirical research report.

STRUCTURE AND FUNCTION: THE RESEARCH REPORT'S "ANATOMY" AND "PHYSIOLOGY"

The structure, or "anatomy," of an empirical research article is a rather standard feature of this form of scientific or technical writing. Because the obvious intent is to enhance communication among professionals across various disciplines and professions, the sections and subsections that constitute a research report must not be left to the preferences or idiosyncrasies of individual researchers.

The various sections and subsections that guide the structure of the research report have the express purpose of accomplishing certain functions, which may be considered the "physiology" of the report.

The combination of a research article's structure and function sets the stage for identifying several criteria that might be used to determine whether a research report provides appropriate information. When appropriate information is provided, the merit of the research effort can be evaluated with regard to its potential for advancing the knowledge base and, eventually, the evidence-based practice massage therapists provide for clients and patients.

The following parts of this section provide you with an overview of the six major sections and their corresponding sub-sections that constitute a research article.

Preliminary Section: Title and Abstract

The first section of the research article, the **preliminary section,** contains the title and abstract of the study. Although a study's title is fairly self-explanatory, it must be formulated such that a potential reader (perhaps scanning a list of studies by bibliographic citation only) can determine such information as the type of study, the major variables, and the participants who were the focal point of the researchers' efforts.

In the **abstract** (or summary), the authors must synthesize the main body of the report (i.e., introduction, method, results, and discussion sections) as efficiently and effectively as possible. A correctly written abstract gives readers a precise idea of the functions the study accomplished, allowing them to decide whether to read the entire report.

Introductory Section

The introduction of the report provides the context within which the remainder of the report is to be considered. Specifically, the **introductory section** has five subsections: (1) the general literature review, (2) the specific literature review, (3) the purpose statement (through identification of the research question), (4) the rationale for the study's research hypothesis, and (5) the statement of the research hypothesis.

The *general literature review* identifies the broader context of the study's major research problem area. The appeal here is at a general level to earlier researchers and authors who have contributed to the research problem area. Following this overview, the *specific literature review* provides a more detailed treatment of related sources in the professional literature. This subsection allows the reader to become considerably more familiar with the earlier literature that informs the current study. These two subsections serve a dual purpose: (1) to establish the credibility of the current study's authors in the minds of readers with regard to the researchers' familiarity with existing sources of information in the research problem area and (2) to provide readers with pertinent information and insight that they should have to better comprehend the current report.

In the *purpose statement* (through identification of the research question), the research question at the very least must be implied, although an explicit formulation of it is strongly preferred. This subsection presents to the reader the true starting point in the study, because any research endeavor bases its many decisions precisely on the research question, which represents the reason the study was conducted. In considering a research question, readers must keep in mind that it is never formulated in a vacuum; this simply means that researchers must have some degree of familiarity with the relevant literature to identify the question. At the same time, they must have at least the beginnings of a research question to know exactly where to search in the literature.

The *rationale for the research hypothesis* relies on and may even expand upon the earlier subsections that dealt with the literature review. A study's authors must rely on the available research literature in a given problem area to acknowledge the rationale or justification for what becomes the study's research hypothesis. Readers must remember that the research hypothesis is basically the predicted answer to the study's research question; it is *not* an "educated guess." It is a predicted answer to the research question that is informed or justified primarily by concepts, theories, and/or existing empirical research contained in the professional literature. Therefore the rationale for the research hypothesis should be presented immediately before the statement of the research hypothesis. In this way, a context is already in place that clarifies the reasons the researchers are predicting a certain answer to the study's question. Although the rationale usually is only implied, the preferred approach is to identify it explicitly, for the reader's benefit.

The *statement of the research hypothesis* sometimes is given less care than it deserves. Unfortunately, far too many authors fail to provide an explicit statement, with justification, of the anticipated outcome of the study (i.e., the answer to the study's research question). The tendency is to allow the research hypothesis simply to be implied. The major advantage of an explicit statement of the hypothesis is that it alerts the reader to several critical features of the study, such as the research category, strategy, and method used; the variables investigated and their predicted relationship; the participants studied; and the context or setting of the study. Knowledge of the research hypothesis sets the stage for a more informed consideration of the study's methodology, the next major section in the research report.

Method Section

Just as its name suggests, the **method section** of the research report provides a detailed account of the methodology used in carrying out the study. It identifies the various research procedures used at different stages of the study and operationalizes them at such a specific level that the study could be replicated. The method section also gives readers as complete a basis as possible for determining whether the implementation of the study in any way justifies or compromises the results and conclusions reached.

To accomplish these objectives, the method section must address several issues, such as the participants and how they were chosen; the instruments used for measuring variables; and the procedures by which the study was implemented. Accordingly, standard subsections that constitute the method section are (1) the participants and sampling procedures; (2) the research method and design; (3) the variables; and (4) the instrumentation. These four subsections provide the report's authors with ample opportunity to specify precisely "what was done" in carrying out the study. Some slight variation in the labeling of these subsections may be seen across different studies. The important point is that the sections address the themes of participants, measuring instruments, and procedures.

The first subsection, typically labeled *participants and sampling procedures,* identifies for the reader the characteristics of the participants used in the study and the activities used to select and assign them. The researchers identify and justify the inclusion criteria and exclusion criteria used as the bases for determining who did and did not qualify as study participants. Researchers also use this subsection to provide information about the power analysis done to determine the optimal sample size for a given study. In addition, the researchers must acknowledge here the extent to which random selection of sample participants from an accessible population was used, as well as the random assignment of subjects to comparison groups. If the researchers used procedures other than random selection and random assignment, they must specify the alternatives employed. These issues are critical, given the nature of the bases for and importance of a study's external and internal validity. Finally, this subsection should specify the ethical provisions taken to ensure the protection of participants, the overall integrity of the study, and prior approval from the appropriate IRB.

In the second subsection, labeled *research method and design,* the focus on these two intermediate points in the research continuum is strategic, because it allows the reader to recognize the research category, strategy, and procedures that, by implication, the researchers used in the study. These factors also have implications regarding the external and internal validity of the study.

The third subsection addresses the *variables* investigated in the study. Although this obviously is not the first time the variables are mentioned in the report, the important feature here is that the researchers operationalize the variables as specifically as possible. In this subsection the reader learns all the details of how the researchers identified, defined, characterized, controlled, manipulated, and/or measured the study's variables.

The fourth and last subsection, *instrumentation,* deals primarily with the measuring instruments used to generate numeric and/or verbal data. This subsection may also refer to a type or model of equipment or apparatus that played a role in the study. Technical characteristics, such as the validity and reliability of instruments, are crucial and therefore are prominent features of the information provided in this subsection.

Results Section

The **results section** provides the reader with a full accounting of the outcomes or results of the data analysis performed in the study. This is accomplished mainly by disclosure of the descriptive and/or inferential statistical techniques used to analyze the study's data, the results of the analysis, and their interpretation. This section is also where the researchers acknowledge, usually by implication, the study's null (statistical) hypothesis, along with their explicit decision to reject or fail to reject it. Based on the decision about the null hypothesis, the researchers then develop the inferences to be drawn about the alternative and research hypotheses.

The results section provides researchers the opportunity to specify other statistical findings beyond hypothesis testing if the study included such findings. For example, researchers may include the establishment of confidence intervals and the citing of effect sizes in this section in an attempt to augment traditional null hypothesis significance testing (NHST).

Discussion Section

The **discussion section,** the final section of the report's main body, presents the authors' discussion of the study's findings. This section gives the researchers the opportunity to (1) reflect on the manner in which the study was conducted, inclusive of its limitations and delimitations (boundaries); (2) elaborate on the interpretation of the study's findings begun in the results section; (3) acknowledge the significance of the study's results, as well as their relationship to earlier research findings in the problem area; (4) theorize as to why the results were forthcoming (i.e., which intervening variables might have come into play during the conduct of the study); and (5) suggest areas of further research that would be logical sequels to the current study.

Concluding Section

The **concluding section** of the research report begins with a list of the bibliographic citations for each of the sources cited in the research report. This list constitutes the references for the report, which are very important because they not only give detailed credit to sources used in the study, they also provide the reader with the necessary information for accessing the sources cited. The research report may provide additional information in the form of appendices, authors' notes, and footnotes.

IMPLIED CRITERIA FOR CRITIQUING A RESEARCH ARTICLE: REFLECTIONS OF STRUCTURE AND FUNCTION

The structure and function of the sections and subsections that constitute a research report provide the foundation for identifying certain criteria or standards that can be used to critique the merits of a report. This approach also gives readers an organizational framework for systematically working through the process of reflecting on the contents of a report. Box 2-2 provides a comprehensive list of specific questions that are relevant to evaluation of the specific sections and subsections of a research report. It is important for you to recognize that this particular list of criteria is geared primarily, though not exclusively, to the types of studies considered thus far, namely, studies that fall into the research continuum at two points: the quantitative research category and the difference-oriented research strategy.

A BRIEF LOOK AT SINGLE-SUBJECT/ SINGLE-CASE RESEARCH METHODS

As mentioned earlier, several types of research methods focus on a single subject or case of interest. The four **single-subject/single-case research methods** and their affiliated research strategies and categories are (1) the **single-case experimental method;** (2) the **single-case quantitative analysis method;** (3) the **case report method;** and (4) the **case study method.** The first of these four research methods represents the difference-oriented research strategy within the quantitative research category; the second and third methods represent the descriptive-oriented research strategy that is likewise within the quantitative research category; and the fourth method represents the contextual/interpretive-oriented research strategy within the qualitative research category. Figure 2-13 shows the four research methods in their respective contexts.

- Quantitative Research Category
  - Difference-Oriented Research Strategy
    - Single-Case Experimental Method
  - Descriptive-Oriented Research Strategy
    - Single-Case Quantitative Analysis Method
    - Case Report Method
- Qualitative Research Category
  - Contextual/Interpretive-Oriented Research Strategy
    - Case Study Method

FIGURE 2-13 ■ Single-subject/case research methods in the context of their affiliated research strategies and categories.

The single-subject/single-case research methods are particularly relevant for massage therapists because they typically represent a twofold opportunity for professional growth. As informed consumers of this type of research literature, practitioners can gain insight about specific client populations and conditions and pertinent interventions that have resulted in certain outcomes. For practitioners who may want to become involved in massage therapy research, these methods afford an opportunity to relate one's clinical experience to the research process.

The textbook's Evolve website gives an overview of the essential features of the four single-subject/single-case research methods, providing an introduction to the similarities and distinctions across these research methods. However, the case report method should be highlighted as being of particular importance and relevance to massage therapists. This research method has recently gained increased recognition among massage therapists as an important entry point in the research process. For example, in 2005 the Massage Therapy Foundation inaugurated an annual student case report competition as a means of promoting student interest in and familiarity with the research process. The first winner of this competition was a study by Hamm (2006), "Impact of Massage Therapy in the Treatment of

Box 2-2 Criteria for Critiquing a Research Study

Preliminary Section

1 Does the title of the study provide a basis for identifying the type of study, major variables, and participants?

2 Does the abstract synthesize the main body of the report (i.e., the introduction, method, results, and discussion) with a particular focus on the research question, research hypothesis, participants, research method and design, major variables, instruments, statistical techniques, principal findings, and conclusions?

Introductory Section

3 Is the reader introduced to the relevant professional literature bearing on the study being reported by way of a general overview of the research problem area, as well as more specific coverage of individual studies?

4 Is the purpose of the study identified by means of formulation of the research question at an operational level?

5 Is a rationale or justification that is based on various features of the professional literature presented as a context or framework for the study's research hypothesis?

6 Do the authors state the study's research hypothesis in such a way that the predicted answer to the research question is clear and unambiguous?

Method Section

7 Are the study's participants clearly characterized, along with the inclusion and exclusion criteria used to identify them?

8 Did the researchers justify the number of participants constituting the sample size by means of a power analysis?

9 Was an accessible population of potential participants acknowledged and an indication given of how the sample was derived from such a population, whether through random selection or some other procedure?

10 Did the authors specify the manner in which the participants were assigned to the two or more comparison groups, whether through random assignment or some other means?

11 Was any clarification provided as to how the ethical aspects of the study were governed, particularly in reference to the protection of the participants, the overall integrity of the research, and the earlier approval of the study by an Institutional Review Board?

12 Was the nature of the research effort adequately characterized in terms of its position in the research continuum (i.e., its position regarding research category, strategy, method, design, and defining procedures)?

13 Were the study's variables operationalized in a comprehensive fashion so that their manipulation and/or measurement could be replicated?

14 Did the authors clearly specify the equipment and instruments used in the study for variable manipulation or measurement purposes, along with documentation of the technical characteristic of such, including validity and reliability?

Results Section

15 Were the data analysis techniques used identified and justified?

16 Were the results of the study communicated by an appeal to descriptive and/or inferential statistics consistent with the nature of the research question and the research method and measurement scales used?

17 Were the results of the data analysis related to an appropriate decision regarding the study's null (statistical) hypothesis?

18 Was the decision on the null hypothesis acknowledged as a basis for inferring decisions concerning the alternative and research hypotheses?

19 If hypothesis testing was performed, were the analyses augmented with other statistical techniques, such as confidence interval estimation or effect size calculations (or both)?

20 Were tables and figures used appropriately to make the data analyses more comprehensible?

Discussion Section

21 Did the researchers reflect on the manner in which the study was designed and conducted with regard to any limitations or delimitations (i.e., intentional or unintentional boundaries)?

22 Did the authors elaborate on the interpretation of the study's findings beyond the interpretation started in the results section?

23 Did the researchers address the significance of the study and its findings, particularly as they relate to earlier studies in the problem area investigated?

24 Were possible intervening variables in the study addressed that might explain why the results obtained were forthcoming?

25 Were recommendations made to the reader about needed follow-up studies that might fully or partly replicate, or at least augment, the current study?

Concluding Section

26 Does the list of references accurately reflect each of the sources cited in the research report, with a consistent bibliographic citation style used?

27 Does the research report have any appendices that provide greater detail on information presented earlier in the article?

28 Are authors' notes included that provide insight into funding support for the study, contact directives for communicating with the authors as a follow up, and collegial assistance in completing the study?

29 Are any footnotes provided that elaborate on one or more aspects of the study that would have been misplaced or distracting if they had been embedded in the main body of the report?

Linked Pathologies: Scoliosis, Costovertebral Dysfunction, and Thoracic Outlet Syndrome," which appeared in the July 2006 issue of the *Journal of Bodywork and Movement Therapies.* The current plan is to extend this type of competition to practitioners beginning in 2007.

In brief, the case report method focuses on a detailed description of a clinical practice issue that defines a recommended treatment plan in the context of the client's profile and the justification for the selected intervention. Against this backdrop, the case report describes the sequence of clinical visits and the continual and final results of the treatment's effectiveness. This focused and detailed description of clinical practice can be developed from either of two possible perspectives, namely, a *retrospective perspective* or a *prospective view.* As distinguished by Dumholdt (2000):

Retrospective case reports are developed when a practitioner realizes that there are valuable lessons to be shared from a case in which the . . . therapy episode has been completed. Prospective case reports are developed when a practitioner, on initial contact with a patient or sometime early in the course of treatment, recognizes that the case is likely to produce interesting findings that should be shared. When a case report is developed prospectively, there is the potential for excellent control of measurement techniques and complete description of the treatments and responses as they unfold. Unfortunately, the prospective case report suffers from the possibility that the case was managed differently from usual because of the desire to publish the results in the future (p. 148).

With regard to the format of a case report, the generic coverage found in more standard research reports is appropriate in that introductory, method, results, and discussion sections typically allow for the clinical practice features to be reported adequately. *Writing Case Reports* (McEwen, 2001) is a helpful resource that includes, among many valuable features, a detailed checklist organized around the components essential to a comprehensive case report.

The Massage Therapy Foundation provides a set of guidelines for structuring a case report that can be accessed at http://massagetherapyfoundation.org/grants_education.html. Consistent with the standard content of research reports, the format for a case report includes a cover/title page, acknowledgments, abstract, key words, introduction (including the literature review), method (including the client profile and treatment plan), results, discussion, and references.

Stylistic requirements for manuscript preparation typically are specified in author guidelines provided by the journal or organization to which the manuscript will be submitted. The two stylistic formats most often used are found in the *Uniform Requirements for Manuscripts Submitted to Biomedical Journals,* prepared by the International Committee of Medical Journal Editors (ICMJE, 2003), and in the *Publication Manual of the American Psychological Association* (American Psychological Association, 2001).

RESEARCH MATRIX OF REPRESENTATIVE STUDIES IN CLINICAL MASSAGE THERAPY AND RELATED LITERATURE

The concepts and procedures covered in this chapter are intended to provide at least the beginning of a familiarity with the research process and its terminology. This initial step, in turn, should allow you to start examining the research literature currently available in clinical/medical massage and related areas. To encourage this process, the textbook's Evolve website presents a research matrix that crosses authors or studies with various client and patient systems, conditions, and populations. The specific information needed to locate the studies is found on the website, as are full bibliographic citations.

The focus here is not on exhaustive coverage and interpretation of the pertinent research literature, but rather on the identification of representative studies of probable interest to you as you work your way through the remaining chapters of this book. In subsequent chapters you will have ample opportunity to revisit in greater detail many of the studies cited in the research matrix as we discuss the various patient conditions and populations that define the scope of clinical/medical massage.

The resources primarily used to compile the research matrix were (1) electronic searches of standard databases, such as **PubMed,** PsycInfo, and CINAHL; (2) integrative literature reviews of the traditional narrative and meta-analytic types by Field (1998) and Moyer et al. (2004), respectively; and (3) the works on therapeutic and medical massage by Turchaninov (2000) and Turchaninov and Cox (1998). Of particular note among these resources are the two works by Turchaninov and colleagues because they provide exhaustive coverage spanning several decades of Russian and Eastern European research on therapeutic and medical massage.

evolve 2-1

The following terms and expressions specific to Chapter 2 have already been used to search PubMed for the latest research literature available. The *Click Here for Massage* feature associated with this chapter on your textbook's Evolve website allows you to hyperlink to a continually updated PubMed search of research literature that corresponds to this subject.

Hyperlink Search Terms

Massage case report
Massage randomized controlled trial
Massage research
Massage research methods

SUMMARY

This chapter provided an overview of the research process to provide a basis for a better understanding of the topics covered in the remainder of this book. In so doing, the emphasis was on surveying the various research categories, strategies, methods, designs, and procedures that represent the various options available to researchers. Particular emphasis was given to the true experimental—or randomized controlled trial (RCT)—research method as well as the concepts, principles, and procedures that constitute the foundations of scientific investigation. This knowledge base should allow at least the following capabilities at a more informed level: (1) the critical reading of available research on massage and its relationship to healthcare, (2) possible participation as one of several members of a research team, and (3) collaborative communication with other healthcare professionals on issues of mutual interest.

REFERENCES

American Psychological Association: *Publication manual of the American Psychological Association,* ed 5, Washington, DC, 2001, The Association.

Chang MY, Wang SY, Chen CH: Effects of massage on pain and anxiety during labour: a randomized controlled trial in Taiwan, *J Adv Nurs* 38:68-73, 2002.

Cherkin DC, Eisenberg D, Sherman KJ et al: Randomized trial comparing traditional Chinese medical acupuncture, therapeutic massage, and self-care education for chronic low back pain, *Arch Intern Med* 161:1081-1088, 2001.

Crewswell JW: *Qualitative inquiry and research design: choosing among five traditions,* Thousand Oaks, Calif, 1998, Sage.

Dumholdt E: *Physical therapy research: principles and applications,* ed 2, Philadelphia, 2000, WB Saunders.

Ernst E: Evidence-based massage therapy: a contradiction in terms? In Rich GJ, editor: *Massage therapy: the evidence for practice,* New York, 2002, Elsevier.

Field T: Massage therapy effects, *Am Psychol* 53:1270-1281, 1998.

Field T: *Touch therapy,* New York, 2000, Churchill Livingstone.

Field T, Hernandez-Reif M, Taylor S et al: Labor pain is reduced by massage therapy, *J Psychosom Obstet Gynaecol* 18:286-291, 1997.

Finfgeld DL: Metasynthesis: the state of the art—so far, *Qual Health Res* 13:893-904, 2003.

Gehlbach SH: *Interpreting the medical literature,* ed 4, New York, 2002, McGraw-Hill.

Hagino C: *How to appraise research: a guide for chiropractic students and practitioners,* New York, 2003, Churchill Livingstone.

Hamm M: Impact of massage therapy in the treatment of linked pathologies: scoliosis, costovertebral dysfunction, and thoracic outlet syndrome, *J Bodywork Move Ther* 10:12-20, 2006.

Hulley SB, Cummings SR, Browner WS et al: *Designing clinical research: an epidemiologic approach,* ed 2, Philadelphia, 2001, Lippincott Williams & Wilkins.

Hymel GM: *Research methods for massage and holistic therapies,* St Louis, 2006, Mosby.

International Committee of Medical Journal Editors. *Uniform requirements for manuscripts submitted to biomedical journals: writing and editing for biomedical publication,* Philadelphia, 2003, American College of Physicians.

Marks DF, Sykes CM: Synthesizing evidence: systematic reviews, meta-analysis and preference analysis. In Marks DF, Yardley L, editors: *Research methods for clinical and health psychology,* Thousand Oaks, Calif, 2004, Sage.

McEwen I, editor: *Writing case reports: a how-to manual for clinicians,* ed 2, Alexandria, Va, 2001, American Physical Therapy Association.

Moyer CA, Rounds J, Hannum JW: A meta-analysis of massage therapy research, *Psychol Bull* 130:3-18, 2004.

Mulrow C, Cook D, editors: *Systematic reviews: synthesis of best evidence for healthcare decisions,* Philadelphia, 1998, American College of Physicians.

Patterson BL, Thorne SE, Canam C, Jillings C: Meta-study of qualitative health research: a practical guide to meta-analysis and meta-synthesis, Thousand Oaks, Calif, 2001, Sage.

Peat JK, Mellis C, Williams K, Xuan W: (2002). Health science research: a handbook of quantitative methods, Thousand Oaks, Calif, 2002, Sage.

Portney LG, Watkins MP: Foundations of clinical research: applications to practice, ed 2, Upper Saddle River, NJ, 2000, Prentice-Hall Health.

Preyde M: Effectiveness of massage therapy for subacute low-back pain: a randomized controlled trial, Can Med Assoc J 162:1815-1820, 2000.

Sandelowski M, Barroso J: Creating metasummaries of qualitative findings, *Nurs Res* 52:226-233, 2003.

Stommel M, Wills CE: *Clinical research: concepts and principles for advanced practice nurses,* Philadelphia, 2004, Lippincott Williams & Wilkins.

Turchaninov R: *Therapeutic massage: a scientific approach,* Phoenix, Ariz, 2000, Aesculapius Books.

Turchaninov R, Cox CA: *Medical massage,* vol 1, Phoenix, Ariz, 1998, Aesculapius Books.

WORKBOOK

1. The research process comprises five levels of specificity: *research strategies, research categories, research designs, research methods,* and *research procedures.* List these five levels in the proper order, from most general to most specific, according to the chapter's discussion of the research continuum. Briefly explain and justify this order.

2. Explain the function of each of the four major sections of a research report: (1) introduction, (2) method, (3) results, and (4) discussion.

3. Distinguish between (a) the randomized controlled trial and (b) the case report research methods.

4. Using the Evolve 2-1 box, specifically the hyperlink *Massage randomized controlled trial,* perform the following tasks: (a) locate and obtain a copy, electronic or print, of a massage therapy research study of your choice that used this particular research method and (b) provide a schematic illustration or flowchart of the procedures used in your selected study, as demonstrated in the investigation by Chang et al. (2002) in Box 2-1 and Figure 2-12.

5. Perform the following tasks: (a) formulate a research question that is operational, of interest to you, and potentially beneficial to the profession; (b) identify and justify the research category to which the question belongs, as well as the most appropriate research strategy for implementing your investigation.

Chapter 3 Concept Map

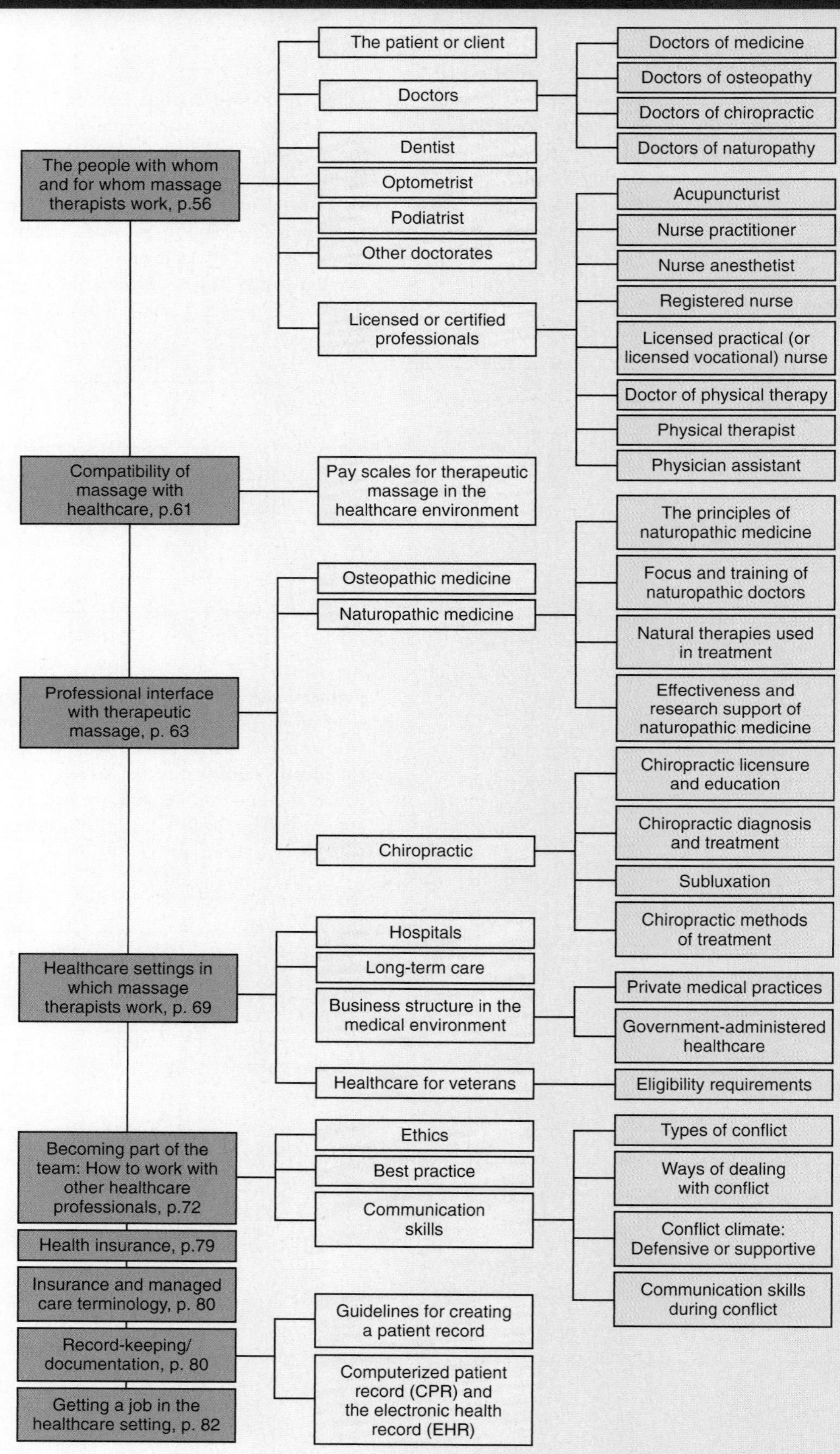

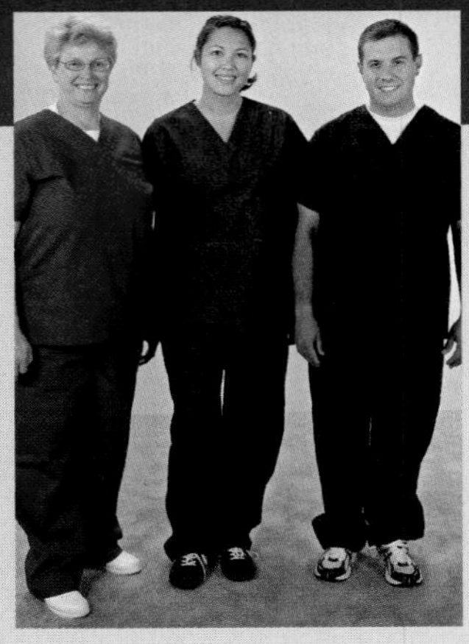

CHAPTER 3

MEDICAL AND HEALTH-RELATED PROFESSIONS*

Key Terms

Adjustment	Confidentiality	Ethics	Rights
Best practice	Ethical dilemma	Etiquette	Subluxation
Chiropractic	Ethical distress	Informed consent	Tenderness

For definitions of key terms, refer to the Evolve website.

OBJECTIVES

Upon completion of this chapter, the reader will have the information necessary to:

1. Develop a mission statement for yourself and incorporate the patient or client into it.
2. Explain how medical doctors differentiate their specialties and describe the education needed for these specialties.
3. Explain how a medical doctor differs from a doctor of chiropractic and a naturopath.
4. Name the different types of health centers that most likely would use massage therapy.
5. Describe various healthcare professions, along with the job responsibilities and scope of practice for each.
6. Describe and perform insurance-related issues and activities.

*Contributions and review of this chapter provided by W. Randy Snyder.

Chapter 1 described massage from author Sandy Fritz's perspective as a massage therapist and explained conventional, complementary, alternative, and integrated healthcare. (Thanks to Dr. Leon Chaitow for his continued knowledge and support.) Chapter 2 (and the Evolve site) written by Glenn M. Hymel, presented essential research that supports the use of massage as a justifiable and beneficial intervention.

This chapter presents the diverse world of healthcare. Massage professionals who want to be a successful part of an interdisciplinary team in the integrated healthcare environment must learn about the types of healthcare professionals and their roles in a variety of healthcare delivery systems. This information can teach the massage therapist how to integrate massage professionally into the healthcare world. The first section describes types of healthcare professionals and then various healthcare systems. The next section covers unique skills, such as working with insurance coverage and necessary record-keeping. Finally, strategies for becoming a contributing member of the healthcare team are described.

In any professional environment, it is important to understand how the environment and those in it develop the structure that forms and is formed by these elements: the professionals, the environments, and the unique skills. It is similar to how the body functions: form follows function, and function determines the form.

The healthcare world is as dynamic as the human body. Demands on the system eventually change the structure. This is one reason for the increase in massage as part of the healthcare delivery system. Demands from the public have begun the process of changing the form of healthcare. These changes do not happen quickly, and transitional times can be difficult, because the preexisting structure is no longer as effective, but the new form is not ready to assume function completely. This is the state of healthcare today. What seems to be a mess is actually the dynamics of change based on demand. The massage therapist in this environment must understand the preexisting form, the demands causing the change, and what is needed to support the transition. Massage therapists must be patient, as well as persistent, in developing their careers during these active transitional periods. They must also be progressive; they must anticipate the skills and qualities that will be required in the future and train for them *now,* so that they are ready when opportunities become available.

Currently healthcare is organized into a *hierarchy,* or top-down system. Health insurance coverage and managed healthcare systems have cast the top role of the hierarchy into question. At the top of the hierarchy is the doctor, then come levels of support professionals, typically based on training, with the least-trained at the bottom of the hierarchy. Traditionally, healthcare administration (the management and business) is in a struggle with the doctor for the top position in the hierarchy. When this type of power shift occurs, conflict is common until some sort of resolution occurs. The healthcare delivery system in the United States is trying to figure out how to achieve this resolution. Other countries, such as Canada and the United Kingdom, are involved in their own struggles to provide effective government-administered healthcare. It is not the goal of this text to solve these problems.

In these healthcare delivery environments, various complementary health methods are becoming part of the healthcare system, and the transition is clumsy. The biggest hurdle truly seems to be economic issues. Healthcare insurance providers are exploring ways to include methods such as therapeutic massage in their reimbursement policies. Where therapeutic massage has been incorporated, the transition has been smooth. However, because few studies have confirmed the cost-saving benefits of therapeutic massage, the justification for payment is elusive. Again, this text is not going to resolve that issue; in time, it will resolve itself. The massage professional needs to prepare now to be ready as the transition occurs.

THE PEOPLE WITH WHOM AND FOR WHOM MASSAGE THERAPISTS WORK

THE PATIENT OR CLIENT

The intent of healthcare is to help people with medical concerns. The patient should always be the most important person in the medical environment. The term *patient* is a bit controversial. To some it denotes submissiveness and seems demoralizing. The use of respectful terminology is important. The person is recognized first. A person *has* a disease; he or she is not the disease. A person may be physically disabled, but the individual is not a disabled person. In some healthcare environments the term *client* is used, which is the term typically used by massage therapists. Medical spa professionals tend to think of people as clients, denoting a partnership in care. This text tends to use the current term *patient* but occasionally uses *client.* Whichever term is used, people (individuals, patients, clients) are receiving a service from healthcare professionals and are paying for it, either directly (i.e., out of pocket) or indirectly (i.e., through insurance premiums or taxes), and they have **rights** of their own (Box 3-1). They deserve to receive what is called *best practice* in

BOX 3-1 **The Patient Care Partnership: Understanding Expectations, Rights and Responsibilities**

Our goal is for you and your family to have the same care and attention we would want for our families and ourselves. The sections explain some of the basics about how you can expect to be treated during your hospital stay. They also cover what we will need from you to care for you better. If you have questions at any time, please ask them. Unasked or unanswered questions can add to the stress of being in the hospital.

What to Expect During Your Hospital Stay

- **High quality hospital care.** Our first priority is to provide you the care you need, when you need it, with skill, compassion, and respect. Tell your caregivers if you have concerns about your care or if you have pain. You have the right to know the identity of doctors, nurses and others involved in your care.
- **A clean and safe environment.** We use special policies and procedures to avoid mistakes in your care and keep you free from abuse or neglect. If anything unexpected and significant happens during your hospital stay, you will be told what happened, and any resulting changes in your care will be discussed with you.
- **Involvement in your care.** Please tell your caregivers if you need more information about treatment choices. When decision-making takes place, it should include:
  - *Discussing your medical condition and information about medically appropriate treatment choices.* To make informed decisions with your doctor, you need to understand:
    - The benefits and risks of each treatment, and whether the treatment is experimental or part of a research study.
    - What you can reasonably expect from your treatment and any long-term effects it might have on your quality of life.
    - What you and your family will need to do after you leave the hospital.
    - The financial consequences of using uncovered services or out-of-network providers.
  - *Discussing your treatment plan.* When you enter the hospital, you sign a general consent to treatment. In some cases, such as surgery or experimental treatment, you may be asked to confirm in writing that you understand what is planned and agree to it.
  - *Getting information from you.* Your caregivers need complete and correct information about your health and coverage so that they can make good decisions about your care. That includes:
    - Past illnesses, surgeries or hospital stays; past allergic reactions; any medicines or dietary supplements (such as vitamins and herbs) that you are taking; and any network or admission requirements under your health plan.
  - *Understanding your health care goals and values.* Make sure your doctor, your family and your care team know your wishes.
  - *Understanding who should make decisions when you cannot.* If you have signed a health care power of attorney stating who should speak for you if you become unable to make health care decisions for yourself, or a "living will" or "advance directive" that states your wishes about end-of-life care; give copies to your doctor, your family and your care team.
- **Protection of your privacy.** State and federal laws and hospital operating policies protect the privacy of your medical information. You will receive a Notice of Privacy Practices that describes the ways that we use, disclose and safeguard patient information and that explains how you can obtain a copy of information from our records about your care.
- **Preparing you and your family for when you leave the hospital.** The success of your treatment often depends on your efforts to follow medication, diet and therapy plans. You can expect us to help you identify sources of follow-up care and to let you know if our hospital has a financial interest in any referrals. You can also expect to receive information and, where possible, training about the self-care you will need when you go home.
- **Help with your bill and filing insurance claims.** Our staff will file claims for you with health care insurers or other programs, such as Medicare and Medicaid. If you have questions about your bill, contact our business office. If you need help understanding your insurance coverage or health plan, start with your insurance company or health benefits manager. If you do not have health coverage, we will try to help you and your family find financial help or make other arrangements.

(This is an abridged text. Full text is available at www.aha.org).

medical care. **Best practice** is the most effective, least risky treatment delivered with respect from qualified, competent practitioners in a safe, supportive environment.

DOCTORS

Of the professionals in the medical system, the doctor has the most extensive training and therefore becomes accountable and responsible for the outcomes in the healthcare process. The services of the healthcare system are based on the doctor's decisions and instructions. Various types of doctors work in the healthcare environment.

Doctor of Medicine

Medical doctors (MDs) diagnose illness and disease, recommend treatment, write prescriptions, and perform surgeries. They also teach patients about preventive healthcare, which means that doctors must keep up-to-date on new health information. A person who wants to become a doctor must first complete 4 years of undergraduate training (premed) and then 4 years of medical school. After medical school, the individual must complete an internship and residency program, which lasts 3 to 8 years. Interns treat patients under the supervision of licensed doctors. After the internship, the graduate is called a *resident;* he or she most often chooses a specialty in a hospital and is paid while completing training. Certain specialties require more training than others. The training that doctors undergo is lengthy and comprehensive compared to that for many other professions.

An MD must have a state license to practice, and continuing education is required to retain the license. Graduates of foreign medical schools usually can obtain a license after passing a medical board examination and completing a residency program.

Doctor of Osteopathy

The philosophies and treatment approaches of the MD and the doctor of osteopathy (DO) do not differ as much as they did in the past. Osteopaths tend to have a greater awareness of the influence of biomechanical factors on health than do typical MDs. Another major difference is that osteopaths use osteopathic manipulative therapy, along with medicine and surgery. This type of therapy involves soft tissue manipulation, mobilization, and high-velocity adjustments (as in chiropractic). Methods commonly used by massage therapists, such as muscle energy techniques and positional release techniques, originated in osteopathic medicine, as did craniosacral therapy. Osteopathic physicians must meet requirements similar to those for medical doctors to graduate and practice medicine, and they must pursue continuing education to retain their license.

Both MDs and DOs can obtain board certification in one or more of 24 specialty areas recognized by the American Board of Medical Specialties (ABMS).

JUST BETWEEN YOU AND ME

If you add up the educational requirements for a doctor (MD or DO), they come to at least 8 years of formal, university-based education and 3 years of internships, for a total of 11 years of education, before the individual is considered eligible to practice independently as a doctor. Most practitioners devote 15 years of their life to preparing to be a healthcare professional. It should serve as a reality check when these requirements are compared to the current educational requirements for the practice of therapeutic massage. Doctors and massage therapists deserve mutual respect and support.

evolve 3-1

See the Evolve website for a description of these 24 medical specialties.

Doctor of Chiropractic

Doctors of chiropractic (DCs), or chiropractors, focus their attention on the nervous system and examine the bones to detect any hindrance to the nervous system. The science of **chiropractic** deals with the relationship between the articulations of the skeleton and the nervous system and the role this relationship plays in the restoration and maintenance of health.

Chiropractic colleges require undergraduate studies in biology, organic and inorganic chemistry, physics, English, and the humanities, followed by 3 years of study in chiropractic. Each state has its own licensing requirements, and continuing education is required for relicensure. Some chiropractors devote their practice to a specific specialty, but most practice general chiropractic. Chiropractors are a source of employment opportunities for massage therapists, who therefore must understand the nature of chiropractic care.

evolve 3-2

The Evolve website provides a comprehensive description of the theory and practice of chiropractic.

Chiropractors use a wide variety of manual procedures to treat a subluxation. A properly applied **adjustment,** or manipulation, is specific, induces joint separation, and is painless. The position of the patient creates preadjustive tension, and then a specific, controlled force is applied. The procedure should not cause joint compression, injury, or distractive forces at adjacent, unaffected segmental levels of the spine.

Doctor of Naturopathy

Naturopathic medicine is defined primarily by its fundamental principles. The doctor of naturopathy (ND), or naturopath, selects and applies methods and treatments based on these principles according to the individual needs of each patient. Diagnostic and therapeutic methods are selected from various sources and systems and continue to evolve with the progress of knowledge.[1]

Diagnostic and treatment methods used by NDs include all clinical and laboratory diagnostic testing procedures, including diagnostic radiology and other imaging techniques; nutritional medicine, dietetics, and therapeutic fasting; medicines of mineral, animal, and botanical origin; hygiene and public health measures; homeopathy, acupuncture, and traditional Chinese medicine (TCM); psychotherapy and counseling; minor surgery and naturopathic obstetrics (natural childbirth); naturopathic physical medicine, including naturopathic manipulative therapies; hydrotherapies; heat, cold, and ultrasound techniques; and therapeutic exercise. Naturopathic practice excludes major surgery and the use of most synthetic drugs.

DENTIST

Dentists are doctors of dental medicine (DMD) or dental surgery (DDS). Dentistry is the study of the prevention and treatment of problems involving the teeth and gums and the tissue surrounding the teeth. Dentists perform oral surgery and can prescribe medications such as antibiotics and analgesics. As with medical school, dental school is completed after undergraduate studies and usually lasts 4 years. Dentists must meet licensing requirements. An increasing number of dentists are incorporating holistic methods (e.g., craniosacral work and soft tissue techniques) into the care they provide for some dental conditions, such as temporomandibular joint (TMJ) problems.

OPTOMETRIST

A doctor of optometry (OD), or optometrist, examines the eyes to test visual acuity and treats vision defects by prescribing correctional lenses and other optical aids. An optometrist is different from an ophthalmologist, who is a licensed MD or DO. Optometrists study at accredited optometry schools for 4 years after completing undergraduate studies in the sciences, mathematics, and English. Optometrists must be licensed in the state in which they practice.

PODIATRIST

Podiatrists, or doctors of podiatric medicine (DPMs), are trained and educated in the care of the feet, including surgical treatment. Podiatrists train for 4 years at an accredited college after completing undergraduate studies in the sciences.

OTHER DOCTORATES

Massage therapists may encounter other medical professionals who are referred to as "doctor" because of the degree they have earned. For example, a person with an advanced degree in his or her field (e.g., the doctor of philosophy, or PhD, degree) may be addressed as "Doctor." A person with a PsyD degree is a doctor of psychology, and an individual with an EdD degree is a doctor of education.

LICENSED OR CERTIFIED PROFESSIONALS

Acupuncturist

According to the American Academy of Medical Acupuncturists, a physician must have a minimum of 300 hours of systematic acupuncture training to be certified as a medical acupuncturist. However, in many states physicians can practice acupuncture without any certification at all. Licensed acupuncturists primarily study TCM, along with the basics of Western medicine. Schooling averages 4 years.

Nurse Practitioner

Nurse practitioners (NPs) are registered nurses (RNs) with additional education and clinical experience that enable them to diagnose and prescribe medications for common illnesses, along with providing basic patient care services. Nurse practitioners usually focus on preventive care and health maintenance. In some areas, they are allowed to practice independently but are usually part of a team of healthcare professionals with physician oversight. A nurse practitioner's education involves programs that grant a certificate or a master's degree beyond the registered nurse degree, as well as clinical experience. An intensive preceptorship under the direct supervision of a physician or an experienced nurse practitioner and instruction in nursing theory are key components of most NP programs. The scope of an NP's practice varies, depending on the regulations in each state. Specifics can be obtained at the website www.nurse.org.

Nurse Anesthetist

Nurse anesthetists can be found in many different medical settings, from plastic surgery centers to hospitals. The nurse anesthetist is a registered nurse who administers anesthetics to patients during medical care. This level of practice is quite advanced, and nurse anesthetists can be found in both metropolitan and rural communities.

Nurse anesthetists, or certified registered nurse anesthetists (CRNAs), are licensed professional nurses (registered nurses, or RNs) who undergo extensive training and are nationally certified by examination after graduation. They provide services similar to those provided by an anesthesiologist. CRNAs can be licensed and practice in all 50 states.

Nurse anesthetist programs run 24 to 36 months (the average is 28 months) and are provided on the master's degree level. To enter the program, a prospective student must be a registered nurse, must have a degree in science or nursing (BSN) from a 4-year college, and must have at least 1 year of acute care nursing experience.[2]

Registered Nurse

Registered nurses provide patient care and are the keystone of the healthcare system, because they are in continual direct contact with the patient and closely evaluate the patient's condition. The work settings in healthcare available to registered nurses seem endless. They include nursing homes, hospice care, hospitals, and private medical practices, to name but a few. A prospective nursing student first must acquire an associate's or bachelor's degree from a trade school, community college, or university. Some hospitals offer RN courses to individuals who already have a bachelor's degree.

Licensed Practical (or Licensed Vocational) Nurse

Licensed practical nurses (LPNs), sometimes called licensed vocational nurses (LVNs), take vital signs, chart patients' progress, administer medications and intravenous fluids when allowed by law, and provide overall patient care. LPNs are trained and educated one level above a certified nurse assistant (CNA). LPN programs include emergency care, biology, physical education, and hands-on clinical work. The program takes 1 year of training through a community college, trade school, or local hospital, after which the graduate can sit for the National Council Licensure Examination for licensed practical nurses.

Doctor of Physical Therapy

A doctor of physical therapy (DPT) works toward the restoration of function in individuals of all ages who are impaired. An integral member of the healthcare team, the doctor of physical therapy is a skilled practitioner who plans, organizes, and directs patient care and preventive programs.[3] Doctors of physical therapy provide patient care in hospitals, nursing homes, schools, rehabilitation centers, community and public health centers and agencies, private practices, research centers, industry, and sports medicine centers. They also serve educators in colleges and universities offering programs in physical therapy.

Physical Therapist

Physical therapists (PTs) help people with injuries or impairments to regain physical function. The physical therapist performs a patient assessment and then works with a physician to develop a treatment plan. To sit for the licensing examination, the individual must have graduated from an accredited master's degree or higher program in physical therapy. Licensing is required by all states.

Physician Assistant

Physician assistants (PAs) provide direct patient care services under the supervision of licensed physicians. They are trained to identify conditions and care for patients as directed by the physician, and in 46 states and the District of Columbia, they are allowed to write prescriptions. Physician assistants are qualified by graduation from an accredited physician assistant educational program and/or certification by the National Commission on Certification of Physician Assistants. These professionals take patient histories, order and interpret tests, perform physical examinations, and even make diagnostic decisions. PA practice is centered on patient care and may include educational, research, and administrative activities. Physician assistants can be found in physicians' offices, hospitals, military bases, and other healthcare facilities.

evolve 3-3

For further information on medical professionals, see the Evolve website.

COMPATIBILITY OF MASSAGE WITH HEALTHCARE

As you can see, the list of healthcare professionals (provided in this chapter and on the Evolve website) who make up the healthcare staff is extensive. Increased specialization is driven both by increases in available information and by advances in technology. It is almost impossible anymore to be a generalist in any field; there is just too much to know. This textbook describes a specialization for massage, and the authors believe that the massage therapist should be part of the healthcare team.

Are the current massage education and credentialing requirements compatible with the education and credentialing required for those who work in the healthcare system? This is a good question. An overview of the education required for all medically trained professionals reveals some commonalities, the most obvious being the study of anatomy and physiology. Where in the hierarchy does massage fit? Who will be the supervisors? Is it possible to justify massage as a beneficial modality in the healthcare system? What will be the extent of responsibility and accountability? A comparison of the most typical massage education programs in the United States shows little availability of an associate's degree in massage at this time, although this is improving. Opportunities to obtain a bachelor's degree in massage therapy are even more rare. Some in the massage profession do not believe that a degree is necessary. This is a valid viewpoint, because some medical jobs require only certification, not a degree (e.g., the emergency medical technician [EMT], an example discussed in detail on the Evolve website).

The most common level of education for massage is the entry level, which requires 500 to 750 contact hours. On the next level, this can be combined with specialized clinical massage training (such as that provided by this textbook) involving a minimum of 250 contact hours plus a minimum of 250 additional hours of clinical experience, for a total of about 1200 contact hours. This number of contact hours can be compared to about 36 credit hours, typical of 1 year of college (three terms of 12 credits each). The comparable educational level in healthcare would be that of a certified technician, nondegreed but vocationally trained.

Future educational requirements for clinically based massage may rise to the associate's degree level. What does this mean for the massage therapist working in the medical setting? The simple answer is status, responsibilities, and pay comparable to those of others at this level of professional development. It implies that massage therapists will recognize their comparative level of training and abide by their limited scope of practice. In this milieu of other professionals with much more extensive training and much greater responsibility, humility and a cooperative attitude will be important. To get respect, we must first give it.

evolve 3-4

See the Evolve website for the pay scales for various healthcare professionals.

PAY SCALES FOR THERAPEUTIC MASSAGE IN THE HEALTHCARE ENVIRONMENT

Let's be logical. Concrete data that compare similar training levels and degrees of responsibility and that are limited to a highly focused medical intervention should provide at least the basis for assessing how massage therapists will fit into the healthcare system. Let's consider the EMT. The educational requirements and the professional responsibilities of an EMT include the following:

- Have a high school diploma, have successfully completed EMT training, have registered with the National Registry of Emergency Medical Technicians (NREMT), have obtained licensure by the state EMS authority, and have 2 to 4 years of related experience
- Respond to an emergency call, assess the situation, obtain a basic medical history and perform a physical examination of the patient, and provide emergency care at the scene and during transit to the hospital
- Use necessary medical equipment to treat the patient and ascertain the extent of the injuries or illness
- Communicate with the medical facility receiving the patient about the person's condition, status, and arrival time
- Be familiar with standard concepts, practices, and procedures in a particular field
- Rely on experience and judgment to plan and accomplish goals
- Maintain certification (certification standards vary by state)

A comparison of educational requirements for adjunctive healthcare professionals shows that those who provide direct, hands-on patient care usually have an associate's degree (although this is not required for EMTs).[4] Health professionals whose level of training is similar to that of a massage therapist include phlebotomists, dental assistants, EMTs, and occupational therapy assistants. The requirements listed for massage therapists in one source[4] include a high school diploma plus a training program and certification (i.e., by the National Certification Board for Therapeutic Massage and Bodywork [NCBTMB]), just about like an EMT.

Based on these data, entry level salaries for clinical/medical massage therapists can be expected

JUST BETWEEN YOU AND ME

If you are a really, really good massage therapist with a solid retention client base, you will make more money in private practice than in an hourly paid or a salary position in healthcare. The information in units 2, 3, and 4, will increase your skills, making you an even better massage therapist. However, there is the issue of the stability of a career track in the healthcare world, as well as an important path of service. I believe that younger massage therapists, especially men, will find more career opportunities in healthcare. Traditionally massage has been primarily a female career, although this is changing, just as nursing has changed.

Therapeutic massage needs to find its identity in the medical world, and you and I will be the groundbreakers in this endeavor. Once we understand where we fit, the next issue is where we will practice.

to range from $22,000 to $30,000 a year. Typical benefits packages, including healthcare, would also be offered. If a massage therapist has an associate's degree or higher or previous healthcare experience or is dually trained (e.g., as an LPN), the pay rate may be $35,000 per year.

PROFESSIONAL INTERFACE WITH THERAPEUTIC MASSAGE

Massage theory and application complement other healthcare disciplines that have roots in manual therapy. Three areas in particular, osteopathy, naturopathy, and chiropractic, have great potential for the integration of massage therapy. Professionals in these disciplines are active employers of massage therapists, therefore the massage therapist must have an in-depth understanding of the philosophy, language, and methodology that are unique to each and of the aspects that they share.

evolve 3-5

To support this understanding, comprehensive descriptions of osteopathy, chiropractic, and naturopathy are presented on the Evolve website.

OSTEOPATHIC MEDICINE

More than 130 years after its introduction as a distinctively American approach to healthcare, osteopathic medicine has become an integral segment of the U.S. healthcare system. It is one of two fully licensed, comprehensive systems of medical care in the United States. Andrew Taylor Still, an MD who is considered the father of osteopathic medicine, developed the discipline in 1874. Still was an early proponent of "wellness"—now a common term among healthcare professionals. He identified the musculoskeletal system as an essential element of health, stressed the body's ability to heal itself, and advocated the use of preventive medicine, exercise, and nutrition.

As mentioned previously, practitioners of osteopathic medicine are identified by the letters *DO* (allopathic physicians are identified by the letters *MD*). Osteopathic medicine provides all the benefits of modern medicine, including prescription drugs, surgery, and the use of technology to diagnose disease and evaluate injury. It also offers a distinctive educational and practice pathway to becoming a physician. Although this pathway and the infrastructure of the osteopathic system are different from those of allopathic medicine, osteopathic medical graduates earn "parallel" status and opportunities for clinical practice.

Doctors of osteopathy are licensed to practice the full scope of medicine in the United States and many other countries. They practice in all types of environments, including the military, and in all types of specialties, from family medicine to obstetrics, surgery, and aerospace medicine. DOs have a strong history of serving rural and underserved areas, often providing their unique brand of compassionate, patient-centered care to some of the most economically disadvantaged members of society.

In addition to studying all the typical subjects that allopathic physicians are expected to master, osteopathic medical students take approximately 200 hours of training in the art of osteopathic manipulative medicine. This system of hands-on diagnostic and treatment techniques helps to alleviate pain, restore motion, support the body's natural functions, and influence the body's structure to help it function more efficiently. Osteopathic physicians consider the impact that lifestyle and community have on the health of each individual, and they work to erase barriers to good health.

As mentioned earlier, the popularity of osteopathic medicine has grown in recent years. Each year approximately 100 million patient visits are made to doctors of osteopathy, and the number of DOs has increased 67% since 1990. According to the American Osteopathic Association, DOs account for about 6% of all physicians (and more than 8% of military physicians). An important factor that differentiates DOs from MDs is the former's approach to a medical or surgical problem. The osteopathic approach is rooted in the philosophy of that discipline. DOs believe that all the systems in the body operate in an integrated fashion. Perhaps the most significant difference between DOs and MDs is that DOs consider the role of the musculoskeletal system in the development of symptoms and illness. They have special training in recognizing and correcting structural problems through various manual techniques, called *osteopathic manipulative therapy (OMT)*. This concern with muscle and bone leads many DOs to practice in sports medicine, as well as in physical medicine and rehabilitation. It also explains why they may be more supportive of manual methods such as massage.[5]

In the United States most DOs are almost indistinguishable from conventional MDs. It is not surprising that the two disciplines share so much common ground. MDs increasingly have embraced a whole person (holistic) approach to medicine, such as recognizing the effect of stress on physical health. DOs have embraced the diagnostic and therapeutic approaches used by MDs, including the use of medication. Most DOs use the same medical therapies and medications as MDs.[5]

Because of the underlying philosophy of osteopathy, DOs appreciate the importance of a thorough understanding of the correct position and function of each of the structures in the body. Osteopaths can be considered specialists in the biomechanics of the human machine.

The self-healing mechanism is the main principle and application of osteopathy. Belief in the self-healing capacity of the body is ancient; in the Western medical tradition, it can be traced back to Hippocrates. *Homeostasis* is the process by which every living thing makes continual adjustments to keep itself in a stable condition and function to the best of its ability. It is a self-regulating activity, with preset limits. The body is constantly readjusting to maintain this balance.[6]

Osteopaths believe that disease comes primarily from within the individual, therefore they concentrate on the person who is suffering rather than on the microorganisms that are thought to cause disease. In some stages of disease, however, the changes the disease has brought about have gone beyond the point of return. In these cases, osteopathy helps the person to function to the best of his or her ability, given the circumstances. When necessary, osteopaths refer a patient for further examination and treatment by a specialist.[6]

A key concept that osteopathic medical students learn is that structure influences function. Therefore a problem in one part of the body's structure may affect function in that area and possibly in others. For example, restriction of motion in the lower ribs, lumbar spine, and abdomen can cause stomach pain with symptoms that mimic irritable bowel syndrome. By using osteopathic manipulative medicine techniques, DOs can help restore motion to these areas, improving gastrointestinal function and often restoring it to normal.[7]

The osteopathic philosophy, central to all physicians practicing this approach to medicine, has four major tenets:

- Each patient is a unique unit consisting of an integrated mind, body, and spirit.
- Each patient has within the innate ability for self-healing and inner reserves important in maintaining and maximizing health.
- Structures of the body affect function; likewise, functional demands determine structure.
- Every osteopathic encounter involves an approach that incorporates consideration and appropriate application of the three preceding tenets.

The high-touch aspect of osteopathic medicine is an important distinction that motivates many of the students who apply to osteopathic medical schools.

Most OMT is performed by osteopathic family practice physicians and specialists in neuromusculoskeletal medicine, but all osteopathic specialists are taught to be generalists first and are encouraged to integrate palpatory diagnosis and treatment into their specialty whenever possible.

NATUROPATHIC MEDICINE

As a distinct healthcare profession, naturopathic medicine is almost 100 years old. It is rooted in the philosophy of Hippocrates and the healing wisdom of many cultures. Benedict Lust introduced naturopathic medicine to New York in 1896. In the early 1900s, practitioners of a variety of medical disciplines joined to form the first naturopathic medical societies. Naturopathic medical conventions attracted more than 10,000 practitioners. Between the 1900s and 1930s, more than 20 naturopathic colleges had been established, and naturopathic physicians were licensed in most states.[8]

Naturopathic medicine experienced a decline in the 1940s and 1950s with the increase in popularity of pharmaceutical drugs and technologic medicine, which was accompanied by a widespread belief that these therapies could eliminate all disease. However, over the past 20 years, a health-conscious public has sought alternatives to conventional medicine, and naturopathic medicine has experienced a resurgence.[8]

Naturopathy continues to grow and evolve as a body of knowledge. Naturopathic medicine, as an organized profession, is committed to ongoing research and the development of its science. It incorporates many elements of scientific modern medicine.[8]

The Principles of Naturopathic Medicine[9,10]

The Healing Power of Nature (Vis Medicatrix Naturae). Naturopathic medicine recognizes in the body an inherent ability that is ordered and intelligent. Naturopaths identify and remove obstacles to recovery and facilitate and augment this healing ability.

Identify and Treat the Causes (Tolle Causam). Naturopathic doctors seek to identify and remove the underlying causes of illness rather than eliminate or suppress its symptoms.

First, Do No Harm (Primum Non Nocere). Naturopathic medicine follows three principles to avoid harming the patient: (1) methods and medicinal substances are used that minimize the risk of harmful side effects; (2) when possible, the harmful suppression of symptoms is avoided; and (3) the individual's healing process is acknowledged and respected, and the least force necessary to diagnose and treat illness is used.

The Doctor as Teacher (Docere). Naturopathic doctors educate the patient and encourage self-responsibility for health. They also acknowledge the therapeutic value inherent in the doctor-patient relationship.

Treat the Whole Person. Naturopathic doctors treat each patient individually, taking into account the person's physical, mental, and emotional state, as well as genetic, environmental, and social factors. Because total health includes spiritual health, naturopathic doctors encourage individuals to pursue their own spiritual paths.

Prevention. Naturopathic doctors emphasize disease prevention. They assess the patient's risk factors and hereditary susceptibility to disease and make appropriate interventions to prevent illness. Naturopathic medicine seeks to improve conditions through preventive measures so that individuals may live healthier lives.

Maintain Wellness. Wellness follows the establishment and maintenance of optimum health and balance. It is a state of being healthy and is characterized by positive emotion, thought, and action. Wellness is inherent in everyone, no matter what disease or diseases the person may have. If this fact is recognized and experienced by an individual, the person will heal quicker than if the disease were only treated.

The guiding principles of naturopathy can be summarized as follows[11]:

- A life force exists that, given the right conditions, will self-heal or self-correct. This life force is stimulated by factors that promote health and is suppressed by excesses and deficiencies.
- Prevention is preferable to cure.
- The underlying cause is identified, not just the disease.
- The whole person is treated, physically, mentally, emotionally, and spiritually.
- The person is treated, not the disease.
- The individual is unique; each person responds in a different way.
- Ill health is a result of the internal disorder of the body rather than of external influences of the environment or "disease-causing agents."

Focus and Training of Naturopathic Doctors

Naturopathic doctors hold a doctorate in naturopathic medicine from one of five accredited naturopathic medical schools. This degree confers the title of doctor and allows the holder of the degree to guarantee to the public that he or she has the requisite didactic and clinical training to practice naturopathic medicine. The doctorate prepares NDs to be primary care general practitioners and to work with other medical providers.[12]

Naturopathic doctors are experts in the use of natural therapies and drug/nutrient, drug/herb interactions. For this reason, naturopathic doctors increasingly are being asked to serve as experts in the field of complementary and alternative medicine (CAM). They are members of the White House Commission on CAM; they are researchers and members of the advisory board for the National Institutes of Health (NIH) and the National Center for Complementary and Alternative Medicine (NCCAM); and they serve on the Medicare Coverage Advisory Committee.

Naturopathic doctors use a variety of natural and noninvasive therapies, including clinical nutrition, herbal medicine, homeopathy, physical medicine, counseling, and hydrotherapy. Many naturopathic doctors receive additional training in disciplines or treatments such as natural childbirth (midwifery), acupuncture and Oriental medicine, and Ayurvedic medicine. Naturopathic doctors are able to work in integrated settings with other medical providers. The result is a patient-centered approach that strives to provide the most appropriate treatment for an individual's needs.[13]

The training of a naturopathic doctor involves an accredited, 4-year, postgraduate, residential naturopathic medical program. It consists of comprehensive study of the conventional medical sciences, including anatomy, physiology, pathology, microbiology, immunology, clinical and physical diagnosis, laboratory diagnosis, cardiology, gastroenterology, gynecology, and so on. The naturopathic education is unique in that these doctors complete an extensive academic and clinical course of study in the use of natural medicines based on the principles of naturopathic medicine. Naturopathic doctors are trained to perform physical examinations, laboratory tests, gynecologic exams, nutritional and dietary assessments, allergy testing, imaging, and other diagnostic techniques. Naturopathic doctors refer patients to other specialists and healthcare providers for diagnosis and treatment when indicated.[13]

The Council on Naturopathic Medical Education (CNME) is the recognized authority for establishing and maintaining the educational standards for the profession. Naturopathic doctors take a national board examination, the Naturopathic Physicians Licensing Examination (NPLEX), and obtain a state license where it is available. Thirteen states and the District of Columbia license naturopathic doctors; the states are Alaska, Arizona, California, Connecticut, Hawaii, Kansas, Maine, Montana, New Hampshire, Oregon, Utah, Vermont, and Washington.[13]

In licensing states, NDs practice as independent primary care general practitioners; they are allowed to diagnose and treat medical conditions, perform physical examinations, and order laboratory tests. In these states, many healthcare consumers specifically choose NDs as their primary care providers. In nonlicensing states, such as New York, naturopathic doctors are not able to offer all the services they are trained to provide.[13]

Natural Therapies Used in Treatment

Clinical Nutrition. Nutrition and the therapeutic use of food form a cornerstone of naturopathic medicine. The naturopathic approach to diet and nutrition has been validated in many scientifically based professional journals on nutrition and dietary sciences. Many medical conditions can be treated as effectively with foods and nutritional supplements as by other means, with fewer complications and side effects. Most medical doctors have fewer than 20 classroom hours in clinical nutrition, but naturopathic physicians have more than 140 hours.[14]

Homeopathic Medicine. Homeopathy, a powerful system of medicine that is more than 200 years old, is widely accepted in many countries. When properly prescribed, homeopathic medicines affect the body's "vital force" and strengthen its innate ability to heal. Homeopathic remedies function on both the physical and emotional levels, with few side effects. Some conditions that do not respond well to conventional medicine respond effectively to homeopathy.

Botanical Medicine. Many plant substances are highly effective in the right dosage and when used correctly with other herbs and treatments. Herbs can be prepared in many forms, such as teas, tinctures, and capsules. Naturopathic doctors are trained in both the art and science of botanical medicine.

Physical Medicine. Physical medicine offers treatment for musculoskeletal concerns. Treatments can include soft tissue work (including therapeutic massage), spinal adjustments, physiotherapy using heat and cold, gentle electrical impulses, ultrasound, diathermy, hydrotherapy, and exercise therapy.

Counseling. Mental attitudes and emotional states are important elements in healing and disease. Naturopathic doctors are trained in various approaches, such as short-term situational counseling, couples counseling, and mind-body techniques.

Effectiveness and Research Support of Naturopathic Medicine

The effectiveness of naturopathic diagnosis and therapeutics is supported by scientific research drawn from peer-reviewed journals from many disciplines, including naturopathic medicine, conventional medicine, European complementary medicine, clinical nutrition, phytotherapy, pharmacognosy, homeopathy, psychology, and spirituality.

Information technology and new concepts in clinical outcomes assessment are particularly well suited to evaluation of the effectiveness of naturopathic treatments, and these are being used in research, both at naturopathic medical schools and in the offices of practicing physicians. Clinical research into natural therapies has become an increasingly important focus for naturopathic doctors.

CHIROPRACTIC

Chiropractic is a healthcare discipline that emphasizes the inherent recuperative powers of the body to heal itself without the use of drugs or surgery. Chiropractors study the relationship between structure and function in the human body and believe that it is a significant health factor; if those relationships are hindered, so is one's health.[15]

The practice of chiropractic focuses on the relationship between structure (primarily of the spine) and function (as coordinated by the nervous system) and how that relationship affects the preservation and restoration of health.[15]

Doctors of chiropractic recognize the value and responsibility of working in cooperation with other health care practitioners when in the best interest of the patient.[15]

Chiropractic Licensure and Education

There are currently 16 chiropractic colleges in the United States, 10 of which were established before 1945. Since 1974, standards for chiropractic education have been established and monitored by the Council on Chiropractic Education (CCE), a nonprofit organization located in Scottsdale, Arizona. Recognized by the U.S. Department of Education as the specialized accrediting agency for chiropractic education, the CCE sets the standards for the curriculum, faculty and staff, facilities, patient care, and research.[16]

Sixty credits or more must be completed before admission to a chiropractic college. Two colleges currently require 75 units, and one college requires 90 units. Currently, six state licensing boards require a bachelor's degree in addition to the doctor of chiropractic degree for licensure, and that number is continually on the rise.[16]

A chiropractic program consists of 4 academic years of professional education averaging a total of 4822 hours of course work. Several areas of study are emphasized during the course of chiropractic education:

1. Adjustive techniques/spinal analysis
2. Principles/practices of chiropractic
3. Physiologic therapeutics
4. Biomechanics

The practice of chiropractic is licensed and regulated in all 50 states in the United States and in more than 30 countries worldwide. State licensing boards regulate, among other factors, the education, experience, and moral character of candidates for licensure, and protect the public health, safety, and welfare.[16]

The practice of chiropractic means the practice of that branch of the healing arts consisting of the science of adjustment, manipulation, and treatment of the human body in which vertebral subluxations and other malpositioned articulations and structures that may interfere with the normal generation, transmission, and expression of nerve impulse between the brain, organs, and tissue cells of the body, which may be a cause of disease, are adjusted, manipulated, or treated.

Adjustment means the application of a precisely controlled force applied by hand or by mechanical device to a specific focal point on the anatomy for the express purpose of creating a desired angular movement in skeletal joint structures to eliminate or decrease interference with neural transmission and to correct or attempt to correct a subluxation complex.[17] This is also termed a *high velocity, low amplitude (HVLA) thrust.*

Chiropractors are trained to locate subluxations using palpation as well as x-ray and remove them, thereby restoring the normal flow of nerve energy so that the entire body functions in an optimal fashion. They believe that the same innate inner intelligence that grows the body from a single cell into a complex human being can also heal the body if it is free of disturbance to the nervous system. The philosophy is that health, not merely absence of symptoms, comes from within the body, not from the outside. The subluxation complex includes any alteration of the biomechanical and physiological dynamics of contiguous spinal structures, which can cause neuronal disturbances.

Chiropractic Diagnosis and Treatment

Since many chiropractors employ or work with massage therapists, it is important to understand the process of diagnosis and treatment in chiropractic care. The doctor of chiropractic uses observation, palpation, percussion, and auscultation during assessment. The acronym *PARTS* (Pain and tenderness; Asymmetry; Range-of-motion abnormality; Tissue tone, texture, and temperature abnormality; and Special tests) modified from the osteopathic profession describes five diagnostic criteria for identifying joint subluxation or dysfunction.

Subluxation

A **subluxation** is a complex of functional, structural, and/or pathological articular changes that compromise neural integrity and may influence organ system function and general health.[18] The vertebral subluxation complex presents subluxation as a complex clinical entity comprising one or more of the following components: neuropathophysiology, kinesiopathology, myopathology, histopathology, and a biochemical component. A central element of this concept is that subluxation results in pathophysiologic conditions, which can then lead to frank pathologic changes. Moreover, correction of a subluxation is considered to lead to the restoration of normal physiologic processes, thus allowing the reversal of reversible pathologic changes.

A subluxation is evaluated, diagnosed, and managed through the use of chiropractic procedures based on the best available rational and empirical evidence. The preservation and restoration of health are enhanced through the correction of the subluxation to 80% range of normal mobility. Once the chiropractor has identified the hypomobility, adjustive procedures are used to mobilize the fixation. The therapeutic objective is to deliver a dynamic thrust, employing a specific contact and line of drive with the intention of freeing restricted vertebral joint motion altering specific symptomology.

Physiologic and Pathologic Components of Subluxation

1. Neuropathophysiologic component. Biomechanical insult to nerve tissue leads to neural dysfunction in the following way:
   a. Irritation (sustained hyperactivity) of nerve receptors or nerve tissue. This irritation results in facilitating (lowering threshold of excitability) of afferent nerve cells, which is exhibited as hypertonicity or spasm of muscles.
   b. Compression or mechanical insult (pressure, stretching, angulation, or distortion) to neural elements in or about the intervertebral foramina, within fascial layers, or short muscles.
   c. Decreased axoplasmic transport may alter the development, growth, and maintenance of cells or structures that are dependent on this trophic (growth) influence expressed via the nerve.
2. Kinesiopathologic component. Hypomobility, diminished or absent joint play, or compensatory segmental kinematic hypermobility leads to a variety of nociceptive and mecha-

noreceptive reflex functions that include proprioception. In addition, an early manifestation of a chronically fixated vertebral articulation is shortening of ligaments as an adaptation to limited range of motion.

3. Myopathologic component. Spasm or hypertonicity of muscles as a result of compensation, facilitation, Hilton's Law, or any combination. The nerve supplying a joint also supplies the muscles, which move the joint and the skin covering the articular insertion of those muscles, which results in functional muscle imbalance.
4. Histopathologic component. Inflammation can develop from trauma, hypermobile irritation, or as part of the repair process, resulting in osseous tissue changes in the joint.
5. Biochemical component. Hormonal and chemical effects or imbalance related to the preinflammatory stress syndrome and the production of histamine, prostaglandin, and bradykinin. This component is a result of trauma or fixation of the spinal articulation and is proposed to affect nociceptive impulses, resulting in aberrant (deviating from the usual or normal) somatic afferent input into the segmental spinal cord.

Chiropractic Methods of Treatment

- Adjustment (HVLT)
- Manipulation and mobilization of joints (including positional release methods)
- Manual traction or distraction
- Mechanical devices to aid adjustment

Adjustive Manual (Soft Tissues) Procedures

- Mobilization
- Point pressure techniques
- Massage
- Therapeutic muscle stretching or relaxation
- Visceral techniques

HEALTHCARE SETTINGS IN WHICH MASSAGE THERAPISTS WORK

HOSPITALS

Hospitals are classified according to the type of care and services they provide. A hospital may be designated as a community, regional, acute, subacute, specialty, teaching, private, or nonprofit facility. Community hospitals and regional hospitals are very similar in the ways they provide care for most types of injuries and illnesses (e.g., both types have emergency departments). Regional hospitals usually are acute care facilities that serve a large area. Acute care hospitals have intensive care units and emergency or trauma departments for the severely injured or ill, and some provide transitional care for patients recovering from an illness who still need hospital supervision and treatment. A specialty hospital deals with a specific type of illness, such as cancer or mental health. Teaching hospitals are full of interns, residents, and other medical students and provide the medical student with a hands-on learning environment.

An individual, corporation, or organization may open a private hospital, which means that the facility is designed to provide the owner or owners with an income. With a nonprofit hospital, the intention is to serve the community, and these hospitals generally are run by a board of directors. The term *nonprofit* can be misleading, because there is a difference between "profit" and "making money." A nonprofit hospital or organization may make money in a campaign or fund-raiser, but all of the money is returned to the organization.

A hospital is like any business in that different departments are designed to complete certain tasks to provide a service. In a hospital, the top of the hierarchy is the board of directors or president, followed by the financial department, human resources, medical records, nursing services, laboratory, hospice, and so on. The medical staff committee, led by the hospital's chief of staff, assists in the management of the facility and the credentialing process for the physicians who have staff privileges at the hospital.

When a patient arrives at a hospital, the admissions department gathers information from the patient to be used by the medical staff. The nursing staff provides services to patients, making them comfortable, taking their vital signs, and supervising the routine aspects of patient care. The laboratory takes care of medical tests. All the information is gathered into a patient's record, for which the medical records department is responsible. The radiology or nuclear medicine department offers diagnostic imaging and x-ray services. The physical medicine and rehabilitation department offers both physical and occupational therapy. Hospice is part of the social services department, which works with patients to ensure continuity of care, patient education, and social intervention to assist patients with emotional, economic, and social concerns. Chaplains also serve in hospitals to provide patients with spiritual support.

Accreditation is considered the utmost recognition of the quality of care a facility or institution provides. Hospitals and other healthcare facilities supply evidence to an accrediting organization to prove that they provide a certain quality of care and uphold certain standards. In the United States, hospitals often are accredited by the Joint Commission on Accreditation of Healthcare Organizations (JCAHO). Areas examined include the assessment and care of patients; the use of medication; facility, technology, and safety management; orientation, education, and training of staff; medical staff qualifications; and patient rights. Ratings from 1 to 5 are given to the facility on its performance in specific areas. A "1" rating means that the facility is in full compliance with the standards for that specific area; the other ratings indicate different levels of noncompliance. The Department of Health and Human Services (DHHS) also regulates healthcare facilities, as does the Occupational Safety and Health Administration (OSHA). Other countries have similar requirements and organizations.

evolve 3-6

See the Evolve website for a description of the many services provided by hospitals.

LONG-TERM CARE

Many options are available for helping those who need assistance with day-to-day activities. The latest development is retirement communities that provide emergency call buttons and assistance when needed. Some also offer social activities, restaurants, computer access, housekeeping, beauty salons, and other such services.

Nursing homes serve those who need more than just help with day-to-day activities. One of the most popular forms of care is the assisted living facility. Most assisted living facilities provide 24-hour supervision of residents, all meals, and a broad range of services, such as transportation to doctors' appointments, exercise programs, social services, laundry and linen service, and housekeeping. Many new assisted living facilities are designed specifically for individuals with Alzheimer's disease or other memory-care disorders.

Home healthcare offers patient care in the person's home, therapy services, assistance with medications, and other services so that patients can remain in their homes yet still obtain the care they need.

BUSINESS STRUCTURE IN THE MEDICAL ENVIRONMENT

Healthcare is a business, and the business structure can take many forms. The most common types are private practice, nonprofit, and government forms of healthcare.

Private Medical Practices

Private medical practices generally follow one of three models: the sole proprietorship, the partnership, or the corporation.

The Sole Proprietorship. A sole proprietor is an individual who holds exclusive right and title to all aspects of the medical practice. The sole proprietor may employ other physicians and medical staff to participate in the practice. The owner is potentially liable for all the acts of his or her professional employees and staff members. Although practicing alone has many advantages, including flexibility and independence, it also has significant disadvantages, such as total responsibility for the practice 24 hours a day, 7 days a week. Many physicians do not see a sole proprietorship as an avenue for a decent income as a doctor, because so many of the managed care companies have selectively chosen to offer participation to group practices over the single-practice physician. Some doctors organize associate practices. In these arrangements, physicians share office space and often equipment and employees, but they operate their practices as sole proprietorships.

Medical Practice Partnership. Physicians may decide to practice medicine with another doctor and form a partnership. The benefits normally outweigh the potential for liability for the other physician's actions. Both doctors have more freedom, because they rotate an on-call schedule so that each has some time away from the office. The medical associates often alternate weekends and nights and share employees, equipment, insurance, facilities, and even profits; these resources are divided according to the specifications of the partnership agreement or contract.

A group practice has at least three licensed physicians who form either a partnership or a corporation. The group may share income and expenses, equipment, records, and personnel and may combine patient care and business management. The group practice may be an association of practitioners in the same specialty or a multispecialty organization.

The Corporation. A *corporation* may be defined as an artificial entity having a legal and business status that is independent of its shareholders or employees. Corporations are regulated by the laws of the state in which the incorporation takes place. In most cases the physician shareholders are employees of the corporation. Corporations usually are able to offer better benefits packages, such as pension and profit-sharing plans, medical expense reimbursement, life insurance, and disability income insurance.

Government-Administered Healthcare

Your state, along with every state in the nation, has a health insurance program for infants, children, and teens (Box 3-2). The insurance is available to children in working families, including families in which members' immigration status varies. For little or no cost, this insurance pays for doctor visits, prescription medicines, hospitalizations, and much more. Children who do not currently have health insurance are likely to be eligible, even if the parent or parents are working. Eligibility rules vary from state to state, but in most states, uninsured children 18 years old or younger whose families earn up to $34,100 a year (for a family of four) are eligible. This is called *means testing,* because eligibility depends on the household income (means).

BOX 3-2 The Origins of Medicare and Medicaid

In 1965 the Social Security Act established both Medicare and Medicaid. Medicare was a responsibility of the Social Security Administration (SSA), whereas federal assistance to the state Medicaid programs was administered by the Social and Rehabilitation Service (SRS). These two agencies were part of the Department of Health, Education, and Welfare (HEW). In 1977 the Healthcare Financing Administration (HCFA) was created under HEW to coordinate Medicare and Medicaid. In 1980 HEW was divided into the Department of Education and the Department of Health and Human Services (HHS). In 2001, HCFA was renamed the Centers for Medicare and Medicaid Services (CMS).

CMS is the federal agency that administers the Medicare program. Medicare currently provides coverage to approximately 40 million Americans. It is the national health insurance program for the following people:

- Individuals age 65 or older
- Some people under age 65 with disabilities
- People with end-stage renal disease (ESRD), a condition of permanent kidney failure that requires dialysis or a kidney transplant

Medicaid

Medicaid is a program that pays for medical assistance for certain individuals and families with low incomes and resources (means-tested eligibility). The program is jointly funded by the federal and state governments to assist the states in providing medical long-term care assistance to people who meet the eligibility criteria. Medicaid is the largest source of funding for medical and health-related services for people with a limited income.

HEALTHCARE FOR VETERANS

The Department of Veterans Affairs (still known as the VA, it formerly was the Veterans Administration) provides a medical benefits package, a standard enhanced health benefits plan, which is available to all enrolled veterans. This plan emphasizes preventive and primary care and offers a full range of outpatient and inpatient services within the VA healthcare system.

The VA maintains an annual enrollment system to manage the provision of quality hospital and outpatient medical care and treatment to all enrolled veterans. A priority system ensures that veterans with service-connected disabilities and those below the low-income threshold can enroll in the VA's healthcare system.

Eligibility Requirements

Eligibility for most veterans' healthcare benefits is based solely on active military service in the Army, Navy, Air Force, Marines, or Coast Guard (or Merchant Marine during World War II) and discharge under other than dishonorable conditions.

Reservists and members of the National Guard who are called to active duty by a federal Executive Order may qualify for VA healthcare benefits. Returning service members, including reservists and National Guard members, who served on active duty in a theater of combat operations have special eligibility for hospital care, medical services, and nursing home care for 2 years after discharge from active duty. Veterans' healthcare facilities are not just for men only; the VA offers full-service healthcare to women veterans. Also, healthcare eligibility is not just for those who have served in combat.

BECOMING PART OF THE TEAM: HOW TO WORK WITH OTHER HEALTHCARE PROFESSIONALS

In 1994 the Bureau of Health Professions* released the findings of a task force that had studied the use of interdisciplinary teams in healthcare. The task force identified six characteristics of successful interdisciplinary teams:

- Team members provide care to a common group of patients.
- Team members develop common goals for performance outcomes and work together toward these goals.
- Appropriate roles and functions are assigned to each team member.
- Members understand and respect the roles of others.
- All members contribute and share essential information about both tasks and group process.
- The team has a mechanism to ensure that plans are implemented, services are coordinated, and the performance of the team is evaluated.

*U.S. Department of Health and Human Services, Health Resources and Services Administration, bhpr.hrsa.gov

An interdisciplinary medical team functions as a whole, which requires the understanding and involvement of all team members. Individual tasks may lend themselves to one team member or another with specialized skills, but the final outcome is a team effort. Typically, the physician is responsible for deciding on the diagnostic and therapeutic criteria that must be met for optimal treatment of the patient.

Behaving in a professional manner in the medical environment creates trust, and trust is one of the most important factors that can help avoid problems of medical professional liability. *Professionalism* is the characteristic of conforming to the technical or ethical standards of a profession. It involves showing courtesy, being conscientious, and conducting oneself in a businesslike manner in the workplace. Professionalism is vital in the medical setting. Some of the characteristics of professionalism are loyalty, dependability, courtesy, initiative, flexibility, credibility, confidentiality, and a good attitude.

ETHICS

Ethics are judgments of right and wrong or actions on issues that have implications in a professional setting. **Etiquette** deals with courtesy, customs, and manners. **Rights** are claims that are made by a person or group on society, a group, or an individual. Although these terms have different definitions, the concepts are interrelated, and often all are involved in ethical questions.

Ethical distress is a problem to which an obvious solution exists, but some type of barrier hinders the action that needs to be taken. An **ethical dilemma** is a situation in which two or more solutions are possible, but in the choice of one, something of value is lost by failing to choose the other (or others). Often an ethical problem has several aspects, and more than one type of problem is presented.

Making an ethical decision is easier when a problem is approached logically, using a process based on the clinical reasoning model:

- First, gather relevant factual information and identify the problem, then generate possibilities and explore alternative solutions.
- Next, analyze each alternative and identify the pros and cons of each potential solution.
- Finally, make a decision and develop a plan to implement it.

Confidentiality is vital in the medical profession. Because it is such a critical aspect of patient care, revealing any information about a patient to anyone else is considered highly unethical. All massage therapists are required and expected to uphold the confidentiality of any information that comes their way.

Informed consent gives the patient a full understanding of the condition that has been diagnosed, including what could happen if the patient undergoes treatment, refuses treatment, or delays treatment. It provides the patient with information about the advantages and risks of a medical procedure and alternative or complementary treatments (including massage) that the patient may wish to consider. Informed consent places control in the hands of the patient, who is given the opportunity to make the decisions about his or her healthcare. Patients can never be forced to undergo any type of procedure or treatment.

Several disclosures must be made with regard to a patient's health that do not require patient consent. Information about births and deaths, injuries or illnesses caused by violence, accidental or suspicious deaths, sexually transmitted diseases, and any type of abuse are examples of legal disclosures that must be made by healthcare professionals.

The Health Insurance Portability and Accountability Act of 1996 (HIPAA) established extensive privacy rules and regulations governing patient information, including the electronic transfer of such information (Box 3-3).

BEST PRACTICE

The world of health services appears to be changing gradually from one in which individual doctors

BOX 3-3 The Health Insurance Portability and Accountability Act of 1996 (HIPAA)

The Health Insurance Portability and Accountability Act of 1996 is more commonly known by its acronym, *HIPAA*. A federal agency, the Centers for Medicare and Medicaid Services (CMS), is responsible for implementing various unrelated provisions of HIPAA, which therefore may mean different things to different people. HIPAA has had a significant impact in a number of areas of healthcare.

Health Insurance Reform

Title I of HIPAA protects health insurance coverage for workers and their families when they change or lose their jobs. This is known as the *portability* of health insurance coverage.

Administrative Simplification

Title II of HIPAA, the administrative simplification provisions, require the Department of Health and Human Services to establish national standards for electronic healthcare transactions and national identifiers for providers, health plans, and employers. It also addresses the security and privacy of health data. Adoption of these standards will improve the efficiency of the nation's healthcare system by encouraging widespread use of electronic data interchange in healthcare.

Pre-existing Condition Exclusions

Under HIPAA regulations, a group health plan or a health insurer offering group health coverage may impose a pre-existing condition exclusion with respect to a participant or beneficiary only if the following requirements are satisfied:

- The pre-existing condition exclusion must relate to a condition for which medical advice, diagnosis, care, or treatment was recommended or received during the 6-month period before an individual's enrollment date.
- The pre-existing condition exclusion may not last longer than 12 months (18 months for late enrollees) after an individual's enrollment date.
- The 12-month or 18-month period must be reduced by the number of days of the individual's previous creditable coverage, excluding coverage before any break in coverage of 63 days or longer.

Other HIPAA Effects

Besides limiting administrative costs by supporting the use of electronic transfer of information, HIPAA established guidelines for preventing fraud and abuse. The privacy issues arising from HIPAA have been the most discussed and debated topics related to this law. Massage therapists should receive in-service training in procedures relating to HIPPA requirements and the ways they are implemented in a specific healthcare environment.

U.S. Department of Health and Human Services.

provide care one-on-one to a limited number of patients to a world in which physician-led interdisciplinary teams provide a wide array of services to populations of patients. The activities of teams of the future will be founded on evidence-based interventions as much as possible, and team members will closely monitor their own performance as they seek to improve their team's outcomes, as measured by clinical quality, service quality, and cost.

The massage therapist can become a contributing member of the healthcare team by knowing his or her limitations and working with physician supervision, according to quality medical practice and effective risk management (best practice). Because most patients are not at their best when visiting the physician's office, the attitude of the staff plays an important role in the patient's attitude. Massage therapists need patience and understanding when working with people who are injured or ill.

Teamwork makes any job easier to complete. If you are willing to help coworkers who may be overwhelmed with duties, they will return the favor when the situation is reversed. Straightening up the waiting room or stuffing envelopes may not be part of your job description, but if you are not busy with massage-related activities, a team player helps out where and when he or she can. Never participate in gossip. If you take part in gossip, others are likely to gossip about you, too; it's just not constructive or acceptable professional behavior. Make a good attempt to get along with all employees.

Insubordination is being disobedient to any type of authority figure, usually the supervisor, and can be grounds for immediate or eventual dismissal. When given a task, you should complete the work unless it is unlawful or unethical. If you have concerns about tasks not in your job description, speak with a supervisor. Discuss the issue and attempt to reach an agreement about the appropriateness of performing the task in the future.

First impressions are critical in the medical environment. Dress, attitude, and appearance all influence the credibility of the massage therapist. Typically you will wear scrubs; flat, closed-toed, rubber-soled shoes; little or no jewelry; little or no makeup; no fragrances; and a modest hair style with the hair pulled away from your face. Your finger nails will be short and unpolished, and you will be generally clean and neat. Visible tattoos and other forms of body art may be a concern, so make sure these can be concealed by the typical professional clothing (Figure 3-1).

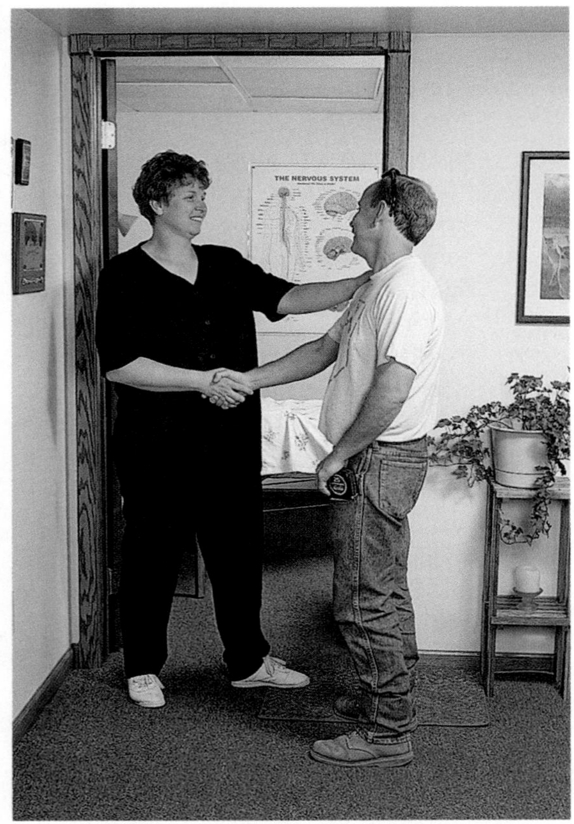

FIGURE 3-1 ■ A professional healthcare worker greeting a client. (From Fritz S: *Mosby's fundamentals of therapeutic massage*, ed 3, St Louis, 2004, Mosby.)

COMMUNICATION SKILLS

Clear, concise, and friendly communication is essential. Communication is difficult if a person is behaving in a defensive way. Defense mechanisms are psychological methods of dealing with stressful situations; they include sarcasm, denial, making excuses, blaming, and other forms of ineffective communication. Listening is one of the most important skills in communication. Listening involves not only silence, but also active feedback. Open-ended questions help restate what the patient, coworker, or supervisor is saying, so that the listener can be sure that he or she understands the message clearly.

Everyone experiences conflict in daily living, therefore we must develop skills in dealing with conflict in the most positive way. Conflict is not always negative and can be quite beneficial in professional relationships. *Conflict* is an expressed struggle between at least two interdependent parties who perceive incompatible goals, scarce resources, and/or interference from the other party in achieving their goals. Clinical massage in the healthcare environment involves working as part of a group; this is different from independent massage practice. Because clinical massage therapists work in partnership with other healthcare professionals, the potential for conflicts exists. Conflict arises from a number of factors, such as:

- Varied perspectives on a situation
- Differing belief systems and values, derived from the involved parties' accumulated life experience and conditioning
- Differing objectives and interests

Conflict and conflict resolution play important roles in individual and social evolution and development. Healthcare is a very culturally diverse environment, and massage therapists must be culturally aware and sensitive to how conflict is perceived and managed. Many cultures value harmony, compatibility, satisfaction, and independence, which may lead to a tendency to avoid conflict. Other cultures are more direct in the management of conflict. However, in all situations involving conflict, cultural influence plays a role only in the individual's response; people must never be stereotyped.

Conflict arises when one or more people view the current system as not working and when the distress of the situation reaches a critical point. At least one person is sufficiently dissatisfied with the status quo to speak up, in the hope of improving the condition. Through conflict, people have opportunities to do things differently in the future.

Conflict exists at two levels. In addition to the obvious interpersonal dispute among individuals, some measure of conflict almost always exists within ourselves. This intrapersonal conflict may manifest as confusion, inconsistency, or lack of congruity. The personal reflection necessary to identify and manage internal conflict is part of professional behavior. At times this internal conflict is stressful enough that the individual may benefit from professional counseling to resolve issues.

Successful resolution of conflict begins with the awareness that people in conflict share common ground as well as differences. These areas of common ground include:

- Overlapping interests
- Interdependence
- Points of agreement

The common ground can serve as the starting point for conflict resolution. Conflict resolution does not necessarily resolve tensions between people. It may simply identify or align matters sufficiently to allow each person to make progress toward his or her goals rather than stall in the uncertain and stressful state of disagreement.

Many people have long believed the myth that the best way to resolve conflict is to "do battle," and the one who "wins" ends the conflict. This approach is more about power and control than about conflict resolution. Doing battle and winning or losing supports the corresponding belief that every situation has a "right" and a "wrong." If we respond to conflict this way, we have limited our understanding of the nature of conflict and alternative means of responding to it, such as mediation and negotiation. Factors and influences necessary for mediation and negotiation are:

- Concerns about the impact of the dispute on the relationship among those involved
- Time concerns
- Expense
- Impact on affected others
- Lost opportunities
- Stress
- Lack of closure
- Uncertain compliance
- Areas of existing common ground

The decision-making process in this text presents a format for this type of conflict resolution.

JUST BETWEEN YOU AND ME

Years ago I contracted to provide massage to a group of leaders in an organization that was undergoing a vast change in management. The chief executive officer (CEO), a client of mine, came up with the idea that if everyone involved got a massage and was relaxed and less stressed, the discussions would be more productive. And that is exactly what happened. I provided massage all day, and then a nice dinner was provided for the group. By the end of the evening, the major issues had been resolved. Smart CEO.

Types of Conflict

Various types of conflict can arise, and if the type of conflict can be pinpointed, those involved are more likely to be able to resolve it.

Relationship Conflicts. Relationship conflicts, often called *personality conflicts,* occur because of the presence of strong negative emotions, misperceptions or stereotypes, poor communication or miscommunication, or repetitive negative behaviors. Relationship problems often lead to an unnecessary escalation in destructive conflict. Conflict resolution supports a safe, balanced expression of the perspectives and emotions of each person involved, leading to acknowledgment and understanding of that individual's point of view. Gaining a broader perspective on diversity of culture and individual operational style is very helpful. Evaluation tools that identify different personality styles can be helpful. One of the most frequently used evaluation tools is the Myers-Briggs Type Indicator. These evaluations help individuals with opposite perspectives interact well rather than allowing conflict to develop. The more we personalize a person's operational style, the more likely it is that conflict will develop.

JUST BETWEEN YOU AND ME

Relationship conflicts are tough to manage. They are full of the "trauma-drama" stuff we all tend to enjoy at some level, otherwise soap operas wouldn't be so popular. However, relationship conflicts tend to spread to uninvolved people, who often think that they need to take sides. *Don't do that.* Mind your own business. It could be you in that position one day.

Data Conflicts. Data conflicts occur when people lack the information necessary to make wise decisions, are misinformed, disagree on which data are relevant, interpret information differently, or have collected data differently. Some data conflicts may be unnecessary because they are caused by poor communication between the people in conflict. Other data conflicts may be incompatibilities associated with data collection, interpretation, or communication. Most data conflicts have "data solutions," and once the information has been corrected, the conflict will resolve unless it has developed into a relationship conflict.

Interest Conflicts. Interest conflicts are caused by competition over perceived incompatible needs. Conflicts of interest result when one or more people believe that to satisfy their needs, the needs and interests of an opponent must be sacrificed. This often occurs during times of scarcity or when it is perceived that there is not enough to go around. Interest-based conflicts may occur over such things as money, physical resources, or time; over procedural issues, such as the way a dispute is to be resolved; or over psychological issues, such as perceptions of trust and fairness and the desire for participation and respect. To resolve an interest-based dispute, those involved must define and express their individual interests so that all interests may be addressed jointly. Interest-based conflict is best resolved through maximum integration of the parties' respective interests, positive intentions, and desired experiential outcomes. A third person, such as a mediator, often is needed to resolve this type of conflict.

Values Conflicts. Values give meaning to our lives; they explain what is "just" or "unjust." Differing values need not cause conflict. People can live together in harmony with different value systems. Values disputes arise only when people try to force one set of values on others or lay claim to exclusive value systems that do not allow for divergent paths. Trying to change values and systems during relatively short and strategic mediation interventions is useless. However, supporting each participant's expression of his or her values and beliefs for acknowledgment by the other party can be helpful. Belief systems are more amiable to change. Values are like ethical principles and deeply ingrained. Belief systems often are superimposed on us during our developmental childhood years. We are taught what is right or wrong, good or bad. Because we learn our belief systems, we can change them through education and willingness to be open to new possibilities.

Ways of Dealing with Conflict

There are five common ways of dealing with conflict. Learning about the alternative means of handling conflict gives us a wider choice of actions in any given situation and makes us better able to respond to the situation. Although the methods listed below are the common ways of increasing the chance of success, the reality is that we use each of these ways of dealing with conflict at least some of the time. We approach conflict in the way that we believe will be most helpful to us. Our style for dealing with conflict changes with the circumstances. Conflict-handling behavior is not a static procedure; rather, it is a process that requires flexibility and constant evaluation to be truly productive and effective.

Denial or Withdrawal. In the denial or withdrawal approach, a person tries to eliminate conflict by denying that it exists and refusing to acknowledge it. Usually, however, the conflict does not go away but grows to the point that it becomes unmanageable. If the issue and the timing are not critical, and if the issue is short-lived and will resolve itself, denial may be a productive way of dealing with the conflict. The effectiveness of this approach depends on the person's knowing when to use denial.

JUST BETWEEN YOU AND ME

I love denial, and sometimes it works really well (other times, not so well). I remember a small group of students who, for some reason (relationship conflict), decided not to like a particular instructor. No problems had ever arisen with this instructor before, and even though others demanded that I take action, I chose denial instead. Why? Because that group of students would be graduating in a month, and that would likely solve the problem. It did, and the issue has never cropped up again. One method of treating prostate cancer is "watchful waiting" to see what happens, because many times the cancer does not progress or progresses so slowly that the person eventually dies from something else. I like that term, *watchful waiting,* and it sounds better than denial.

Suppression or Smoothing Over. A person using suppression plays down differences and does not recognize the positive aspects of handling the conflict openly. Instead, the situation is acknowledged (unlike denial) but glossed over. The source of the conflict rarely goes away. However, suppression may be used when preserving a relationship is more important than dealing with a relatively insignificant issue.

JUST BETWEEN YOU AND ME

Smoothing over works sometimes. One of my key people, who has worked with me for years, can be, let's say, abrasive on occasion. Yet I know she is just kind of like that and not likely to change. Certainly the positives of this relationship outweigh this particular personality quirk. It can bother others much more than it bothers me, but the people it bothers tend to move through the system in a natural career progression and leave. She stays.

Power or Dominance. Power often is used to settle differences. Power may be inherent in a person's authority or position. Power may take the form of a majority (as in voting) or a persuasive

JUST BETWEEN YOU AND ME

Personally, I like to say "because I said so." It's easy, and I sometimes have the power to get away with it. Also, there are times when relationship boundaries are necessary in both the professional and personal worlds. Some time ago, I became truly convinced that massage education has to evolve, and I undertook a wide-ranging curriculum revamp at my school. The science, assessment documentation, and clinical reasoning, based on the patient's individual circumstances, not protocols, focused on outcome-based massage practice. Needless to say, staff members were resistant, because change is difficult for some people, and most of them would need major upgrading on their skills. When I announced the changes formally at a staff meeting, I used power and got away with it only because I have that power as the owner of the school. Two instructors quit on the spot. Others whined some but came around, and the rest embraced the change. The outcome has been great.

minority. Power strategies result in winners and losers. The losers do not support a final decision in the same way the winners do. Future meetings of a group may be marred by the conscious or unconscious renewal of the struggle previously "settled" by the use of power. In some instances, especially when other forms of handling conflict are not effective, power strategies may be necessary. Parents often say to children, "Because I said so." This use of power works in the short term, but over time results in deeper relationship conflict.

Compromise or Negotiation. Compromise ("You give a little, I'll give a little, and we'll meet each other half-way") has some serious drawbacks. Such bargaining often causes both sides to assume initial inflated positions, because they are aware that they are going to have to "give a little" and want to reduce the loss. The compromise solution may be watered down or weakened to the point that it is ineffective. There may be little real commitment by any of the parties. Still, at times compromise makes sense, such as when resources are limited or a speedy decision must be made.

Integration or Collaboration. The integration or collaboration approach suggests that all parties to the conflict recognize the interests and abilities of the others. Each individual's interests, positive intentions, and desired outcomes are thoroughly explored in an effort to solve the problems in the best possible way. Participants are expected to modify and develop their original views as work progresses. This sounds like the ideal way to manage and resolve conflict; however, for collaboration to succeed, those involved need an unthreatening, collectively supportive system. This process takes time, openness, and energy.

JUST BETWEEN YOU AND ME

Negotiation is a lose-lose situation, but don't discount it. The summer that I was working on this text, I was in negotiation with a hummingbird. The feeder is near my home office window, so I can watch the birds while I work. This particular bird would not eat when I was outside on the porch, but instead buzzed around my head. I didn't want to move the feeder, but having a hummingbird diving at and bumping me wasn't pleasant. So I guess we have compromised. The feeder stayed put, I go in while he eats, and he waits for me to leave if I'm outside. It would have been nice to have collaborated with this beautiful creature, but I don't have the time, and he really doesn't care!

Conflict Climate: Defensive or Supportive

The defensive climate reflects the type of atmosphere characteristic of competition; that is, an atmosphere that inhibits the mutual trust required for effective conflict management. The supportive climate reflects collaboration; that is, an environment that leads to mutual trust and to an atmosphere conducive to managing differences. Participants in conflict resolution hopefully come to appreciate that the apparent presenting problem does not need to limit their discussions. Participants are encouraged to express the full breadth and depth of their interests, with each participant seeking to identify a "value" that he or she can bring to the discussion and the maximized satisfaction of underlying interests and intentions.

Conflict is important. If managed well, it identifies and supports effective change. Conflict can foster avoidance, or it can expand our experiences. Making good decisions about managing and resolving conflict can pave the way for greater understanding and well-being.

In the resolution of conflict, written documentation should be kept about the nature of the conflict, the type of resolution attempted, the success of the conflict resolution, and the outcome. Because conflict already exists, interpretation of the requirement for resolution can become confused. Objective documentation that is agreed upon by the parties helps maintain clarity. If the conflict cannot be resolved independently, documentation of the nature of the conflict is extremely important, in case the situation escalates to legal action. This is a major concern in healthcare. Each organization has a procedure for conflict management and documentation; all must be familiar with this process and follow it meticulously if the need arises.

Communication Skills During Conflict

To resolve conflict we need to communicate. Communication is more difficult than we might believe. It is very subjective; information shared is open to interpretation based on current situations, emotional states, and sense of importance, as well as past influences. Verbal communication provides no concrete record (unless recorded), therefore accuracy can be a real problem. Written communication can be reviewed, which is why written records (computer or otherwise) are necessary in healthcare. Interpersonal communication can range from factual dispensing of information to highly charged emotional exchanges. Effective communication is important and can be compromised by various circumstances such as time, old patterns, and avoidance. All these concerns escalate during conflict.

Barriers to Effective Communication

Time. Communicating effectively takes time. This is why writing sometimes is a more effective form of communication. When writing, we should make time to consider the words and reflect on what is being said. The person responding to the written message also has time to reread and reflect on the message.

Old Patterns. Falling into old patterns and old conditioning limits effective communication. "Know thyself" is an important rule, and we must recognize personal triggers to old reactionary patterns in communication. Sometimes we need to leave a situation and come back to it so that we can respond instead of react emotionally.

Avoidance. People generally avoid communicating about conflict until it is unavoidable, and they avoid people who display strong emotion because it makes them feel uncomfortable. Effective communication is a skill that can be learned, and it is essential in the therapeutic relationship. Professionals must work diligently to improve their communication skills.

HEALTH INSURANCE

Reimbursement for services by health insurance companies is common in healthcare. Currently, reliable reimbursement is one of the main obstacles to inclusion of many complementary methods, such as massage. in the healthcare process. This situation likely will improve as more research identifies a positive risk/benefit/cost value for massage services to justify healthcare insurance reimbursement.

In the healthcare environment, the infrastructure already exists for billing insurance companies for payment for services rendered. Large facilities, such as hospitals, have billing departments; small medical practices usually designate a person to take charge of health insurance billing. In the typical healthcare setting, massage therapists would not be billing directly for services rendered; therefore their responsibility is to make sure that all record-keeping, as well as preauthorization treatment plans, are in the patient record. Although some massage therapists bill insurance companies directly in some areas, this is not a common practice. The massage therapist with a career in healthcare needs to understand enough about health insurance and reimbursement to support the specialist in this area (i.e., the insurance biller and health information management professionals) (Box 3-4).

BOX 3-4 Billing and Coding Responsibilities

- Assign Current Procedural Terminology (CPT) when required for facility and professional fee billing.
- Assign CPT for services and procedures and HCPCS billing codes for medical equipment and devices, with appropriate modifiers, when required for facility and professional fee billing and statistical indices.
- Assign codes to each diagnosis ICD9CM identify and code the providers who ordered or provided services (ICD-9-CM Codes/ Diagnostic) in each healthcare encounter as required for facility and professional fee billing.
- Assemble the patient's health information by making sure that initial medical charts are complete, including the member ID number and group number to verify eligibility of benefits.
- Follow federal and state regulations governing the assignment of any of the above codes for reimbursement.
- Work with insurance companies on issues such as prior approval and medical necessity to ensure payment.

Health insurance is a type of third-party payer system. This means that the consumer pays for insurance, and when medical expenses occur, the costs are billed and possibly covered by the insurance. Numerous third-party payers base reimbursements on the *allowable charge,* which has been influenced by managed care organizations and the government. Many forms of health insurance are available. People can buy individual policies, but most get health insurance by being a member of a group that pools its resources to buy the health insurance. Group access to health insurance may include arrangements such as employees of a business (often the employer offers health insurance as a benefit); the Chamber of Commerce, where small business owners can obtain coverage; and, for the massage profession, professional associations, such as the American Massage Therapy Association (AMTA) and the Associated Bodywork and Massage Professionals (ABMP). Insurance policies have many coverage options, from minimal coverage to maximum coverage that includes independent nursing facilities, and some now include alternative and complementary care coverage.

Because of the rising cost of health insurance, a growing number of people do not have it and therefore do not receive medical care when necessary. Some countries have government-based healthcare. Others have combined processes, in which most people carry some sort of private insurance, and certain at-risk groups, such as children, the poor, and the elderly, are eligible for government programs (e.g., Medicare and Medicaid).

Healthcare in the United States has changed tremendously in recent years, and the cost of quality healthcare has skyrocketed. Efforts have been made in both the public and private sectors to introduce various healthcare reforms to contain these costs. Unfortunately, healthcare reform has had little success on the national level; however, state legislatures are beginning to pass laws that have brought improvement. *Managed care* is a broad term used to describe a variety of healthcare plans developed to provide services at a lower cost. However, many are confused about exactly what managed care entails. Managed care has had both positive and negative effects on healthcare delivery.

Massage therapists should become familiar with the major third-party payers, including major medical group insurers, Aetna, United HealthCare, Blue Cross/Blue Shield, Medicaid, Medicare, CHAMPVA, TRICARE, and workers' compensation. Medicare, the largest third-party insurer in the United States, makes quality healthcare affordable for the elderly and other select groups. Medicaid, a joint program of the federal and state governments, provides healthcare for individuals who qualify for benefits based on income limitations and/or disability (see Box 3-2). Workers' compensation covers employees who are injured or who become ill as a result of accidents or adverse conditions in the workplace. Disability programs reimburse individuals for monetary losses incurred as a result of an inability to work for reasons other than those covered under workers' compensation.

Automobile insurance coverage operates in many different ways, has different requirements, and may or may not cover personal injury.

INSURANCE AND MANAGED CARE TERMINOLOGY

Insurance and managed care terminology is unique. You need to learn the language. Refer to the Evolve website for information on terminology.

evolve 3-7

The Evolve website defines and discusses the components of health insurance and presents definitions for terms, which are listed in alphabetical order.

RECORD-KEEPING/DOCUMENTATION

Record-keeping is the recording of relevant data. In medical settings, especially, it is extremely important. Record-keeping is a skill that needs to be practiced and perfected. Unfortunately, this is an area in which massage therapy training often is lax, therefore it must be diligently and thoroughly addressed by massage therapists who want a career in healthcare. (Unit Two presents specific record-keeping procedures that are relevant to massage.)

> **evolve 3-8**
>
> The Evolve website provides examples of various types of medical records.

Quality health data have the following nine hallmarks:

- *Validity* (the information is accurate)
- *Reliability* (the information can be counted on to be accurate, and medical decisions can be made based on it)
- *Completeness* (the information is available in its entirety)
- *Recognizability* (the information can be understood by those who need to use it)
- *Timeliness* (the information is the latest available data on which the provider can make decisions about a patient or treatment)
- *Relevance* (the information is useful)
- *Accessibility* (the information is easily available to the provider when it is needed)
- *Security* (steps have been taken to prevent unauthorized people from accessing the information)
- *Legality* (the correctness of the information is authenticated by the healthcare provider)

GUIDELINES FOR CREATING A PATIENT RECORD

Practitioners can create a credible patient record by following some general guidelines.

- Each page of the record should identify the patient by name, hospital, clinic, or private physician clinical record number.
- Each entry should include the date and time the entry was made and the signature and credential of the individual making the entry.
- No blank spaces should be left between entries.
- All entries should be written in ink or produced on a printer or typewriter.
- The record must not be altered in any way. Erasures, use of correction fluid, and marked-out areas are not appropriate.
- Errors should be corrected in a manner that allows the reader to see and understand the error. The recommended procedure involves the following steps:
  1. A single line is drawn through the error, and the legibility of the previous entry is checked.
  2. The correct information is inserted.
  3. The correction is dated and initialed.
  4. If there is not enough room for the correction to be made legibly at the error, a note should be made indicating where the corrected entry can be found and the reference dated and initialed. The correct information is entered in the proper chronologic order for the date the error was discovered and corrected.
- All information should be recorded as soon as possible. Memories can fade, and important facts can be omitted.
- Abbreviations should be used sparingly and should include only those that have been approved by the organization, with an abbreviation code located on the document. A single abbreviation otherwise can have different meanings, which can be misleading.
- All entries must be written legibly. It is embarrassing and can be expensive when caregivers cannot read their own entries in court. Because so many clinicians use the patient record to provide care, the legibility of the record is important to the quality of care given to the patient.
- All entries must be consistent with one another. The assessment must agree with the diagnostic testing, or an explanation must be given as to why it does not.
- Entries should be factual accounts. Criticism of the patient or a colleague should never be

included. Records that blame or belittle others can be damning evidence in a lawsuit.

- All information given to the patient before any procedure should be recorded. This ensures and verifies that the patient was properly informed of the benefits and risks before he or she gave consent to the procedure.
- Telephone contacts with the patient should be entered in the record immediately.
- Some method of organization (e.g., the SOAP format, which is explained more in Unit II) must be used to ensure that the entries are comprehensive and reflect the thought process used in making decisions about the patient's care.

When these rules are followed, the result is a record that is accurate, timely, specific, objective, concise, consistent, comprehensive, logical, and legible and that reflects the thought processes of the healthcare providers.

evolve 3-9

The Evolve website shows an example of a correctly completed healthcare record.

COMPUTERIZED PATIENT RECORD (CPR) AND THE ELECTRONIC HEALTH RECORD (EHR)

The paper medical record is fast becoming a thing of the past. A paper record is difficult to access, often lacks information, and must be in a single location for a single user. Over the past three decades, significant advances have been made in automating the record-keeping process. Technology has improved, allowing the design and implementation of electronic record-keeping systems that are easy to use. Many different terms are used for automated record-keeping systems, such as computerized patient record, electronic patient record, computerized medical record, and electronic record. Massage therapists must be able to use whatever electronic record-keeping system is in place in the setting where they work. The thought process is the same, the data record is the same. Jotting paper notes may be necessary while working with the patient, but eventually those notes must be entered into the electronic system.

evolve 3-10

An example of a computerized patient record (CPR) can be found on the Evolve website.

Patient healthcare records are confidential. Most healthcare providers, and certainly hospitals, have policies governing the release of any information about a patient. Massage therapists must be aware of such policies. Most healthcare providers have implemented policies and procedures that incorporate HIPAA requirements.

All states have laws about which diseases, conditions, and events must be reported to the appropriate agencies. Examples of such incidents include births, deaths, gunshot wounds, communicable diseases, and evidence of child abuse. If any such condition becomes an issue for massage therapists in the healthcare setting, they should report the situation to their supervisor, who will deal with it. Massage therapists should ask the supervisor if there are any specific reportable circumstances they should expect to encounter. When reporting is required by law, confidentiality is no longer an issue. However, the format of the report may or may not include the patient's identity, therefore the massage therapist should be sure to ask about the proper method of reporting. Reporting such incidents to anyone other than the responsible agency is a breach of confidentiality.

GETTING A JOB IN THE HEALTHCARE SETTING

Career development for massage therapists in healthcare is in its infancy. The two main obstacles are a lack of appropriately trained massage therapists and difficulty obtaining health insurance reimbursement for massage treatments.

Because you are reading this text, you have at least some interest in, and perhaps are dedicated and committed to, professional excellence. My personal hope is that in the next 5 years, a qualified pool of massage therapists who are able to perform well in the healthcare environment will develop.

The financial issues are more of a concern, but trends point to coverage that will allow healthcare organizations and professionals to provide massage therapy and receive reimbursement for it. Health insurance currently covers massage if it is supervised by an approved gatekeeper, billed correctly, and provided in the appropriate environment. In some cases a massage therapist may participate in specific insurance networks in which direct billing is possible. However, this situation is not common in a healthcare environment such as a hospital or a physician's office.

As with any job search, the two most effective tactics are networking and contacting employers directly. Networking involves developing a wide-ranging group of individuals who can help you find employment. This group may include business contacts, coworkers, relatives, or friends who can provide leads to potential employers. Contacting employers directly involves taking resumés to specific offices and setting appointments to learn about the facility before using that knowledge during the job search. An important point: Make double-sure your resumé is error free. Make sure everything is spelled correctly, and do not rely solely on your computer's spell-checker. Proofread the document and have someone else who is knowledgeable proofread it to catch errors that may have been overlooked. Salary expectations should never be stated on the resumé, nor should a photograph be included. Do not include personal information, such as height and weight.

Employers in the healthcare setting have basic expectations of their employees. They want individuals who are well trained, have a good appearance, and look as if they fit in the medical profession (Figure 3-2). A massage therapist must also be dependable and have the skills to do the job for which he or she is hired.

Employers seek three types of skill strengths:

- *Job skills* are the actual skills needed to perform a job, such as the ability to give a beneficial massage based on outcomes.
- *Self-management skills* usually are part of your personality. They include honesty, dependability, a sense of humor, tolerance, and flexibility, to name a few.
- *Transferable skills* are skills that can be taken from one job to another or used on any job, such as the ability to maintain appropriate records, communicate effectively, and lead and manage individuals.

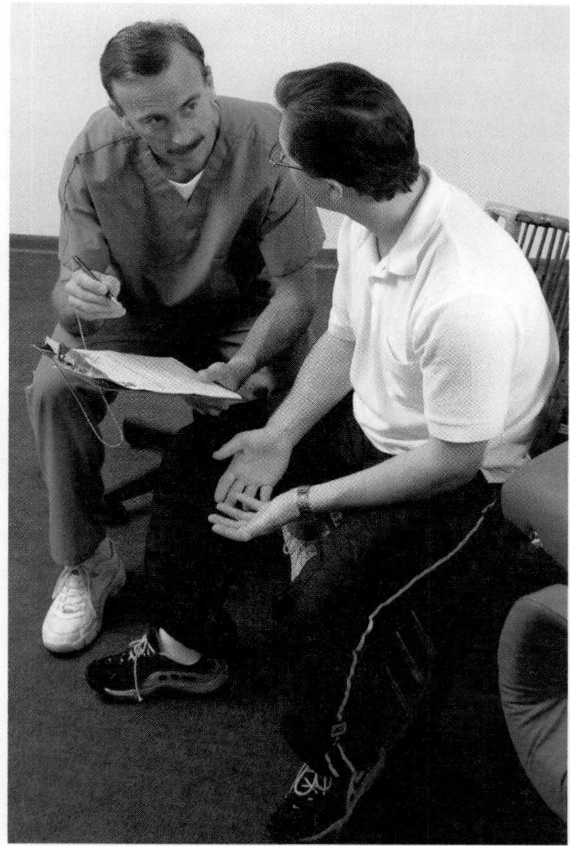

FIGURE 3-2 ■ A professional massage therapist. (From Salvo S: *Massage therapy: principles and practice,* ed. 3, St. Louis, 2007, Saunders.)

The ways in which massage therapy will be provided in the healthcare environment are evolving. Therefore volunteering in various healthcare settings can serve two purposes: It can create awareness of the benefits of massage, and it can put you in a position where potential employers can observe your performance. Volunteer opportunities are available in most hospitals, cancer centers, hospices, and similar facilities. Volunteering to work with medical staff (e.g., doctors, nurses, and others) offers another opportunity. For massage therapists in private practice, gaining the respect of the medical community by following the guidelines in this text and networking with healthcare professionals can promote referrals.

JUST BETWEEN YOU AND ME

I know of a committed massage therapist who volunteered to work with surgical staff members after operations. The surgeon was so impressed with how he felt after massage that he personally paid the massage therapist's salary for a year. I think that was a pretty good strategy on the therapist's part.

evolve 3-11

See the Evolve website for detailed information on how massage therapy is moving into mainstream healthcare.

evolve 3-12

The following terms and expressions specific to Chapter 3 have already been used to search PubMed for the latest research literature available. The *Click Here for Massage* feature associated with this chapter on your textbook's Evolve website allows you to hyperlink to a continually updated PubMed search of research literature that corresponds to this subject.

Hyperlink Search Terms

Massage doctors
Massage healthcare sites
Massage insurance business issues
Massage long-term care
Massage patient client
Massage team

SUMMARY

This chapter covered many aspects of the healthcare environment. Complying with all these rules and regulations while acquiring the skill base to provide therapeutic massage successfully may seem like an overwhelming task. In reality, it is already happening, and the integration of massage into the various healthcare settings will continue to evolve. Teamwork and cooperation are necessary for any group process. Respect for other professionals and the people served are the foundations of ethical and professional behavior. There is no such thing as "clinical" or "medical" massage. Instead, there is beneficial therapeutic massage provided within the structure of the healthcare setting.

REFERENCES

1. www.healthy.net: Naturopathic Therapeutics.
2. www.anesthesia-nursing.com: "What is a CRNA? Part II"
3. www.gradschools.com: Touro College
4. Venes D, Thomas CL, Taber CW, editors: *Tabor's cyclopedic medical dictionary.* Philadelphia, 2005, FA Davis.
5. National Women's Health Resource Center (www.healthywomen.org): Osteopathic Medicine.
6. www.innerself.com: Discovering Osteopathy.
7. www.aacom.org: Osteopathic Medicine.
8. www.globalnpac.org: Naturopathic Medicine.
9. www.amfoundation.org/naturopathinfo.htm#: Principles
10. CCNM: www.whidbeynaturopathic.com/naturopathic_medicine/seven_principles.
11. www.naturopathy_anp.com
12. www.mand.org
13. www.calnd.org/education.asp
14. www.naturodocs.com: Principles
15. www.chirocolleges.org/paradigm_scopet.html: Association of Chiropractic Colleges.
16. www.chiroweb.com
17. Alaska Statues
18. www.chiro.org

WORKBOOK

1. Based on the discussion of the various physician specialties (e.g., chiropractic, physical therapy, family practice), pick three you would consider potential avenues for a successful massage career. Write a proposal to a fictitious physician in each of the three specialties, explaining why massage would be beneficial as an aspect of the care offered.

2. Choose one of the medical environments in which you would most enjoy working (e.g., hospital, ambulatory medical center, long-term care). Then choose a specific area within that setting (e.g., labor and delivery unit in a hospital) and explain what motivates you to develop the skills to provide massage in this specific area.

3. Investigate the educational and licensing standards in your state and the pay ranges for various healthcare professions. Pick one of these professions and write a resumé for yourself that is currently accurate; compare it with your state's requirements and the information provided in this text with regard to education and experience. Finally, write a cover letter with a requested pay range and justify the salary you are seeking.

4. Review the discussion on health insurance reimbursement. Then, using your list of three specialties from question 1 in this section, write a proposal to one of the main third-party insurance providers supporting the inclusion of massage as a reimbursable service within a particular medical specialty.

5. Review the section on best practices. Identify three areas in which you consider yourself strong and at least one area in which you need improvement. Write a self-improvement plan for the weaker area.

6. Objectively evaluate your current charting skills based on the information provided in the chapter and on the Evolve website. Develop a self-improvement plan that would bring your charting skills up to the standard required in the healthcare setting.

Chapter 4 Concept Map

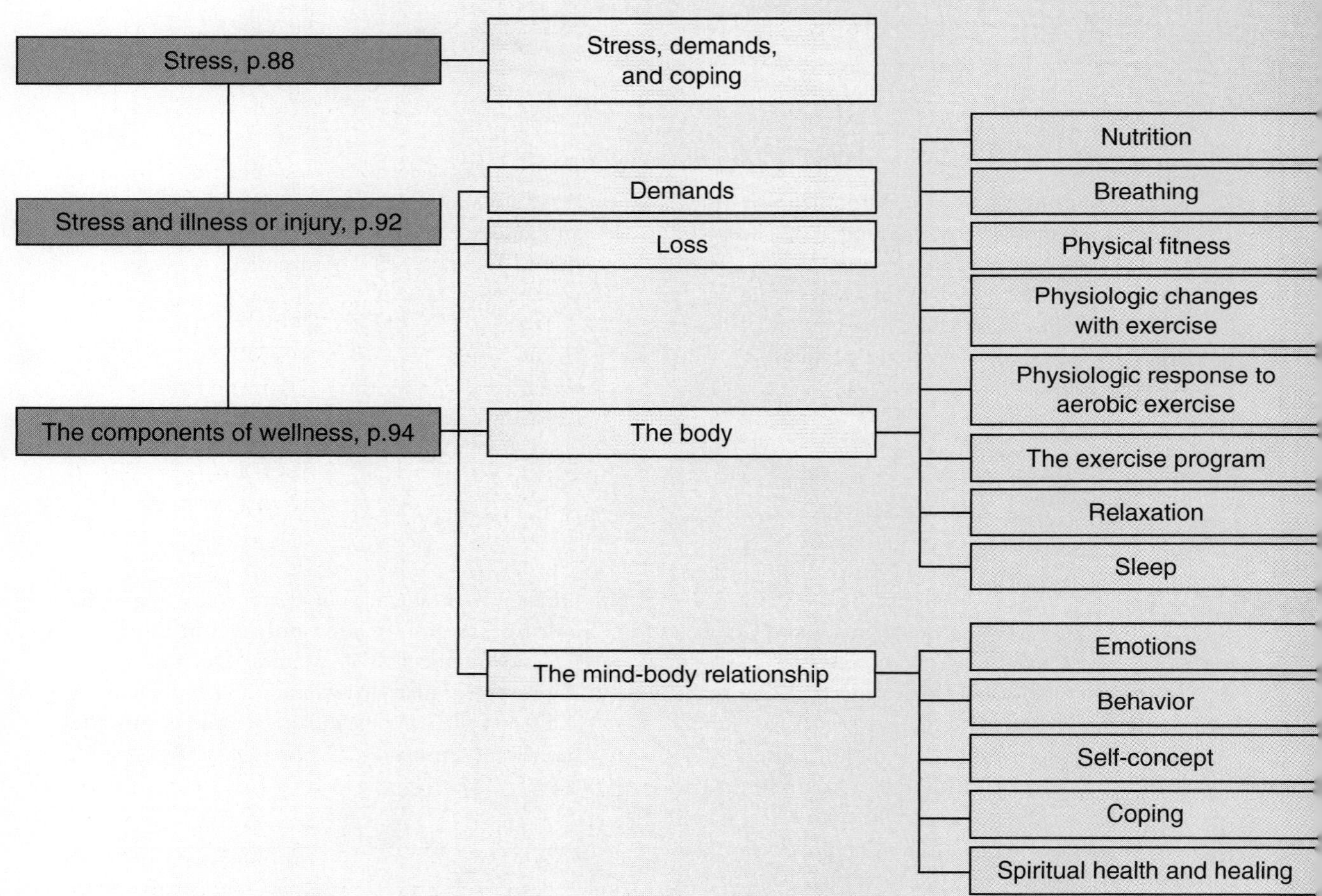

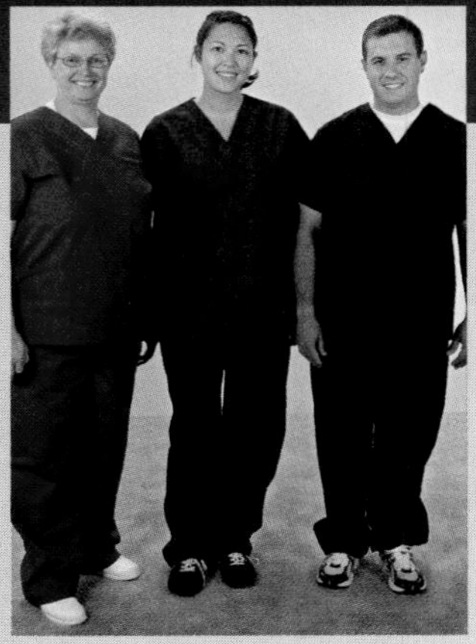

CHAPTER 4

PREVENTIVE MEDICINE, WELLNESS, AND LIFESTYLE

Key Terms

Adaptation
Adaptive capacity
Aerobic exercise training
Aerobic system
Anaerobic system
Behavior
Cardiovascular changes
Deconditioning
Defensive measures
Duration
Emotions
Endurance
External control
Faith
Feelings
Fitness
Flexibility
Frequency
Hope
Intensity
Internal control
Love
Mindfulness
Relaxation
Stress
Stressors
Stretching
Training stimulus threshold
Wellness

For definitions of key terms, refer to the Evolve website.

OBJECTIVES

Upon completion of this chapter, the reader will have the information necessary to:

1 Identify the basic components of a wellness program.
2 Locate resources to develop a wellness program.
3 Develop a personal wellness program.
4 Provide patients with general wellness guidelines.
5 Provide massage as part of a wellness program.

This chapter focuses on the general concepts of wellness that form the basis for the trend toward preventive medicine. It also is about how we, as massage professionals, take care of ourselves. Life is stressful, and working in healthcare settings adds to that stress. At the very least, we can be thankful that giving massage is a stress-reducing activity. Just imagine the stress levels of coworkers! To understand wellness and the concepts of preventive healthcare, massage therapists must understand dysfunctional responses to stress and how stress influences health and healing. This chapter is not about mental disease (which is discussed in Unit Three), but about how we cope with the stressors of life in general. We are considered well when body, mind, and spirit are in ideal balance; we are not well when imbalance exists and balance cannot be restored.

In the words of a renowned nutrition scientist, Professor Jeffrey Bland, many people are "vertically ill." They are not sick enough to lie down, but they are certainly not well. This situation is brought about not just by the type of stress involved, but also by the amount of stress that accumulates, until the breakdown begins. Then, it is only a matter of time before physical health, the mind, or the person's quality of life simply falls apart under the accumulation of multiple stressors.

People in this condition often see their doctors about subclinical symptoms that are difficult to diagnose. When told they are experiencing stress responses, they may become frustrated with the medical professionals, and they often resist instruction in changing their lifestyle. The management of stress requires participation by the patient, who must make lifestyle changes. No medical cure exists for stress, and long-term use of medication can produce side effects. The patient wants the doctor to "fix it"; but that is something the doctor cannot do. Approaches such as yoga, meditation, support groups, exercise, and good nutrition are helpful and beneficial, but they require effort from the patient. If a program is complicated, compliance by the individual often is poor.

Massage is a method that avoids this trap. It is mostly passive (from the client's perspective), pleasant, and effective. The person need only show up for appointments. Typically, as clients begin to feel better, they become more committed to the real "cure," which is a change in lifestyle. This assumes that recovery is possible. However, that is not the case for all clients. Therefore, for treatment purposes, massage therapists must categorize clients as (1) those who will recover whatever treatment is offered or even without treatment; (2) those who can improve and possibly recover fully; and (3) those who will not recover, for whom massage at best can slow the decline and keep the person as comfortable as possible.

Wellness is about the whole person; it is not about the diagnosed condition of the person. Wellness methods (prevention) typically are beneficial for everyone, regardless of what ails them. Prevention is about staying healthy and not getting sick or hurt in the first place. Steps on the path to wellness can have a domino effect. Simple changes in lifestyle may become synergistic and create a chain reaction throughout a person's entire life. For this reason, a person may need to commit to just a few carefully planned lifestyle changes, increase his or her awareness of and intent to achieve wellness, and then allow the rest of the "pieces" to fall into place.

The concept of self-regulation also comes into play; for example, broken bones mend, cuts heal, and most infections (more than 95%) resolve without intervention. The body heals itself, given the chance. The formula for supporting self-regulation is: reduce adaptive load, enhance adaptive capacity, and modulate symptoms if appropriate (many, such as inflammation, are part of the recovery process). The body does the rest.

Making a change to wellness takes determination. Letting go of behavioral patterns is difficult. This process is very hard to work through alone, therefore relationships with others who are supportive (e.g., through support groups or professional therapy) are helpful.

STRESS

In and of itself, **stress** is not a bad thing. It is a reaction to any demand on the body or mind to respond, adapt, or alter. It is a state of readiness to survive, a hypervigilance of the body and mind. Our emotional reaction to stress and the defensive measures the body uses to counter it may make the difference between positive action and destructive breakdown, especially if many of the stressors are beyond our control.

Stressors are any internal perceptions or external stimuli that demand a change in the body. A person's **adaptive capacity** is the amount of stress the individual can handle successfully. As the stress response increases, adaptive capacity decreases. As adaptive capacity diminishes, symptoms begin to appear, and when the person can no longer adapt physically or emotionally, illness occurs. Adaptive capacity is restored and maintained by reducing sympathetic autonomic nervous system dominance, getting sufficient restorative sleep, maintaining appropriate nutrition, drawing support from healthy relationships, and having some sort of empowering spiritual practice.

Defensive measures are the ways our bodies defend against a stressor (e.g., the production of antibodies and white blood cells) or behavioral and emotional defenses. Sometimes defending is not the best way to deal with stress. It is important and resourceful to know when to quit or surrender and move on. Hormonal and nervous stimuli encourage the body to retreat and ignore stressors. On an emotional level, this is sometimes called *denial,* which can be an important method of coping with stress.

People need to maintain a balance between external stressors and their unique physical, biochemical, and psychosocial attributes, both inherited and acquired. This adaptation depends on the stress load (how much and how long) and the individual's ability to compensate for and adapt to it. Adaptation is an individualized process. Two people can experience the same stress load, with two different outcomes. Therefore, when stress is a problem, an important consideration is not just the stress load, but also what factors make the individual, at this time, unable to cope (i.e., handle the load), and what is the least invasive, least demanding way to modify those factors. The body deals with stress load by activating a physiologic series of events described by Hans Selye as the general adaptation syndrome. The three phases are alarm, resistance, and exhaustion.

Mental excitement and physical stressors cause an initial exhilaration that is followed by a secondary phase of depression. Similarly, a law of physics states that for every action, there is an equal and opposite reaction. Certain chemical compounds, such as the hormones produced during the acute alarm reaction phase of the general adaptation syndrome, are able first to key up the body for action and then to cause a depression. Both effects may provide great protective value. The body must be keyed up for peak accomplishment, but it is equally important for it to relax and restore during the secondary phase of depression. This prevents the body from operating too long at top speed. According to noted stress researcher Hans Selye:

> The fact is that a person can be intoxicated with his own stress hormones. I venture to say that this sort of drunkenness has caused much more harm to society than the alcoholic kind. We are on our guard against external toxicants, but hormones are parts of our bodies; it takes more wisdom to recognize and overcome the foe which fights from within. In all our actions throughout the day, we must consciously look for signs of being keyed up too much, and we must learn to stop in time. To watch our critical stress level is just as important as to watch our critical quota of cocktails. More so; intoxication by stress is sometimes unavoidable and usually insidious. You can quit alcohol and, even if you do take some, at least you can count the glasses; but it is impossible to avoid stress as long as you live, and your conscious thoughts often cannot gauge its alarm signals accurately. Curiously, the pituitary is a much better judge of stress than the intellect. People can learn to recognize the danger signals fairly well, if they know what to look for (Box 4-1).

STRESS, DEMANDS, AND COPING

As well as addressing a patient's illness or injury, a clinical/medical massage therapist must understand the demands placed on the whole person. Psychological stress has been shown to predict increases in illness or injury. Stress is thought to increase the risk of illness and injury through suppression of the immune response, disruption of concentration or attention, and increased muscle tension. People especially prone to illness and injury seem to be those who experience considerable life stress, especially if they have little social support and few psychological coping skills and are apprehensive, detached, and overly sensitive. Poor coping mechanisms allow the system to be overwhelmed, therefore the goal is to reduce the stress load and/or enhance adaptability (coping).

Stress often is associated with situations or events that are difficult to handle. How a person views events also affects the level of stress. Unrealistic or high expectations increase the stress response. Psychologists use cognitive behavioral therapy to help people change how they view events by altering the stress response.

Stress may be linked to a number of external factors, such as:

- Community
- Unpredictable events

Box 4-1 Common Stress Responses

Stress and the body's response to it produce a number of common signs, which arise from fluctuations in the autonomic nervous system and resulting endogenous chemical shifts. These signs include:

- General irritability, hyperexcitation, or depression
- Pounding of the heart
- Dryness of the throat and mouth
- Impulsive behavior and emotional instability
- Overpowering urge to cry, run, or hide
- Inability to concentrate
- Weakness or dizziness
- Fatigue
- Tension and extreme alertness
- Trembling and nervous tics
- Intermittent anxiety
- Tendency to be easily startled
- High-pitched, nervous laughter
- Stuttering and other speech difficulties
- Grinding of the teeth
- Insomnia
- Inability to sit still or physically relax
- Sweating
- Frequent need to urinate
- Diarrhea, indigestion, queasiness, and vomiting
- Migraine and other tension headaches
- Premenstrual tension or missed menstrual cycles
- Pain in the neck or lower back
- Loss of or excessive appetite
- Increased use of chemicals, including tobacco, caffeine, and alcohol
- Nightmares
- Neurotic behavior
- Psychosis
- Proneness to accidents

From Fritz S: *Mosby's fundamentals of therapeutic massage,* ed 3, St Louis, 2004, Mosby

- Environment
- Work
- Family

Stress also can be caused by internal factors, such as:

- Irresponsible behavior
- Poor health habits
- Negative attitudes and feelings
- Unrealistic expectations
- Perfectionism

It's one thing to be aware of stress in daily life, but it's another to know how to change or manage it. Stress is not something that is "all in your head." It is a physical response to an overwhelming situation, and it has the potential to control a person's life. As we've shown, stress has many sources. Getting caught in a traffic jam, standing in line at a store, or getting a parking ticket can be causes of mild stress. Stress also can be severe and cause major health problems. Divorce, family problems, and the death of a loved one can be devastating.

Stress can be short term (acute) or long term (chronic). Acute stress is a reaction to an immediate threat or perceived threat. However, everyday life often poses problems that are not short-lived, such as relationship difficulties, loneliness, or financial or health worries. The pressures may seem unrelenting and can cause chronic stress.

When a person's coping behavior is ineffective, a physical stress response occurs to meet the energy demands of the situation. First, the stress hormone adrenaline is released. As a result, the heart beats faster, the breath quickens, and the blood pressure rises. The liver increases its output of blood sugar, and blood flow is diverted to the brain and large muscles. The massage therapist would recognize the signs and symptoms of nonproductive sympathetic dominance. After the threat or anger has passed, the body relaxes again. People usually are able to handle an occasional stressful event, but if such events occur repeatedly, as occurs with chronic stress, the effects multiply and compound over time.

When people face more stress than they are able to cope with, six telltale signs appear:

- Irritability
- Sleep problems (sleeping all the time or inability to sleep)
- Lack of joy
- Loss of appetite (or inability to stop eating)
- Trouble with relationships and inability to get along with friends and family
- Illness, infertility, and fatigue

Chronic stress can damage overall well-being, producing the following signs:

- Uneasiness and vigilance
- Anxiety and panic attacks

- Sadness or a heightened sense of energy
- Depression or melancholia
- Anorexia or overeating
- Hyperalertness
- Irritability
- Suppression of the immune system
- Impaired resistance to infection
- Increased metabolism and use of body fats
- Diabetes
- Hypertension
- Infertility
- Fatigue
- Absence of menstruation (amenorrhea) or loss of sex drive and impotence

People can take a number of steps to help themselves better cope with stressors that cannot be controlled.

- Sleep is very important and can provide a person with the energy needed to face each day. Going to sleep and awakening at a consistent time also may help a person sleep more soundly. Restorative sleep should be a major goal for massage.
- A balanced diet that includes a variety of foods provides the right mix of nutrients to keep body systems working well. A diet that reduces the potential for inflammation is valuable. When healthy, a person is better able to control stress and pain.
- Changing the pace of the daily routine. Allow the day to progress more slowly.
- Keeping a positive attitude is vital. This is easier to do if the individual spends time with people who have a positive outlook and a sense of humor. Laughter actually helps to ease pain, because it causes the release of chemicals in the brain that provide a sense of well-being.

Physical relaxation aids in the management of stress in several ways:

- It reduces anxiety and conserves energy.
- It increases a person's self-control in dealing with stress.
- It helps a person recognize the difference between tense muscles and relaxed ones.
- It helps a person remain alert, energetic, and productive.

Massage is a major relaxation therapy. Other activities also can be helpful for patients, such as the following:

- Deep breathing (see p. 96). Massage supports optimal breathing function.
- Progressive muscle relaxation. This technique involves relaxing a series of muscles, one at a time. First, the patient increases the tension level in a group of muscles (e.g., a leg or an arm) by tightening the muscles; then, the muscles are relaxed. The patient should concentrate on letting the tension go out of each muscle. Then the next muscle group is worked. Muscles near pain sites should not be tensed. Massage supports the practice of progressive muscle relaxation.
- Word repetition. With this technique, the patient chooses a word or phrase that is a cue to relax and then repeats it. While repeating the word or phrase, the patient should try to breathe deeply and slowly and think of something that provides pleasant sensations of warmth and heaviness.
- Guided imagery. Also known as *visualization,* this method involves lying quietly and picturing oneself in a pleasant, peaceful setting. The patient should experience the setting with all the senses, as if actually there. For instance, the individual should imagine lying on the beach. He or she should picture the beautiful blue sky, smell the saltwater, hear the waves, and feel the warm breeze on the skin. The messages the brain receives as the patient experiences these senses aid relaxation.

People can better cope with stressors by making a few lifestyle adjustments. For example, they should:

- Simplify life.
- View negative situations as positive and a chance to improve life.
- Use humor to reduce or relieve tension.
- Exercise and stretch.
- Get more sleep.
- Eat a good breakfast and lunch.
- Reduce or eliminate caffeine in the diet (caffeine is a stimulant).
- Get a regular massage.
- Don't take work problems home or home problems to work.

- Strengthen or establish a support network.
- Hug family and friends.
- Do volunteer work or start a hobby.
- Pray or meditate.
- Practice relaxation techniques (e.g., deep breathing, progressive muscle relaxation, self-hypnosis)

Physical stress patterns, whether occupational or athletic (e.g., poor posture, poor working position, repetitive activities), often result in progressive changes that can arise in local areas (shoulders or knees) or affect the whole body. These can include changes in soft tissues and joints, and dysfunctional patterns may emerge that add to the stress load (pain disability) and further reduce adaptive capacity. The solution lies in the previously stated formula: reduce load, enhance functionality.

STRESS AND ILLNESS OR INJURY

Recovering from an illness or injury or coping with chronic conditions can present many challenges. How a patient understands and responds to fatigue, pain, and limitation is a very individual experience based on many factors. However, certain responses and psychological skills can help most people take an active role in their coping and recovery plan.

People often initially feel overwhelmed by an illness or injury. The ability to cope greatly improves if the patient works closely with the doctor and other healthcare providers to develop a clear intervention plan. The process begins with the patient becoming informed about the situation. It is important that the person know the extent of the condition, the anticipated prognosis, the effective treatments, and the potential side effects of treatment.

Patients must see themselves as active participants in the process of treatment planning. They may not understand the scientific aspects of their condition or treatment options, but they are the experts about their own experience—a reality that may either help or hinder the treatment process.

Patients should try to maintain a sense of identity and importance by engaging in activities that help them feel good, such as massage. They should express their needs and concerns to the healthcare team. A helpful technique is to identify any nonproductive mental responses and then reframe them to promote a positive approach to healing the various aspects of body, mind, and spirit. The patient must be able to acknowledge his or her current level of function and what function has been lost and then move beyond those limitations to envision the future as a healthy, productive individual. Patients need to ask for and receive help, and they should be surrounded with emotionally and physically supportive people. Interaction with people who hinder the healing process should be eliminated or minimized. Some people know how to deal successfully with being ill or injured; others have a hard time coping, which increases their already high stress load. The patient may need professional help processing the life changes he or she faces; the massage therapist must be supportive but must not assume the role of psychologist.

Signs that a person is having problems coping with healthcare issues include:

- Depression
- Feeling helpless
- Mood swings
- Dwelling on minor complaints
- Denial

Illness and injury affect patients in many ways:

- The patient's status with regard to peers may change.
- Pain may be a constant presence or a dominant element.
- The patient may need to develop the discipline to comply with healing and rehabilitation programs.
- The patient's level of independence and control may be decreased.
- Financial worries may develop.
- The patient's self-esteem or self-image may suffer.

Generally speaking, ill or injured patients often experience feelings of vulnerability, isolation, and low self-worth. Denial of the reality of the illness or injury also can come into play. All these feelings can have an adverse effect on the patient and the healing process. The individual may experience a number of personal reactions, including physical, emotional, and social reactions. A fairly predictable response to significant health concerns and injury occurs in five sequential stages: (1) denial, (2) anger, (3) grief, (4) depression, and (5) reintegration. These responses are normal, and the massage therapist needs to remain nurturing and compassionate in a quiet, nonjudgmental way while maintaining a neutral response to the patient's coping pattern. Patients who fail to move through these five stages may suffer adverse psychological effects related to the health condition. These adverse effects are more likely to occur if the illness or injury is severe enough to cause major life changes.

Most people who suffer a serious injury or are diagnosed with a life-changing illness experience some degree of psychological distress and discomfort. However, more serious problems of poor psychological adjustment to illness and injury often are preceded by the following warning signs:

- Feelings of anger and confusion
- Obsession with the question of when the person will be well
- Denial of the illness or injury
- Guilt about letting family, friends, or peers down
- Withdrawal from significant others
- Rapid mood swings
- Pessimistic attitude about the prognosis for recovery

The severity of the condition usually determines how long healing and/or rehabilitation will take. Regardless of how long that is, the patient must deal with three reactive phases of the healing and rehabilitation process:

- Reaction to illness and injury
- Reaction to healing and rehabilitation
- Reaction to return to previous responsibilities

Not all patients have all these reactions, nor do the reactions necessarily follow this sequence. Other factors that influence a patient's reactions to illness and injury and to healing and rehabilitation are the person's coping skills, past history, social support, and personality traits.

People who deal with their feelings and focus on the future rather than the past have a tendency to advance through treatment more rapidly. Individuals who have a high degree of hardiness, a good self-concept, coping strategies, mental skills, and spiritual strength are more likely to recover quickly and fully than patients who lack these qualities. Patients who lack motivation and are depressed or in denial more often have difficulty with the healing and rehabilitation process.

The medical team is responsible for care relating to the person's health condition and often becomes the primary mechanism of social support. The massage therapist can play an important part in this support process only if the various health professionals work together. Conflict among professionals can make the situation worse.

After an illness or injury, particularly one that requires long-term healing and rehabilitation, the patient may have problems adjusting socially and may feel alienated. The person may believe that he or she has received little help from social and work support systems. Injuries and illness also can create *secondary gain,* which develops when the health condition results in the following:

- A beneficial "timeout"
- Time to rest and refocus
- Reduction of pressures and expectations
- Becoming the center of others' attention

Secondary gain can both support and interfere with the healing process.

Psychologists use strategies and communication skills to help the patient move successfully through the healing and rehabilitation process. Care must be taken to maintain appropriate boundaries during this vulnerable time for the patient. The medical staff uses a number of strategies, and the extent of the massage therapist's involvement in these strategies varies.

- *Coping skills.* The massage professional has a limited role in this area; teaching self-help is appropriate as long as it does not conflict with other treatments.
- *Education about the condition.* Before sharing such information, the massage therapist must make sure that it is correct and does not conflict with that provided by other professionals.
- *Management of emotional reactions to the health issue (e.g., depression, anxiety, anger)*

and regaining a sense of control. The massage therapist can target the massage to address the physical effects of emotional turmoil and can refer the patient to the psychologist or social worker for additional mental support.
- *Pain management for coping with pain related to the condition and various treatments.* The massage therapist can play an active role in pain management.

The six emotional demands of treatment are:

- Compliance (doing what the patient is supposed to do)
- Maintaining motivation
- Tolerating pain
- Goal-setting and achievement
- Consulting with medical staff as needed
- Coping with chronic pain

Massage therapists can play an important role in healing and rehabilitation by developing an understanding of patients' emotional response to health problems and by helping to manage the stress response.

THE COMPONENTS OF WELLNESS

Wellness is a way of being. Even those who are ill or injured can have an attitude of wellness. Many professionals are involved in specific therapeutic interventions that make up the components of a wellness program. Doctors, counselors, other healthcare providers, educators, and religious and spiritual advisors all play an important part in helping an individual become well again or maintain wellness. Ultimately, people must do the work and take responsibility for who, what, and where they are, but it is important to use whatever help is available. For example, if a person has a large tumor and a surgeon can remove it safely, then the doctor's help gives the body a head start on healing.

The appropriate wellness components and medical and therapeutic treatments work synergistically. This produces a much better outcome than relying strictly on one or the other approach. A balance exists between intuition and science in wellness. In the development of a wellness program, it is important to consider these two very important sources of information. Hippocrates advised, "Do no harm." A wellness program is based on this advice; it is a balance between what science knows and what a person knows he or she needs. A wellness program must evolve and change as the status of the individual changes. In following a synergistic wellness program, the individual can look forward to getting back to living life to the fullest and, at the appropriate time, to dying with dignity.

Wellness programs require considerable information about diet, exercise, lifestyle, and behavior patterns. It is important to seek out those with experience to obtain that information. In the healthcare environment, many professionals are available to help people develop a wellness program. In this development process, the individual's spiritual, mental, and physical history must be considered. The sense of self in relation to others is also important. If this connection with others is not respected and nurtured, the result is a strain that interferes with spiritual, emotional, and physical health.

DEMANDS

In modern life, many of the demands placed on us exceed the designed capacity of the body; we have too much to know, too much to do, too many responsibilities, and too many places to be. Our lives have become hurried, mired in a constant battle for time. There are too many options with too many choices, and it all costs too much. Wellness often revolves around simplification of

JUST BETWEEN YOU AND ME

If you are *really* good at what you do, you will become busy. The demand for your time and expertise will grow. We often consider only the more "negative" aspect of demands, but success also creates many demands. I am very good at what I do. Often, there's not enough of me to go around. I'm at a point in my life now where I need to simplify things to support my own wellness. The intention of this text (and of all the books I write) is that its readers will pursue their personal goals and become excellent massage therapists. You, too, will be *really* good at what you do, and the time will arrive when you will need to make your own decisions on simplifying things.

a person's lifestyle. Simplification requires the individual to make choices, set boundaries, practice discipline, and let go in many dimensions.

LOSS

Sometimes an event in life results in the loss of some part of an individual. It could be a body part, a body function, a relationship, a member of the family, or a job. Loss heals though grieving. Grief is a physiologic response that involves stimulation of the sympathetic autonomic nervous system. The emotional response is first alarm, then disbelief and denial, which progress to anger and guilt. The process continues to the finding of a source of comfort and culminates in adjustment to the loss. To heal, people need to reconstruct the aspect that was lost or learn to live resourcefully without it.

JUST BETWEEN YOU AND ME

Loss is tough. My family experienced a major fire, in which we lost a lot of tangible items. Thankfully, it was all replaceable, just stuff. I have also lost irreplaceable people and pets—or have I? Their memories still have an impact on many lives, inspiring others to do good and to be better people, tender reminders of lessons about life and love.

THE BODY

The care of our bodies is an important part of any wellness program. Areas that require attention in a wellness program include nutrition, breathing, physical fitness (e.g., exercise and stretching), relaxation, and sleep.

Nutrition

Proper nutrition is easy to explain. However, people do not always follow recommendations, because nutrition involves more than just eating. Eating affects the mood; mood influences feelings; and behavior supports feelings. The issue of food therefore becomes an emotional topic.

The basics of balanced nutrition are explained in the Department of Agriculture's new guide to good eating, called MyPyramid. This food pyramid includes the original four food group recommendations, suggesting a diet high in vegetables, whole grains, legumes, and fruit. The requirement for protein from animal sources has been reduced. Dairy needs are moderate to small. It is prudent to buy hormone- and antibiotic-free products that come from naturally raised animals.

evolve 4-1

Because the food pyramid (currently called MyPyramid) is an ever-changing chart, please refer to the Evolve website for the latest version.

Although fat and sugar requirements in the diet are minimal, human beings have a strong urge for sweets and fats. This instinctive craving contributes to many dietary problems. In early eras of human existence, fats and sweets were difficult to find. Human beings had to have a deep instinctual desire to fight the bees for their honey, and the animals for their fat, or to gather fatty seeds. Today fats and sugar are abundantly available, but our primitive nature still functions as though we need to store up for a future famine. Weight management is a major healthcare concern, and obesity is epidemic. Many healthcare programs target weight-related issues, and massage is a beneficial component in this area.

An ideal diet avoids trans fats completely and reduces animal-based saturated fats, sugars, and artificial ingredients as much as possible. The diet should include a moderate amount of high-quality protein, but most of the dietary calories should come from complex carbohydrates (fruits and vegetables). Consuming a small amount of good fat (e.g., olive oil) also is important. Some nutritional experts recommend diets that are higher in protein and lower in carbohydrates. An antiinflammatory diet emphasizes whole foods that are colorful, because colorful foods are high in antioxidants, which help reduce inflammation. Essential fatty acids, such as those found in cold water fish (e.g., sardines, salmon), nuts and seeds, and extra virgin olive oil, are important. Cultured dairy products, such as yogurt and kefir with active cultures, are beneficial.

Drinking enough pure water is very important to a wellness program. Because our bodies are more than 70% water, most diets recommend at least 64 ounces of water per day for efficient body function. Adequate fiber and water in the diet promote the bladder and bowel habits that support wellness. Eating on a regular schedule is important to maintain body rhythms, which in turn support wellness. Portion control is as important as a regular schedule of food intake. Most experts recommend three moderate meals and three small snacks each day. Certain herbs used in cooking (e.g., turmeric, ginger, and cinnamon) seem to have a beneficial effect on inflammation and insulin balance.

Cycles of high and low blood sugar are caused by unbalanced diets, aggravated by improper spacing between meals, and supported by caffeinated fluids such as coffee, tea, alcohol, and cola drinks. These fluids stimulate the production of adrenaline, which forces the release of sugar into the blood. The body then pushes sugar levels down again with insulin. This rise and fall in insulin (also called *glycemic demand* or *glycemic load*) is a contributing factor in the development of diabetes, another major health concern.

Nutritional Supplements. Many people take nutritional supplements, and experts disagree on the value of these supplements. Food sources of vitamins and minerals can be compromised by growth in soil depleted through conventional farming practices, such as the use of artificial fertilizers, pesticides, and other chemicals, and by the addition of antibiotics and growth hormones to livestock feed. (The increasing availability of organic food is encouraging.) Nutritional value also is compromised by long-term storage and preservation. Obtaining optimal nutritional value from the food we eat is difficult without extraordinary attention to the diet, which requires time, dedication, and discipline.

Reasonable supplementation is a plausible answer to this problem. The closer a supplement is to a "real food," the better the body is able to use it. Unless the instructions say otherwise, supplements should be taken with food to enhance absorption.

Herbs, which are very powerful, should not be used as nutritional supplements or medicines without the guidance of a professional knowledgeable about their effects. Using herbs or high doses of various vitamins and supplements should be considered the same thing as taking medication. There is value but danger as well, and the use of supplements to treat medical conditions should be managed by a trained professional. The patient should discuss with the doctor, the doctor's assistant (physician assistant [PA]), or the nurse practitioner (NP) all herbs and supplements the person is taking, because they may affect the action of medication or pose a risk before and after surgery and during other forms of treatment. Massage therapists should *never* recommend nutritional supplements; rather, they should refer the patient to the appropriate healthcare professional, naturopathic doctor, or possibly a trained herbalist who is part of the multidisciplinary team.

JUST BETWEEN YOU AND ME

Body stuff is easy, really. Because making body changes is easy, many people begin a wellness journey at this point. However, sooner or later, the rest—demands, loss, spiritual empowerment based on love, gratitude, and peace—become aspects of wellness. Success in making body changes often provides the energy and motivation to address the more complex issues.

Breathing

Breathing patterns present a direct means of altering autonomic nervous system patterns, which in turn affect mood, feelings, and behavior. Almost every meditation or relaxation system uses breathing patterns. The ancient Sanskrit word *prana* means both *breath* and *life energy*. Breathing can also be modulated through singing and chanting.

Proper breathing is important, but most of us do not breathe efficiently. For many, the air quality is poor. In our homes, the outgassing of chemicals from furniture, carpeting, building materials, artificial air fresheners, and so forth makes for poor air quality and possibly tainted air. Environmentally, air quality is compromised by pollutants. Unfortunately, the elements that sustain life—food, water, and air—are in significant danger of becoming health risks through pollution and depletion. Fortunately, the global community is becoming aware of this major health concern.

We have to get the air inside us to make use of it. The simple bellows breathing mechanism is a body-wide coordination of muscle contraction and relaxation. The shoulders should not move during normal, relaxed breathing. The accessory muscles of respiration in the neck area should be activated only when increased oxygen is required for the fight-or-flight response, which is the pattern for sympathetic dominance breathing. The accessory muscles of respiration (e.g., the scalenes, sternocleidomastoid, serratus posterior superior, levator scapulae, rhomboids, abdominals, and quadratus lumborum) may be constantly activated for breathing when forced inhalation and expiration are not needed; this results in dysfunctional muscle patterns. Tightness in the quadratus lumborum or shoulder pain often is not identified as an inefficient breathing pattern during assessment by the massage professional.

Phases of Breathing. The process of breathing can be divided into three phases of *inspiration* (bringing air into the body) and two phases of *expiration* (moving air out of the body) (Figure 4-1, *A*). Quiet inspiration takes place when an individual is resting or sitting quietly. The diaphragm and external intercostals are the prime movers. During deep inspiration, the actions of quiet inspiration are intensified. When people need more oxygen, they breathe harder. Any muscles that can pull the ribs up are called into action. Forced inspiration occurs when an individual is working very hard and needs a great deal of oxygen. Not only are the muscles of quiet and deep inspiration working, but also the muscles that stabilize and/or elevate the shoulder girdle to elevate the ribs directly or indirectly.

One of the two phases of expiration, quiet expiration, is mostly a passive action (Figure 4-1, *B*). It occurs through relaxation of the external intercostals and the elastic recoil of the thoracic wall and tissue of the lungs and bronchi, with gravity pulling the rib cage down from its elevated position. Essentially, no muscle action occurs. Forced expiration brings in muscles that can pull down the ribs and muscles that compress the abdomen, forcing the diaphragm upward.

Normal breathing consists of a shorter inhale with a longer exhale. The ratio of inhale duration to exhale duration is one count inhale and four counts exhale. The ideal pattern ranges from two to four counts for the inhale to eight to 16 counts for the exhale. The reverse of this pattern (i.e., shorter exhale, longer inhale) is the basis for breathing pattern disorders.

Breathing well is very difficult if the mechanisms are not working efficiently. Therapeutic massage can normalize many of these conditions and support more effective breathing. Many who have attempted breathing retraining have become frustrated by their inability to accomplish the pattern. They may find more success if the status of the body and the mechanism of breathing are first normalized.

JUST BETWEEN YOU AND ME

Breathing is a big deal. It's amazing how many physiologic processes in the body are influenced by the breathing function. Disordered breathing is a common factor in most illnesses and injuries. Pain, stress, and anxiety can cause or be caused by disordered breathing. Breathing is discussed in detail later in the text, because massage can specifically and effectively address disordered breathing.

Physical Fitness

Fitness is a general term for the ability to perform physical work. Physical work requires cardiorespiratory functioning, muscular strength and endurance, and musculoskeletal **flexibility.** To become physically fit, people must participate regularly in some form of physical activity that challenges all the large muscle groups and the cardiorespiratory system and promotes postural balance.

Exercise and **stretching** are integral parts of any wellness program because they provide the activity our bodies were designed to have. Fitness programs need to be appropriate; it is important to modify exercise systems and stretching

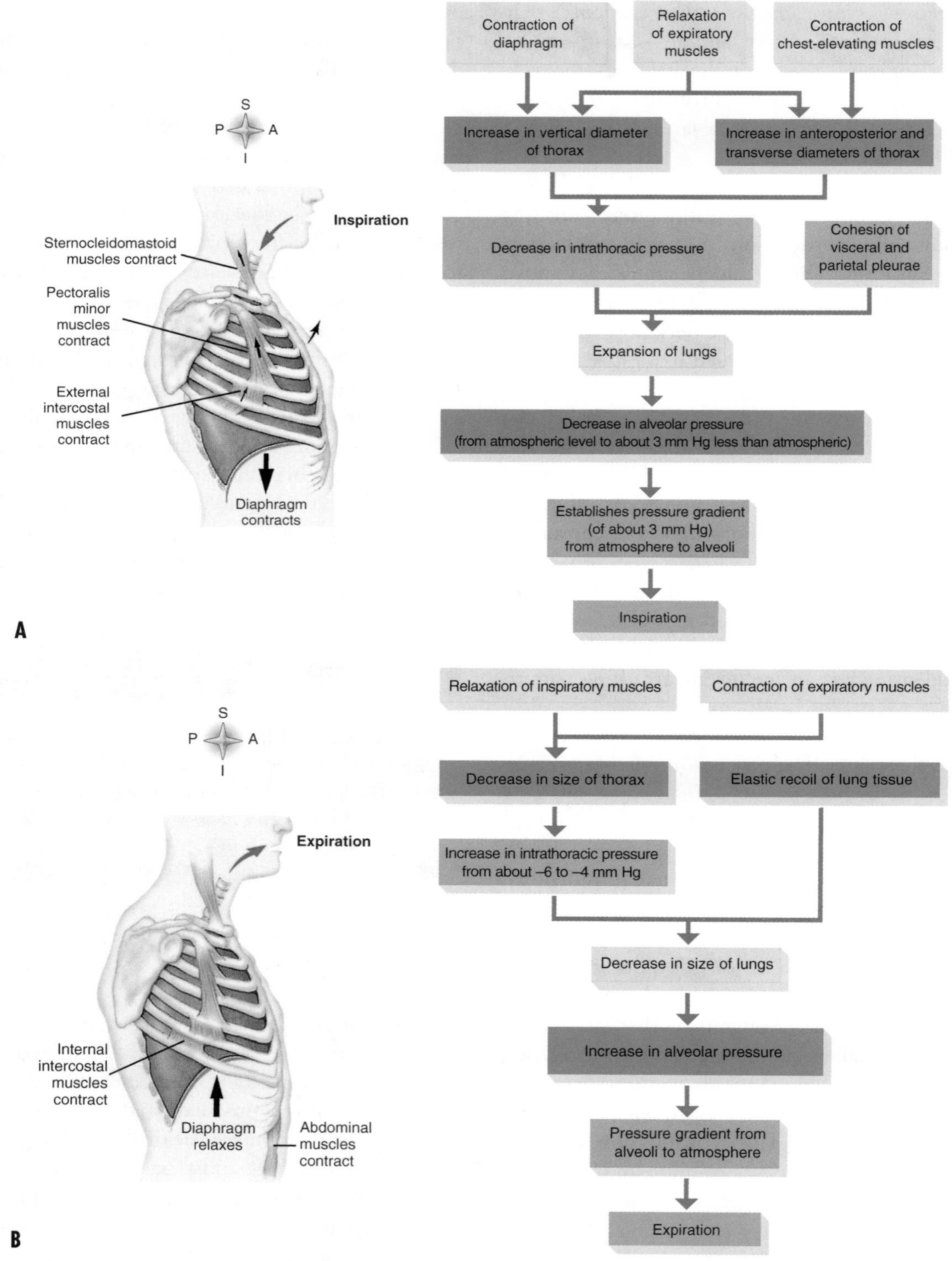

FIGURE 4-1 ■ **A,** Mechanism of inspiration. **B,** Mechanism of expiration. (From Thibodeau GA, Patton KT: *Anatomy and physiology,* ed 5, St Louis, 2003, Mosby.)

programs to fit the individual. An exercise and stretching program must begin slowly. Activity levels can be increased gradually each week. It takes about 7 weeks for those who are new to movement to reach a level of comfort. Massage can help manage the discomfort of exercise programs and thereby support compliance. New activities may be added slowly, once the body has adapted.

Endurance is a measure of fitness. It is the ability to work for prolonged periods and to resist fatigue. It includes muscular endurance and cardiovascular endurance. *Muscular endurance* refers to the ability of an isolated muscle group to perform repeated contractions over a designated period, whereas *cardiovascular endurance* refers to the ability to perform large muscle, dynamic exercise (e.g., walking, swimming, or biking) for long periods.

Deconditioning occurs with prolonged bed rest or reduced activity, and its effects frequently are seen in a person who has had an extended illness. Maximal oxygen consumption, cardiac output, and muscular strength decline very rapidly. These effects also are seen, although possibly to a lesser degree, in an individual who has spent some time on bed rest without any accompanying disease process and in individuals who are sedentary as a result of lifestyle or increasing age.

Aerobic Exercise Training. **Aerobic exercise training** is an exercise program that focuses on increasing fitness and endurance. This type of training depends on exercise of sufficient intensity, duration, and frequency to produce cardiovascular and muscular adaptation in the person's endurance. This is different from training for a particular sport, in which a person improves in the exercise task specific for the sport but may not improve in other tasks or in whole body conditioning.

Adaptation. **Adaptation** results in increased efficiency of body function as long as the demand does not overwhelm the person's adaptive potential. It represents a variety of neurologic, physical, and biochemical changes in the cardiovascular, neuromuscular, and myofascial systems. Performance improves as a result of these changes, and the systems adapt to the training stimulus over time. Significant changes in fitness can be measured in 10 to 12 weeks. Positive results are achieved if adaptive demands match adaptation potential; otherwise, there is no gain, but rather increased dysfunction, which can lead to exercise-related injuries and problems.

A person with a low level of fitness has more potential to improve than one who has a high level of fitness. This is reflected in the **training stimulus threshold,** which is the stimulus that elicits a training response. The higher the initial level of fitness, the greater the intensity of exercise needed to elicit a significant change.

Energy Expenditure. Energy is expended when the body engages in physical activity. Activities can be characterized as light or heavy by determining the energy cost. Most daily activities are categorized as light activity, with energy supplied by the **aerobic system** (oxygen based) because they require little power but occur over prolonged periods. Heavy work usually requires energy supplied by both the aerobic system and the **anaerobic system** (nonoxygen based).

Intensity. The **intensity** of exercise is based on the overload principle. *Overload* is a stress on an organism that is greater than the one regularly encountered during everyday life. To improve cardiovascular and muscular endurance, an overload must be applied to these systems. For adaptation to occur, the exercise intensity load must be just above the training stimulus threshold. Once adaptation to a given load has occurred, the individual can achieve further improvement only by increasing the training intensity (exercise load). Increasing intensity too quickly can result in injury. Training stimulus thresholds vary, depending on the individual's health status, level of activity, age, and gender. Physical therapists and exercise physiologists are best trained to develop and monitor therapeutic exercise programs.

Duration. The optimal **duration** of exercise for cardiovascular conditioning depends on the total work done, the intensity and frequency of the exercise, and the individual's fitness level. Generally speaking, the greater the intensity of the exercise, the shorter the duration needed for adaptation. The lower the intensity of exercise, the longer the duration needed. A 20- to 30-minute session at 70% of the person's maximum heart rate is considered optimal. If the intensity is below the heart rate threshold, a 45-minute continuous exercise period may provide the appropriate overload. With high-intensity exercise, 10- to 15-minute exercise periods are adequate. Three 5-minute daily periods may be effective in those who are deconditioned. Prolonging an exercise session beyond 45 minutes increases the risk of musculoskeletal injury and soreness, and the benefit does not justify the risk.

Frequency. The optimal **frequency** for fitness training generally is considered to be three to four times a week. Frequency can vary, however, depending on a person's health and age. If training is done at a low intensity, greater frequency may be beneficial. A frequency of two times a week does not generally evoke cardiovascular changes, although individuals who are deconditioned initially may benefit from a program of this frequency. As frequency increases beyond the optimal range, the risk of musculoskeletal injury and soreness increases. For individuals in good general health, exercising 30 to 45 minutes at least three times a week appears to protect against coronary heart disease.

Maintaining Fitness. The frequency or duration of physical activity required to maintain a certain level of aerobic fitness is less than that required to improve it. However, the beneficial effects of exercise training are reversible. The process of deconditioning occurs rapidly when a person stops exercising. After only 2 weeks of reduced activity, significant reductions in work capacity can be measured, and improvements can be lost within several months.

Physiologic Changes with Exercise

Changes in the cardiovascular and respiratory systems, as well as changes in muscle metabolism, occur with endurance training. These changes happen both at rest and with exercise. It is important to note that one training program cannot achieve all of the important training effects. A regular, ongoing process of exercise using a variety of activities is necessary to achieve and maintain fitness.

Physiologic Response to Aerobic Exercise

The rapid increase in energy demands during exercise requires equally rapid circulatory adjustments to meet the increased need for oxygen and nutrients; to remove the end products of metabolism (e.g., carbon dioxide and lactic acid); and to dissipate excess heat. The shift in body metabolism occurs through coordinated activity of all body systems (i.e., the cardiovascular, respiratory, metabolic, neuromuscular, and hormonal systems). Effective endurance training must produce a conditioning or cardiovascular response. As noted earlier, conditioning depends on the three critical elements of exercise: intensity, duration, and frequency.

Cardiovascular Changes. A number of **cardiovascular changes** occur as a result of exercise. Changes at rest involve a reduction in the resting pulse rate with a decrease in sympathetic dominance and lower levels of norepinephrine and epinephrine. Parasympathetic restorative mechanisms increase, and a decrease in blood pressure can occur. Blood volume and hemoglobin often increase, which improves the oxygen delivery capacity of the system.

Changes during exercise include a reduction in the pulse rate and a decrease of norepinephrine and epinephrine. Cardiac function increases, as does extraction of oxygen by the working muscle.

Respiratory Changes. Respiratory changes are observed at rest and with exercise after endurance training. One change noted at rest is a greater lung volume as a result of improved pulmonary function. Changes with exercise occur because of a larger diffusion capacity in the lungs based on the larger lung volumes and greater alveolar-capillary surface area. Breathing is deeper and more efficient.

Metabolic Changes. Muscle hypertrophy and increased capillary density are observed at rest and with exercise after endurance training. At rest, a noticeable increase is seen in the number and size of mitochondria; this increases the capacity to generate adenosine triphosphate (ATP) aerobically.

During exercise, the muscle glycogen depletion rate declines and lower blood lactate levels are seen at submaximal work levels as a result of an increased capacity to mobilize and oxidize fat, which arises from an increase in enzymes that mobilize and metabolize fat.

Other System Changes. Changes in other systems that occur with exercise training include a decrease in body fat and blood cholesterol and triglyceride levels, as well as an increase in heat acclimatization and in the breaking strength of bones, ligaments, and tendons.

JUST BETWEEN YOU AND ME

Okay. We must get appropriate exercise. If our lifestyle were still based on the hunter/gatherer society or on farming with manual labor, we wouldn't need to dedicate additional time to exercise. However, in most of the developed countries, heavy labor is no longer required. Nevertheless, our bodies are designed to move, not sit. My brain works like crazy when I'm writing a book, and my body sits still. I think I've expended a lot of energy, so I eat. The end result may be a great book, a weight gain of 10 to 15 pounds, and loss of physical fitness; and I know better. This helps me to be more compassionate toward others.

The Exercise Program

An appropriate exercise program can result in a higher level of fitness for a healthy person. It also can slow the decline in functional capacity in the elderly and recondition individuals who have been ill or who have a chronic disease or a sedentary lifestyle. An exercise program has three important components: a warm up, aerobic exercise, and a cool down. A flexibility and strength training program is also important. Some individuals used certified personal trainers to help them pursue the wellness-based exercise program.

evolve 4-2

See the Evolve website for the specifics of the exercise program.

Appropriate exercise is necessary for wellness. The components of an exercise program can be accomplished in many ways, through many activities that support health. One day you can walk for about an hour, and the next day you can strengthen your core muscles with activities on an exercise ball or a movement program, such as tai chi. Climbing stairs is a great exercise, and yoga supports flexibility. When the body has the movement it needs, relaxation activities are more effective.

JUST BETWEEN YOU AND ME

Physical fitness is very important, and massage can support the physical fitness program. I work with a lot of professional athletes. They have to perform. But performance is more than fitness. Performance is a strain on the systems, which means that the body has to recover. Fitness, which supports wellness, is necessary for recovery. When we demand performance of our bodies but have not maintained fitness, the result usually is illness or injury. You don't have to be an athlete to get caught in the performance trap.

Relaxation

Methods that promote **relaxation** initiate a parasympathetic response. Because muscle tension patterns are habitual, most successful relaxation methods combine movement, stretching, tensing, and then releasing of muscles (progressive relaxation). The heart rate and breathing rate are synchronized *(entrainment)* while the individual focuses on a quiet or neutral topic, event, or picture *(visualization)*. Slow, rhythmic music can be a beneficial component of a relaxation program. Most meditation and deliberate relaxation processes are built around this pattern. The focus of relaxation is to quiet the body, not to create a spiritual experience; however, many prayer systems use similar patterns, which are beneficial for relaxation as well.

Almost any type of pleasurable, simple, repetitive activity that requires focused attention induces the relaxation response. Gardening, needlepoint, playing music, and watching fish in an aquarium or birds at a bird feeder are all forms of relaxation if no need exists to achieve, compete, or produce results in a specific period. Knitting a sweater for pleasure and having to finish one in a week are two different activities. Relaxation takes time, and when something is urgent, it usually interferes with the ability to relax. **Mindfulness** is a concept of relaxation; it is being attentive to the present moment, letting go of thoughts about the past or future.

Just as tension patterns are habitual, relaxation can become a habit. Typically, 8 to 10 weeks of consistent reinforcement are required to develop a habit. Unlike exercise, which can be varied to prevent boredom, a relaxation sequence needs to be the same to reinforce the conditioned response. It is important to use the same or a similar location, music, time of day, smells, colors, position, and breathing pattern in the sequence. After the conditioned response has been learned, any of the components of the relaxation program can become triggers for relaxation.

People should experiment with relaxation methods until they find the right program, and then they should use it every day for at least 15 minutes. (It takes this long for the body's physiology to shift from an aroused state to a relaxed one.) Many audiocassette programs facilitate progressive relaxation and self-hypnosis and pull together all the components of a relaxation program. This type of resource can be very useful.

Sleep

Restorative sleep is necessary for wellness and absolutely necessary for healing. Lack of quality sleep is becoming a major health concern. Many people do not get enough sleep. An absolute minimum of 6 hours of uninterrupted sleep is required, and most people need 8 to 9 hours.

Numerous things can interrupt sleep, such as pain that repeatedly wakes the person; external, random noise (e.g., traffic noise); the needs of infants and children; varying work schedules; a restless bed partner; sinus or other respiratory difficulties (e.g., coughing); and urinary frequency. The list of possible interruptions is endless. Whatever the cause, sleep is compromised, and the deep sleep stage is seldom achieved.

Other people have disrupted sleep patterns because of insomnia, snoring, sleep apnea, hormone fluctuations, high cortisol (stress hormone) levels, medications, and stimulant intake (e.g., caffeine). Quality sleep is sacrificed.

Light/dark cycles regulate sleep patterns. For effective sleep, we need adequate exposure to daylight, which stimulates serotonin. We also need adequate exposure to darkness. The advent of artificial lighting has meant that we spend less and less time in the dark, and this results in sleep disturbances. Absence of light supports the release of melatonin, a pituitary hormone that is involved in the sleep pattern.

During sleep the body renews, repairs, and generally restores itself. Growth hormone is an important factor in this process, with more than half of its daily secretions taking place during sleep. If the deeper stages of sleep are not sustained, the body's restorative mechanisms are compromised. Sleep disturbances are a major factor in many chronic fatigue and pain syndromes (see Unit Three).

Sleep, especially during dreaming, is the time when we seem to repair, sort, and restore emotionally. Dreaming is still a mystery, but research indicates that it is essential for emotional well-being. Therapeutic massage supports restorative sleep in the following ways:

- It diminishes the activity of the sympathetic autonomic nervous system and reduces cortisol levels.
- It promotes parasympathetic autonomic nervous system dominance.
- It relieves or reduces pain and discomfort that may interrupt sleep.
- It raises levels of serotonin, which both elevates mood and serves as a precursor chemical for the body's manufacture of melatonin.

A number of self-help measures can help you make sure you are getting sufficient restorative sleep.

- Maintain a regular sleep/wake cycle. Get up and go to bed at the same times every day, including days off.
- Get at least 30 minutes of daylight exposure by going outside or by placing yourself in front of an open window (this also causes the body to naturally produce more serotonin).

- Exercise moderately on a regular basis, but do not exercise aerobically 4 hours before sleeping.
- Reduce your stimulant intake substantially, and be sure to avoid taking any stimulants for 10 hours before sleeping. For example, if you go to bed at 11 PM, do not drink colas or coffee after 1 PM.
- Concentrate protein food intake 6 hours before going to sleep. Eat carbohydrates after this time. Do not eat a heavy meal before going to bed. Do not go to bed hungry. Eat a small snack of complex carbohydrates (without sugar) with some dairy product (e.g., yogurt) 30 minutes before bed if you are hungry. Although a protein, turkey is high in tryptophan, which encourages sleep. A small turkey sandwich is a possible bedtime snack.
- Stretch gently 1 hour before retiring. A slow, rhythmic pattern is best.
- Get into the dark or soft lighting (only enough light for safe movement) 1 hour before bedtime. Stretching in the dim light is an excellent way to begin the wind-down process to prepare for sleep.
- Develop a bedtime ritual that you follow consistently. The ritual should begin 30 minutes before going to bed. Make sure to stay in dim lighting. This ritual should last 15 minutes. It can include hygiene practices such as washing your face and brushing your teeth, but it should not consist of full body application of water, because both hot and cold application can stimulate the body. (A warm bath 1 hour before sleep is relaxing.) Meditating or reading something that is gentle and can be finished in 5 or 10 minutes may be helpful. Listening to soft, gentle music is soothing. Various aromas are considered relaxing and are available in such forms as scented candles, incense, and essential oil diffusers. Drinking a cup of relaxing herbal tea is soothing. Meditation, prayer, and/or rituals are appropriate. The ritual needs to be reinforced and should be done every night. Eventually the ritual will signal the body to move into a sleep pattern.
- When drowsiness occurs, immediately relax into sleep. The drowsy pattern lasts only about 15 minutes, and then a new body rhythm cycle begins, which lasts about 90 minutes.
- If you miss the sleep window, continue with calm activities until the sense of drowsiness occurs again. Then go to bed.
- Sleep in the dark. Especially do not sleep with the television on.
- Get up at the same time in the morning regardless of when you went to bed.
- Avoid taking long naps. A short nap (i.e., 15 to 30 minutes) usually is alright for midday fatigue.

JUST BETWEEN YOU AND ME

Restorative sleep is a great healer. Nutritious food, clean air, and effective breathing, along with physical fitness and restorative sleep, are all part of the regimen of a healthy body. Seems simple, doesn't it? But often it isn't. What are the things that interfere with this regimen? Too many demands, lack of resources and support, and misunderstanding the importance of these necessary wellness components. I certainly have not consistently resolved these issues for myself, let alone anyone else. I do believe this, though: a massage helps.

THE MIND/BODY RELATIONSHIP

The mind is the part of us that reasons, understands, remembers, thinks, and adapts. It coordinates the conscious and subconscious parts of us that influence and direct mental and physical behavior. The mind processes what we believe. We can change our mind (beliefs) fairly quickly, although habitual belief patterns are difficult to overcome. Belief changes need to be supported over time to be reflected in lifestyle and wellness programs. The body responds to mind changes, but more time may be required for the effects of that response to manifest in the body's anatomy and physiology. Patience is required to identify body changes that have occurred in response to mind changes. This interaction between mind and body is the basis for current approaches to mind/body medicine. The mind involves emotions, behavior, self-concept, and coping.

Emotions

Emotions are feelings driven by thoughts. They lead to actions that represent the consequences of how we think and what we do. What we think and feel and how we live are all inextricably linked. As human beings, we learn to be helpless and addictive and to have low self-esteem. We learn to hate. The important point to remember is that if we learned the maladaptive behavior in the first place, we can also learn a more resourceful behavior to use instead.

Emotions can be very powerful. If used resourcefully, they can provide each of us with the empowerment to reach our goals. Many good things have come from an emotion turned into resourceful behavior.

Wellness behavior encompasses a full range of emotions. Some people pride themselves on not feeling certain emotions; however, if we can experience an emotion in a resourceful way, it is not healthy to deny its expression. For example, turning something as powerful as anger inward does not lead to positive outcomes. However, if the anger is expressed resourcefully, to the person or others involved, a sense of resolution develops, and we can get on with our lives, free of the anger.

Wellness comes from using the emotion instead of allowing the emotion to use us. Used resourcefully, emotions can provide the motivation to achieve wellness; used otherwise, they can make us ill and become destructive to those who share our lives.

Feelings are the body's interpretation of emotions. They occur as a response to the effect of hormones, neurotransmitters, and other endogenous chemicals. People use chemical substances such as food, nicotine, alcohol, and drugs to create feelings. Behaviors, such as the need to create crises, eating disorders, accident proneness, hypervigilance, panic, illness, and codependent relationships, all generate feelings. By choosing instead behaviors such as gentle caregiving, giving simple presents, and appreciating beauty, we can generate feelings of compassion, nurturing, and belonging.

Often, if a person's physiology can be changed, the individual's feelings also can be changed. The easiest way to change the physiology is to move, as in exercising or breathing. A massage also changes the physiology, which perhaps is why it feels so good. Being touched in a resourceful way supports wellness. Sensory stimulation is essential for the body to thrive. Many people are deprived of touch, and many adults exchange touch only in the context of a sexual relationship. Touch is essential for wellness. Touching generates and expresses feelings. Compassionate, nurturing, nonjudgmental touch supports wellness and healing.

When feelings are unresourceful, an opposing response must be activated to restore a balance. For example, if a person feels weighed down with too much thinking, simply moving around and pulling some weeds in the garden may create a balance. If we feel angry, finding a way to laugh is balancing. If we feel sad, helping someone else feel better restores balance. If we feel anxious and alone, receiving a hug or a massage is helpful.

JUST BETWEEN YOU AND ME

As I sit outside writing this section of the book, a monarch butterfly is fluttering around in my flower garden. What a beautiful creature it is, and what a healing moment I have experienced by taking the time to be mindful of this. Healing environments should be beautiful. Research has shown that patients who have hospital rooms with windows do better.

Behavior

Behavior is what we do in response to feelings, to trigger thoughts and feelings, and occasionally to avoid feelings. Resourceful behavior results in our feeling good about what has happened. Unresourceful behavior still results in at least a temporary good feeling (or we would not do it), but often, we later feel bad about what happened and/or others feel bad.

Addictive behavior can take many forms. A person who is addicted to food, drugs, alcohol, exercise, pain, crisis, or loss develops a lifestyle that both protects and supports the substance or behavior of choice. Addictions require a great deal of time and energy and often stress the body to the point that healthcare intervention is required. Hard work and lots of support are needed to change an addictive behavior. Sometimes a less damaging addiction can replace a more damaging one, and vice-versa. A person may resolve a food habit by creating an exercise dependency. Behavior changes that are at least steps in the resourceful direction should be encouraged. Behavior modification programs are found in various healthcare settings, and massage as a stress management intervention is appropriate. This is partly because massage generates changes in endogenous blood chemicals (hormones) and brain chemicals (neurotransmitters) that can help stabilize behavior by reducing addictive urges.

Self-Concept

Another threat to wellness is misjudging our self-worth. It is important to have a good **self-concept.** Everyone is good at something; no one is good at everything. If people measured success and self-worth by their accomplishments rather than by the amount of money or the degree of fame they have, society would be healthier. Especially with massage, an inner sense of accomplishment is important. Massage is a quiet, unpretentious profession. It does not usually receive a lot of public glory. Nevertheless, massage is an important service, and some of its benefits cannot be objectively measured. As with any type of prevention activity, it is difficult to know what did not happen because someone took preventive measures.

When we have developed a healthy relationship with ourselves, we can develop and sustain healthy relationships with others. Supportive relationships are important to wellness. A relationship is supportive when we are empowered in a relationship and free to give and receive with a balance of energy exchanged. Sometimes one gives more and other times one receives more, but the total long-term outcome is mutual support for one another's highest good, and that supports wellness.

Coping

Resourceful **coping** consists of commitment, control, and challenge. Commitment is the ability and willingness to be involved in what is happening around us, to have a purpose for being. This purpose is more than what we do; it is how we serve. It is possible to serve in many ways. A career in massage can be a path of service or just a job. Purpose and service have nothing to do with the task. Picking up garbage is as much a service as is being a doctor. Cleaning house, cutting hair, building houses, and packing cartons can all be paths of service, contributing to the greater good.

Control is characterized by the belief that we can influence events by the way we feel, think, and act. This is **internal control,** which involves adjusting ourselves to the situation and looking for ways to respond resourcefully. Those who instead try to exert **external control** attempt to direct circumstances and people. It is impossible to control the weather, most circumstances, and most people. Relying on external control is a poor coping mechanism. The eternal wisdom expressed in the saying, "Grant me the serenity to accept the things I cannot change, the courage to change the things I can, and the wisdom to know the difference," speaks to self-concept and internal versus external control.

Living each day as a challenge filled with things to learn, skills to practice, tasks to accomplish, and obstacles to overcome supports wellness. Those who see change as a challenge cope much better than those who do not. Using available resourceful coping mechanisms to adjust to changes in life allows the individual to welcome change as a process that leads to personal development.

Poor stress-coping skills (e.g., attempts at external control) and unproductive emotions (e.g., unresolved anger) suppress the immune system and predispose us to infection and poor health. The individual's response to a stressor, not the stressor itself, determines the effect on immunity. Wellness includes learning more efficient ways to cope with life (through counseling and behavior modification programs if needed).

To improve your coping skills, pay attention to people who cope well and ask them to share how they cope. Attend seminars and read books on effective coping, assertiveness, and the development of internal control. Professional counseling and support groups also can be helpful.

Spiritual Health and Healing

Our spirit is the part of us that transcends. Spirituality is empowering and personal. It is not religion; spirituality is larger than the limits of a religious practice. Religious practice is a way to nurture spirituality. Our spiritual selves "know our truth." Spiritual wellness consists of faith, hope, and love.

Faith is the ability to believe, trust, and know certain things that science cannot prove. Faith is the strength of wellness and involves the expression of that connecting strength each day through faith in ourselves, our partners, our families, and humanity as a whole. Faith is essential to wellness

Hope is the belief, assurance, conviction, and confidence that our future will somehow be okay. It is the belief that the choices we make now will be the most resourceful choices as we create our future. Without hope, we have no sense of continuity.

Love has no concrete explanation. It is a prerequisite for wholeness, and wholeness is necessary for wellness. This is not romantic love; it is bigger, stronger, more empowering, and mightier. It is quiet, gentle, tolerant, compassionate, empathic, forgiving, and nonjudgmental. This type of love celebrates the irrepressible process of life. This is the love of wellness.

evolve 4-3

The following terms and expressions specific to Chapter 4 have already been used to search PubMed for the latest research literature available. The *Click Here for Massage* feature associated with this chapter on your textbook's Evolve website allows you to hyperlink to a continually updated PubMed search of research literature that corresponds to this subject.

Hyperlink Search Terms
Massage and stress
Massage mental health
Massage mind body
Massage preventive medicine
Massage wellness lifestyle

SUMMARY

Wellness is more than the components discussed in this chapter. Wellness is living life in a simple, gentle, respectful way for ourselves and with others. Wellness is the result of the healing that takes place on multiple levels when we take care of ourselves, and that sense of wellness then extends to caring for others and the planet in general. A competent massage therapist practices self-care, as well as educating patients about the basic components of wellness. Wellness is peace within and sharing that peace in simple ways. Sharing this peace consistently with respect and compassion can support the wellness of all.

WORKBOOK

1. Consider a situation in which you personally felt excessively stressed. What physiologic changes did you experience (e.g., pounding heart, fatigue, anxiety, upset stomach, headache; see Box 4-1 for more examples)?

2. Identify a time when you became ill after a stressful period. Develop a time line that starts before the stress event and ends when you recovered from the illness. List major events that led to the illness and contributed to your recovery. For example:

Decided to go back to school
Made a change in job schedule
Had to move in with parents
Car broke down
Got a cold
Rested for 3 days
Went back to work
Had a relapse
Took over-the-counter medication to relieve symptoms
Got an upset stomach
Went to the doctor
Rested for a week
Wrote in a journal about what is important
Set reasonable goals

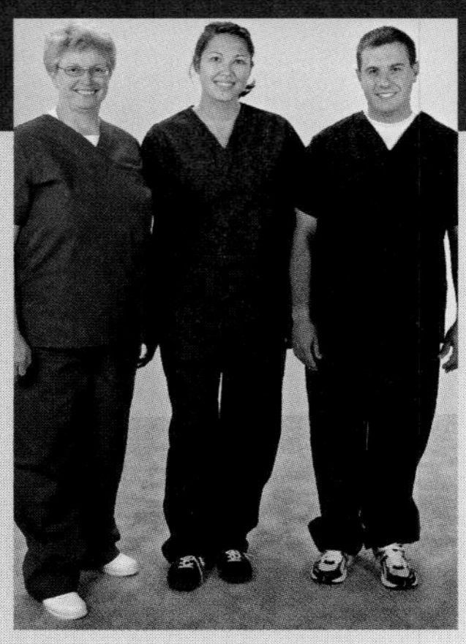

UNIT ONE REFERENCES

Abrams SM: Attention-deficit/hyperactivity disordered children and adolescents benefit from massage therapy, doctoral dissertation, Miami, 1999, University of Miami.

Acolet D, Modi M, Giannakoulopoulos X et al: Changes in plasma cortisol and catecholamine concentration in response to massage in preterm infants, *Arch Dis Child* 68:29-31, 1993.

Ahles TA, Tope DM, Pinkson B et al: Massage therapy for patients undergoing autologous bone marrow transplantation, *J Pain Symptom Manage* 18:157-163, 1999.

Akmedzhanov MY, Leshchinskaya NP, Arkhangelsky VV et al: Pericardiac massage and its adaptive effect in rehabilitation therapy with dosed physical exercises in patients who had myocardial infarction [translation], *Vopr Kurortol Fizioter Lech Fiz Kult* 4:21-23, 1981.

Aksenova AM: New method of deep reflex–muscular massage [translation], *Vopr Kurortol Fizioter Lech Fiz Kult* 6:24-26, 1997.

American Massage Therapy Association [1999a]: AMTA definition of massage therapy [1999a]. Accessed April 6, 2003, at www.amtamassage.org/about/definition.html

American Massage Therapy Association [1999b]: Enhancing your health with therapeutic massage. Accessed April 6, 2003, at www.amtamassage.org/publications/enhancing-health.htm

American Psychological Association: *Publication manual of the American Psychological Association,* ed 5, Washington, DC, 2001, The Association.

Anderson S, Lundeberg T: Acupuncture: from empiricism to science—functional background to acupuncture effects in pain and disease, *Med Hypotheses* 45:271-281, 1995.

Andrade CK, Clifford P: *Outcome-based massage,* Baltimore, 2001, Lippincott Williams & Wilkins.

Antoniev AA, Belaya LV: Physical therapy, massage and self-massage in dermatological practice [translation], *Vopr Kurortol Fizioter Lech Fiz Kult* 1:34-37, 1985.

Aorell M, Skoog M, Carleson J: Effects of Swedish massage on blood pressure, *Complement Ther Clin Pract* 11:242-246, 2005.

Arkko PJ, Pakarinen AJ, Kari-Koshinen O: Effect of whole body massage on serum protein, electrolyte and hormone concentrations, enzyme activities and hematological parameters, *Int J Sports Med* 4:265-267, 1983.

Asdonik J: Physical lymph drainage and therapy of edema in chronic venous insufficiency [translation], *Z Lymphol* 5:107-111, 1981.

Ask N, Oxelbeck T, Lundeberg T et al: The influence of massage on quadriceps function after exhaustive exercise, *Med Sci Sports Exerc* 19: 53, 1987.

Askenova AM, Romanova MM: Influence of reflex-muscular massage on metabolism of patients with complicated gastric ulcers [translation], *Vopr Kurortol Fizioter Lech Fiz Kult* 6:24-26, 1998.

Askew LJ, Beckett VL, Kai Nan An, Chao EYS: Objective evaluation of hand function in scleroderma patients to assess effectiveness of physical therapy, *Br J Rheumatol* 22:224-232, 1983.

Astin JA, Shapiro SL, Eisenberg DM et al: Mind-body medicine: state of the science, implications for practice, *J Am Board Fam Pract* 16:131-147, 2003.

Avery M, Van Arsdale L: Perineal massage: effect on the incidence of episiotomy and perineal laceration in nulliparous population, *J Nurse Midwifery* 32:181-184, 1987.

Ballweg R, Stolberg S, Sullivan E: *Physician assistant: a guide to clinical practice,* ed 3, Philadelphia, 2003, WB Saunders.

Beck MF. *Theory and practice of therapeutic massage,* ed 4, New York, 2006, Thomson Delmar Learning.

Braverman DL: Schulman rheumatoid arthritis: Massage techniques in rehabilitation medicine, *Phys Med Rehabil Clin N Am* 10:631-649, 1999.

Cannon WB: *The wisdom of the body,* New York, 1932, Norton.

Chaitow L: *The acupuncture treatment of pain,* Rochester, Vt, 1976, Healing Art Press.

Chaitow L: *The acupuncture treatment of pain,* ed 2, Rochester, Vt, 1983, Healing Art Press.

Chaitow L: *The acupuncture treatment of pain,* ed 3, Rochester, Vt, 1990, Healing Art Press.

Chaitow L: *The body/mind purification program,* New York, 1991, Fireside.

Chaitow L, Delany J: *Clinical application of neuromuscular techniques: the upper body,* vol 1, London, 2000, Churchill Livingstone.

Chaitow L, Delany J: *Clinical application of neuromuscular techniques: the lower body,* vol 2, London, 2002, Churchill Livingstone.

Chang MY, Wang SY, Chen CH: Effects of massage on pain and anxiety during labour: a randomized controlled trial in Taiwan, *J Adv Nurs* 38:68-73, 1996.

Cherkin DC, Deyo RA, Sherman KJ et al: Characteristics of licensed acupuncturists, chiropractors, massage therapists, and naturopathic physicians, *J Am Board Fam Pract* 15:378-390, 2002.

Cherkin DC, Eisenberg D, Sherman KJ et al: Randomized trial comparing traditional Chinese medical acupuncture, therapeutic massage, and self-care education for chronic low back pain, *Arch Intern Med* 161:1081-1088, 2001.

Cherry B, Jacob S: *Contemporary nursing: issues, trends, and management,* ed 2, St Louis, 2002, Mosby.

CO: Federation of Chiropractic Licensing Boards; Retrieved Jan 2007 5401 W. 10st Greely CO USA fclb.org.

Crewswell JW: *Qualitative inquiry and research design: choosing among five traditions,* Thousand Oaks, Calif, 1998, Sage.

Davidson RJ, Kabat-Zinn J, Schumacher J et al: Alterations in brain and immune function produced by mindfulness meditation, *Psychosomatic Medicine* 65:564-570, 2003.

Dumholdt E: *Physical therapy research: principles and applications,* ed 2, Philadelphia, 2000, WB Sanders.

Eisenberg DM: Advising patients who seek alternative medical therapies, *Ann Intern Med* 127:61-69, 1997.

Eisenberg DM, Cohen MH, Hrbek A et al: Cooper rheumatoid arthritis: credentialing complementary and alternative medical providers, *Ann Intern Med* 137:965-973, 2002.

Ernst E: Evidence-based massage therapy: a contradiction in terms? In Rich GJ, editor: *Massage therapy: the evidence for practice,* New York, 2002, Elsevier.

Field T: Massage therapy effects, *Am Psychol* 53:1270-1281, 1998.

Field T: *Touch therapy,* New York, 2000, Churchill Livingstone.

Field T, Hernandez-Reif M, Taylor S et al: Labor pain is reduced by massage therapy, *J Psychosom Obstet Gynaecol* 18:286-291, 1997.

Finfgeld DL: Metasynthesis: the state of the art—so far, *Qual Health Res* 13:893-904, 2003.

Fukuda K, Straus SE, Hickie I et al: The chronic fatigue syndrome: a comprehensive approach to its definition and study, International Chronic Fatigue Syndrome Study Group, *Ann Intern Med* 121:953-959, 1994.

Goats C: Massage: the scientific basis of an ancient art. Part 1. The techniques, *Br J Sports Med* 28:149-156, 1994.

Gehlbach SH: *Interpreting the medical literature,* ed 4, New York, 2002, McGraw-Hill.

Given B, Given CW, McCorkle R et al: Pain and fatigue management: results of a nursing randomized clinical trial, *Oncol Nurs Forum* 29:949-956, 2002.

Gulick DT, Kimura I: Delayed onset muscle soreness: what is it and how do we treat it? *J Sport Rehabil* 5:234-243, 1996.

Hagino C: *How to appraise research: a guide for chiropractic students and practitioners,* New York, 2003, Churchill Livingstone.

Hamm M: Impact of massage therapy in the treatment of linked pathologies: scoliosis, costovertebral dysfunction, and thoracic outlet syndrome, *J Bodywork Move Ther* 10:12-20, 2006.

Hasson D, Arnetz B, Jelveus L, Edelstam B: A randomized clinical trial of the treatment effects of massage compared to relaxation tape recordings on diffuse long-term pain, *Psychother Psychosom* 73:17-24, 2004.

Hulley SB, Cummings SR, Browner WS et al: *Designing clinical research: an epidemiologic approach,* ed 2, Philadelphia, 2001, Lippincott Williams & Wilkins.

Hymel GM: *Research methods for massage and holistic therapies,* St Louis, 2006, Mosby.

International Committee of Medical Journal Editors: *Uniform requirements for manuscripts submitted to biomedical journals: writing and editing for biomedical publication,* Philadelphia, 2003, American College of Physicians.

Irnich D, Behrens N, Molzen H et al: Randomised trial of acupuncture compared with conventional massage and "sham" laser acupuncture for treatment of chronic neck pain, *Br Med J* 322:1574-1578, 2001.

Joint Commission on Accreditation of Healthcare Organizations (JCAHO): *Dictionary of health care terms, organizations, and acronyms,* Oakbrook Terrace, Ill, 1998, JCAHO.

Jonas WB, Crawford CC: *Healing intention and energy medicine,* Philadelphia, 2003, Churchill Livingstone.

Kisner C, Colby LA: *Therapeutic exercise: foundations and techniques,* ed 5, Philadelphia, 2007, FA Davis.

Lederman E: *Fundamentals of manual therapy: physiology, neurology and psychology,* New York, 1997, Churchill Livingstone.

Lee AC, Kemper KJ: Practice patterns of massage therapists, *J Altern Complement Med* 6:527-529, 2000.

Levine AS, Levine VJ: *The bodywork and massage sourcebook,* Los Angeles, 1999, Lowell House.

Lippert L: *Clinical kinesiology for physical therapist assistants,* Portland, Ore, 1991, The Author.

Lippincott Manual of Nursing Practic *practice nurses.* Philadelphia, PA: Lippincott Williams & Wilkins. 2005.

Maitland GD: *Peripheral manipulation,* ed 3, Boston, 1991, Butterworth.

Marks DF, Sykes CM: Synthesizing evidence: systematic reviews, meta-analysis and preference analysis. In Marks DF, Yardley L, editors: *Research methods for clinical and health psychology* Thousand Oaks, Calif, 2004, Sage.

McEwen I, editor: *Writing case reports: a how-to manual for clinicians,* ed 2, Alexandria, Va, 2001, American Physical Therapy Association.

Moyer CA, Rounds J, Hannum JW: A meta-analysis of massage therapy research, *Psychol Bull* 130:3-18, 2004.

Mulrow C, Cook D, editors: *Systematic reviews: synthesis of best evidence for health care decisions,* Philadelphia, 1998, American College of Physicians.

National Center for Complementary and Alternative Medicine: Manipulative and body-based practices: an overview, Publication No D238, October, 2004. Accessed August, 2005, at http://nccam.nih.gov

Nixon P, Andrews J: A study of anaerobic threshold in chronic fatigue syndrome (CFS), *Biol Psychol* 43:264, 1996.

Official Directory: Chiropractic Licensure and Practice Statistics. Greeley, see Chiropractic Federation.

Patterson BL, Thorne SE, Canam C, Jillings C: *Meta-study of qualitative health research: a practical guide to meta-analysis and meta-synthesis,* Thousand Oaks, Calif, 2001, Sage.

Peat JK, Mellis C, Williams K, Xuan W: *Health science research: a handbook of quantitative method,* Thousand Oaks, Calif, 2002, Sage.

Petty NJ, Moore AP: *Neuromusculoskeletal examination and assessment: a handbook for therapists,* ed 3, London, 2006, Elsevier Science.

Portney LG, Watkins MP: *Foundations of clinical research: applications to practice,* ed 2, Upper Saddle River, NJ, 2000, Prentice-Hall Health.

Preyde M: Effectiveness of massage therapy for subacute low-back pain: a randomized controlled trial, *Can Med Assoc J* 162:1815-1820, 2000.

Price S, Price L: *Aromatherapy for health professionals,* London, 1999, Churchill Livingstone.

Rattray F, Ludwig L: *Clinical massage therapy: understanding, assessing and treating over 70 conditions,* Elora ontorio canada, 2000, Talus. Elova Ontario Canada.

Redwood D, Cleveland CS III: *Fundamentals of chiropractic,* St Louis, 2003, Mosby.

Rich GJ, editor: *Massage therapy: the evidence for practice,* St Louis, 2002, Elsevier.

Robbins DA: Weaving wellness into mainstream medicine, *Managed Healthcare* Aug:38-39, 2000.

Sacks O: a neurologist notebodk An anthropologist on Mars, *The New Yorker* 27-Dec: 106-125, 1993.

Saidoff DC, McDonough AL: *Critical pathways in therapeutic intervention: extremities and spine,* St Louis, 2002, Mosby.

Sandelowski M, Barroso J: Creating metasummaries of qualitative findings, *Nurs Res* 52:226-233, 2003.

Selye H: *The stress of life,* ed 2, New York, 1978, McGraw-Hill.

Simons D: Understanding effective treatments of myofascial trigger points, *J Bodywork Move Ther* 6:177-182, 2002.

Simons D, Travell J, Simons L: *Myofascial pain and dysfunction*: upper body, ed 2, Baltimore, 1999, Williams & Wilkins.

Spector M: Connective tissue cells with muscle: expression of muscle action in and contraction of fibroblasts, chondrocytes, and osteoblasts. Accessed August 2, 2004, at http://healthcare.partners.org

Stommel M, Wills CE: (2004). *Clinical research: concepts and principles for advanced practice nurses,* Philadelphia, 2004, Williams & Wilkins.

Sunshine W, Field T, Quintino O et al: Fibromyalgia benefits from massage therapy and transcutaneous electrical stimulation, *J Clin Rheumatol* 2:18-22, Sunshine W, Field T, Quintino et al. 1996.

Turchaninov R: *Therapeutic massage: a scientific approach,* Phoenix, Ariz, 2000, Aesculapius Books.

Turchaninov R, Cox CA: *Medical massage,* vol 1, Phoenix, Ariz, 1998, Aesculapius Books.

van den Dolder PA, Roberts DL: A trial of the effectiveness of soft tissue massage in the treatment of shoulder pain, *Aust J Physiother* 49:183-188, 2003.

Wolsko PM, Eisenberg DM, Davis RB et al: Use of mind-body medical therapies, *J Gen Intern Med* 19:43-50, 2004.

Yates J: *A physician's guide to therapeutic massage,* ed 3, Toronto, 2004, Curties-Overzet.

Additional Resources

Acupuncture and Oriental Medicine Alliance

States with statutes, regulations, and bills in progress

www.acuall.org/current.htm

Agency for Healthcare Research and Quality (AHRQ)

The AHRQ is an agency of the Public Health Service, part of the U.S. Department of Health and Human Services (DHHS). It is the lead agency charged with supporting research designed to improve the quality of health care, reduce its cost, and broaden access to essential services. One of the AHRQ's highest priorities is providing consumers with science-based, easily understandable information that will help them make informed decisions about their health care, including the selection of the highest quality health plans and the most appropriate healthcare services.
www.ahrq.gov

AHRQ Publications Clearinghouse
P.O. Box 8547
Silver Spring, MD 20907
Telephone toll-free in the US: 1-800-358-9295
Telephone outside the US: 410-381-3150
TDD toll-free telephone: 1-888-586-6340
AHRQ InstantFAX: Call 301-594-2800 for instructions.

American Massage Therapy Association: Massage Practice Laws Information Guide
www.amsa.org/humed/CAM/
www.amtamassage.org/pdf/2005_StateLaws.pdf

Bureau of Labor Statistics
www.bls.gov

Evanston Northwestern Healthcare, Hospitals and Health
www.enh.org

Life and Health Insurance Foundation for Education
hsl.mcmaster.ca/tomflem/ill.html
hsl.mcmaster.ca/tomflem/top.html

National Center for Complementary and Alternative Medicine (NCCAM)
http://nccam.nih.gov

NCCAM Clearinghouse
Toll-free: 1-888-644-6226
TTY/TDY: 1-888-644-6226
e-mail: nccamc@altmedinfo.org

The Virtual Hospital
www.vh.radiology.uiowa.edu

The World Health Organization (WHO)
www.who.com

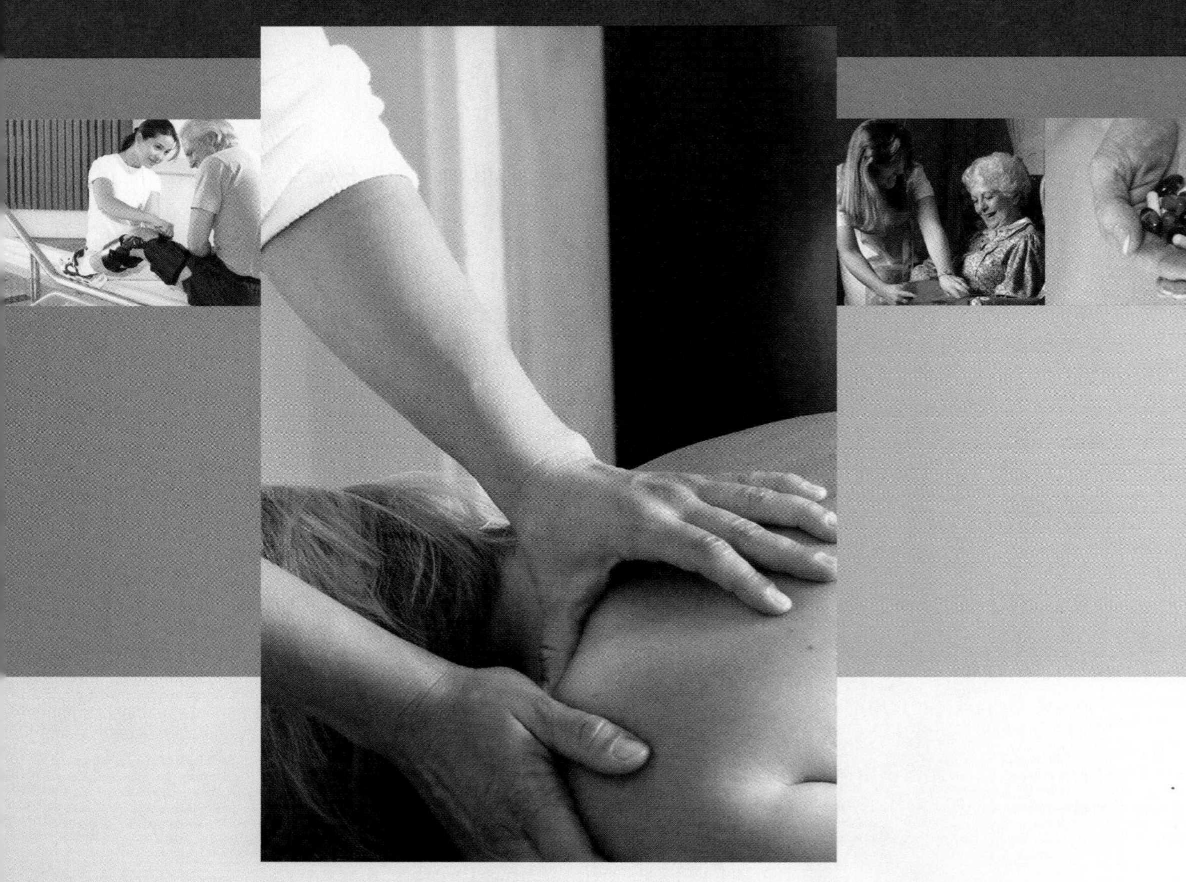

5 *Indications and Contraindications to Massage, 116*

6 *Review of Pertinent Anatomy and Physiology, 140*

7 *Sanitation, 196*

8 *Review and Application of Massage, 208*

9 *Massage Application Assessment for Physical Healing and Rehabilitation, 248*

10 *Focused Massage Application, 314*

11 *General Massage Protocol and Palliative Variation, 380*

12 *Unique Circumstances and Adjunct Therapies, 432*

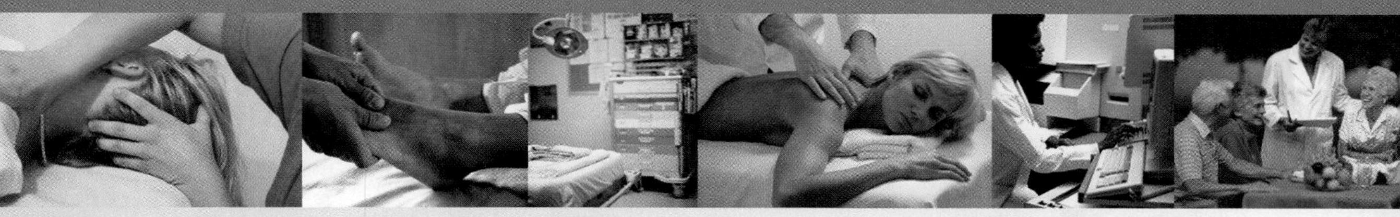

Unit Two

MASSAGE APPLICATION FOR HEALTHCARE BENEFIT

This unit targets the application of massage in the healthcare environment. Just as Unit One targeted healthcare in general, this unit focuses almost entirely on massage as it relates to people receiving services in various healthcare settings. It is necessary to identify indications for and contraindications to massage, to understand the physiologic mechanisms of massage in order to determine massage interactions with other treatments (e.g., medication or physical therapy), and to make good decisions about changes in massage application that may be necessary to benefit the patient and to do no harm. Sanitation is extremely important to prevent the spread of pathogens and to protect both the patient and the massage therapist. Medical patients often are immunocompromised, and the massage therapist may be in contact with individuals who have a contagious disease.

The actual massage methods are reviewed and expanded, and various protocols are offered as starting points for massage application. Protocols always need to be individualized according to the needs of the patient. Adjunct methods that combine effectively with massage, such as aromatherapy and hydrotherapy, are discussed. Finally, special considerations are explored, such as patients who are sleeping, bedridden, or using medical devices such as drainage tubes and catheters. The DVD demonstration brings the methods alive, and the Evolve site is used to expand the content in this unit.

The primary outcomes of massage for people receiving healthcare are increased body stamina, stability, mobility, flexibility, agility, reduced soft tissue tension and binding, normalized fluid movement (blood and lymph), management of pain, reduction of suffering, support of healing mechanisms, alteration of mood, increase in physical and mental performance, and experience of pleasure. Although almost all massage experts agree that massage has both indications and contraindications, obtaining a consensus on such information is difficult, because the experts do not all agree on the specifics. Clinical reasoning, development of a treatment plan, and justification of the approaches used are necessary.

Chapter 5 Concept Map

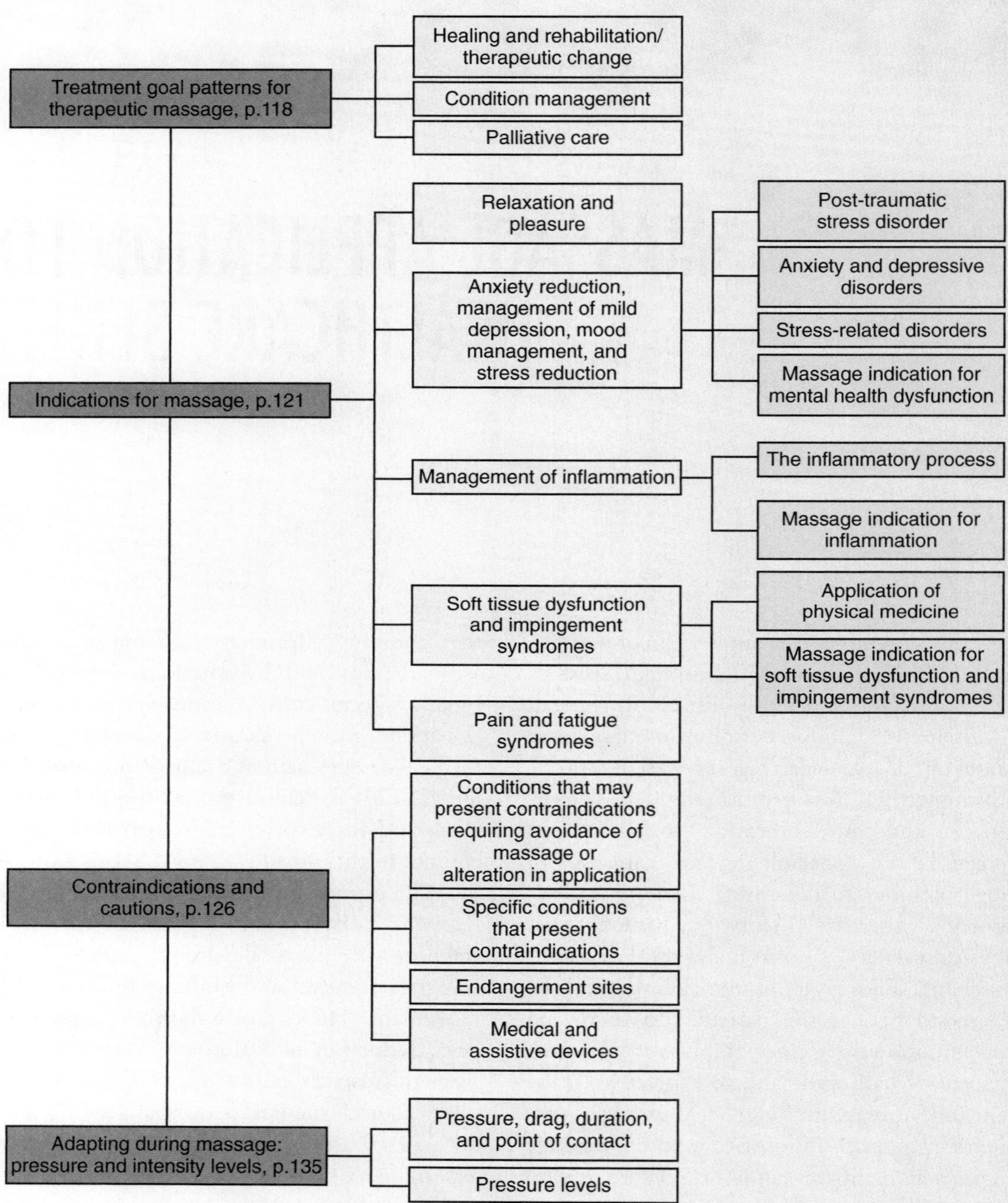

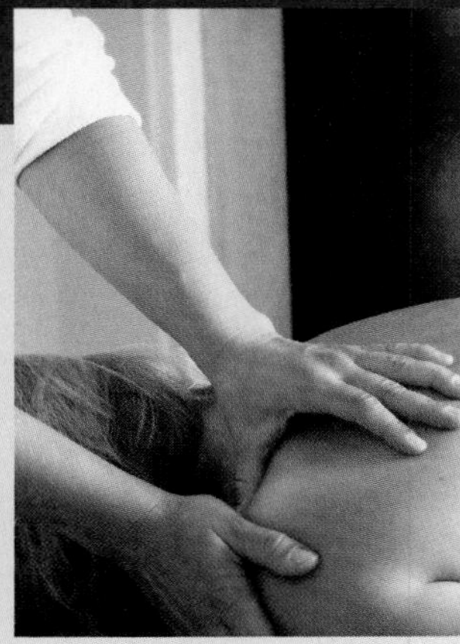

CHAPTER 5

INDICATIONS AND CONTRAINDICATIONS TO MASSAGE

Key Terms

Anxiety
Chemotaxis
Depression
Lymphadenopathy
Phagocytosis
Post-traumatic stress disorder
Trauma

For definitions of key terms, refer to the Evolve website.

OBJECTIVES

Upon completion of this chapter, the reader will have the information necessary to:

1 List the indications for massage in the context of healthcare.
2 Describe illness and injury and how they predispose a person to contraindications and cautions for massage.
3 Evaluate various medications for possible effects on massage application.
4 Identify and avoid endangerment sites and medical devices.

Normal physiologic mechanisms protect us by inhibiting the tendency to function at the body's anatomic and physiologic limits. We usually do not run as fast as we can, work as long as we can, or exert all of our energy to complete a task. Instead, the body signals fatigue, pain, or strain before the anatomic or physiologic limits are reached, and activity is reduced. This very important protective mechanism allows us to live within a healthy range of energy expenditure while maintaining functioning energy reserves in case of emergency or extraordinary demand. This aspect of homeostatic balance is often strained when people are ill or injured. Illness can be described as the breakdown of the protective mechanisms of homeostasis. Injury places demands on the body to heal. Massage can support the restorative process to help people maximize healing processes.

The benefits of massage are most effectively focused on assisting people to stay within the healthy range of physical functioning and supporting those who want to achieve fitness. It's best for people to be proactive in managing stress and keeping the body healthy. Massage can be a very beneficial part of the health maintenance process, and it also is indicated for preventive healthcare.

People receiving some sort of medical care typically are already ill or injured. *Illness* occurs when a normal body process breaks down. A person whose immune system did not effectively fight off a cold virus becomes ill with a cold. A person with diabetes is ill. Chronic fatigue syndrome, ulcers, cancer, and multiple sclerosis are all examples of illness. *Injury* occurs when tissue is damaged. Cuts, bruises, burns, contusions, fractured bones, sprains, and strains are examples of injuries. Inflammation is a factor in both illness and injury, because healing for both involves appropriate activation of the inflammatory response system. Paradoxically, unproductive and inappropriate inflammation can be the cause of illness and can predispose a person to injury.

The healing of illness and injury taxes the body and strains restorative mechanisms. If an injured person is not in a state of health to begin with, the stress of the injury commonly compromises the immune system, and the person then becomes susceptible to illness or can experience a worsening of symptoms if chronic illness is present.

Illness tends to produce general cautions and contraindications that require massage to be avoided entirely or altered based on the condition. Injury more often creates regional cautions and contraindications, and massage can proceed as normal, although avoiding the injured areas, as long as adaptive capacity is not strained. For massage treatment planning, surgical areas can be considered injuries. Even though surgery is a treatment for a medical condition, the actual procedures involve incisions, which are wounds (a type of injury). Endoscopy, arthroscopy, and microsurgery, which allow the surgical procedure to be performed through small incisions, have proved a great medical advancement. Because the incisions are so much smaller, the trauma they cause is much less than even 5 or 6 years ago. For example, the ability to work with the heart with these types of procedures has reduced the need for open heart surgery, in which the opening of the chest to get to the heart produces significant trauma.

To understand the indications and contraindications for massage, you must understand how massage affects the body. Massage application clusters into reflex and mechanical methods, with a large degree of overlap effect. Reflex response results from stimulus to the nervous system to activate feedback loops; the therapeutic intent is adjustment of neuromuscular, neurotransmitter, endocrine, or autonomic nervous system homeostatic mechanisms. Mechanical methods impose various forces, such as tension, compression, rotation or torsion, bending, and shearing, as well as the combination of these forces, to change body structure or function.

Therapeutic massage is indicated for both illness and injury. Massage techniques for illness involve a very general application of massage to support the body's healing responses (e.g., stress management, pain control, and restorative sleep). This approach to massage, sometimes called *general constitutional application,* is more reflexive in nature and is used to reduce the stress load so that the body can heal or cope more effectively. Massage for injury incorporates aspects of general constitutional massage, because healing is necessary for tissue repair. In addition, the more mechanical application of lymphatic drainage is used to control edema. Gliding methods are used to approximate (bring close together) the ends of some types of tissue injuries (e.g., minor muscle tears, strains, and sprains), which supports healing. Hyperstimulation analgesia and counterirritation can reduce acute pain perception. Methods to increase circulation to the injured area support tissue healing. Connective tissue applications are used to manage scar tissue formation. With the proper training and supervision, massage therapists can use their skills to aid recovery or maintenance (or both) for most health concerns (Table 5-1).

TREATMENT GOAL PATTERNS FOR THERAPEUTIC MASSAGE

The typical outcomes of massage application are to influence the adaptive, restorative, and healing capacity of the body. All of these outcomes can be appropriately applied to wellness and preventive healthcare or used to support the healing and rehabilitation of a pathologic condition, especially in the context of a multidisciplinary healthcare

TABLE 5-1 Stages of Tissue Healing and Associated Massage Interventions

Stage 1 (3 to 7 Days) Acute Stage (Inflammatory Reaction)	Stage 2 (14 to 21 Days) Subacute Stage (Repair and Healing)	Stage 3 (3 to 12 Months) Chronic Stage (Maturation and Remodeling)
Vascular changes	Growth of capillary beds into area	Maturation and remodeling of scar
Inflammatory exudates	Collagen formation	Contracture of scar tissue
Clot formation	Granulation tissue; caution necessary with massage	Alignment of collagen along lines of stress force (tensegrity)
Phagocytosis, neutralization of irritants	Tissue fragile, easily injured	Absence of inflammation
Early fibroblastic activity	Inflammation diminished	Pain after tissue resistance
Inflammation	Pain during tissue resistance	Return to function
Pain before tissue resistance	Controlled motion	Increased strength and alignment of scar tissue
Protection	Promote development of mobile scar	*Massage intervention:* Cross-fiber friction of scar tissue, coupled with directional stroking along lines of tension away from injury
Control and support effects of inflammation: protection, rest, ice, compression, elevation (PRICE)	*Massage intervention:* Cautious, controlled soft tissue mobilization of scar tissue along fiber direction toward injury	Progressive stretching and active motion; full-range
Promote healing and prevent compensation patterns	*Massage intervention:* Active and passive, open- and closed-chain range of body massage motion, midrange	*Massage intervention:* Support rehabilitation activities with full body massage
Massage intervention: Passive movement, midrange	*Massage intervention:* Support healing with full body massage	
Massage intervention: General massage and lymphatic drainage, with caution		
Massage intervention: Support rest with full body massage		

From Fritz S: *Mosby's fundamentals of therapeutic massage,* ed 3, St Louis, 2004, Mosby.

system. These outcomes can be classified into three main goal patterns:

- Healing and rehabilitation/therapeutic change (fix it)
- Condition management (contain and cope)
- Palliative care (reduce suffering and provide compassionate support)

HEALING AND REHABILITATION/THERAPEUTIC CHANGE

Healing and rehabilitation together result in the return to normal function from a state of illness or injury. Massage for this goal pattern is complex and requires the most training. Also, the benefit of massage in this context is limited. Massage cannot "fix" things, as surgery can, but it can support the healing process.

Unit Three of this text and the accompanying Evolve website present specific information on massage strategies for various illnesses and injuries. The specific massage applications are then integrated into the general massage protocols described here. Massage can support physical rehabilitation by managing postexercise soreness, reducing pain awareness, and supporting sleep. If the condition is primarily of soft tissue origin (which is very rare), massage may be suggested as a primary care modality.

JUST BETWEEN YOU AND ME

I can't think of a health condition that is solely a soft tissue concern; perhaps a repetitive strain injury, but in those cases, inflammation is a factor. Even trigger points involve metabolic and nutritional factors. Maybe scar tissue management would be just soft tissue work, although if I thought about it enough, I bet that could be disputed. The point is, massage has limited use as a primary rehabilitative intervention (i.e., to cure or fix a condition). I wouldn't be surprised if that statement shook up a few belief systems about massage!

CONDITION MANAGEMENT

Unfortunately, many health conditions are chronic. In these cases, the goal for healthcare professionals, including massage therapists, is to manage symptoms, stabilize the condition, stop or slow its progression, and increase functioning (i.e., contain and cope) This approach is used for disorders such as diabetes, depression, migraine headache, arthritis, fibromyalgia, chronic pain syndrome, irritable bowel syndrome, and conditions of aging.

JUST BETWEEN YOU AND ME

Management of chronic conditions is an aspect of healthcare in which massage can be very beneficial. It is important to really study this area of massage application. Working with patients who have chronic conditions can get discouraging, because the results are less apparent. People typically cycle through good and bad phases, and just about the time things seem to be improving, the condition takes a turn for the worse, only to improve a bit again. Slowing the progression of a condition is a success. I tell students that most of my clients have been satisfied with getting worse slower and suffering less. Then, I end up discussing the importance of empathy and a nonjudgmental attitude.

PALLIATIVE CARE

Palliative care massage reduces suffering and provides pleasurable, soothing sensations. These may be the most important outcomes of massage in the healthcare environment. Comfort, support, nurturing, pleasure, and soothing are essential in the care of people, regardless of their condition. Attention to creating a warm and inviting environment, atmosphere, and ambience is part of the caring experience. The massage application is slow, painless, rhythmic, and general, with sufficient pressure to produce relaxation (remember, light touch is arousing). History taking and assessment should reveal any contraindications and cautions, including areas to avoid and changes that should be made in the massage application. Palliative care massage is different from massage provided to achieve therapeutic change or condition management, which requires specific treatment plans. In palliative care massage, palliative care *is* the treatment plan, and it involves methods to ease suffering and produce pleasurable sensations.

Patience, flexibility, and commitment are necessary when palliative care is the goal. Injured, ill, fragile, or elderly patients may be tired, discouraged, and in pain. Periods of exhilaration and disappointment occur within complex life experiences; reducing suffering and offering pleasurable sensations are invaluable for supporting beneficial psychological and physical responses to these stresses.

During healing and rehabilitation, a patient's progress can plateau. The satisfaction of seeing ongoing change is diminished, and palliative care may help support the patient during these times. Patients undergoing medical care can experience diminished progress or setbacks. These individuals can be comforted temporarily by a nurturing touch. Sometimes there is just too much pain and discomfort to endure, regardless of the outcome goals, and palliative massage is the recommended approach when a "vacation" from treatment would be beneficial. A specific protocol for palliative massage and methods are demonstrated in the accompanying DVD, as are suggested protocols. The approaches must be modified according to the patient's circumstances.

JUST BETWEEN YOU AND ME

Massage encompasses aspects of the body, mind, and spirit. Of all the applications of massage, I think that providing palliative care (i.e., reducing suffering and providing pleasure) is truly an expression of the spirit.

Each of the three common outcomes for massage just discussed supports healing, rehabilitation, and recovery, as well as condition management and reduction of suffering. The three generalized outcomes provide the combination of the following massage benefits:

- Local tissue repair, such as a sprain or contusion
- Connective tissue normalization, which affects elasticity, stiffness, strength, pliability, and overall flexibility, as well as the neurologic influence of various mechanoreceptors in the fascia
- Shifts in pressure gradients to influence body fluid movement
- Neuromuscular function interfacing with muscle tension-length relationships; motor tone of muscles; concentric, eccentric, and isometric functions; and contraction-activation patterns of muscles working together to support efficient movement (firing pattern, muscle activation sequences, and force couple relationship)
- Mood and pain modulation through shifts in autonomic nervous system function, resulting in neurochemical and neuroendocrine responses
- Increased immune response to support systemic health and healing

INDICATIONS FOR MASSAGE

Massage offers much as an aspect of healthcare treatment. Massage methods are generally safe and have few side effects when applied properly. Massage supports many other medical treatments, enhancing their effects and reducing their side effects. In general, massage is indicated for a number of purposes.

RELAXATION AND PLEASURE

The relaxation and pleasure aspects of massage are often discounted, and this is a huge mistake. In fact, the purpose of palliative care is to reduce suffering, and massage can accomplish this outcome by creating relaxation and pleasure. With a fragile patient, regardless of the diagnosis or prognosis, massage that targets relaxation and pleasure is perhaps the most important outcome in the medical environment. Massage in general should feel good. Some methods that are targeted to a specific adaptation can be intense but should still "hurt good."

JUST BETWEEN YOU AND ME

A general massage that feels good and nurtures the person is your most important tool in the healthcare system. I get very impatient with students and therapists who discount the importance of these outcomes for the patient. They are the gifts of massage. What other professional can provide them for a person who is hurting?

ANXIETY REDUCTION, MANAGEMENT OF MILD DEPRESSION, MOOD MANAGEMENT, AND STRESS REDUCTION

Science has validated the body/mind link in terms of health and disease. Many risk factors for the development of physical (body) pathology are mentally (mind) influenced, such as a person's stress level and lifestyle choices. The same is true for mental health and pathology. The physical state of an individual has a strong influence on mental functioning. Usually, when people feel well physically, they also feel well mentally; the reverse, too, often is true—feeling bad mentally results in physical dysfunctions. Neurochemicals, such as serotonin and dopamine, exert a strong influence on a person's mental state.

The major mental health dysfunctions affecting Western society are trauma, post-traumatic stress disorder, pain and fatigue syndromes coupled with anxiety and depression, and stress-related illness. **Trauma** is defined as a physical illness or injury caused by violent or disruptive action or by a toxic substance. Psychic illness and injury can result from a severe emotional shock, either short term or long term.

Post-Traumatic Stress Disorder

Post-traumatic stress disorder, as defined by the *Diagnostic and Statistical Manual of Mental Disorders (DSM-IV),* includes flashback memory experiences, state-dependent memory, somatization, anxiety, irritability, sleep disturbance, concentration difficulties, times of melancholy or depression, grief, fear, worry, anger, and avoidance behavior. Post-traumatic stress disorder can have long-term effects.

Anxiety and Depressive Disorders

Anxiety is an uneasy feeling usually connected with increased sympathetic arousal responses. **Depression** is characterized by a decrease in vital functional activity and mood disturbances of exaggerated emptiness, hopelessness, and melancholy, or periods of high energy with no purpose or outcome. Anxiety and depressive disorders are commonly seen in conjunction with fatigue and pain syndromes. Panic behavior, phobias, and a sense of impending doom, along with a sense of hopelessness and of being overwhelmed, are common with these conditions. Mood swings, breathing pattern disorders, sleep disturbances, concentration difficulties, memory disturbances, outbursts of anger, fatigue, and changes in habits of daily living, appetite, and activity levels are symptoms of these disorders.

Stress-Related Disorders

Stress-related disorder is defined as an increased stress load or reduced ability to adapt that depletes the reserve capacity of individuals, increasing their vulnerability to health problems. Stress-related illness can encompass the previously mentioned conditions as the primary cause of dysfunction or as the result of the stress of the dysfunction. Excessive stress sometimes manifests as cardiovascular problems, including hypertension; digestive difficulties, including heartburn, ulcer, and bowel syndromes; respiratory illness and susceptibility to bacterial and viral illness; endocrine dysfunction, particularly adrenal or thyroid dysfunction and delayed or reduced cellular repair; sleep disorders; and breathing pattern disorders, just to mention a few conditions.

Massage Indication for Mental Health Dysfunction

Massage intervention has a strong physiologic effect through the comfort of compassionate touch, as well as a physical influence on mental state through the effect on the autonomic nervous system (ANS) and neurochemicals. Individuals experiencing mental health problems, therefore, may derive benefits from massage. Soothing of any ANS hyperactivity or hypoactivity provides a sense of inner balance. Normalization of the breathing mechanism allows the individual to breathe more efficiently and can reduce the tendency to adopt a disordered breathing pattern. This is important, because breathing abnormalities increase the tendency for anxiety and panic.

Therapeutic massage can provide intervention on a physical level to restore a more normal function to the body, which supports appropriate interventions by qualified mental health professionals. Certainly strong and appropriate indications exist for the use of massage therapy in the restoration of mental health, but caution is indicated in terms of the establishment of dual roles and boundary difficulties. Working in conjunction with mental health providers is very important in these situations.

JUST BETWEEN YOU AND ME

I often warn students about getting involved in the trauma/drama of people's physical, emotional, and spiritual events. I wonder if so many TV programs about medical environments are popular because of our natural attraction to trauma and drama. Remember, too much trauma and drama lead to stress, which is a risk factor for developing an illness or injury. If you become emotionally involved with other people's trauma/drama, it could very well make you sick. You can be empathetic without becoming involved.

Stress management outcomes for massage include supporting homeostasis and restorative mechanisms, such as:

- Enhanced immune function
- Efficient circulation of body fluids
- Effective digestion and elimination
- Enhanced growth, development, and regeneration

These outcomes typically are achieved by reducing stress and enhancing restorative sleep. Many factors can cause sleep interruptions, such as pain that repeatedly wakes a person, external random noise (e.g., traffic noise), interruptions from medical staff, the need to tend to infants and children, varied work schedules, a restless or snoring bed partner or roommate, and sinus or other respiratory difficulties (e.g., coughing and urinary frequency). Other people have disrupted sleep patterns because of insomnia, sleep apnea, hormone fluctuations, high cortisol (stress hormone) levels, medications, and stimulant intake (e.g., caffeine). Traveling across time zones also interferes with sleep.

Light/dark cycles regulate sleep patterns. For effective sleep, we need adequate exposure to daylight, which stimulates serotonin. We also need adequate exposure to darkness. With the advent of artificial lighting, we have come to spend less and less time in the dark, which disturbs sleep. Absence of light supports the release of melatonin, a pineal gland hormone that is involved with the sleep pattern. The bottom line is, we need dark as much as light to sleep well.

During sleep the body renews, repairs, and generally restores itself. Growth hormone is an important factor in this process, and more than half of its daily secretion takes place during sleep. If the deeper stages of sleep are not sustained, the body's restorative mechanisms are compromised. Sleep disturbances are a major factor in many chronic fatigue and pain syndromes; in diminished work and skill-based performance; in a predisposition to illness and injury; and in delayed recovery. Massage is very effective at supporting restorative sleep.

MANAGEMENT OF INFLAMMATION

When trauma or invasion by a pathogen occurs, the body responds in a predictable manner, a process called *inflammation.* To defend itself, the body initiates specific responses to destroy and remove pathogenic organisms and their byproducts or, if this is impossible, to limit the extent of damage caused by pathogenic organisms and byproducts. This process produces the four classic symptoms of inflammation: redness, swelling or edema, pain, and heat. When the body is exposed to an infectious agent or a foreign substance, cellular damage occurs at the site. Inflammatory mediators (e.g., histamine, prostaglandins, and kinins) are released, producing three different responses at the cellular level. All three actions are designed either to increase the number of white blood cells (WBCs) at the injury site or to increase the number of WBCs available to attack infectious agents systematically.

The Inflammatory Process

With a local injury, the inflammatory process proceeds as follows:

1. Blood vessels at the site dilate, causing an increase in local blood flow that results in redness and heat.
2. Blood vessel walls become more permeable. This assists the movement of WBCs to the area so that they can begin forming a fibrous capsule around the injury to protect surrounding cells from the damage caused by the source of infection. Blood plasma also filters out of the more permeable vessel walls, resulting in edema, which puts pressure on the nerves and causes pain.
3. **Chemotaxis** (the release of chemical agents) occurs, attracting WBCs to the site. This results in **phagocytosis,** or the engulfment and destruction of microorganisms and damaged cells. Destroyed pathogens, cells, and WBCs collect in the area and form a thick, white substance called *pus.*

If the inflammatory response is more systemic, as may occur with a viral infection, the result is fever, fatigue, stiffness, and activation of the lymphatic system (Figure 5-1).

If the pathogenic invasion cannot be controlled by the previously described process, the pathogens may collect in the lymph nodes, where more WBCs are present to help fight the battle. This causes swollen lymph nodes, or **lymphadenopathy.** If the body is too weak or the number of pathogens is too great, the infection may spread to the bloodstream. A systemic infection, called *septicemia* (also *pyemia* or *blood poisoning*), may occur, which ultimately could affect the entire body. Without appropriate medical intervention, death can result.

In the acute phase of healing, the inflammatory response is beneficial and should be supported. Massage is most beneficial during the subacute inflammatory response for managing edema and supporting healing. Nonproductive chronic inflammation causes many of the chronic diseases that plague people. Autoimmune diseases, cardiovascular disease, degenerative joint disease, and more can be directly linked to nonproactive

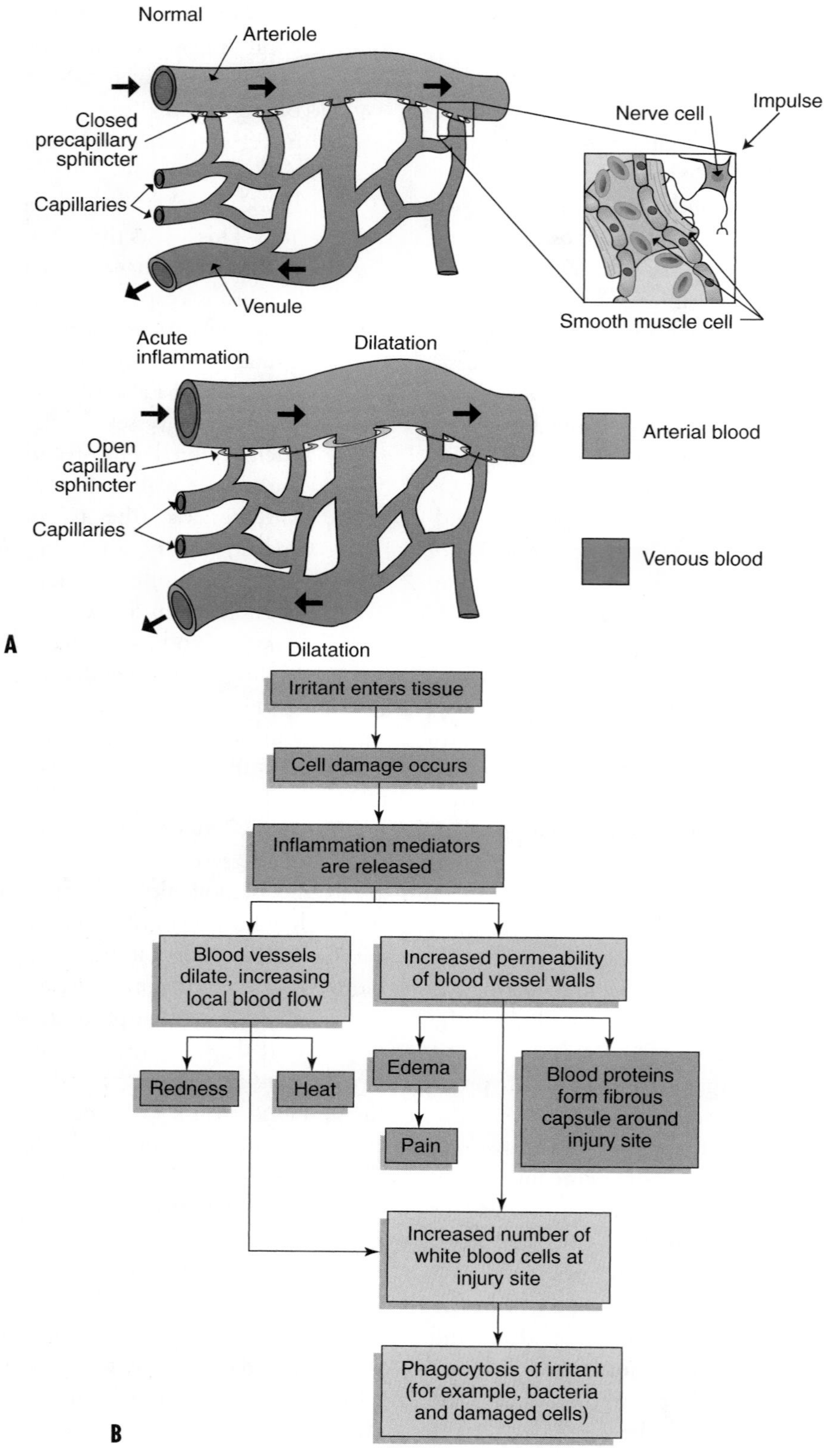

FIGURE 5-1 ■ **A,** Circulatory changes with inflammation. Relaxation of the precapillary sphincter in the arterioles results in flooding of the capillary network and dilation of capillaries and postcapillary venules. **B,** Inflammatory response. (**A** modified from Damjanov I: *Pathology for the health professions,* ed 3, St Louis, 2006, Mosby; **B** modified from Fritz S: *Mosby's essential sciences for therapeutic massage: anatomy, physiology biomechanics, and pathology,* ed 2, St Louis, 2004, Mosby.)

inflammation (this is discussed in detail later in the chapter) (Table 5-2).

Massage Indication for Inflammation

Massage has only a limited influence on chronic inflammation. Sympathetic arousal and the stress response tend to make these conditions worse. Massage seems to have a general normalizing influence on the body. Through its ability to reduce sympathetic arousal, support sleep, and promote effective fluid movement, massage may also support the body's ability to deal with chronic inflammation. The influences are indirect. The general, nonspecific, restorative type of massage (the mechanisms of which we still do not fully understand) is the approach that seems to have the most benefit.

TABLE 5-2 Disorders Related to Chronic Inflammation*

Disorder	Mechanism
Allergy	Inflammatory mediators induce autoimmune reactions.
Alzheimer's disease	Chronic inflammation destroys brain cells.
Anemia	Inflammatory mediators disrupt erythropoietin production.
Aortic valve stenosis	Chronic inflammation damages heart valves.
Arthritis	Inflammatory mediators destroy joint cartilage and synovial fluid.
Asthma	Inflammatory mediators induce swelling that closes the airways.
Cancer	Chronic inflammation causes most cancers.
Congestive heart failure	Chronic inflammation causes heart muscle wasting.
Fibromyalgia	Inflammatory mediators are elevated in fibromyalgia patients.
Fibrosis	Inflammatory mediators attack traumatized tissue.
Heart attack	Chronic inflammation contributes to coronary atherosclerosis.
Kidney failure	Inflammatory mediators cause restriction of circulation and damage nephrons.
Lupus	Inflammatory mediators induce an autoimmune attack.
Pancreatitis	Inflammatory mediators cause pancreatic cell injury.
Psoriasis	Inflammatory mediators induce dermatitis.
Stroke	Chronic inflammation promotes thromboembolic events.
Surgical complications	Inflammatory mediators prevent healing.

*Seemingly unrelated disorders often have a common link: inflammation. This is a partial list of common medical problems associated with chronic inflammation.

From Fritz S: *Mosby's fundamentals of therapeutic massage,* ed 3, St Louis, 2004, Mosby.

SOFT TISSUE DYSFUNCTION AND IMPINGEMENT SYNDROMES

Various types of soft tissue dysfunction can be similarly categorized as disruption of motor tone and disruption of muscle tone. Motor tone is the control of the nervous system over muscle tension-length relationships. Disruption of muscle tone is caused by fluid (hydrostatic pressure) connective tissue tautness and tissue pliability. The two types of nerve impingement syndromes are compression and entrapment. *Compression* is the exertion of pressure on a nerve by a bony structure, and *entrapment* is the exertion of pressure on a nerve by soft tissue. Both can be effectively addressed with massage application.

Application of Physical Medicine

Physical medicine methods (i.e., osteopathy, physical therapy, chiropractic, naturopathy, and massage) are often the treatment of choice for soft tissue dysfunction and impingement syndromes. In these conditions, the specific muscle releases, connective tissue methods, trigger point application, and so on have the most direct effect and may be indicated.

Massage Indication for Soft Tissue Dysfunction and Impingement Syndromes

Massage methods can soften and stretch connective tissues that may be impinging upon nerves. They also can normalize muscle tone and motor tone disturbances, restoring a more normal resting length to shortened muscles, thereby reducing pressure on nerves. Massage is beneficial for entrapment and can manage some symptoms of nerve compression, even though the direct causal factor is not addressed.

PAIN AND FATIGUE SYNDROMES

Pain and fatigue syndromes are defined as multicausal and often chronic nonproductive patterns that interfere with well-being, activities of daily living, and productivity. Some conditions in this category are fibromyalgia, chronic fatigue syndrome, Epstein-Barr viral infection, sympathetic reflex dystrophy (now known as *complex regional pain syndrome*), headache, arthritis, chronic cancer pain, neuropathy, low back syndrome, idiopathic pain, somatization disorder, and intractable pain syndrome. Acute pain can be a factor, as can acute episodes of chronic conditions.

The management of pain is an important element of healthcare. Because therapeutic massage often offers symptomatic relief from chronic pain, the helplessness that accompanies these conditions may dissipate as the person realizes that management methods are available.

JUST BETWEEN YOU AND ME

Pain is a complex issue. Most of us have experienced acute pain from some sort of injury. Pain teaches us to be aware of things that will harm us. It is chronic pain that drives people nuts. One of my best teachers was Dr. David Gurevich, a Russian physician. He had endured war, pain, and other awful things, and as a doctor he especially tried to help those who were suffering. He came into my life as a refugee during the collapse of the Soviet Union. At that point, I was in chronic pain from a compressed disk and a pelvic injury I had suffered giving birth to my last child. I was a miserable wretch when he began to work with me using physical medicine skills. One day I was whining, and I guess he had had enough of it. This dear old doctor, who had experienced real suffering, took my face in his hands, looked me in the eye, and firmly but compassionately said, "Sandy, it is only pain. You will not die. Your life may not be good, but you will not die." I tell this story a lot, because it was a moment of deep realization for me and a truth worth sharing. The experience of the injury, the pain, the understanding of the pain, and living despite the pain have made me more compassionate toward and tolerant of others in pain. Massage helps (but does not cure) those in pain. I lived this reality again in 2006, when I had open heart surgery and a triple bypass for coronary artery disease. The postsurgical pain was intense, to say the least. Dr. Gurevich's words again gave me strength. I could understand that the hurt of the surgery did not harm me but the harm of clogged arteries and heart attack could kill me. Dr. Chaitow and I discussed this about 12 weeks after my surgery, during a conference at which we were making presentations. We became aware of the importance of people experiencing pain to understand the difference between hurt and harm. Yes, the surgical site hurt a lot, but it did not harm me, and the surgical procedure and the skills of the medical staff saved my life. Massage eased my pain.

CONTRAINDICATIONS AND CAUTIONS

A *contraindication* means that some element of the patient's condition makes a type of treatment more harmful than beneficial, therefore the treatment should not be used. A *caution* means that a treatment (e.g., massage application) needs to be adjusted to provide benefit without doing harm. Massage is totally contraindicated in some instances, such as end stage kidney failure. However, most contraindications require a change in the massage application rather than the elimination of massage; this usually is described as massage with caution. The massage therapist must adjust the technique or avoid a particular area to apply methods safely.

Massage may be totally contraindicated if the patient's condition is critical or acute or if the body could be damaged by the results of the massage. However, there are very few total contraindications to massage if the application is changed appropriately.

The complex and fragile nature of the condition of many individuals in the healthcare system makes identifying contraindications especially important. Contraindications and cautions are unique to each situation. The ability to reason clinically is essential for making appropriate decisions about modifying or forgoing massage interventions.

Contraindications and cautions can be categorized as regional (local) or general (systemic). Regional contraindications pertain to a specific area of the body. For our purposes, the existence of a regional contraindication means that massage may be provided, but the application must be altered or the problematic area must be avoided. Examples of situations involving regional contraindications include a skin wound, a fracture, or a tumor site where some sort of medical device is used.

With general contraindications, a doctor's evaluation is required before any massage can be provided. If the doctor recommends massage, he or she must advise the massage therapist about cautions. The doctor also will probably preapprove a comprehensive treatment plan for massage that incorporates those cautions. Examples of this type of situation include renal failure, congestive heart failure, high fever, and infection.

People with any vague or unexplained symptoms of fatigue, muscle weakness, and general aches and pains should be referred immediately to the doctor or supervising nurse. Many disease processes share these symptoms. This recommendation may seem overly cautious, but in the early stages of some very serious illnesses, the symptoms are not well defined. If the doctor can detect a disease process early in its development, a more successful treatment outcome often is possible. A specific diagnosis is essential for effective treatment (Figure 5-2).

Massage should be avoided during the acute phase of infectious diseases involving fever, nausea, and lethargy until a diagnosis has been made and the doctor's recommendations can be followed.

Recommendations on contraindications are provided in the sections on specific health conditions in Unit Three. However, remember that every situation is unique, and every patient's condition needs to be evaluated individually using effective assessment and critical reasoning skills.

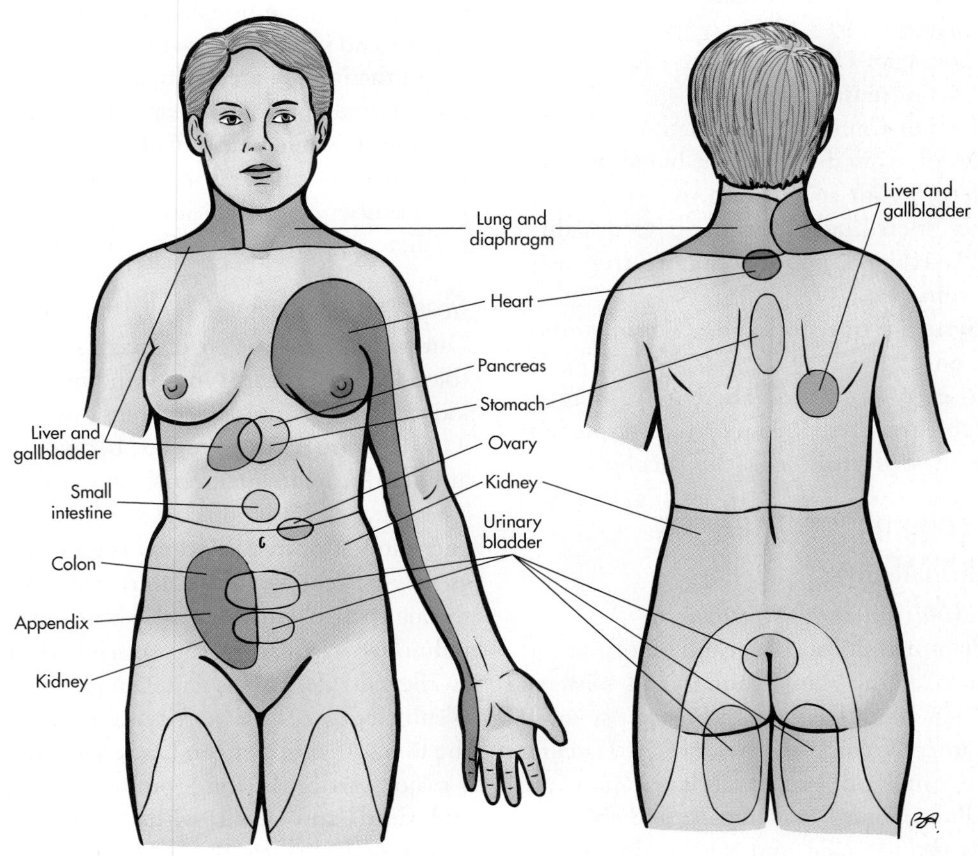

FIGURE 5-2 ■ Referred pain. The diagram indicates cutaneous areas to which visceral pain may be referred. A massage professional who encounters pain in these areas should refer the client for diagnosis to rule out visceral dysfunction. (From Fritz S: *Mosby's fundamentals of therapeutic massage*, ed 2, St Louis, 2004, Mosby.)

It is absolutely necessary to seek recommendations about the appropriateness of massage from the supervising healthcare professional. When contraindications exist and massage is indicated, the interaction should be monitored by a healthcare professional such as the doctor, nurse, physical therapist, or other qualified personnel. The general massage recommendation is to be cautious and not to take risks.

CONDITIONS THAT MAY PRESENT CONTRAINDICATIONS REQUIRING AVOIDANCE OF MASSAGE OR ALTERATION IN APPLICATION

A number of conditions may give rise to contraindications that require the massage therapist to change the method of application or forgo massage entirely:

- Acute illness and injury
- Acute or severe cardiac, liver, or kidney disease
- Contagious condition
- Loss of sensation
- Loss of voluntary movement
- Medication that thins the blood by interfering with coagulation, whether a prescription drug (e.g., warfarin [Coumadin], Plavix) or a nonprescription drug (e.g., aspirin)
- Systemic infection and acute inflammation
- Use of sensation-altering substances, whether prescribed (e.g., pain medication) or recreational (e.g., alcohol).

SPECIFIC CONDITIONS THAT PRESENT CONTRAINDICATIONS

Acute Local Soft Tissue Inflammation

Acute inflammation can occur in any of the soft tissues, such as the skin (wounds and blisters), muscles, tendons, ligaments, bursae, synovial capsule, intervertebral disks, and periosteum. Common causes of acute inflammation are overuse, illness, injury, and surgery, and common symptoms include pain and dysfunction in the affected area, heat and redness, and swelling local to the injury.

Superficial signs and symptoms usually are easy to identify. However, when inflammation occurs in deep tissues, the symptoms may not be visible, but only palpable. Upon palpation, areas of acute inflammation deep in the tissues feel hard and denser than surrounding tissue. Focused pressure may cause a sharp pain. These symptoms could indicate an acute problem that requires caution in massage application with a focus on lymphatic drainage.

To test for acute inflammation, apply enough pressure to the area to cause mild discomfort. Maintain this fixed pressure for up to 10 seconds. If the discomfort increases, this suggests that the tissues are in an acute state; if it decreases, it generally is safe to apply massage.

Bone and Joint Injuries

Fractures tend to cause pain and tenderness around the injury site with any movement or weight bearing. Stress fractures are very difficult to diagnose. Be especially concerned if the pain persists and is accompanied by swelling and bruising in the injured area. Massage is obviously contraindicated in the acute stage of these conditions, because it would cause further damage. Surgery that involves the cutting of bone (e.g., joint replacement or open heart surgery) creates fracturelike conditions.

Deep Vein Thrombosis (DVT)

During the application of massage, a thrombus (blood clot) can form in a vein and become dislodged, or a fragment (embolus) may break off. This is a rare occurrence, but because the results are life-threatening, extreme caution is required. The veins typically affected are those in the calf and hamstring areas. Because the veins get larger as they travel toward the heart, the clot can pass through the chambers of the heart and into the pulmonary circulation. The vessels become smaller as they divide up into the lungs, and the clot eventually blocks the vessels, occluding an area of the lung. A large clot can block the circulation to a major part of the lung (pulmonary embolism), and death can result within minutes. Factors that could lead to this condition include the following:

- Long periods of immobility or bed rest, which reduces circulation and can compress the veins

- Recent major surgery
- Varicose veins
- Heart disease
- Diabetes
- Use of the contraceptive pill
- Impact trauma, which can cause damage inside the vein

DVT can occur in seemingly healthy people as a result of these predisposing factors. Acute pain and hard swelling may be felt when minimal pressure is applied, which can be confused with an acute muscle strain. Some general swelling and discoloration of the distal part of the limb may be noted as a result of restricted circulation. The person may feel more pain and aching in the area when resting than would be expected with a muscle strain, and nothing in the history would suggest an injury. *These individuals must be referred to a doctor immediately; this is a medical emergency. Do not massage.*

Diabetes

Diabetes can affect the peripheral circulation, especially in the feet, causing the tissues to become more brittle and fragile. It can also affect the nerves and reduce a patient's sensitivity to pressure. Deep massage techniques or methods with excessive drag can damage the brittle tissues, and with an impaired pain response, which is common in diabetes, feedback mechanisms become ineffective.

The stimulating effect of massage on the circulation sometimes seems to have the same effect as exercise on the blood sugar level of a person with diabetes. Clients with diabetes should be informed of this possibility so that they can alter their medication and/or diet accordingly. Although caution is required, if massage is applied correctly, it is extremely beneficial for individuals with diabetes. Caution is advised around common injection sites (Figure 5-3).

Local Infection

Bacterial Infection. Boils are superficial abscesses. A boil appears on the skin as a localized swelling that eventually ruptures and discharges pus. Folliculitis, a condition in which the hair follicles become inflamed, appears as a rash of very small blisters. Massage can break the blisters, leaving the skin open to further infection. These areas are local contraindications.

Fungal Infection. Ringworm and athlete's foot are the most common fungal infections. They can affect warm, moist areas, such as the skin between the toes, the armpits, or the area under the breast. The affected area may appear red and have white, flaky skin. Although massage does not worsen the problem, it can cause irritation, and the infection could be transmitted to the therapist's hands. For these reasons, treatment of the area is avoided.

Lymphangitis. Bacteria can invade the lymphatic system through open wounds. The wound itself may be minor, but the area around it appears red and swollen. Sometimes a dark line can be seen running up the limb toward the lymph nodes, which may also be swollen and tender. Massage could spread the infection. *These individuals should be referred immediately for medical treatment.*

Viral Infection

Herpes is a virus that affects DNA and currently has no cure. The infection is communicable, and the sores recur from time to time. Herpes is a local contraindication. Cold sores, the most common symptom of herpes, usually appear on the face and on or near mucous membranes in the general area. Before the sores erupt, the skin usually feels hypersensitive and tingles.

Other viral infections, such as warts and verrucae, should also be considered contraindications, because the infection could be transmitted.

Myositis Ossificans

A large hematoma that occurs with a deep bruise and that goes untreated for a long time may ossify and form small pieces of bone material in the soft tissues. This is more likely to happen when a fracture is also involved, because osteoblasts move into the tissues and can serve as the catalyst for calcification. Massage over the area could cause the pieces of bone to damage the surrounding soft tissues. This is a local contraindication, therefore the area should be avoided. Although myositis ossificans is a rare condition, it should be

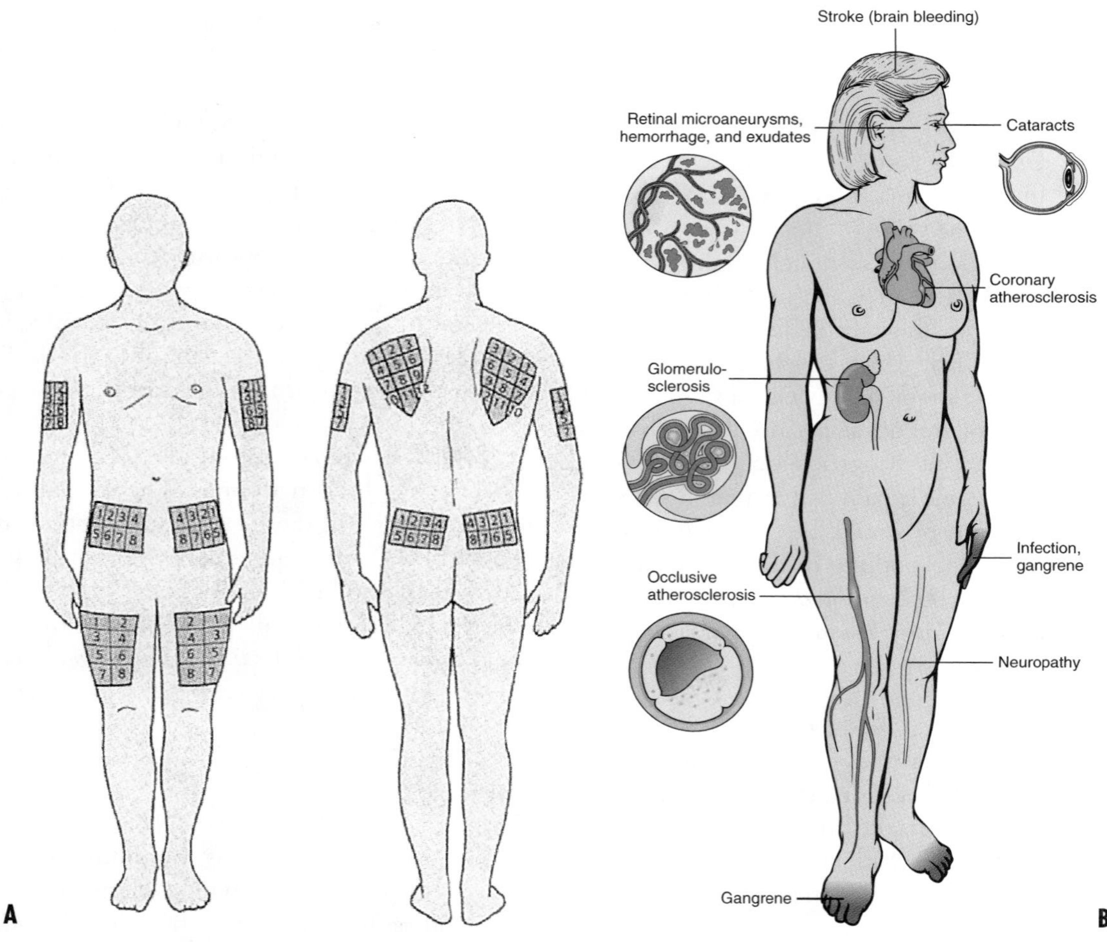

FIGURE 5-3 ■ **A,** Insulin injection sites. **B,** Complications of diabetes mellitus. (**A** from Potter PA, Perry AG: *Fundamentals of nursing,* ed 4, St Louis, 1997, Mosby; **B** from Damjanov I: *Pathology for the health professions,* ed 3, St Louis, 2006, WB Saunders.)

considered a possibility in patients who have had a long recovery from a serious fracture or other major impact trauma.

Open Wounds

An open wound is the most obvious contraindication and should be a matter of common sense. After a large wound has healed, a residual problem caused by scar tissue may exist, which can be treated by massage.

Tumors

Undiagnosed tumors should be referred to a doctor for diagnosis. Massage of a tumor, particularly friction, could stimulate its development and help it spread to other areas. If a tumor is diagnosed as benign, the tumor area is locally contraindicated. If the area is malignant, massage application follows the doctor's recommendation.

Massage should not be applied directly to any tumor, and the area should be avoided. Benign tumors are usually encapsulated, but malignant tumors are much less isolated and more apt to have cells break away. Massage of a malignant tumor could increase the potential for cells breaking away from tumor mass.

If malignancy exists, contraindications to massage include patient fatigue, possible fragile bones in areas of radiation treatment, tissue damaged by radiation, fragile skin from chemotherapy, and a suppressed immune system.

Bleeding Disorders

Hemophilia is a hereditary disease that inhibits the blood's ability to clot. Several different forms of the disease exist, and it varies in severity. Males are primarily affected. Also, many people take anticoagulant medication that predisposes them to bleeding.

In individuals with bleeding disorders, anything that could cause trauma to the tissues, on any level, must be avoided. The person's doctor will be able to advise the massage therapist on what is safe and possible.

Varicose Veins

Varicose veins usually develop at the back of the leg. In this condition, the valves in the veins that prevent circulatory backflow break down and stop functioning. In minor cases, light, superficial stroking over the area should do no harm and may in fact ease the pressure off the vein and aid repair. Deep pressure and drag should not be applied, because they can further damage the walls of the blood vessels. In advanced cases, even superficial stroking should be avoided because of the added risk of DVT. This contraindication affects only the actual location of the vein. The tissues adjacent to the area can be massaged, which can improve circulation away from the varicose vein and relieve some of the pressure in it.

Kidney Disease

Massage moves fluid, helping it to pass through the kidneys, and increased fluid movement strains the kidneys. Massage methods that target fluid movement, such as lymphatic drainage, need to be used very cautiously and only with a doctor's supervision. Massage may be appropriate with impaired kidney function, depending on the severity of the impairment. It is impossible to do massage and not at least temporarily increase fluid movement. Energy-based methods that sooth and relax, using entrainment, may be appropriate.

Cardiac Disease

The term *heart failure* seems to imply that the heart no longer works at all, and nothing can be done. Actually, *heart failure* means that the heart is not pumping as well as it should be. This results in fatigue and shortness of breath. Everyday activities such as walking, climbing stairs, and carrying groceries can become very difficult.

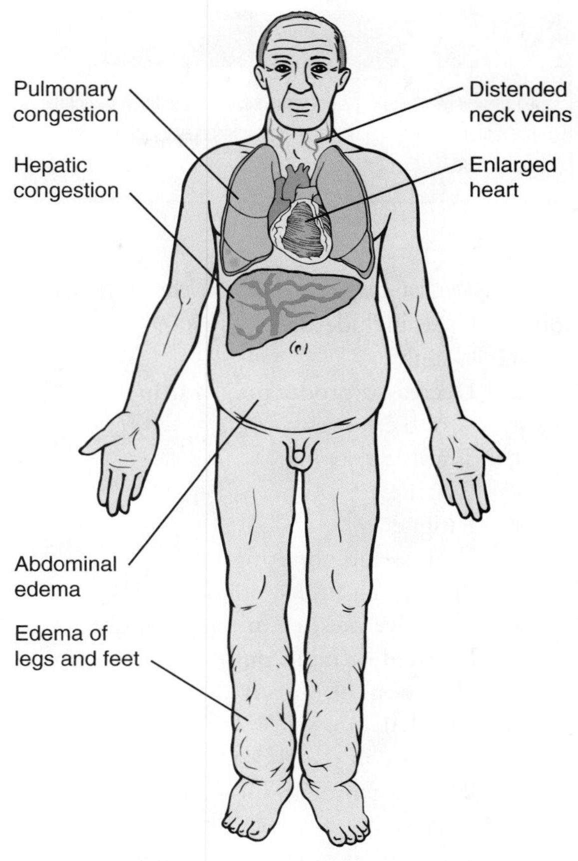

FIGURE 5-4 ■ Signs of congestive heart failure. (From Frazier MS, Drzymkowski JW: *Essentials of human diseases and conditions,* ed 2, Philadelphia, 2000, WB Saunders.)

Congestive Heart Failure. Congestive heart failure (CHF) occurs when the heart is unable to pump blood efficiently throughout the body, and circulatory needs are not met (Figure 5-4). The two types of CHF are left-side damage and right-side damage. When the left side of the heart is damaged, blood backs up into the lung area, making breathing difficult. The kidneys also are damaged, and sudden weight gain can occur. With right-side damage, blood and other fluids accumulate in the ankles, bloating occurs in the abdominal area, and the person has extreme fatigue.

evolve 5-1

See the Evolve website that accompanies this textbook for further information on the pathophysiologic mechanisms of congestive heart failure.

Symptoms of Congestive Heart Failure. The symptoms of CHF include the following:

- Cough
- Decreased production of urine
- Trouble focusing
- Trouble sleeping
- Dizziness
- Fatigue
- Nausea and vomiting
- Protruding neck veins
- Excessive need to urinate at night
- Elevated or rapid pulse
- Shortness of breath after exertion and after lying down
- Swelling in the abdominal area
- Weight gain without a change in diet or exercise

Because massage moves the blood and changes the fluid pressure in the body, compromised cardiac function can be unduly strained. General massage typically is beneficial for those with cardiac conditions, but cautions are indicated. If the patient has been diagnosed with CHF, massage is contraindicated except for gentle energy-based and gentle palliative methods.

JUST BETWEEN YOU AND ME

Contraindications can be scary. It is good to be cautious and respectful of conditions that present contraindications, but being afraid limits your ability to develop into a confident massage therapist. Replace fear with knowledge. Get support and direction from other healthcare professionals who know more than you about the pathologic condition. Trust your gut instinct. I asked a psychologist once how he knew when a patient was becoming psychotic, and he gave me a list of signs and symptoms. However, he then said," The final test is the gut test." If something feels wrong, then it probably is. At least in the healthcare setting, you are not isolated; other professionals are present who can help you in providing a massage that is beneficial (indicated) and not harmful (contraindicated).

ENDANGERMENT SITES

Endangerment sites are areas in which nerves and blood vessels surface close to the skin and are not well protected by muscle or connective tissue. Therefore deep, sustained pressure into these areas could damage the vessels and nerves. Areas that have fragile bony projections that could be broken off are also considered endangerment sites (i.e., xiphoid process). The kidney area is considered an endangerment site because the kidneys are loosely suspended in fat and connective tissue; heavy pounding is contraindicated in this area.

To prevent damage, massage therapists should avoid endangerment sites or use only light pressure in these areas. The areas shown in Figure 5-5 are commonly considered endangerment sites for massage therapists.

Other endangerment sites and activities that should be avoided include the following:

- Eyes
- Inferior to the ear (fascial nerve, styloid process, external carotid artery)
- Posterior cervical area (spinous processes, cervical plexus)
- Lymph nodes
- Medial brachium (between the biceps and triceps)
- Musculocutaneous, median, and ulnar nerves
- Brachial artery
- Basilic vein
- Cubital (anterior) area of the median nerve, radial and ulnar arteries, and median cubital vein
- Deep stripping over a vein in a direction away from the heart (contraindicated because of possible damage to the valve system)
- Application of lateral pressure to the knees

MEDICAL AND ASSISTIVE DEVICES

A *device* is an apparatus, such as a machine or an object, that performs some sort of function. Examples include cervical collars, intravenous lines, various tubes, pacemakers, ports for chemotherapy, cosmetic implants, colostomy bags, catheters, intrauterine devices, prostheses, and various

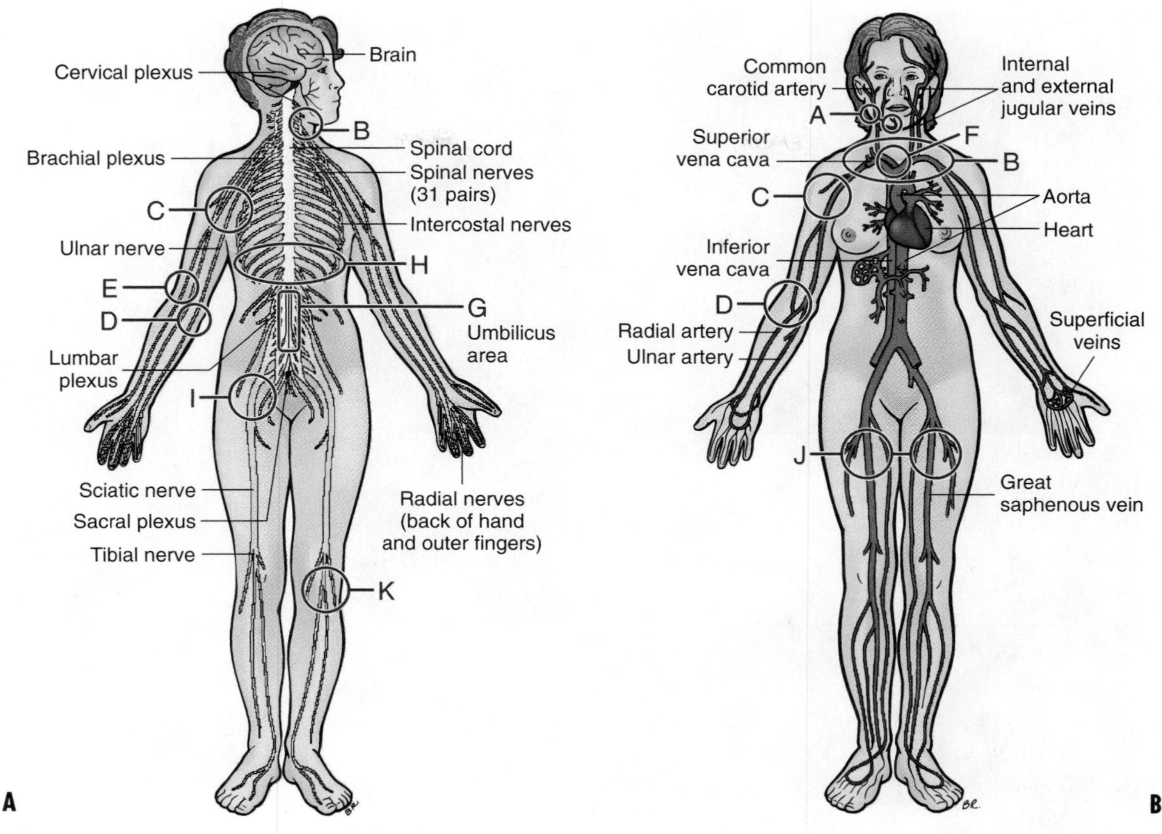

FIGURE 5-5 ■ Endangerment sites of the nervous system **(A)** and cardiovascular system **(B)**. **A,** Anterior triangle of the neck: carotid artery, jugular vein, and vagus nerve, which are located deep to the sternocleidomastoid muscle. **B,** Posterior triangle of the neck: the nerves of the brachial plexus, the brachiocephalic artery and vein superior to the clavicle, and the subclavian arteries and vein. **C,** Axillary area: the brachial artery, axillary vein and artery, cephalic vein, and nerves of the brachial plexus. **D,** Medial epicondyle of the humerus: the ulnar nerve, also the radial and ulnar arteries. **E,** Lateral epicondyle: the radial nerve. **F,** Area of the sternal notch and anterior throat: nerves and vessels to the thyroid gland and the vagus nerve. **G,** Umbilical area: descending aorta and abdominal aorta. **H,** Twelfth rib, dorsal body: location of the kidney. **I,** Sciatic notch: sciatic nerve. **J,** Inguinal triangle located lateral and inferior to the pubis: medial to the sartorius, external iliac artery, great saphenous vein, femoral vein, and femoral nerve. **K,** Popliteal fossa: popliteal artery and vein and tibial nerve. (From Fritz S: *Mosby's fundamentals of therapeutic massage,* ed 2, St. Louis, 2004, Mosby.)

types of monitoring equipment (Figure 5-6). These devices, whether temporary or permanent, create local areas of contraindication similar to endangerment sites. An added concern is sanitation, especially in areas where a line or catheter is located.

evolve 5-2

An explanation and illustrations of renal dialysis, with massage considerations, are posted on the Evolve website that accompanies this textbook.

Medical devices must not be disturbed by the massage application. The massage therapist may be instructed to address scar tissue development around an implant, but the massage application is targeted to the area around the device, not on the device. To reduce the chance of contamination in the area of a device, the massage therapist should reduce or eliminate the use of lubrication and stay about 6 inches away from the area.

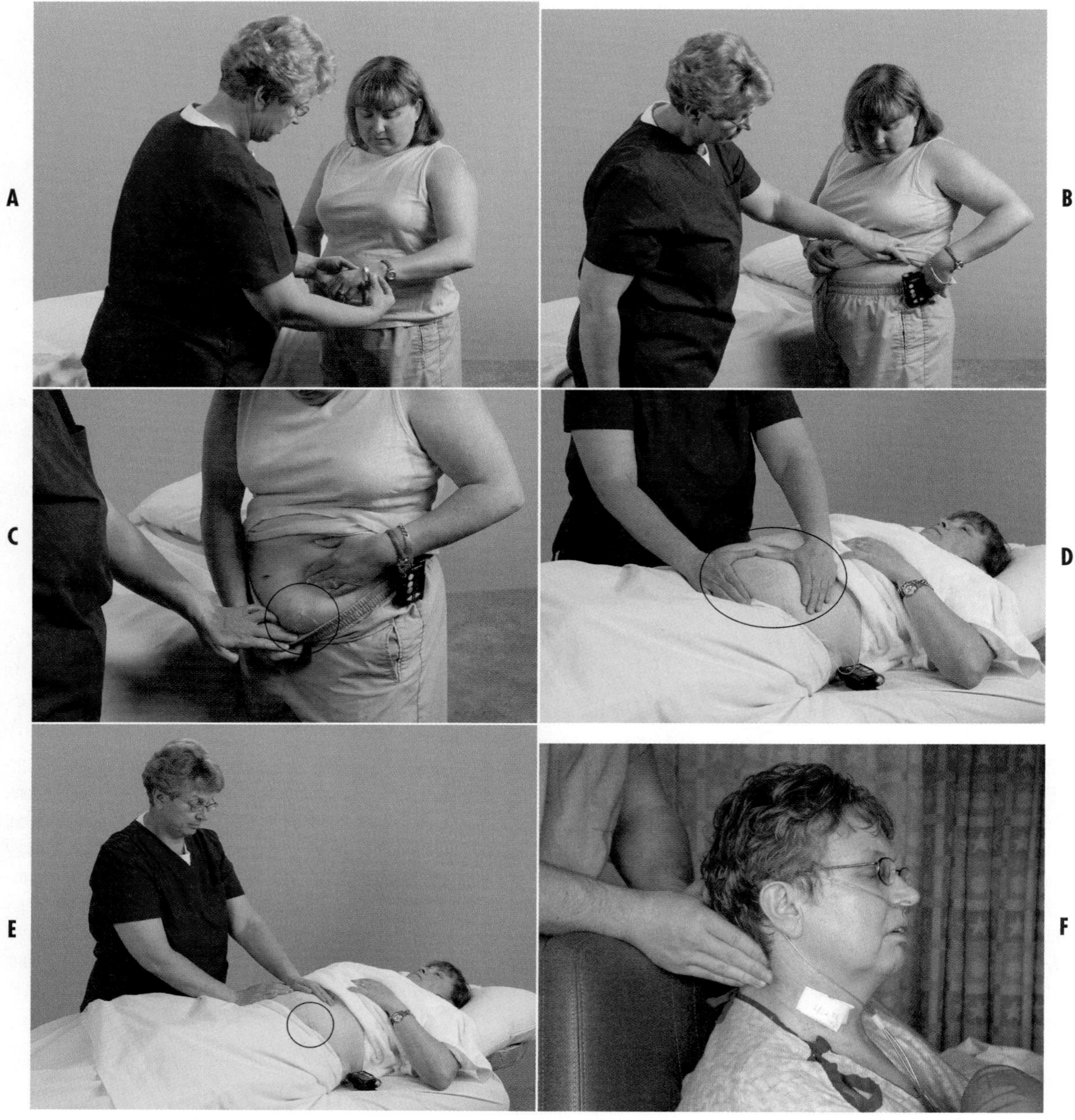

FIGURE 5-6 ■ Medical devices. **A,** Be aware of medical alert bracelets or necklaces. **B,** Ask questions; this patient uses an insulin pump. **C,** Identify areas of regional contraindications. **D,** Locate areas to avoid during massage. **E,** Massage a safe distance from the area. **F,** Note the medical devices surrounding this patient recovering in the hospital. (**F,** Courtesy Sandy Fritz.)

JUST BETWEEN YOU AND ME

Medical and assistive devices can be intimidating. Remember, these things are not the person. Tubes, bags, monitors, equipment (e.g., wheelchairs, braces), and prostheses (replacement parts) can get in the way of a massage. Instead of being intimidated, realize that devices can be cumbersome and can complicate the massage application. Ask patients with such equipment to teach you about any permanent devices they use, and let them move it out of the way. The same goes for temporary devices. Ask the nurse or other appropriate person to move the device. If it can't be moved, work around it, but don't be overwhelmed by it. It is the person to whom the device is attached who is getting the massage.

ADAPTING DURING MASSAGE: PRESSURE AND INTENSITY LEVELS

Most changes in the application of massage to accommodate contraindications involve changes in the depth of pressure (i.e., drag, speed, and duration) and avoiding areas with regional contraindications. With study and practice, the massage practitioner can determine the elements of safe massage application.

PRESSURE, DRAG, DURATION, AND POINT OF CONTACT

Attempting to describe various pressures and drag intensities is difficult. Many authors and teachers (including myself) have presented a number of approaches to teach massage students to gauge the most beneficial and safe pressure and drag intensity.

Pressure has been defined in numerous ways, such as compressive force, force application depth, tight, light, medium depth, deep, and so forth. For the purposes of this text, *pressure* means compressive force exerted downward into the tissue at a 90-degree angle.

Drag is the resistance to glide. *Glide* moves horizontal to the tissues. If you apply tension force to tissues to stretch them, the angle of force can be anything more than 180 degrees to just less than 90 degrees and away from the point of contact. Therefore, by combining pressure with drag, you can create a multitude of intensities. For example, light pressure with extensive drag significantly stretches the skin. Increase the pressure slightly and maintain significant drag, and the superficial fascia is stretched (tension force applied).

If you factor in *duration* (how long), the intensity can be modified. Long duration is more intense, and short duration is less intense.

Another factor is the size of the point of contact. A large contact area is less intense than a small contact point. More pressure can be applied safely with a broad base of contact (e.g., the forearm or full hand) than with a small point of contact (e.g., the thumb).

The factors that gauge the intensity of a massage application, therefore, are compressive force, drag, duration, and the size of the contact point. In addition, a fast rhythmic application is more intense than a slow rhythmic application. As you can see, determining the right pressure is more difficult than it appears.

PRESSURE LEVELS

Let's begin with compressive force. If we consider that increasing force is necessary to affect various layers of soft tissue (taking into account physiologic factors), and if we hypothetically simplify the fleshy areas of the body (typically between the joints) into seven layers, we can describe seven levels of compressive force. The seven tissue layers, progressing from the skin surface to deep tissue, would be as follows (Figure 5-7):

1. Skin surface
2. Skin
3. Superficial fascia
4. First muscle layer with deep fascia
5. Second muscle layer with deep fascia
6. Third muscle layer with deep fascia
7. Bone

The seven levels of pressure can be described as follows:

- Level 1 pressure just touches the skin, without denting it; it slides on the skin and cannot produce drag or tension of the skin. The therapist's fingertips do not blanch (change color). A bathroom scale or other type of scale would not register this pressure (Figure 5-7, *A*).
- Level 2 pressure slightly dents the skin, moves (drags) the skin to bind, but cannot apply a tension force to stretch the skin past bind.

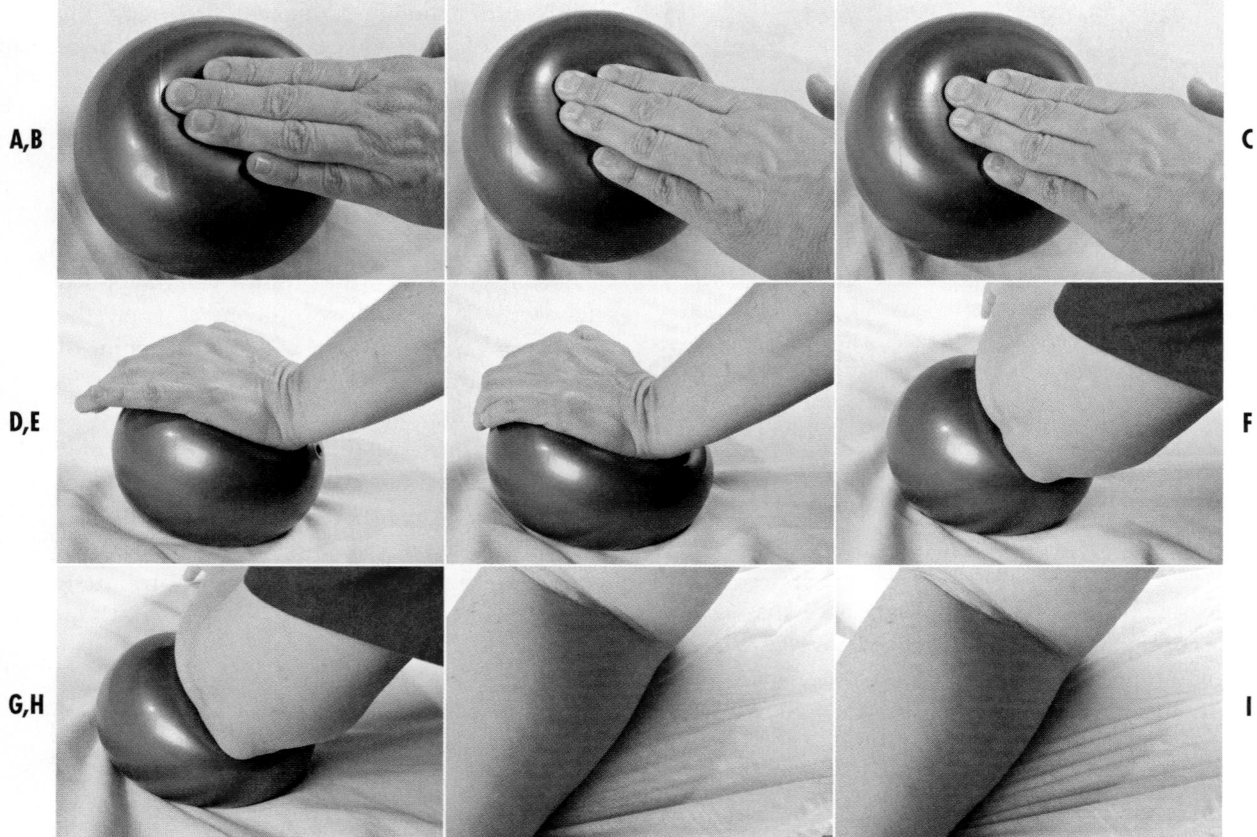

FIGURE 5-7 ■ Pressure level and drag application. **A,** Level 1. **B,** Level 2. **C,** Level 3. **D,** Level 4. **E,** Level 5. **F,** Level 6. **G,** Level 7. **H,** Drag-level 1 and 2. **I,** Drag-level 3.

The therapist's fingertips blanch, but the nail beds do not change color. A scale would barely register this pressure (0 to 5 pounds), depending on the density of the client's skin (Figure 5-7, *B*).

- Level 3 pressure is the compressive force needed to penetrate through the skin but not to the muscle. Palpation of muscle structure indicates that the force is too intense. The therapist's fingertips and nail beds blanch, and a scale would register 3 to 10 pounds. Body mechanics for the therapist involve slight leaning into the tissue (Figure 5-7, *C*).
- Level 4 pressure is the compressive force needed to penetrate through the skin and superficial fascia (Figure 5-7, *D*). The skin layer is displaced (pressed away), and the therapist should be able to palpate muscle, especially if the muscle is contracting. A scale would register 7 to 16 pounds, depending on the client's tissue density. Body mechanics for the therapist involve moderate leaning into the tissue.
- Level 5 pressure is the compressive force needed to displace surface tissue (i.e., the skin fascia and the first muscle layer) and penetrate to the middle muscle layer. A narrow or small contact would feel "pokey." A scale would register 12 to 35 pounds, depending on the client's tissue density and the bulk of the first muscle layer. Broad-base contact and leaning body mechanics typically are used (Figure 5-7, *E*).
- Level 6 pressure is the compressive force needed to displace surface tissue (i.e., the skin fascia and the first and second muscle layers)

and penetrate to the third muscle layer (Figure 5-7, *F*). This layer of muscle, which is smaller than the first and second layers, lies next to the bone, and force applied compresses the muscle against the bone. If bone is felt, the force is too intense. A scale would register 25 to 60 pounds (sometimes higher), depending on the client's muscle bulk and tissue density. Broad-base contact is required, or pain and protective guarding will occur in the first and second muscle layers. The therapist may need to use full leaning body mechanics and simultaneous counterpressure to reach this layer.

- Level 7 pressure, or bone application, is slightly more intense than level 6 pressure. The therapist feels bone pressing against tissue. The exception is around the joints, where the muscle layers are not prominent and the bone is beneath the skin and superficial fascia (Figure 5-7, *G*).

Drag can be described on an arbitrary scale, such as the following:

0—No drag
1—Moves tissue but not to bind
2—Moves tissue to bind (Figure 5-7, *H*)
3—Moves tissue past bind (Figure 5-7, *I*)

The duration of specific work is described as follows:

Short: 1 to 5 seconds
Moderate: 5 to 15 seconds
Long: 15 to 60 seconds

Similarly, session length is categorized as follows:

Short: 10 to 15 minutes
Moderate: 15 to 30 minutes
Long: 30 to 60 minutes

When pressure, drag, duration, and speed (slow, moderate, fast) are all considered in combination, the general guidelines shown in Table 5-3 apply.

TABLE 5-3 General Guidelines for Pressure, Drag, Speed, and Duration in Massage Applications for Various Conditions

Desired Outcome	Pressure	Drag	Speed	Duration
Fragile patient (to provide comfort and to soothe)	1 to 2	0	Slow	Short to moderate
Palliative, pleasure based (nonfragile patient; to stimulate parasympathetic dominance)	2, 3, or 4	1	Slow	Moderate
Lymphatic drainage, surface	2 to 3	2	Slow	Moderate to long
Lymphatic drainage, deep	4 to 5	2	Slow	Moderate
Myofascial release (superficial fascia)	3	3	Slow	Long
General relaxation (to inhibit sympathetic arousal)	4 to 5	2	Slow	Moderate
Trigger point inhibition	4 to 6 (depending on location)	0	Moderate	Moderate
Scar tissue surface (mature scar)	2 to 3	2 to 3	Slow	Moderate
Adhesion of muscle layer or layers	4 to 6	3	Slow	Moderate
Arterial support	4 to 5	0	Moderate to fast at location over artery	Short to moderate
Venous return support	3	1	Slow	Moderate
Anticoagulant use	1 to 2	0 to start (monitor results)	Varies	Varies
Fragile bones (osteoporosis)	1 to 4 (depending on muscle bulk and density)	0 to 3	Varies	Varies
Stimulation of sympathetic autonomic nervous system (ANS) dominance	2 to 5	0 to 1	Moderate to fast	Short to moderate

The safe application of massage and the benefits it confers are determined by the combination of methods used, including compressive force, drag, speed, duration, and rhythm, as well as the location, outcome, client's condition, tissue density, superficial factors, and muscle bulk. Protocols and recommendations for massage application are important, but the correct approach more specifically depends on all the factors taken together.

evolve 5-3

The following terms and expressions specific to Chapter 5 have already been used to search PubMed for the latest research literature available. The *Click Here for Massage* feature associated with this chapter on your textbook's Evolve website allows you to hyperlink to a continually updated PubMed search of research literature that corresponds to this subject.

Hyperlink Search Terms

- Massage anxiety
- Massage cautions
- Massage condition management
- Massage contraindications cautions
- Massage depression
- Massage healing rehabilitation
- Massage impingement syndromes
- Massage indications
- Massage mood
- Massage pain fatigue management
- Massage relaxation
- Massage soft tissue dysfunction
- Massage stress
- Massage therapeutic change
- Massage treatment goals

SUMMARY

Massage is a valuable treatment option for most conditions, including generalized stress related to illness or an injury, but it must be applied intelligently based on the current state of the patient. People who need healthcare and rehabilitation have some sort of illness or injury, and contraindications and cautions come with the territory when working with these individuals. It is important not to assume that minor symptoms are signs of minor causes. Nothing is lost by being cautious.

As we've discussed, massage is indicated for musculoskeletal discomfort, circulation enhancement, relaxation, stress reduction, and pain control, as well as in situations in which analgesics, antiinflammatory drugs, muscle relaxants, and blood pressure, anxiety, and antidepressant medications may be prescribed. Therapeutic massage, appropriately provided, can support the use of these medications, manage some side effects, and in mild cases may be able to replace them, particularly pain medication and muscle relaxants. The general effects of stress and pain reduction and increased circulation, as well as the physical comfort derived from therapeutic massage, complement most other medical and mental health treatment methods. However, when other therapies, including medication, are used, the doctor must be able to evaluate accurately the effectiveness of each treatment the patient is receiving. If the doctor, physical therapist, or other healthcare provider is unaware that the patient is receiving massage or that the massage is different from the agreed upon treatment plan, the effects of other therapies may be misinterpreted. Therefore a supervising medical professional (e.g., the doctor or physician assistant) is important for case management, so that all the professionals working with the patient and all the methods used can be evaluated in the appropriate context. Omitting this supervisory function can be dangerous, especially with regard to medication dosages or when a treatment may mask the symptoms of a serious underlying condition. Massage can temporarily alleviate symptoms of aching, pain, fatigue, and anxiety, thereby preventing or delaying effective treatments such as medication and surgery. This is a major concern of healthcare professionals and the reason massage patients with medical conditions are best managed through a multidisciplinary team approach.

Working in the healthcare setting has a big advantage over private practice. In the healthcare setting, the massage therapist is part of a multidisciplinary team that is supervised by healthcare professionals who can discuss and offer advice on both indications and contraindications for massage and monitor the progress of the person receiving care.

WORKBOOK

1. Compare the indications for massage with those given in Chapter 2 (both text and Evolve website material). Match the various research findings with the conditions indicated for massage.

   Example: Anxiety reduction (research findings and study referenced)

   ____
   ____
   ____
   ____
   ____
   ____
   ____
   ____
   ____
   ____

2. Choose one area of interest for professional development from your indications list in question 1. Identify the healthcare environment in which you might work if this were your specialty (e.g., anxiety reduction—private practice, clinical psychologist). Then, using the information from question 1, write a proposal that includes massage in the healthcare process for that specific medical specialty. Include the indications justified by research and discuss possible changes in massage application based on any identified contraindications.

   ____
   ____
   ____
   ____
   ____
   ____

Chapter 6 Concept Map

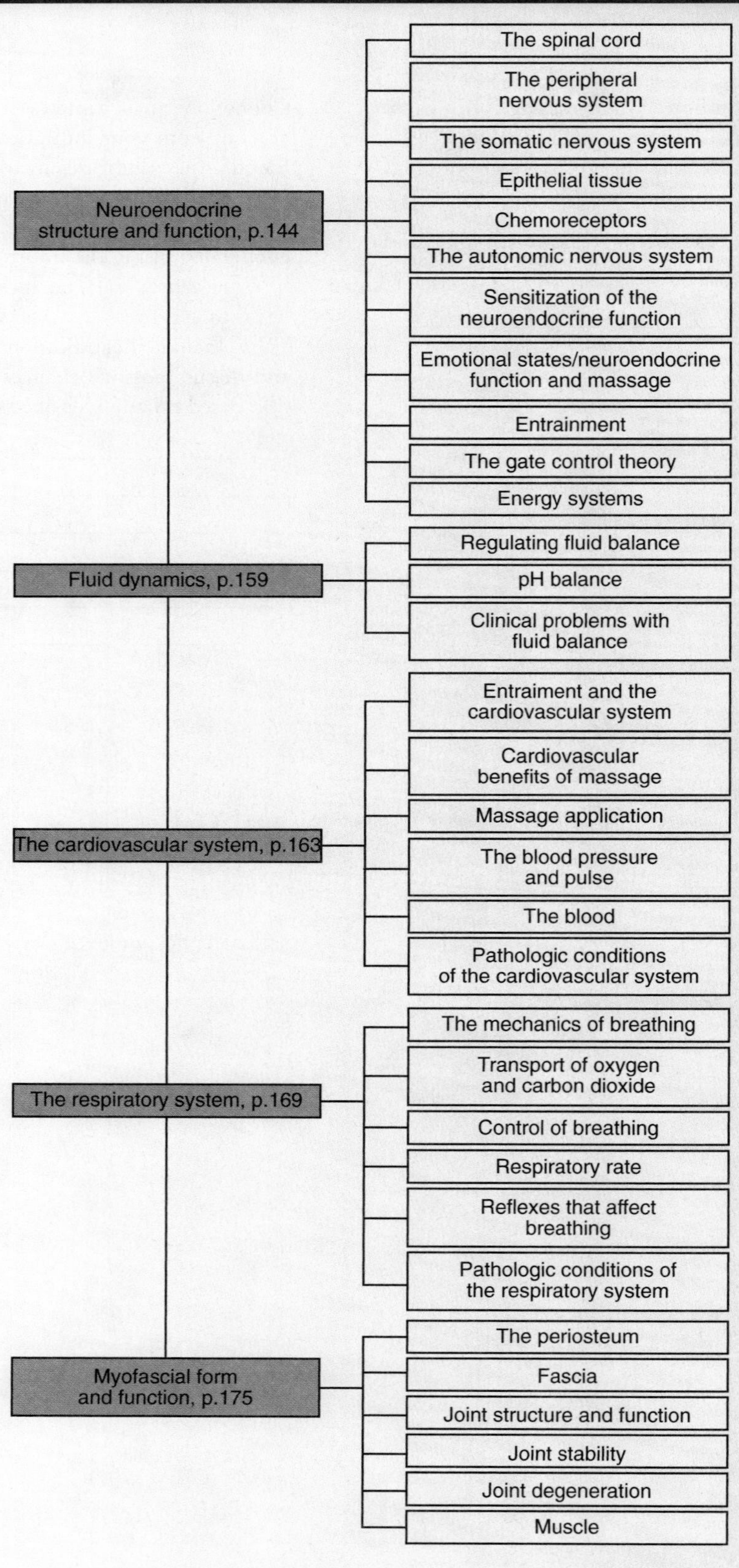
Neuroendocrine structure and function, p.144
The spinal cord
The peripheral nervous system
The somatic nervous system
Epithelial tissue
Chemoreceptors
The autonomic nervous system
Sensitization of the neuroendocrine function
Emotional states/neuroendocrine function and massage
Entrainment
The gate control theory
Energy systems
Fluid dynamics, p.159
Regulating fluid balance
pH balance
Clinical problems with fluid balance
The cardiovascular system, p.163
Entraiment and the cardiovascular system
Cardiovascular benefits of massage
Massage application
The blood pressure and pulse
The blood
Pathologic conditions of the cardiovascular system
The respiratory system, p.169
The mechanics of breathing
Transport of oxygen and carbon dioxide
Control of breathing
Respiratory rate
Reflexes that affect breathing
Pathologic conditions of the respiratory system
Myofascial form and function, p.175
The periosteum
Fascia
Joint structure and function
Joint stability
Joint degeneration
Muscle

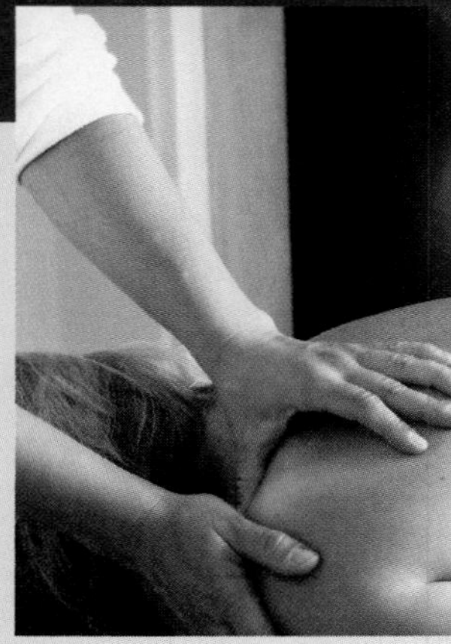

CHAPTER 6

REVIEW OF PERTINENT ANATOMY AND PHYSIOLOGY

Key Terms

Acidosis
Adhesions
Agonists
Alkalosis
Amygdala
Antagonists
Apnea
Arteriole tone
Arterioles
Atria
Autonomic nervous system
Basal ganglia
Blood pressure
Bradycardia
Bradypnea
Brainstem
Breathing
Breathing pattern disorder
Bursae
Capillaries
Cartilage
Central nervous system (CNS)
Cerebellum
Chemoreceptors
Chondrocytes
Co-contraction
Collagen
Concentric action
Core
Cortisol
Counterirritation
Dehydration
Diastolic pressure
Dopamine
Eccentric action
Edema
Elasticity
Elastin fibers
Electrolytes
Endocardium
Enkephalins
Entrainment
Epinephrine
Expiratory reserve volume
Fascia
Fibrosis
Fibrous joint capsule
Force couples
Force stability
Form stability
Frontal plane movement
Full body pronation
Functional movement patterns
Gate control theory
Global muscles
Golgi tendon organs
Growth hormone
Guarding
Heart rate
Hippocampus
Hyaline (articular) cartilage
Hydrostatic pressure
Hyperpnea
Hyperstimulation analgesia
Hypertension
Hypothalamus
Inspiratory reserve volume
Isometric contraction action
Joint arthrokinematics
Joint play
Length-tension relationship
Ligaments
Ligand-gated channel
Limbic system
Local muscles
Mechanoreceptors
Motor tone
Muscle spindles
Muscle tone
Musculotendinous junction
Neurons
Nociceptors
Norepinephrine
Oxytocin
Parasympathetic nervous system
Peripheral nervous system (PNS)
Phasic/mover muscles
Piezoelectricity
Plasma
Plasticity
Platelets
Proprioceptors
Pulse
Red blood cells
Reserve volume
Resistance
Respiration
Sagittal plane movement
Serial distortion pattern
Serotonin
Skin
Somatic motor nerves
Somatic sensory nerves
Spinal cord
Spurs
Strain

Supination	Systolic pressure	Tonic/postural stabilizing muscles	Ventricles
Sympathetic nervous system	Tachycardia	Transverse plane rotational movement	Venules
Synapses	Tachypnea	Vascular system	Vestibular apparatus
Synergist	Tendons	Venous system	Viscosity
Synergistic dominance	Tenoperiosteal junction		Vital capacity
Synovial joints	Tidal volume		White blood cells

For definitions of key terms, refer to the Evolve website.

OBJECTIVES

Upon completion of this chapter, the reader will have the information necessary to:

1 Describe neuroendocrine control of the body and create outcome goals for massage application that support the effects of neuroendocrine function.
2 Describe the fluid content of the body and create outcome goals for massage application that support beneficial fluid dynamics.
3 Describe the tensegrity and spiral design of the body as it is influenced by connective tissue and explain the relationship of muscle function to predictable patterns of dysfunction.
4 Describe joint function and its interrelationship with muscular balance.
5 Explain illness and injury in relation to the tensegrity and spiral patterns of the body.
6 Explain how the kinetic chain relates to assessment and the development of treatment goals.
7 Create outcome goals for massage that support myofascial function.

This chapter reviews and then briefly expands on the anatomy and physiology relevant to indications and contraindications for therapeutic massage in the healthcare environment. The chapter is extensively supported by the Evolve website, which provides a more comprehensive review. To make reading easier, the Evolve site also includes the textbook content so that the information is presented in context. The research described in Chapter 2 supports the information in this chapter.

Before we discuss massage in technical terms, it is important to remember that touch is a multidimensional experience, encompassing both the individual receiving care and the massage therapist's body/mind/spirit experience. The interplay of these three realms forms the therapeutic relationship. Even though massage application can be explained in terms of stimuli and forces, the more abstract, integrated experience of nurturance, compassion, and respect is just as important to an understanding of the effects of massage. Although research has identified most of the physiologic mechanisms of the effects of massage, there remains the mystery of the unknown that is to be honored.

Effective, intelligent application of massage in the healthcare environment is founded on a knowledge of anatomy, physiology, kinesiology, biomechanics, pathology, and medical treatments. This chapter and the Evolve website review and discuss information on anatomy and physiology

JUST BETWEEN YOU AND ME

I have been teaching a long time, have had many students, and almost all of them grumble about learning anatomy and physiology. This is what I tell them, with passion and concern for their professional development: "Get over it, because understanding and being able to use this information is what makes an excellent massage therapist. Stop whining and figure out a way to learn it and strive to love it. You might as well decide to like this stuff, because you can't really be a good massage therapist without it." I truly love anatomy and physiology. It is the foundation of what we do as massage therapists. In my opinion, you can't learn enough about the body. When I'm asked what continuing education I recommend, first on my list is always more "A&P" (anatomy and physiology), followed by health and disease mechanisms. I rarely recommend modality classes. Understand the body, and you can figure out the appropriate method once you have mastered massage application.

Box 6-1 Recommended Reading for Anatomy and Physiology

Chaitow L, DeLany J: *Clinical application of neuromuscular techniques,* vol. 1 and 2
Chaitow L: *Maintaining body balance, flexibility and stability: a practical guide to the prevention and treatment of musculoskeletal pain and dysfunction*
Chaitow L: *Multidisciplinary approaches to breathing pattern disorders*
Fritz S: *Mosby's fundamentals of therapeutic massage*
Fritz S: *Mosby's essential science for soft tissue and movement therapies*
Horrigan B: *Voices of integrated medicine*
Macciocia Foundations of Chinese Medicine
Muscolino J: *Kinesiology: the skeletal system and muscle function*
Muscolino J: *The muscular system manual: the skeletal muscles of the human body,* ed 2
Muscolino J: *The musculoskeletal anatomy* (coloring book)
Muscolino J: *The musculoskeletal anatomy* (flashcards)
Muscolino J: *Flashcards for bones, joints and actions of the human body*
Myers T: *Anatomy trains: myofascial meridians for manual and movement therapists*
Neuman D: *Kinesiology of the musculoskeletal system: foundation for physical rehabilitation*
Pizzorno J, Murray M: *Textbook of natural medicine,* ed 3, Churchill Livingstone
Salvo S: *Mosby's pathology for massage therapists*

as it relates to commonly targeted massage outcomes for healthcare patients. This section should be used in conjunction with the recommended readings (Box 6-1) and the Evolve website.

Anatomy can be thought of as structure and physiology as function. Most massage outcomes influence physiology through both reflexive and mechanical application. Some massage applications can shift structure, primarily through the influence of the connective tissue of the body. Massage always has a physiologic result because of the adaptation required by the presence of the massage therapist, the sensory stimulation of various touch receptors, and the patient's perception of the therapeutic interaction. Therefore massage can achieve primarily physiologic responses from the body. However, massage results cannot be isolated strictly to structural outcomes. This is an important concept in the synergistic and multidisciplinary use of various methods to support the person receiving healthcare.

During entry level education, you probably studied the human body by individual systems, learning the various parts of the body and how they work together. In this textbook, and the accompanying Evolve website, the information is presented in a more conceptual and integrated form. This perspective should enhance and expand on your current foundation of body structure and function.

The massage therapist works mostly with the structural fluid and fiber aspects of the body and the functional interplay of body systems coordinated by chemicals and electrical signals. The chemicals and electrical signals control the body, and the fluid and fibers make up the bone and soft tissue. Soft tissue includes the skin, fascia, muscles, **tendons, ligaments, cartilage, bursae,** joint capsules, nerves, vascular and lymphatic tubes, and the various body fluids, such as blood, lymph, and synovial fluid. Fibers (mostly connective tissue) provide structure for the body, similar to the framework of a building. They provide the tension force to keep the body upright in gravity and transmit the forces from muscle cell contraction to create movement.

In general, the application of massage has been described in terms of methods and techniques rather than the physiologic response of the body to the various stimuli and forces applied. To better understand the synergistic interface of massage and various types of health and medical care, we must move beyond the classic description of massage in terms of techniques, such as effleurage (gliding strokes), petrissage (kneading), compression, friction, vibration, rocking, shaking (oscillation), tapotement (percussion), and joint movement. For that matter, neither methods (e.g., reflexology and deep tissue massage) nor population-focused applications (e.g., sports massage, prenatal massage, and geriatric massage) describe the mechanisms of outcomes and benefits.

For healthcare purposes, massage application must be described according to which stimulus is applied to which receptor or what force is applied to affect what tissue type or physiologic function;

then, we must explain how the stimulus and force produce the desired outcome.

Massage can be described as a manual application to the body that influences multiple body responses. Variations in depth of pressure, drag on the tissue, speed of application, direction of movement, frequency of application, duration of application, and rhythm allow for a wide range of application options based on treatment plan outcomes. Research has shown that massage influences body structure and function (see Chapter 2). Outcomes are achieved through the body's ability to respond and adapt to stimuli and forces applied to it. This is important information if the massage therapist is going to make intelligent decisions about massage application.

As discussed in Chapter 2 and on the Evolve website, research data are beginning to identify patterns of the underlying physiologic mechanisms that massage addresses. The research results identify a pattern of physiologic effects regardless of the philosophy of the system used, and they indicate that the benefits of soft tissue methods seem to be attributable to a cluster of physiologic effects. It is important to remember that continuing research will change how the effects of massage are understood. Future research findings will either confirm or conflict with our current understanding of massage effects. Either case is fine, as research continues to clarify the factors that make therapeutic massage beneficial. The current consensus is that the effects of massage are produced by a combination of neural, chemical, mechanical, and psychological factors. Our current understanding is that the effects of massage are achieved through the interrelationship of the peripheral and central nervous systems (and their reflex patterns and multiple pathways), the autonomic nervous system, neuroendocrine control, and the responsiveness of the fascial network to mechanical forces applied during massage.

NEUROENDROCRINE STRUCTURE AND FUNCTION

Massage influences central nervous system processing of cognitive perception and the peripheral somatic and autonomic nervous systems, including fluctuations in neurotransmitters and hormones that influence nervous system response. Massage can affect the nervous system in several ways. For example, it stimulates the nerve receptors in the tissues. On a sensory level, it stimulates the mechanoreceptors that respond to touch, pressure, warmth and so on. A reflex effect generally leads to relaxation of the tissues and a reduction in pain (although the opposite can happen).

The nervous system is anatomically and functionally connected throughout the body. However, structurally it can be divided into the **central nervous system (CNS)** and the peripheral nervous system; the peripheral nervous system, in turn, can be functionally divided into the somatic (or motor) nervous system and the autonomic nervous system. Endocrine hormone functions are interrelated as a mechanism of communication for homeostatic function. Massage affects every part of the nervous and endocrine systems. Massage targets all aspects of these functions. Proper functioning of the nervous and endocrine systems is especially important for healthcare patients, because most injuries and disease processes involve these systems at some level.

evolve 6-1

The Evolve website expands on this information on neuroendocrine structure and function.

The cerebrum is the largest part of the brain. The cerebrum, with the **limbic system** and **hypothalamus,** integrates emotional states, visceral responses, and the muscular system through endocrine and neurotransmitter chemicals. Emotions can alter muscle tension by increasing motor tone, primarily through increased sympathetic dominance in the autonomic nervous system. States of anxiety and depression create a sustained increase in muscle tension. Individuals who deal with health issues often experience anxiety and depression; this includes not only the patient but also family and friends.

The workings of the brain depend on the ability of nerve cells to communicate with each other. Communication occurs at small, specialized structures called **synapses.**

evolve 6-2

Further information on synapses can be found on the Evolve website.

The usual form of communication involves electrical signals that travel within neurons, giving rise to chemical signals that cross synapses, which in turn give rise to new electrical signals in the postsynaptic neuron. Each neuron, on average, makes more than 1000 synaptic connections with other neurons. Purkinje cells may make 100,000 to 200,000 connections. The brain has been estimated to contain 100 trillion to 1 quadrillion synapses. These synapses are not randomly located. Each region of the brain has an exquisite architecture consisting of layers and other anatomic substructures in which synaptic connections are formed. Ultimately, the pattern of synaptic connections gives rise to "circuits" in the brain. At the integrative level, large- and small-scale circuits are the substrates of behavior and mental life. One of the most awe-inspiring mysteries of brain science is how neuronal activity within circuits influences behavior and consciousness.

The complexity of the brain is such that a single neuron may be part of more than one circuit. The organization of circuits in the brain reveals that the brain is a massive information processor. For example, the circuits involved in vision receive information from the retina. After initial processing, these circuits categorize information into different streams, so that one stream of information identifies and describes the visual object, and another determines where the object is in space. The information stream related to the identity of the object is actually broken down into several more refined, parallel streams. One stream analyzes shape, and another analyzes color. Ultimately, the visual world is resynthesized with information about the tactile world and the auditory world and with information from memory, all of which is combined with emotional meaning. With its massively parallel design, this integrative processing mechanism is a great pattern recognizer and very tolerant of failure in individual elements. This is why a brain made up of neurons is still a better and longer lasting information processor than a computer.

To some degree, the specific connectivity of circuits is stereotyped (i.e., set in expected patterns) in the brain, which leads to the notion that certain places in the brain are specialized for certain functions. Thus the cerebral cortex (the mantle of neurons in which the enormous surface area is increased by outpouchings, called *gyri,* and indentations, called *sulci*) can be functionally subdivided. For example, the back portion of the cerebral cortex (i.e., the occipital lobe) is involved in the initial stages of visual processing. Just behind the central sulcus is the part of the cerebral cortex involved in the processing of tactile information (i.e., the parietal lobe). Just in front of the central sulcus is a part of the cerebral cortex involved in motor behavior (i.e., the frontal lobe). In the front of the brain is a region called the *prefrontal cortex,* which is involved in some of the highest integrated functions of the human being, including the ability to plan and to integrate cognitive and emotional streams of information.

Beneath the cerebral cortex are enormous numbers of **axons** sheathed in an insulating substance called *myelin.* This subcortical *white matter* (so called because of its appearance on freshly cut brain sections) surrounds groups of **neurons,** or *gray matter* (like the cortex, it appears gray because of the presence of neuronal cell bodies). The white matter can be thought of as the wiring that conveys information from one region to another. The brain processes information in the gray matter.

Gray matter regions include the **basal ganglia,** which is involved in the initiation of motion (affected in Parkinson's disease) and also the integration of motivational states; it is the part of the brain that becomes dysfunctional with addictive disorders. Other important gray matter structures are the amygdala and the hippocampus. The **amygdala** appears to play a special role in aversive or negative emotions, such as fear, and is involved in determining the emotional meaning of events and objects. The **hippocampus** initially encodes and consolidates specific memories of people, places, and things.

The brain is chemically complex as well as structurally complex. As explained previously, electrical signals within neurons are converted at synapses into chemical signals that create electrical signals on the other side of the synapse. These chemical signals are molecules called *neurotransmitters.* Two primary types of molecules serve as neurotransmitters: small molecules, some quite well known (i.e., **dopamine, serotonin,** and **norepinephrine**) and large molecules, which are essentially protein chains called *peptides.* The peptides include the endogenous opiates, such as endorphins, dynorphins substance P, and corticotropin-releasing factor (CRF), among others. Currently, researchers have found more than 100 different neurotransmitters that seem to be at work in the brain.

A neurotransmitter can exert a biologic effect in a postsynaptic neuron by binding to a protein known as a *neurotransmitter receptor.* The job of the neurotransmitter receptor is to pass the information contained in the neurotransmitter from the synapse to the inside of the receiving cell. Apparently, almost every known neurotransmitter has multiple receptors that can accept different signals on the receiving neuron. Dopamine has five known neurotransmitter receptors; serotonin has at least 14. This is one reason developing medications to specifically address a neurotransmitter dysfunction is so difficult.

evolve 6-3

More information on selected neurotransmitters that are important in psychopharmacology is available on the Evolve website.

Although the brain has many kinds of receptors with many different signaling functions, most neurotransmitter receptors can be divided into two general classes: excitatory neurotransmitter receptors and inhibitory neurotransmitter receptors. An excitatory neurotransmitter receptor may also be called a **ligand-gated channel.** In this term, *ligand* simply means a molecule (i.e., a neurotransmitter) that binds to a receptor. When neurotransmitters interact with this kind of receptor, a pore in the receptor molecule itself opens and positive or negative charges enter the cell. The entry of a positive charge may activate additional ion channels, allowing more positive charges to enter. At a certain threshold, this causes a cell to fire an *action potential,* an electrical event that ultimately leads to the release of neurotransmitter. By definition, therefore, receptors that admit a positive charge are excitatory neurotransmitter receptors. The classic excitatory neurotransmitter receptors in the brain use the excitatory amino acids glutamate and, to a lesser degree, aspartate as neurotransmitters.

Inhibitory neurotransmitters act by permitting negative charges into the cell, taking the cell farther away from firing. The classic inhibitory neurotransmitters in the brain are the amino acids gamma aminobutyric acid (GABA) and, to a lesser degree, glycine.

The interaction between excitatory and inhibitory neurotransmitters is like the control exerted on a car by using the brake and the gas pedal. The gas pedal (excitatory) accelerates and the brake (inhibitory) slows down. By working the two pedals, the driver maintains control of the car.

Most of the other neurotransmitters in the brain (e.g., dopamine, serotonin, and norepinephrine) are neither precisely excitatory nor inhibitory; rather, they produce complex biochemical changes in the receiving cell, altering the way receiving neurons can process signals from glutamate (excitatory) or GABA (inhibitory).

evolve 6-4

See the Evolve website for more information on neurotransmitters in the brain.

The neuroendocrine substances carry messages that regulate physiologic functions. Neuroendocrine regulation is a continuous, ever-changing chemical mix that fluctuates with each external and internal demand on the body to respond, adapt, or maintain a functional degree of homeostasis. The immune system also produces and responds to these communication substances. The substances that make up this "chemical soup" remain the same, but the proportion and ratio change with each regulating

Box 6-2 The Importance of Cortisol

It is important to remember that cortisol is an essential hormone. Health is threatened only when the body sustains excessively high levels of cortisol. Fibromyalgia apparently is characterized by very low levels of cortisol; when patients with fibromyalgia show improvement in symptoms, their cortisol levels inevitably are on the rise.

Modified from Reidel W, Schlapp U, Leck S et al: Blunted ACTH and cortisol responses to systemic injection of corticotropin-releasing hormone (CRH) in fibromyalgia: role of somatostatin and CRH-binding protein, *Ann NY Acad Sci* 966:483-490, 2002.

function or message transmission. The "flavor" of the soup, which is determined by the ratio of the chemical mix, affects such factors as mood, attentiveness, arousal, passiveness, vigilance, calmness, ability to sleep, receptivity to touch, response to touch, anger, pessimism, optimism, connectedness, loneliness, depression, desire, hunger, love, and commitment.

Research now indicates that most problems in behavior, mood, and the perception of stress and pain, as well as other so-called mental and emotional disorders, are caused by dysregulation or failure of the biochemical components. Problem behaviors, symptoms, and emotional and physical states often are normal chemical mixes that occur at inappropriate times (Box 6-2).

The effects of neurotransmitters that are influenced during massage may explain and validate the use of sensory stimulation methods to treat chronic pain, anxiety, and depression. Much of the research on massage, especially the research done at the University of Miami School of Medicine's Touch Research Institute* revolves around shifts brought about by massage in the proportion and ratio of the components of the body's "chemical soup."

evolve 6-5

For a more detailed discussion of some of the main neurotransmitters influenced by massage, see the Evolve website.

*Touch Research Institute, University of Miami School of Medicine, P.O. Box 016820, Miami, FL, 33101.

Therapeutic massage seems to support balance of the blood levels of these neurochemicals, which in turn facilitates the production of natural killer cells in the immune system and regulates moods. This response indicates that massage can be a beneficial component of a total treatment program for people with an illness or injury. Massage tends to increase levels of the hormone **oxytocin,** which supports feelings of connectedness. It also stimulates vagal nerve function, reduces cortisol, and regulates **epinephrine** and norepinephrine, facilitating the action of **growth hormone.** It has been well documented that a patient's emotional state influences his or her health, healing, rehabilitation, efforts to cope with pain, and ability to die gently and with dignity and peace.

THE SPINAL CORD

The **spinal cord,** a continuation of the medulla of the brain, travels through the vertebral canal from the foramen magnum to the lumbar spine. The spinal cord divides into individual spinal nerves as it exits the vertebral column through openings between the sides of the vertebrae, called the *intervertebral foramina.* Anatomically this is where the peripheral nervous system begins.

All four classes of sensory receptors (i.e., mechanoreceptors, **proprioceptors,** chemoreceptors, and **nociceptors**) send information to the spinal cord, which stimulates countless reflexive adjustments in the body to maintain homeostasis.

THE PERIPHERAL NERVOUS SYSTEM

The **peripheral nervous system (PNS)** consists of 12 pairs of cranial nerves and 31 pairs of spinal nerves. The nerves are lubricated, and the fibers, fascicles, and gross nerves are designed to slide within the connective tissue spaces and grooves. The peripheral nerves are vulnerable to compression and irritation at the nerve roots in the area of the intervertebral foramen and to entrapment, irritation, or compression in the extremities. They can become restricted or entrapped by adhesions in the connective tissue spaces or hypertonic muscles through which they travel, and this restriction prevents normal gliding of the nerve. Nerves can become compressed in fibro-osseous tunnels, such as the carpal tunnel. They also can become compressed, restricted, or irritated as a result of pressure caused by increased fluid retention and pooling caused by inflammation arising from overuse, illness, or injury. Nerve pain tends to radiate and follow traceable pathways in the body.

THE SOMATIC NERVOUS SYSTEM

The somatic sensory nerves relay information about pain, temperature, touch, and pressure from the skin to the CNS. These nerves also convey pain signals, proprioceptive information, information about movement and position, and mechanoreceptor information from the muscles, tendons, ligaments, joint capsules, and periosteum.

EPITHELIAL TISSUE

The epithelium and the nervous system derive from the same embryologic tissue, the ectoderm. The **skin,** therefore, is an extension of the nervous system. The skin is the body's largest organ; it contains blood vessels, glands, muscles, connective tissue, and nerve endings.

The skin contains four types of sensory nerve receptors, called **mechanoreceptors,** which communicate with every other part of the body. The mechanoreceptors are sensitive to touch, pressure, movement, superficial proprioception, pain, and temperature. The skin provides sensation, information, and protection; assists with water balance; and regulates temperature.

Sensory information from the skin communicates to the spinal cord, where reflex connections are made to muscles, internal organs, and blood vessels. Skin pain can cause contraction of the skeletal muscles or internal organ symptoms, and skeletal muscle and internal organs can refer pain to the skin. Massage accesses the body through the skin and sends signals (e.g., pressure, movement, and stimulation) for the body to process.

Visceral Sensation

The visceral sensory nerves, which are part of the autonomic nervous system, send pain and pressure information from the internal organs to the CNS. The visceral motor nerves transmit impulses from the autonomic nervous system to the involuntary muscles, such as those found in internal organs, and to glandular tissue.

Somatic Sensory Nerves

The **somatic motor nerves** relay information from the brain, through the spinal cord, and then to the skeletal muscles. The **somatic sensory nerves** are the principal means by which the massage therapist communicates with the body. Each touch and movement sends a message to the CNS (spinal cord and brain), which in turn communicates with every other part of the body, including the centers of the person's emotions.

Soft tissue has four basic categories of sensory nerves. The sensory receptors are:

- Mechanoreceptors, which respond to touch, pressure, and movement
- Proprioceptors, which respond to changes in position and movement
- Chemoreceptors, which are sensitive to acid-base balance, oxygen levels, and so forth
- Nociceptors, which detect irritation and pain

The main proprioceptors influenced by massage are the spindle cells and the Golgi tendon receptors. The mechanoreceptors of the skin and connective tissue are also influenced by stretching, compression, rubbing, and vibration. Stimulation of joint mechanoreceptors affects the adjacent muscles, and stimulation of the skin overlying muscle and joint structures has beneficial effects through shared innervation.

Somatic sensory nerves are specialized receptors that relay information to the CNS about four types of sensation: touch, pressure, position, and movement.

Touch and pressure originate from sensory nerve endings in the superficial and deep layers of the skin. These sensory nerves communicate light touch, deep pressure, temperature, and pain. They also respond to external information from the environment. Massage stimulation of the skin and superficial fascia is an effective means of communication with these sensors.

Proprioceptors and mechanoreceptors, which are located in the fascia, muscles, tendons, and joints, communicate information about body position and movement. Massage interacts with these receptors through muscle energy methods, active and passive movements, and various mechanical forces of bend, shear, torsion, tension, and compression. Dysfunction of these sensory nerves can be caused by irritation, inappropriate compression, and illness or injury.

Muscle Tone and Motor Tone

Muscle tone is the result of fluid pressure and tension and density in the connective tissue elements of the myofascial structure of muscle. The fluid element of muscle tone includes interstitial fluid around the cells, the fluid part of connective tissue ground substance, and the fluid in the various lymph vessels, capillaries, veins, and arteries. Muscle tone is influenced more by mechanical massage applications that target the water and ground substance component of the tissue.

Motor tone arises from motor neuron excitability and is influenced by reflexive massage applications that inhibit or stimulate motor neuron activity. The most common cause of increased motor tone is an increase in sympathetic arousal and sustained sympathetic dominance. Another cause is proactive muscle guarding after injury and nervous system damage. Both situations are common in those receiving medical care.

The basic premises of therapeutic massage to address muscle tone and motor tone are:

- To substitute a different neurologic signal stimulant to support a normal muscle resting length
- To influence muscle and motor tone by lengthening and stretching the muscles and connective tissue
- To normalize fluid dynamics
- To re-educate the muscles involved
- To stimulate neurochemical balance
- To support homeostasis

In general terms, the total sensory input to the CNS affects overall motor tone throughout the body. This is why nonphysical emotional and mental stress can lead to physical symptoms, such as headaches, digestive problems, and muscular discomfort. Massage works on many levels to reduce the symptoms that cause negative sensory input and to increase positive sensory input. This accounts for the general feeling of well-being that people usually have after receiving a massage.

Sensory Nerve Receptors of Muscle

The muscle sensory nerves respond to pain, chemical stimuli, temperature, deep pressure, muscle length and the rate of muscle length changes, and muscle tension and the rate of change in tension. Five types of sensory nerve receptors supply each muscle:

- Type 1a is a primary muscle spindle.
- Type 1b is a Golgi tendon organ (GTO).
- Type 2 is a secondary muscle spindle, including paciniform and pacinian corpuscles, which are sensitive to deep pressure.
- Type 3 are free nerve endings, which are sensitive to pain, chemicals, and temperature.
- Type 4 are nociceptors.

The two classes of sensory receptors that are particularly significant for the massage therapist are the muscle spindles and Golgi tendon organs. They detect the length and tension in the muscle and tendon, set the resting motor tone of the muscle, adjust the motor tone in a muscle for coordination and fine muscular control, and protect the muscles and joints through reflexes that contract or inhibit the muscle automatically. **Muscle spindles** are specialized muscle fibers, called *intrafusal fibers,* that are located in a fluid-filled capsule embedded within the muscle. Muscle spindles respond to slow and rapid changes of muscle length, and the secondary endings respond to slow changes in muscle length and are sensitive to deep pressure. The spindles also play a role in joint position, muscle coordination, muscular control, and muscle tone.

Because muscle spindles detect changes in muscle length, stretching a muscle increases their rate of signal discharge. The more refined the muscle's function, the greater the concentration of spindles. The greatest concentration of spindles is found in the lumbrical muscles of the hand, the suboccipital muscles, and the muscles that move the eyes.

States of anxiety or emotional or psychological tension can increase the firing rate of the spindle cells. As a result, the muscle tone is "set" too high, causing hypertonicity and stiffness. The firing rate can be slowed, causing the muscle to relax (i.e., a decrease in motor tone), in three ways:

- By reducing the muscle length by bringing the proximal and distal attachments toward each other
- By contracting a muscle isometrically (e.g., contract and relax methods), which causes the spindle activity to stop temporarily, allowing the muscle to be set to a new, more relaxed length
- By applying inhibitory compression in the belly of the muscle to slow firing

Golgi tendon organs are sensory receptors in the form of a slender capsule located along the muscle fiber at the **musculotendinous junction.** GTOs sense changes in muscle tension and fire during minute changes in tension. They serve a protective function by preventing damage to a muscle being forcefully contracted. Discharge of the GTO stimulates nerves at the spinal cord (i.e., inhibitory interneurons), causing the muscle to relax.

Abnormal firing of the Golgi tendon organs can set the resting tone of the muscle too high, creating hypertonicity. GTO firing can be influenced in two ways.

- Muscle energy methods can reset the muscle to its resting length and tone, but the exact mechanism by which this occurs is not fully understood. When a muscle voluntarily contracts isometrically, GTO discharges increase, which has an inhibiting effect on the muscle, causing it to relax.
- Inhibiting compression at the tendons also can reduce GTO activity.
- Using one or both of these methods seems to increase the tissue's tolerance to being stretched and supporting a normalization in motor tone.

Dysfunction of soft tissue (muscle and connective tissue) without proprioceptive hyperactivity or hypoactivity is uncommon. Proprioceptive hyperactivity is believed to cause tense or spastic muscles and hypoactivity of opposing muscle groups.

Massage Application. Deep, broad-based massage has a minimal and short-term inhibitory effect on the motor tone of muscle caused by motor neuron activity. This type of massage is used primarily to support a muscle re-education process (e.g., therapeutic exercise) or to reduce motor tone temporarily so that muscle firing patterns can be reset or more mechanical methods can address tissue shortening without causing muscle spasm. Active movements of the body, using techniques such as active assisted joint movement, and/or active muscle contraction and release used during muscle energy methods of tense and relax, reciprocal inhibition, and combined methods of positional release seem to improve motor function by interacting with proprioceptive function.

CHEMORECEPTORS

As mentioned earlier, **chemoreceptors** are sensory receptors that are sensitive to the acid-base balance, oxygen levels, and other factors. Chemoreceptors are irritated when the body is inflamed and when a muscle is in a sustained contraction, which reduces the amount of oxygen in the tissue. The decrease in oxygen content interacts with fibroblasts, mast cells, and other cells to create a neurogenic inflammatory response, called *neurogenic pain.* Massage may purposely use controlled, focused pain to release pain-inhibiting chemicals. Tension in the soft tissues or the stress response can cause overactivity of the sympathetic nervous system. By reducing soft tissue tension, massage can help restore balance and stimulate the parasympathetic system, resulting in a positive effect on both minor and sometimes quite major medical conditions, such as high blood pressure, migraine, insomnia, and digestive disorders.

The usual outcome of reflexive massage that targets neurochemical mechanisms is inhibitory and antiarousal. Antiarousal massage (i.e., relaxation massage) may influence motor tone activity in the same way that pharmaceutical muscle relaxers do, because the main cause of motor tone difficulties is sympathetic arousal.

ARCHIE 6-1 The Vestibular Apparatus and Cerebellum

The **vestibular apparatus** is a complex system composed of sensors in the inner ear (vestibular labyrinth), upper neck (cervical proprioception), eyes (visual motion and three dimensional orientation), and body (somatic proprioception). Information from these sensors is processed in several areas of the brain (i.e., the brainstem, cerebellum, and parietal and temporal cortex). The reflexes associated with the sensory receptors affect the eyes (vestibulo-ocular reflexes), neck (vestibulocollic reflexes), and balance (vestibulospinal reflexes) by sending and receiving information simultaneously about how we are oriented to the environment around us. Many amusement park rides create disorienting sensations that contribute to the effects of the ride.

The vestibular apparatus and the cerebellum are interrelated. Output from the **cerebellum** goes to the motor cortex and the **brainstem.** Stimulation of the cerebellum by means of a change in motor tone, position, and vestibular balance stimulates the hypothalamus to adjust functions to restore homeostasis. This is the point of complex processing of sensory information, and the results of effective mechanical and reflexive massage methods can overlap, making it difficult to determine the mode of effect.

Massage Application. The massage techniques that most strongly affect the vestibular apparatus and therefore the cerebellum are those that produce rhythmic oscillation, including rocking. Rocking produces movement at the neck and head that influences the sense of equilibrium. Rocking stimulates the inner ear balance mechanisms, including the vestibular nuclear complex and the labyrinthine righting reflexes, to keep the head level. Stimulation of these reflexes produces a body-wide effect involving muscle contraction patterns.

Massage can alter body positional sense and the position of the eyes in response to postural change. It can initiate a specific movement pattern that changes sensory input from muscles, tendons, joints, and the skin and stimulates various vestibular reflexes. This feedback information, which adjusts and coordinates movement, is relayed directly to the motor cortex and the cerebellum, allowing the body to integrate the sensory data and adjust to a more efficient postural balance and optimal movement strategies.

If massage application involves vestibular influences, short-term nausea and dizziness can occur while the mechanisms rebalance. The use of massage to restore appropriate muscle activation pattern sequences and gait reflexes is valuable. Influencing the balance of the various force couples in the body can shift the relationship of the eyes, neck, hips, and so on, as well as influencing positional balance, mobility, and agility.

Nerve Impingement

Soft tissue often impinges upon nerves. Tissues that can bind are skin, fascia, muscles, ligaments, joint structures, and bones. An increase in fluid in an area can cause nerve impingement. Shortened muscles and connective tissue (fascia) often impinge upon major and minor nerves, causing discomfort. Tissues that are long and taut can also cause impingement.

The specific nerve root, trunk, or division affected determines the resultant condition (e.g., thoracic outlet syndrome, sciatica, or carpal tunnel syndrome).

The Cervical Plexus. With impingement upon the cervical plexus, a person experiences headaches, neck pain, and breathing difficulties. The muscles most responsible for pressure on the cervical plexus are the suboccipital and sternocleidomastoid muscles. Shortened connective tissues at the cranial base also can press on these nerves.

The cervical plexus is formed by the ventral rami of the upper four cervical nerves. The phrenic nerve, which is part of this plexus, innervates the diaphragm, therefore any disruption of this nerve affects breathing. Many cutaneous (skin) branches of the cervical plexus transmit sensory impulses from the skin of the neck, ear, and shoulder. The motor branches innervate muscles of the anterior neck (Figure 6-1, *A*).

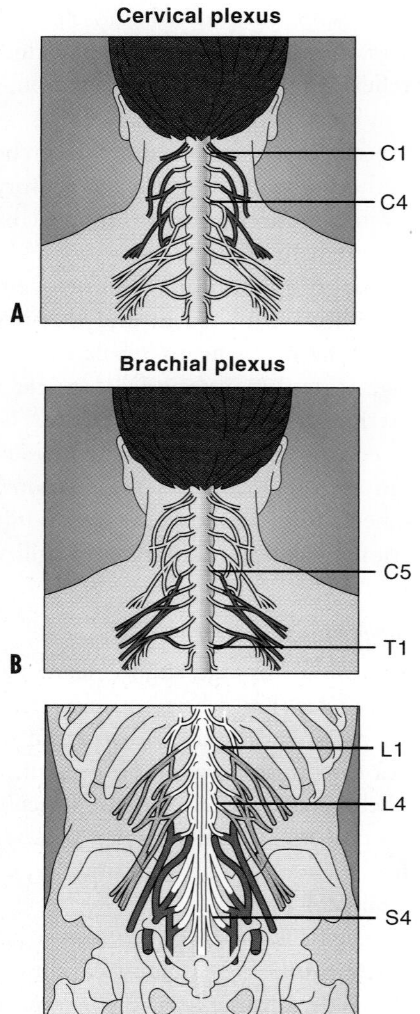

FIGURE 6-1 ■ **A,** The cervical plexus. **B,** The brachial plexus. **C,** The lumbosacral plexus. (From Thibodeau GA, Patton KT: *Anatomy and physiology,* ed 5, St Louis, 2003, Mosby.)

The Brachial Plexus. The brachial plexus, situated partly in the neck and partly in the axilla, provides virtually all the nerves that innervate the upper limb. Any imbalance that brings pressure on this complex of nerves results in shoulder pain, chest pain, arm pain, wrist pain, and hand pain.

The muscles that most often are responsible for impingement upon the brachial plexus are the scalenes, pectoralis minor, and subclavius. Muscles of the arm occasionally impinge upon branches of the brachial plexus. Brachial plexus impingement is responsible for thoracic outlet symptoms (such as pain in the shoulder and numbness in fingers), which often are misdiagnosed as carpal tunnel syndrome. Whiplash injury involves the brachial plexus (Figure 6-1, *B*).

The Lumbar Plexus. Lumbar plexus nerve impingement may cause low back discomfort with a belt-like distribution of pain, as well as pain in the lower abdomen, genitals, thigh, and medial lower leg. The main muscles that impinge upon the lumbar plexus are the quadratus lumborum and the psoas. Shortening of the lumbar dorsal fascia exaggerates a lordosis and causes vertebral impingement upon the lumbar plexus (Figure 6-1, *C*).

The Sacral Plexus. The sacral plexus has approximately a dozen named branches. Almost half of these serve the buttock and lower limb; the others innervate pelvic structures. The main branch is the sciatic nerve. Impingement upon this nerve by the piriformis muscle can cause sciatica.

Ligaments that stabilize the sacroiliac joint can affect the sacral plexus. Pressure on the sacral plexus can cause gluteal pain, leg pain, genital pain, and foot pain.

Massage Application. Therapeutic massage techniques work in many ways to reduce pressure on nerves. Primarily, they:

- Reflexively change the tension pattern of short muscles and lengthen them
- Mechanically stretch and soften connective tissue
- Reduce localized edema
- Interrupt the pain-spasm-pain cycle caused by protective muscle spasms that occur in response to pain
- Support the effectiveness of therapeutic exercise to shift posture and function
- Support the use of medications such as antispasmodics, analgesics, antiinflammatories, and circulation enhancers (e.g., vasodilators).

THE AUTONOMIC NERVOUS SYSTEM

The **autonomic nervous system (ANS)** innervates the heart, blood vessels, diaphragm, internal organs, and endocrine glands. It influences every other part of the body, including the muscular system. The ANS has two main divisions, the sympathetic nervous system and the parasympathetic nervous system (Table 6-1).

The Sympathetic Nervous System

The **sympathetic nervous system** is responsible for the fight-or-flight response, excitement, anticipation, and performance. It is active when a person is under stress. It releases adrenaline into the bloodstream, causes constriction of the peripheral blood vessels, increases the heart rate, and inhibits normal movement of the intestines so that the blood is available to the skeletal muscles. When a person is under stress, the motor tone of the muscles increases because of the effects of the sympathetic nervous system. This process uses energy, and if the pattern is not reversed, fatigue can occur. Stress can lead to sympathetic dominance and a collection of problems such as breathing disorder, slowed healing, emotional agitation, digestive upset, and sleep disturbance, to name a few.

The Parasympathetic Nervous System

The **parasympathetic nervous system** is responsible for energy building, food digestion, and assimilation. It functions to restore homeostasis and is active when the body is at rest and recuperating. It causes a decrease in the heart rate, stimulates the normal peristaltic smooth muscle movement of the intestines, and promotes the secretion of all digestive juices and tropic (tissue building) hormones. A person can be in parasympathetic override (dominance), which would contribute to lethargy, loss of normal motivation, and depression.

Many people have an underactive parasympathetic nervous system and an overactive sympathetic nervous system. One of the primary benefits of massage that is given in a relaxing manner is the stimulation of the parasympathetic nervous system. This induces a state of relaxation and promotes the healing and rejuvenation functions of the parasympathetic nervous system, which supports homeostasis.

SENSITIZATION OF THE NEUROENDOCRINE FUNCTION

The term *sensitization* is used to describe the nervous system phenomenon characterized by an exaggerated response to normal stimuli. Sensitization is common in chronic pain conditions, and it has two principal causes.

- The limbic areas of the brain can cause an emotional exaggeration of pain, which can trigger the CNS to cause the muscles to become either too tight or too loose. Concurrent stimulation of the hypothalamus alters endocrine function. This emotional exaggeration is caused by many factors, including culture, family history, pain history, and individual psychology.
- The area in the spinal cord that receives information about pain is next to the receptive field for movement. Chronic inflammation can cause sensitization of the mechanoreceptors so that normal mechanical stimuli cause the mechanoreceptor to be a pain producer.

Sensitization perpetuates pain patterns, chronic pain, and lingering pain after illness and injury. Massage applied over time may alter these pathways, reducing chronic pain sensations.

EMOTIONAL STATES/NEUROENDOCRINE FUNCTION AND MASSAGE

The body tissues form a unified whole, and each tissue not only influences all other tissues, but also affects the person's emotions and psychological state. Massage affects the ANS, which regulates breathing, blood flow, heart rate, respiration, neurotransmitters, and endocrine functions, all physiologic aspects of emotion.

The emotional roller coaster of living and the physical and emotional effects of trauma, recurring illness, injury, pain, and fatigue all have a psychological impact that can manifest as part of traumatic stress syndrome and state-dependent memory.

The sensory input during massage may trigger a memory pattern of an emotionally charged

TABLE 6-1 Sympathetic and Parasympathetic Effects

Organ Response	Parasympathetic System Response	Sympathetic System Response
Sweat glands	No response at this time	Secretion increased
Arrector pili muscle	No response at this time	Contraction, erection of hairs
Skeletal muscles	No response at this time	Contraction force increased
Radial muscle of iris	No response at this time	Contraction (pupils dilate)
Sphincter muscles of iris	Contraction (pupils constrict)	None identified
Ciliary muscle	Contraction (lenses bulge for near vision)	
Lacrimal (tear) glands	Secretion	None identified
Heart	Heart rate and contraction force decreased	Heart rate and contraction force increased; vasodilation of coronary vessels
Blood vessels	No response at this time	Constriction
Blood coagulation	No response	Coagulation increased
Bronchial muscles	Contraction	Relaxation
Salivary glands	Mucus secretion	Watery, serous secretion
Intestinal motility and tone	Increased	Decreased
Sphincters	Relaxation	Contraction
Digestive secretions	Stimulation	Possible inhibition
Liver	Glycogen synthesis	Glycogen breakdown; glucose synthesis and release
Pancreas	Increased secretion of exocrine and endocrine (insulin)	Exocrine secretion decreased
Kidney	Urine production increased	Urine production decreased
Detrusor muscle	Contraction	Relaxation
Sphincter	Relaxation	Contraction
Mental	Calm	Alertness increased

event. Each memory, including all the sensory information, nervous system functions, and endocrine functions in play at the time of the experience, is stored in a multidimensional way. When the body state changes, the memory becomes vague and less clear. Because massage produces changes in the nervous and endocrine systems and is a source of sensory stimulation, a state that holds a memory pattern for a patient can be altered. This may help a person resolve and integrate a past experience, provided appropriate mental health professional support is available.

Often only pieces of a memory are retrieved, as is common with body memories. The massage may trigger a physiologic response, yet no visual or sequential memory is retrievable. Compassion is required to support the patient during these times. No verbal interaction is necessary. Referral to a psychiatrist or psychologist may be necessary. Addressing the neurochemical aspect of the body-mind interaction is necessary for physical and emotional healing.

Excessive sympathetic output causes most of the stress-related diseases and dysfunction, such as headaches, gastrointestinal difficulties, high blood pressure, anxiety, muscle tension and aches, and sexual dysfunction.

Long-term stress (i.e., stress that cannot be resolved by fleeing or fighting) may also trigger the release of **cortisol,** a hormone manufactured by the body. Long-term high blood levels of cortisol cause side effects similar to those of the drug cortisone, including fluid retention, hypertension, muscle weakness, osteoporosis, breakdown of connective tissue, peptic ulcer, impaired wound healing, vertigo, headache, reduced ability to deal with stress, hypersensitivity, weight gain, nausea, fatigue, and psychic disturbances.

Physical and tactile measures are effective for reducing arousal and promoting self-regulation and therefore result in the perception of comfort. Pleasure is an important experience in health and healing. Pain causes muscular contraction, withdrawal, abrupt movement, breath holding, an increased heart rate, and an increased generalized stress response. The perception of pain is heightened by psychological states such as anxiety and depression. Low self-esteem and apprehension reduce pain tolerance.

Pleasure can counteract the pain response. Massage provides pleasurable sensation. Pleasurable pain often accompanies massage application. Pain sensation generated by manual techniques needs to result in pleasurable outcomes and should never be sharp, bruising, or tearing.

Emotional states such as anticipation, anxiety, anger, depression, and tension usually result in increased muscular motor tone, whereas relaxed states supported by pleasure sensation produce a reduction in muscular motor tone. These responses are modulated by the limbic system. Applications of touch that are perceived as pleasurable usually are sedating and parasympathetic in nature. The initial adaptation to touch and touch perceived as uncomfortable, aggressive, and nonproductive increase sympathetic arousal.

These pleasurable factors during massage are crucial to the support of a patient recovering from illness or injury. One of the biggest mistakes massage therapists make is undervaluing this aspect of massage. Often the massage application is too aggressive and painful, based on the misconception that "medical massage" is "deep tissue" massage (whatever that is). This is not necessarily so. The correct technique depends on the desired outcome and the individual situation.

Because of its generalized effect on the ANS and associated functions, massage can cause changes in mood and excitement levels and can induce the relaxation/restoration response. Massage seems to be a gentle modulator, producing feelings of general well-being and comfort. The pleasure aspect of massage supports these outcomes. The emotional arousal often found in the healthcare environment also is favorably influenced.

Initially, massage stimulates sympathetic functions. The increase in autonomic sympathetic arousal is followed by a decrease if the massage is slowed and sustained with sufficient pleasurable pressure and lasts about 45 to 50 minutes. The pressure levels must be relatively deep and broad based but not painful. Slow, repetitive stroking, broad-based compression, rhythmic oscillation, and movement all initiate relaxation responses. Sufficient pressure applied with a compressive force to the tissues supports serotonin functions and vagal nerve tone. Compression and a fast-paced massage style stimulate sympathetic responses and may lift depression temporarily.

Point holding, such as acupressure or reflexology, releases the body's own painkillers and mood-altering chemicals. These chemicals stimulate the parasympathetic responses of relaxation, restoration, and contentment. These massage methods depend on the creation of a moderate, controlled, acute pain to relieve chronic pain. A greater pain or stress stimulus than the existing perceived pain is required to generate the endorphin response. When the release of substance P triggers pain, **enkephalins** are released, which suppress the pain signal. A negative feedback system activates the release of serotonin and endogenous opiates, which inhibit pain. Therapeutic massage methods can be used to create a controlled, noxious (pain) stimulation that triggers this cycle. Patients often refer to this noxious stimulation as "good pain."

Altering the muscles so that they are more or less tense, or changing the consistency of the connective tissue, affects the ANS through the feedback loop, which in turn affects the powerful body-mind phenomenon.

ENTRAINMENT

Entrainment is the coordination of synchronization to a rhythm. It is an important reflexive effect that seems to be processed through both the ANS and the CNS. You might ask, What body rhythms are entrained, what difference does it make, and how does massage influence entrainment?

Biologic oscillators, such as the heart rate/respiratory rate/thalamus synchronization, combine to support the entrainment process, and the other, subtler body rhythms follow. A synaptic traveling wave results in neural rhythmic synchronization. Synchronization of the rhythms of the heart, respiration, and digestion promotes this balance (i.e., homeostasis) to support a healthy body.

A balance between the sympathetic and parasympathetic divisions of the ANS influences the sinus node of the heart and the **vascular system,** which in turn modulates the heart rate and blood pressure. Our nasal reflexes, stimulated by the movement of air through the nose, rhythmically interact with the heart, lungs, and diaphragm. Thus the entire body is affected because biologic rhythms are interconnected.

The CNS includes a series of rhythms classified by frequency: alpha, beta, gamma, and theta. The effects of massage on these particular rhythms are the subject of current speculation. Entrainment methods that synchronize the motions and rhythms of the body could provide benefit, because these rhythms are associated with sensory processing and cognitive states. Traube-Hering-Mayer waves (THM oscillations) are another factor. These are rhythmic variations in blood pressure that occur at 6 to 10 cycles per minute. THM oscillations can be felt all over the body. Many experts wonder whether these oscillations are the mechanisms upon which craniosacral therapy and biofield/energetic modulations are based. We do know that THM oscillations are interrelated with ANS function.

The body also entrains to external rhythms. Any activity that uses a repetitive motion or sound, depending on its rhythmic speed or pace, quiets or excites the nervous system through entrainment and thereby alters the physiologic process of the body. Sometimes the body rhythms are disrupted. Music and discord can be disruptive, as can multiple rhythms out of sync in the same environment. This can be seen in hectic, noisy healthcare environments. People (patients, family, and medical staff) become fatigued or "out of sorts" in these disharmonic environments.

When a person experiences positive emotional states, the biologic rhythms naturally tend to begin to oscillate together, or *entrain.* To encourage entrainment, massage is provided in a quiet, rhythmic manner. The rhythmic application of massage and the proximity of a centered, compassionate professional's breathing rate and heart rate can support restorative entrainment if body rhythms are out of sync. Focused, centered professionals introduce their own ordered rhythms as part of the environment. They serve as an additional external influence that enables the patient's body rhythms to synchronize. Oscillation, in the form of rhythmic rocking that affects the vestibular mechanism, has an antiarousal effect. When synchronization occurs, homeostatic mechanisms seem to work more efficiently.

THE GATE CONTROL THEORY

In 1965 Melzack and Wall proposed the **gate control theory.** Although some aspects of the original theory have been modified over the past 40-plus years, the basic premise remains viable. According to this theory, a gating mechanism functions at the level of the spinal cord. Pain impulses pass through a "gate" to reach the lateral spinothalamic system. Pain impulses are transmitted by large-diameter and small-diameter nerve fibers. Stimulation of large-diameter fibers prevents the small-diameter fibers from transmitting signals. Stimulation of large-diameter fibers (e.g., through rubbing and massage) helps suppress the sensation of pain, especially sharp or visceral pain.

Hyperstimulation Analgesia

Various massage methods, including pressure, positioning, and lengthening, stimulate the large-diameter nerve fibers at sufficient intensity to activate the gating mechanism and produce **hyperstimulation analgesia.**

Tactile stimulation produced by massage travels through the large-diameter fibers, which also carry a faster signal. In essence, massage sensations win the race to the brain, and the pain sensations are blocked because the gate is closed. Stimulating techniques, such as percussion or vibration of painful areas to activate stimulation-produced analgesia (i.e., hyperstimulation analgesia), also are effective. Pain management in healthcare is essential, therefore these methods are beneficial.

Pain sensation may be reduced by manual analgesia. This can be done by stimulating the sensory gating achieved when multiple sensations are processed at the same time. The reflexology (foot massage) benefit seems to be mediated by hyperstimulation analgesia.

Counterirritation

Counterirritation is a superficial irritation that relieves some irritation of deeper structures. Counterirritation may be explained by the gate control theory. Inhibition of central sensory pathways, produced by rubbing or oscillating (shaking) an area, may explain counterirritation.

All methods of massage can be used to produce counterirritation. Any massage method that introduces a controlled sensory stimulation intense enough to be interpreted by the patient as "good pain" will work to create counterirritation.

Massage therapy in many forms stimulates the skin over an area of discomfort. Techniques that exert friction on the skin and underlying tissue to cause reddening are effective. Many therapeutic ointments contain cooling and warming agents and mild caustic substances (capsicum), which are useful for muscle and joint pain. This is also a form of counterirritation.

ENERGY SYSTEMS

Some methods of massage, especially the more subtle energetic approaches, have not yet been researched enough to be scientifically validated. The effectiveness of various kinds of hands-on bodywork may arise from the entrainment of electrical and magnetic rhythms from therapist to patient.

These methods, based on the subtle electrical energy of the body, have been around for eons. Most ancient healing practices are based on the interaction with these subtle energy fields (Figure 6-2). The concept of the vibratory nature of these bodywork approaches is intriguing. It should not be discounted because science has yet to validate eons of experiential evidence. We cannot measure compassion and respect with the scientific method either, but we know they exist. It has been my experience that individuals in healthcare are very sensitive to and accepting of these methods as long as they are presented in a nonmystical way and applied matter of factly.

Intention and Energy Medicine

Wayne B. Jonas and Cindy C. Crawford present an exhaustive look at the topic of intention and energy healing in their book, *Healing, Intention and Energy Medicine Science: Research Methods and Clinical Implications.** After reviewing more than 2200 published reports, they concluded that evidence suggests that the mind can influence matter and that mental intention is a component of healing practices. The mechanisms of these processes are not yet understood, and more research is needed.

Intention. As used in this text, *intention* is an outcome that is expected or that guides planned actions. Other definitions are:

- What one intends to do or achieve: aim, ambition, design, end, goal†
- Intent, intentionality; purpose‡
- Uses, especially when we speak of purpose, aim, meaning, and the like§
- Action that one intends to follow; an aim that guides action; an objective||

Energy Medicine. The International Society for the Study of Subtle Energies and Energy Medicine (ISSSEEM), an interdisciplinary organization that focuses on the study of the basic sciences and medical and therapeutic applications of subtle energies, defines energy medicine as follows:

> Energy medicine includes all energetic and informational interactions resulting from self-regulation or brought about through other energy linkages to mind and body. In addition to various therapeutic energies which we may use, there are also energy pulses from the environment which influence humans and animals in a variety of ways.

*Jonas WB, Crawford CC: *Healing, intention and energy medicine science: research methods and clinical implications,* 2003 Churchill Livingstone.

†Rogets II: *The new thesaurus,* ed 3, 1995.

‡Mawson, C.O. Sylvester: *Roget's international thesaurus of English words and phrases,* 1992.

§*The Columbia guide to standard American English,* 1993.

||*The American Heritage dictionary of the English language,* ed 4, 2000.

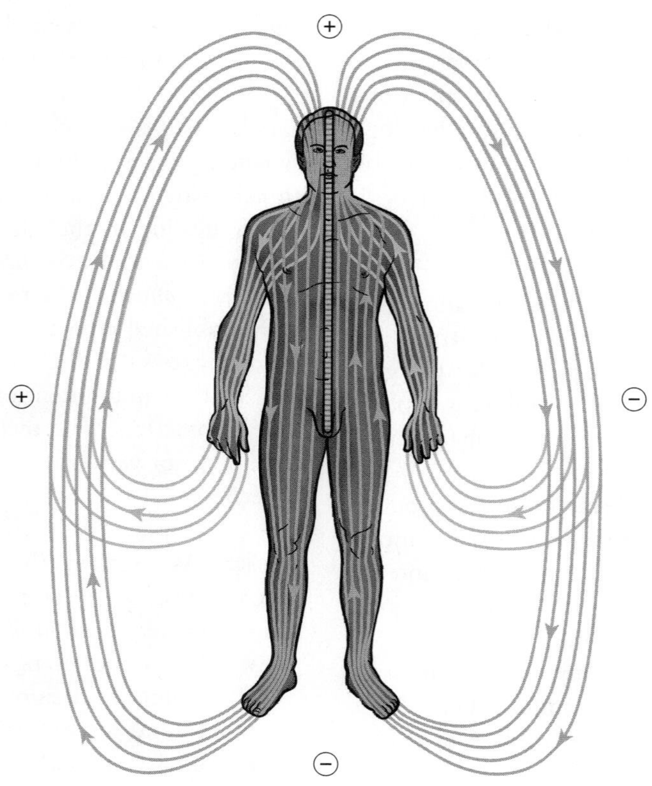

FIGURE 6-2 ■ Electromagnetic currents traveling vertically on the body. (From Fritz S: *Mosby's fundamentals of therapeutic massage,* ed 3, St Louis, 2004, Mosby.)

For instance, low-level changes in magnetic, electric, electromagnetic, acoustic, and gravitational fields often have profound effects on both biology and psychology. In addition to energies originating in the environment, it has been documented that humans are capable of generating and controlling subtle, not-yet-measurable energies that seem to influence both physiological and physical mechanisms.

Subtle energies, compared with 'energy medicine,' is a concept more difficult to define within the current scientific paradigm. Ancient and modern wisdom traditions describe human bioenergies referred to by many names (e.g., chi, ki, prana, etheric energy, fohat, orgone, odic force, mana, homeopathic resonance) that are believed to move throughout the so-called 'etheric' (or subtle) energy body and thus are difficult to measure using conventional instrumentation. In addition, many of the complementary and alternative therapies that are becoming increasingly popular appear to involve the flow of these subtle energies through the dense physical body. In addition, it is traditionally accepted that expansions of consciousness often are related to changes in subtle energies that cannot be quantified. These latter 'energies,' which are said to be associated with interactions and with transcendence, may not, in fact, actually be involved with known physical fields.

Various energy systems overlap in application to support energy, flow, balance, and harmony by tapping, massaging, pinching, twisting, or connecting specific energy points on the skin; by tracing or swirling the hand over the skin along specific energy pathways; by exercises or postures designed for specific energetic effects; by focused use of the mind to move specific energies; and by surrounding an area with healing energies (one person's energies affect the energies of another).

The key to effectiveness in all systems is intention. The prudent massage therapist is clear about the intention of the massage provided and realizes that some interaction among the various energy mechanisms probably is at work when a compassionate, skilled therapist touches another person in a therapeutic way.

FLUID DYNAMICS

The human body is approximately 70% water. This water is named by the tubes or compartments that contain it. Fluids include the blood in the vessels and heart, lymph in the lymph vessels, synovial fluid in the joint capsules and bursa sacs, cerebrospinal fluid in the nervous system, and the interstitial fluid that surrounds all soft tissue cells. Water is found inside all cells (intracellular fluid). Water is bound with glycoproteins in connective tissue ground substance. The amount of water in connective tissue helps to determine the tissue's consistency, pliability, and density.

Water in the body is moved in waves by pumps, which include the heart, the respiratory diaphragm, the smooth muscle of the vascular and lymph systems, and rhythmic movements of muscles and fascia. Water moves along the path of least resistance from high pressure to low pressure and flows downhill with gravity. Water moves at different speeds, depending on other variables. The properties of water must be considered in the application of massage methods.

Water is a constituent of all living things and often is referred to as the universal biologic solvent. It also serves to minimize temperature changes throughout the body. Box 6-3 lists the many important functions of water in the body.

The water content of the body tissues varies. Adipose tissue (fat) has the lowest percentage of water; the skeleton has the second lowest water content. Skeletal muscle, skin, and blood are among the tissues that have the highest water content (Table 6-2).

The total water content of the body decreases most dramatically during the first 10 years and continues to decline through old age, at which time water content may be only 45% of total body weight. Men tend to have a higher percentage of water (about 65%) than women (about 55%), mainly because of their increased muscle mass and smaller amount of subcutaneous fat.

Water is in a constant state of motion inside the body, shifting between the two major fluid compartments, the lymphatic system and the cir-

BOX 6-3 Functions of Water in the Human Body

- Provides a medium for chemical reactions
- Functions as a crucial factor in the regulation of chemical and bioelectric distributions with cells
- Transports substances such as hormones and nutrients
- Aids oxygen transport from body cells to the lungs
- Aids carbon dioxide transport from body cells to the lungs
- Dilutes toxic substances and waste products and transports them to the kidneys and the liver
- Distributes heat around the body

From Fritz S: *Sports & exercise massage: comprehensive care in athletics, physical fitness, & rehabilitation,* St Louis, 2006, Mosby.

TABLE 6-2 Percentage of Water in Body Tissues

Tissue	Percentage of Water
Blood	83.0
Kidneys	82.7
Heart	79.2
Lungs	79.0
Spleen	75.8
Muscle	75.6
Brain	74.8
Intestines	74.5
Skin	72.0
Liver	68.3
Skeleton	22.0
Adipose tissue	10.0

From Fritz S: *Mosby's essential sciences for therapeutic massage: anatomy, physiology, biomechanics, and pathology,* ed 2, St Louis, 2004, Mosby.

culatory system. Water is continuously lost from and taken into the body. In a normal, healthy person, water input equals water output. Maintaining this balance is of prime importance in maintaining health. Approximately 90% of water intake occurs via the gastrointestinal tract (i.e., food and liquids). The remaining 10%, called *metabolic water,* is produced by various chemical reactions in tissue cells. Table 6-3 shows the routes by which a normal, healthy adult loses water.

The amount of water lost via the kidneys is under hormonal control. The average amount of water lost and consumed per day by a healthy adult is around 2.5 L (about $4^1/_4$ pints). Perspiration lost during exercise increases water loss and requires increased water consumption.

The walls of the blood vessels form a barrier to the free passage of fluid between interstitial areas and blood plasma. In the **capillaries,** these walls are only one cell thick. Capillary walls generally are permeable to water and small solutes but impermeable to large organic molecules, such as proteins. Blood plasma tends to have a higher concentration of these molecules than does the interstitial fluid. Water from the blood moves through the capillary walls into spaces around the cells, becoming interstitial fluid. Much of the interstitial fluid is taken up by the lymphatic system and eventually finds its way back into the bloodstream. Increased interstitial fluid is a common form of edema. Lymphatic drainage massage methods support movement of interstitial fluid into the lymph capillaries.

TABLE 6-3 Water Loss from the Body in Healthy Adults

Organs	Mode of Loss	Percentage of Loss
Kidneys	Urine	62
Skin	Diffusion and sweat	19
Lungs	Water vapor	13
Gastrointestinal tract	Feces	6

From Fritz S: *Mosby's essential sciences for therapeutic massage: anatomy, physiology, biomechanics, and pathology,* ed 2, St Louis, 2004, Mosby.

Water and small solutes (e.g., sodium, potassium, and calcium) can be exchanged freely between the blood plasma and the interstitial fluid. The action of the kidneys on the blood regulates these **electrolytes.** This exchange depends mainly on the hydrostatic and osmotic forces of these fluid compartments.

Force exerted by water, called **hydrostatic pressure,** is caused by the weight of water pushing against a surface, such as a dam in a river or the wall of a blood vessel. The pressure of blood in the capillaries serves as a major hydrostatic force in the human body. The capillary hydrostatic pressure is a filtration force, because the pressure of the fluid is higher at the arterial end of the capillary than at the venous end. The pressure of the interstitial fluid is negative (−5 mm Hg), because the lymphatic system continuously takes up the excess fluid forced out of the capillaries.

Osmotic pressure is the attraction of water to large molecules, such as proteins. Because proteins are more abundant in the blood vessels than outside them, the concentration of proteins in the blood tends to attract water from the interstitial space. Overall, near equilibrium exists between fluid forced out of the capillaries and the fluid reabsorbed, because the lymphatic system collects the excess fluid forced out at the arterial end and eventually drains it back into the veins at the base of the neck.

A similar situation exists with the interstitial fluid and the intracellular fluid, although ion pumps and carriers complicate the process. Generally, water movement is substantial in both directions; however, the movement of ions (e.g., potassium, calcium, and sodium) is restricted and depends on active transport via pumps. Nutrients and oxygen, because they are dissolved in water, move passively into cells while waste products and carbon dioxide move out.

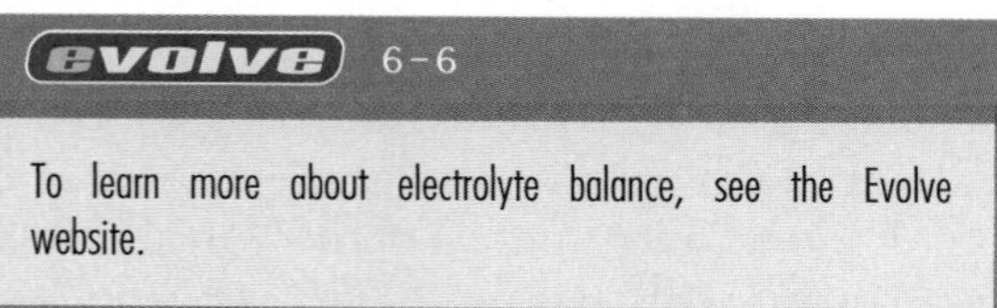
evolve 6-6

To learn more about electrolyte balance, see the Evolve website.

REGULATING FLUID BALANCE

The mechanisms for regulating body fluids are centered in the hypothalamus. The hypothalamus also receives input from the digestive tract that helps to control thirst. Antidiuretic hormone (ADH) regulates body fluid volume and extracellular osmosis. ADH influences many processes in the body. For example, one of its major functions is to increase the permeability of the collecting tubules in the kidneys, which allows more water to be reabsorbed in the kidneys. If the body lacks fluid intake, such as during sleep or heavy exercise, the result is a concentrated, darker urine of reduced volume. Absence of ADH occurs when a person is overhydrated. The urine is dilute, pale, or colorless and of high volume.

Primary factors in the triggering of ADH production are osmoreceptors and baroreceptors (pressure receptors). Secondary factors are stress, pain, hypoxia, and severe exercise.

Dehydration arises from water loss or lack of fluid intake; in relative dehydration, the body loses no overall water content but gains sodium ions, which stimulates osmoreceptors.

The thirst response is connected to the osmoreceptors. How the response actually works is not yet completely understood. Moistening of the mucosal lining of the mouth and pharynx seems to initiate some sort of neurologic response, which sends a message to the thirst center of the hypothalamus. Perhaps more important, stretch receptors in the gastrointestinal tract also appear to transmit nerve messages to the thirst center of the hypothalamus that inhibit the thirst response.

Changes in the circulating volume of body fluid also stimulate ADH secretion, resulting in an increase or a decrease in the internal pressure monitored by baroreceptors.

An 8% to 10% reduction in the normal body volume of water as a result of hemorrhage or excess perspiration causes ADH secretion. Pressure receptors in the **atria** of the heart and the pulmonary artery and vein relay messages to the hypothalamus via the vagus nerve.

pH BALANCE

pH is a measurement of the hydrogen concentration of a solution. Lower pH values indicate a higher hydrogen concentration, or higher acidity. Higher pH values indicate a lower hydrogen concentration, or higher alkalinity. The hydrogen ion balance, therefore, often is referred to as the *pH balance* or *acid-base balance.* Hydrogen ion regulation in the fluid compartments of the body is critical to health. Even a slight change in the hydrogen ion concentration can result in a significant alteration in the rate of chemical reactions. Changes in the hydrogen ion concentration also can affect the distribution of ions such as sodium, potassium, and calcium, as well as the structure and function of proteins.

The normal pH of arterial blood is 7.4, and the normal pH of venous blood is 7.35. The lower pH of venous blood is the result of its higher concentration of carbon dioxide, which dissolves in water to make a weak acid called *carbonic acid.* When the pH changes in the arterial blood, two conditions may result: acidosis or alkalosis. **Acidosis** occurs when the hydrogen ion concentration of the arterial blood increases and therefore the pH decreases. **Alkalosis** occurs when the hydrogen ion concentration in the arterial blood decreases and the pH increases. As in overbreathing, in which excessive carbon dioxide is lost, this results in reduced carbonic acid levels.

Sources of hydrogen ions in the body include carbonic acid (formed as previously mentioned), sulfuric acid (a byproduct of the breakdown of proteins), phosphoric acid (a byproduct of protein and phospholipid metabolism), ketone bodies (from fat metabolism), and lactic acid (a product formed in skeletal muscle during exercise).

About half of all the acid formed by or introduced into the body is neutralized by the ingestion of alkaline foods. (The Evolve website presents more information on this topic.) The remaining acid is neutralized by three mechanisms: chemical buffers, the respiratory system, and the kidneys.

evolve 6-7

The Evolve website provides more information on pH balance and fluid dynamics.

CLINICAL PROBLEMS WITH FLUID BALANCE

The fluid balance of the body can be upset in many ways, resulting in severe problems and even death.

Dehydration

Dehydration obviously occurs in conditions in which water is unavailable (Figure 6-3). However, conditions such as diarrhea, severe vomiting, excessive sweating, bleeding, and surgical removal of body fluids also can result in dehydration.

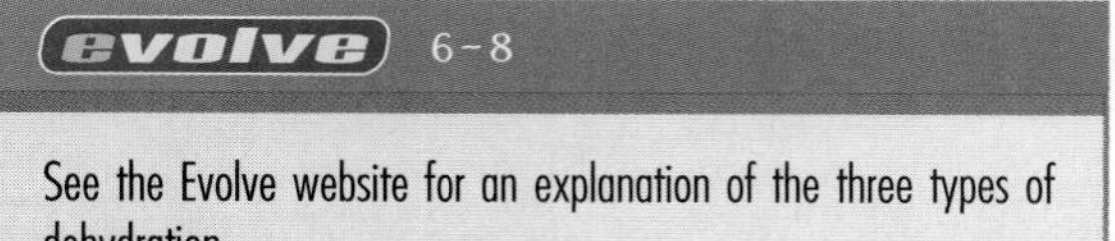

See the Evolve website for an explanation of the three types of dehydration.

Edema

Edema is a condition in which an excess of fluid exists within the interstitial compartment (Figure 6-4). The condition often results in tissue swelling and is common whenever lymphatic blockage occurs or when the lymphatic system cannot drain the area fast enough for some other reason. Renal failure can lead to edema, especially the early stages of acute renal failure and the later stages of chronic renal failure. To test for edema, the thumb is used to apply steady pressure for 10 to 20 seconds to a point on the lower leg or to some other area thought to be affected. If a depression remains in the skin after the thumb is removed, fluid retention is indicated. This is referred to as *pitting edema.*

Edema is also a symptom of liver failure and heart failure. Liver failure can result in inefficient

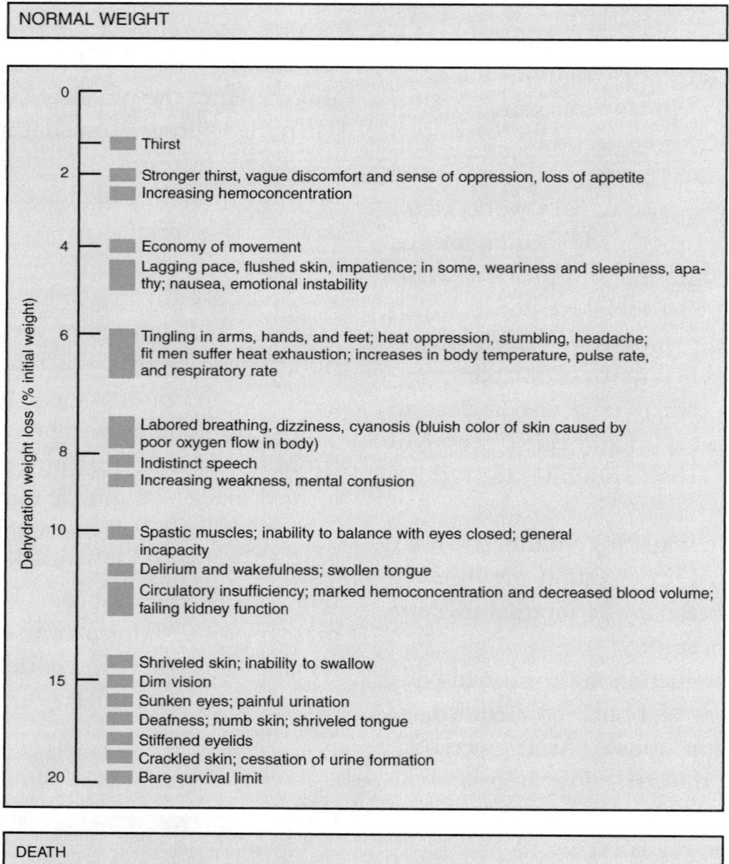

FIGURE 6-3 ■ The effects of dehydration. (From Thibodeau GA, Patton KT: *Anatomy and physiology,* ed 5, St Louis, 2003, Mosby.)

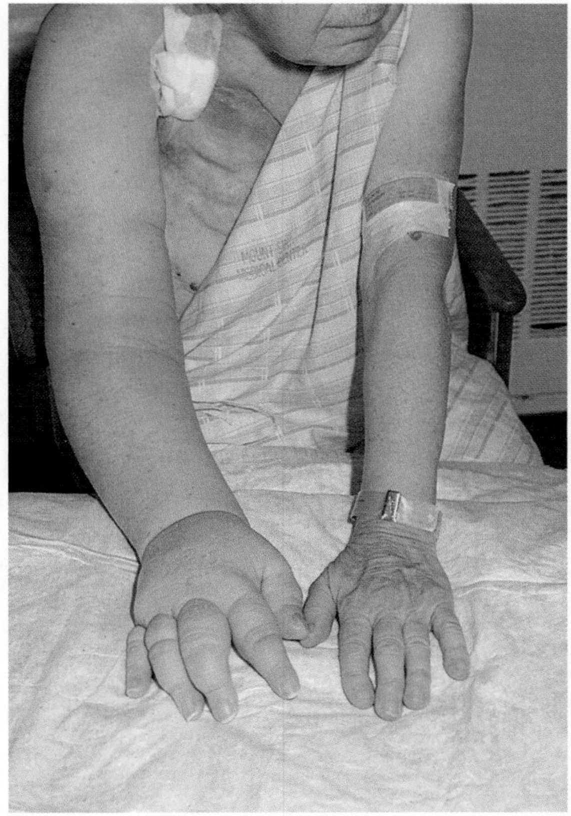

FIGURE 6-4 ■ Lymphedema. (From Swartz M: *Textbook of physical diagnosis: history and examination,* ed 4, Philadelphia, 2002, WB Saunders.)

metabolism of aldosterone, a hormone that controls sodium levels. Heart failure means that the production of aldosterone is enhanced because of the lowering of the blood pressure. The result is the same as in liver failure. Excessive ADH secretion is a rare condition that may occur because of tumors in the lung, brain, or pancreas, resulting in increased reabsorption of water.

Local edema may be part of the inflammatory response or a protective mechanism, especially in joint dysfunction.

A major tenet of massage is support of the body's fluid dynamics. Massage can be targeted to influence blood and lymphatic movement. Important cautions and contraindications apply to massage techniques that target fluid dysfunction. Cardiac and kidney disease are a major concern, as is pre-eclampsia during pregnancy and side effects of medications.

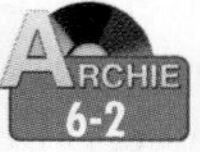

THE CARDIOVASCULAR SYSTEM

The cardiovascular system is a transport system composed of the heart, blood vessels, and blood. The heart is the pump that sends the oxygen and nutrient-rich blood out to the body via the arteries and **arterioles.** The oxygen and nutrients in the blood leave the capillaries and enter the tissues. Carbon dioxide and metabolic wastes leave the tissues, re-enter the capillaries, and pass through the venules and veins on their way to the lungs, liver, and kidneys. The lungs eliminate carbon dioxide, and the liver and kidneys alter or eliminate other waste products.

> **evolve 6-9**
>
> See the Evolve website for a more comprehensive discussion of the cardiovascular system.

ENTRAINMENT AND THE CARDIOVASCULAR SYSTEM

As described previously, entrainment is coordination or synchronization to a rhythm. Research at the Institute of Heart Math and other facilities indicates that the heart rhythm tends to be the guide that the other body rhythms follow. The heart rate, respiratory rate, and thalamus synchronizations combine to support the entrainment process, and the other, more subtle body rhythms follow. Most meditation processes and relaxation methods create an environment in which this entrainment can occur.

> **evolve 6-10**
>
> The Evolve website has more information on entrainment.

CARDIOVASCULAR BENEFITS OF MASSAGE

Massage therapists can increase arterial blood flow in two ways.

- First, by stimulating sympathetic autonomic functions, massage therapists increase the heart rate, providing more push to the blood in the arteries. The action is a reflexive, indirect method that involves the use of homeostatic mechanisms to maintain balance. The massage can be structured to stimulate the sympathetic ANS. In general, the methods used are brisk and involve active contraction of the muscles coupled with an increased respiratory rate; also, parasympathetic influences are enhanced through deep relaxation and by encouraging more relaxed diaphragmatic breathing, thereby reducing pH influences.
- Second, arterial blood flow can be increased mechanically through the pump and tube mechanism of the cardiovascular system, which functions in the same way as the fluid dynamics of hydraulics. Arteries are pliable muscular tubes that carry blood (a fluid) under pressure from the heart pump. Crimping or closing of the tubes causes pressure to build up between the pump (the heart) and the barrier, like water behind a dam. With removal of the barrier, the buildup of pressure provides an initial extra push to the fluid. Compression over more superficial arteries to close off blood flow temporarily results in the same phenomenon. Back pressure builds, and on release of the compression, the blood pushes forward with more force than would have been available from the heart action alone. The massage therapist applies compression against the arteries in the legs and arms to assist peripheral circulation. The rhythm of compression and release is a rate of about 60 beats per minute, to coincide with the heart rhythm. The increase in blood flow is temporary, and in healthy individuals with adequate blood flow, the effect may be negligible.

evolve 6-11

For more information on arterial flow, see the Evolve website.

Maintaining an adequate venous return to the heart at all times is vital, because cardiac output depends on venous return (cardiac input). In most instances, cardiac output equals venous return. Therefore if venous return falls, cardiac output and blood pressure also may drop. Several mechanisms help maintain venous return at all times. Increasing venomotor tone is an important mechanism because it reduces the capacity of the **venous system,** thereby aiding venous return. Long periods of bed rest reduce venomotor tone, because the body is not constantly exposed to the force of gravity, for which the veins are not required to compensate. The massage therapist should remember this when helping a patient up from a session. An essential practice is to move the patient slowly and steadily and to support the person in case he or she becomes dizzy and feels faint.

Two systems, sometimes referred to as the *skeletal muscle pump* and the *respiratory pump,* also assist venous return. Contraction of the skeletal muscles, especially in the limbs, squeezes the veins and pushes blood in the extremities toward the heart; numerous valves prevent backflow. Many communicating channels also allow emptying of blood from the superficial limb veins into the deep veins when rhythmic muscular contractions occur. Consequently, every time a person moves the legs or tenses the muscles, these actions push a certain amount of blood toward the heart. The more frequent and powerful such rhythmic contractions, the more efficient their action. However, unlike rhythmic contractions, sustained, continuous muscle contractions impede blood flow as a result of continuous blocking of the veins. The muscle pump mechanism is an efficient system. When a person stands still for a long period, the muscle pump cannot operate and venous return decreases. As a result, the person may faint because of inadequate cerebral blood flow. Voluntarily contracting and relaxing the muscles of the legs and buttocks aids venous return when standing still for long periods.

Respiration produces variations in the intrapleural and intrathoracic pressures. Each inspiration lowers the pressure in the thorax and the right atrium of the heart, increasing the pressure gradient and aiding blood flow back to the heart.

At the same time, the movement of the diaphragm into the abdomen raises the intraabdominal pressure and increases the gradient to the thorax, again favoring venous return. With expiration, the pressure gradients reverse and blood tends to flow in the opposite direction; fortunately, valves in the medium-size veins prevent this tendency.

Maintaining an adequate circulating blood volume also is necessary. If the blood volume is depleted for some reason (e.g., dehydration or hemorrhage), the body increases the effective circulating volume in the short term through venoconstriction and vasoconstriction in the blood reservoirs of the body, such as the skin, liver, lungs, and spleen. However, restoration of the blood volume eventually requires fluid replacement.

MASSAGE APPLICATION

Massage therapists can incorporate the principles of venous return into massage approaches to encourage venous return flow:

- *Muscle pump:* Rhythmic contraction and relaxation of the muscles during movement encourages venous return flow. Restoring normal muscle function and reducing muscle tension supports venous return.
- *Gravity:* Positioning the limbs higher than the heart passively assists venous return flow.
- *Respiratory pump:* Slow, deep, diaphragmatic breathing with the massage modality used enhances venous return flow.
- *Stroking technique:* Stroking over the veins toward the heart passively moves blood in the veins. This method is particularly effective in the limbs.
- *Muscle contraction:* The therapist can encourage rhythmic contraction of the muscles by having the person move the limbs through a complete range of motion against movement resistance in a contract and relax rhythm of about 60 cycles per minute. Short strokes (1 or 2 inches long) then can be applied over the veins toward the heart at sufficient pressure to push the blood in the superficial veins.

evolve 6-12

See the Evolve website for a more detailed description of massage application in venous return.

The capillaries are the most important vessels functionally because they transport essential materials to and from the cells. Efficient exchange between capillary blood and the surrounding tissue fluid occurs because the capillaries are so numerous and so small that blood in the capillaries flows at its slowest rate, which ensures maximum contact time between blood and tissue. This flow of blood through the capillary bed is referred to as the *microcirculation.* The capillary network, whatever its form, drains into a series of vessels with increasing diameter that form **venules** and veins.

The massage therapist can manipulate the network of capillaries, using compression and kneading to encourage movement of blood through the capillaries.

THE BLOOD PRESSURE AND PULSE

The amount of pressure exerted by the blood on the walls of the **blood vessels** is called **blood pressure.** The maximum pressure, called **systolic pressure,** occurs when the **ventricles** contract. **Diastolic pressure** occurs when the ventricles relax. Blood forced into the aorta during systole sets up a pressure wave that travels along the arteries and expands the arterial wall. This expansion can be palpated by pressing the artery against tissue. The number of waves is known as the **pulse,** which is a direct reflection of the **heart rate.**

The pulse rate, measured when a person is at rest, may be regular or irregular, strong or weak. An irregular pulse commonly occurs with atrial fibrillation and premature contractions. A strong pulse occurs with hyperthyroidism; a weak one with shock and myocardial infarction. A resting heart rate above 100 beats per minute is known as **tachycardia;** a heart rate below 50 or 60 beats per minute is known as **bradycardia.**

Massage therapists can monitor the pulses during assessment. In general, the pulses should feel bilaterally equal. If the therapist identifies differences, the patient should be referred for diagnosis. A normal pulse rate ranges from 50 to 70 beats per minute at rest. A rate much slower or faster indicates a need for referral. If the general intent of the massage therapy session is stress management focused on relaxation with parasympathetic predominance, the pulse rate should slow somewhat over the duration of the session. The opposite is true if the goal is increased arousal of the sympathetic system to energize the patient.

Many Asian medical practices use the feel of the pulse in the assessment of the meridian system. Pulse diagnosis takes many years to perfect.

Sympathetic nerves to the arterioles regulate blood pressure. Normally, arterioles are in a state of partial constriction, called **arteriole tone.** Stimulation of the sympathetic system causes further arteriolar constriction and an increase in blood pressure. Nonstimulation results in a decrease in blood pressure. With **hypertension,** the sympathetic system is in a state of continuous stimulation, resulting in constant high blood pressure.

evolve 6-13

See the Evolve website for more information on blood pressure.

Stress management programs, such as movement methods, moderate aerobic exercise, stretching programs, and massage and other soft tissue methods, can be used to influence blood pressure. Although these approaches initially elevate blood pressure, when continued, they activate parasympathetic quieting responses such as slow, deep breathing and progressive relaxation and therefore tend to have a normalizing effect on the blood pressure. These methods are classified as nonspecific constitutional approaches; they allow the homeostatic mechanisms to reset to a more effective functional pattern after disruption.

Hydrostatic Pressure

All fluids in a confined space exert pressure. The term *hydrostatic pressure* refers to the force that a liquid exerts against the walls of its container (Figure 6-5).

As described, the pressure that blood exerts in the vascular system is known as *blood pressure.* If pressure is exerted on a confined fluid, the pressure is transmitted equally in all directions (this is Pascal's principle). If a weak point exists in the wall of the container and the pressure exerted is great enough, the container wall may break. This is what happens when an aneurysm bursts. In a person with hypertension, the blood vessels harden or undergo sclerotic changes (arteriosclerosis) to prevent the vessels from bursting with the increased blood pressure. Hypotension occurs when the blood pressure is excessively low.

The flexibility of a container (e.g., the veins) also influences the hydrostatic pressure that develops; if the container is flexible, the pressure in the fluid is less than in a rigid container.

Fluid Flow

The flow of a fluid through a vessel is determined by the pressure difference between the two ends of the vessel and also the resistance to flow. For any fluid to flow along a vessel, a pressure difference must exist; otherwise, the fluid will not move. In the cardiovascular system, the pumping of the heart generates the "pressure head," or force, and a continuous drop in pressure occurs from the left ventricle of the heart to the tissues and from the tissues back to the right atrium of the heart. Without this drop in blood pressure, no blood would flow through the circulatory system. **Resistance** is a measure of the ease with which a fluid flows through a tube: the easier the flow, the less the resistance to flow, and vice versa. In the circulatory system the resistance usually is

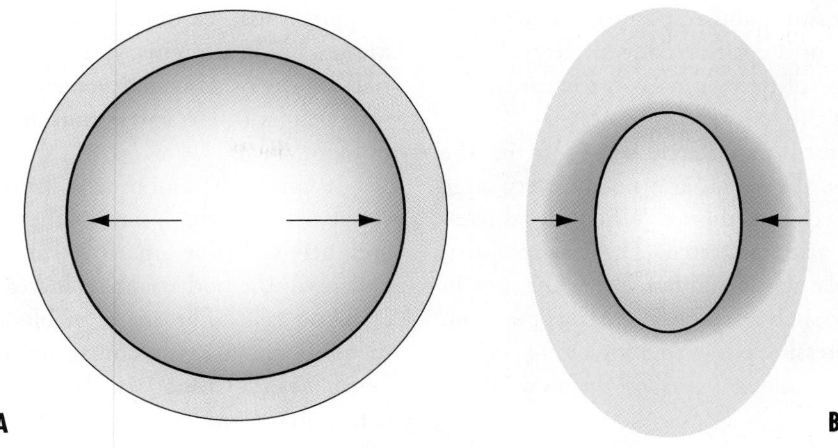

FIGURE 6-5 ■ The effect of hydrostatic pressure. **A,** Enclosed fluid exerts pressure against the interior sides of a container. **B,** External fluid exerts pressure against the outside walls of a container. (Modified from Fritz S: *Sports and exercise massage: comprehensive care in athletics, physical fitness, and rehabilitation,* St Louis, 2006, Mosby.)

described as the *vascular resistance,* because it originates mainly in the peripheral blood vessels; it is also known simply as the *peripheral resistance.*

Resistance is essentially a measure of the friction between the molecules of the fluid and between the tube wall and the fluid. Resistance depends on the viscosity of the fluid and the radius and length of the tube.

Viscosity is a measure of the tendency of a liquid to resist flow. The greater the viscosity (thickness) of a fluid, the greater the force required to move the fluid. For example, water has a lower viscosity than a milkshake.

Normally the viscosity of blood remains constant. However, with polycythemia, a condition in which the red blood cell content is high, the viscosity of the blood can be considerably greater, reducing the blood flow. Severe dehydration, in which loss of plasma occurs, and cooling of the blood can lead to increased viscosity.

The smaller the radius of a vessel, the greater the resistance to the movement of particles. This increased resistance results from a greater probability of the particles of the fluid colliding with the vessel wall. When a particle collides with the wall, some of the kinetic energy (energy of movement) of the particle is lost on impact, resulting in slowing of the particle. In a smaller diameter vessel, a greater number of collisions occur, reducing the energy content and speed of the particles moving through the vessel. The result is a decrease in the hydrostatic pressure.

Small changes in the radius of the blood vessels, particularly the more peripheral vessels, can influence the flow of blood. Changes in the walls of large and medium-size arteries can cause narrowing of the lumen of the vessels and result in increased vascular resistance.

The nature of the lining of a tube or vessel also affects the way fluids flow. If the lining of the blood vessel is smooth, the fluid flows evenly; this is known as *streamline* or *laminar flow.* However, if the lining is rough or uneven or if the fluid flows irregularly, the fluid flow is turbulent. Laminar flow is characteristic of most parts of the vascular system and is silent, whereas turbulent flow is audible, such as during blood pressure measurements with a sphygmomanometer.

The Medulla and Baroreceptors

In the medulla of the brain, the cells of the reticular formation regulate three vital signs: heart rate, blood pressure, and respiration. They work with signals from the various nerve centers in the body. One type of nerve center in the cardiovascular system is the baroreceptor.

Baroreceptors are stretch receptors in the carotid arteries, the aorta, and nearly every large artery of the neck and thorax. When blood pressure increases, arteries stretch. The baroreceptors transmit signals about sudden, brief changes in blood pressure, such as when we change position. When blood pressure is elevated for a long period, the baroreceptor reflex resets to the new blood pressure level.

When blood pressure drops suddenly, the frequency of signals from the baroreceptors declines. This change sets off a response in the cardioregulatory center of the medulla that increases sympathetic stimulation and decreases parasympathetic stimulation, resulting in an increase in the heart rate and blood pressure. Conversely, when blood pressure increases, the signal increases and the medulla changes its output to slow the heart rate and blood pressure by increasing parasympathetic signals. This is an example of how a negative feedback system works in the body.

Stimulation of baroreceptors during therapeutic massage could affect blood pressure. The blood pressure could drop, and the patient may be lightheaded and show other signs of low blood pressure.

evolve 6-14

See the Evolve website for a discussion of the hepatic portal system.

THE BLOOD

Blood transports nutrients to the individual cells and removes waste products. Whole blood consists of solid formed elements and the liquid matrix, or **plasma.**

Red blood cells, white blood cells, and **platelets** are the formed elements of blood that float in the plasma, a thick, straw-colored fluid. Amino acids, carbohydrates, electrolytes, hormones, lipids, proteins, vitamins, and waste materials are the other constituents of blood. A person who weighs 140 to 150 pounds has about 5 quarts of blood.

In an adult, blood cells form mainly in the red marrow of the bones of the chest, vertebrae, and pelvis. Yellow marrow can convert to red marrow if the body requires increased production of blood cells. The stages of blood cell development in red marrow constitute a process called *hematopoiesis.* Blood cells originate from a common precursor cell, called the *stem cell.* Immature blood cells are *blast cells.* When the cells are mature, they move into the bloodstream. In a person with leukemia, blast cells may be seen in peripheral blood because the body sends them out before they are mature.

evolve 6-15

See the Evolve website for specific information on various elements of the blood.

Clotting

Damage to a blood vessel causes the release of chemicals. Special proteins, called *clotting factors,* are activated and then form additional clotting factors. A special protein called *fibrin* forms and seals the damaged blood vessels by trapping red blood cells, platelets, and fluid to form a clot. Fibrin then anchors the clot. The clotting process starts the instant the blood vessel is damaged and takes only a few minutes to complete. Calcium and vitamin K are important to the success and speed of the clotting process.

PATHOLOGIC CONDITIONS OF THE CARDIOVASCULAR SYSTEM

Cardiovascular disease is the leading cause of death in Western societies. Cardiac arrest may occur because of a number of conditions, the most common being a heart attack (myocardial infarction).

evolve 6-16

Detailed information on pathologic conditions is presented on the Evolve website.

Massage Application

In general, cardiovascular disease presents contraindications for therapeutic massage. If the contraindication does not arise from the disease itself, the medication taken to control the disease may pose problems. Anticoagulant medications, for example, increase the possibility of bruising and hemorrhage. Nonetheless, therapeutic massage often is indicated as part of a supervised treatment program. The key is supervision by a qualified healthcare provider, because cardiovascular diseases can be complex in the presenting pathologic condition and the treatment protocols. The general stress management and homeostatic normalization effects of therapeutic massage are desirable for most cardiovascular difficulties, as long as the treatments are supervised as part of a total therapeutic program.

evolve 6-17

For a comprehensive list of cardiovascular pathologic conditions, see the Evolve website.

THE RESPIRATORY SYSTEM

Of all the basic life support systems in the body, the respiratory system is the only one under voluntary and automatic control. The respiratory system functions to obtain the oxygen necessary to create energy for body functions and to eliminate carbon dioxide produced during cellular metabolism. A person can exercise considerable voluntary control over respiratory movements, most often in connection with speech. Respiration and breath are connected intimately to the expression of emotion, as in laughing or crying, the explosive burst in anger, breath holding in fear, and the sigh of relief. This voluntary control of breathing allows a person to regulate the ANS. Control of breathing, therefore, is an important element of many relaxation and meditation practices.

In terms of vital functions, the respiratory system may be considered the most important because the heart and brain require a continuous supply of oxygen to function. **Apnea,** the lack of spontaneous breathing, can cause irreversible brain damage if it lasts longer than 3 or 4 minutes.

Respiration is the movement of air into and out of the lungs, the exchange of oxygen and carbon dioxide between the lungs and blood and between blood and body tissues. **Breathing** is a mechanical action of inhalation and exhalation that draws oxygen into the lungs and releases carbon dioxide into the atmosphere.

External respiration is the exchange of oxygen and carbon dioxide between the lungs and the bloodstream. The exchange of gases between the tissues and blood is called *internal respiration.*

The organs of the respiratory system are divided into upper and lower regions. The upper respiratory tract consists of the nasal cavity, all its structures, and the pharynx; the lower respiratory tract consists of the larynx, the trachea, and the bronchi and alveoli in the lungs.

evolve 6-18

For a comprehensive discussion of the anatomy and physiology of the respiratory system, see the Evolve website.

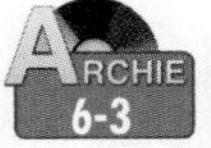

THE MECHANICS OF BREATHING

In the moments before we take a breath, the pressures inside the lungs and outside the body are equal, whereas the pressure inside the pleural space is slightly lower. When we begin to inhale, the external intercostal muscles between the ribs contract, lifting the lower ribs up and out. This creates a vacuum that expands the lungs, causing the pressure inside the lungs to decrease. The diaphragm moves downward, increasing the volume of the pleural cavities and reducing lung pressure even more. Elastic fibers in the alveolar walls stretch, permitting expansion of the air sacs.

The lungs draw in air until the pressures are equal again.

As we exhale, the pressure inside the pleural cavity increases; the external intercostals, diaphragm, and alveolar walls relax; the volume inside the lungs decreases; and the pressure in the lungs increases until it again equals the atmospheric pressure (Figure 6-6).

In diseases such as asthma, bronchitis, and emphysema, the accessory muscles of respiration are often used. Contraction of the sternocleidomastoid muscle and other muscles of the neck aids inspiration, and use of the internal intercostals and abdominal muscles aids expiration (Figures 6-7 to 6-9).

Lung Volumes

Breathing in and out changes the volume of air in the lungs. The four pulmonary volumes can be measured to use as guidelines in health assessments. The **tidal volume** is the amount of air taken in or inhaled in a single breath during normal breathing, usually while the person is resting. The **inspiratory reserve volume** is the amount of air a person can inhale forcefully after normal tidal volume inspiration; the **expiratory reserve volume** is the amount of air a person can exhale forcefully after a normal exhalation. The **reserve volume** is the amount of air that remains in the lungs and passageways after a maximal expiration. **Vital capacity** is the total of the tidal volume, inspiratory reserve volume, and expiratory reserve volume. In a normal healthy adult lung, the vital capacity usually ranges from 3.5 to 5.5 L of air.

In lungs with diseases such as asthma and emphysema, the vital capacity and expiratory reserve volume are abnormal. A person with asthma, for example, may have a normal tidal volume and vital capacity but decreased expiratory reserve volume, whereas a person with emphysema may have a normal (but often decreased) tidal volume and decreased vital capacity and expiratory reserve volume. The end result in both conditions is ineffective exhalation.

TRANSPORT OF OXYGEN AND CARBON DIOXIDE

The exchange of oxygen and carbon dioxide takes place by diffusion. The pulmonary arteries bring oxygen-deficient blood from the right ventricle to the lungs. Carbon dioxide diffuses from the bloodstream through the capillary and alveolar membranes for exhalation by the lungs. Oxygen diffuses in the opposite direction, from the alveoli through both membranes into the bloodstream. The pulmonary veins return oxygen-rich blood to the left atrium.

The amount of oxygen in the blood depends on the amount of oxygen available in the atmosphere. The air in the average room is composed of the following:

- Nitrogen (N_2): 79%
- Oxygen (O_2): 20.96%
- Carbon dioxide (CO_2): 0.04%

Red blood cells transport oxygen in the blood as oxyhemoglobin. Red blood cells move into the capillaries. At the arteriole end of the capillary, oxygen leaves the red blood cell and passes through the capillary membrane into the tissue fluid. It then diffuses through the tissue cell membrane and is used for cellular metabolism.

Carbon dioxide moves out of the tissue cell in the reverse direction through the same membranes and into the red blood cell, where most of it is converted to bicarbonate ion (HCO_3). The plasma transports bicarbonate to the lungs, where the process reverses in the alveolus to allow exhalation of carbon dioxide.

CONTROL OF BREATHING

The respiratory center is a group of nerve cells in the medulla and pons. A variety of stimuli affect the respiratory center. Impulses from the cerebral cortex under voluntary control modify respiration, as do changes in the carbon dioxide content and acidity of blood and cerebrospinal fluid. Chemoreceptors, nerve cells found near the baroreceptors, are sensitive to the oxygen level and to a lesser extent to the carbon dioxide level and pH (acid-base balance) of the bloodstream. Two chemoreceptors are located near the arch of the aorta (aortic bodies), and one is in each carotid artery (carotid bodies). The aortic bodies transmit impulses to the respiratory center in the medulla through the vagus nerve; the carotid bodies transmit by way of the glossopharyngeal nerve. A low concentration of oxygen in the body stimulates the chemoreceptors, and the respiratory rate increases.

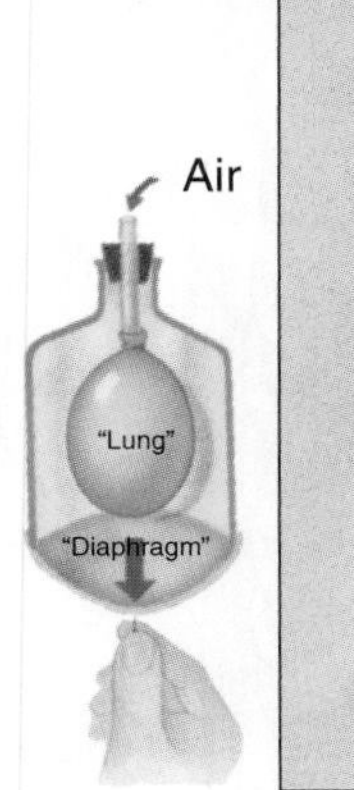

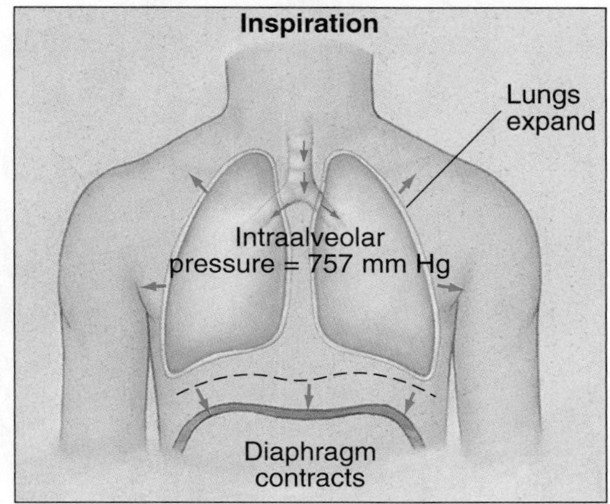

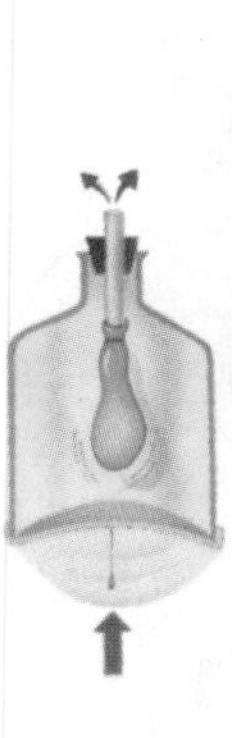

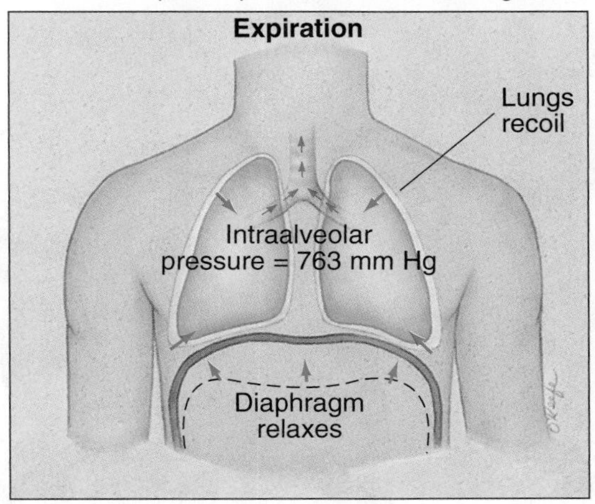

FIGURE 6-6 ■ The mechanics of breathing. During *inspiration,* the diaphragm contracts, increasing the volume of the thoracic cavity. This increase in volume results in a decrease in pressure, which causes air to rush into the lungs. During *expiration,* the diaphragm returns to an upward position, reducing the volume in the thoracic cavity. Air pressure increases, forcing air out of the lungs. Insets show the classic model in which a jar represents the rib cage, a rubber sheet represents the diaphragm, and a balloon represents the lungs. (From Thibodeau GA, Patton KT: *Anatomy and physiology,* ed 5, St Louis, 2003, Mosby.)

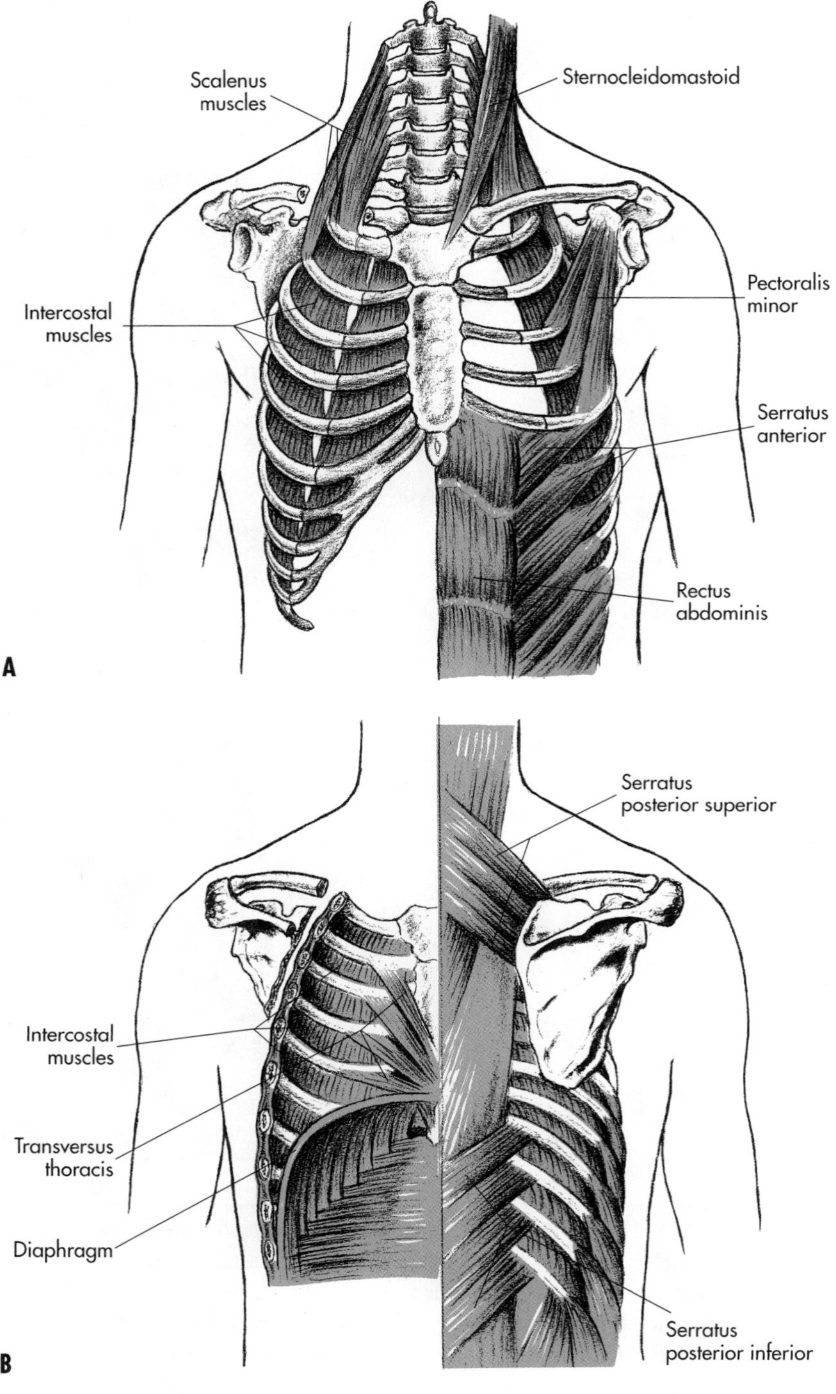

FIGURE 6-7 ■ The muscles of respiration. **A,** Anterior view. **B,** Posterior view. (From Seidel HM et al: *Mosby's guide to physical examination,* ed 5, St Louis, 2003, Mosby.)

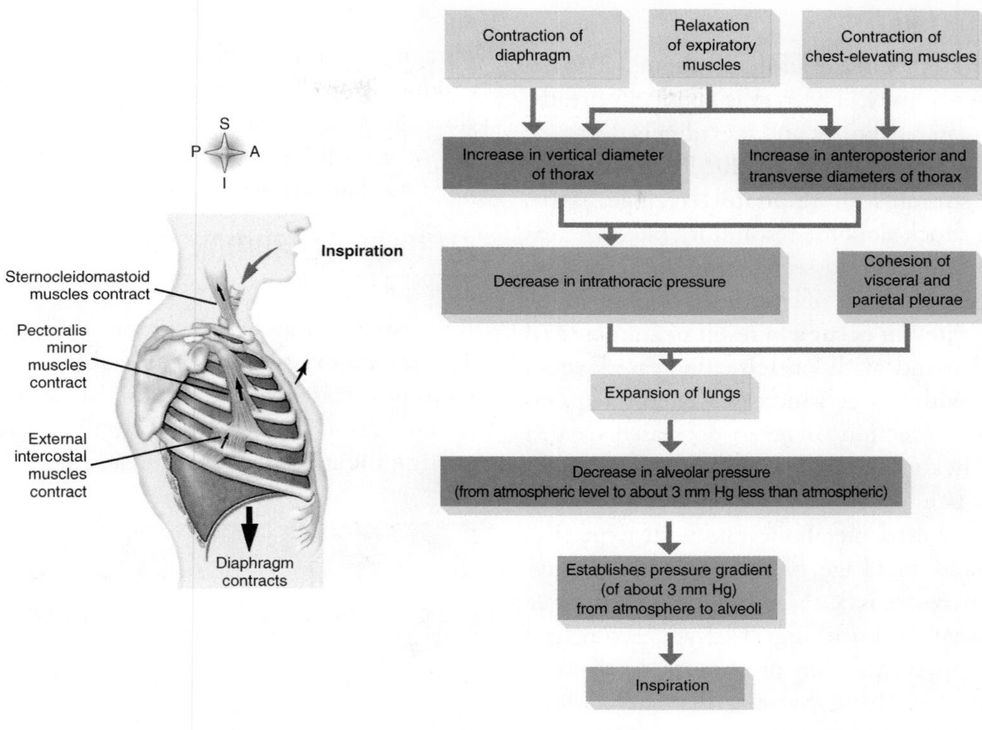

FIGURE 6-8 ■ The mechanism of inspiration. (From Thibodeau GA, Patton KT: *Anatomy and physiology,* ed 5, St Louis, 2003, Mosby.)

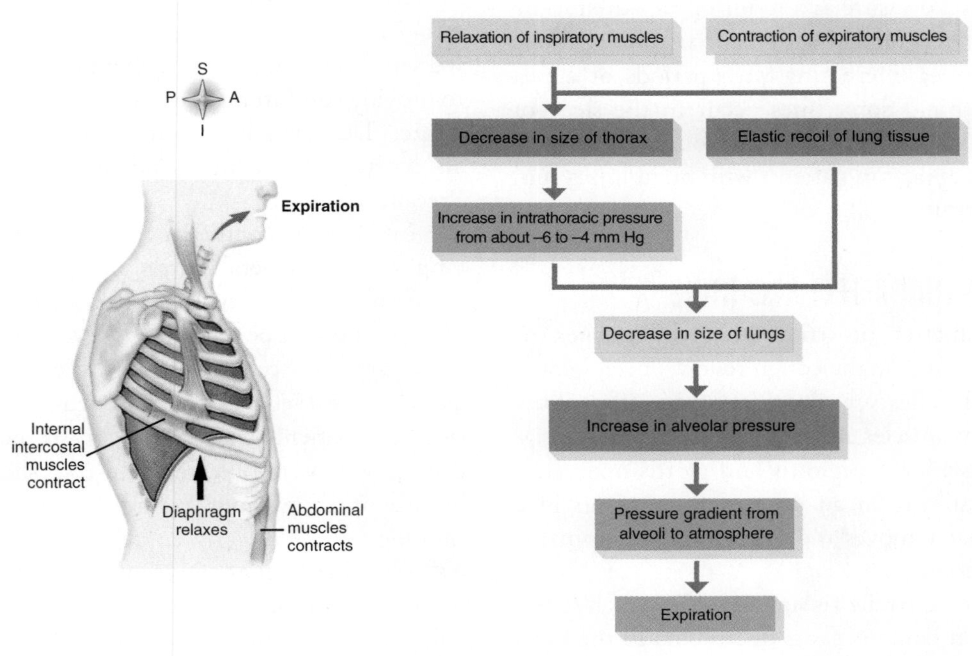

FIGURE 6-9 ■ The mechanism of expiration. (From Thibodeau GA, Patton KT: *Anatomy and physiology,* ed 5, St Louis, 2003, Mosby.)

RESPIRATORY RATE

The respiratory rate in adults is about 12 to 16 breaths per minute. The rate is about 35 breaths per minute in newborns, and it gradually decreases to adult values by about age 20. Emotions are a powerful stimulus for respiratory changes. Fear, grief, and shock slow the respiratory rate, whereas excitement, anger, and sexual arousal increase it.

Besides the effects of emotions, changes in the breathing rate can occur as a result of an increased oxygen demand with exercise; increased vessel resistance with obesity; increased energy requirements with infection or fever; decreased oxygen flow with heart failure; increased nervous stimulation with pain; decreased oxygen transport with anemia; increased metabolic rate with hyperthyroidism; and blockage of oxygen with emphysema. **Hyperpnea** is fast breathing, and **tachypnea** is rapid, shallow breathing. Tachypnea can lead to acute hyperventilation or chronic overbreathing, called **breathing pattern disorder,** which causes a variety of signs and symptoms (discussed later in this section). **Bradypnea,** or slow breathing, occurs with alcohol and other depressant drug intoxication because of the depressant action on the brain. Bradypnea also occurs with increased intracranial pressure as a result of pressure on the respiratory center and with diabetic coma. Periods of hyperpnea alternating with periods of apnea (no breathing) sometimes occur in the sleep of infants, particularly premature ones. These patterns also appear in patients with brain injury and in the terminally ill.

REFLEXES THAT AFFECT BREATHING

Foreign matter or irritants in the trachea or bronchi stimulate the cough reflex. The epiglottis and glottis reflexively close, and contraction of the expiratory muscles causes air pressure in the lungs to increase. The epiglottis and glottis open suddenly, resulting in an upward force of air in a cough that removes the offending contaminants in the throat.

The sneeze reflex is similar to the cough reflex, except that contaminants or irritants in the nasal cavity provide the stimulus. A burst of air moves through the nose and mouth, forcing the contaminants out of the respiratory tract. A hiccup is an involuntary, spasmodic contraction of the diaphragm that causes the glottis to close suddenly, producing a characteristic sound. A yawn is a slow, deep inspiration through the open mouth. Scientists still have not found the actual physiologic mechanism for yawning.

PATHOLOGIC CONDITIONS OF THE RESPIRATORY SYSTEM

Respiratory disease is a major healthcare concern. The respiratory system is vulnerable to infection. Chronic disease is also common. Massage application for respiratory disease typically involves supporting the mechanisms of breathing.

evolve 6-19

See the Evolve website for a discussion of respiratory pathology.

Massage Application

A viral or bacterial cause of any respiratory system disorder usually is a contraindication to therapeutic massage until the disease runs its course. Whenever the body is under stress, as with a respiratory infection, further stress in the system can worsen the condition. Simple palliative measures to provide comfort and encourage sleep are appropriate. The massage practitioner should follow all sanitary procedures and observe Standard Precautions.

In chronic conditions, such as asthma or emphysema, general stress management and maintenance of normal function of the muscles of respiration are beneficial. However, the massage therapist must carefully gauge the appropriate added stress levels caused by the massage stimulation. For patients with cystic fibrosis, percussion can help loosen phlegm, but this should not be attempted without medical supervision and training.

Therapeutic massage approaches and moderate application of movement therapies such as tai chi, yoga, or aerobic exercise often help breathing pattern disorder. Almost every meditation or relaxation system uses breathing patterns because they are a direct means of altering ANS patterns, which in turn alters mood, feelings, and behavior. Other ways to modulate breathing are through singing and chanting.

The shoulders should not move during normal breathing. The accessory muscles of respiration in the neck area should be activated only when increased oxygen is required for fight or flight. This is the pattern for sympathetic breathing. If the person does not use the additional oxygen through increased activity levels, blood gas levels change and symptoms appear. Constant activation of the accessory muscles of respiration for breathing (e.g., the scalenes, sternocleidomastoid, serratus posterior superior, levator scapulae, rhomboids, abdominals, and quadratus lumborum) when forced inhalation and expiration are not required results in dysfunctional muscle patterns. Therapeutic massage can bring balance into these areas to encourage a more effective breathing pattern. General stress management reduces anxiety and helps to normalize the breathing pattern.

Although detailed discussion of the many types of meditation, breathing modulation, and retraining measures is beyond the scope of this text, two basic systems exist: one leads to physiologic hyperarousal, and the other leads to hypoarousal. Both processes facilitate re-establishment of homeostasis, just as a muscle can be encouraged to relax by tensing it first and then releasing it or by using the antagonist pattern to initiate reciprocal inhibition to allow the muscle to relax. Hyperarousal systems increase sympathetic activity with a secondary parasympathetic balance. Aerobic exercise is an example of this system. Hypoarousal systems directly activate parasympathetic responses. Examples are quiet reflection or meditative prayer combined with a chant to promote exhalation. Many resources use retraining programs to improve breathing patterns, and an individual should find one that is comfortable and use it regularly.

Herbs such as eucalyptus give off a vapor that is soothing to the respiratory system. Aromatherapy uses different scents that are taken into the body through the respiratory system. Some scents have a stimulating effect, and others have a more calming effect. The efficacy of aromatherapy is valid when we understand the influence of the sense of smell on physiology. Like most forms of therapeutic massage, aromatherapy is nonspecific, supporting the body in balanced function.

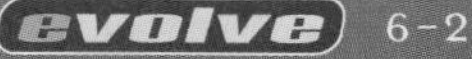

6-20

Log on to the Evolve website for extensive information on breathing pattern disorders.

MYOFASCIAL FORM AND FUNCTION

Buckminster Fuller coined the word *tensegrity* to describe a structure that consists of tension parts (e.g., tent ropes and the tent canvas) and compression units (e.g., the tent poles). In the body, the myofascial unit is the tension part of the tensegrity form that transmits the force of muscle contraction to the connective tissue in order to move the body and dynamically stabilize posture. The bones are the compression units, which cannot keep the body upright without the muscle and connective tissues. The tension aspects of the structure, not the compression aspect, hold the body upright. The human body depends on the soft tissues, including the tendons, ligaments, and joint capsules, for both stability and mobility. Dysfunction results in hypermobility, hypomobility, and instability.

The spiral is also an essential pattern in the universe and is represented extensively in human form and function. The spiral form, coupled with the elements of tensegrity, conceptually unifies the form and function of the body. An understanding of this principle is critical, because efficient movement is composed of twisting and untwisting of the body (Figure 6-10). Muscles are composed of parallel fibers organized in spirals. Actin and myosin, the basic proteins that compose muscle fiber, form a double helix spiral. Microscopically, tendons, ligaments, joint capsules, and the fascia of muscles are composed of collagen molecules, which form a triple helix spiral. Soft tissue is organized around the joint in a spiral. Even deoxyribonucleic acid (DNA), the code of instructions for cellular reproduction, is a double helix spiral.

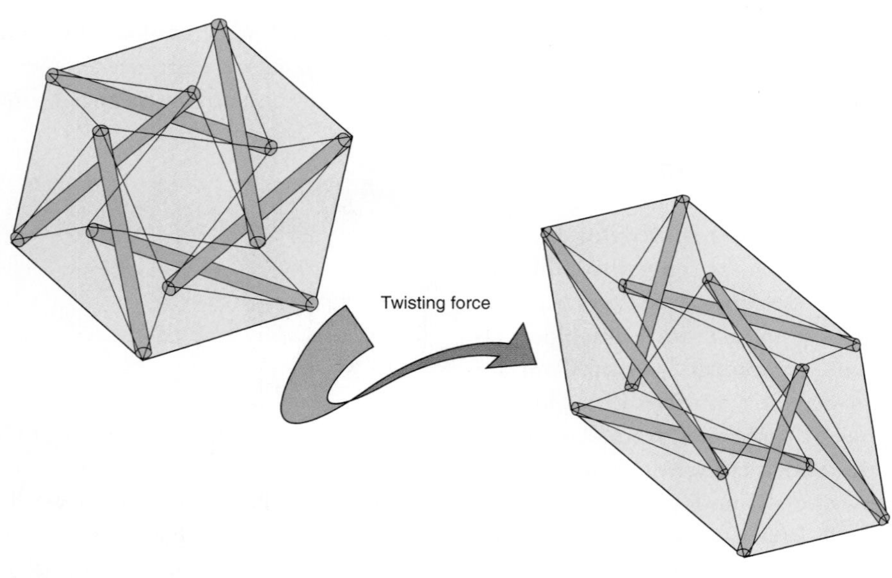

FIGURE 6-10 ■ A demonstration of a cell reacting to a twisting force. (From Fritz S: *Mosby's fundamentals of therapeutic massage,* ed 3, St Louis, 2004, Mosby.)

Soft tissue injury and dysfunction change the normal alignment of the soft tissue in multiple areas because of the tensegrity and spiral interconnective relationships of the body. These shifts influence function first and then form. Distortions in the tension units (soft tissues) create imbalances in the forces moving through the body, creating dysfunction. Muscles, tendons, and ligaments can misalign from illness, injury, repetitive use, and abnormal demands, such as changes in movement secondary to some other illness or injury (e.g., being bedridden or having to use a walker). If the soft tissue develops an abnormal position from dysfunction, illness, or injury, it introduces an abnormal torsion or twist into the tissue. The abnormal force reduces the water content of the tissue. If body fluids stagnate, the mobility of the cells is decreased. The swelling that occurs after acute illness and injury prevents normal fluid exchange.

Sustained muscle contraction and adhesions in chronic soft tissue dysfunction caused by illness or injury also create stagnation in the tissue. Stagnation reduces the tissue's ability to repair itself because of decreased cellular activity, decreased nutrition, and the accumulation of waste products. The tissue becomes fibrotic, nonpliable, and unelastic, which alters its ability to stretch and recoil. Adhesions and abnormal function in the soft tissue and an associated joint may develop as a result of a decrease in water content. Layers of tissue begin to stick together, and function becomes strained and limited. The network of nerves can be embedded within collagen, creating bind and impingement. Adhesions, loss of the normal parallel alignment of the soft tissue fibers, abnormal position, torsion, and fluid stagnation all cause pain and create abnormal neurologic reflexes, which in turn affect the function of somatic structures and internal organs.

When soft tissue is injured, the collagen fibers suffer both microscopic and macroscopic tears. The fibers are repaired during the acute and subacute healing phases with new collagen that is deposited in a random orientation. If managed and appropriate remodeling of the fiber accumulation does not occur in the final stage of healing, the bundles of fibers, or fascicles, lose their ability to slide relative to each other, and adhesions can form. These adhesions prevent the normal broadening of the muscle fibers that occurs during muscle contraction.

Abnormal position and torsion of the soft tissue contribute to the movement of abnormal forces through the joint, creating **strain,** compensation, and eventually degeneration. Joint dysfunction and degeneration cause irritation to the sensory nerve receptors in the soft tissue surrounding the joint. This irritation can create neurologic reflexes that either inhibit or create hypertonicity in the surrounding muscles. For a patient, this outcome compromises the ability to perform daily life activities, as well as work and recreational activities, and contributes to continued illness, injury, and fatigue.

The soft tissues that can restrict joint motion are muscles, connective tissue, and skin. When stretching procedures are applied to these soft tissues, the speed, intensity, and duration of the stretch force, as well as the temperature of the tissues, all affect the response of the different types of soft tissues. These elements are described as different qualities of touch applied during massage: depth of pressure, direction, duration, rhythm, speed, frequency, and drag.

The mechanical characteristics of contractile and noncontractile tissue, as well as the neurophysiologic properties of contractile tissue, all affect soft tissue lengthening.

When soft tissue is stretched, either elastic or plastic changes occur. **Elasticity** is the ability of soft tissue to return to its resting length after passive stretch. **Plasticity** is the tendency of soft tissue to assume a new and greater length after the stretch force has been removed. Both contractile and noncontractile tissues have elastic and plastic qualities. Muscle is primarily composed of contractile tissue, but it is attached to and interwoven with the noncontractile tissue of tendons and fascia. The connective tissue framework in muscle, not active contractile components, is the primary source of resistance to passive elongation of muscle. Adhesions in the skin can develop after an impact injury, wounds, or surgery. Because the superficial fascia in the dermis is connected to the underlying deep fascia coverings of the muscles, these adhesions reduce the mobility of the soft tissue. Adhesions in the superficial fascia can also entrap the cutaneous nerves, leading to pain, numbness, and tingling. Cumulative changes in skin pliability are problematic and can be managed with massage.

How massage and stretching increase tissue pliability and length is still not fully understood. The response of the tissue to imposed mechanical force can result in soft tissue and body injury. However, if these same mechanical forces are applied in a purposeful, controlled manner during massage, benefits are achieved.

evolve 6-21

See the Evolve website for a comprehensive anatomy and physiology of connective tissue.

Collagen makes up approximately 80% of tendons, ligaments, and joint capsules and a large percentage of cartilage and bone, providing shape to the soft tissue. It forms the structural support for the skin, muscles, blood vessels, and nerve fibers. Normal stresses in the form of exercise and the activities of daily living increase collagen synthesis and strengthen connective tissue. This is an important aspect of fitness, especially for the elderly.

Collagen stabilizes the joints through the ligaments, joint capsules, and periosteum by resisting the tension or pulling force transmitted through the joints by movement or gravity. Collagen transmits the pulling force of muscle contraction through the fascia within the muscle and the tendon attachment. The collagen fibers tend to orient to parallel and longitudinal alignment along the lines of mechanical stress imposed through loading of the tissue during activity. Normal gliding of collagen fibers is maintained by movement and lubrication from connective tissue ground substance.

Immobilization or lack of use reduces collagen production, leading to atrophy in the connective tissue and osteoporosis in the bone. Without movement, collagen is laid down in a random orientation, and the fibers are packed close together, forming microadhesions. **Adhesions** are abnormal deposits of connective tissue between gliding surfaces. This atrophy and random orientation of the fibers creates weakness in the tissue and instability of the associated joint. This condition is more common in those who are just beginning a fitness regimen, and it increases the potential for injury. The aging process reduces the amount and quality of the collagen structure, therefore exercise helps prevent age-related soft tissue dysfunction.

Too much mechanical and repetitive stress results in excessive deposits of collagen, causing abnormal cross-fiber links and adhesions. The fibers pack closer together, lubrication is decreased, and the water content of ground substance is reduced. This reduces the ability of the fibers and fascicles to slide relative to each other. This condition is often called **fibrosis.** Adhesions and fibrosis create a resistance to normal electrical flow, and the decrease in electrical currents conducted in the connective tissues interferes with the normal repair and rejuvenation process.

People are prone to excessive mechanical stress during daily living activities, work, and recreation. Massage mechanically deforms the collagen fibers by introducing bind, shear, torsion, compression, and tension forces. **Piezoelectricity** is the ability of a tissue to generate electrical potentials in response to the pressure of mechanical deformation. Piezoelectricity is a property of most, if not all, living tissues. Electric potentials are generated during the formation of collagen fiber. Piezoelectric current also increases the negative charge in the soft tissue, which has a strong proliferative effect, stimulating the creation of new cells to repair the body.

Injury results in an acute inflammatory response. During the acute and subacute repair phases of the healing process, connective tissue fibers are laid down in a random orientation instead of in normal tissue configuration. In essentially the same process of fibrotic change discussed above, the fibers pack closer together, forming abnormal cross-fiber links and adhesions. These adhesions can occur at every level of the soft tissue, including the ligament or tendon adhering to the bone, between the fascicles, between the fibers themselves, or in individual muscle layers. First and second layer muscle adhesion is common, such as with the gastrocnemius and soleus or the pectoralis major and pectoralis minor.

Because adhesions reduce tissue extensibility, the tissue becomes less elastic, thicker, and shorter. People often feel stiff in the area of adhered and fibrotic tissue.

evolve 6-22

For more information on adhesions and fibrotic tissue, log on to the Evolve website.

Because tendons and ligaments stabilize joints and act as neurosensory structures, injuries to these structures can cause dysfunction of the joint and surrounding soft tissue. A reflex connection exists between the ligaments of a joint and the surrounding muscles that affects muscle tone. If ligaments are lax or excessively loose, tone in the involved muscles and tendons reflexively increases to provide joint stability.

The joint capsule and ligaments typically respond to injury by becoming stretched, resulting in joint instability. These structures can also shorten, causing loss of a joint's normal range of motion and joint stiffness. Immobilization causes ligaments to atrophy and weaken, which changes the normal gliding motion of the joint. Ligaments can twist into abnormal position. Irritation or injury of the ligaments usually causes a reflexive contraction or inhibition in the surrounding muscles. Muscle energy methods that address gait and muscle activation sequence firing patterns can help restore normal function temporarily, because the muscle is connected to the ligaments by a neurologic reflex. However, the condition will recur because the instability of the joint is the underlying cause.

Injured ligaments can become thick and fibrous from increased collagen formation, abnormal cross-fiber links, and adhesions. This is especially common if inflammatory responses are slow to resolve or have remained chronic.

Massage applied to ligaments that have developed adhesions is performed across the direction of fiber to increase pliability and realign fiber structure. If ligaments are too lax, exercise and rehabilitation can stimulate the production of new collagen and help restore normal joint integrity. External stabilization, such as braces and other types of supports, can be used if necessary. Friction massage can be used to create small, controlled inflammation in the ligament structure to stimulate collagen production. However, because the process is tedious and uncomfortable for the client, compliance is reduced.

THE PERIOSTEUM

The periosteum is a dense, fibrous connective tissue sheath that covers the bones. The outer layer, made up of collagen fibers oriented parallel to the bone, contains arteries, veins, lymphatics, and sensory nerves. The inner layer contains *osteoblasts* (i.e., cells that generate new bone formation). Repetitive stress can stimulate the inner layer of the periosteum to create bone outgrowths, called **spurs.** This often occurs at the heel when the plantar fascia is short.

The periosteum weaves into ligaments and the joint capsule. Stretching of the periosteum provides mechanoreceptor information about joint function at these junctions.

The periosteum also blends with the tendons, forming the **tenoperiosteal junction** (Figure 6-11), where the muscle pulls on the bone during joint movement. The sensory nerves in the periosteum are sensitive to tension forces. The tenoperiosteal junction is a common site of soft tissue injury. An acute tear or cumulative microtearing of the periosteum can result in random orientation of the collagen in the area, leading to the development of abnormal cross-fiber links and adhesions. Massage can address this abnormal fibrotic development at the tenoperiosteal junction. Friction is used to introduce small amounts of controlled inflammation, which results in an active acute healing process. With appropriate healing and rehabilitation, a more functional outcome is achieved.

FASCIA

Fascia is a fibrous connective tissue arranged as sheets or tubes. It can be thick and dense (like duct tape) or take the form of thin, filmy membranes (like plastic wrap). Fascia is connected throughout the body, creating a unified form. Superficial fascia lies under the dermis of the skin and is composed of loose, fatty connective tissue. Deep fascia is dense connective tissue that surrounds muscles and forms fascial compartments, called *septa,* that contain muscles with similar functions. In the healthy state, these compartments are well lubricated, which allows the muscles inside to move freely.

Fascia can tear, adhere, torque, shorten, or become lax, just as other connective tissue structures can (Figure 6-12). It responds well to

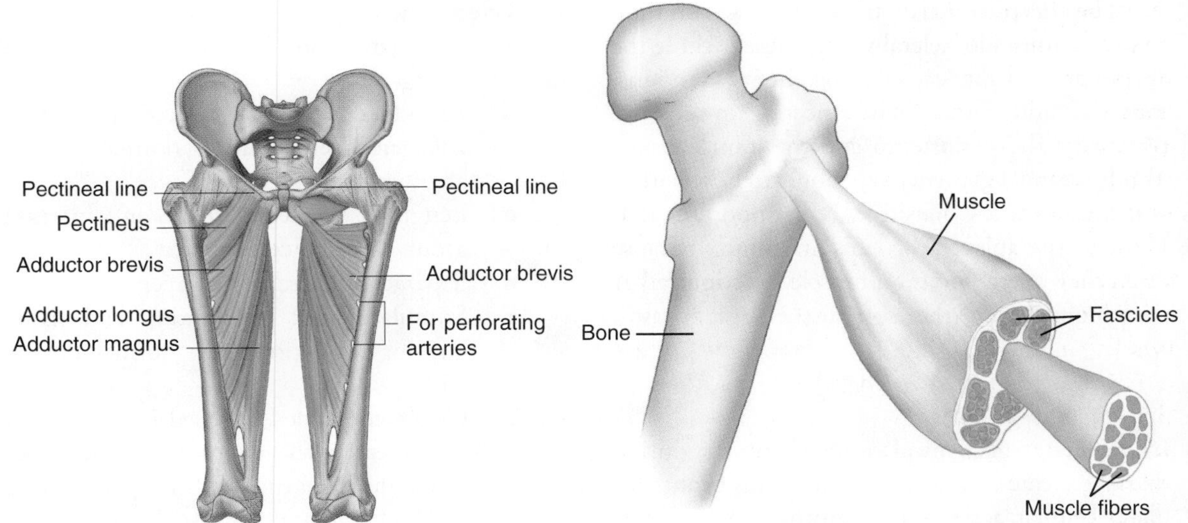

FIGURE 6-11 ■ **A, B,** Tenoperiosteal junctions. (**A** from Drake R, Vogl W, Mitchell A: *Gray's anatomy for students,* Edinburgh, 2005, Churchill Livingstone; **B** from Muscolino JE: *Kinesiology: the skeletal system and muscle function,* enhanced edition, St Louis, 2006, Mosby.)

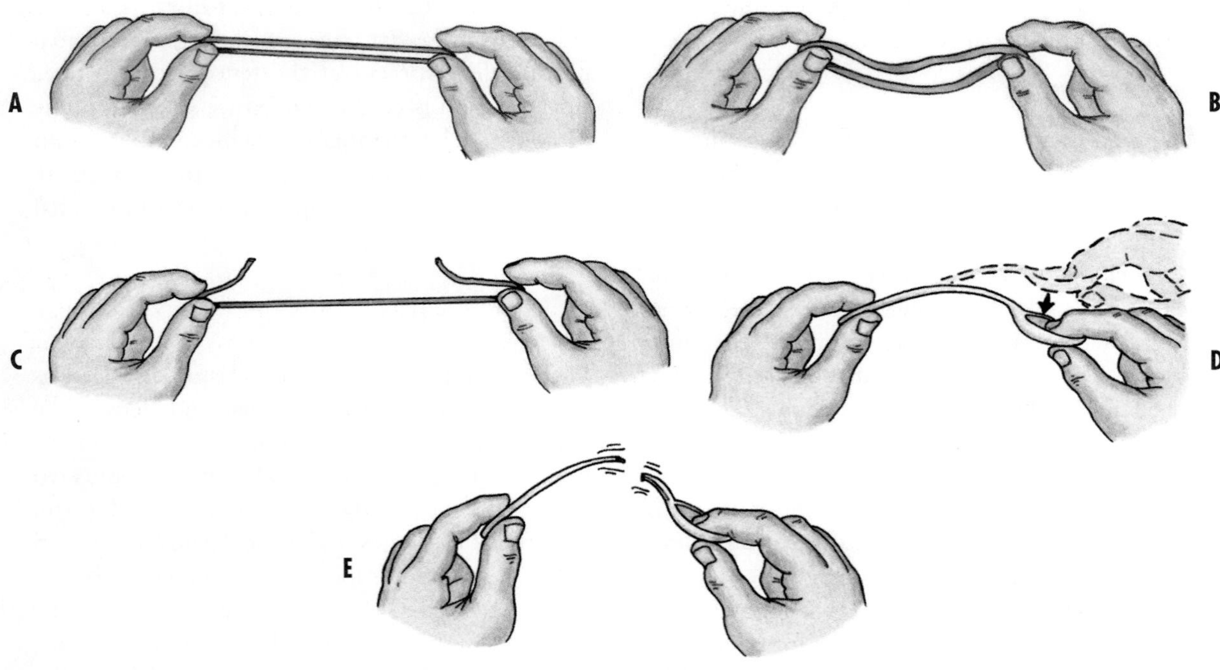

FIGURE 6-12 ■ The properties of connective tissue. **A** to **C**, Elastic deformation. Stress applied to a rubber band. When stress is removed, the rubber band returns to its original length. If the stress exceeds the band's strain capabilities, the band will break. **D** and **E**, Plastic deformation. A low degree of stress is applied to a plastic spoon. The spoon deforms slowly and accommodates to a new shape. If stress is applied suddenly and with great force, the spoon breaks. (Modified from Shankman GA: *Fundamental orthopedic management for the physical therapist assistant*, ed 2, St Louis, 2004, Mosby.)

connective tissue massage methods, which are described later in this unit.

The deep somatic tissues are a common source of musculoskeletal pain. These include the periosteum, joint capsule, ligaments, tendons, muscles, and fascia. The most pain-sensitive tissues are the periosteum and the joint capsule. Tendons and ligaments are moderately sensitive, and muscle is less sensitive. It is important that massage therapists keep this in mind, because often they overly focus on muscle function rather than considering the soft tissue system as a whole.

Massage Application

In general, mechanical forces applied during massage create heat in the tissues. This heat stimulates cellular activity and improves the lubrication of the fibers by making the ground substance more fluid. Fascia is embedded with mechanoreceptors and smooth muscle bundles that respond to the mechanical forces applied during massage to reduce fascial tone and increase pliability.

Effectively focused massage can:

- Stimulate fibroblasts to repair injured collagen
- Introduce mechanical forces to realign collagen fibers in their normal parallel alignment
- Lengthen shortened tissue and increase ground substance pliability
- Separate adhered tissue layers
- Stimulate fluid distribution and tissue layering to promote normal tissue gliding
- Create controlled, focused inflammation to increase collagen proliferation, especially in lax structures (proper healing and rehabilitation must be combined with this approach for a beneficial outcome, otherwise increased adherence and scar tissue formation can result)

- Alter fascial tone through mechanical stimulation of embedded nerves and smooth muscle

JOINT STRUCTURE AND FUNCTION

Joints are innervated by the articular nerves, which are branches of the peripheral nervous system. Branches of these nerves also supply the muscles controlling the joint. This is important in understanding how muscles can cause joint dysfunction and how joint dysfunction can cause muscle problems.

Many sensory receptors surround the joint. The four types of joint receptors are located in the joint capsule, ligaments, periosteum, and articular fat pads.

- Type 1 receptors are located in the superficial layers of the superficial joint capsule. These are mechanoreceptors that provide information about the static and dynamic position of the joint.
- Type 2 receptors are located in the deep layers of the **fibrous joint capsule.** They are dynamic mechanoreceptors that provide information about acceleration and deceleration movement.
- Type 3 receptors are located in the intrinsic and extrinsic joint ligaments. These are dynamic mechanoreceptors that monitor the direction of movement and have a reflex effect on muscle tone to provide deceleration.
- Type 4 receptors are located in joint capsules, ligaments, and the periosteum. They are pain receptors.

These receptors send information to the CNS on the functional status of the joint and its surrounding soft tissue. The reflex control of the muscles surrounding the joint is called the *arthrokinematic reflex.* The CNS creates contraction or relaxation of the muscles to protect the joint. The arthrokinematic reflex coordinates agonists, antagonists, and synergists around the joint and in other jointed areas for large movements and fine muscular control.

Proper function of these reflex mechanisms is extremely important in posture, coordination, and balance; direction and speed of movement; position of the joint and body; and pain in the joint. With irritation of the pain receptors and mechanoreceptors, the joint flexors typically are facilitated (i.e., they become short, tight, and hypertonic) and the joint extensors are inhibited (i.e., they become weak, long, and taut).

Irritation of the joint receptors can also lead to abnormalities in posture, muscle coordination, and control of movement, balance, and awareness of body position. This is a major concern for patients. Assessment and treatment of gait patterns and firing patterns through the use of massage and muscle energy methods can support normal reflex functions.

evolve 6-23

See the Evolve website for more detailed information about joint structure and function.

Irritation and injury to the joint capsule can create muscle contractions designed to protect the joint; this muscle response is called **guarding.**

evolve 6-24

For more information on guarding, see the Evolve website.

Fibrosis, or thickening of the outer layer of the joint capsule, is caused by acute inflammation, irritation or inflammation caused by imbalanced stresses on the joint, and/or immobilization. A tight, fibrotic joint capsule results in compression of certain areas of the cartilage and degeneration of the joint surfaces. The capsule and supporting ligaments may also be overstretched because of injury or excessive stretching during activities such as dancing and gymnastics. If immobilization causes a loss of adequate motion, the fibrous layer of the joint capsule atrophies, resulting in joint instability.

The synovial membrane can also be injured or become dysfunctional as a result of immobilization, acute trauma to the joint, or cumulative stress from chronic irritation caused by imbalanced forces on the joint. Joint swelling occurs during inflammation. The swelling typically causes abnormal function of the muscle controlling the joint. During immobilization, the synovial fluid thickens with disuse, and the amount of synovial fluid secreted decreases. This leads to the development of adhesions between the capsule and the articular cartilage, tendon sheaths, and bursae, which contributes to stiffness and joint degeneration.

Massage Application

With a fibrotic joint capsule, massage is used to introduce mechanical forces into the tissue to increase pliability. The fibrotic capsule is treated with manual pressure on the capsule itself. The massage strokes are oriented in all directions, addressing the irregular alignment of the collagen. Active and passive movement and stretching are used to reduce intraarticular adhesions.

A capsule that is too loose needs exercise rehabilitation to help lay down new collagen fibers and proprioception exercises to help restore neurologic function. Appropriate friction massage can stimulate an acute inflammatory response that stimulates collagen formation.

An acute, swollen joint capsule is treated with gentle, rhythmic compression and decompression of the joint and lymphatic drainage to pump the excess fluid out of the capsule. Pain-free, passive range of motion is also used in the flexion-extension pattern to act as a mechanical pump. If the joint has too little fluid, passive and active movements help stimulate the synovial membrane, increasing the production and movement of synovial fluid and thereby supporting lubrication and nutrition.

evolve 6-25

See the Evolve website for more detailed information on massage application with regard to joint movement.

Synovial joints generate compression and decompression through movement, intermittent contraction of the muscles, and twisting and untwisting of the joint capsule. Massage application that includes passive joint movement introduces compression and decompression and supports joint health.

Cartilage damage is common. An arthritic joint is a joint with degeneration of the cartilage. Damage to articular cartilage may be caused by acute trauma or cumulative stress. These stresses often are the result of imbalances in the muscles surrounding the joint, a tight joint capsule, or a loose joint capsule. A tight capsule creates a high-contact area of the cartilage and decreased lubrication. A loose capsule allows inappropriate joint laxity and rubbing. Dysfunction of the muscles that move the joint create excessive pressure on the cartilage. The cartilage degenerates, beginning with damage to the collagen fibers and depletion of the ground substance.

Recent studies show that cartilage cells can create new cartilage. The joint must be moved to stimulate the synthesis of **chondrocytes** and the secretion of synovial fluid. Compression followed by decompression of the joint capsule pumps synovial fluid into and out of the cartilage, rehydrating it. In addition to appropriate exercise, massage and muscle energy methods support joint health through the use of techniques such as contract, relax, reciprocal inhibition, pulsed muscle, or a combination of these methods. Both active and passive movement of the joint, as well as compression and decompression, promote fluid exchange.

JOINT STABILITY

To perform a full and painless range of motion, a joint must be stable. A rule to follow for joint health is stability before mobility, mobility before agility. Otherwise, abnormal forces move through the joint, leading to excessive wear and tear on the articular surfaces. Joint stability is determined by several key factors:

- The shape of the bones that make up the joint; this is called **form stability** (e.g., the hip joint)
- The passive stability provided by the ligaments and joint capsule; this is also called *form stability* (e.g., the sternoclavicular joint)
- The dynamic stability provided by the muscles; this is called **force stability** (e.g., the glenohumeral joint)

If the joint instability is a form instability (e.g., arising from the bones and ligaments), soft tissue massage methods focus on condition management and palliation. However, if force instability is the cause, joint function can be improved with exercise and massage.

The motor tone of the muscles that cross a joint must be balanced, or the forces on the joint will create uneven stresses, leading to dysfunction and eventual degeneration of the cartilage.

When a joint is in the close-packed position, the capsule and ligaments are tightest. In the loose-packed position, the joint is most open and the capsule and ligaments are somewhat lax. Generally, extension closes and flexion opens the joint surfaces. Midrange of the joint typically is the least-packed position, which is when the joint is most vulnerable to injury. For most traction methods, the joint should be positioned in the midrange (Tables 6-4 and 6-5).

Dr. John Mennell introduced the concept of "joint play," which describes movements in a joint that can be produced passively but not voluntarily. In most joint positions, a joint has some "play" in it that is essential for normal joint function.

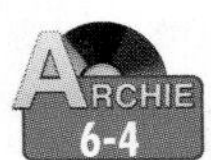

JOINT DEGENERATION

A common cause of joint degeneration is loss of normal function of the joint. This altered function can occur as a result of a prior trauma or cumulative stress on the joint. Most conditions called "arthritis" no longer involve an active inflammatory response; for accuracy, these conditions should be referred to as *arthrosis,* which means joint degeneration. The terms *osteoarthritis* and *degenerative joint disease* typically are used interchangeably to describe chronic degeneration of a joint, although *osteoarthritis* may be used to describe a true inflammatory joint condition. Many people develop arthritis and arthrosis. Technical advances in joint replacement surgery have increased the success of joint replacement and rehabilitation (Figure 6-13).

Massage Application

Appropriate massage addresses adhesions and tightening of the joint capsule or ligaments, sustained contraction of the muscle surrounding the joint, muscle tone imbalances (muscle and motor types) across a joint, and irregular muscle activation sequences (firing patterns) of the muscles moving the joint. Short, tight muscles must be lengthened and relaxed, and muscles that are weak and inhibited need to be re-educated and exercised to regain their normal strength. Also, firing patterns need to be normalized.

Joint mobilization is any active or passive attempt to increase movement at a joint. Joint mobilization within the normal range of motion is within the scope of practice for the massage therapist. The movement must not be forcefully abrupt or painful. The goals of joint mobilization are to:

TABLE 6-4 Least-Packed Positions of Joints

Joints	Position
Spine	Midway between flexion and extension
Temporomandibular	Mouth slightly open
Glenohumeral	55 degrees abduction, 30 degrees horizontal adduction
Acromioclavicular	Arm resting by side in normal physiologic position
Sternoclavicular	Arm resting by side in normal physiologic position
Elbow	70 degrees flexion, 10 degrees supination
Radiohumeral	Full extension and full supination
Proximal radioulnar	70 degrees flexion, 35 degrees supination
Distal radioulnar	10 degrees supination
Wrist	Neutral with slight ulnar deviation
Carpometacarpal	Midway between abduction/adduction and flexion/extension
Thumb	Slight flexion
Interphalangeal	Slight flexion
Hip	30 degrees flexion, 30 degrees abduction and slight lateral rotation
Knee	25 degrees flexion
Ankle	10 degrees plantar flexion, midway between maximum inversion and eversion
Subtalar	Midway between extremes of range of motion
Midtarsal	Midway between extremes of range of motion
Tarsometatarsal	Midway between extremes of range of motion
Metatarsophalangeal	Neutral
Interphalangeal	Slight flexion

From Magee D: *Orthopedic physical assessment,* ed 4, Philadelphia, 2002, Saunders.

TABLE 6-5 Close-Packed Positions of Joints

Joints	Position
Spine	Extension
Temporomandibular	Clenched teeth
Glenohumeral	Abduction and lateral rotation
Acromioclavicular	Arm abducted to 30 degrees
Sternoclavicular	Maximum shoulder elevation
Elbow	Extension
Radiohumeral	Elbow flexed 90 degrees, 5 degrees forearm supination
Proximal radioulnar	5 degrees supination
Distal radioulnar	5 degrees supination
Wrist	Extension with ulnar deviation
Carpometacarpal	Full flexion
Thumb	Full opposition
Interphalangeal	Full extension and medial rotation*
Hip	Full extension and lateral rotation of femur
Knee	Maximum extension
Ankle	10 degrees plantar flexion, midway between maximum inversion and eversion
Subtalar	Supination
Midtarsal	Supination
Tarsometatarsal	Supination
Metatarsophalangeal	Full extension
Interphalangeal	Full extension

*Some authors include abduction.
From Magee D: *Orthopedic physical assessment*, ed 4, Philadelphia, 2002, Saunders.

- Restore the normal joint play
- Promote joint repair and regeneration
- Stimulate normal lubrication by stimulating the synovial membrane to promote rehydration of articular cartilage
- Normalize neurologic function
- Reduce swelling
- Diminish pain

Joint manipulation can be valuable. Osteopathic physicians, chiropractors, and physical therapists are a few of the healthcare professionals trained to manipulate the joint structure.

MUSCLE

The structural unit of skeletal muscle is the muscle fiber. The fibers are arranged in parallel bundles, called *fascicles.* Each fascicle is composed of many myofibrils. A myofibril is composed of thousands of strands of proteins, also arranged in parallel bundles, called *myofilaments;* these are further divided into actin and myosin, the basic proteins of contraction. Muscles contain satellite cells that can regenerate muscle fibers.

The muscle fibers are so interwoven with connective tissue that separating the two is difficult. A more appropriate term may be *myofascia.*

The connective tissue of muscle transmits the pulling force of the contracting muscle cells to the bones and gives the muscle fibers organization and support. The collagen fibers found in the epimysium, perimysium, endomysium, and other connective tissue components of muscle converge to form the tendon. The tendon fibers weave into the connective tissue of the periosteum, joint capsule, and ligaments. In the healthy state, all these connective tissue layers are lubricated so that muscles can slide over each other during movement. If this does not happen, function is altered. This commonly occurs as part of the aging process or as a result of adhesions that form during the injury repair process.

Muscles are dynamic stabilizers of the joints because they actively hold the joints in a stable position for posture and movement. Proprioceptors in muscle tissue sense joint movement and body position. Muscles are connected to the nerves in the skin, and the nerves in the neighboring joint's capsule and ligaments through neurologic reflexes. If the skin or joint is irritated or injured, the associated muscles may go into a reflexive spasm, may be inhibited, or may attempt whatever could best protect the area. Muscles have pain receptors that fire with chemical or mechanical irritation.

The muscles act as a musculovenous pump because the contracting skeletal muscle compresses the veins and moves blood toward the heart. A similar process assists lymphatic movement.

Types of Muscle Actions

Muscles exert a pulling force when actin and myosin are stimulated to contract. Muscle functions can be divided into three types:

- Isometric: In an **isometric action** the muscle contracts, but its constant length

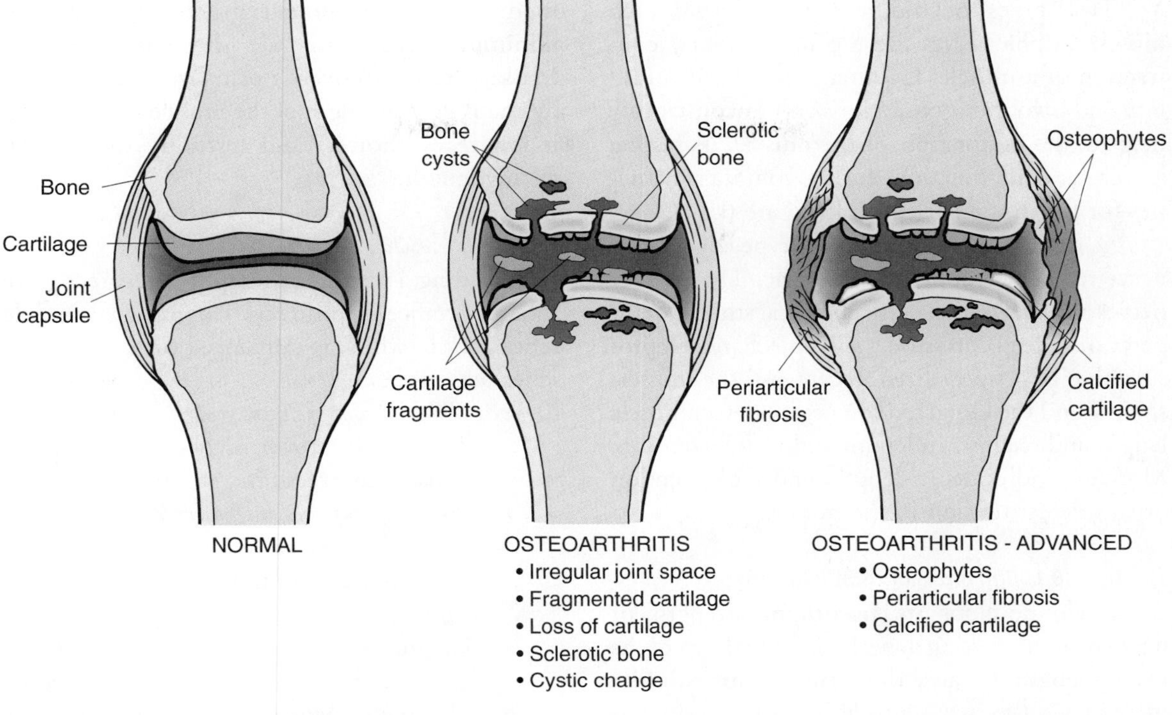

FIGURE 6-13 ■ An example of degenerative joint disease. (From Damjanov I: *Pathology for the health professions,* ed 3, St Louis, 2006, Mosby.)

is maintained. The main outcome is stabilization.

- Concentric: In a **concentric action,** the muscle shortens as it contracts. The main outcome is movement/acceleration.
- Eccentric: In **eccentric action,** the proximal and distal attachments move apart. The main outcome is control of movement and deceleration.

All movements in the body are accomplished by more than one muscle. The muscles that contract concentrically to perform a certain movement are called the **agonists.** This action is called *acceleration,* and the muscle is also called the *prime mover.* For example, the biceps is an agonist for elbow flexion. The muscles that perform the opposite movement of the agonists are called the **antagonists;** they provide control through deceleration during eccentric function. The triceps is the antagonist for the biceps, because the triceps both extends the elbow and controls flexion of the elbow. A muscle that works with another muscle to accomplish a certain motion is a **synergist.** The synergists include stabilizers and neutralizers.

Typically, when the agonist is working concentrically, the antagonist is functioning eccentrically. Sherrington's law of reciprocal inhibition states that a neurologic inhibition of the antagonist occurs when the agonist is working. When the biceps is contracted to flex the elbow, the triceps is neurologically inhibited, which allows it to lengthen during elbow flexion. Co-contraction is an exception to this rule. **Co-contraction** occurs when the agonist and antagonist work together. For example, when you make a fist, the flexors and extensors of the wrist co-contract to keep the wrist in a position that ensures the greatest strength of the fingers.

Human movement seldom involves pure forms of isolated concentric, eccentric, or isometric actions. This is because the body segments are periodically subjected to impact forces, as in running or jumping, or because some external force (e.g., gravity) causes the muscle to lengthen. In many situations, the muscles first act eccentrically, and a concentric action follows immediately, mixed in with isometric stability function.

Two types of motor nerves supply each muscle. Alpha nerves fire during voluntary contraction of a muscle. Gamma nerves have voluntary and involuntary functions and unconsciously help set the motor tone of the muscle, its resting length, and its function during voluntary activities for fine muscular control (Figure 6-14).

As discussed previously, five types of sensory nerve receptors supply each muscle. The sensory nerves are sensitive to pain, chemical stimuli, temperature, deep pressure, and mechanoreceptor stimuli. Two specialized receptors, the muscle spindle and the Golgi tendon organ, detect muscle length and changes in length and muscle tension. Muscle spindles detect length, and Golgi tendon organs detect tension in the muscle.

The Muscle Length-Tension Relationship

A muscle develops its maximum strength or tension at its resting length or just short of its resting length, because the actin and myosin filaments have the maximum ability to slide in this position. When a muscle is excessively shortened or lengthened, it loses its ability to perform a strong contraction. This is called the **length-tension relationship.** A muscle can develop only moderate tension in the lengthened position and minimum tension in the shortened position. Massage can effectively normalize this situation by changing the length of the muscle (i.e., making it longer or shorter) and restoring the normal resting length.

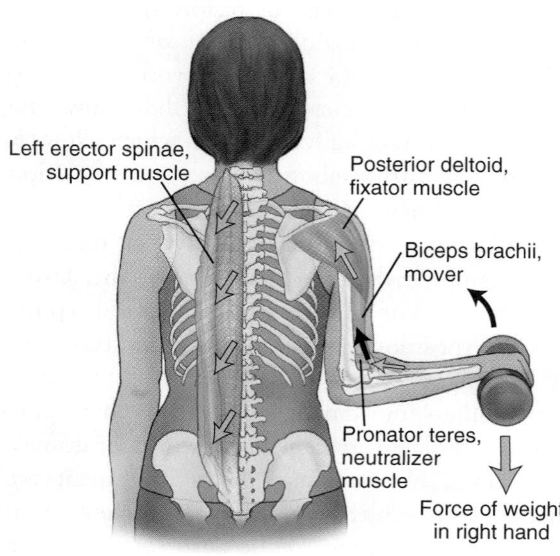

FIGURE 6-14 ■ The roles of muscles. A muscle may perform six major roles: mover, antagonist, fixator, neutralizer, support, and synergist. (From Muscolino JE: *Kinesiology: the skeletal system and muscle function,* enhanced edition, St Louis, 2006, Mosby.)

Reflexive Muscle Action

In providing a massage, therapists must recognize the importance of protective coordinated muscle reflex action, which is influenced by a number of reflex actions.

- *Withdrawal reflexes* (e.g., pulling away from a hot stove) involve instantaneous muscle contraction.
- *Righting reflexes* and *occulopelvic reflexes from the eyes, ears, ligaments, and joint capsules* are communicated to the muscle and stimulate instantaneous contraction to protect the joints and associated soft tissue and to support upright posture.
- *Arthrokinematic reflexes* are unconscious contractions of the muscles surrounding a joint, caused by irritation in the joint.
- *Splinting, guarding,* or *involuntary muscle contraction* can be caused by various types of muscle pathology.
- *Viscerosomatic reflexes* occur when irritation or inflammation in a visceral organ causes muscle spasm.
- Emotional or psychological stress causes excessive and sustained muscle tension.

The Kinetic Chain

Muscles do not function independently; rather, a body-wide, interactive network is involved. This network has been labeled the *kinetic chain* (Figure 6-15).

The kinetic chain influences training, conditioning, healing and rehabilitation, and massage application. The kinetic chain consists of the muscle/fascia system (functional anatomy), the articular joint system (functional biomechanics), and the neural/chemical system (motor behavior). These systems work interdependently to allow structural and functional efficiency. If any one of the systems does not work efficiently, compensation and adaptation occur in the other systems. Compensation and adaptation lead to tissue over-

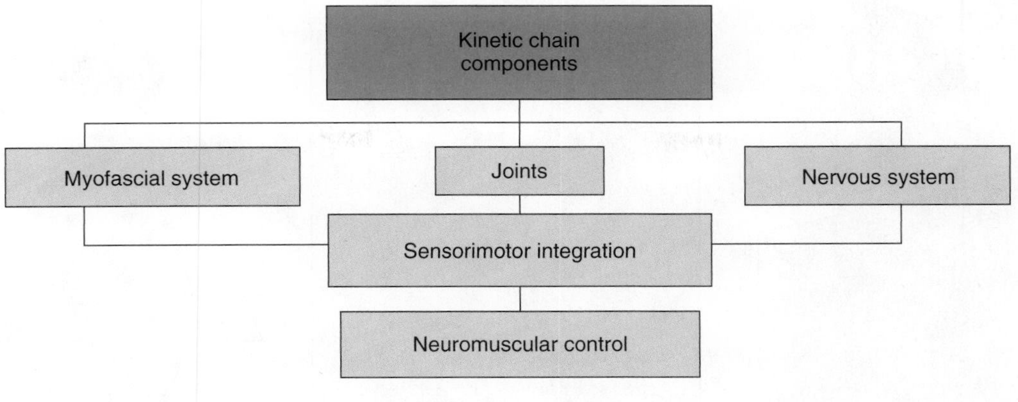

FIGURE 6-15 ■ The components of the kinetic chain. (Modified from Fritz S: *Mosby's essential sciences for therapeutic massage: anatomy, physiology, biomechanics, and pathology,* ed 2, St Louis, 2004, Mosby.)

load, diminished ability to function, and predictable patterns of dysfunction.

Efficient motor function is an effectively integrated, multiplanar (frontal, sagittal, and transverse planes) movement process that involves acceleration, deceleration, and stabilization of muscle and fascial tissue and joint structures. Many exercise programs involve only a uniplanar force movement (e.g., weight lifting machines). Very little time is spent on core stabilization, neuromuscular stabilization, and eccentric training in all three planes of motion. This situation sets up a patient for neuromuscular dysfunction. The massage professional must manage or assist in the reversal of the dysfunctional patterns that develop.

Physical fitness protocols should follow a sequence. Stability must develop before effective mobility. The **core** is made up of the lumbo-pelvic-hip complex, the thoracic spine, and the cervical spine. The core operates as an integrated unit to dynamically stabilize the body during functional movements. The stabilization system must function optimally to utilize the strength and power in the prime movers effectively. Many low back pain conditions are directly related to problems with core stability.

Functional movement patterns involve acceleration, stabilization, and deceleration, which occur at every joint. **Frontal plane movement** includes adduction and abduction. **Sagittal plane movement** includes flexion and extension, and **transverse plane rotational movement** includes internal and external rotation (Figure 6-16).

During functional movement, the transverse abdominis, internal oblique, multifidi, and deep erector spinae muscles stabilize the lumbopelvichip complex while the prime movers perform the actual functional activities.

Muscles function synergistically in groups, called *force couples,* to produce force, reduce force, and dynamically stabilize the kinetic chain. **Force couples** are integrated muscle groups that provide neuromuscular control during functional movements. The various movements of the scapula are the result of force couple action (Figure 6-17).

If the movement of the body is viewed as an integrated functional system, muscles can be classified as either local or global. Muscles that cross one joint are considered **local muscles** and form the inner unit. **Global muscles** cross multiple joints and form the outer unit.

The local musculature and connective tissue (inner unit) structurally consist of soft tissue that is predominately involved in joint support or stabilization. The joint support system of the core (lumbo-pelvic-hip complex) are muscles that either originate from or insert into the lumbar spine. These include the transverse abdominis, lumbar multifidi, and internal oblique muscles, the diaphragm, and the muscles of the pelvic floor.

Local musculature also forms the peripheral joint support systems of the shoulder and pelvic girdles and the limbs. These systems consist of muscles that are not movement specific but that provide stability to allow movement of a joint. These muscles also have attachments to the joint's

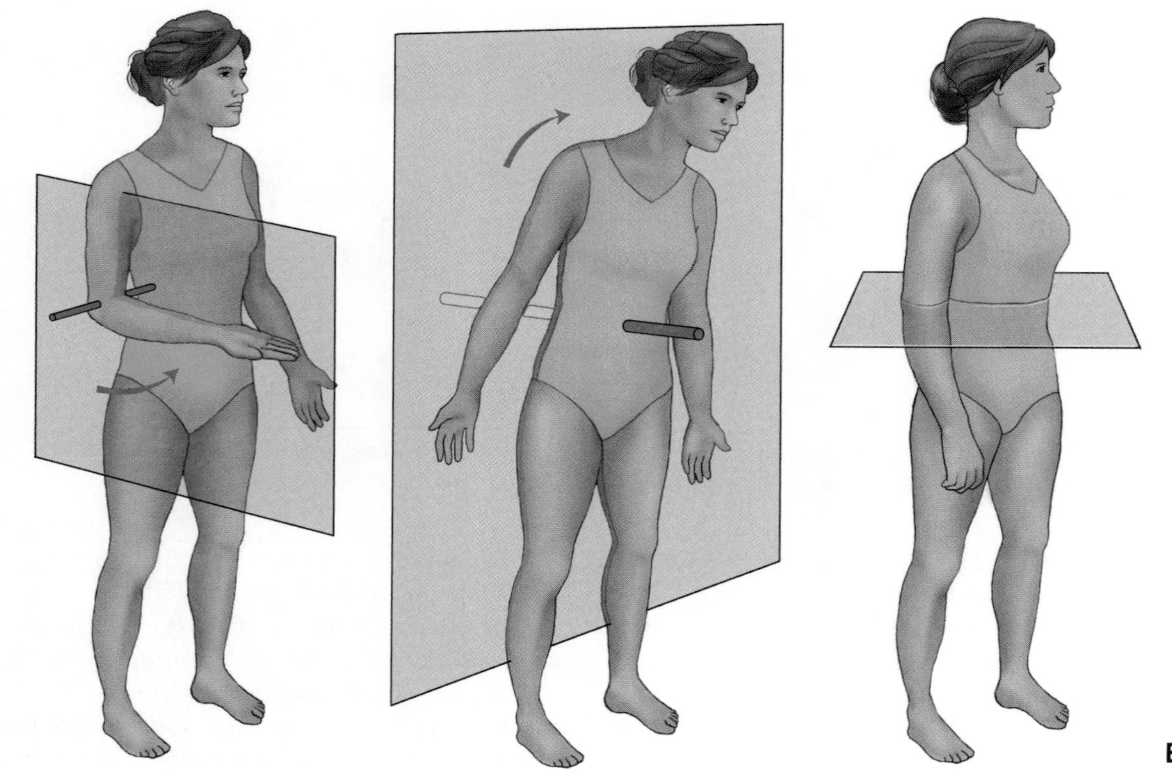

FIGURE 6-16 ■ The corresponding axes for the three cardinal planes (the axes are shown as red tubes). **A,** Sagittal plane. **B,** Frontal plane. **C,** Transverse plane. (From Muscolino JE: *Kinesiology: the skeletal system and muscle function,* enhanced edition, St Louis, 2006, Mosby.)

passive elements (e.g., ligaments and capsules) that make them ideal for increasing joint stability. A common example of a peripheral joint support system (local muscles/inner unit) is the rotator cuff of the glenohumeral joint, which provides dynamic stabilization for the humeral head in relation to the glenoid fossa during movement. Other joint support systems include the posterior fibers of the gluteus medius and the external rotators of the hip, which perform pelvic-femoral stabilization, and the vastus medialis obliquus (VMO), which provides patellar stabilization at the knee.

As mentioned, the global muscles (outer unit) cross multiple joints and are predominately responsible for movement. This group consists of more superficial muscles. The outer unit muscles typically are larger than inner unit muscles. They are associated with movement of the trunk and limbs, and they equalize external loads placed on the body. The major global muscles include the rectus abdominis, external obliques, erector spinae, gluteus maximus, latissimus dorsi, adductors, hamstrings, quadriceps, biceps, and triceps brachii. They are also important because they work together in complementary patterns to transfer and absorb forces from the upper and lower extremities to the pelvis.

evolve 6-26

For more information on the major global muscles, see the Evolve website.

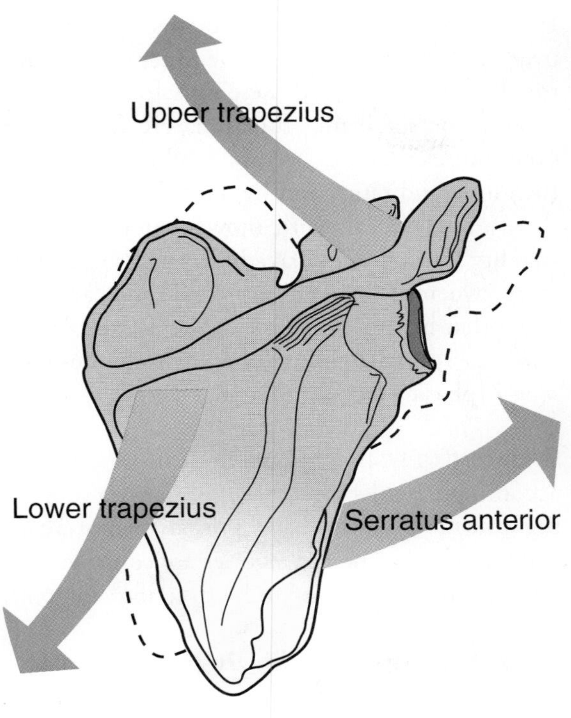

FIGURE 6-17 ■ The upper trapezius, lower trapezius, and serratus anterior pull in three different directions to achieve one type of motion—upward rotation of the scapula. This is called a *force couple.* (Modified from Fritz S: *Mosby's essential sciences for therapeutic massage: anatomy, physiology, biomechanics, and pathology,* ed 2, St Louis, 2004, Mosby.)

Functional Movement

During functional movement patterns, almost every muscle has the same synergistic function: to eccentrically decelerate pronation or to concentrically accelerate supination. The CNS recruits the appropriate muscles in an optimal firing pattern during specific movement patterns.

When the body is in a closed kinematic chain (standing upright), **full body pronation** is multiplanar (frontal, sagittal, and transverse planes), synchronized joint motion that occurs with eccentric muscle function. **Supination** is multiplanar (frontal, sagittal, and transverse planes), synchronized joint motion that occurs with concentric muscle function. This means that for one joint pattern to move effectively, all the involved joints must move. Movement can be initiated at any joint in the pattern, and restriction of any joint in the pattern restricts or increases motion in interconnected joints (Box 6-4).

Box 6-4 Joint Movement in Pronation and Supination

Body Part	Pronation	Supination
Foot	1. Dorsiflexion 2. Eversion 3. Abduction	1. Plantar flexion 2. Inversion 3. Adduction
Ankle	1. Dorsiflexion 2. Eversion 3. Abduction	1. Plantar flexion 2. Inversion 3. Adduction
Knee	1. Flexion 2. Adduction 3. Internal rotation	1. Extension 2. Abduction 3. External rotation
Hip	1. Flexion 2. Adduction 3. Internal rotation	1. Extension 2. Abduction 3. External rotation

To briefly describe functional biomechanics, we now review the gait cycle. During walking or other locomotor activities (e.g., running), motion at the subtalar joint is linked to the transverse plane rotations of the bone segments of the entire lower extremity. During the initial contact phase of gait, the subtalar joint pronates, which creates internal rotation of the tibia, femur, and pelvis. At midstance the subtalar joint supinates, which creates external rotation of the tibia, femur, and pelvis. Poor control of pronation reduces the ability to eccentrically decelerate multisegmental motion and can lead to muscle imbalances, joint dysfunction, and injury. Poor production of supination reduces the ability of the kinetic chain to concentrically produce the appropriate force during functional activities and can lead to synergistic dominance.

The term **joint arthrokinematics** refers to the roll, slide, glide, and translation that occur between two articular partners. **Joint play** is defined as the involuntary movement between articular surfaces that is separate from the range of motion produced by muscles. This is an essential component of joint motion and must occur for normal functioning of the joint. Predictable patterns of joint arthrokinematics occur during normal movement patterns. Optimal length-tension and force couple relationships ensure maintenance of normal joint kinematics.

Optimal muscle posture supports the development of high levels of functional strength and neuromuscular efficiency. *Functional strength* is the ability of the neuromuscular system to perform dynamic eccentric, isometric, and concentric actions efficiently in a multiplanar environment. This process allows the appropriate muscle activation sequence to be chosen to perform an activity and ensures that the right muscle contracts at the right joint, with the right amount of force, and at the right time. If any component of the kinetic chain is dysfunctional (e.g., short muscle, weak muscle, or joint dysfunction), neuromuscular control is altered, which increases the potential for injury.

When the kinetic chain is not functioning optimally, the result is a decrease in structural efficiency, functional efficiency, and performance. For example, if one muscle is short and tight (altered length-tension relationships), the force couples around that particular joint are altered. If the force couples are altered, the normal arthrokinematics are altered, and joint pain can occur.

Arthrokinematic inhibition is the neuromuscular phenomenon that occurs when a joint dysfunction inhibits the muscles that surround the joint. For example, a sacroiliac joint dysfunction causes arthrokinematic inhibition to the deep stabilization mechanism of the lumbo-pelvic-hip complex (transverse abdominis, internal oblique, multifidus, and the lumbar transversospinalis muscles). All these neuromuscular phenomena occur as a result of postural dysfunctions. Various movement systems, such as the Feldenkrais method and the Alexander technique, interact with this mechanism.

Development of Muscle Imbalances

Muscle imbalances are caused by postural stress, pattern overload, repetitive movement, lack of core stability, and lack of neuromuscular efficiency.

Serial Distortion Patterns. Kinetic chain dysfunction typically results in predictable patterns. These patterns differ somewhat from individual to individual, but an overview provides a means of understanding integrated function and dysfunction.

Vladimir Janda discovered that muscles react to pain or excessive stress in predictable patterns. He found that certain muscles tend to become overactive, short, and tight (i.e., increased motor tone), and he described these muscles as having a postural or stabilizing function. He found that other muscles tend to become inhibited and weak (i.e., long and taut), and he noticed that most of these muscles dealt with movement rather than stability. Many terms have been used to describe these two muscle functions. The more accurate terms that have been suggested are *tightness-prone stabilizer* (postural) muscles and *inhibition-prone mover* (phasic) muscles (Box 6-5).

Muscle Function Types. The muscles can be classified according to which ones have primarily a stabilizing role and which have primarily movement roles. However, these categories are controversial, because most muscles can function in both roles.

Tonic/postural stabilizing muscles play a primary role in the maintenance of posture and joint stability. The primary role of **phasic/mover muscles** is quick movement. Tonic/postural stabilizing muscles have been found to react to stress by becoming short and tight, whereas phasic/mover muscles react to stress by becoming inhibited and weak.

Box 6-5 Mover and Stabilizer Muscles of the Body

Movers	Stabilizers
Gastrocnemius/soleus	Peroneals
Adductors	Anterior tibialis
Hamstrings	Posterior tibialis
Psoas	Vastus medialis oblique
Tensor fasciae latae	Gluteus maximus/medius
Rectus femoris	Transversus abdominis
Piriformis	Internal oblique
Erector spinae	Multifidus
Pectoralis minor/major	Deep erector spinae
Latissimus dorsi	Transversospinalis
Teres major	Serratus anterior
Upper trapezius	Middle/lower trapezius
Levator scapulae	Rhomboids
Sternocleidomastoid	Teres minor
Scalenes	Infraspinatus
Teres major	Posterior deltoid
	Longus colli/capitis
	Deep cervical stabilizers

The movement group is characterized as being prone to developing tightness, readily activated during most functional movements, and overactive in fatigue situations or during new movement patterns. The stabilization group is prone to weakness and inhibition, less activated in most functional movement patterns, and fatigues easily during dynamic activities. As discussed, if the movement group is prone to tightness, shortening, and overuse, the muscles can cause reciprocal inhibition to their functional antagonists. This inhibition leads to poor neuromuscular efficiency and further postural dysfunction. If the stabilization group is prone to weakness, these muscles allow synergistic dominance and altered muscle activation sequences (firing patterns).

An important difference between the two muscle groups is that a small reduction of strength in an inhibition-prone muscle initiates a disproportionately larger contraction of the antagonist tightness-prone (shortening) muscle. Work and recreational activities favor tightness-prone muscles getting stronger, tighter, and shorter as the inhibition-prone muscle become weaker and more inhibited (long). Unless fitness programs (both physical and rehabilitative) are balanced, dysfunctional patterns are exacerbated. This is one reason the length-tension relationship is important. Some muscles, such as the quadratus lumborum and the scalenes, can react with either tightness or weakness.

Muscle dysfunction caused by illness or injury, job or exercise activity, reduced recovery time, chronic pain, or inflammation creates disturbances in normal muscle function and may stimulate a neurologically based tightness (shortening) or weakness (long and inhibited) in a muscle. Force couple occurs when muscles work together to produce movement or dynamic force joint stability. Serial distortion patterns in the kinetic chain disrupt force couple relationships.

A **serial distortion pattern** is a state in which the functional and structural integrity of the kinetic chain is altered, resulting in compensation and adaptation. These distortion patterns can be described as upper crossed syndrome (Figure 6-18), lower crossed syndrome (Figure 6-19), and pronation distortion syndrome (Figure 6-20).

JUST BETWEEN YOU AND ME

Let's simplify things a bit: Muscles that curl you toward your belly button (flexors, adductors, and internal rotators) shorten and pull the posture forward (make a cave). In response, the opposite muscles, which would uncurl you (extensors, abductors, and external rotators), are pulled long and become stretched (taut) over the "hills." These muscles feel taut and tight and often hurt, but only because they are fighting the ones that curl you forward, trying to maintain some aspect of upright posture. An effective, two-prong treatment approach involves using massage to lengthen the muscles in the "cave" and therapeutic exercise to strengthen the muscles on the "hills" (see the Evolve website for more information).

A short, tight muscle is held in a sustained contraction. The muscle is constantly working, and it consumes more oxygen and energy and generates more waste products than a muscle at rest. Circulation diminishes because the muscle is not performing its normal function as a pump; this leads to ischemia, which causes the pain receptors to fire. The sustained tension pulls on the muscle's attachments to the periosteum, joint capsule, and ligaments, creating increased pressure, uneven forces, and excessive wear in the joint.

Short, tight muscles often compress nerves between the muscles or through a muscle, which is a form of impingement syndrome. Weak, long muscles (i.e., they feel tight but are taut) are unable to support joint stability and contribute to poor posture, excessive tension and compression of adjunct structures, and abnormal joint movements. Firing patterns (muscle activation sequences) and gait reflexes are disturbed.

Inhibited muscles interfere with vascular and lymphatic movement. *Reciprocal inhibition* is the process by which a tight muscle (e.g., the psoas) causes decreased neural stimulus in its functional antagonist (in this case, the gluteus maximus). The result is decreased force production by the prime mover, leading to compensation by the synergists, a condition called *synergistic dominance.* **Synergistic dominance** occurs when synergists compensate for weak or inhibited prime mover patterns. It is the process by which a synergist compensates for a prime mover to maintain force production. For example, if a patient has a weak

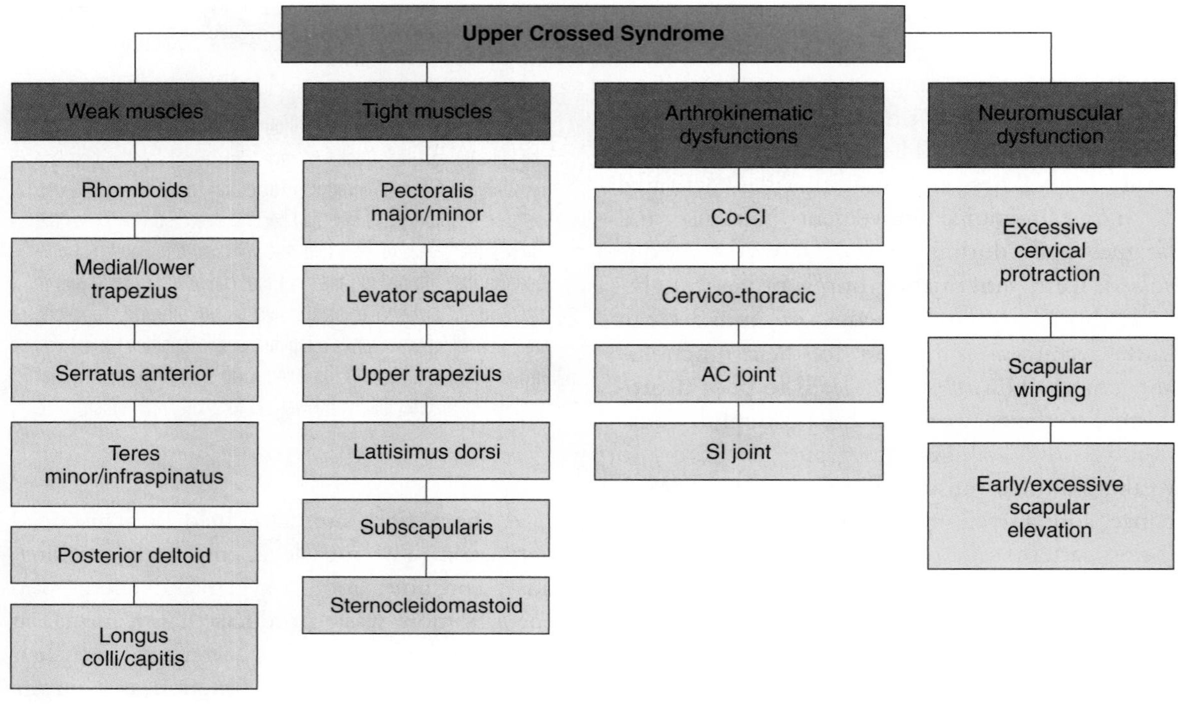

FIGURE 6-18 ■ An upper crossed syndrome flowchart. (Data from Chaitow L, Delany JW: *Clinical applications of neuromuscular techniques, vol 1, The upper body,* Edinburgh, 2001, Churchill Livingstone.)

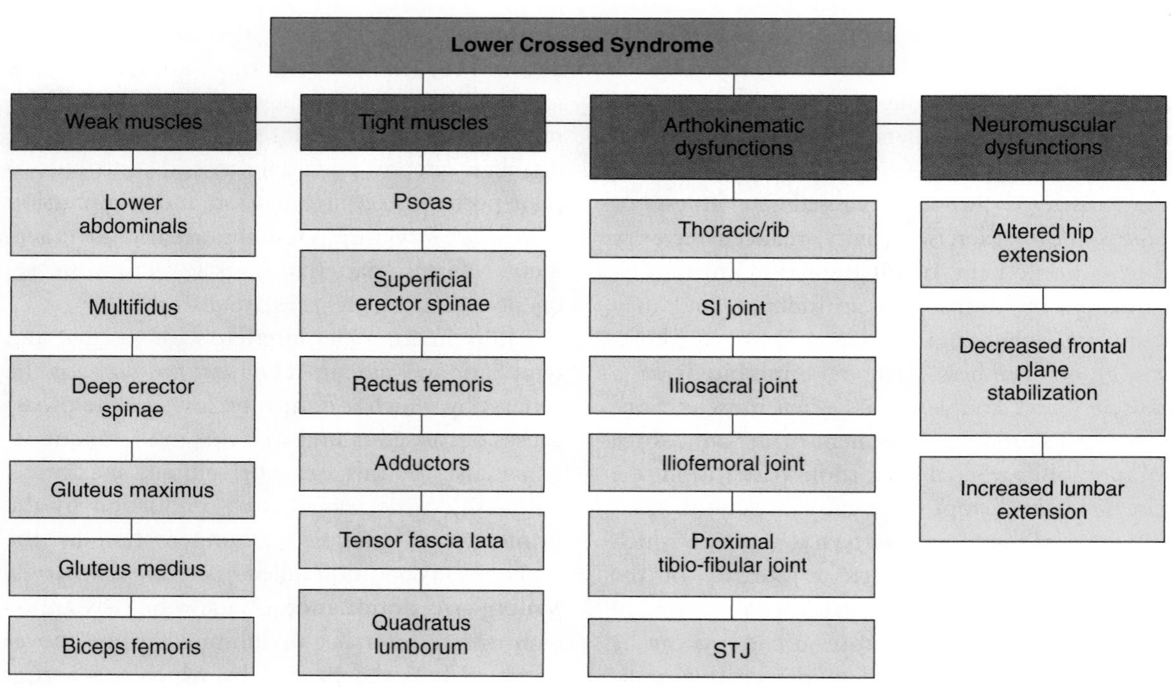

FIGURE 6-19 ■ A lower crossed syndrome flowchart. (Data from Chaitow L, Delany JW: *Clinical applications of neuromuscular techniques, vol 1, The upper body,* Edinburgh, 2001, Churchill Livingstone.)

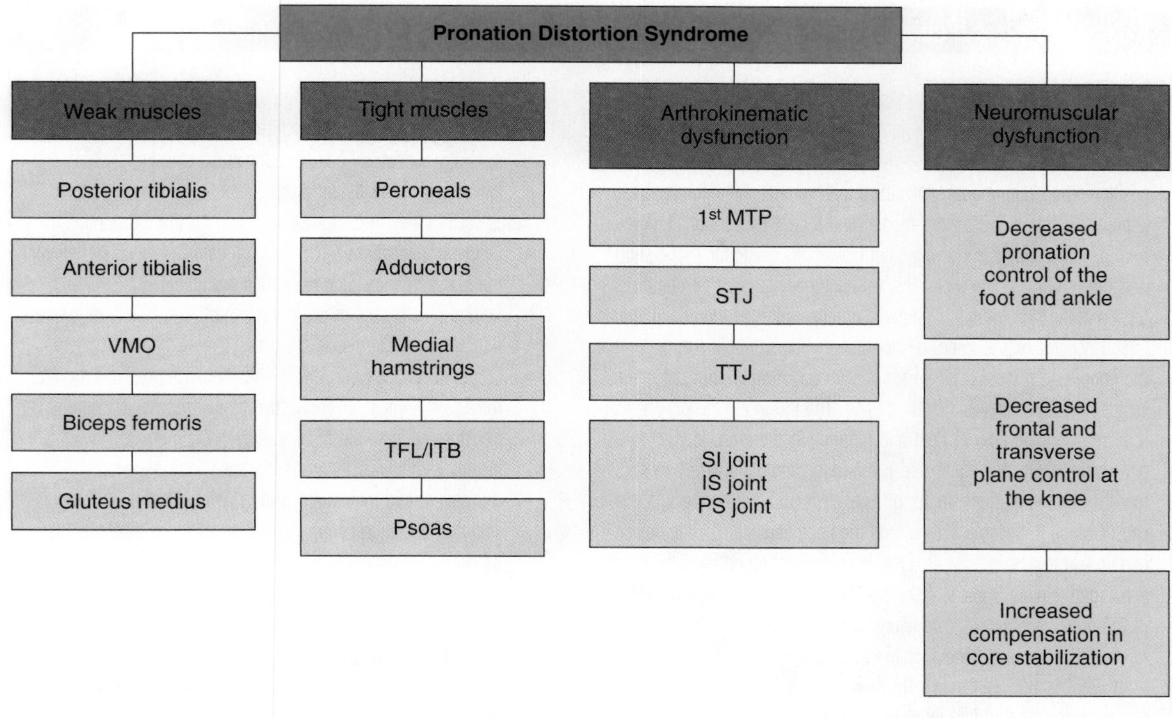

FIGURE 6-20 ■ Pronation distortion syndrome. (Data from Chaitow L, Delany JW: *Clinical applications of neuromuscular techniques, vol 1, The upper body,* Edinburgh, 2001, Churchill Livingstone.)

gluteus medius, synergists (i.e., the tensor fasciae latae, adductor complex, and quadratus lumborum) become dominant to compensate for the weakness. This alters normal joint alignment, which further alters the normal length-tension relationships around the joint where the muscles attach. This process leads to altered movement patterns, which are assessed and treated with firing pattern sequences. Synergistic dominance often occurs when a person performs an activity while fatigued. The individual will complain of heavy or labored movement.

The process by which poor posture and muscle imbalances cause reciprocal inhibition and synergistic dominance also causes altered joint alignment. This condition arises from muscle shortening and muscle weakness. Altered arthrokinematics (joint movement) is further altered as a result of altered force couple relationships. If the synergists are dominant, normal joint movements are altered because different muscles are activating out of sequence. This is a continuous and cyclic process. Muscle shortening, muscle weakness, joint dysfunction, or decreased neuromuscular efficiency all can initiate this dysfunctional pattern.

Massage Application

As described in this text, massage is particularly effective in dealing with muscle dysfunction conditions and in supporting other professional treatments. Primarily, massage lengthens short, tight muscles, normalizes firing patterns, and increases tissue pliability. These benefits support therapeutic exercise to treat the long (taut), weak, inhibited muscles. In other words, treatment involves massage and stretching of short, tight muscles and exercise for long, weak muscles. Put another way, the goal is to massage and stretch the "cave" and strengthen the "hills" (Box 6-6).

Massage targets both the connective tissue and neuromuscular aspects of muscle function, because tension in a muscle and its fascia is created by active and passive elements. The passive elements include the collagen fibers and ground substance, which are influenced by massage with the introduction of various mechanical forces. Because muscle contains ground substance, it demonstrates viscous behavior. It becomes thicker and stiff when stretched quickly, cold, or immobilized. It becomes more fluidlike when stretched slowly or warmed up. Active components of

BOX 6-6 Putting It Together

Consider the knee, one of the most used and abused joints. An injury to the knee typically causes the joint to be held in a sustained midrange flexion during the acute phase. This position is the least packed joint position, can accommodate increased fluid, and is most comfortable. It pulls the soft tissue on the medial and lateral aspects of the knee into an abnormal posterior alignment, with the posterior tissue short and the anterior tissue long. This misalignment creates an abnormal torsion in the skin, muscles, tendons, and ligaments of the medial and lateral aspects of the knee, a shortening of structure at the back of the knee, and a weakening of the medial quadriceps, particularly the vastus medialis obliquus (VMO) muscle. The increased torsion causes a decrease in the flow of fluid and nutrition in the area, leading to a diminished ability for repair and a tendency for tissue layers to stick together and adhesions to form. The sustained position eventually causes tissue to become fibrotic, and the knee ends up stuck in flexion and unable to extend fully. Body-wide compensation patterns begin to occur, and reinjury is likely. Also, areas of compensation in other parts of the body become prone to injury, with a tendency for tissue layers to stick together and adhesions to develop.

So what is the next step? No defined recipe is available. Clinical reasoning is essential and revolves around two elements:

- Applying therapeutic massage with an intelligent focus
- Normalizing soft tissue structures by reintroducing the normal spiral orientation to the soft tissue and increasing pliability and separation of the tissue layers

In cases such as this, massage can accomplish the following:

- Create a mechanical force, tension, bind, shear, or torsion on the fibers to encourage relaxation and pliability
- Reintroduce control of acute inflammation to signal regeneration of connective tissue structures
- Create a piezoelectric effect with application of mechanical force to dysfunctional connective tissue (mechanical energy is transformed into electrical energy); the piezoelectric effect increases cellular activity, tissue repair, and alignment
- Normalize fluid movement using rhythmic cycles of compression and decompression, rocking, and specific methods, such as lymphatic drainage, to restore the natural rhythmic movement of the body's fluids
- Normalize autonomic nervous system, neurotransmitter, and endocrine functioning (deliberate use of stimulation or inhibition and pressure levels encourages appropriate neurochemical function)

evolve 6-27

The following terms and expressions specific to Chapter 6 have already been used to search PubMed for the latest research literature available. The *Click Here for Massage* feature associated with this chapter on your textbook's Evolve website allows you to hyperlink to a continually updated PubMed search of research literature that corresponds to this subject.

Hyperlink Search Terms

Massage autonomic nervous system
Massage cardiovascular system
Massage central nervous system
Massage emotion neuroendocrine
Massage energy systems
Massage fluid dynamics
Massage gate control theory
Massage myofascial
Massage neuroendocrine
Massage parasympathetic nervous system
Massage respiratory system
Massage sensitization neuroendocrine function
Massage somatic nervous system
Massage sympathetic nervous system

muscle include the contractile proteins, actin and myosin, and nerves, and massage interaction causes the neurochemical stimulus.

SUMMARY

To provide massage intelligently, you must understand the principles of anatomy and physiology. This knowledge is essential for developing treatment plans based on indications, contraindications, and outcomes in the healthcare environment. If massage is to be taken seriously in the healthcare setting, you must be able to speak intelligently and concisely with other healthcare professionals, and the foundation of communication is the commonality of anatomy and physiology. Also, you must have a thorough understanding of these two areas to maintain medical records. Anatomy and physiology form the foundation on which therapeutic massage is based, and continuing study of these fascinating principles is one of the elements of professional excellence.

WORKBOOK

1. Locate and summarize the various discussions throughout the textbook that relate to fluid dynamics. Include concepts of assessment, treatment outcomes, contraindications, and benefits. List page numbers.

____

____

____

____

____

2. Locate and summarize the various discussions throughout the textbook that relate to neuroendocrine control of the body. Include concepts of assessment, treatment outcomes, contraindications, and benefits. List page numbers.

____

____

____

____

____

3. Locate and summarize the various discussions throughout the textbook that relate to connective tissue and its function. Include concepts of assessment, treatment outcomes, contraindications, and benefits. List page numbers.

____

____

____

____

____

4. Locate and summarize the various discussions throughout the textbook that relate to joint function. Include concepts of assessment, treatment outcomes, contraindications, and benefits. List page numbers.

____

____

____

____

____

5. Locate and summarize the various discussions throughout the textbook and the Evolve website that relate to muscular function. Include concepts of assessment, treatment outcomes, contraindications, and benefits. List page numbers.

____

____

____

____

____

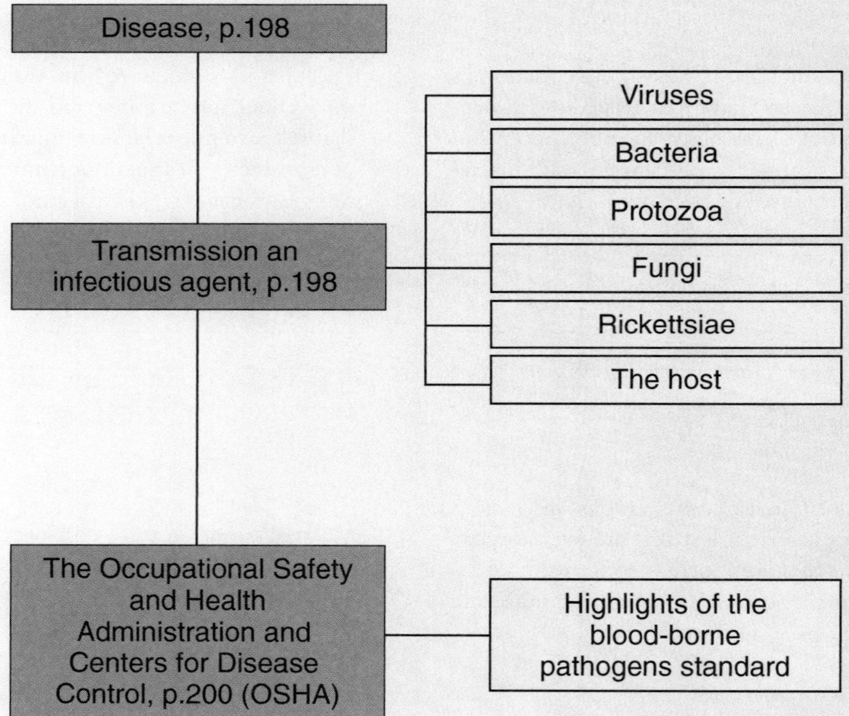
Disease, p.198
Transmission an infectious agent, p.198
Viruses
Bacteria
Protozoa
Fungi
Rickettsiae
The host
The Occupational Safety and Health Administration and Centers for Disease Control, p.200 (OSHA)
Highlights of the blood-borne pathogens standard

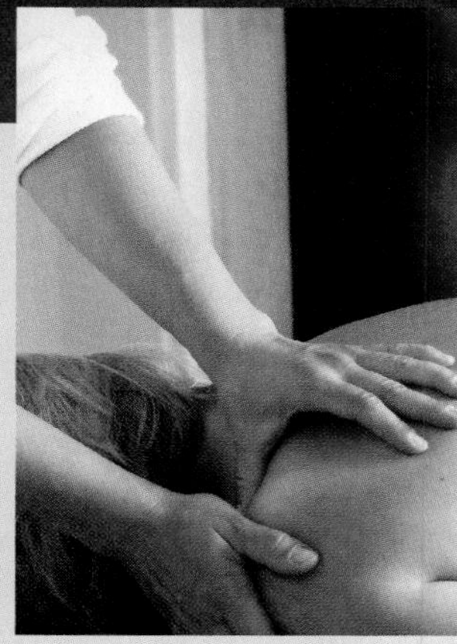

CHAPTER 7

SANITATION

Key Terms

Acute infections	Disease	Infectious diseases	Sanitation
Carrier	Fungi	Latent infection	Slow infections
Chronic infections	Hand hygiene	Portal of entry	Susceptible host
Direct transmission	Indirect transmission	Protozoa	Vectors

For definitions of key terms, refer to the Evolve website.

OBJECTIVES

Upon completion of this chapter, the reader will have the information necessary to:

1 Maintain sanitary practices in the healthcare setting.
2 Maintain compliance with Standard Precautions.
3 Recognize transmission routes for pathogens.

Massage therapists should *always* be meticulous about hygiene and sanitation. However, this behavior is even more important in the medical setting, in which exposure to disease is increased and patients are more susceptible to pathogens. The concepts of disease transmission and the response to infection form the basis for understanding the importance of the first line of defense in preventing disease. Before we can assist in the prevention of disease, we have to look at methods we can use to minimize the chances of being a carrier of disease. One of the simplest techniques for preventing the spread of disease is hand washing. In medical practice, every procedure begins and ends with hand washing, both because of the need for infection control and because of the impact of guidelines established by the Occupational Safety and Health Administration (OSHA). The concepts presented in this chapter and on the Evolve website are basic to infection control; by following them scrupulously, you can reduce the transmission of disease, lessen the severity of disease, and possibly save the life of a patient or co-worker, or even your own life.

DISEASE

Disease is defined as any sustained, harmful alteration of the normal structure, function, or metabolism of an organism or a cell that manifests as a group of clinical signs, symptoms, and laboratory findings. Diseases have been categorized into many different types, such as hereditary (genetic), drug induced, autoimmune, degenerative, communicable, and infectious, to name only a few. Sometimes a specific disease may fit into two or more categories.

The goal of **sanitation** is to prevent the spread of infectious (communicable) disease. Any disease caused by the growth of pathogenic microorganisms in the body falls into the category of infectious disease. Microorganisms are present almost everywhere. The only places free of microorganisms are the insides of sterilized containers and the tissues of certain internal body organs. In the normal state, organs and tissues that are not connected to the outside of the body by mucus-lined membranes are free of all living microorganisms.

The mere entrance of a living microbe into the body does not constitute disease, because until the infected cell shows a harmful alteration of its structure, physiology, or biochemistry, disease is either not detected or not considered present. In fact, a living microbe may be ingested, injected, or inhaled and never cause disease in an individual. However, an unaffected person (i.e., a carrier) can transmit the infection to another person.

Acute infections have a rapid onset of symptoms but last a relatively short time. The *prodromal period* is the interval when the patient first exhibits vague, nonspecific symptoms of the disease. In an acute viral infection, the host cell typically dies within hours or days. Not until after the tissue damage begins do symptoms appear, and the virus usually can be isolated only shortly before or after the prodromal period. In most acute infections, such as the common cold, the body's defense mechanisms eliminate the virus within 2 to 3 weeks.

Chronic infections endure for a long period, in some cases for a lifetime. With chronic viral hepatitis B (HBV), the individual is asymptomatic but the virus is detectable through blood tests and remains transmissible throughout the person's life. Hepatitis B, or serum hepatitis, is transmitted by blood, blood products, and all body fluids. It is a serious health hazard to medical personnel. All individuals employed in a healthcare setting should consider being immunized against HBV.

A **latent infection** is a persistent infection in which the symptoms cycle through periods of relapse and remission. Cold sores (oral herpes simplex) and genital herpes are latent viral infections. The virus enters the body and causes a lesion. It then lies dormant, in a nerve cell away from the surface, until a certain provocation (e.g., illness with fever, sunburn, or stress) causes it to leave the nerve cell and seek the surface again. Once the virus reaches the superficial tissues, it becomes detectable for a short time and causes another outbreak at the original site. The herpes zoster virus may lie dormant along a nerve pathway for years and later erupt as the painful disease shingles.

Slow infections progress over very long periods. These conditions include the degenerative neurologic diseases, such as progressive Lyme disease or advanced syphilis.

TRANSMISSION OF AN INFECTIOUS AGENT

Infectious diseases can spread only under certain circumstances. Infection starts with the infectious agent. The five groups of potentially pathogenic organisms are viruses, bacteria, protozoa, fungi, and rickettsiae. For infection to occur, an infectious microorganism must be present. Therefore the best way to prevent the spread of disease is to use adequate infection control procedures; these include consistent hand washing, proper use of antiseptics, and disinfection and sterilization methods.

VIRUSES

The smallest of all pathogens, viruses, lead the list of important disease-causing agents. Viral microorganisms are intracellular parasites that take over the deoxyribonucleic acid (DNA) of the invaded cell. Viral invasion may not cause significant immediate symptoms, because host cells infected with viruses can produce a substance called *interferon,* which protects nearby cells. Antibiotics are unable to destroy viral invaders that enter a normal cell and multiply within the cell. Therefore the treatment for viral infections typically focuses on relief of symptoms or palliative treatment. To counteract and destroy the viral invaders, interferon and antiviral agents, such as acyclovir (Zovirax), amantadine (Symmetrel), and zidovudine (Retrovir), may be prescribed.

BACTERIA

Bacteria are tiny, primitive cells that produce disease in a variety of ways. Every person has normal *flora* (nonpathogenic bacteria) that reside in various body systems, especially the digestive tract. These "friendly" bacteria provide protection from disease by competing for nutrients that pathogenic bacteria require to grow and multiply. Pathogenic bacteria can secrete toxic substances that damage human tissues; they can act as parasites inside human cells; or they can form colonies in the body that disrupt normal human functions. Bacteria are classified according to their shape, or *morphology.* Spherical bacteria are known as *cocci,* rod-shaped bacteria are *bacilli,* and spiral-shaped bacteria are *spirilla.* Some bacteria can produce resistant forms, called *spores,* that make treatment difficult.

A bacterial infection can be treated in a number of ways. The most common approach is to use antibiotics to destroy or inhibit the growth of the invader. Unfortunately, overuse and incorrect use of antibiotics have resulted in mutated forms of bacteria that are resistant to antibiotics. In addition, antibiotics can also kill the beneficial bacteria, increasing the person's susceptibility to infection. This is a major healthcare concern, and research is underway to find new antibiotics that can deal with these resistant strains.

PROTOZOA

Protozoa are unicellular parasites that can replicate and multiply rapidly once inside the host. Diseases caused by protozoa include giardiasis, which is confined to the gastrointestinal tract, and malaria, in which the organism invades the blood system. Protozoal infections are frequently seen in tropical climates because vectors (transmission process) are needed to transmit the disease. For example, the mosquito is the vector for the transmission of malaria.

FUNGI

Fungi are a division of plants that may be unicellular or multicellular. They include such growths as mushrooms, molds, and yeasts. Many types of fungi are pathogenic and can cause disease, such as candidiasis and *Tinea* infection (e.g., athlete's foot). Fungi grow best in dark, moist environments. Treatment with antifungal agents includes the application of topical preparations for *Tinea* infections (e.g., Lotrimin or Nizoral [ketoconazole]); the use of vaginal suppositories for candidiasis (e.g., Monistat [miconazole]); or the administration of oral mediations (e.g., Diflucan [Fluconazole] and nystatin). Fungal infections are also called *mycotic infections.*

RICKETTSIAE

Rickettsiae are a group of microorganisms that have some of the characteristics of both bacteria and viruses. Like viruses, they are parasites that require living host cells for growth. However, they are larger than viruses and can be viewed with a microscope. Vectors such as fleas, ticks, and mites usually transmit pathogenic forms of rickettsiae. Diseases caused by rickettsiae can be treated with antibiotics. These diseases include Lyme disease and Rocky Mountain spotted fever, which are both transmitted by ticks.

THE HOST

Most pathogens must gain entrance into a host or else they die. A *reservoir host* supplies nutrition to the organism, allowing it to multiply. Reservoir hosts may be people, insects, animals, water, food, or contaminated instruments. The pathogen either causes infection in the host or, in the case of vector-borne diseases, exits the host in great enough numbers to cause disease in another host.

Infection is spread according to how the pathogen escapes the reservoir host. Exits include the mouth, nose, eyes, ears, intestines, urinary tract, reproductive tract, and open wounds. The use of Standard Precautions, such as wearing latex gloves, using masks, ensuring proper wound management and correct disposal of contaminated products, and hand washing, helps control the ability of the infectious material to spread from one host to another.

After exiting the reservoir host, organisms spread by transmission, either direct or indirect. **Direct transmission** occurs through contact with an infected person or with the discharges of an infected person, such as feces or urine. **Indirect transmission** occurs in a number of ways, including airborne droplets expelled through coughing, speaking, or sneezing; **vectors** that harbor pathogens; contaminated food or drink; and contaminated objects (called *fomites*). Measures that help control the transmission of pathogens include proper sanitation of food and water; proper use of sanitization, disinfection, and sterilization procedures; and the use of germicides (e.g., Wave Cide and Cidex).

The Portal of Entry

The **portal of entry** is the route by which a transmitted pathogen gains entry into a new host. Like the means of exit, the means of entry may be the mouth, nose, eyes, intestines, urinary tract, reproductive tract, or an open wound.

The first line of defense against pathogenic invasion is an intact integumentary system (i.e., the skin), which serves as a mechanical barrier to infection. Other anatomic defense mechanisms include integumentary secretions, tears, cilia, mucous membranes, and the pH of body fluids.

The body's second line of defense includes the inflammatory process and the immune system response. The immune system responds to an invader by producing antibodies specifically designed to combat the presence of a foreign substance or antigen. This process is called *humoral immunity.* The immune system also reacts at the cellular level with *cell-mediated immunity,* causing the destruction of pathogenic cells at the site of invasion. An example of cell-mediated immunity is *phagocytosis,* a process in which specialized immune system cells, called *macrophages,* ingest and destroy pathogenic microbes.

If the host is a *susceptible host* (i.e., one that can support the growth of the infecting organism), the organism multiplies. Factors that affect a host's susceptibility include the location of entry, the dose of organisms, and the condition of the individual. If the conditions are favorable, the organisms reach infectious levels, the susceptible host becomes a reservoir host, and the cycle begins again.

Individuals who are effectively immunized against a disease (e.g., HBV) are not susceptible to the disease even if exposed to the pathogen, because their immune systems have created antibodies to protect them. In addition to immunization, people can reduce their susceptibility to disease by getting proper nutrition and following a healthy lifestyle.

THE OCCUPATIONAL SAFETY AND HEALTH ADMINISTRATION AND CENTERS FOR DISEASE CONTROL

The mission of the Occupational Safety and Health Administration (OSHA), a federal agency, is to "ensure the safety and health of America's workers by setting and enforcing standards; providing training, outreach, and education; establishing partnerships; and encouraging continual improvement in workplace safety and health."

In 1987, concern about the increasing prevalence of human immunodeficiency virus (HIV) and HBV infection prompted the Centers for Disease Control (now called the Centers for Disease Control and Prevention [CDC]) to recommend a new approach to dealing with potentially infectious materials called *Universal Precautions* (these are now called *Standard Precautions*). The underlying concept of Standard Precautions is this: because it is impossible for healthcare workers to know whether a patient has an infectious disorder, all blood and certain body fluids must be treated as if they are known to be infectious for blood-borne pathogens. Precautions therefore should be implemented for all patients, regardless of the healthcare professional's knowledge of the person's individual health history. Universal Precautions also protect the patient from any blood-borne infection the healthcare worker may have.

OSHA recognizes that employees face significant health risks from occupational exposure to blood or other potentially infectious materials that may contain HBV, hepatitis C (HCV), or HIV. In July, 1992, OSHA began enforcing work practice controls to reduce or eliminate occupational exposure to blood-borne pathogens. Employers whose workers are at risk of occupational exposure to blood or other infectious materials must implement an Exposure Control Plan that details employee protection procedures. The plan must describe how an employer will use a combination of controls, including personal protective equipment, training, medical surveillance, HBV immunization, record keeping for occupational injuries, and labeling of hazardous materials. Engineering controls (e.g., safer medical equipment, puncture-proof sharps containers, and shielded needle devices) are recommended as the primary means of reducing or eliminating employee exposure.

The revised standard also clarifies the use of washing or flushing of any exposed body area or mucous membranes immediately after or as soon as possible after exposure to potentially infectious materials. This includes hand washing after the removal of gloves or other personal protective equipment.

HIGHLIGHTS OF THE BLOOD-BORNE PATHOGENS STANDARD

Because the pathogen standards are written to cover employees in all health fields, only some of the regulations apply to the practice of therapeutic massage. The information presented here is that which most applies to the massage therapist.

NOTE: Massage therapists must use hand-washing techniques that are applied up past the elbows, because the forearm often is used during massage application.

A good antimicrobial soap with chlorhexidine (e.g., Hibiclens) that has antiseptic residual action that lasts several hours should be used for hand washing in the healthcare environment. Each sink should be equipped with a liquid soap dispenser. A water-soluble lotion may be rubbed into the hands after they have been washed and dried. Dry, cracked, chapped skin is an interruption of the skin's integrity and can result in the transmission of disease.

Proper hand washing involves two crucial elements: running water and friction. The water should be warm, because water that is too hot or too cold causes the skin to become chapped. Friction involves firmly rubbing all surfaces of the hands, wrists, and forearms. Remember that fingers have four sides and fingernails have two sides. All jewelry is removed for medical hand washing. The hands and forearms are washed under running water, with the fingertips pointing downward. Soap and friction are applied to the hands, wrists, and forearms because these areas are used for massage application. Allow the water to wash away debris from the elbows down toward the fingertips (Figure 7-1).

Remember, the goals of aseptic hand washing are to protect you from infection and to prevent cross-contamination through the transfer of microorganisms from one patient to another. It is important to use this hand-washing technique as follows:

- After you finish with one patient and before you attend to another
- Before and after you use toilet facilities
- Whenever you touch something that causes your hands to become contaminated
- When you arrive at work and before you leave the office
- Before and after eating
- At the end of the day

evolve 7-1

Hand Washing

It is impossible to sterilize your hands; therefore the goal of hand washing is to reduce the number of bacteria on the skin by using mechanical friction, antimicrobial soaps, and warm, running water. Normally, two types of bacteria can be found on the skin: transient bacteria, which are surface bacteria that remain a short time, and resident bacteria, which are found under the fingernails, in hair follicles, in the openings of the sebaceous glands, and in the deeper layers of the skin. The goal of thorough hand washing is to eliminate or reduce the number of transient bacteria on the skin surface, preventing transient bacteria from becoming resident bacteria. The most effective barrier against infection is unbroken skin.

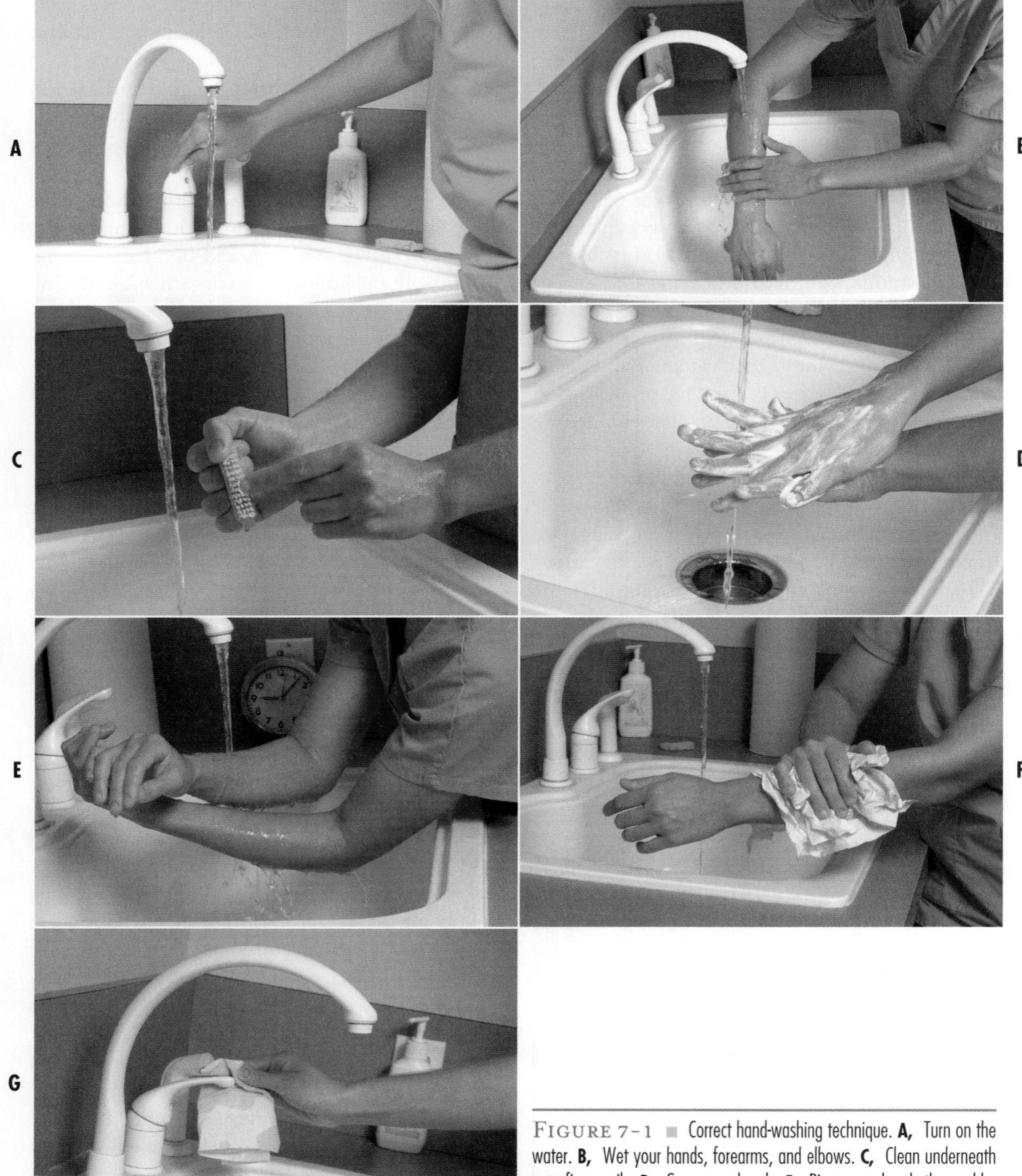

FIGURE 7-1 ■ Correct hand-washing technique. **A,** Turn on the water. **B,** Wet your hands, forearms, and elbows. **C,** Clean underneath your fingernails. **D,** Soap your hands. **E,** Rinse your hands thoroughly. **F,** Dry your hands. **G,** Turn off the water. (From Salvo S: *Massage therapy: principles and practice,* ed 2, St Louis, 2003, WB Saunders.)

The CDC recently released new recommendations for hand hygiene in healthcare settings. The term **hand hygiene** applies to hand washing, the use of an antiseptic hand rub, or surgical hand antisepsis. Evidence suggests that hand antisepsis (i.e., cleaning the hands with an antiseptic hand rub) is more effective at reducing nosocomial infections than plain hand washing.

When you use an alcohol-based hand rub, apply the product to the palm of one hand and rub the hands together, covering all surfaces of the hands and fingers, until the hands are dry. Follow the manufacturer's recommendations on the amount of hand rub to use. Hands that are visibly soiled should still be washed with soap and water.

Routinely use an alcohol-based hand rub to decontaminate your hands (1) before and after patient contact and (2) immediately after touching blood, body fluids, secretions, excretions, mucous membranes, skin that is not intact, and contaminated items (e.g., wound dressings), regardless of whether you wore gloves.

Further guidelines established by the CDC include the following:

- Wash the hands with soap and water before eating and after using a restroom. Antimicrobial-impregnated wipes (i.e., towelettes) are not a substitute for using an alcohol-based hand rub or antimicrobial soap.
- Wear clean, nonsterile gloves when touching blood, body fluids, secretions, excretions, mucous membranes, skin that is not intact, and contaminated items.
- Change gloves between procedures on the same patient after exposure to potentially infectious material.
- Remove gloves immediately after patient contact and wash your hands (Figure 7-2).
- Use plain soap for routine hand washing and an antimicrobial or antiseptic agent for specified situations.
- Wear protective barrier equipment (e.g., mask, goggles, face shield, gown) as necessary to protect the mucous membranes of your eyes, nose, and mouth, and to avoid soiling of your clothes when performing cleanup procedures that may generate splashes or sprays of blood, body fluids, secretions, or excretions.

As improved procedures are developed, safety and sanitation recommendations and requirements change. It is the responsibility of each professional to remain current on sanitation procedures.

evolve 7-2

See the Evolve website for a list of common diseases caused by pathogens.

Environmental Protection

The environmental protection section of the compliance guidelines covers controls to minimize the risk of occupational injury by isolating or removing any physical or mechanical health hazard in the medical workplace. Massage therapists must follow these and any other safety rules when working in the healthcare system.

- Observe warning labels on biohazard containers and equipment.
- Minimize splashing, spraying, and spattering of drops of potentially infectious materials. Splattering of blood onto skin or mucous membranes is a proven mode of transmission of HBV.
- Bandage any breaks or lesions on your hands before gloving.
- If exposed body surfaces, such as the eyes, come in contact with body fluids, flush with water and/or scrub with soap and water as soon as possible. For massage therapists this is most likely to happen during cleanup procedures.
- Equipment (including linens) that has been contaminated with blood or body fluids should be decontaminated.
- Smoking, eating, drinking, applying cosmetics or lip balm, and handling contact lenses are prohibited in work areas where

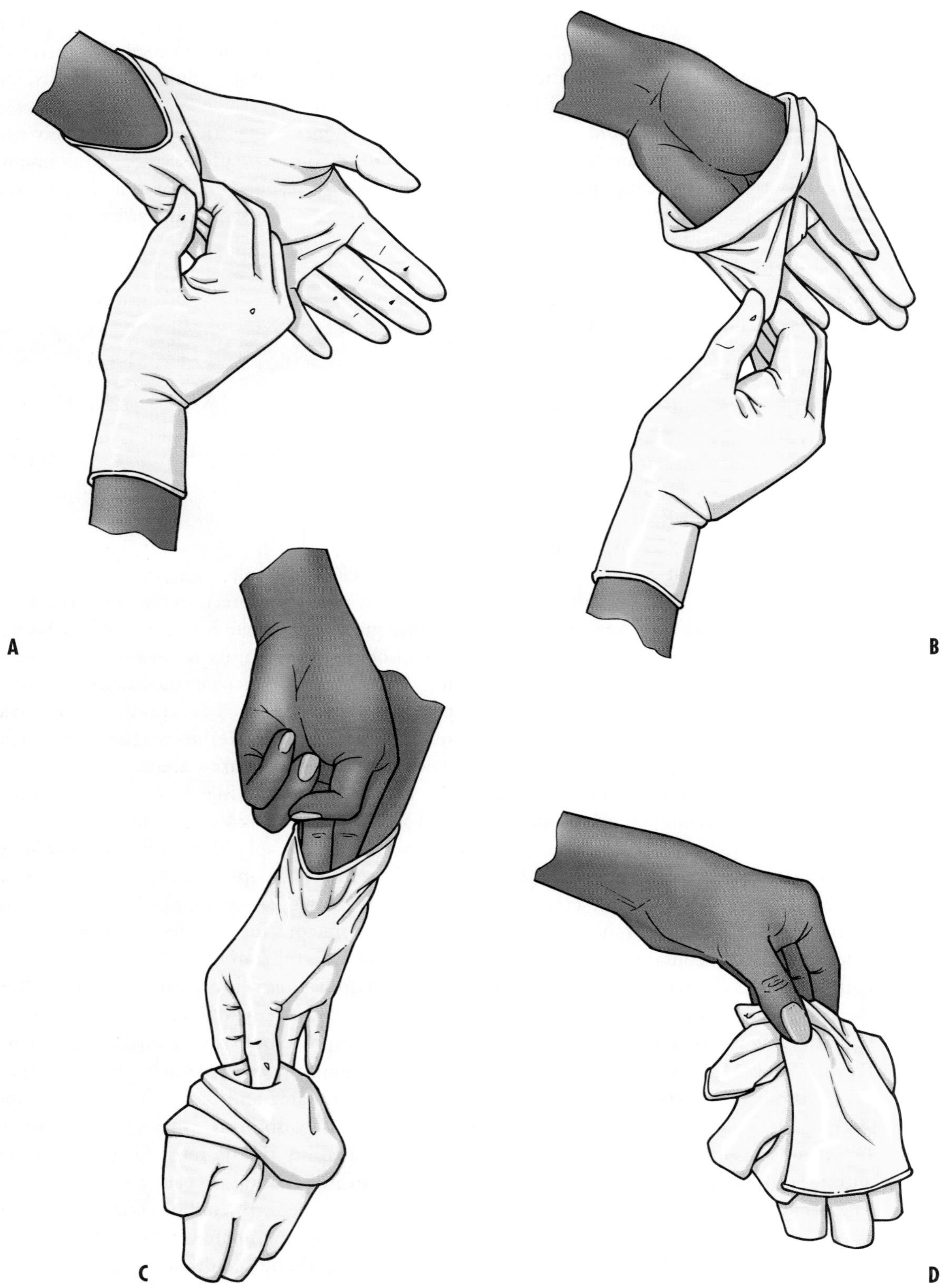

FIGURE 7–2 ■ Proper removal of disposable gloves. **A,** Pull off one glove. **B,** Put the removed glove in the palm of your gloved hand. **C,** Remove the other glove with the first glove inside. **D,** Dispose of the used gloves. (From Salvo S: *Massage therapy: principles and practice,* ed 2, St Louis, 2003, WB Saunders.)

a reasonable likelihood of contamination from blood-borne pathogens exists.

- Food and drink cannot be kept in refrigerators, freezers, shelves, or cabinets, or on countertops where blood or other potentially infectious materials could be present.

Housekeeping Controls

The OSHA standard specifies certain housekeeping measures to be followed to promote a clean, sanitary work area. One requirement is a posted schedule for cleaning and decontaminating each work area where exposure could occur. This documentation must be specific and must include information on the surface cleaned, the type of waste encountered, and procedures performed in the designated area.

- Work surfaces must be decontaminated with a disinfectant (e.g., a 1 : 10 solution of sodium hypochlorite or chlorine bleach) immediately after accidental spills of blood or body fluids and at the end of each procedure.
- All reusable containers must be disinfected and decontaminated on a routine basis.
- Spilled material and broken glassware should never be picked up with the hands. Brooms, brushes, dustpans, and pickup tongs or forceps should be used, and the material should be placed immediately in an impervious biohazard bag or container at the spill site. An absorbent, professional biohazard spill preparation should be used as directed on the label to decontaminate the site.
- Soiled linen should be handled as little as possible and always while wearing gloves or other protective equipment. Linens soiled with blood or body fluids should be double-bagged and transported in labeled, leakproof biohazard bags.
- Contaminated materials and/or infectious waste must be handled with extreme caution to prevent exposure. Biohazardous waste must be collected in impermeable red, polyethylene or polypropylene, biohazard-labeled bags or containers and sealed. This waste must be disposed of in accordance with all applicable federal, state, and local regulations. Disposal methods include treatment by heat, incineration, steam sterilization, chemical treatment, or other equivalent methods that render the waste inactive before it can be placed in a landfill.

Hepatitis B Vaccination

Hepatitis B vaccine must be available free of charge to all employees who are at risk for occupational exposure to blood-borne pathogens, whether they are full-time or part-time workers, within 10 days of starting employment. The vaccine is administered by intramuscular injection in three doses. The second injection is administered 4 weeks after the first, and the third injection 6 months after the first.

Although the effectiveness rate for the vaccine is almost 96%, employees should have a blood titer done after completing the injection cycle to determine whether they have created antibodies against the virus. If the employee did not respond to the first series or if the series was not completed, revaccination with another three-dose series is recommended. If antibodies still do not develop, no further vaccination is given.

Employees may decline the immunization process, but they must sign a declination form that is kept on file as a record of worker refusal. Employees who decline may receive the vaccine at a later date free of charge.

Postexposure Follow-up

If a worker is exposed through an accidental needle stick, a human bite, contact with broken skin, or a splash or splatter onto mucous membranes (e.g., the eyes), certain procedures must be followed.

- Immediately or as soon as possible after exposure, the exposed area should be washed or flushed.
- The exposure incident must be reported immediately to the supervisor.
- The employee must immediately receive a confidential medical evaluation.
- An incident report must be filed that documents the details of the exposure

incident, the route or type of exposure, and the identity, if known, of the source individual. The source individual is the person, living or dead, whose blood or potentially infectious material was the source of the occupational exposure.

- All documentation related to the incident must remain confidential; it cannot be disclosed to any individual without the employee's express written permission. The documentation must be kept for at least the duration of the worker's employment plus 30 years.
- The exposed worker should be tested for HBV and HIV if consent is given. If the employee refuses the tests but blood is drawn, the sample must be stored for 90 days, which allows the worker to decide later whether to consent to screening.
- The source individual, if known and if consent is given, is also screened for HBV and HIV. Depending on state regulations, the employee may be told the results of the source individual's tests.
- If the employee has not been vaccinated against HBV, vaccination is offered. The physician may recommend administration of gamma globulin as a preventive measure. It should be administered within 24 hours of exposure.
- The employee must receive a copy of the healthcare provider's written opinion within 15 days of completion of the evaluation.
- The employee must receive health counseling about the risk of illness or other adverse outcomes of exposure. He or she also must be advised of the potential for transmission of the disease to family members, patients, and others, as well as the consequences of such transmission.

A complete, unabridged copy of OSHA's bloodborne pathogens standard may be obtained at the agency's website: www.osha.gov.

evolve 7-3

The following terms and expressions specific to Chapter 7 have already been used to search PubMed for the latest research literature available. The *Click Here for Massage* feature associated with this chapter on your textbook's Evolve website allows you to hyperlink to a continually updated PubMed search of research literature that corresponds to this subject.

Hyperlink Search Terms
Massage disease
Massage hazard
Massage infection
Massage infectious agent
Massage occupational safety
Massage sanitation

SUMMARY

This textbook focuses on the use of massage therapy in healthcare settings. This chapter has specifically described the standard practice for disease prevention in medical settings. Just like any other healthcare professional, the massage therapist must comply with sanitation and safety requirements. Massage therapists who are offered employment in a healthcare setting should receive specific training in sanitary practices and in the implementation of OSHA and CDC guidelines for safe practice.

WORKBOOK

1. Develop a pre-massage and postmassage standard precautions protocol in a checklist style.

Premassage Standard Precautions Protocol

Post-massage Standard Precautions Protocol

Chapter 8 Concept Map

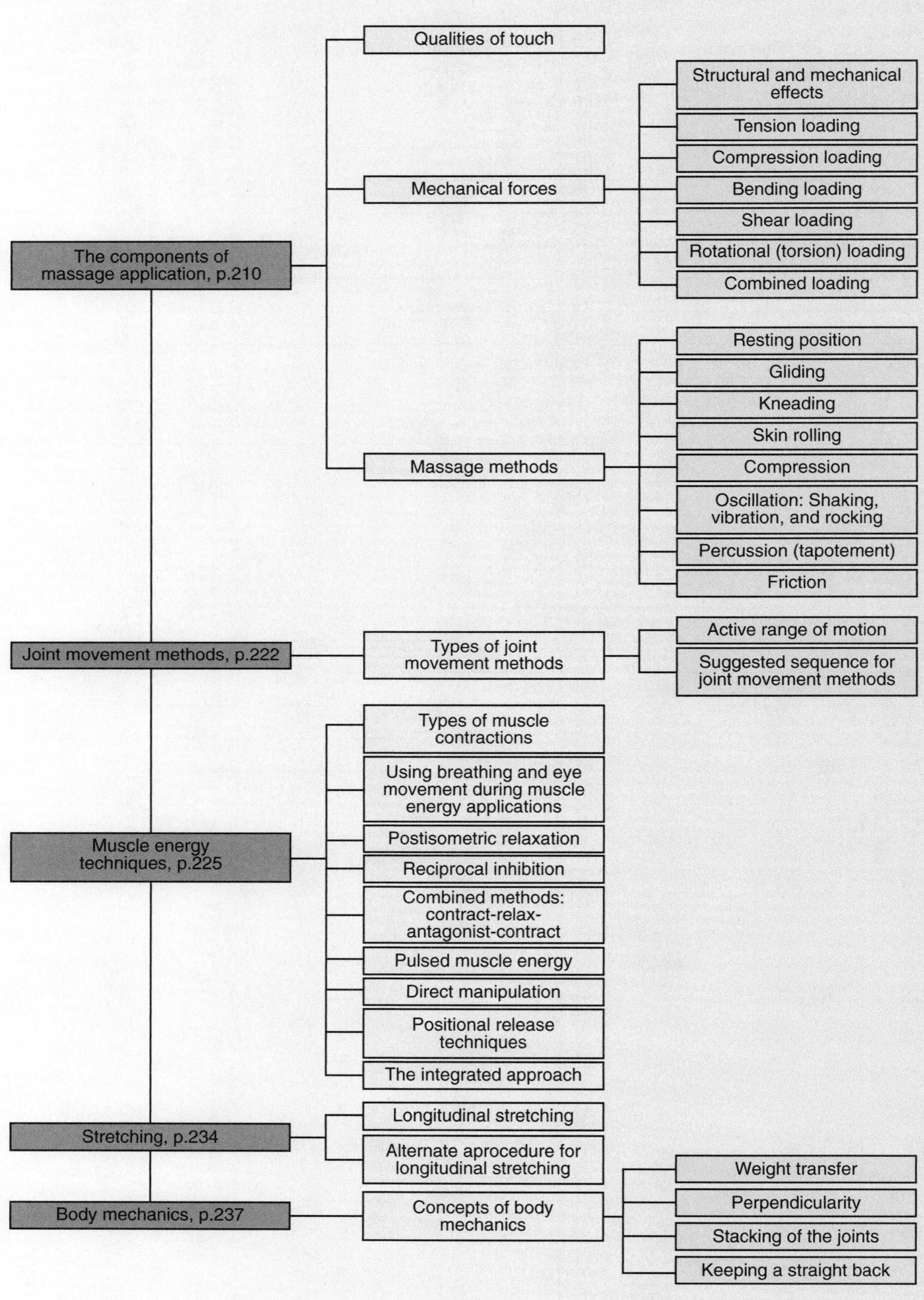

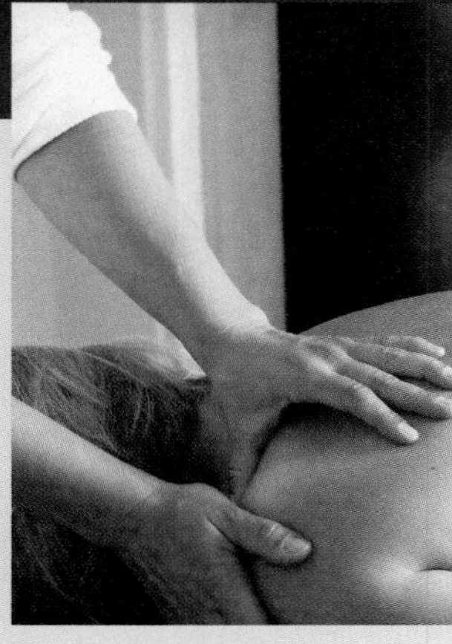

CHAPTER 8

REVIEW AND APPLICATION OF MASSAGE

Key Terms

Bending force
Combined loading
Compression
Compressive force
Concentric isotonic contraction
Cross-directional tissue stretching
Depth of pressure
Direction
Drag
Duration
Eccentric isotonic movement
Frequency
Friction
Gliding stroke
Isometric contraction
Isotonic contraction
Joint movement
Kneading
Mechanical force
Multiple isotonic contractions
Muscle energy techniques
Oscillation
Percussion
Positional release
Postisometric relaxation (PIR)
Pulsed muscle energy procedures
Reciprocal inhibition (RI)
Resting position
Rhythm
Shear force
Skin rolling
Speed of manipulation
Stretching
Tapotement
Tension force
Torsion force
Weight transfer

For definitions of key terms, refer to the Evolve website.

OBJECTIVES

Upon completion of this chapter, the reader will have the information necessary to:

1 Provide all massage applications.
2 Achieve determined outcomes by adjusting the depth of pressure, drag, duration, frequency, direction, speed, and rhythm of all massage applications.
3 Choose appropriate methods to achieve targeted outcomes.
4 Explain all massage methods in terms of physiologic mechanisms.
5 Perform all massage applications using proper body mechanics.

This chapter reviews the fundamentals of massage application. Simple massage methods exert **mechanical force** to alter tissue structures or to stimulate reflexive responses in the nervous system with the intent of creating beneficial structural and physiologic changes in the body. Even though massage can be explained in this simple way, the actual application is seldom simple. Mechanical massage application can feel intense and can be interpreted as painful; however, comforting measures that are more reflexive can support acceptance of the method. A reflexive stimulus usually results from a mechanical force applied to the body. A skilled therapist recognizes the complexity of touch interaction. The following reductionist descriptions of massage can simplify the thought processes necessary during clinical reasoning, treatment plan development, and charting.

Expert application of massage is a complex interaction of the subtle influences of pressure changes, drag, duration, rhythm, and speed; it is more like playing a musical instrument than using a tool. The goal of the massage in some way guides the gliding, kneading, compression, and other techniques that come together to create the experience that people find so beneficial. Becoming an expert takes practice, practice, and more practice, along with the ability to analyze one's own performance. This chapter reminds you of the basics that must be truly absorbed if you are to become an expert.

This textbook assumes that you already have a solid foundation in therapeutic massage skills. Therefore this chapter presents only a brief review of massage application. It is strongly suggested that you reread or read for the first time *Mosby's Fundamentals of Therapeutic Massage* and *Mosby's Essential Sciences for Therapeutic Massage.* The DVD that accompanies this text demonstrates all the applications in this chapter.

Performing massage methods is actually pretty simple. The manner in which a massage is given depends on your ability to execute the various movements using efficient body mechanics, because massage is manual labor. The performance of massage procedures is perfected by practice. The more difficult questions that the massage therapist must learn to answer are why the massage is being given and what it is supposed to accomplish. This chapter is about both how and why.

THE COMPONENTS OF MASSAGE APPLICATION

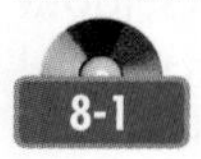

QUALITIES OF TOUCH

Massage is the manual manipulation of the soft tissues. If you analyze the various aspects of manual manipulation, this means that massage therapists use some part of their body (i.e., hands, arms, legs, feet) to alter the soft tissue of the person receiving the massage. Massage involves physical contact. Some methods apply a stimulus to the body without touching it. Typically called *energy-based modalities,* these methods are not massage, even though they are easily incorporated into a massage as an adjunct method. All massage consists of a combination of the following qualities of touch:

- **Depth of pressure (compressive force),** which can be light, moderate, deep, or variable. Depth of pressure is extremely important. Most soft tissue areas of the body consist of three to seven layers of tissue, which include the skin; the superficial fascia; the superficial, middle, and deep layers of muscle; and the various fascial sheaths and connective tissue structures. Pressure must be delivered through each successive layer to reach the deeper tissue layers without damage and discomfort to the more superficial tissues. The deeper the pressure, the broader the base of contact required with the surface of the body. Otherwise, the surface tissue tightens and guards against compression injury. It takes more pressure to address thick, dense tissue than delicate tissue.
- **Drag** is the amount of pull (stretch) on the tissue (tensile force). Many structural and functional tissue changes depend on the amount of drag on the tissue. Connective tissue changes, in particular, are obtained during massage applied with drag on the tissues.
- **Direction** can move outward from the center of the body (centrifugal) or inward from the extremities toward the center of the body (centripetal). It can proceed from proximal to distal attachment (or vice versa) of the muscle, following the muscle fibers, transverse to the tissue fibers, or in circular motions. Direction is particularly important in addressing fluid movement in the body and stretching methods.
- **Speed of manipulation** can be fast, slow, or variable. Typically, slow movements are used to create mechanical changes in

the body and to achieve general relaxation, whereas fast movements can increase motor tone and stimulate sympathetic arousal.

- **Rhythm** is the regularity of application of a technique. If the method is applied at regular intervals, it is considered even, or rhythmic. If the method is disjointed or irregular, it is considered uneven, or nonrhythmic. Massage is usually applied in a rhythmic fashion, especially if fluid movement and relaxation are the goals.
- **Frequency** is the rate at which a method repeats itself in a given time frame. Typically, the massage therapist repeats each method about three times before moving or switching to a different approach. In general, the first application is assessment, the second is treatment, and the third is postassessment. If the postassessment indicates remaining dysfunction, the frequency is increased to repeat the treatment and postassessment until the desired results have been achieved.
- **Duration** is the length of time a method lasts or a manipulation stays in the same location. Typically, the duration should not be longer than 30 to 60 seconds if the nervous system is being targeted. A connective tissue application may be sustained longer but usually not longer than 2 or 3 minutes.

Through these varied qualities of touch, simple massage methods are adapted to the patient's desired outcomes. The qualities of touch provide the therapeutic benefit. The mode of application (e.g., gliding, kneading) provides the most efficient application. Each mode of application can be varied, depending on the desired outcome, by adjusting depth, drag, direction, speed, rhythm, frequency, and duration. In perfecting massage application, the quality of touch is more important than the method. Quality of touch is altered when a contraindication or caution exists for massage. For example, when a patient is fatigued, the duration of the application often is reduced; if a patient has a fragile bone structure, the depth of pressure is altered (Figure 8-1).

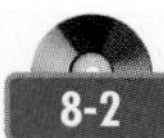

8-2 MECHANICAL FORCES

All massage manipulations introduce mechanical forces into the soft tissues. These forces stimulate various physiologic responses. Force may be perceived as mechanical force, which we are going to discuss in this chapter, or as a field force, such as gravity or magnetism. Examples of actions that create mechanical forces are those that involve pushing, pulling, friction, or sudden loading (e.g., a direct blow). Mechanical forces can act on the body in a variety of ways. They can cause injury, or they can be beneficial if applied appropriately.

It is helpful to identify the different types of mechanical forces and to understand the ways in which mechanical forces applied during massage act therapeutically on the body. Mechanical applications are discussed first, followed by a discussion of reflexive approaches.

Structural and Mechanical Effects

Manual methods of massage that most specifically affect body structure involve the application of mechanical forces to the body to load the tissue. Connective tissue and fluid dynamics are most affected by mechanical force. Mechanical forces influence connective tissue by changing its pliability, orientation, and length. The movement of fluids in the body is a mechanical process. Forces applied to the body mimic various pumping mechanisms of the heart, arteries, veins, lymphatics, muscles, respiratory system, and digestive tract.

The forces created by massage are tension loading, compression loading, bending loading, shear loading, rotational (torsion) loading, and combined loading.

Tension Loading

Tension force (also called tensile force) occurs when two ends of a structure are pulled apart from one another. This is different from muscle tension. Muscle tension is created by excessive muscular contraction or by an increase in fluid pressure, not by strong levels of pulling force applied to the tissue. Tissues elongate under tension loading during massage, which fulfills the

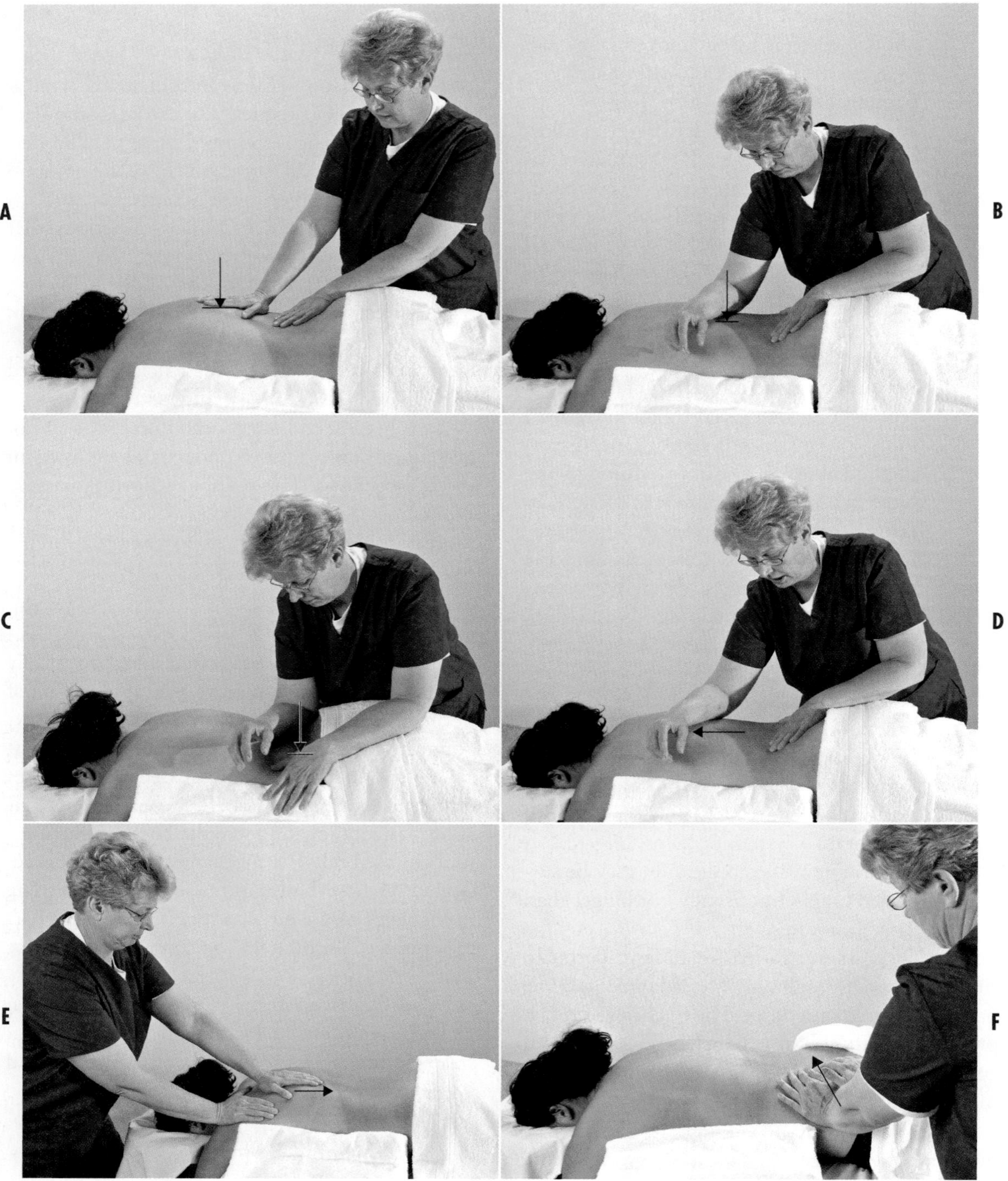

FIGURE 8-1 ■ Qualities of touch. Variations in massage applications occur as the qualities of touch are manipulated. **A,** Depth of pressure, light. **B,** Depth of pressure, medium. **C,** Depth of pressure, deep. **D,** Drag, slight with lubricant. **E,** Drag, extensive with no lubricant. **F,** Direction.

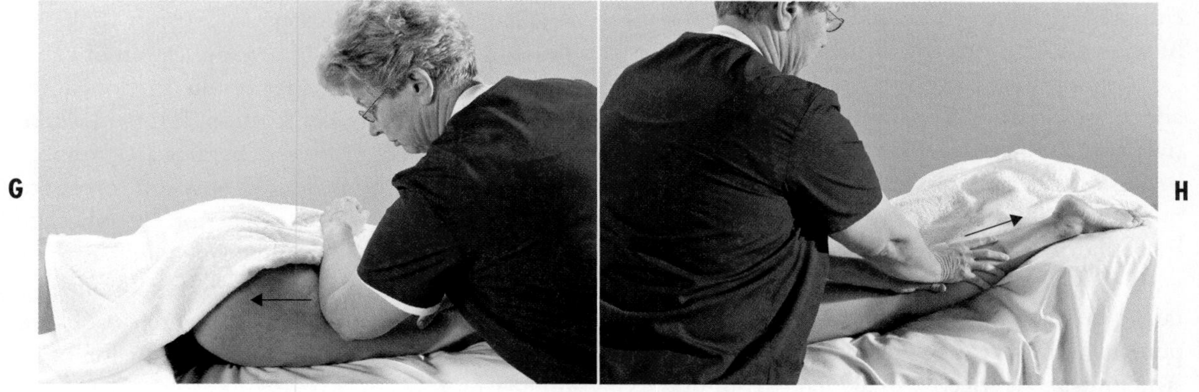

FIGURE 8-1, cont'd ■ **G,** Direction. **H,** Direction.

intent of lengthening shortened tissues. Tension force is created by methods such as traction, longitudinal stretching, and stroking with tissue drag. Tensile forces also cause an aggregation of collagen, resulting in thicker, denser tissue; this improves the direction of fiber development, stiffness, and strength. Tension loading is effective during the secondary phase of healing, after the acute inflammatory stage has begun to dissipate. It also is effective in moving body fluids.

Certain tissues, such as bone, are highly resistant to tensile forces. An extreme amount of force would be needed to break or damage a bone by pulling its two ends apart. However, soft tissues are very susceptible to tension injuries. In fact, tensile stress injuries are the most common soft tissue injuries. Examples of such injuries include muscle strains, ligament sprains, tendonitis, fascial pulling or tearing, and nerve traction injuries (i.e., sudden stretching of nerves, such as occurs in whiplash). Muscles and other soft tissues that are long yet taut are being pulled apart by tensile force. However, this taut condition is often mistaken for short, contracted tissue because it palpates as "tight," when actually the tissue is overstretched, much like an overstretched rubber band.

Do not apply tension force to tissues that are long and taut; this will result in further stretching and dysfunctional tissue. Tension force is used during massage with applications that drag, glide, lengthen, and stretch tissue to elongate connective tissues and lengthen short muscles.

Compression Loading

Compressive force occurs when two structures are pressed together. In massage applications, compressive force is described as depth of pressure. This kind of force may be sudden and strong, as with a direct blow (tapotement), or it may be slow and gradual, as with gliding strokes. The magnitude and duration of the force are important in determining the outcome of the application of compression. Some tissues are quite resilient to compressive forces, whereas others are more susceptible. Nerve tissue is an interesting example. Nerve tissue can withstand a moderately strong compressive force if the force does not last long (e.g., a sudden blow to the back of your elbow that hits your "funny bone"). However, even slight compressive force applied for a long time (as occurs with carpal tunnel syndrome) can cause severe nerve damage. The massage therapist needs to consider this when determining the duration of a massage application that uses compression, especially over areas of nerves.

Ligaments and tendons are quite sturdy and resistant to strong compressive loads. Muscle tissue, on the other hand, with its extensive vascular structure, is not as resistant to compressive forces. Excessive compressive force will rupture or tear muscle tissue, causing bruising and connective tissue damage. This is a concern when pressure is applied to deeper layers of tissue. To avoid tissue damage, the massage therapist must distribute the compressive force of massage over a broad contact area on the body. The more compressive force that is used, the broader should be the base of contact with the tissue.

Compressive force is used therapeutically to affect circulation, nerve stimulation, and connective tissue pliability. **Compression** is effective because it acts as a rhythmic, pumplike method to facilitate fluid dynamics. With this technique, tissue shortens and widens, increasing the pressure within the tissue and affecting fluid flow. Sustained compression, especially with a drag component, results in more pliable connective tissue structures and is effective in reducing tissue density and binding.

Bending Loading

Bending force is a combination of compression and tension. One side of a structure is exposed to compressive forces while the other side is exposed to tensile forces. Bending occurs during many massage applications. Pressure is applied to the tissue, or force is applied across the fiber or across the direction of the muscles, tendons or ligaments, and fascial sheaths. Bending forces rarely damage soft tissues; however, they are a common cause of bone fractures. Bending force is very effective in increasing connective tissue pliability and affecting proprioceptors in the tendons and belly of the muscles.

The massage therapist applies combined forces of tension to the convex side and compression on the concave side of the tissue. Bending is used where the combined effects of lengthening and shortening and an increase in pliability are desired.

Shear Loading

Shear force moves tissue back and forth, creating a combined pattern of compression and elongation of tissue. Shearing is a sliding force; as a result, significant friction often is created between the structures sliding against each other. The massage method of friction uses shear force to generate physiologic change by increasing connective tissue pliability and creating therapeutic inflammation and to ensure that tissue layers slide over one another instead of adhering to underlying layers, creating bind. Excessive friction (shearing force) may result in an inflammatory irritation that causes many soft tissue problems.

Rotational (Torsion) Loading

Torsion force is a combined application of compression and wringing that results in elongation of tissue along the axis of rotation. It is used where a combined effect of fluid dynamics and connective tissue pliability is desired. Torsion forces are best thought of as twisting forces. Massage methods that use kneading introduce torsion forces. Torsion force is not very often applied to a single soft tissue structure and is rarely the cause of significant tissue injury. However, torsion force applied to a group of structures (e.g., a joint) is much more likely to be the cause of significant illness and injury. For example, when the foot is on the floor and the person turns the body, the knee as a whole is exposed to significant torsion force.

Combined Loading

Combined loading blends two or more forces to effectively load tissues. The more forces applied to tissue, the more intense the response. Tension and compression underlie all the different modes of loading, therefore any form of manipulation is either tension, compression, or a combination of the two. Tension is important when tissue needs to be elongated, and compression is important when fluid flow needs to be affected. Oscillation of tissue can be considered combined loading (Figure 8-2).

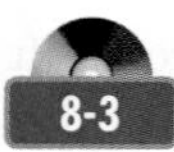

MASSAGE METHODS

The methods of massage described next introduce to the body one or a combination of the forces just discussed for therapeutic benefit. This process is influenced by the qualities of application; that is, depth of pressure, drag, direction, duration, speed, rhythm, and frequency. Appropriate use of force is necessary. If insufficient force or the wrong mechanical force is used, the application will not be effective; conversely, excessive force or the wrong mechanical force can cause tissue damage.

Resting Position

The initial contact with the patient must be made with respect and with a patient-centered focus that includes a clear intention and understanding

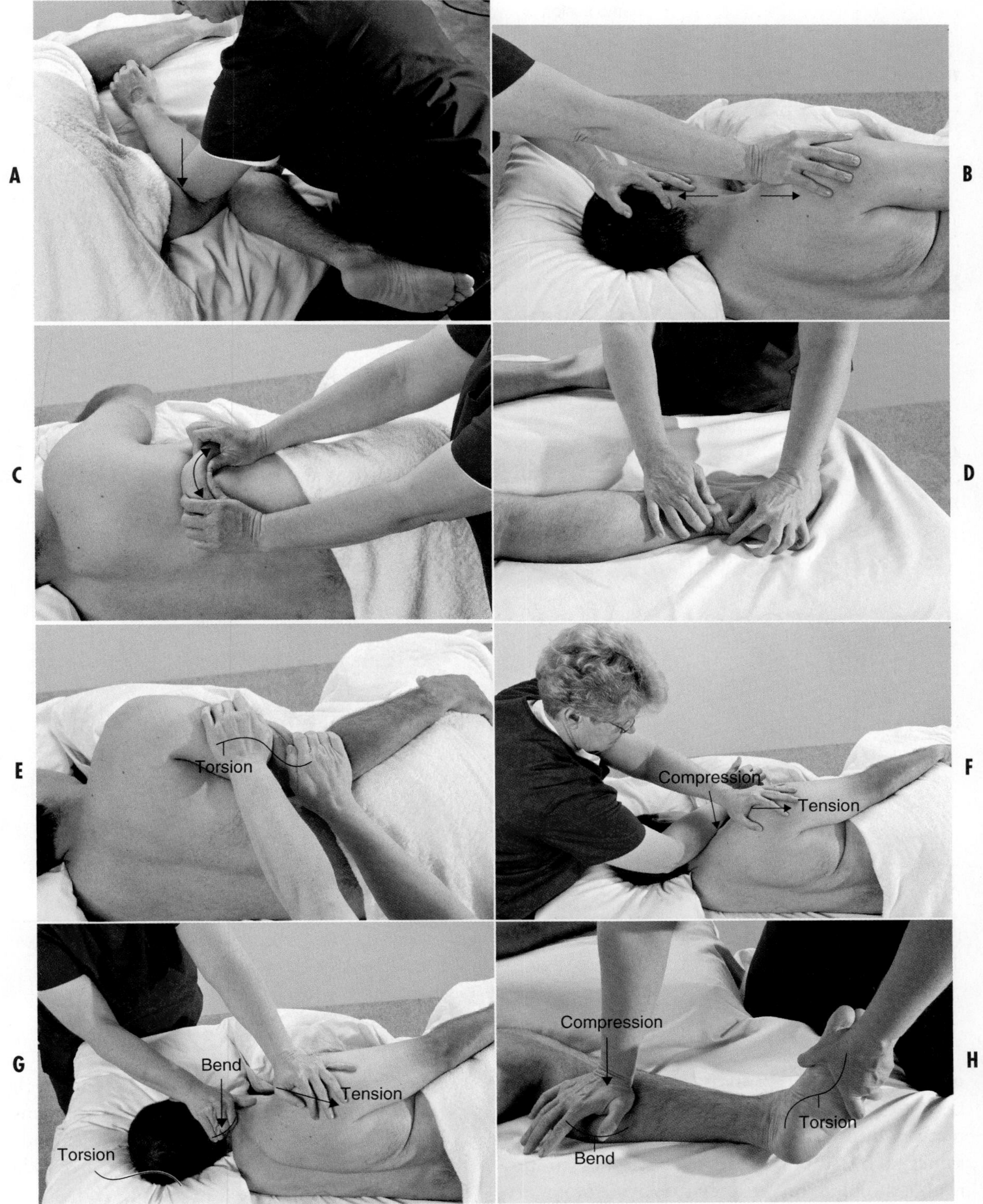

FIGURE 8-2 ■ Application of mechanical forces during massage. **A,** Compression. **B,** Tension. **C,** Bending. **D,** Shear. **E,** Torsion. **F,** Combined loading: compression + tension. **G,** Combined loading: tension + bend + torsion. **H,** Combined loading: compression + bend + torsion.

Continued

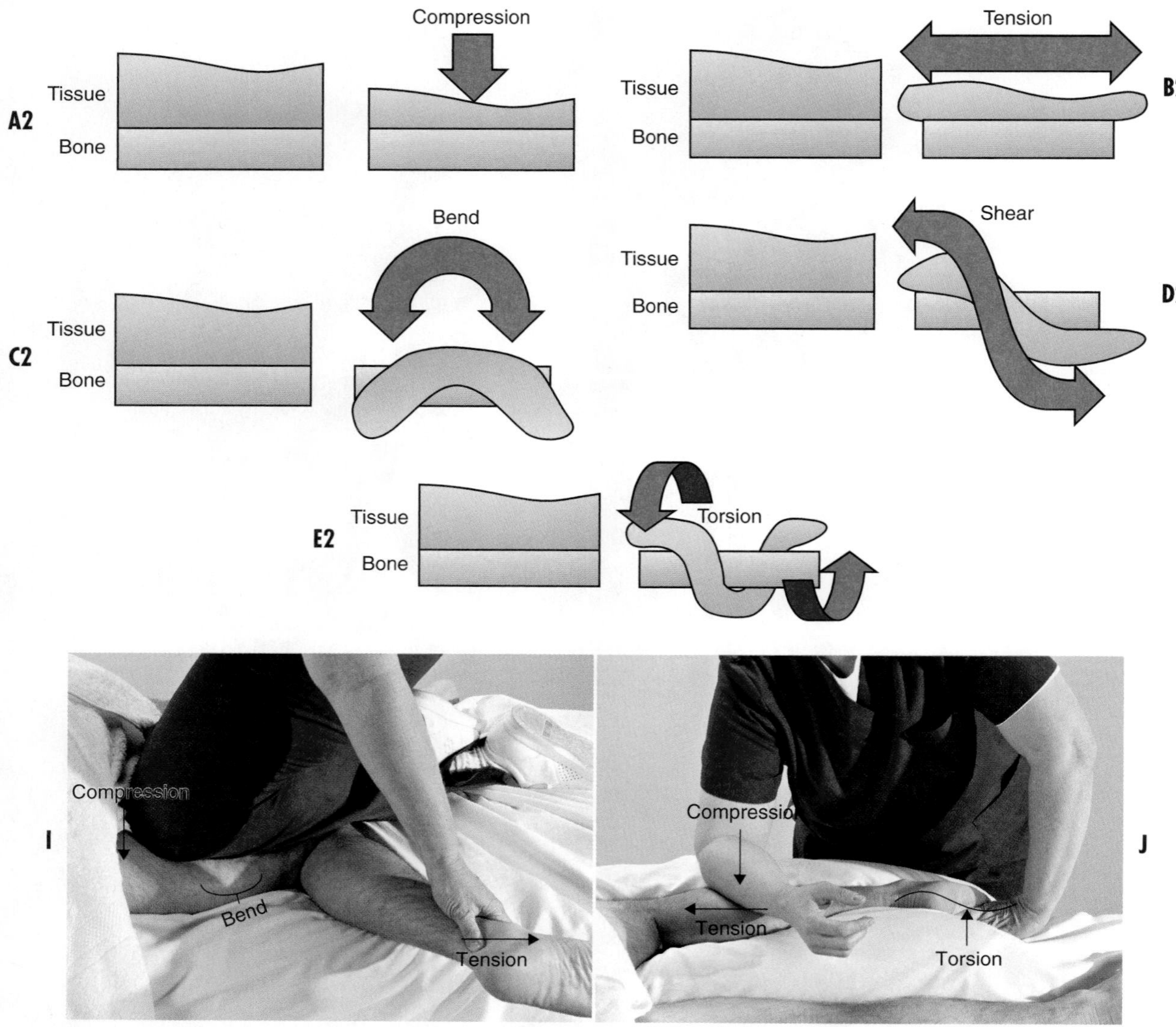

FIGURE 8-2, cont'd ■ **I,** Combined loading: compression + bend + torsion. **J,** Combined loading: tension + compression + torsion. (Drawings from Fritz S: *Mosby's fundamentals of therapeutic massage,* ed 3, St. Louis, 2004, Mosby/Elsevier.)

of the outcome of the massage. The body needs time to process all the sensory information it receives during a massage. **Resting position** is achieved by stopping the motions and simply resting the hands on the body to provide moments of integration (Figure 8-3, *A*).

Gliding

The distinguishing characteristic of gliding strokes is that they are applied horizontally in relation to the tissues, generating a tensile force (Figure 8-3, *B*). During a **gliding stroke,** light pressure remains on the skin, and moderate pressure extends through the subcutaneous layer to reach muscle tissue but does not penetrate deeply enough to compress the tissue against the underlying bony structure. Moderate to heavy pressure that puts sufficient drag on the tissue mechanically affects the connective tissue and the proprioceptors (spindle cells and Golgi tendon organs) found in

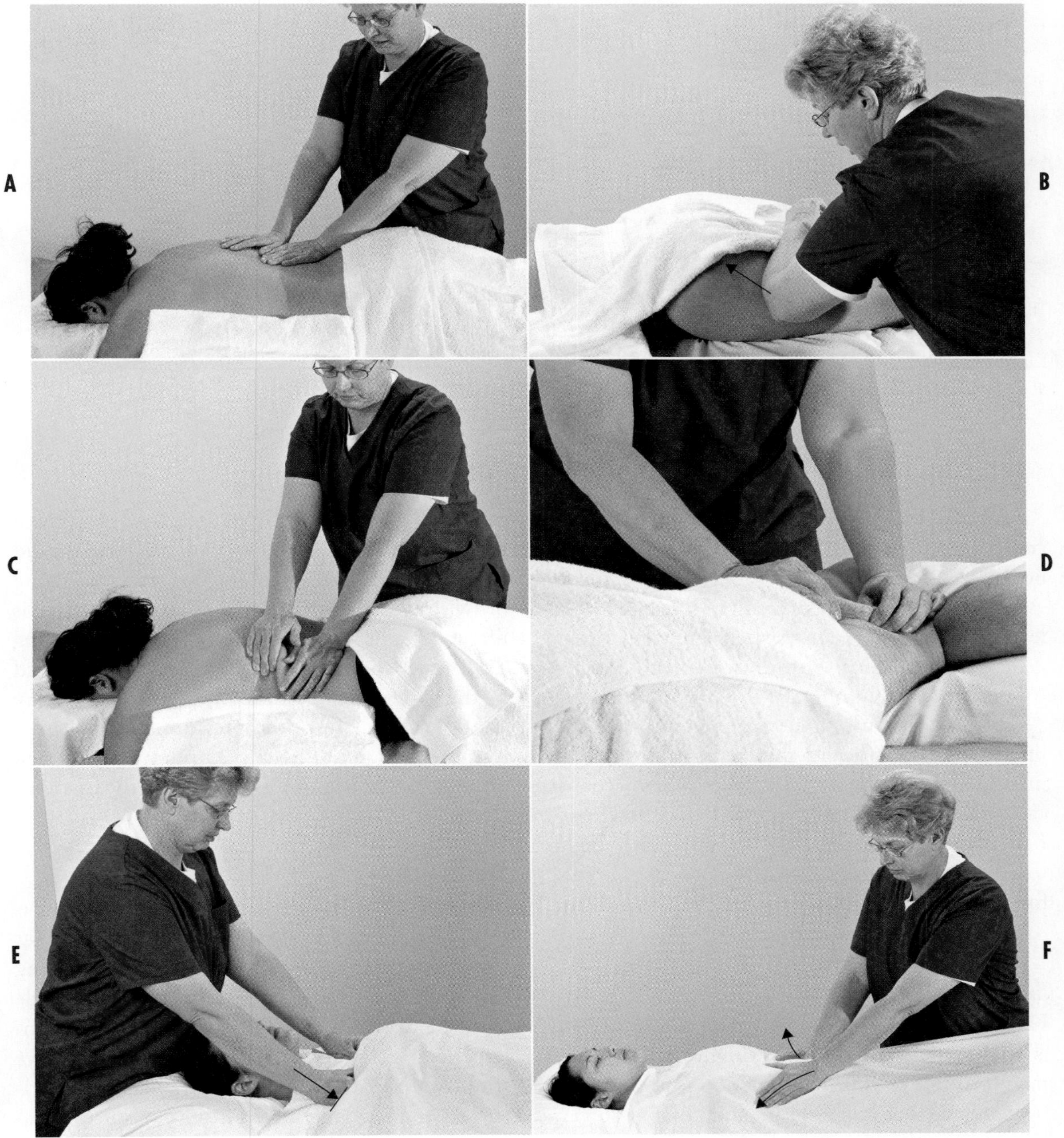

Figure 8-3 ■ Massage methods. **A,** Resting position. **B,** Gliding stroke. **C,** Kneading. **D,** Skin rolling. **E,** Compression with 90-degree contact. **F,** Oscillation: rocking.

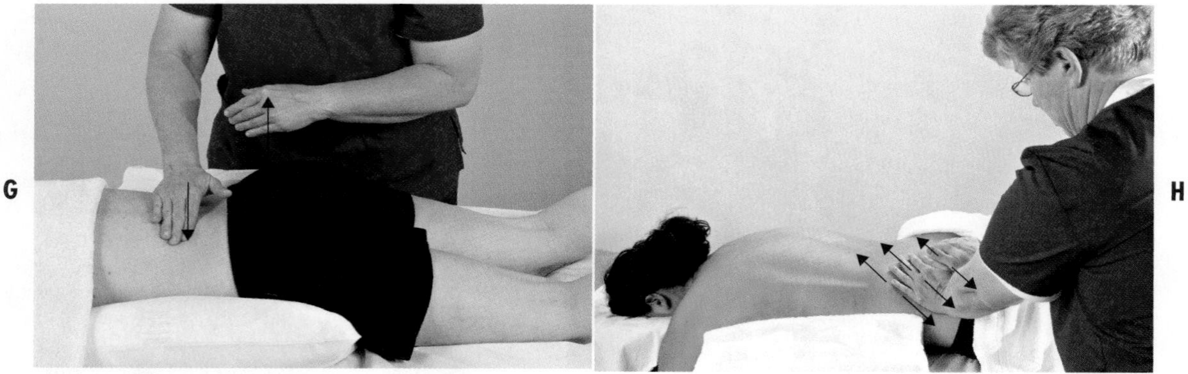

FIGURE 8-3, cont'd ■ **G,** Percussion: slapping. **H,** Broad-based friction.

the muscle. Heavy pressure produces a distinctive compressive force of the soft tissue against the bone.

Depth of pressure is a result of leverage and of leaning on the body. Increases in pressure are not achieved by pushing with muscle strength. Pressure increases as the angle of the lean increases.

Strokes that use moderate pressure from the fingers and toes toward the heart, following the muscle fiber direction, are excellent for mechanical and reflexive stimulation of blood flow, particularly venous return and the lymphatics. Light to moderate pressure with short, repetitive gliding, following the patterns for the lymph vessels, is the basis for manual lymph drainage.

Kneading

Kneading is a technique in which the soft tissue is lifted, rolled, and squeezed (Figure 8-3, *C*). The main purpose of this manipulation is to lift tissue by applying bending, shear, and torsion forces. Kneading is effective for reducing muscle tension. The lifting, rolling, and squeezing action affects the spindle cell proprioceptors in the muscle belly. As the belly of the muscle is squeezed (thus squeezing the spindle cells), the muscle feels less tense. When lifted, the tendons are stretched, thus increasing tension in both the tendons and the Golgi tendon receptors, which have a protective function.

Kneading is very good for mechanically softening the superficial fascia. Kneading methods are effective in supporting circulation by squeezing the capillary beds in tissues and supporting fluid exchange. Kneading may incorporate a wringing or twisting component (torsion) after the tissue is lifted. Changes in depth of pressure and drag determine whether the manipulation is perceived by the patient as superficial or deep. By the nature of the manipulation, the pressure and pull peak when the tissue is lifted to its maximum and then decrease at the beginning and end of the manipulation.

Skin Rolling

Skin rolling is a variation of the lifting manipulation. Deep kneading attempts to lift the muscular component away from the bone, but skin rolling lifts only the skin from the underlying muscle layer (Figure 8-3, *D*). It has a warming and softening effect on the superficial fascia, causes reflexive stimulation of the spinal nerves, and is an excellent assessment method. Areas of "stuck" skin often suggest underlying problems. Skin rolling is one of the very few massage methods that is safe to use directly over the spine. Because only the skin is accessed and the direction of pull to the skin is up and away from the underlying bones, little risk of injury to the spine exists, unlike when any type of downward pressure is used.

Sometimes a person's tissue does not lift. This may be a result of excessive edema (swollen tissue), a heavy fat layer, scarring that extends into the deeper body layers, or thickened areas of connective tissue, especially over aponeuroses (flat sheets of superficial connective tissue). If these conditions exist, applications of kneading or skin rolling are uncomfortable for the patient. Shifting to gliding and compression with drag may soften the tissue enough that kneading can be used more effectively later in the massage session.

Compression

Compression applies forces then moves down into the tissues, with varying depths of pressure adding bending and compressive forces. The manipulations of compression usually penetrate the subcutaneous layer, whereas in the resting position they stay on the skin surface. Much of the effect of compression results from pressing tissue against the underlying structures, causing it to spread. This can be called *tissue displacement.*

Compression used in the belly of the muscle spreads the spindle cells, causing the muscle to sense that it is stretching. To protect the muscle from overstretching, the spindle cells signal for the muscle to contract. The lift-press application stimulates the muscle and nerve tissue. The combination of these two effects makes compression a good method for stimulating muscles and the nervous system. However, because of this stimulation, compression is a little less desirable for a relaxing or soothing massage.

Compression is an excellent method for enhancing circulation. The pressure against the capillary beds changes the pressure inside the vessels and encourages fluid exchange. Compression appropriately applied to arteries allows back pressure to build, and release of the compression encourages increased arterial flow.

Compression can be done with the point of the thumb or with a stabilized finger; with the palm and heel of the hand, the fist, the knuckles, and the forearm; and in some systems with the knee and the heel of the foot. Even though the compressive pressure is exerted perpendicular to the tissue, the position of the forearm in relation to the wrist is about 120 to 130 degrees. Application against a 45-degree angle of the body (hill) plus the 45-degree angle of the therapist's hand and forearm results in 90-degree contact on the tissue. If you are using your knuckles or fist, make sure the forearm is in a direct line with the wrist. Use of the thumb should be avoided if possible, because the thumb joints can be damaged by extensive use, especially on large muscle masses.

The tip (radioulnar side) of the elbow should not be used for compression, because the ulnar nerve passes just under the skin, and extensive compression can result in injury for the massage therapist. Instead, use the forearm near the elbow to apply compression. The massage professional's arm and hand must be relaxed, or neck and shoulder tension will develop. Leverage applied through appropriate body mechanics does the work, not muscle strength.

Compression proceeds downward into the tissues; the depth is determined by what is to be accomplished, where compression is to be applied, and how broad or specific the contact with the individual's body is. Deep compression presses tissue against the underlying bone. Because of the diagonal pattern of the muscles, the massage therapist should stay perpendicular (i.e., at a 90-degree angle) to the bone, with actual compression somewhere between a 60- and 90-degree angle to the body (Figure 8-3, *E*). Beyond those angles, the stroke may slip and turn into a glide.

Oscillation: Shaking, Vibration, and Rocking

Oscillation is the rhythmic or dysrhythmic movement of tissues on a body part. Oscillation is one of the most effective methods of normalizing the motor tone of muscles. Shaking is a massage method that is effective in relaxing muscle groups or an entire limb. Shaking manipulations confuse the positional proprioceptors, because the sensory input is too disorganized for the integrating systems of the brain to interpret; muscle relaxation is the natural response in such situations. Most patients respond well to shaking.

Shaking warms and prepares the body for deeper bodywork and addresses the joints in a nonspecific manner. Shaking is effective when the muscles seem extremely tight because motor tone has increased. This technique is reflexive in effect, but a small mechanical influence may be exerted on the connective tissue as well, because of the lift-and-pull component of the method. Shaking begins with a lift-and-pull component. Either a muscle group or a limb is grasped, lifted, and shaken.

Shaking is not a manipulation to be used on the skin or superficial fascia, nor is it effective for use on the entire body. Rather, it is best applied to any large muscle groups that can be grasped and to the synovial joints of the limbs. Good areas for shaking are the upper trapezius and shoulder area, biceps and triceps groups, hamstrings, quadriceps, gastrocnemius, and, in some cases, the abdominals and the pectoralis muscles close to the axilla. The joints of the shoulders, hips, and extremities also respond well to shaking.

The larger the muscle or joint, the more intense the method must be to be effective. If the movements are performed with all the slack out of the tissue, the focus point of the shake is very small, and the technique is extremely effective. The more purposeful the approach, the smaller the focus of the shaking applied. You should always stay within the limits of both range of motion of a joint and the elastic give of the tissue.

Vibration is a smaller, more focused oscillation that involves very fast, small movements.

Rocking is a soothing, rhythmic method that is used to calm people. Its effects are both reflexive and chemical (Figure 8-3, *F*). Rocking also works through the vestibular system of the inner ear and feeds sensory input directly into the cerebellum. Other reflex mechanisms probably are affected as well. Because of this, rocking is one of the most productive massage methods for achieving entrainment. For rocking to be most effective, the patient's body must move so that the fluid in the semicircular canals of the inner ear is affected, initiating parasympathetic mechanisms.

Rocking is rhythmic and should be applied with a deliberate, full body movement. This attunement to the patient's rhythm is a powerful interface point for synchronizing entrainment. The easiest way to do this is to take the patient's pulse and match the rhythm to that of the pulse. The massage therapist works within the rhythm to maintain and amplify it by attempting to gently extend the limits of movement or by slowing the rhythm if it is too fast. Incorporation of a rocking movement that supports this entrainment process into all massage applications effectively individualizes the application and speed of the method. The patient seems to relax more easily when a subtle rocking movement, matching the person's innate rhythm pattern, is used as part of the generalized massage approach, along with such techniques as gliding, kneading, compression, joint movement, and, especially, passive movements.

Percussion (Tapotement)

Percussion, also called **tapotement,** is classified as light or heavy (i.e., surface or deep). The difference between light and heavy tapotement is whether the compressive force of the blows penetrates only to the superficial tissue of the skin and subcutaneous layers (light) or deeper into the muscles, tendons, and visceral structures, such as the pleura in the chest cavity (heavy).

Percussion is a stimulating manipulation that operates through the response of the nerves. Because of its intense stimulating effect on the nervous system, percussion initiates or enhances sympathetic activity of the autonomic nervous system. The effects of the manipulations are reflexive except for the mechanical results of percussion in loosening and moving mucus in the chest.

When applied to the joints, percussion affects the joint kinesthetic receptors responsible for determining the position and movement of the body. The quick blows confuse the system, similar to the effect of joint-focused rocking and shaking, but the body muscles tone instead of inhibit. This method is useful for stimulating weak muscles. The force used must move the joint but should not be strong enough to damage the joint. For example, one finger may be used over the carpal joints, whereas the fist may be used over the sacroiliac joint.

Percussion is very effective when used at motor points that are usually located in the same area as the traditional acupuncture points. The repetitive stimulation causes the nerve to fire repeatedly, stimulating the nerve tract (Figure 8-3, *G*).

Percussion focused primarily on the skin affects the superficial blood vessels of the skin, initially causing them to contract. Heavy percussion or prolonged lighter application dilates the vessels as a result of the release of histamine, a vasodilator. Although prolonged percussion seems to increase blood flow, surface application enhances the effect of cold application used in hydrotherapy.

Heavy percussion should not be done over the kidneys or other endangerment site areas or anywhere pain or discomfort is present.

Friction

Friction consists of small, deep movements performed on a local area. It creates shear force to the tissue. Friction burns may result if the fingers are allowed to slide back and forth over the skin. Friction creates therapeutic inflammation. Friction manipulation prevents and breaks up local adhesions in connective tissue, especially over tendons, ligaments, and scars, by creating therapeutic inflammation. This method is not used over an acute injury or fresh scar and should only be used if the patient's adaptive capacity can respond to superimposed tissue trauma.

Modified use of friction after a scar has stabilized or the acute phase has passed may prevent adhesions and can promote a more normal healing process. This application also reduces pain through the mechanisms of counterirritation and hyperstimulation analgesia.

The movement in friction usually is transverse to the fiber direction, and the technique generally is applied for 30 seconds to 10 minutes. This type of friction initiates a small, controlled inflammatory response. The chemicals released during inflammation result in activation of tissue repair mechanisms, with reorganization of connective tissue. This type of work, coupled with proper healing and rehabilitation, is very valuable.

Friction is a mechanical approach best applied to areas of high connective tissue concentration, such as the musculotendinous junction. Microtrauma caused by repetitive movement and overstretching is common in this area. Microtrauma predisposes the musculotendinous junction to inflammatory problems, connective tissue changes, and adhesion.

Experts disagree on whether an area that is to receive friction should be stretched or relaxed. Because both ways have merit, both positions should be included when frictioning.

Another use for friction is to combine it with compression, thereby adding a small stretch component. The movement includes no slide. This application has mechanical, chemical, and reflexive effects and is the most common approach for the use of friction.

Remember that the main focus when using friction is to move tissue under the skin. Do not use lubricant, because the tissues must not slide. Place the area to be frictioned in a soft or slack position. To produce the movement, begin with a specific and moderate to deep compression using the fingers, the palm, or the flat part of the forearm near the elbow. After reaching the depth of pressure required to contact the target tissue, move the upper tissue back and forth across the grain or fiber of the undertissue for transverse or cross-fiber friction or around in a circle for circular friction.

As the tissue responds to the friction, gradually begin to stretch the area and increase the pressure. The feeling for the patient may be intense, but if it is painful, modify the application to a tolerable level so that the patient reports the sensation as a "good hurt." The recommended way to work within the patient's comfort zone is to use pressure sufficient for the person to feel the specific area but not to complain of pain. Continue applying friction until the sensation diminishes. Gradually increase the pressure until the patient again feels the specific area. Begin applying friction again, and repeat the sequence for up to 10 minutes.

The area frictioned typically is tender to the touch for 48 hours after the session. The sensation should be similar to a mild after-exercise soreness. Because the focus of friction is the controlled application of a small inflammatory response, heat and redness are caused by the release of histamine. Also, increased circulation results in a small amount of puffiness as more water binds with the connective tissue. The area should not bruise.

Application of Deep Transverse Friction. Deep transverse friction can be applied in the following manner:

1. Place the patient in a suitable position that ensures the appropriate degree of tension or relaxation of the tissues to be frictioned.

2. Identify the exact location to be treated.
3. Make sure your fingers and the patient's skin move as one. Take care not to cause a blister. The patient must understand that deep friction massage can be intense during application, and the area will be tender to the touch for a few days after treatment.
4. Apply the friction across the fibers composing the affected structure.
5. Apply the friction with sufficient sweep. Pressure only accesses the tender area; it does not replace the friction.
6. Make sure the friction reaches deeply enough. If it does not reach the lesion, it is of no value.
7. Keep tendons with a sheath taut during friction massage.
8. Use broadening contractions between sessions to promote circulation and mobilize scar development during the healing process (Figure 8-3, *H*).

Another effective way to apply friction involves a combination of compression and passive joint movement, using the bone under the point of compression to produce the friction. The process begins with compression as just described, but instead of moving the tissue back and forth, the massage therapist moves the patient's body under the compression. This automatically adds the slack and stretch positions for the friction methods. The result is the same. This method is much easier for the massage professional to perform and may be more comfortable for the patient as well. The movement of the joint provides a distraction from the specific application of the pressure and generalizes the sensation. Broad general methods can be used with a greater degree of intensity than can pinpointed, specific treatments.

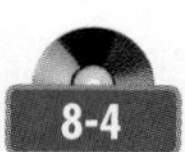

JOINT MOVEMENT METHODS

Joint movement is effective because it provides a means of controlled stimulation to the joint mechanoreceptors. Movement initiates motor tone readjustment through the reflex center of the spinal cord and lower brain centers. As positions change, the supported movement gives the nervous system an entirely different set of signals to process. The joint sensory receptors are able to learn not to be so hypersensitive. As a result, the protective spasm and movement restriction may lessen.

Joint movement also encourages lubrication of the joint and contributes an important enhancement to the lymphatic and venous circulatory systems. Much of the pumping action that moves these fluids in the vessels results from compression of the lymph and blood vessels during joint movement and muscle contraction. The tendons, ligaments, and joint capsule are warmed by the movement. This mechanical effect helps keep these tissues pliable.

TYPES OF JOINT MOVEMENT METHODS

Joint movement involves moving the jointed areas within the physiologic limits of the patient's range of motion. The two types of joint movement are active movement and passive movement. In active joint movement, the patient moves the joint by means of active contraction of muscle groups. Active joint movement is subcategorized as *active assisted movement,* which occurs when both the patient and the massage therapist move the area, and *active resistive movement,* which occurs when the patient actively moves the joint against a resistance provided by the massage therapist.

In passive joint movement, the patient's muscles remain relaxed and the massage therapist moves the joint with no assistance from the patient. For example, joint oscillation is a passive joint movement. With passive joint movement, the massage therapist should assess for the soft or hard end-feel of the joint range of motion. This is an important evaluation.

Whether active or passive, joint movements are always done within the comfortable limits of the patient's range of motion. The patient's body must always be stabilized, allowing only the joint being worked on to move. Occasionally the entire limb is moved to allow for coordinated interaction among all the joints of the area, but the rest of the body is stabilized. *It is essential to move slowly, because quick changes or abrupt moves may cause the muscles to initiate protective contractions.*

As a massage therapist, working within the physiologic range of motion for a particular patient is within your scope of practice. The physician, physical therapist, or chiropractor deal directly with joint pathology. The specific method section describes a simple joint play method based on indirect functional techniques, which are very safe when the principles of tissue ease and bind are used. These techniques are applied to joints by identifying the ease position and then having the patient move the joint into and out of bind.

Joint movement becomes part of the application of muscle energy techniques to lengthen muscles and of stretching methods to elongate connective tissues. Therefore the massage professional should concentrate on developing the ability to use joint movement efficiently and effectively.

Hand placement is very important in joint movement. The therapist should make sure the area is not squeezed, pinched, or restricted in its movement pattern. The therapist should place one hand close to the joint to be moved, both to act as a stabilizer and for evaluation. The other hand is placed at the distal end of the bone; this is the hand that actually provides the movement. Proper use of body mechanics is essential when performing joint movement. The stabilizing hand must remain in contact with the patient and must be placed near the affected joint (Figure 8-4).

Another method for determining the placement of the stabilizing hand is to move the jointed area without stabilization and observe where the patient's body moves most in response to the range-of-motion action. The stabilizing hand is placed at this point. Avoid working cross-body. Usually, the hand closest to the joint is the stabilizing hand.

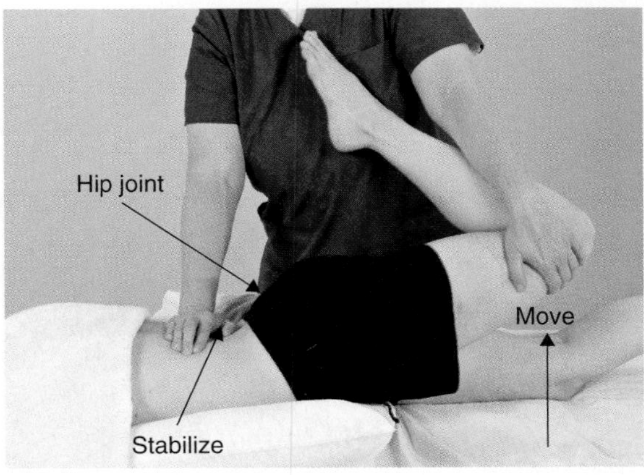

FIGURE 8-4 ■ Hand positions for joint movement.

Before joint movement begins, the moving hand lifts and leans back to produce the slight traction necessary to put a small stretch on the joint capsule. The technique is much less effective if this is not done. When tractioning has been mastered and the joint is moved simultaneously, the size of the movement becomes smaller and the effectiveness increases. It is not necessary or desirable to have the patient's limbs flailing about in the air. Joint oscillation simply means that the joint is rhythmically moved in small, controlled, rhythmic movement.

Active Range of Motion

In active range of motion, the patient moves the area without any type of interaction by the massage therapist. This is a good assessment method and should be used before and after any type of joint work because it provides information about the limits of range of motion (preassessment) and the improvement after the work is complete (postassessment). As mentioned previously, the two variations of active range-of-motion methods are active assisted range of motion and active resistive range of motion.

Active Assisted Range of Motion. In active assisted range of motion, the patient moves the joint through the range of motion and the massage therapist helps or assists the movement. This approach is very useful in cases of weakness or pain with movement. The action remains within the comfortable limits of movement for the patient. The focus is to create movement within the joint capsule, encouraging synovial fluid movement to warm and soften connective tissue and support muscle function.

Active Resistive Range of Motion. In active resistive range of motion, the massage therapist firmly grasps and holds the end of the bone just distal to the joint being addressed. The therapist leans back slightly to place a small traction on the limb to take up the slack in the tissue. Then the therapist instructs the patient to push slowly against a stabilizing hand or arm while moving the joint through its entire range. A tap or light slap against the limb to begin the movement works well to focus the patient's attention.

Another method is to stabilize the entire circumference of the limb and instruct the patient to pull gently or move the area. The job of the massage therapist is to maintain a gentle traction to prevent slack in the tissue, keep the movement slow, and give the patient something to push or pull against.

The counterforce applied by the massage therapist in active resistive methods does not exceed the patient's pushing or pulling action, but rather matches it and then allows movement against the resistance.

After a form of active range of motion has been completed, the patient's body is more apt to accept passive range of motion.

Suggested Sequence for Joint Movement Methods (Figure 8-5)

To incorporate joint movement into a massage, follow these basic suggestions:

- If possible, perform active joint movement first. Assess range of motion by having the patient move the area without your participation.
- Have the patient move the area against a stabilizing force you supply to increase the intensity of the signals from the contracting muscles.
- Incorporate any or all of the previously discussed massage methods.

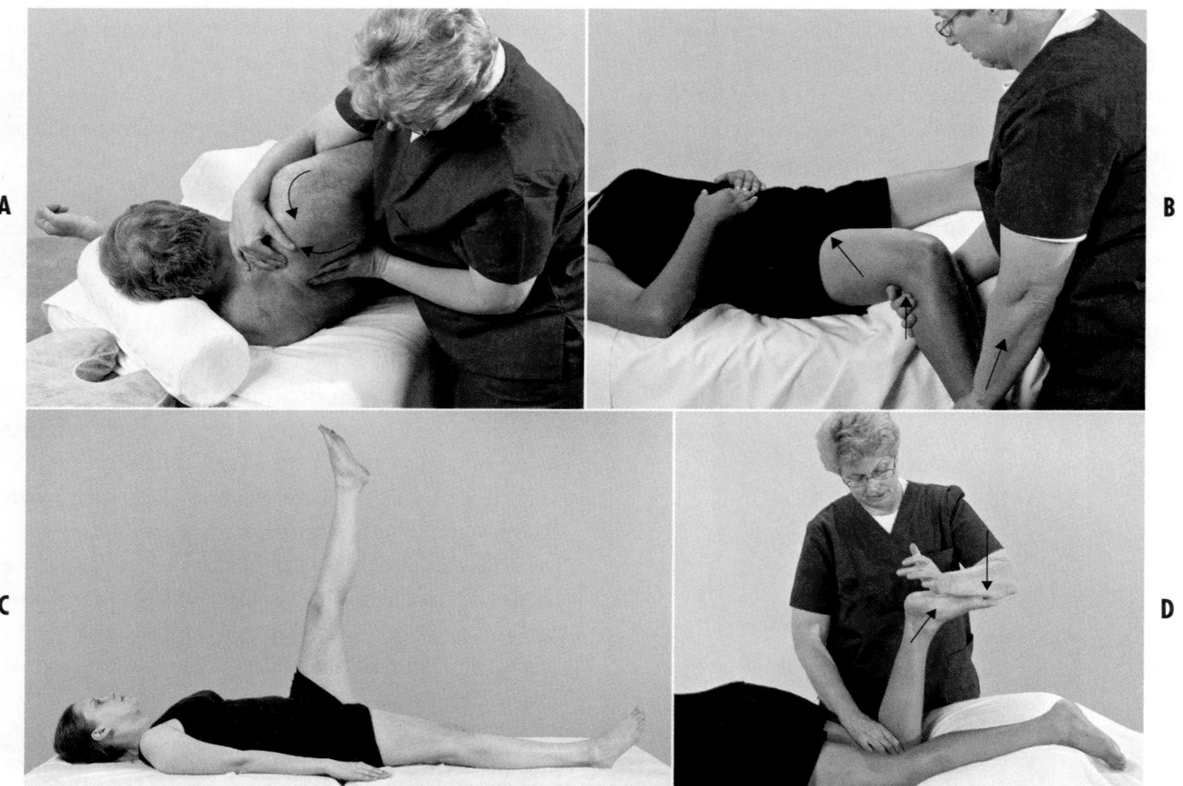

FIGURE 8-5 ■ Four types of joint movement (range of motion). **A,** Passive movement: the patient does not assist; the massage therapist moves the area. **B,** Active assisted movement: both the patient and therapist move the area. **C,** Active movement: the patient moves the area with no help from the therapist. **D,** Active resistive movement: the patient moves against resistance provided by the therapist.

- After the tissue is warm and the nervous system normalized, perform the passive range of motion/joint movement.
- Try to move every joint approximately three times during a massage session. Each time, take up any slack in the tissues and gently encourage an increase in the range of motion (Figure 8-6).

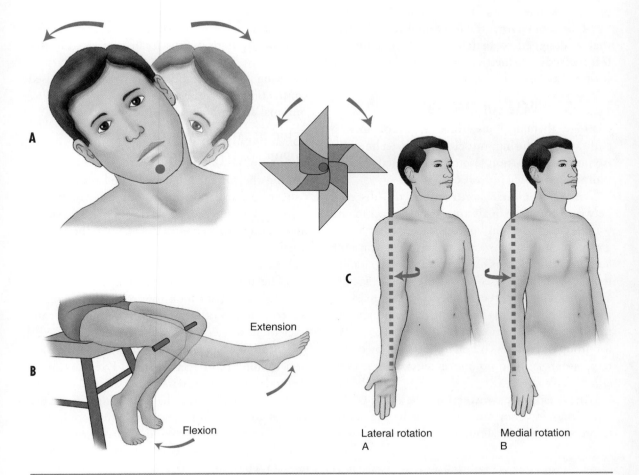

8-5 MUSCLE ENERGY TECHNIQUES

Muscle energy techniques involve a voluntary contraction of the patient's muscles in a specific and controlled direction, at varying levels of intensity, against a specific counterforce applied by the massage therapist. Muscle energy procedures have a variety of applications and are considered active techniques in which the patient contributes the corrective force. The amount of effort may vary from a small muscle twitch to a maximum muscle contraction. The duration may be a fraction of a second to several seconds. All contractions begin and end slowly, gradually building to the desired intensity.

> **evolve 8-1**
>
> Movements of the body are concepts that should have been learned in previous classes. For a refresher on the subject, see the Evolve website for additional illustrations of movements of the body.

The focus of muscle energy techniques is to stimulate the nervous system to allow a more normal muscle resting length. To describe what

FIGURE 8-6 ■ Movements of the body. **A,** Frontal plane movement. **B,** Sagittal plane movement. **C,** Transverse plane movement. (From Muscolino JE: *Kinesiology: the skeletal system and muscle function,* enhanced edition, St Louis, 2006, Mosby.)

happens, the term *lengthening* is used because lengthening is more of a neurologic response that allows the muscle cells to stop contracting and restore a normal resting length. Stretching is more correctly defined as a mechanical force applied to elongate connective tissue. Muscle energy methods often are used in conjunction with stretching. These methods seem to increase the patient's tolerance to stretching.

Muscle energy techniques focus on specific muscles or muscle groups. It is important to be able to position muscles so that the muscle attachments are either close together or in a lengthening phase with the attachments separated. Study muscle charts until you understand the configuration of the muscle patterns and practice isolating as many muscles as possible, keeping in mind that proper positioning is very important. When practicing, make sure the muscles can be isolated regardless of whether the patient is in a supine, prone, side-lying, or seated position.*

Counterpressure is the force applied to an area that is designed to match the exerted effort or force exactly (isometric contraction) or partially (isotonic contraction).

TYPES OF MUSCLE CONTRACTIONS

Massage therapists use three types of muscle contractions during muscle energy techniques: isometric contraction, isotonic contraction, and multiple isotonic contractions.

In an **isometric contraction,** the distance between the proximal and distal attachments (origin and insertion) of the target muscle (or group of muscles) is maintained at a constant length. A fixed tension develops in the target muscle as the patient contracts the muscle against an equal counterforce applied by the massage therapist, preventing shortening of the muscle. In this type of contraction, the effort of the muscle (or group of muscles) is exactly matched by counterpressure so that no movement occurs, only effort.

In an **isotonic contraction,** the effort of the target muscle is not quite matched by the counterpressure, which allows a degree of resisted movement to occur. With a **concentric isotonic contraction,** the massage therapist applies a counterforce but allows the patient to move the proximal and distal attachments of the target muscle together against the pressure. In an **eccentric isotonic movement,** the massage therapist applies a counterforce but allows the patient to move the jointed area such that the origin and insertion of the target muscle separate as the muscle lengthens against the pressure.

Multiple isotonic contractions require the patient to move the joint through a full range of motion against partial resistance applied by the massage therapist.

Muscle energy techniques usually do not use the patient's full contraction strength. With most isometric work, the contraction should start at about 25% of the strength of the muscle. Subsequent contractions can involve progressively greater degrees of effort, but never more than 50% of the available strength.

Many experts use only about 10% of the available strength in muscles being treated in this way and find that they can increase effectiveness by using longer periods of contraction. Pulsed contractions (a rapid series of repetitions) using minimal strength are also effective.

USING BREATHING AND EYE MOVEMENT DURING MUSCLE ENERGY APPLICATIONS

Having the patient use coordinated breathing to enhance particular directions of muscular effort is helpful. During muscle energy applications, all muscular effort is enhanced by having the patient inhale as the effort is made and exhale on the lengthening phase.

The use of eye movement is also effective. Having the patient look toward the direction of the contraction causes the target muscles to contract or facilitates their contraction. Having the patient look away from the direction of contraction inhibits the target muscles. Eye movement methods are very valuable for patients who are prone to cramping, who have difficulty using only a small contraction force, or who are fatigued or weak. Eye movement should be used first, before active target muscle contraction. The following are common examples of the use of eye movement:

*The author strongly suggests that the reader obtain Dr. Leon Chaitow's book, *Muscle Energy Techniques,* ed 3, New York, 2005, Churchill Livingstone.

- To increase tension in neck flexors (tense and then relax), have the patient look toward the belly, rolling the eyes down.
- To reduce tension in the neck flexors, have the patient look up over the head, rolling the eyes up.
- To increase tension in the left neck rotators or lateral flexors, have the patient look left.
- To reduce tension in the left neck rotators or lateral flexors, have the patient look right.
- Reverse for right rotator or lateral flexor patterns.
- Almost all flexor patterns (i.e., the trunk, hip, knee, ankle, shoulder, arm, and wrist) are increased in tone (facilitated) when the patient looks toward the abdomen and are inhibited when the patient rolls the eyes up.
- Extensor patterns (e.g., the trunk, hip, knee, and ankle) are facilitated when the patient looks up and inhibited when the patient rolls the eyes down.
- When in doubt about the position, instruct the patient to slowly and deliberately roll the eyes in big circles; this results in a contract-relax antagonist contraction pattern.
- The eye movement replaces the contraction of the target muscles, or it can enhance the contraction being used with muscle energy techniques.

A successful application involves lengthening the target area to bind and holding it there. The eye movement (usually big circles) then is started (Figure 8-7). As facilitation (contraction) and inhibition (relaxation) of the muscles take place, the lengthening force on the target muscles is slowly increased until a more normal resting length is achieved.

POSTISOMETRIC RELAXATION

Postisometric relaxation (PIR), also called *tense and relax* and *contract/relax,* occurs after isometric contraction of a muscle or when the patient's eye movements are directed as previously described. PIR results from the activity of the Golgi tendon bodies. In the brief latent period of 10 seconds or so after such a contraction, the muscle can be lengthened painlessly, farther than it could before the contraction. The comfort barrier is the first point of resistance just before the patient perceives any discomfort at either the physiologic or pathologic barrier. The isometric contraction involves minimal effort lasting 7 to 10 seconds. Repetitions continue until no further gain is noted. The procedure for PIR is as follows (Figure 8-8):

1. Lengthen the target muscle to the comfort barrier where tissue begins to bind. Back off slightly.
2. Tense (contact) the target muscle for 7 to 10 seconds, or use eye position, or both.
3. Stop the contraction and lengthen the target muscle.
4. Repeat steps 1 through 3 until normal full resting length is obtained.

RECIPROCAL INHIBITION

Reciprocal inhibition (RI) occurs when a muscle contracts, causing its antagonist to relax to allow for more normal movement. Generally, isometric contraction of the antagonist of a shortened target muscle allows the muscle to relax and be taken to a new resting length. Such contractions usually begin in the midrange rather than near the barrier of resistance and last 7 to 10 seconds. RI targets muscle as the tone increases in its antagonist. This response works through the central nervous system, which cannot allow the prime movers and the antagonists to tighten at the same time in this reflex arc pattern. The procedure for RI is as follows (Figure 8-9):

1. Isolate the target muscles by putting them in passive contraction (the massage therapist moves the proximal and distal attachments of the muscles together using joint positioning).
2. Contract the antagonist muscle group, or activate eye movement, or both (the muscle in extension).
3. Stop the contraction and slowly bring the target muscle into a lengthened state, stopping at resistance (bind).
4. Place the target muscle slightly into passive contraction again.

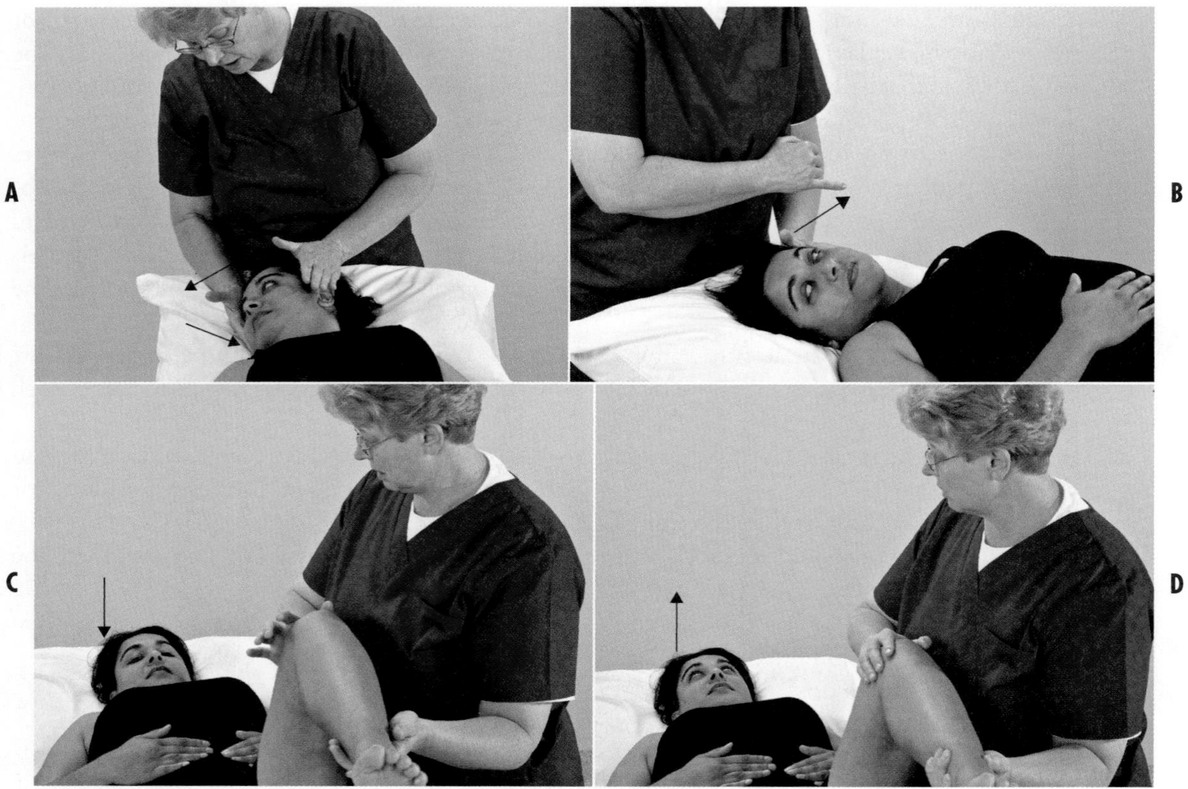

FIGURE 8-7 ■ The use of eye movements during muscle energy techniques. **A,** Having the patient look toward the direction of contraction causes the target muscles to contract. **B,** Having the patient look away inhibits the target muscles and facilitates lengthening. **C,** In general, having the patient look down toward the abdomen facilitates concentrated contractions in flexors, adductors, and internal rotators; this can be used during muscle energy methods to enhance the target muscle antagonist or to replace target muscle contraction. **D,** In general, having the patient look back up over his or her head facilitates concentric contraction in extensors, abductors, and external rotators; this can be used during muscle energy methods instead of direct target muscle contraction.

5. Repeat steps 2 through 4 until normal full resting length is obtained.

COMBINED METHODS: CONTRACT-RELAX-ANTAGONIST-CONTRACT

Tense and relax and RI can be combined to enhance the lengthening effects. This method can be called contract-relax-antagonist-contract. The procedure for contract-relax-antagonist-contract is as follows (Figure 8-10):

1. Position the target muscle as in tense and relax procedures.
2. Lengthen the target muscle to the barrier where tissues begin to bind. Back off slightly.
3. Contract the target muscle for 7 to 10 seconds, or have the patient roll the eyes in a big circle, or both.
4. Contract the antagonist as in RI, or have the patient roll the eyes in a big circle, or both.
5. Stop the contraction of the antagonist.
6. Lengthen the muscle to a more normal resting length.

PULSED MUSCLE ENERGY

Pulsed muscle energy procedures involve engaging the comfort barrier where tissues begin to

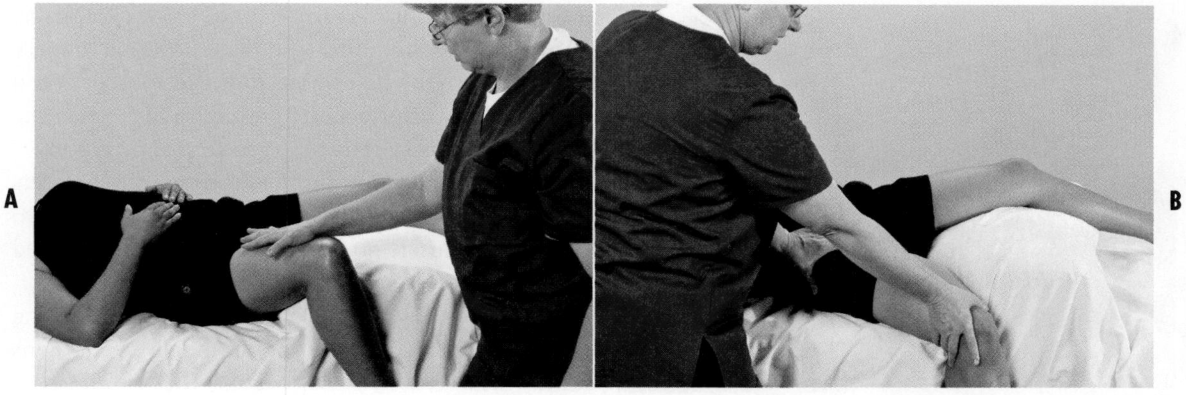

FIGURE 8-8 ■ Postisometric relaxation (tense and relax). **A,** Muscle energy: target the quadriceps and contract. **B,** Relax and lengthen the quadriceps.

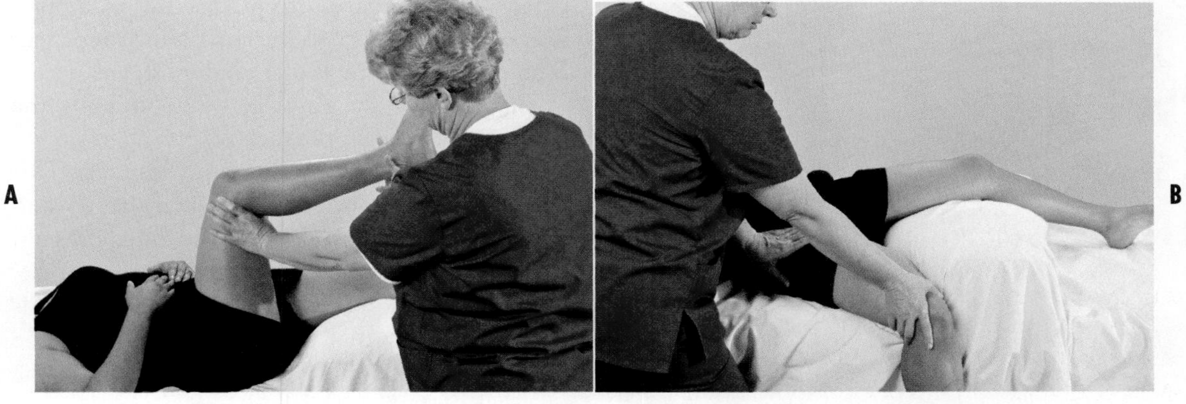

FIGURE 8-9 ■ Reciprocal inhibition. **A,** Target the quadriceps; contract the hamstrings. **B,** Lengthen the quadriceps.

bind and using small, resisted contractions (usually 20 in 10 seconds); this introduces mechanical pumping as well as PIR or RI, depending on the muscles used. The procedure for pulsed muscle energy is as follows (Figure 8-11):

1. Isolate the target muscle by putting it into a passive contraction.
2. Apply counterpressure for the contraction.
3. Instruct the patient to contract the target muscle rapidly in very small movements for about 20 repetitions. Then go on to step 4, or use this variation: maintain the position, but switch the counterpressure location to the opposite side and have the patient contract the antagonist muscles for 20 repetitions. Rapid eye movement can replace the pulses or enhance the action.
4. Slowly lengthen the target muscle.
5. Repeat steps 2 through 4 until normal full resting length is obtained.

NOTE: All contraction and resistance efforts should start and finish gently.

DIRECT MANIPULATION

In some circumstances a patient cannot or does not want to participate actively in the massage. Direction manipulation, a variation of the muscle

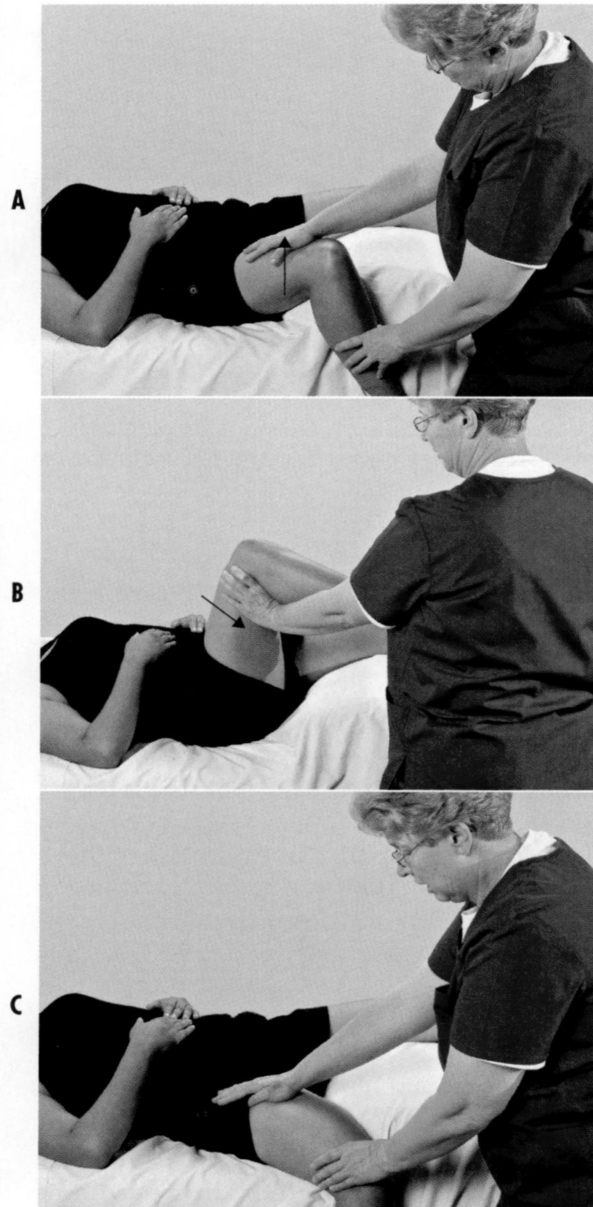

FIGURE 8-10 ■ **A,** Target the quadriceps; contract and relax. **B,** Contract the antagonist. **C,** Lengthen the quadriceps.

energy technique, can be used for these patients and also when a patient is sleeping (Figure 8-12). The principles of muscle energy techniques can still be used by direct manipulation of the spindle cells or Golgi tendons. Pushing muscle fibers together in the direction of the fibers in the belly of a muscle weakens the muscle by working with the spindle cells. As the fibers of the muscle are pushed together, the spindle cells (which sense muscle length) determine that the muscle is too short. The proprioceptive response is to relax the muscle fibers so that the muscle can be comfortable in its chosen position. Pushing muscle fibers together in the belly of the muscle is a way to relieve a muscle cramp. This is sometimes called *approximation.*

Separating the muscle fibers in the belly of a muscle in the direction of the fibers strengthens the muscle. When this occurs, the spindle cells determine that the muscle is too long; they signal the brain's proprioception center to shorten the muscle so that the muscle can do the job it is supposed to do.

The same responses can be obtained using the Golgi tendon organs, except that the manipulation of the proprioception signal cells is reversed. Manipulation of the Golgi tendon organs occurs at the ends of the muscle, where it joins the tendons. To weaken the muscle, pull apart on the tendon attachments of the target muscle. This tells the body's proprioception center that tension on the tendon is excessive and the muscle should loosen to be in balance. To strengthen the muscle, push the tendon attachments together. This signals the body that too little tension is on the tendon (in relation to the tension within the muscle belly). The muscle therefore contracts.

The pressure levels used to elicit the response need to be sufficient to contact the muscle fibers. Pressure that is too light does not access the proprioceptors. Excessive pressure negates the response by activating protective reflexes. Moderate pressure, by which the muscle itself can be palpated, is most effective.

The procedure for direct manipulation of the spindle cells to initiate the relaxation and lengthening response is as follows:

1. Place the target muscle in comfortable passive extension.
2. Press the spindle cells together on the target muscle.
3. Pull the spindle cells apart on the antagonist muscle.
4. Lengthen the target muscle.
5. Repeat steps 2 through 4 until normal full resting length is obtained.

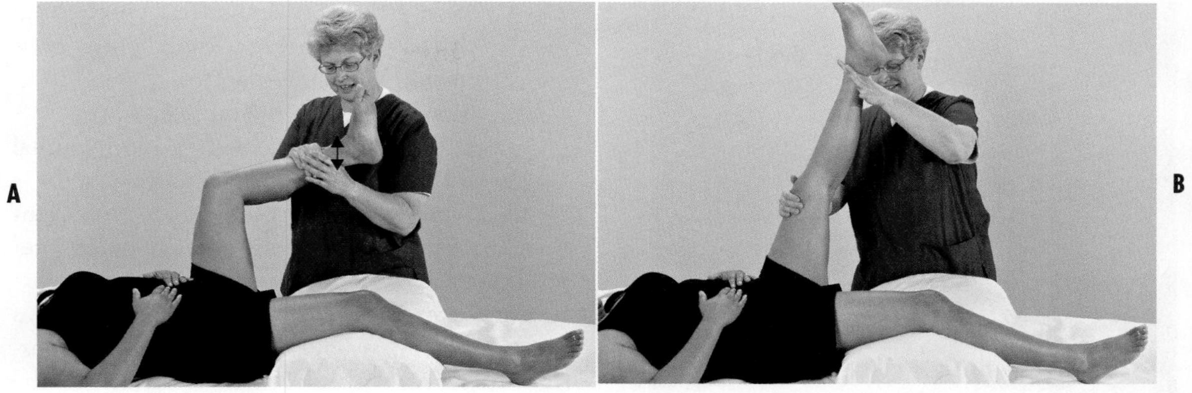

FIGURE 8-11 ■ Pulsed muscle energy. **A,** Target the hamstring (small, controlled contractions). **B,** Lengthen the target muscle.

The procedure for direct manipulation of the Golgi tendon organs to initiate the PIR response is as follows:

1. Place the target muscle in comfortable passive extension.
2. Pull apart on the tendon attachments of the target muscle.
3. Push the tendon attachments together on the antagonist muscle.
4. Lengthen the target muscle.
5. Repeat steps 2 through 4 until normal full resting length is obtained.

POSITIONAL RELEASE TECHNIQUES

According to Dr. Leon Chaitow, during positional release techniques, a muscle's spindles are influenced by methods that take them into an "ease" state and that theoretically allow them an opportunity to "reset" and reduce hypertonic status. Strain-counterstrain and other positional release methods use the slow, controlled return of distressed tissues to the position of strain as a means of offering spindles a chance to reset and so normalize function. This is particularly effective if the spindles have inappropriately held an area in just such protective splinting.

Positional release is a more generic term used to describe these methods. Positional release methods are used on painful areas, especially recent strains, before, after, or instead of muscle energy methods. The tender points often are located in the antagonist of the tight muscle because of the diagonal balancing process the body uses to maintain an upright posture in gravity.

Repositioning of the body into the original strain (often the position of a prior injury) allows proprioceptors to reset and stop firing protective signals. By moving the body into the direction of ease (i.e., the way the body wants to go and out of the position that causes the pain), the proprioception is taken into a state of safety. Remaining in this state for a time allows the neuromuscular mechanism to reset itself. The massage therapist then gently and slowly repositions the area into neutral. If the condition is extremely painful, the body is gently held in the neutral position. If the condition is chronic and not acutely painful, the body can be positioned from neutral into a lengthening phase by slowly positioning at bind, engaging the resistance barrier, and holding in this position, gradually taking up any slack as the tissues lengthen.

The positioning used during positional release is a full body process. Remember, an injury or loss of balance is a full body experience. For this reason, areas distant to the tender point must be considered during the positioning process. The position of the feet may very well have an effect on a tender point in the neck. Eye position is almost always a factor. Often the ease position can be found just with eye movement. The procedure for positional release is as follows (Figure 8-13):

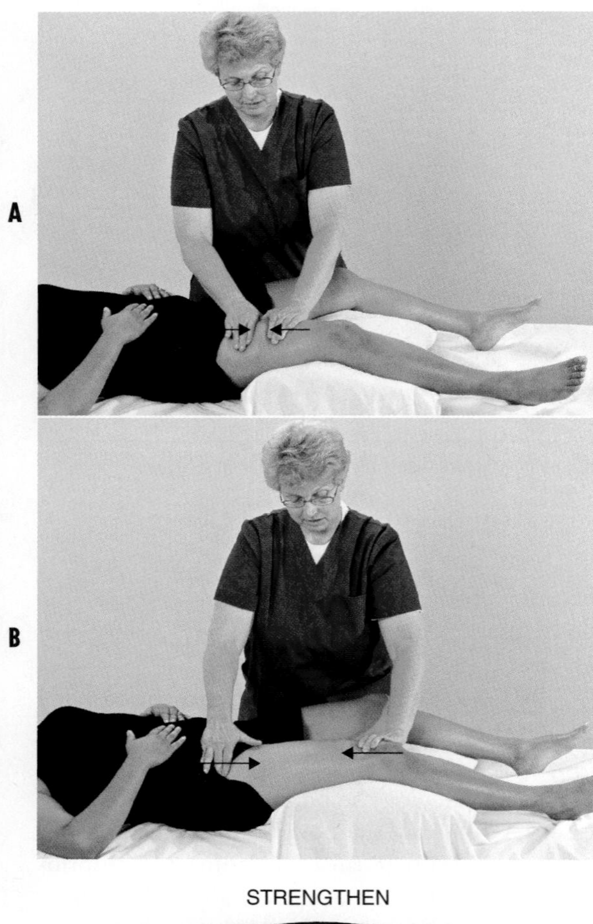

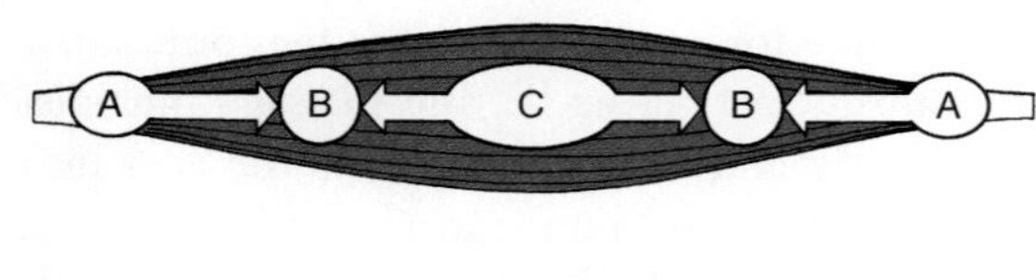

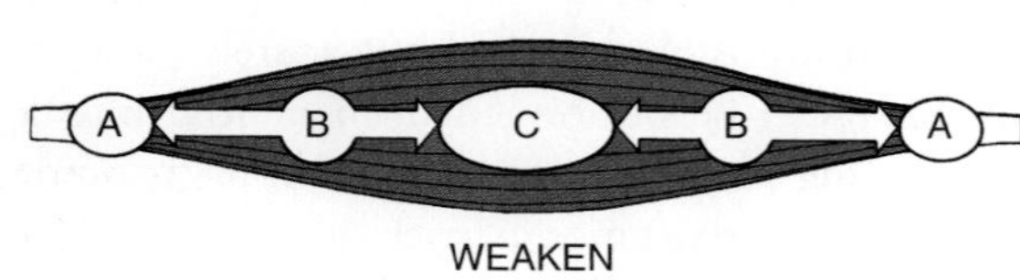

FIGURE 8-12 ■ Direct manipulation. **A,** Weaken the quadriceps by pushing the muscle fibers together in the belly of the muscle. **B,** Target the quadriceps and strengthen it by pushing together the tendon attachments of the muscle. **C,** Overview. (**C** from Fritz S: *Sports & exercise massage: comprehensive care in athletics, fitness, & rehabilitation,* St Louis, 2006, Mosby.)

1. Locate the tender point.
2. Gently initiate the pain response with direct pressure. Remember, the sensation of pain is a guide.
3. Slowly position the body until the pain subsides. Include eye position.
4. Wait at least 30 seconds or longer until the patient feels the release, lightly monitoring the tender point.
5. Slowly lengthen the muscle.
6. Repeat steps 1 through 5 until normal full resting length is obtained.

Positional release techniques are important because they gently allow the body to reposition and restore balance. They also are highly effective ways of dealing with tender areas regardless of the pathology. Sometimes it is impossible to know why the point is tender to the touch. However, if tenderness is present, a protective muscle spasm surrounds it. Positional release is an excellent way to release these small areas of muscle spasm without inducing additional pain.

THE INTEGRATED APPROACH

Muscle energy methods can be used together or in a sequence to enhance their effects. Muscle tension in one area of the body often indicates imbalance and compensation patterns in other areas of the body. Tension patterns can be self-perpetuating. Often, using an integrated approach introduces the type of information the nervous system needs to self-correct. The procedure outlined here relies on the body's innate knowledge of what is out of balance and how to restore a more normal functioning pattern.

The procedure for an integrated approach is as follows (use the position from either option A, steps 1 and 2, or option B, steps 1 and 2, as the starting point for the rest of the process, which begins at step 3, p. 233):

Option A (Figure 8-14)

1. Identify the most obvious of the postural distortion symptoms.
2. Exaggerate the pattern by increasing the distortion, moving the body into ease. This position becomes the pattern of isolation of various muscles that are addressed in the next part of the procedure (e.g., if the left shoulder is elevated and rotated forward, exaggerate and increase the elevation and rotation pattern). Continue with step 3, p. 233.

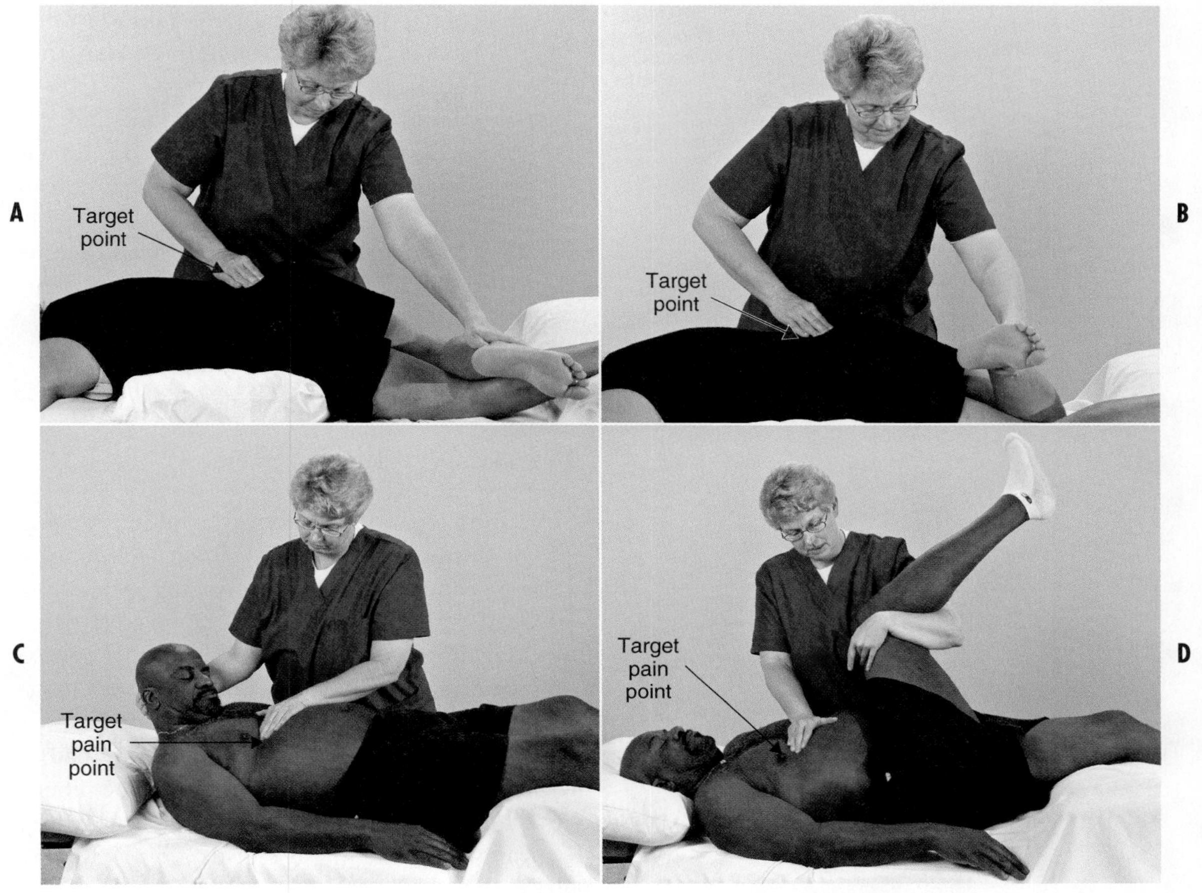

FIGURE 8-13 ■ Two examples of positional release. **A,** 50% reduction in pain. **B,** Modifying the position results in a 90% reduction in pain. **C,** 50% reduction in pain. **D,** Modifying the position results in a 90% to 100% reduction in pain.

Option B

1. Identify a painful point.
2. Use positional release to move the body into ease until the point is substantially less tender to pressure. The position of ease found becomes the pattern of isolation of various muscles that are addressed in the next part of the procedure. Continue with step 3.

After choosing from option A or option B, continue the procedure as follows:

3. Stabilize the patient in as many different directions as possible.
4. Instruct the patient to move out of the pattern. Be as vague as possible and do not guide the patient, because it is important for the patient to identify the resistance pattern.
5. Provide resistance for the patient to push or pull against.
6. Modify the resistance angle as necessary to achieve the most solid resistance pattern for the patient.
7. Spend a few moments noticing when the patient's breathing changes; then, while still providing modified resistance, allow the patient to move through the pattern slowly.
8. When the patient has achieved as much extension as possible on his or her own, recognize that the patient has achieved the lengthening pattern and has moved

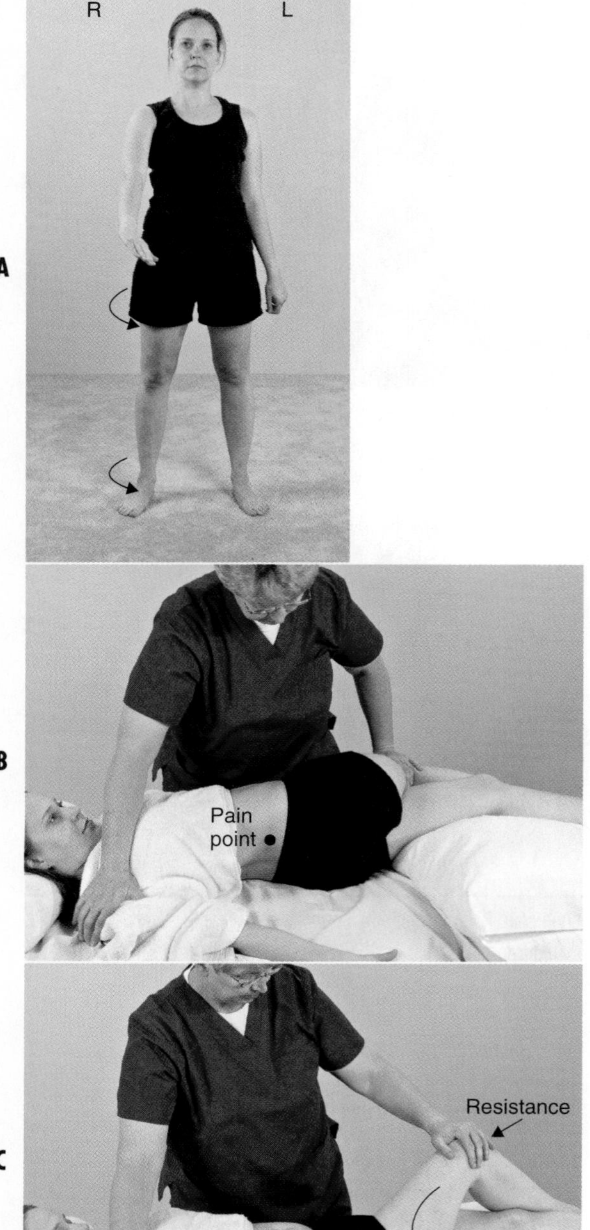

FIGURE 8-14 ■ Integrated muscle energy. **A,** Target internal rotation of the right hip. **B,** Increase the distortion pattern (ease) or use positional release to find a position of ease. Internal rotation. **C,** Instruct the patient to move out of the position, against applied resistance from the massage therapist, into the opposite position (in this case, from internal rotation to external rotation).

from a position of ease to a position that has engaged the binding resistance barrier.

9. Gently increase the lengthening. If additional elongation in this position is desired, connective tissue stretching can be achieved.
10. Pay attention to what body areas become involved besides the one addressed. This is your guide to the next position.

STRETCHING

Stretching is a mechanical method of introducing various forces into connective tissue to elongate areas of connective tissue shortening. Stretching affects the fiber component of connective tissue by elongating the fibers past their normal give so that they can enter the plastic range past the existing bind. This results in either freeing and unraveling of fibers or a small therapeutic inflammatory response that signals for change in the fibers. Stretching also affects the ground substance, warming and softening it and thereby increasing pliability.

Because fascial sheaths provide structural support, it is important to work with a sense of three dimensional awareness, realizing that shifts in structure have more than a localized effect. The body supports stability before mobility, and compensation patterns are body wide, therefore changes in structure need to be balanced with either lengthening or strengthening activities that allow the body to maintain a sense of perpendicular orientation in gravity.

If the stability/mobility factor is not considered, the body's method of reacting to changes in structure is to increase muscle spasm and acute pain. This results in a decreased ability to adapt effectively to the changes introduced; it reduces the effectiveness of the methods. Stretching introduces forces of bend, torsion, and tension that mechanically affect connective tissue.

As explained previously, stretching and lengthening are different. Before stretching, muscles should be lengthened through massage and muscle energy techniques, or the muscles of the area may develop protective spasms; this occurs because stretching often moves the tissue into pathologic barriers formed by connective tissue changes. The connective tissue component cannot be accessed until the muscle has been lengthened. Without stretching, any neuromuscular lengthening may be restricted by shortened connective tissue. Lengthening can be done without stretching (this is sometimes even desirable); however, if stretching is used, lengthening must always be done *before* stretching. During stretching, muscle energy techniques are used to prepare muscles to stretch by activating lengthening responses.

Longitudinal stretching pulls connective tissue in the direction of the fiber configuration. Cross-directional stretching pulls the connective tissue against the fiber direction. The two techniques accomplish the same thing, but longitudinal stretching is done in conjunction with movement at the joint. If longitudinal stretching is not advisable, if it is ineffective in situations of hypermobility of a joint, or if the area to be stretched is not effectively stretched longitudinally, cross-directional stretching is a better choice. Cross-directional stretching focuses on the tissue itself and does not depend on joint movement. Various forces can be combined to increase stretching effectiveness. In a method called *pin and stretch,* the short tissue is compressed and immobilized ("pinned") and at the same time a tension force is used to stretch it. In a similar approach, called *active release techniques,* the massage therapist compresses and holds the short tissue and the patient moves the area to stretch the tissue.

The direction of ease is the way the body allows for postural changes and muscle shortening or weakening compensation patterns, depending on its balance in gravity. Although compensation patterns may be inefficient, the patterns developed serve a purpose and need to be respected. It may seem logical to locate a shortened muscle group or a rotated movement pattern and use direct methods to reverse the pattern. However, this may not be the best approach. Protective sensory receptors prevent any forced stretch out of a compensation pattern. Instead, the pattern of compensation is respected, and the body position is exaggerated and coaxed into a more efficient position.

For example, let's say you have a patient with shortened pectoralis muscles that pull the shoulders forward, creating a gorilla-like appearance. Instead of pulling the pectoralis muscles into a stretch by forcing the arms back, curl the shoulders and arms more into adduction, providing slack and space to the receptors in the pectoralis muscles. Begin corrective action from this point, slowly stretching the binding tissue.

Developing good stretching techniques is perhaps as much an art as a science, because many variables are involved. An individual muscle needs to be carefully isolated by positioning and stabilizing so that the stretch is focused. With the muscles that work one joint only, this is usually quite simple; however, with two-joint muscles, it becomes more complicated. One joint needs to be fixed so that it prestretches the muscle, whereas the other joint is moved to increase the stretch. This means that two different techniques may be used for the same muscle to focus the stretch at either end.

Within each stretch some fine tuning needs to be done, through careful adjustments in the position, to try to focus the stretch into the target area. The muscle must be fully relaxed and non-weight bearing, otherwise it will not stretch fully, even though the patient may feel a sensation of stretch.

When a muscle is stretched, it first should be taken slowly to the point where the patient feels a mild discomfort; this is the restrictive barrier. It should be held firmly but comfortably in that binding position. The patient should not feel any pain, tearing, or burning, which would indicate that the fibers are being overstretched and torn. After a period of time the tissues may begin to ease and the stretch can be gently increased. Expert opinion varies on how long a stretch should be held, but it is generally accepted that the duration of a stretch is more significant than its intensity. Short, ballistic-type stretches or the use of too much force can increase tension through a reflex action. Long, sustained, progressive stretching seems to produce the best results.

LONGITUDINAL STRETCHING

The procedure for longitudinal stretching is as follows:

1. Position the target muscle in the direction of ease. Stabilize and isolate a muscle group.
2. Choose a method to prepare the target muscle to stretch (e.g., gliding, kneading, PIR, RI, pulsed muscle energy, direct application).
3. After the target muscle has been prepared, stretch the muscle to its physiologic or pathologic barrier or to wherever protective contraction is engaged (bind). Back off slightly to prevent muscle spasm. Stay in line with the muscle fibers. Exert effort or movement with the inhalation. Stretch just past bind on the exhalation.

The following two approaches are used for the actual stretch phase:

1. Hold the position just off the physiologic or pathologic barrier for at least 10 seconds and up to 30 to 60 seconds to allow for the neurologic reset. This is the lengthening phase. Feel for secondary response (a small give in the muscle).
2. Take up slack and hold for 20 to 30 seconds to create longitudinal pull (tension force) on the connective tissue. You must hold the muscle stretch as instructed to allow for changes in the connective tissue component of the muscle.

ALTERNATE PROCEDURE FOR LONGITUDINAL STRETCHING

If only a small section of muscle needs to be stretched, if the muscle does not lend itself to stretching with joint movement, or if the joints are so flexible that not enough pull (tension force) is put on the muscles to achieve an effective stretch to the tissues, the following alternate procedure for longitudinal stretching should be used:

1. Locate the fibers or muscle to be stretched.
2. Place the hands, fingers, or forearms in the belly of the muscle or directly over the area to be stretched.
3. Contact the muscle with sufficient pressure to reset the neuromuscular mechanism.
4. Separate the fingers, hands, or forearms (tension force) or lift the tissue with pressure sufficient to stretch the muscle (bending or torsion force). Take up all slack from lengthening until you feel the tissues bind, then increase the intensity slightly and wait for the connective tissue component to respond (this may take as long as 30 seconds).

NOTE: All requirements for preparation of the muscle and for the direction of stretch are the same as those described for the previous longitudinal stretching procedure.

The procedure for active assisted longitudinal stretching is as follows:

1. Identify and isolate the muscle, making sure it is not working against gravity in this position. Remind the patient to exhale during the stretching phase of this technique.
2. Lengthen the muscle to its physiologic or pathologic barrier (bind), move slightly beyond this point, and stretch gently for 1 to 2 seconds.
3. Return the muscle to its starting position.
4. Repeat this process in a rhythmic, pulse-like fashion for 5 to 20 repetitions.
5. The patient will benefit from doing a contraction with the antagonist while the target muscle is lengthened and then stretched. As in all proper lengthening and stretching movements, attention must be paid to the stretch reflex; bouncing is never done, because it initiates this reflex.

Cross-directional tissue stretching uses a pull-and-twist component, introducing torsion and bend forces. The procedure for cross-directional stretching is as follows:

1. Access the area to be stretched by moving against the fiber direction.
2. Lift or deform the area slightly and hold for 30 to 60 seconds until the area warms or seems to soften.

The following procedure is used for skin and superficial connective tissue:

1. Locate the area of restriction.
2. Lift and pull (like taffy), first moving into the restriction and then pulling and twisting out of it, keeping a constant tension on the tissue (think plastic wrap) (Figure 8-15).

JUST BETWEEN YOU AND ME

Okay, you should now understand the hows and whys of massage application. There should be no more mindless rubbing posing as therapeutic massage. Massage is a deliberate application with a specific purpose in mind. You should be able to answer these questions while giving a massage:

- How do you perform the specific method? Demonstrate and explain (show and tell).
- How do you alter the method through variations in qualities of touch. Demonstrate and explain (show and tell).
- Why did you choose to use this particular method?
- What is the expected result or results of the application of this method?
- How do these results pertain to the outcome of the massage based on the goals for the patient?

My students really get flustered when I walk around and expect them to provide relatively intelligent responses to these questions. How would you answer them?

BODY MECHANICS

The DVD that accompanies this text demonstrates body mechanics. Carefully watch the body mechanics used during all demonstrations on the DVD. As appropriate during a demonstration, a narrator identifies correct and effective body mechanics and points out ineffective body mechanics and correction procedures.

Effective body mechanics is essential for the massage therapist. In general, the therapeutic massage community does a poor job of teaching and practicing proper body mechanics. The concept of massage as a fluid, dancelike movement involving flexed knees and arms is not effective and can result in injury to the massage therapist. Concepts of yoga, martial arts, and tai chi do not translate into effective body mechanics during massage. Contrary to common perception, massage is *not* a dynamic movement system. It is a repeated series of static activities. If you want a long, successful career, effective and ergonomically correct body mechanics is essential. The patient does not want to be poked, prodded, or dug into, but this is what happens if the therapist uses ineffective body mechanics.

The massage therapist needs to provide a sustained, restrained, and somewhat static movement with pressure focused downward and forward to deliver the various levels of compressive force. The forearms, wrists, hands, fingers, thumbs, knees, and foot can be used to deliver the compressive force effectively. In the healthcare environment, massage application may need to be modified for work in a hospital bed. It is even more important to use effective body mechanics in less than ideal situations.

JUST BETWEEN YOU AND ME

As far as actually giving a massage goes, body mechanics is the most important aspect for both the therapist and the patient. There is a lot of confusion over the correct way to give a massage. The truth is, we don't know the definitive answer, because no targeted ergonomic studies have ever been done to determine the most efficient way to perform the massage methods at various pressure depths, speeds, and so on.

Please pay attention to the strategies described for body mechanics in this section. They are based on solid information obtained from physical therapists, athletic trainers, ergonomic specialists in industrial settings, and years and years of my professional practice, which includes teaching thousands of students. If you hurt after giving a massage, you're not doing it right. You should be able to perform 6 to 7 hours of massage application without undue pain or fatigue. If you cannot do this, something about your body mechanics is less than efficient. You may have to "unlearn" your current approach and learn this more effective method.

CONCEPTS OF BODY MECHANICS

Four basic concepts pertaining to body mechanics are common to all techniques used to apply compressive force to body tissues during massage application. These concepts are:

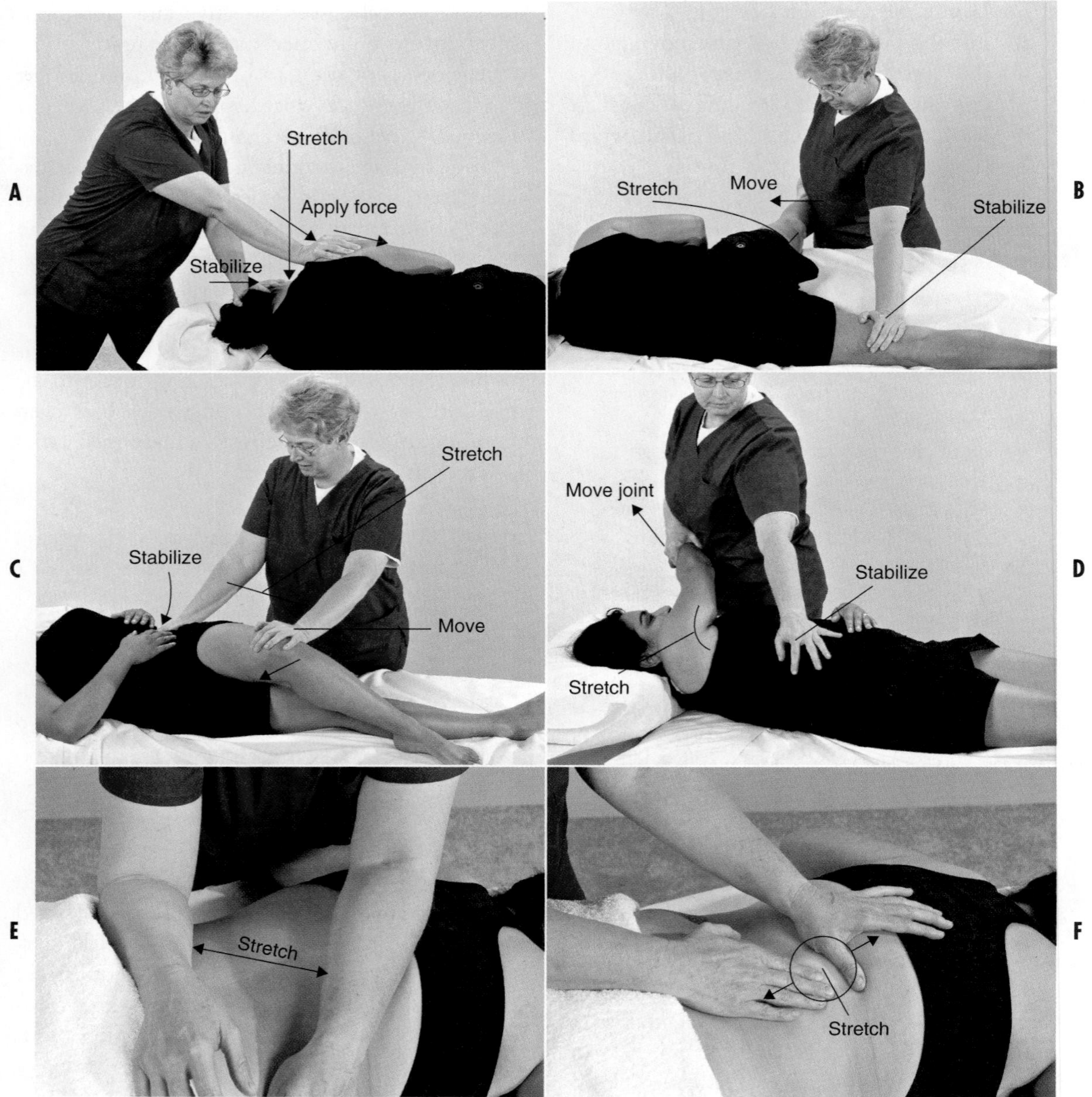

FIGURE 8-15 ■ Stretching. Mechanical forces to move tissue to just past the binding barrier can be applied by moving joints apart or by directly stretching tissue. **A,** Stabilize and move the area. **B,** Stabilize and move the area. **C,** Stabilize and move the joint. **D,** Stabilize and move the joint. **E,** Stretching of a large area with direct tension force application. **F,** Stretching a small area with direct tension force application.

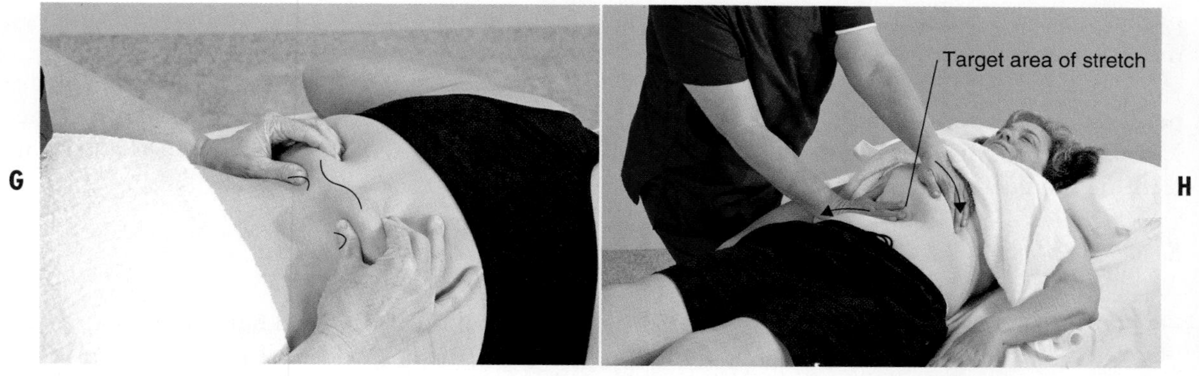

FIGURE 8-15, cont'd ■ **G,** Direct stretching of tissue with bend and shear forces. **H,** Specific local application of combined mechanical forces to produce stretch.

- Weight transfer
- Perpendicularity
- Stacking of the joints in close-packed position
- Keeping the back straight

Weight Transfer

Weight transfer allows the massage therapist to transfer his or her body weight by shifting the center of gravity forward to achieve a pressure that is comfortable for the patient. To transfer weight, the therapist stands (or kneels) with one foot forward and the other foot (or knee) back in an asymmetric stance; the feet are under the hips and about 1 to 1½ feet apart, never wider than the shoulders. In the standing position, the front leg is in a relaxed knee flexion with the foot forward enough to be in front of the knee. The back leg is straight. This means that the knee is at 0 degrees of flexion and, in the normal knee, screw home position for stability. The knee is not hyperextended, and the hips and shoulders are aligned so that the back is straight. The transfer is accomplished by taking the weight off the front leg and moving it to the heels of the hands, thumbs, or whichever part of the arm is used to apply pressure. The weight of the body is distributed (whole foot included) to the heel of the weight-bearing leg, not the toes.

Pressure is increased by moving the back leg farther away from the patient; it is decreased by moving the back leg closer to the patient. When moving away from the patient to increase pressure, always stay on flat feet. Do not move up on the toes.

Perpendicularity

Perpendicularity is an important principle that ensures that the pressure exerted sinks straight into the tissues. The line from the shoulders to the point of contact (e.g., the forearm or heel of the hand) must be 90 degrees to the plane of the contact point on the patient's body. The patient should be positioned such that the pressure is applied against a 45-degree incline whenever possible. The massage therapist's feet should be pointed toward the point of contact; they should not be in a T-stance or externally rotated.

Stacking of the Joints

Stacking of the joints one atop another is essential to the concepts of perpendicularity and weight transfer. The therapist's body must be in a straight line from the heel of the weight-bearing rear foot through the knee, hip, and shoulder, and then from the shoulder to the forearm, or through the elbow acting as an extension of the shoulder, to the heels of the hands. The ankle, knee, hip of the back leg, and spine are stacked and stable in a close-packed joint position. The pelvic girdle and the shoulder girdle are lined up. The shoulder is stacked over the elbow, which in turn is stacked over the wrist. Stacking the joints in this way allows the pressure exerted by the massage therapist to travel straight and effortlessly into the patient's body as the therapist's center of gravity moves forward.

The weak point is the shoulder, which must be flexed forward at no more than 45 degrees. Maintaining a straight back and straight arm protects the shoulder.

Keeping a Straight Back

A straight back and a weight-bearing leg are essential components of body mechanics. If the back is not straight, the therapist often ends up pushing with the upper body instead of using the more effortless feeling of transferred weight. The muscles of the torso, especially the abdomen, are considered the core. Core stability is necessary for back stability. Most massage therapists need to develop core stability.

The therapist's weight should be borne on the back leg on the heel and flat of the foot, never on the toes. At first this may feel uncomfortable; however, some of the biggest muscles in the body are in the legs. The ankles must be in at least 15 degrees of dorsiflexion. Many massage therapists may need to increase their ankle flexibility.

Massage uses primarily a force generated forward and downward with a 90-degree contact against the body. The combination of a 45-degree slant from the contours of the patient's body (hills) plus the 45-degree angle of force used during appropriate body mechanics results in the 90-degree contact. The patient therefore must be positioned such that the 45-degree angles are accessible. The side-lying position is the most accessible. The seated position is a viable option that is seldom used and may be one of the most effective positions in various healthcare settings.

The center of gravity and the weight force are redistributed by keeping the weight on the back foot (heels and flat of the foot, not on the toes); the back knee is maintained 0 to 10 degrees of flexion and stable, with the back straight; the weight distribution coming from the abdomen; and the balance point at the object-contact point. The joints of the wrist, arm, shoulder, back, hip, weight-bearing knee, and ankle are stacked for effective delivery of force. The arm generating the pressure is opposite the weight-bearing leg, which allows proper counterbalance and prevents twisting of the body at the shoulder and pelvic girdle. The shoulder girdle must stay in line with the pelvic girdle, with the head held up and the eyes forward.

Creative use of the massage therapist's body is essential in working with patients. When the situation allows, use of the knee/leg and foot during massage can be helpful.

COUNTERPRESSURE

Because of the density and bulk of some patients' muscle structure, you may need to use a body mechanics strategy that allows you to apply very deep compressive force. By using counterpressure, the massage therapist can safely reach the deep tissue layers without poking the patient. The principle is simple: Combining the forward weight transfer with a pull-back motion squeezes the forces together. The technique is as follows:

1. Apply compressive force as presented by leaning and weight transfer.
2. Make sure the weight is on the heel of the back foot.
3. Use the arm that is not exerting pressure to hold the table, and pull up to squeeze the forces together (a body part also may be used).

The thumb is seldom used during massage. The proper application involves a braced hand and supported fingers, because hinge joints effectively move into a stable, close-packed position (Figure 8-16).

Use of a Mat During Massage

Some patients are more comfortable on a mat, especially large patients who really do not fit on a standard massage table. Nevertheless, the body mechanics principles do not change. The only difference is that the weight-bearing contacts on the floor most often are the back knee and shin, whereas the forward upper limb (e.g., hand or forearm) used to apply massage becomes the point of contact. Also, use of the leg and foot is easier when working on a mat (Figure 8-17).

In the healthcare setting, some people who are ill or injured cannot be placed on a massage table, or a patient may be unable to assume certain positions that are most efficient for massage. In such cases, creativity and experimentation are required of the massage therapist. Typically, a

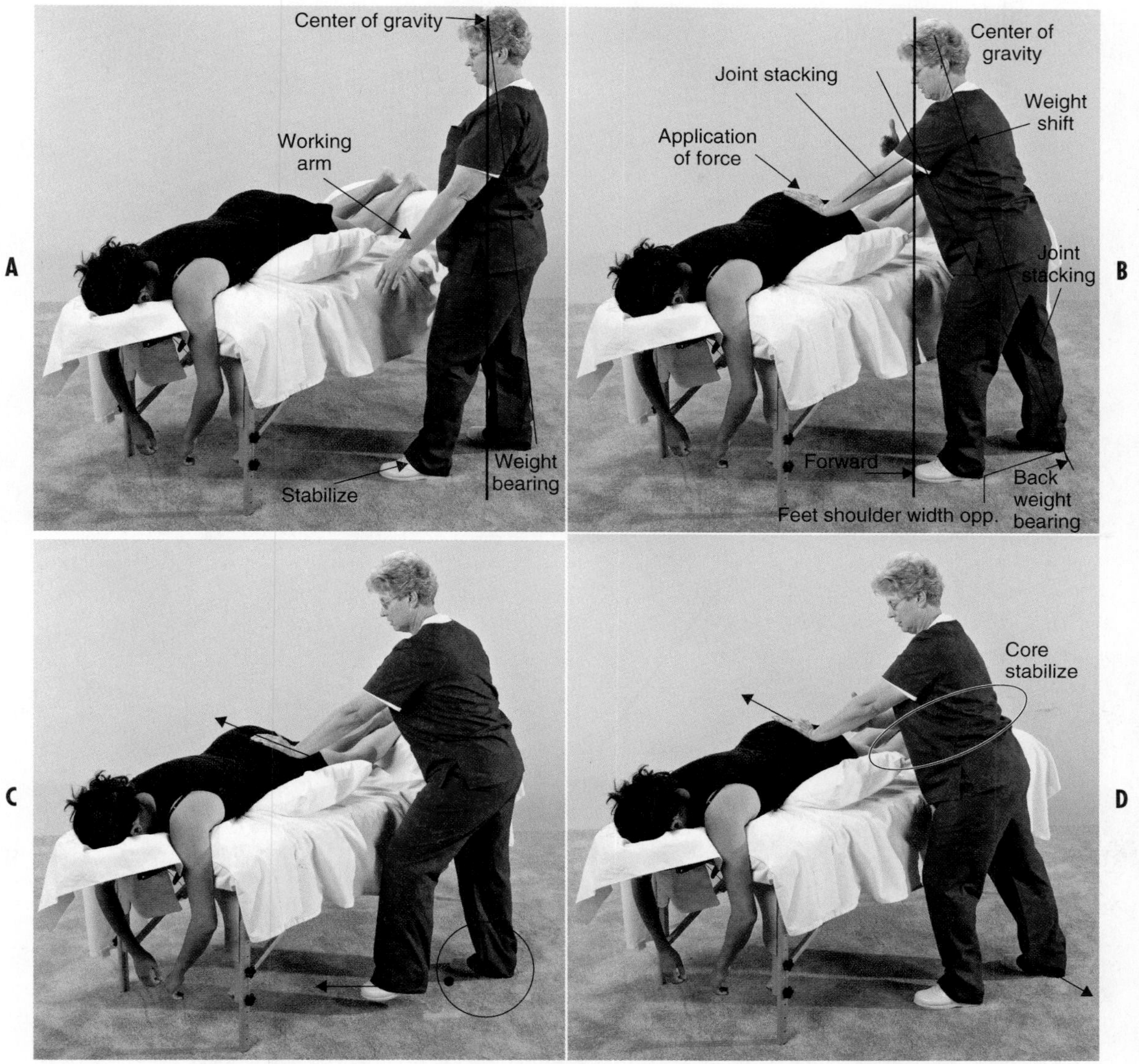

FIGURE 8-16 ■ The fundamentals of body mechanics (make sure you observe the body mechanics in all photographs in this book and on the DVD). **A,** Begin. **B,** Lean, weight shift, stabilization, joint stacking. **C,** Glide: when weight from your back foot moves forward, from the heel to the ball of your foot and your toes, it is time to reposition by taking a step. **D,** After taking the step, re-establish core stabilization and the leaning posture.

Continued

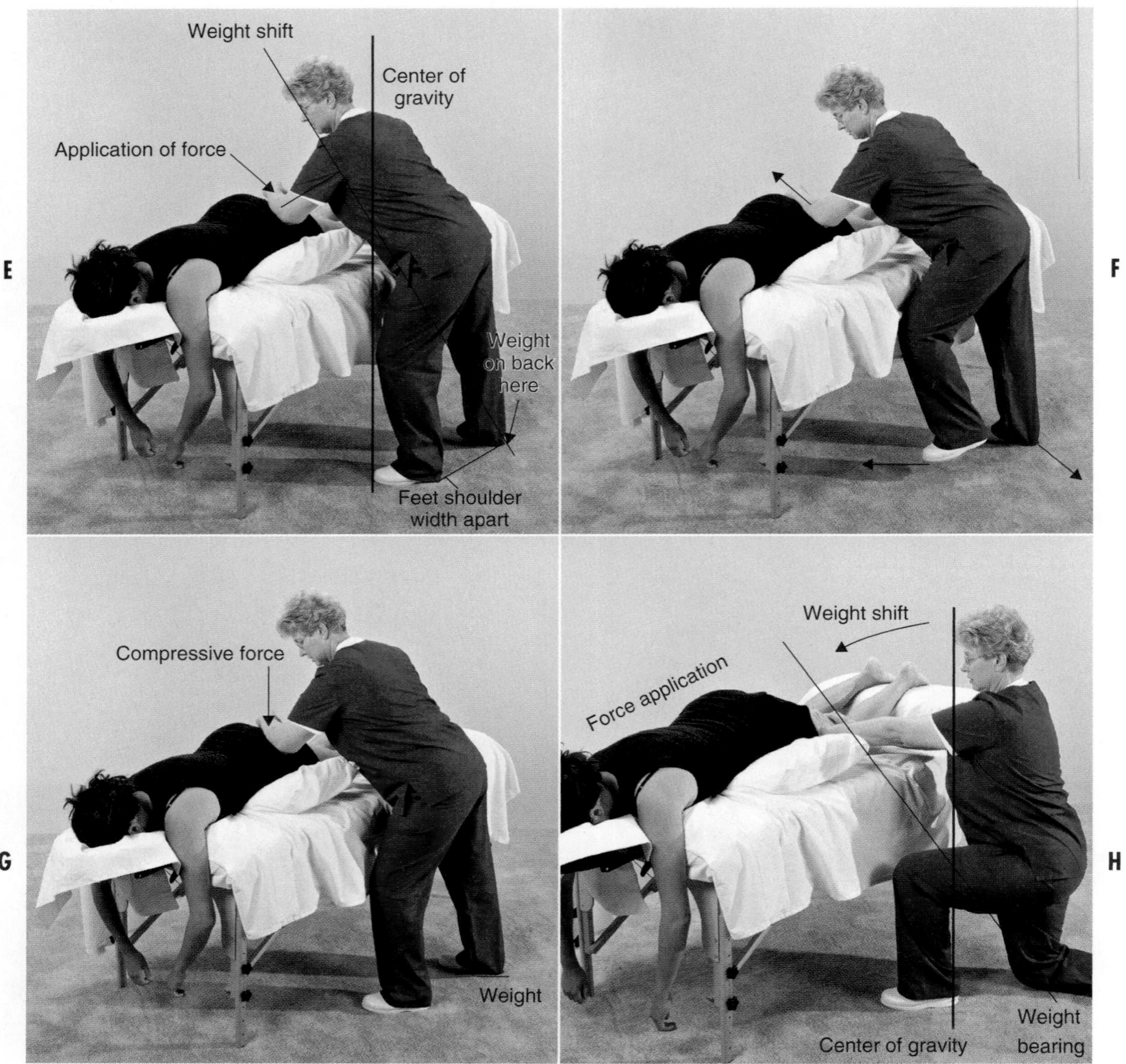

FIGURE 8-16, cont'd ■ **E,** The same sequence is followed when you use your forearm. **F,** To glide, push your heel into the floor, and your forearm will move forward. When the glide distance shifts your weight from the back of your heel to the ball of your foot and your toes, it is time to take a step. **G,** Reposition in the leaning stance with core stabilization. **H,** Kneeling is efficient body mechanics, especially for kneading.

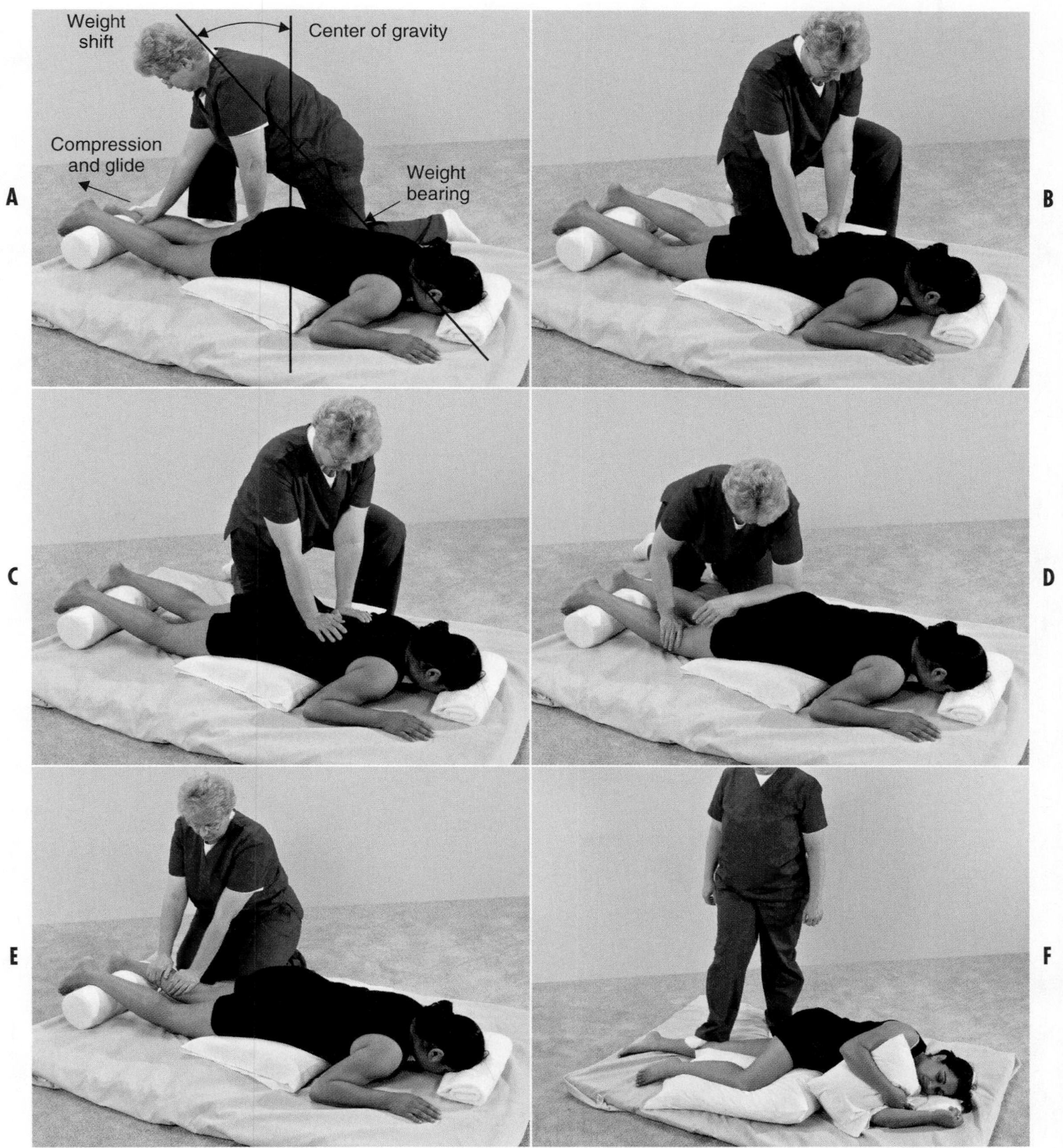

FIGURE 8-17 ■ Examples of body mechanics, client positioning, and massage application when working on a mat (additional examples can be found on the DVD). **A,** Example of body mechanics. **B,** Position of bolsters for supine position, application of compression. **C,** Position for gliding or compression using the palms. **D,** Position for forearm glide or compression. **E,** Position for kneading. **F,** Using the foot to apply mechanical faces; position for side lying.

Continued

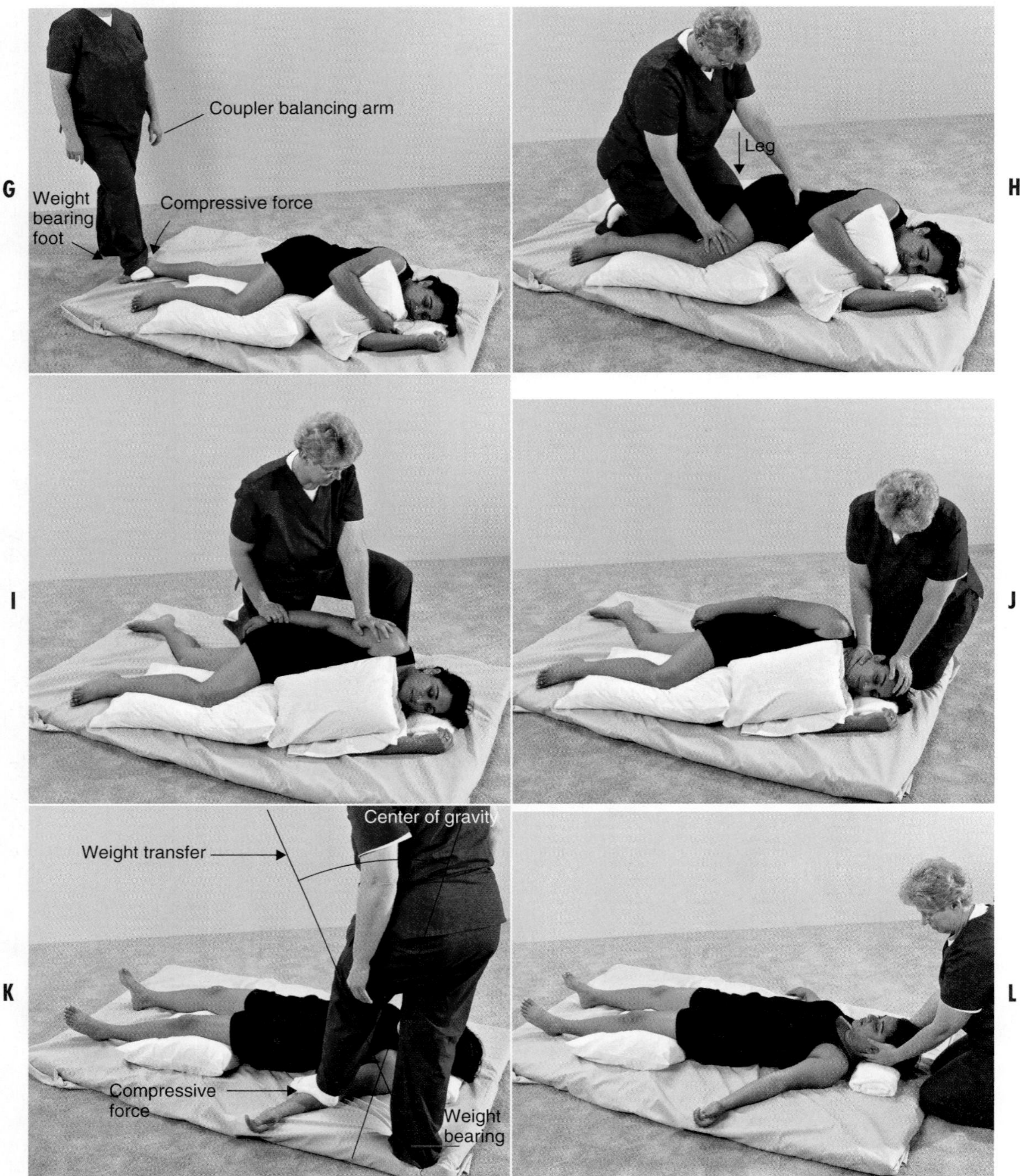

FIGURE 8-17, cont'd ■ **G,** Body mechanics, standing. **H,** Compression using therapist's leg in side-lying position. **I,** Massage of the arm in side-lying position. **J,** Massage of the neck and head in side-lying position. **K,** Compression using the foot. **L,** Massage of the shoulder, neck, head, and face.

person who is bedridden does not require excessive compressive force; this is helpful to the massage therapist, because pressure delivery is the most tasking aspect of massage application. Nevertheless, if you perfect the basic skills of body mechanics presented in this text, you should be able to adapt even when significant pressure delivery is required.

evolve 8-2

The following terms and expressions specific to Chapter 8 have already been used to search PubMed for the latest research literature available. The *Click Here for Massage* feature associated with this chapter on your textbook's Evolve website allows you to hyperlink to a continually updated PubMed search of research literature that corresponds to this subject.

Hyperlink Search Terms

Massage body mechanics
Massage joint movement methods
Massage loading
Massage mechanical force
Massage methods
Massage muscle energy techniques
Massage stretching
Massage touch quality

SUMMARY

This chapter provided a review of massage methods for patients under medical care. In this unit, the general protocol found in Chapter 11 and the focused massage applications described in Chapter 6 are both based on the methods in this chapter. Almost all the methods described in the chapter are also assessment methods. Indeed, most massage is a form of assessment, which is described in the next chapter.

The actual massage is a weaving of palpation and movement assessment with treatment and then postassessment. Gliding is palpation that can first discern surface edema and then become a method to move the fluid. Kneading is assessment to identify connective tissue bind and then becomes a method to introduce forces into the tissue to reduce bind, and so on. Active and passive joint movement serves as range-of-motion assessment that then can become some type of application of a muscle energy technique to lengthen and stretch an area of restricted movement. Postassessment also is active and passive joint movement. One thing becomes the other and then back again in the assessment, treatment, and postassessment continuum.

Effective body mechanics is the key to massage application. Massage therapists who do not consistently practice proper body mechanics eventually suffer an injury. This is unacceptable. Body mechanics as presented in this chapter, if applied correctly, can protect the massage therapist and can ensure that the patient benefits from the quality of the therapist's touch.

WORKBOOK

1. Choose a current bodywork method with which you are familiar (e.g., Swedish massage, reflexology, shiatsu, deep tissue massage) and describe it in terms of stimulus and forces.

   Example: Deep tissue massage (my personal pet peeve; there is no such modality, really)

   Depth of pressure—Moderate to deep
   Drag—Moderate to intense
   Duration—Intermediate (60 seconds)
   Frequency—Two or three repetitions
   Speed—Slow
   Rhythm—Even
   Consists of mechanical force application to affect connective tissue structures.
   Stimulus to deep muscles by inhibition of pressure, either to belly or attachment.
   Muscle energy methods are appropriate with primary application of localized tissue lengthening and cross-fiber stretching.

   ____
   ____
   ____
   ____
   ____
   ____
   ____
   ____

2. Watch someone give a massage (can be a video or DVD) and describe the application in terms of stimulus and force.

   Example: The massage began with superficial glide to assess skin temperature, texture, and bind. The glide assessment identified an area of bind in the midscapular region. Compressive force was increased to moderate and the direction was changed, which moved tissue into the ease position. The tissue was held for 30 seconds and then moved into the bind direction. At bind, drag was increased and sustained for 30 seconds. The tissue then was kneaded.

   ____
   ____
   ____
   ____
   ____
   ____
   ____
   ____
   ____
   ____
   ____
   ____
   ____

WORKBOOK

3. Perform a massage. Provide a continuous narrative during the process, describing the application using terminology from this chapter.

   Example: I am beginning the massage with a palpation assessment using near touch to identify heat. Now, I am gently touching the skin and using a light pressure with drag to assess for areas of ease and bind.

4. Do a comprehensive evaluation of your body mechanics while giving a massage. Identify areas of strength and weakness and develop a corrective action plan.

Chapter 9 Concept Map

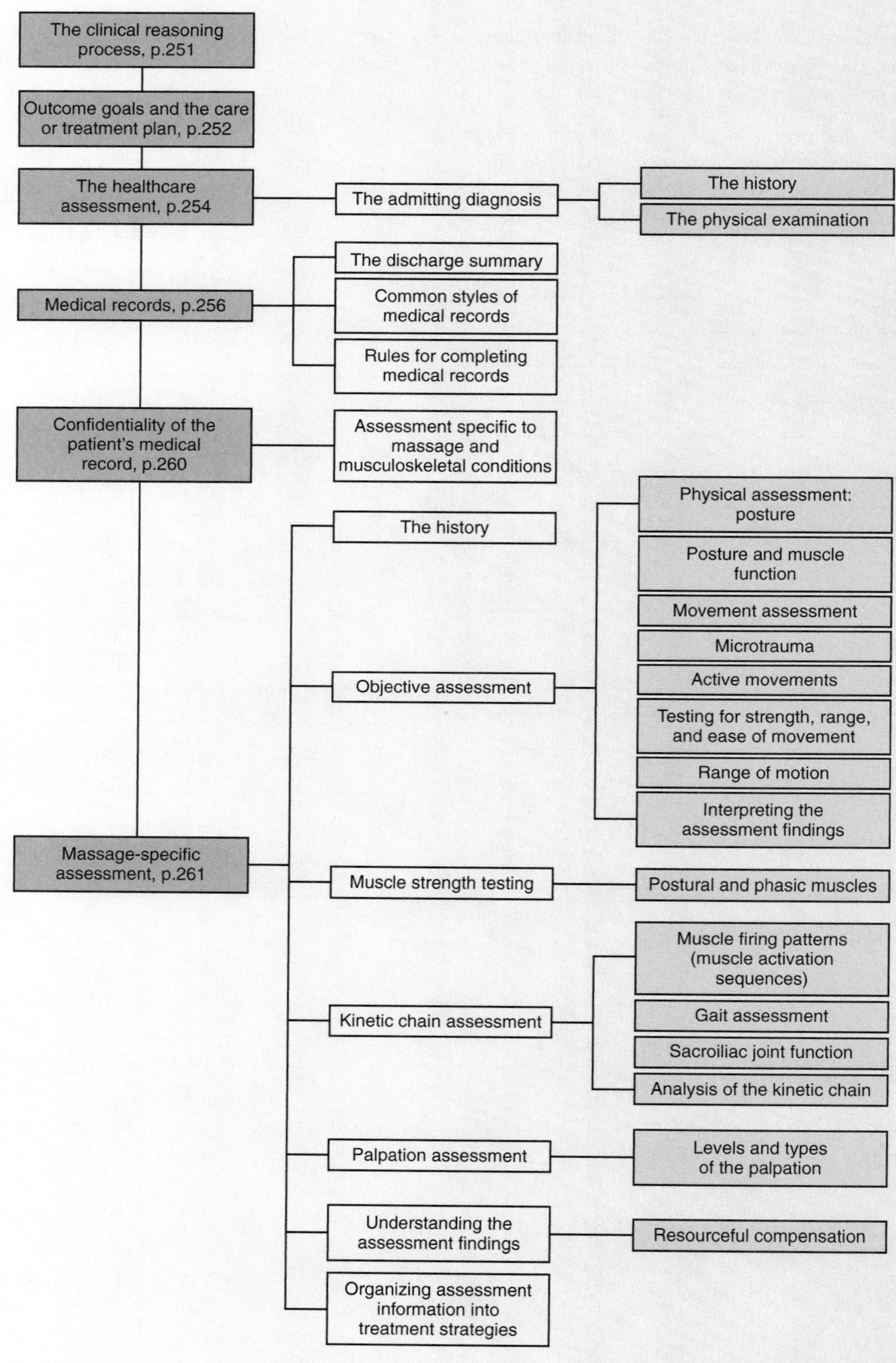

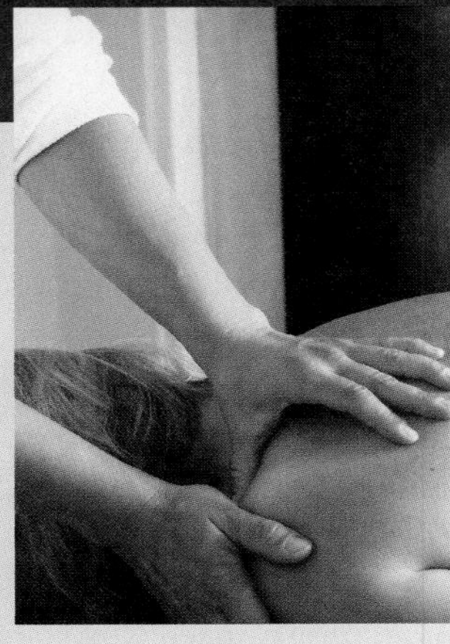

CHAPTER 9

MASSAGE APPLICATION ASSESSMENT FOR PHYSICAL HEALING AND REHABILITATION

Key Terms

Assessment
Anatomic barriers
Boggy end-feel
Bony (hard) end-feel
Capsular stretch (leathery) end-feel
Clinical reasoning
Documentation
Empty end-feel
Justification
Long-term goals
Muscle spasm end-feel
Muscular (tissue stretch) end-feel
Outcome goals
Overpressure
Pathologic barriers
Phasic (mover) muscles
Physician's orders
Physiologic barriers
Postural (stabilizer) muscles
Qualifiable
Quantifiable
Resourceful compensation
Routine (standing) orders
Short-term goals
Soft tissue approximation end-feel
Springy block (internal derangement) end-feel
Treatment plans

For definitions of key terms, refer to the Evolve website.

OBJECTIVES

Upon completion of this chapter, the reader will have the information necessary to:

1. Apply a clinical reasoning process to the development of a treatment plan.
2. Complete a comprehensive history.
3. Complete a comprehensive physical assessment.
4. Relate assessment data to first-, second-, and third-degree dysfunction and categorize the adaptation response to stage 1, 2, or 3 pathology.
5. Integrate ongoing assessment data into appropriate massage treatment strategies.

Massage therapists who work with patients in active medical care have an expanded assessment responsibility. Not only do they need to collect and apply assessment data relevant to massage application, they also must be able to understand the medical team's assessment process and treatment orders. Massage therapists must be able to contribute assessment data to the medical team and to develop and justify appropriate massage applications based on the requested massage outcomes. (Make sure to visit the Evolve website where indicated throughout the chapter for more detailed information.)

JUST BETWEEN YOU AND ME

Like the review of anatomy and physiology, the information in this chapter can seem overwhelming, and it is. There is too much for any one person to know, and that is why the trend toward multidisciplinary medical teams has developed. You have to understand the type of information that medical professionals collect and how that information influences the massage application. Thankfully, a whole group of specially trained support staff participates in the assessment process. The doctor is held accountable for making sure the information is accurate and for making sense of it all to guide an effective course of treatment that benefits the patient. I have a tremendous respect for doctors (e.g., MDs, DOs, chiropractors, naturopaths, psychiatrists, dentists, and so on). It is your job to assist them, not hinder them. Can they sometimes be difficult to talk to or seem impatient with you? Yes, and so what? Get over it. We all get that way at one time or another. When I get overloaded, I'm not very nice, either. Remember the vastness of a doctor's responsibility—often life or death.

Assessment identifies the structures with which work needs to be done, establishes a clear intention with regard to treatment goals, provides a baseline of objective information for measuring the effectiveness of treatments, and helps identify conditions in which a particular treatment may be contraindicated. Information from the physician and other healthcare professionals provides the foundation for patient treatment. As a massage therapist, you must understand and apply assessment information provided by the doctor, physical therapist, nurse, and other healthcare providers. If at any time you do not understand the information or instructions, make sure to ask questions to clarify the issue. Information gathered by the massage therapist should be shared with the physician or other appropriate member of the medical team in a concise, intelligent manner. Once the comprehensive treatment plan has been determined, the massage therapist must develop strategies for achieving the goals pertaining to therapeutic massage. Teamwork is essential and is based on cooperation and consensus among the various professionals attending to the patient.

The massage therapist needs to gather specific information about treatment goals, both long-term and short-term, as well as data that are pertinent to the massage treatment. Each massage treatment plan reflects the outcomes determined by the comprehensive medical treatment plan. For example:

- A plan based on efficient biomechanical movement would focus on re-establishing or supporting effective movement patterns. Efficient biomechanical movement is smooth, bilaterally symmetric, and coordinated, marked by an easy, effortless use of the body. Functional assessment measures the efficiency of coordinated movement. During the assessment, noticeable variations need to be considered.
- A plan based on pain management needs to determine the location, duration, and intensity of the pain. The reason for the pain must be found in order to determine whether it results from soft tissue dysfunction, which massage can directly address, or from other causes, in which case massage may be used to reduce sensation and the patient's perception of the painful condition.
- A plan based on mood management involves targeting neurochemical balance and normalization of autonomic nervous system function. Stress reduction often is a major outcome.
- A plan based on scar tissue management involves assessment to determine the reason for and type of scarring and the age of the scar; the assessment then proceeds with determining the best treatment approach, how aggressively to work the tissue, and supportive measures to aid the reorganization of the tissue.
- A presurgery plan is based on relaxation, whereas a postsurgery plan targets sleep support and pain management.

The general protocol presented in Chapter 11, in the Appendix, and on the Evolve website is both an assessment and a treatment process. It is written as a full body comprehensive approach, and you should practice it that way during the learning process. Once you have perfected these skills and have gained an understanding of the process of massage assessment and treatment, the protocol can be used as an approach to care. However, it must always be adapted to the patient's individual needs as directed by the supervising medical staff.

THE CLINICAL REASONING PROCESS

No standardized massage protocols have been developed for treating medical patients (or anyone else for that matter). This and any other textbook can only offer organized suggestions that have been effective when adapted to the individual receiving the massage. Similarities in application exist, but there is no one-size-fits-all "massage recipe" to follow. The condition of medical patients is complex, and each case must be addressed uniquely. Clinical reasoning and justification are essential to this approach. **Clinical reasoning** is the process of collecting data, analyzing the data, and developing appropriate treatment plans based on the outcomes required relative to the data. **Justification** is the process of explaining the validity of a particular method of treatment. Justification describes the expected benefits of massage in relation to the potential harm (i.e., the harm versus benefit ratio). (In Unit Four, case studies are used to model the clinical reasoning process to help you increase your proficiency.)

It would be much easier if a specific treatment protocol were applicable, but unfortunately, this is not the case. The practice of medicine is educated trial and error based on a process of gathering facts, identifying possible causes and treatments, making educated decisions on treatments, continually reassessing the effectiveness of chosen treatments, and adjusting treatment plans to better achieve the determined outcomes. Massage is a similar process.

As the volume of knowledge increases and as soft tissue modalities, such as massage, are integrated into medical care, the ability to think or reason through an intervention process and justify the effectiveness of a therapeutic intervention is becoming increasingly important. Therapeutic massage therapists must be able to gather information effectively, analyze that information to make decisions about the type and appropriateness of a therapeutic intervention, and evaluate and justify the benefits derived from the intervention.

Effective assessment, analysis, and decision making are essential to meeting the needs of each patient. Routines or a recipe-type application of therapeutic massage do not work for this group, because each person's set of presenting circumstances and outcome goals is so varied. The mark of an experienced massage professional is effective use of clinical reasoning skills devoted to working with this group of individuals with complex health issues.

JUST BETWEEN YOU AND ME

In the process of education, information needs to be delivered at least three different ways. It goes like this: Describe what you are going to teach; teach it; and review what you taught. The brain likes this kind of repetition. Therefore the material just presented was delivered three times. I know that information in this text is repeated over and over and over. As I write this, I wonder if the information gets assimilated. Has it been repeated enough in a variety of different ways? It took me a long time to get it, with lots of repetition. (Writing textbooks and teaching involve repetition.) Therefore, here it is again in simple, direct language: You have to learn to think.

Assessment is fact gathering. Fact gathering is the first part of the clinical reasoning process. Each situation is unique and needs to be researched thoroughly. This text provides only a portion of the information needed. Further investigation into medical conditions and treatments is almost always necessary.

Every massage professional needs to have a comprehensive medical dictionary, a comprehensive pathology text, resources on the patient's particular illness or injury, and references on medication and nutritional supplements. (Recommendations for these can be found in the text's resource list. The Internet is also a vast resource, especially this text's Evolve website and the related links it provides.)

If valid treatment decisions are to be made, the information collected must be accurate. The massage therapist need not be an expert in all illnesses or injuries. Massage therapists do not diagnose; this is the role of the physician or other members of the medical team. The massage therapist gathers information to develop massage strategies so that the massage outcomes support the interventions of the other members of the medical team.

During fact gathering, the various healthcare professionals use increasingly sophisticated assessment procedures, such as blood and tissue tests, x-ray studies, magnetic resonance imaging (MRI) and positron emission tomography (PET) scans, and so many more. Massage therapists typically use history taking and physical assessment, which includes observation, palpation, and muscle tests. In the medical setting, much of the assessment information is gathered by various healthcare professionals (which would include the massage therapist), and the doctor then analyzes the data to determine the diagnosis and the most beneficial course of treatment. Ongoing assessment of the patient's progress in response to treatment helps the doctor monitor and adjust the treatment plan as needed.

OUTCOME GOALS AND THE CARE OR TREATMENT PLAN

Outcome goals are the targeted objectives that should be achieved as a result of treatment. **Treatment plans** are the "map" that directs the approach to care to achieve the outcome goals. Outcome goals need to be **quantifiable.** This means that they must be able to be measured according to objective criteria, such as time, frequency, a scale of 1 to 10, an increase or a decrease in the ability to perform an activity, or an increase or a decrease in a sensation (e.g., relaxation or pain).

Goals also need to be **qualifiable.** How will the medical team know when a goal is achieved? What will the patient be able to do after a goal has been reached that the person is not able to do now? (e.g., What daily activities will the patient be able to do? What work skills will the patient be able to perform?)

Quantifiable and qualifiable goals are absolutely essential to determining the course of treatment. They also often determine the qualification for and the extent of insurance coverage. The common expectation is that medical treatment will end and the patient will be able to function. However, this is not the case with chronic conditions that require long-term care. Long-term care issues are putting the most strain on the medical system. Healthcare insurance and the current state of medical care support the "fix it" model, an approach that would naturally control the demands on the healthcare system. Healthcare systems require some sort of end-point for the delivery of care, and the quantifiable and qualifiable goals provide this. The goals need to be realistic, as concrete as possible, and obtainable within a determined time frame.

Some examples of quantifiable and qualifiable goals are as follows:

> Patient A will be able to perform all activities of daily living to maintain independent living (qualifiable goal). Patient A will be able to walk ¼ of a mile at a slow pace without needing to rest, will be able to walk up and down one flight of stairs with only moderate pain, and will be able to lift 10 pounds with only mild pain (quantifiable goals). The rehabilitation program will last 12 weeks and consist of five 2-hour segments per week (time frame and frequency).

If outcome goals are not achieved as described in the treatment plan, the reason for treatment failure needs to be determined and an adjusted treatment plan developed and implemented. Eventually, if the treatment fails, the insurer will not justify the cost of treatment and will discontinue funding.

You can see how important the assessment is, because without accurate data, the analysis of the information will be flawed, the treatment plan will be inappropriate, and the patient will not be able to achieve the stated goals.

After the analysis of the history and the assessment data is complete and the problems and goals have been established, decisions need to be made about the care or treatment plan. The medical professional supervising the case (e.g., the doctor, a nurse, or a physical therapist) either will provide the massage therapist with specific treatment orders or will ask the massage therapist to develop a massage treatment plan, including determining the appropriate approach. Depending on the situation, the massage treatment plan may need to be approved by the appropriate supervising personnel.

THE PHYSICIAN'S TREATMENT ORDERS

Physician's orders provide specific directions to others on the healthcare team. Patient records include a section for these orders. To be effective, the physician's treatment orders must be complete, legible, and written without abbreviations. In some cases a few easily recognized abbreviations—and only those approved by the organization—may be used. Orders usually are written or authenticated by the physician when they are given. Occasionally orders may be given by telephone to approved personnel. State regulations and medical staff rules and regulations determine who is allowed to record or accept verbal orders given orally. Verbal orders are to be signed by the physician at the next visit, but no later than 24 hours after being given in most cases. Because of the legal risks incurred when potentially hazardous treatments are carried out without proper authority, many healthcare organizations prohibit the use of verbal orders given orally. Physicians may ask a physician assistant or nurse practitioner to write orders, and these orders typically are countersigned by the physician.

Routine (standing) orders can be used for certain diagnoses or procedures. It is important to note that standing orders can be used only for services that are standard and for which little or no deviation is possible. Standing orders, which generally are preprinted, are placed in the patient's record and must be signed and dated by the supervising or attending physician. Many healthcare organizations limit the use of standing orders because they do not allow for the special needs of individual patients.

MASSAGE TREATMENT ORDERS

The massage therapist receives treatment advice based on the treatment goals that will be influenced by massage. An example of specific treatment orders for a massage therapist might be:

> Use lymphatic drainage and range of motion on the left upper limb to reduce edema in the elbow by 50%. Provide in 30-minute sessions 5 times per week for 2 weeks and then re-evaluate.

In this example, the massage therapist has been informed of the outcome and the methods to be used.

An example of treatment orders in which the massage therapist is asked to submit a treatment plan for approval would be as follows:

> Treatment orders: Reduce edema in left elbow.
>
> Massage therapist responds with: Use lymphatic drainage on left upper limb. Duration of session—30 minutes; frequency—5 times per week for 2 weeks, for a total of 10 sessions, to achieve 50% reduction of edema in target area.

In the first example, the massage therapist is told what to do. In the second example, the outcome is the treatment order, and the massage therapist responds with the specific treatment plan.

SHORT-TERM AND LONG-TERM OUTCOME GOALS

Outcome goals are divided into short-term and long-term goals. **Short-term goals** typically support a session-by-session process and depend on the patient's current status. **Long-term goals** typically support recovery, performance, or healing and rehabilitation. Long-term goals focus on the result toward which treatment is targeted. Short-term goals work on the patient's current status and serve as incremental steps toward achieving the long-term goals. Short-term goals should not conflict with long-term goals.

As an example, let's take a patient who is involved in a cardiac rehabilitation program. She has been working on cardiovascular fitness with the cardiac rehabilitation specialist. The long-term goals for this patient are that she will achieve and maintain cardiovascular conditioning and stress management. Massage is used for stress management and to manage postexercise soreness. For this particular session, the patient indicates that she has muscle soreness and is a bit anxious. The focus of the current massage must consider both short-term and long-term goals. In this case, the short-term goal is to reduce the patient's muscle soreness and sympathetic arousal as part of her existing long-term treatment plan, which is directed toward cardiac fitness and stress management.

The time allocated for achieving each goal depends on the patient's adaptive capacity. In the previous example of the cardiac patient, the stress management element of the massage treatment (the long-term goal) may be reduced or eliminated on days the patient has muscle soreness, because managing the soreness may take priority.

As you can see, the ever-changing dynamic of past history, current conditions, and future outcomes makes any sort of massage routine useless. Each and every session is uniquely developed and applied based on multiple factors. Assessment is the identification of all these influences. Clinical reasoning is the sorting of this information and the development of an appropriate treatment session based on the assessment. Effective charting (discussed later) records the session-by-session massage application and the results. Everything begins with an assessment to gather clinically relevant information.

THE HEALTHCARE ASSESSMENT

Various assessment procedures are used in the healthcare setting. Massage therapists do not perform these assessments, but they may need to review the results to develop beneficial and safe massage application. The clinical information required for a patient varies according to the nature of the illness or injury and the treatment required. If the patient is to be admitted to the hospital, an admitting procedure is followed. Outpatient records should include details for items that are pertinent to each visit.

JUST BETWEEN YOU AND ME

The discussions under The Healthcare Assessment introduce tons of terms. You need to have your medical dictionary ready. As always, look up any words for which you do not know the meaning. No whining. Remember, this level of assessment is the responsibility of the doctor or the designated assistant, such as a physician assistant or nurse practitioner. Appreciate how much they are required to know.

THE ADMITTING DIAGNOSIS

When a patient is admitted to a healthcare facility, the physician admitting the person provides the admitting (or provisional) diagnosis. This generally is included in the admission orders on the patient's arrival.

With outpatient visits, a reason for the patient's visit must be stated. The patient provides this information to the physician, physician assistant (PA), nurse, or other caregiver, and it is documented in the patient record. The reason the patient gives for the visit (i.e., the reason for care) is important, because it identifies why the patient requires treatment and it helps justify the services provided to the patient.

The History

A complete history is required for the first outpatient visit and for inpatient admission. This history is completed at the time of the visit or as soon as possible after admission, but no longer than 24 hours later. The parts of a history are as follows:

- **Chief complaint:** Usually, the chief complaint is the exact reason the patient sought medical attention, stated in the patient's own words. Both the nature and the duration of the symptom or symptoms are recorded.
- **Present illness or injury:** This information is a detailed recording of the patient's exact signs, symptoms, and reactions. It can be collected in different ways. One approach is the "serial 7s" format: quantity, quality, onset, duration, chronology, alleviation, and aggravation. The information also can be collected chronologically, starting from the first sign of the problem up to the hospital admission or clinic visit.
- **Past medical history:** The past medical history consists of the patient's general health, childhood illnesses, allergies, medical hospitalizations, surgical procedures, accidents, psychiatric history, medications, immunizations, blood transfusions, and pregnancies.
- **Psychosocial or personal history:** This section normally includes the patient's residence; education; marital status; dietary habits; typical day; stresses; sexual activity; use of drugs, alcohol, and tobacco; occupations; religion; hobbies; and outlook on life.
- **Family history:** The diseases among the patient's relatives in which heredity or personal contact may play a role are noted here. Allergies, infections, neoplasms, and mental, metabolic, endocrine, cardiovascular, and

renal diseases are included. The health status, ages, ages at death, and causes of death should be recorded for grandparents, parents, siblings, spouses, and children.

- **Review of body systems:** A review of the common symptoms of each body system is completed both to jog the patient's memory and to further define the present illness. The following format can be used to review common parts of each system:
  1. *General:* Weight changes, fatigue, weakness, fever, chills, heat or cold intolerance, fainting.
  2. *Integumentary system:* Ecchymosis; rashes; lesions; wheals; cyanosis; jaundice; erythema; changes in hair, nails, or skin.
  3. *Head, eyes, ears, nose, and throat (HEENT):* Cephalgia, blurred or double vision, blindness, glaucoma, cataracts, hearing loss, otalgia, tinnitus, roaring in the ears, vertigo, discharge from ear or eye, epistaxis, rhinorrhea, deviated septum, postnasal drainage, sinus pain, bleeding gums, hoarseness, trouble swallowing, sore throat, bad taste in the mouth, frequent tonsillitis.
  4. *Respiratory system:* Shortness of breath, wheezing, sputum production, repeated respiratory infections, cough, hemoptysis, asthma, bronchitis, emphysema, tuberculosis or fungal infection, abnormal chest x-ray, history of lung cancer, radiation therapy.
  5. *Cardiovascular system:* Chest pain, syncope, shortness of breath, orthopnea, paroxysmal nocturnal dyspnea, dyspnea on exertion, edema, abnormal electrocardiogram or echocardiogram, previous stress testing, rheumatic fever, scarlet fever, palpitations, thrombophlebitis, varicose veins, history of hypertension.
  6. *Gastrointestinal system:* Dyspepsia, history of ulcer, melena, hematochezia, hematemesis, stool color, nausea, vomiting, diarrhea, constipation, changes in bowel habits, appetite, thirst, rectal bleeding, flatus, food intolerance, hemorrhoids, jaundice, ruptured spleen, colon cancer, abdominal surgery.
  7. *Urinary system:* Dysuria, hematuria, nocturia, frequency, hesitancy, urgency, suprapubic distention.
  8. *Reproductive system:* Dyspareunia, discharge from genitals, venereal disease, high-risk sexual behavior, herpes, genital lesion, sexual activity.
     - Men: Penile abnormalities, hernia, testicular swelling or pain, vasectomy.
     - Women: Age at menarche; menstrual history; menstrual frequency and duration; use of pads; dysmenorrhea; menorrhagia; menopause symptoms; contraception; pregnancies; deliveries; abortions; Pap smears; abnormal Pap smears; breast examination; breast retraction, discharges, masses, or tenderness.
  9. *Neurologic system:* Seizures, syncope, vertigo, suicide plans or tendencies, weakness of extremity, painful spine and radiation of pain, memory loss, cephalgia, visual disturbances, stroke, head injury, depression, mental disorder with treatment, anxiety, insomnia, mood changes, nightmares.

The Physical Examination

The physical examination also should be completed at the time of the visit or as soon as possible after hospital admission, but no longer than 24 hours later. The physical examination often is detailed in the following format:

- **General:** This section gives a description of the patient, including the person's age, gender, general state of health, stature, habits, gait, dress, grooming, personal hygiene, sexual development, motor activity, mood, manner, affect, speech, level of consciousness, and signs of distress.
- **Vital signs:** The patient's blood pressure, pulse, respirations, temperature, and weight are measured and recorded.
- **Skin:** Lesions, color changes, erythema, dry or moist skin, rashes, ecchymosis, hair or nail changes, vascularity, edema, temperature, turgor, mobility, and the thickness or thinness of the skin are noted.

- **HEENT:** This examination includes the hair, scalp, skull, and face; visual acuity, visual fields, eye alignment, sclerae, conjunctivae, pupillary reaction to light, extraocular movements, fundus, accommodation to light, pupil size and shape, iris, eyelids, lacrimal apparatus, and eyebrows; tympanic membranes, hearing, ear discharge, auricles, and canals; external nose, septum, turbinates, nasal mucosa, frontal and maxillary sinuses, smell, discharge, and epistaxis; lips, buccal mucosa, gums, teeth, roof of the mouth, pharynx, tonsils, tongue, and salivary ducts.
- **Neck:** Observations include stiffness, ranges of motion, carotid pulse, adenopathy, jugular venous distention, masses, midline position of the trachea, thyroid, salivary glands, and pulsations.
- **Chest:** The results of anterior and posterior examinations for symmetry, dullness, expansion, ventilation, chest sounds, wheezing, rales, and costovertebral angle tenderness and bruit are recorded.
- **Breasts:** The breasts are palpated for nodularity, masses, tenderness, and discharge and observed for retraction, masses, drainage, nipple shape, and skin texture and color.
- **Heart:** This examination includes assessment for heaves or lifts, thrills, the point of maximum intensity, murmurs, heart sounds, gallops, murmur radiation, displaced heart friction rubs, venous hum, carotid artery pulse, and jugular venous distention.
- **Abdomen:** The abdomen is examined and palpated for scars, asymmetry, bulges, peristalsis, bowel sounds, organ size, rebound tenderness, rigidity, hernia, tenderness, masses, and ascites; also assessed are the liver, spleen, kidneys, femoral pulses and nodes, and suprapubic fullness of masses.
- **Extremities:** This examination, which focuses on the arms and legs, documents skin condition and color, edema, hair, size of the extremity (compared with the opposite limb), pulses, venous patterns, lymph nodes, range of motion, muscular strength, nails, erythema or swollen joints, pain, numbness or weakness of limbs, and deformities, as well as the results of palpation of joints and muscles and specific orthopedic tests.
- **Genitals:** For male patients, features of the penis, scrotum, testes, urethra, rectum, and prostate are recorded. The results of stool tests are also noted, as are scars, lesions, varicoceles, hydroceles, fissures, fistulas, hemorrhoids, sphincter tone, and rectal masses. For female patients, the results of the pelvic examination are noted: external pubic area, Skene's and Bartholin's glands, vagina, cervix, uterus, anal sphincter, rectal fissures, fistulas, hemorrhoids, rectal masses, and results of stool test.
- **Neurologic factors:** The patient's mental status, cranial nerves, reflexes, and muscle strength are noted. The results of ankle clonus tests, cerebellar tests, Babinski's reflex, Romberg's test, and temperature and vibration tests are also recorded.

MEDICAL RECORDS

All assessment findings and the results of diagnostic tests are kept in the medical record; this is called **documentation.** These data also include interpretations of blood test results, medical images, the results of specimen testing, and recordings and interpretations of electrical impulses.

JUST BETWEEN YOU AND ME

Pay attention. Medical records are very important. If you are going to practice therapeutic massage in any healthcare system, you must understand how to interpret a medical record and correctly record massage data in the record. No whining. I teach lots of students this stuff, and typically they whine. It doesn't matter, because you have to do this well.

Reports of any procedures performed are also placed in the patient's medical record; these serve as a historical record for the person performing the procedure and help the healthcare team more easily communicate information among team members and to other caregivers.

For hospital patients, the nursing section of the inpatient record provides valuable information about the patient's daily condition and status. In this section, the patient's vital signs are recorded, the administration of medication is documented, and nursing assessments of the patient are noted. These data can be valuable for assessing changes in the patient's condition.

Other professionals who may enter their assessments and treatments in the patient record include physical therapists, occupational therapists, dietitians, and medical technologists. This is the area in which massage therapists likely would be asked to record the information they collect and the results of massage treatment. Because the information from massage therapists becomes part of the patient's medical record, massage therapists must be able to describe clearly and concisely what they found during the assessment specific to massage, the massage application performed, and the outcomes of that treatment.

THE DISCHARGE SUMMARY

Discharge summaries are used for inpatients. The discharge summary reviews the patient's entire hospital stay. It must include the admitting or provisional diagnosis and the diagnosis (or diagnoses) at the time of discharge. The principal diagnosis (the diagnosis that, after study, best explains the reason the patient was hospitalized) should be listed first and noted as such. All other secondary diagnoses should be listed as well. The discharge summary includes the reason for admission, significant findings of examinations and tests, discussion of any therapies or procedures provided and the patient's response to them, and the information given to the patient at the time of discharge (including medications, physical activity, diet, and follow-up care, which may include massage). Similar procedures are used for outpatient treatment.

COMMON STYLES OF MEDICAL RECORDS

Flow Charts

Flow charts are a method of organizing data from a patient's record. They frequently are used for patients with specific diseases (e.g., diabetes and hypertension) and in special care units. Flow charts may be kept by hand, but when a computer-based patient record is used, the flow chart is generated automatically at each visit, along with a problem list.

Problem-Oriented Medical Records

As the name implies, in the problem-oriented medical record system, the format is organized around the patient's problems. The total historical data are broken into clinical diagnoses, called *problems.* The first page in the patient's record presents a list of all problems; that is, the medical, social, and psychological problems that may relate to physical findings; personal or social issues; treatments (e.g., radiation therapy); and organ or prosthetic implants.

The record then is organized around the various problems using the SOAP format (*s*ubjective, *o*bjective, *a*ssessment/analyze, and *p*lan) (see Box 9-1). The chief complaint and history portion of the record are, of course, subjective information collected from the patient or a significant other and from old records. For each problem, the applicable parts of a traditional history (present illness, past medical history, personal/social history, family history and review of systems) are summarized in a paragraph placed directly under the problem heading.

The objective data, which include the findings on physical examination and the results of any tests, follow the list of problems. The physical examination usually is recorded in the traditional format (i.e., the results are listed by the parts of the body). After the initial assessment, this section includes any changes in the physical findings and the results of any tests or treatments.

The next section in a problem-oriented record is the assessment, or the conclusions reached by the examiner on the basis of subjective and objective data. (Another word for this process is *analysis*). Assessments (i.e., the results of analysis) are listed separately for each problem. When exact diagnoses are unknown, a problem may be stated as a symptom with cause unknown. The differential diagnosis is listed in such cases to show the thinking of the caregiver.

Next comes the plan for each problem. A plan consists of three parts: diagnosis, treatment, and patient education. In this case the term *diagnosis* means the diagnostic tests needed to identify the cause or to follow the case. Treatment can include

Box 9-1 SOAP Method of Charting

Four elements are required to organize progress notes according to the SOAP method:

- Subjective data: The patient's expression of his or her condition, pain, complaints, reactions, and so forth.
- Objective data: The physical examination findings, results of tests, laboratory findings, observations, and so on. This also includes treatments used.
- Assessment (think of this as an analysis): The healthcare professional's evaluation of the situation, which is based on both the subjective and objective information.
- Plan: The details of the course of treatment chosen.

special therapy, drugs, radiation therapy, chemotherapy, or other modalities, such as massage. Patient education is the information given to the patient about the specific problem.

Organizing patient data in this way shows exactly what the medical caregiver is thinking. Each problem can be followed easily through the record. This saves valuable time for the caregiver and enables others to take over the patient's care if necessary.

Progress Notes

Progress notes chart each patient visit. They should follow some systematic method of organizing the information for decision making. As mentioned previously, the SOAP method of organization, taken from the problem-oriented medical record, is commonly used (Box 9-1).

The SOAP approach to recording progress notes provides an outline for logical progression and completeness of thought processes. Use of this system leads therapists to externalize their reasoning and justify their actions. Progress notes should be recorded at least daily for inpatients. For an outpatient or a discharged inpatient, a comprehensive progress note must be recorded for each follow-up clinic visit.

The SOAP process should have been learned in entry level massage training. If the reader is unclear, the appropriate information can be found in Sandy Fritz's text, *Mosby's Fundamentals of Therapeutic Massage* (Mosby, 2004). Various charting methods are used in the healthcare environment. Regardless of the particular style, the basic plan based on SOAP can be easily modified to other charting styles.

Another important point: Most medical facilities are using some degree of computer record keeping, and it is the wave of the future. Therefore, if you do not have basic computer skills, you need to take some classes.

Good record-keeping skills enable the massage therapist to better communicate information to other healthcare personnel and to create an accurate record of the specified treatment goals, the methods of massage used, and the effectiveness of the treatments.

JUST BETWEEN YOU AND ME

When healthcare professionals discuss the performance of massage therapists with me, they almost always complain about record-keeping skills. If you want to work in the healthcare setting, poor record-keeping skills won't cut it. Practice, practice, practice. Learn the medical terminology. Explain things concisely. Use explanations for massage methods and benefits as presented in this text. Record only the facts. Do not use abbreviations unless specifically instructed to do so. Also, you will have to become proficient in computer-based record keeping.

This text assumes that the reader already has completed a comprehensive course of study in therapeutic massage that included assessment procedures such as history taking, physical assessment, treatment plan development, and charting. (See *Mosby's Fundamentals of Therapeutic Massage* and *Mosby's Essential Sciences for Therapeutic Massage* for more detailed information.)

Technologic Advances in Record Keeping

The paper medical record is an impediment to effective delivery of high-quality healthcare. Paper records are difficult to access, often lack information, and must be in a single location for a single use. Paper record forms have changed little over the past 50 years, whereas expectations for use of the data the record contains have changed significantly. Because of these increased demands, healthcare systems and providers have had to search for alternative ways to deliver information effectively.

Improvements in technology over the past 10 years have allowed the design and implementation of electronic record-keeping systems. These automated systems have a variety of names, including *computerized patient record (CPR), electronic patient record (EPR), computerized medical record,* and *electronic health record (HER).* These systems have numerous benefits. For example, they allow more than one user to access a record at the same time. Test results are available in the record as soon as the test is completed. Handwriting legibility is no longer a problem. The data are organized quickly in ways that enhance the caregiver's skills. Problem lists are updated easily, and lists of medications the patient is receiving can be easily maintained.

Many technologic systems are available to providers for clinical use, such as digital dictation systems, document imaging and scanning systems, voice recognition systems, and automated coding systems. Health information networks, Internet sites for the exchange of information, and telemedicine applications also are widely available.

As use of the CPR becomes more common, quality of care will improve, because more complete information will be easily available to everyone providing medical care to the patient. After all, managing information to reach the correct decision results in quality healthcare. However, regardless of whether the record-keeping system is electronic or paper, it is expertise in collecting the information and the ability to interpret it that result in high-quality patient care. The clinical reasoning process is facilitated, not replaced, by electronic record keeping.

evolve 9-1

See the Evolve website for practice using computer-based medical records.

RULES FOR COMPLETING MEDICAL RECORDS

Medical records must be maintained in a specific way.

- Each page of the record must identify the patient by name and by hospital, clinic, or by the private physician clinical record number.
- Each entry in the record must include the date and time the entry was made and the signature and credential of the individual making the entry.
- No blank spaces should be left between entries.
- All entries must be written in ink, produced on a printer or typewriter or, in the electronic format, recorded appropriately.
- The record must not be altered in any way. Erasures, use of correction fluid, and marked-out areas are not appropriate.
- Errors must be corrected in a manner that allows the reader to see and understand the error. Errors are corrected as follows:
  1. A single line is drawn through the error, and the legibility of the previous entry is checked.
  2. The correct information is inserted.
  3. The correction is dated and initialed by the person recording the data.
  4. If there is not enough room for the correction to be made legibly at the error, a note should be made indicating where the corrected entry can be found, and the reference is dated and initialed. The correct information is entered in the proper chronologic order for the date the error was discovered and corrected.
- All information must be recorded as soon as possible. Memories can fade, and important facts can be omitted.
- Abbreviations should be used sparingly. Only those that have been approved by the organization are appropriate. The same abbreviation can have different meanings, which can be misleading. It is always better to write out the information than to use abbreviations that can be misinterpreted.
- Healthcare providers must write legibly. Because the patient record is used by so many other clinicians, it is important to the quality of care that the record be legible. Electronic formats help with this problem.
- All entries must be consistent with one another. The assessment must agree with the diagnostic testing, or an explanation must be given as to why it does not.
- Entries must be factual accounts.

- All information given to the patient before any procedure must be recorded. This ensures and verifies that the patient was properly informed of the benefits and risks before the person gave consent to the procedure.
- Telephone contacts with the patient must be immediately entered into the record.
- Some method of organizing entries (e.g., the SOAP format) must be used to ensure that they are comprehensive and reflect the thought processes used in making decisions about the patient's care.

When these rules are followed, the result is a record that is accurate, timely, specific, objective, concise, consistent, comprehensive, logical, legible, and reflective of the thought processes of the healthcare providers (including massage therapists). Not only will such a record be the best defense in a lawsuit, it also will result in the best care for the patient.

JUST BETWEEN YOU AND ME

I am going to be very direct: If you are not committed to becoming proficient in assessment and record keeping, you should not pursue a massage career in the medical environment.

CONFIDENTIALITY OF THE PATIENT'S MEDICAL RECORD

The patient's right to privacy has traditionally imposed an ethical responsibility on the people involved in the care of that patient. Many different people may see and treat a patient, and each of them needs particular information. How to protect the patient's right to privacy and yet keep all caregivers informed can be a dilemma. With passage of the Health Insurance Portability and Accountability Act (HIPAA) in 1996, the patient's right to privacy was strengthened even more.

HIPAA's privacy standards protect patients' individually identifiable data. These rules apply to health plans, healthcare clearinghouses, and other healthcare providers. Protection applies to a broad range of information in many different formats, including electronic files (Internet, Intranet, private networks, and data moved from one location to another via disk, magnetic tape, or compact disk), paper records, and verbal information. Individually identifiable data are designated as protected health information (PHI). Generally speaking, PHI relates to information that identifies a patient and his or her health status.

Most healthcare providers, and certainly hospitals, have policies governing the release of any information about a patient. Massage therapists must keep informed about those policies. Generally, policies regulating the release of information include components such as the following:

- The patient must consent to the release of any information to any outside entity, and any exceptions are outlined.
- Special considerations apply with regard to the release of information about sensitive conditions (e.g., alcohol, drug, or psychiatric diagnoses) or conditions related to infection by the human immunodeficiency virus (HIV).
- Specific elements are required for a proper consent form, and how long the form is valid must be stated.
- The individuals who can release information to outside parties must be identified.
- Appropriate fees or charges may be made for copies of the information requested.

Other issues should be addressed in separate policies. One such policy may establish the individuals by title who may release information to the media. Another policy might determine what information hospital employees may disclose to telephone callers about the condition of a patient during hospitalization.

Massage therapists who work for healthcare providers should be specifically trained in the HIPAA requirements that apply to the medical environment. This should be in-house training. If it is not offered as part of the orientation training, massage therapists should ask for specific information on how they are expected to comply with these regulations.

All states have laws about which diseases, conditions, and events must be reported to appropriate agencies. These include births, deaths, gunshot wounds, communicable diseases, and evidence of child abuse. When reporting is required by law, confidentiality is no longer an issue. Reporting such incidents to anyone other than the responsible agency, however, is a breach of confidentiality.

ASSESSMENT SPECIFIC TO MASSAGE AND MUSCULOSKELETAL CONDITIONS

Because therapeutic massage often is used to address musculoskeletal conditions, it seems prudent to expand upon that assessment if the outcomes of massage are related to that area of function. The extensiveness of the assessment depends on whether you are working under the direction of a doctor or other healthcare provider or are working independently. This textbook assumes that in a healthcare environment, supervisory medical staff members are involved.

The primary care provider is responsible for taking a thorough history, performing a complete examination, and informing the massage therapist about the patient's condition and the desired outcomes for the massage. If you are working independently with patients who have medical conditions, you are responsible for performing the appropriate comprehensive assessment, especially ruling out contraindications and clarifying treatment goals.

JUST BETWEEN YOU AND ME

It has been my experience that when massage therapists work with patients with really complex medical issues, it is much easier on the therapist to provide the massage as part of a multidisciplinary team. When the other professionals, especially the doctor, are not involved, the burden of responsibility for the benefit versus risk ratio falls on the massage therapist. I personally do not think that most massage therapists are sufficiently trained to be accountable for this type of responsibility. I know I am not.

In the medical care system, the doctor, physician assistant, physical therapist, or some other healthcare professional performs a specific musculoskeletal assessment. Massage therapists must be able both to interpret the information from this assessment and to contribute the information they collect.

evolve 9-2

The information typically found on assessment forms is provided on the Evolve website so that it can be printed and used. A comprehensive assessment normally is performed by a doctor, physician assistant, physical therapist, or some other healthcare professional, but the massage therapist also can do a comprehensive assessment and then report the findings to the physician. See the Evolve website for more information on evaluation versus diagnosis and additional assessment methods.

MASSAGE-SPECIFIC ASSESSMENT

In the assessment process, massage therapists are responsible for reviewing the information from the medical assessment and then completing an additional assessment targeted specifically for a massage treatment plan. This treatment plan typically must be approved by the appropriate healthcare professional to ensure that it is consistent with the comprehensive treatment plan developed by the multidisciplinary team.

evolve 9-3

See the Evolve website for further information on the subject of massage-specific assessment.

THE HISTORY

The patient history sometimes can give the massage therapist an indication of where problems exist in the body without a visual or physical examination. The massage therapist should obtain the following information from the patient:

- Why is the patient receiving a massage?
- What is the history of the current condition?
- Has the patient had any past illnesses or injuries that are related to the current condition?
- Does the patient know of any current contraindications to massage?
- What is the patient's past health history, including any family illnesses?

- What are the patient's current health practices?

In addition to the general history, the massage therapist should explore the following factors with each patient:

- Surgery or medical procedures
- Use of medications and supplements
- Use of hydrotherapy
- Use of electrostimulation
- Therapeutic exercise activities
- Physical therapy intervention
- Nutrition
- Sleep patterns
- Breathing patterns
- Mood
- Cognitive load (mental demands)
- Previous massage experience
- Use of alternative therapies (e.g., essential oils, magnets)

The patient's history may vary, depending on whether the problem is the result of acute illness or trauma, chronic injury or illness, or wellness care.

Massage provided during acute care is non-specific and supports the treatment of the medical team. Condition-specific assessment usually is not required. Massage is more likely to be used during the subacute and remodeling stages of healing or to help manage chronic conditions that require a comprehensive assessment.

Wellness care often involves minor aches and dysfunction. In these cases, the following questions, which provide an overview of the condition, are appropriate:

- What was the nature of the illness or injury?
- How much does it hurt? (Use a scale of 0 to 10, or have the patient characterize the pain as "mild," "moderate," or "severe") (Figure 9-1)
- Where does it hurt?
- What is the nature of the pain (e.g., hot, poking, sharp)?
- Does it hurt when you touch it?
- Does it hurt when you move?
- When does the pain occur? At rest? When bearing weight? During or after activity?
- When did you first notice this condition?
- Have you experienced any previous incidents, illnesses, or injuries that might relate to the current condition?

Once the general information has been collected, the assessment focuses on the current condition. Some questions for this purpose include the following:

- What are the details of the onset of the condition?
- Did the condition arise suddenly or gradually?
- Was there a specific illness and injury?

Typically, a gradual onset without a specific incident suggests an overuse syndrome, postural stresses, or somatic manifestations of emotional or psychological stresses that are common in medical patients.

- Where is the area that hurts? Show me. Ask the patient to point to as well as describe the area of complaint. Pay attention to gestures. The general guidelines for gestures that follow are not written in stone. Professional experience shows that

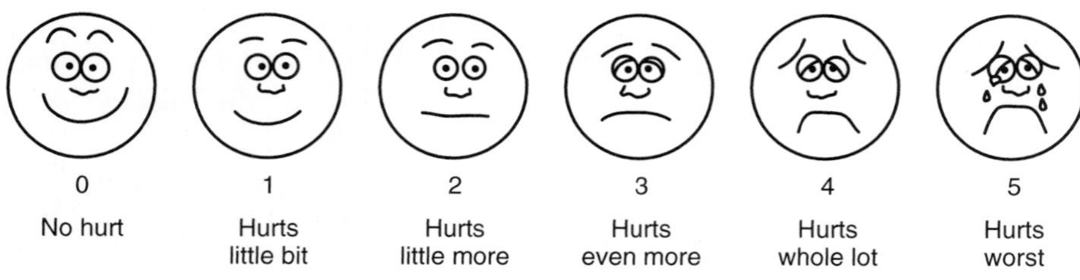

FIGURE 9-1 ■ Pain scale. Point to each face using the words to describe the pain intensity. Ask the patient to choose face that best describes his or her pain and record the appropriate number. (From Hockenberry MJ: *Wong's nursing care of infants and children,* ed 7, St Louis, 2003, Mosby. Reprinted by permission.)

these are fairly dependable starting points when interpreting an individual's body language, but it is the professional's responsibility to understand what a gesture means for a particular individual.

1. A finger pointing to a specific area suggests acupressure or motor point hyperactivity or a joint problem. What the pointing means depends on the area indicated.
2. If the finger points to a specific area but the hand then swipes in a certain direction, a trigger point problem may be the cause.
3. If the area is grabbed, pulled, or held and moved as if being stretched, muscle or fascial shortening often is indicated.
4. If the patient uses a kneading movement while indicating the area of concern, the area may need muscle lengthening combined with muscle energy work to prepare for stretching and for resetting of neuromuscular patterns.
5. If the patient moves into a position and then seems to be stuck there, the area may need connective tissue stretching.
6. If the patient draws lines on the body, nerve entrapment in the fascial planes or grooves is a possibility.

- What is the frequency of the discomfort? Does it occur once a day, once a week, 2 or 3 days a week, or is it constant?

It is important to determine how often the patient notices the dysfunction or disability. With grade 1 and grade 2 sprains and strains of the muscles, tendons, and ligaments, pain usually occurs when these structures are used and is relieved with rest. Constant pain may be associated with a severe illness, injury, or underlying pathologic condition.

- How long have you had the condition? The more serious the condition, the longer it will last.
- What is the nature of the symptoms?

Terms typically used to describe the symptoms include the following:

- *Stiff, achy, tight, fat, stuck, heavy:* These words are associated with muscles, tendons, ligaments, and joint capsules and their associated connective tissue, and they usually describe a simple tension or mild overuse of the soft tissue or edema. An ache that is more than mild, frequent, and lasts a long time is more serious and indicates inflammation. Typically, "tight" means an increase in neuromuscular activity. "Achy" and "fat" often indicate fluid retention or swelling. "Stiff" often indicates a problem with connective tissue pliability. A heavy sensation in the limbs often indicates a firing pattern or gait reflex problem. "Stuck" sensations often mean a joint problem.
- *Sharp, stabbing, tearing:* These terms describe a more severe illness or injury to the musculoskeletal system or a nerve root condition. These types of sensations are experienced with muscle or ligament tears, especially when the muscle or ligament is used. The sensation usually is relieved by rest. A nerve root inflammation can elicit a sharp or stabbing pain independent of movement.
- *Tingling, numbing, picking:* These words describe a nerve compression, either near the spine or in the extremities, or a circulation impairment.
- *Throbbing, hot:* These sensations are associated with acute illness or injury marked by inflammation and swelling, such as an abrasion, a puncture wound, or acute bursitis. Severe throbbing is a contraindication to massage.
- *Gripping, cramping:* These words typically are used to describe a serious condition, often a nerve root injury or visceral problem. Gripping or cramping pain is a contraindication to massage and requires immediate attention from the doctor.

- Does the symptom radiate?

With injury to the soft tissues, referred pain can arise in the extremities as diffuse pain and aching. Nerve entrapment and trigger point pain can radiate. Sharp, well-localized pain in the extremities that manifests even at rest typically indicates a nerve root problem. Visceral referred pain patterns may seem to radiate.

- How severe are the symptoms?

Ask the patient to rate the pain on a scale of 0 to 10, with 10 being the worst pain ever experienced and 0 being no pain. Incapacitating pain should be designated a 10. Moderate pain (5 to 9) interferes with a person's ability to perform sports-related activities. Mild pain (1 to 4) does not interfere with a person's activities of daily living but may interfere with sports performance.

- What are the aggravating factors? What activities make the condition worse (e.g., moving, sitting, standing, walking, running, or resting)?

The simplest strains and sprains of the musculoskeletal system are irritated by too much movement and relieved by rest. A condition that hurts more with rest indicates either inflammation or nerve pathology.

- What relieves the symptoms? What activities make the condition better (e.g., resting, moving, or applying ice or heat)?

Acute injuries involving the soft tissue are painful with large movements and are relieved by rest. Muscle guarding makes stretching painful. As the soft tissue heals, moving the injured area feels good. Stretching tight muscles, shortened ligaments, and joint capsules feels good despite some mild discomfort.

- When do the symptoms occur?

Inflammation and tumors cause more pain at night and during sleep. Constant, gripping pain that is worse at night or during sleep requires immediate referral to the doctor. Pain that arises during rest but is relieved by movement usually indicates inflammation. Joint pain and stiffness with fascial shortening usually are worse in the morning or just after a rest period.

- What previous treatments have you tried, and what were their effects?

Have the patient describe the type of therapy, medication, surgery, or treatment that was prescribed. What was the outcome? It also is important to know whether the patient has had massage therapy before, the type of massage application, and whether it was helpful.

- What medications are you taking?

If the patient has taken pain medication within 4 hours of assessment and treatment, the medication may give the patient a false sense of comfort during the assessment and massage. Massage therapists must have some knowledge of the effects of antiinflammatory drugs, muscle relaxers, anticoagulants, and so on.

- What diagnostic studies have been performed?

Find out whether x-ray studies, MRI scans, or other diagnostic studies have been done and what their results were.

- What is the nature of the progress?

Is the patient getting better, getting worse, or showing no change?

In some cases, the massage therapist may need to ask additional questions to clarify the patient's responses or to better understand the person's condition. Some of these questions might be:

- What can you do? Show me.
- What can't you do? Show me.
- What do you want to improve? Show me.
- What does it feel like?
    - Sore
    - Tight
    - Stiff
    - Weak
    - Stuck
    - Knotted
    - Balled up
    - Fat
    - Cold
    - More painful in the morning or at night
    - Heavy
    - Tired
    - Burning
    - Cramping
    - Poking
    - Twisting

- Painful to touch
- Painful during movement
- Pinching

It is helpful if the patient can draw a picture of the condition (Figure 9-2). When the patient draws the symptom pattern, give as few directions as possible; just let the person do it. Evaluate the drawing for the location and intensity of the symptom. Does the patient use colored, hard, zigzag lines or perhaps small or large circles? Then ask the patient to explain the drawing.

- Ask the patient, "If you could fix the problem, what would you do?"

The patient should demonstrate this for the massage therapist. Trust patients' impressions; they usually are right. Then translate what the patient has said into a massage application.

All the history information is consolidated and then considered with the objective assessment to develop treatment plans and establish session outcomes.

OBJECTIVE ASSESSMENT

After the history is completed, the physical assessment is performed. An accurate physical assessment is best achieved by using a sequence and a checklist to make sure that all relevant information is gathered. A major element of a massage session is a palpation assessment.

In general, the physical assessment includes the following evaluations:

- Visual assessment (blisters, bruises, rash)
- Palpation
- Stability
- Firing patterns
- Gait assessment
- Range of motion
- Tissue pliability
- Mobility
- Agility
- Stamina
- Strength

Scars indicate either previous surgery or previous illness and injury and reveal that the area is compromised. Ask the patient to describe how he or she received the scar.

An area of atrophy has become deconditioned either through lack of use or because of a neurologic involvement. Simple atrophy can be a result

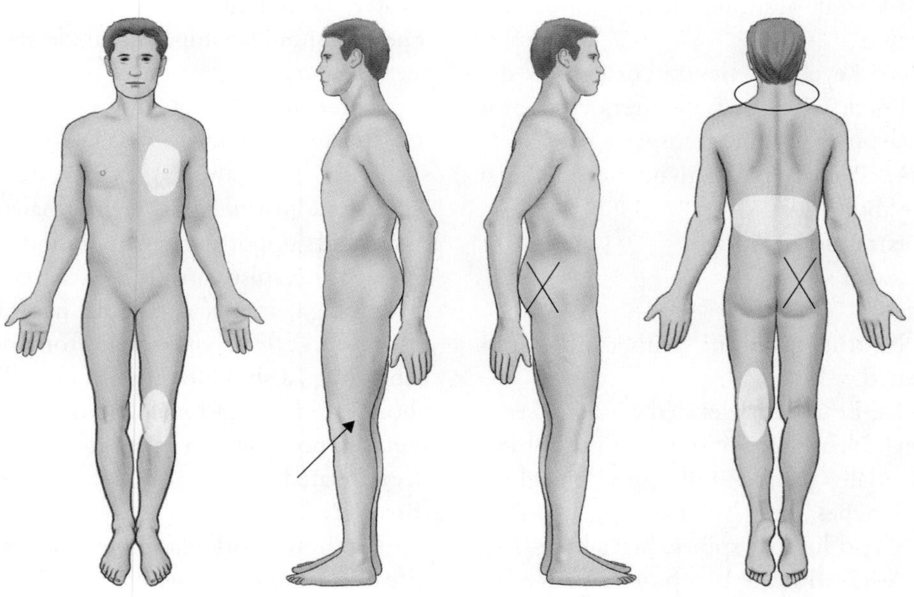

FIGURE 9-2 ■ Self-interpretation: sample analysis. The patient draws on blank human figures to communicate his or her pain. In this case, the left knee is a major focus, with most discomfort in the back. There is an intensity in the area indicated on the chest. The posterior cervical area is less of a concern to the patient, and the X in the right gluteal area is the most specific indicator (i.e., X marks the spot.)

of immobilization caused by a previous fracture or of lack of use caused by pain.

Notice the patient's posture in both the standing and seated positions, as well as the posture or position of the area of complaint. Look for areas of asymmetry. Observe the patient during general movement as opposed to formal assessment. Then perform a structured standing assessment and compare the findings.

9-1 *Physical Assessment: Posture*

Asymmetry usually results when overly tense muscles or shortened connective tissue pulls the body out of alignment. Direct trauma pushes joints out of alignment. Weak stabilizing mechanisms, such as overstretched ligaments or inhibited antagonist muscles, contribute to the problem (Figure 9-3). In these situations a chiropractor, an osteopath, or another trained medical professional skilled in skeletal manipulation is needed. Often a multidisciplinary approach to patient care is necessary.

The standard posture should be assessed as follows:

- Front view
  Head: Neutral position, neither tilted nor rotated
  Shoulders: Level, not elevated or depressed
  Pelvis: Level, with the two anterior superior iliac spines in same transverse plane
  Hip joints: Neutral position, neither adducted nor abducted
  Lower extremities: Straight
  Feet: Parallel
- Back view
  Head: Neutral position, neither tilted nor rotated
  Shoulders: Level, not elevated or depressed
  Scapulae: Neutral position, medial borders essentially parallel and approximately 3 to 4 inches apart
  Thoracic and lumbar spines: Straight
  Pelvis: Level, with the two posterior superior iliac spines in same transverse plane
  Hip joints: Neutral position, neither adducted nor abducted
  Lower extremities: Straight
  Feet: Parallel
- Side view
  Head: Neutral position, not tilted forward or backward
  Cervical spine: Normal curve, slightly convex to anterior
  Scapulae: Flat against upper back
  Thoracic spine: Normal curve, slightly convex to posterior
  Lumbar spine: Normal curve, slightly convex to anterior
  Pelvis: Neutral position, anterior superior iliac spine in same vertical plane as symphysis pubis
  Hip joints: Neutral position, leg vertical at right angle in sole of foot
  NOTE: An imaginary line should run slightly behind the lateral malleolus, through the middle of the femur.

The findings should be charted and related to the patient's history. For the physical assessment, the main considerations are body balance, efficient function, and basic symmetry.

People are not perfectly symmetric, but the right and left halves of the body should be similar in shape, range of motion, and ability to function. The greater the discrepancy in symmetry, the greater the potential for soft tissue dysfunction. The ear, shoulder, hip, and ankle should be in a vertical line.

Three major factors influence posture: heredity, disease, and habit. These factors must be considered in the evaluation of posture. The easiest factor to adjust is habit. By normalizing the soft tissue and supporting rehabilitation exercise, the massage therapist can play a very beneficial role in helping patients overcome habitual postural distortion. Effects may arise from occupational habits (e.g., a shoulder raised from talking on the phone) and recreational habits (e.g., a forward shoulder position in a bike rider), or they may be sleep related (long-term use of high pillows) (Box 9-2).

Clothing, work equipment, shoes, and furniture affect the way a person uses the body. Tight clothing and equipment around the neck restrict breathing and contribute to neck and shoulder problems. Restrictive belts and tight pants also limit breathing and affect the neck, shoulders, and midback. Shoes that have high heels or that do

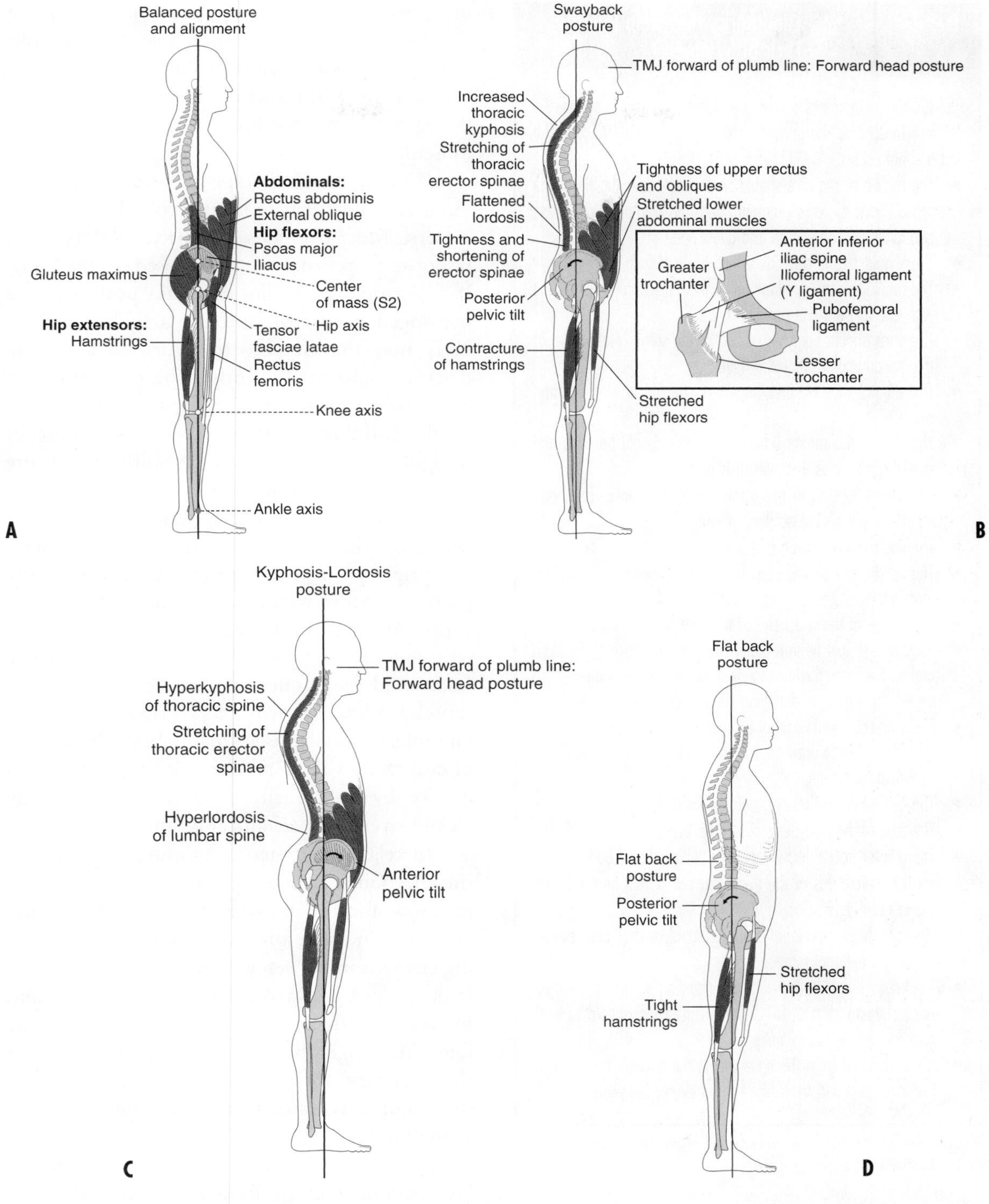

FIGURE 9-3 ■ The effects of postural imbalance. **A,** Ideal posture. **B,** Swayback posture. **C,** Kyphosis-lordosis posture. **D,** Flat back posture. (Modified from Saidoff DC, McDonough AL: *Critical pathways in therapeutic intervention: extremities and spine,* St Louis, 2002, Mosby.)

BOX 9-2 Landmarks That Help Identify Lack of Symmetry

The following landmarks can be used for comparison of symmetry. Be sure to observe the patient from the back, the front, and the left and right sides.

- The middle of the chin should sit directly under the tip of the nose. Check the chin alignment with the sternal notch. These two landmarks should be in a direct line.
- The shoulders and clavicles should be level with each other.
- The shoulders should not roll forward or backward or be rotated with one forward and one backward.
- The arms should hang freely and at the same rotation out of the glenohumeral (shoulder) joint.
- The elbows, wrists, and fingertips should be in the same plane.
- The skin of the thorax (chest and back) should be even and should not look as if it pulls or is puffy.
- The navel, located in the same line as the nose, chin, and sternal notch, should not look pulled.
- The ribs should be even and springy.
- The abdomen should be firm but relaxed and slightly rounded.
- The curves at the waist should be even on both sides.
- The spine should be in a direct line from the base of the skull and on the same plane as the line connecting the nose and the navel. The curves of the spine should not be exaggerated.
- The scapulae should appear even and should move freely. You should be able to draw an imaginary straight line between the tips of the scapulae.
- The gluteal muscle mass should be even.
- The tops of the iliac crests should be even.
- The greater trochanter, knees, and ankles should be level.
- The circumferences of the thigh and calf should be similar on the left and right sides.
- The legs should rotate out of the acetabulum (hip joint) evenly in a slight external rotation.
- The knees should be locked in the standing position but should not be hyperextended. The patellae (kneecaps) should be level and pointed slightly laterally.
- A line dropped from the nose should fall through the sternum and the navel and should be spaced evenly between.

From Fritz S: *Mosby's fundamentals of therapeutic massage,* ed 3, St Louis, 2004, Mosby.

not fit the feet comfortably interfere with postural muscles. Shoes with worn soles imprint the old postural pattern, and the body assumes the dysfunctional pattern if the patient puts the shoes back on after the massage. If postural changes are to be maintained, it is important that the patient change to shoes that do not have a worn sole. Sleep positions also can contribute to a wide range of problems, and furniture that does not support the back or that is too high or too low perpetuates muscular tension.

When massage therapists assess posture, it is important that they note the complete postural pattern. Most compensatory patterns develop in response to external forces imposed on the body. If the patient maintains a certain position for a prolonged period or overuses a body area, the body may not be able to return to a normal dynamic balance efficiently. The balance of the body against the force of gravity is the fundamental determining factor in a person's posture or upright position. Even subtle shifts in posture demand a whole body compensatory pattern.

The cervical, thoracic, lumbar, and sacral curves develop because of the need to maintain an upright position against gravity. The standing posture requires various segments of the body to cooperate mechanically as a whole. The skeleton is supported by passive tension of ligaments, fascia, and the connective tissue elements of the muscles. Muscle activity plays a small but important role. Postural muscles maintain small amounts of contraction that stabilize the body upright in gravity by continually repositioning the body weight over the mechanical balance point.

In relaxed symmetric standing, the hip and the knee joints assume a position of full extension to allow for the most efficient weight-bearing position. The knee joint has an additional stabilizing element in its "screw home" mechanism. The femur rides backward on its medial condyle and rotates medially about its vertical axis to lock the joint for weight bearing. This happens only in the final phase of extension. The hamstrings are the major muscles that resist the force of gravity at the knee.

At the ankle joint, bones and ligaments do little to limit motion. Passive tension of the two-joint gastrocnemius muscle (i.e., the muscle crosses two joints) becomes an important factor. This stabilizing force is diminished if high-heeled shoes are worn. The heel of the shoe puts the gastrocnemius on a slack. If heels are worn constantly, the muscle and the Achilles tendon shorten.

Posture and Muscle Function

Maintaining an upright posture is a complicated process. The ability to stand and move on two legs depends on the integrity of the bone, stability and mobility of the joints, proprioceptive and vestibular balance mechanisms, and coordinated muscle function. Dysfunction in any of these components can cause problems. Typically, it is a combination of factors that leads to impaired function and pain, such as postural strain from occupation, recreational activities, and sleep position that accumulate over time. Inappropriate footwear, restrictive clothing, and obesity are also contributing factors. Most of these factors can be altered with therapeutic exercise, soft tissue treatment (including massage), changes in the work environment, supportive shoes, and better form during recreational activity.

Upright posture is maintained by postural muscles that function in groups. These muscle groups balance each other and work in a coordinated fashion to resist the forces of gravity. Core strength is essential for stability while standing upright. The core muscles are the muscles of the thorax, including the abdominal obliques and paraspinals.

The flexor and adductor muscles of the body are larger than the extensors and abductors; therefore, postural dysfunction typically manifests as a curling forward of the torso with adjustments at the cervical and lumbar areas. This results in changes in the spinal curves, usually with increased kyphosis and lordosis (Figure 9-4).

Movement Assessment

Assessment procedures determine if the muscles in functional units are working within normal parameters. Movement should be fluid and coordinated and able to be performed in a variety of positions (standing, seated, prone, supine, and sidelying) with stability, control, and efficiency. Inability to perform movement effectively indicates dysfunction.

Assessing individual muscle strength alone does not provide sufficient information about how the body really functions. Movement occurs in a system that consists of a network of synchronized events involving the entire body. For example, the nervous system coordinates, the circulatory system provides fuel and removes waste, and the musculoskeletal system functions as a kinetic chain.

Each muscle of the body serves multiple roles, such as agonist, antagonist, and stabilizer. While muscles have multiple functions, they are designed with a mechanical advantage to provide a primary function. This primary function is the main concentric contraction pattern of the muscle, and when researching reference texts, the muscle's function is often described. For example, "The primary function of the hamstrings is to flex the knee."

If soft tissue is overused or overloaded, injury can occur. The muscle/tendon unit is susceptible to fiber tearing called a strain, and the ligament structure becomes vulnerable to injury (sprain) especially in areas with little surrounding muscle, such as the ankle and wrist. Over time these types of injuries can occur on a microscopic level. The isolated injuries may not be significant, but the accumulated effects over time can result in major dysfunction. As with all injury, there is bleeding, swelling, muscle tension, guarding in the surrounding tissues, and the formation of scar tissue. Lack of movement in the muscles also slows blood flow through the area, which can increase congestion and aggravate the problem. Scar tissue can build up gradually with repetitive activity. Adhesions and cross links can form and affect the elasticity within a particular area of the muscle, reducing normal function and making muscles vulnerable to further injury. The delayed onset muscle soreness a person experiences after hard exercise is partly due to this type of trauma. Many authors and researchers have identified this type of damage to the muscle structure.[*†‡§||¶] These

*Hammer: Functional Soft-Tissue Examination and Treatment by Manual Methods, Third Edition, Jones and Bartlett Publishers, Inc., 2007.

†Liebenson: Rehabilitation of the Spine: A Practitioner's Manual, "Emerging evidence indicates the problem of low back pain has been mismanaged," Lippincott Williams & Wilkins, 2nd edition, 2006.

‡Magee: Orthopedic Physical Assessment, 4th Edition, Saunders, 2005.

§Chaitow: Palpation and Assessment Skills, 2nd Edition, Churchill Livingstone, 2003.

||Greenman: Principles of Manual Medicine, 3rd Edition, Lippincott Williams & Wilkins, 2003.

¶Neumann: Kinesiology of the Musculoskeletal System, 2nd Edition, Mosby, 2002.

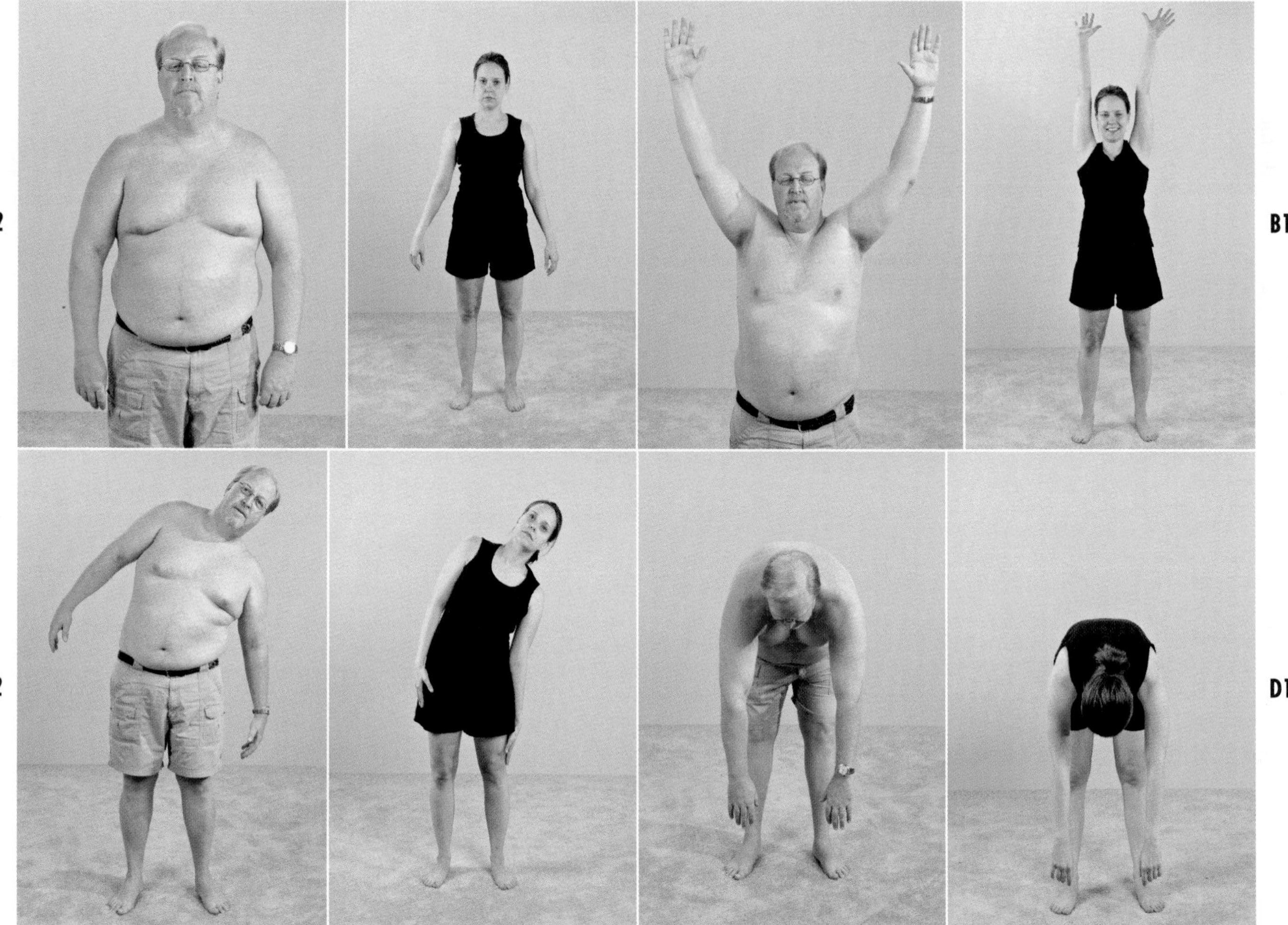

FIGURE 9-4 ■ Physical assessment. Using the photos shown, compare the two individuals for areas of restricted or hypermobile areas. **A1** and **A2,** Comparison of standing assessment. Observe for symmetry and identify differences. **B1** and **B2,** Compare shoulder and scapular movement. **C1** and **C2,** Compare frontal plane movement. **D1** and **D2,** Compare sagittal plane movement, flexion.

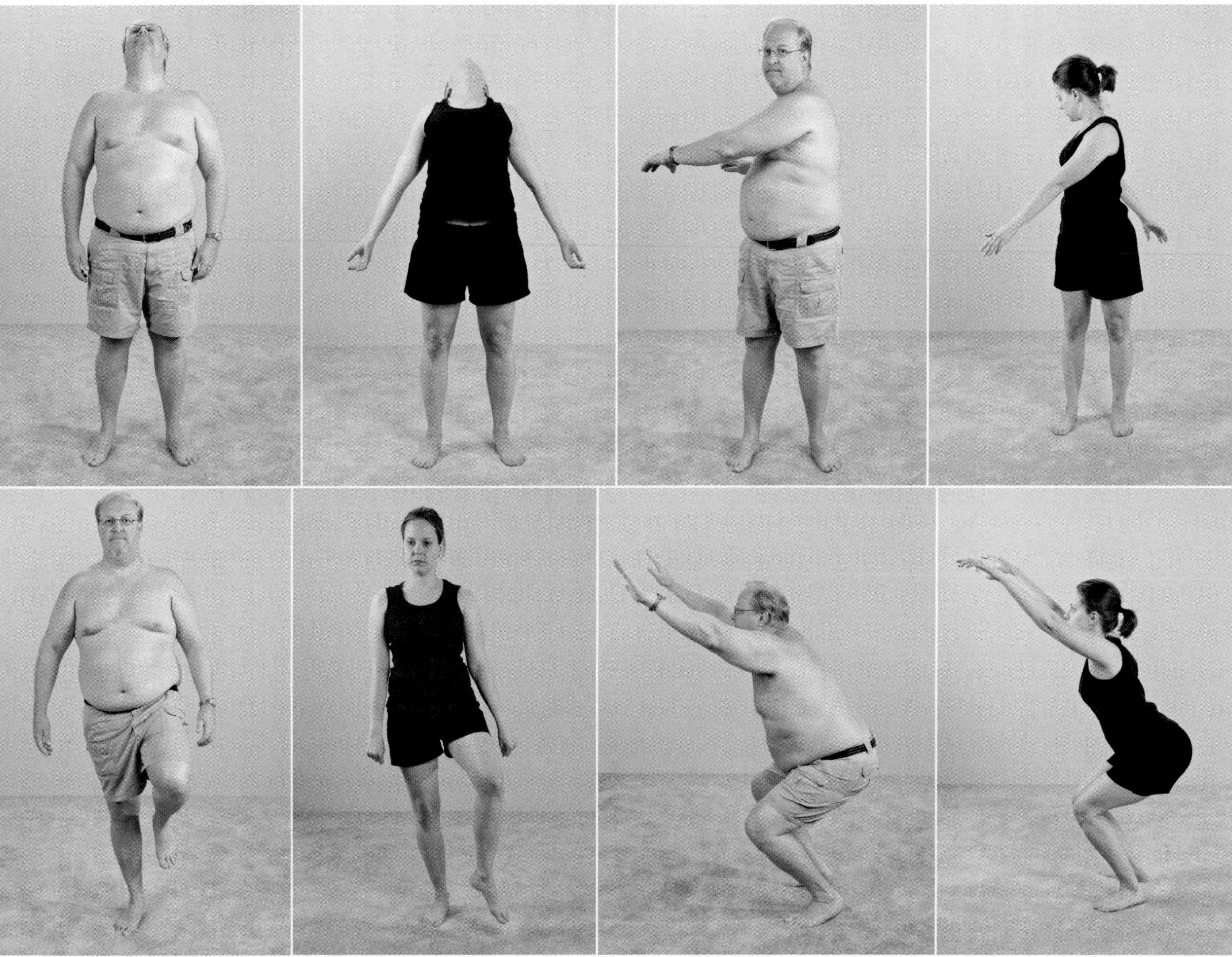

FIGURE 9-4, cont'd ■ **E1** and **E2,** Compare sagittal plane movement, extension. **F1** and **F2,** Compare transverse plane movement. **G1** and **G2,** Compare balance and stability. **H1** and **H2,** Compare multiplanar movement.

areas of microtrauma are treated in much the same way as any chronic muscle injury. Mechanical force is applied to break down the scar tissue to improve flexibility and to realign tangled fibers.

Static positions (e.g., a soldier standing at attention for long periods) put stress on specific tissues, causing microtrauma in a way similar to the active type of overuse; however, this type of overuse is the result of isometric overload rather than eccentric or concentric function. Lack of movement in the muscles also slows blood flow through the area, which can increase congestion and aggravate the problem (Figure 9-5).

Active Movements

A general understanding of biomechanics is important to the massage professional who works with physical rehabilitation patients. The assessment question, "What do you want your body to do?" usually results in answers such as bend, rotate, lift, climb stairs, lie flat, be able to comb one's hair, and so on. The massage therapist needs to break down the movements of the activity, assess for soft tissue changes that interfere with these movements, and identify massage applications that can support the movements. For example, in response to the assessment question, "What do you need to do that you are having problems with?" I often hear something like, "Bend over to tie my shoes" or "Put on my coat." I then ask the person to show me how he or she performs the activity. Observation during the "show me" process begins the physical assessment to target the specific outcomes for the massage.

For example, perhaps the person says, "I can't stand on my left foot with the same balance as on my right foot" (this is necessary for efficient gait). I ask the individual to stand on the right foot, and I observe and palpate to determine the "normal" activity the person can do. This is a general assessment and treatment principle. The least affected movement or structure becomes "normal" for evaluation and comparison purposes. Regardless of the situation, in practical application, this works. I then have the person stand on the left foot, where the problem exists. In this example, I assess by observing, palpating, and comparing the problem area to the more normal function. I then assess for the difference between the two, such as in tissue texture and pliability, ROM, and firing patterns. Choices about treatments to be used are based on the assessment information.

The next part of the examination is divided into two sections. In active movement assessment, the massage therapist asks the patient to perform movements in specific directions in all planes of movement. The squat assessment is particularly beneficial. In passive movement assessment, the massage therapist moves the patient.

Injuries and dysfunctions of the musculoskeletal system are symptomatic when the area is actively moved. More complex conditions (e.g., inflammation of the nervous system), systemic conditions (e.g., heart disease), and pathologic conditions (e.g., tumors) are not significantly affected by movement. If an area does not hurt at rest but does hurt with movement, soft tissue damage likely is a causal factor.

Remember, each individual joint movement pattern is part of an interconnected aspect of the neurologic coordination pattern of muscle movement called the *kinetic chain.* The support system involves the tensegrity of the body's connective design. Both posture and movement dysfunctions identified in an individual joint pattern must be assessed and treated in broader terms of kinetic chain interactions, muscle tension/length relationships, and the effects of stress and strain on the entire system.

When active range of motion is performed, the patient moves the joint through the planes of motion that are normal for that joint. Any pain, crepitus, or limitation noted during the action is charted. This assessment also identifies the patient's ability and willingness to perform the task.

Passive range of motion is performed when the massage therapist moves the joint passively through the planes of motion that are normal for the joint. The assessment identifies limitation (hypomobility) or excessive movement (hypermobility) of the joint. Passive movement is done carefully and gently to allow the patient to fully relax the muscles while the assessment is per-

MASSAGE ASSESSMENT/PHYSICAL PALPATION AND GAIT

PRE
POST

Client Name: ______________________ **Date:** ______________

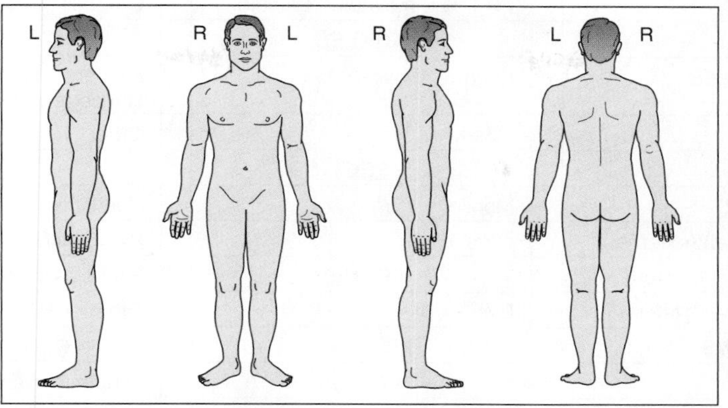

OBSERVATION & PALPATION	OBSERVATION & PALPATION	GAIT ASSESSMENT
ALIGNMENT	**RIBS**	
Chin in line with nose, sternal notch, navel	Even	**HEAD**
Other:	Springy	Remains steady/eyes forward
HEAD	Other:	Other:
Tilted (L)	**ABDOMEN**	**TRUNK**
Tilted (R)	Firm and pliable	Remains vertical
Rotated (L)	Hard areas	Other:
Rotated (R)	Other:	**SHOULDERS**
EYES	**WAIST**	Remain level
Level	Level	Rotate during walking
Equally set in sockets	Other:	Other:
Other:	**SPINE CURVES**	**ARMS**
EARS	Normal	Motion is opposite leg swing
Level	Other:	Motion is even (L) and (R)
Other:	**GLUTEAL MUSCLE MASS**	Other:
SHOULDERS	Even	(L) swings freely
Level	Other:	(R) swings freely
(R) high / (L) low	**ILIAC CREST**	Other:
(L) high / (R) low	Level	**HIPS**
(L) rounded forward	Other:	Remain level
(R) rounded forward	**KNEES**	Other:
Muscle development even	Even/symmetrical	Rotate during walking
Other:	Other:	Other:

FIGURE 9-5 ■ Physical assessment form. This form can be downloaded from Chapter 9 on the Evolve website and used as an assessment tool. (Modified from Fritz S: *Mosby's fundamentals of therapeutic massage,* ed 3, St Louis, 2004, Mosby.)

	SCAPULA		PATELLA		LEGS
	Even		(L) ☐ movable ☐ rigid		Swing freely at hip
	Move freely		(R) ☐ movable ☐ rigid		Other:
	Other:		ANKLES		KNEES
	CLAVICLES		Even		Flex and extend freely through stance and swing phase
	Level		Other:		Other:
	Other:		FEET		FEET
	ARMS		Mobile		Heel strikes first at start of stance
	Hang evenly (internal) (external)		Other:		Plantar flexed at push-off
	(L) rotated ☐ medial ☐ lateral		ARCHES		Foot clears floor during swing phase
	(R) rotated ☐ medial ☐ lateral		Even		Other:
	ELBOWS		Other:		STEP
	Even		TOES		Length is even
	Other:		Straight		Timing is even
	WRISTS		Other:		Other:
	Even		SKIN		OVERALL
	Other:		Moves freely and resilient		Rhythmic
	FINGERTIPS		Pulls/restricted		Other:
	Even		Puffy/baggy		
	Other:		Other:		

FIGURE 9-5, cont'd

formed. The patient reports the point at which pain or bind, if present, occurs. The massage therapist stops the motion at the point of pain or bind unless assessing for joint end-feel. To assess for joint end-feel, a tiny increase in resistance is used to gauge the quality of movement just past the bind. Passive range of motion assessment provides information about the joint capsule and ligaments and other restricting mechanisms, such as muscles.

Range of motion is measured in degrees. Joint movement is measured from the neutral line of anatomic position. Movement of a joint in the sagittal, frontal, or transverse plane is described as the number of degrees of flexion, extension, adduction, abduction, and internal and external rotation. For example, the elbow has approximately 150 degrees of flexion at the end range and 180 degrees of extension at end range. (NOTE: 180 degrees can also be considered 0 degrees). Anything less than this is hypomobility, and anything more is considered hypermobility. (The normal range of motion of joints is found in anatomy texts, such as *Mosby's Essential Sciences for Therapeutic Massage.*)

Each movement pattern (e.g., flexion and extension of the elbow and knee, circumduction and rotation of the shoulder and hip, movement of the trunk and neck) is assessed in sequential positioning of each area in all available movement patterns. As indicated, functional assessment is the combination of all previously described assessments.

Testing for Strength, Range, and Ease of Movement

During strength testing, resistance (counterpressure) applied to the muscles is focused at the end of the lever system. For example, when the function of the shoulder is assessed, resistance is focused at the distal end of the humerus, not at the wrist. When extension of the hip is assessed, resistance is applied at the end of the femur. When flexion of the knee is assessed, resistance is applied at the distal end of the tibia.

Resistance is applied slowly, smoothly, and firmly at an appropriate intensity as determined by the size of the muscle mass. Stabilization is essential to assess movement patterns accurately. Only the area assessed is allowed to move. Movement in any other part of the body must be stabilized. The massage therapist usually applies a stabilizing force; as one hand applies resistance, the other provides the stabilization. Sometimes the patient can provide the stabilization. Some methods use straps to provide stabilization. The easiest way to identify the area to be stabilized is to move the area to be assessed through the range of motion. At the end of the range, some other part of the body begins to move; this is the area of stabilization. Return the body to a neutral position. Provide the appropriate stabilization to the area identified and begin the assessment procedure.

During assessments, muscles should be able to hold against appropriate resistance without strain or pain from the action and without recruiting or using other muscles. As mentioned, appropriate resistance is applied slowly and steadily and with just enough force to cause the muscles to respond to the stimulus. Large muscle groups require more force than small ones. The position should be easy to assume and comfortable to maintain for 10 to 30 seconds. Contraindications to this type of assessment include joint and disk dysfunction, acute pain, recent trauma, and inflammation.

When a movement pattern is evaluated, two types of information are obtained in one functional assessment. First, when a jointed area moves into flexion and the joint angle is decreased, the prime mover and synergists concentrically contract, antagonists eccentrically function while lengthening, and the fixators isometrically contract and stabilize. Body-wide stabilization patterns also come into play to assist in allowing the motion. During assessment, resistance can be applied to load the prime mover groups and synergists to assess for neurologic function of strength and, to a lesser degree, endurance, as the contraction is held for a period of time. At the same time, the antagonist pattern or the tissues that are lengthened when positioning for the functional assessment can be assessed for increased tension patterns or connective tissue shortening.

Dysfunction shows itself in limited range of motion by restricting the movement pattern. Therefore, when placing a jointed area into flexion, the extensors are assessed for shortening. When the jointed area moves into extension, the opposite becomes the case. The same holds for adduction and abduction, internal and external rotation, plantar and dorsiflexion, and so on.

During actual movement assessment, the massage therapist should note the following categories:

- *Range of motion:* Is the motion normal, decreased, increased? Determining normal ROM is more complex than it might seem. You need to consider the patient's age and gender, exercise habits, and muscle texture. ROM declines as we age. Women typically have greater ROM than men. If the complaint is in the extremities, begin with the noninvolved side and always compare the two sides. The least involved side becomes the "normal side" for comparison.
- *Limits to joint movement:* Joints have various degrees of range of motion. Anatomic, physiologic, and pathologic barriers can restrict motion. **Anatomic barriers** are determined by the shape and fit of the bones at the joint. The anatomic barrier is seldom reached because the possibility of injury is greatest in this position. Instead, the body protects the joint by establishing physiologic barriers. **Physiologic barriers** are the result of the limits in range of motion imposed by protective nerve and sensory functions to support optimal function. An adaptation in the physiologic barrier such that the protective function limits instead of supports optimal functioning is called a *pathologic barrier.* **Pathologic barriers**

often are manifested as stiffness, pain, or a "catch." When using joint movement techniques, remain within the physiologic barriers. If a pathologic barrier exists that limits motion, use massage techniques to gently and slowly encourage the joint to increase the limits of the range of motion to the physiologic barrier.

The stretch on the soft tissues, such as muscles, tendons, fascia, and ligaments, and the arrangement of the joint surfaces determine the range of motion of the joint and therefore the joint's normal end-feel. **Overpressure** is the term used when the massage therapist gradually applies more pressure when the end of the available passive range of joint motion has been reached. The sensation transmitted to the therapist's hands by the tissue resistance at the end of the available range is the end-feel of a joint.

Types of End-Feel

Normal End-Feel. **Soft tissue approximation end-feel** occurs when the full range of the joint is restricted by the normal muscle bulk; it is painless and has a feeling of soft compression. **Muscular (tissue stretch) end-feel** occurs at the extremes of muscle stretch, such as in the hamstrings during a straight leg raise; it has a feeling of increasing tension, springiness, or elasticity. **Capsular stretch (leathery) end-feel** occurs when the joint capsule is stretched at the end of its normal range, such as with external rotation of the glenohumeral joint; it is painless and has the sensation of stretching a piece of leather. **Bony (hard) end-feel** occurs when bone contacts bone at the end of normal range, as in extension of the elbow; it is abrupt and hard.

Abnormal End-Feel. **Empty end-feel** occurs when no physical restriction to movement exists except the pain expressed by the patient. **Muscle spasm end-feel** occurs when passive movement stops abruptly because of pain; a springy rebound may occur from reflexive muscle spasm. **Boggy end-feel** occurs when edema is present; it has a mushy, soft quality. **Springy block (internal derangement) end-feel** is a springy or rebounding sensation in a noncapsular pattern; this indicates loose cartilage or meniscal tissue within the joint. Capsular stretch (leathery) end-feel that occurs before normal range indicates capsular fibrosis with no inflammation. Bony (hard) end-feel that occurs before normal range indicates bony changes, degenerative joint disease, or malunion of a joint after a fracture.

An empty end-feel with the absence of bind or stability indicates a seriously damaged joint, and referral is required.

Range of Motion

As mentioned previously, the range of motion of a joint is measured in degrees. A full circle is 360 degrees. A flat, horizontal line is 180 degrees. This flat, horizontal line can also be considered 0 degrees. Two perpendicular lines (as in the shape of a capital L) create a 90-degree angle. Various ranges of motion are possible. For example, when the range of motion of a joint allows 0 to 90 degrees of flexion, anything less is hypomobile and anything more is hypermobile. A great degree of variability exists among individuals as to the actual normal range of motion, and the degrees of normal movement are general guidelines. Range of motion is measured from the anatomic position. Anatomic position is considered 0 degrees of motion, regardless of whether the patient is standing, supine, or side-lying (Figure 9-6).

Decreased ROM is caused by pain, changes in the joint position, or soft tissue bind. If the loss of motion is not a result of pain, more information is needed to determine whether the lack of motion is caused by adhesions in the joint capsule, muscle guarding, joint degeneration, or other factors.

Increased ROM significantly different from that seen on the body's opposite side indicates a moderate to severe illness and injury to the ligaments, the joint capsule, or both. Increased ROM on both sides compared with normal anatomic ROM suggests a generalized hypermobility syndrome and potential instability in the joints.

If active movement is painful, ask the patient to describe the pain's location, quality, and severity. The three stages of healing that elicit pain at different ranges of the movement are as follows:

- Acute conditions cause pain before the normal ROM.

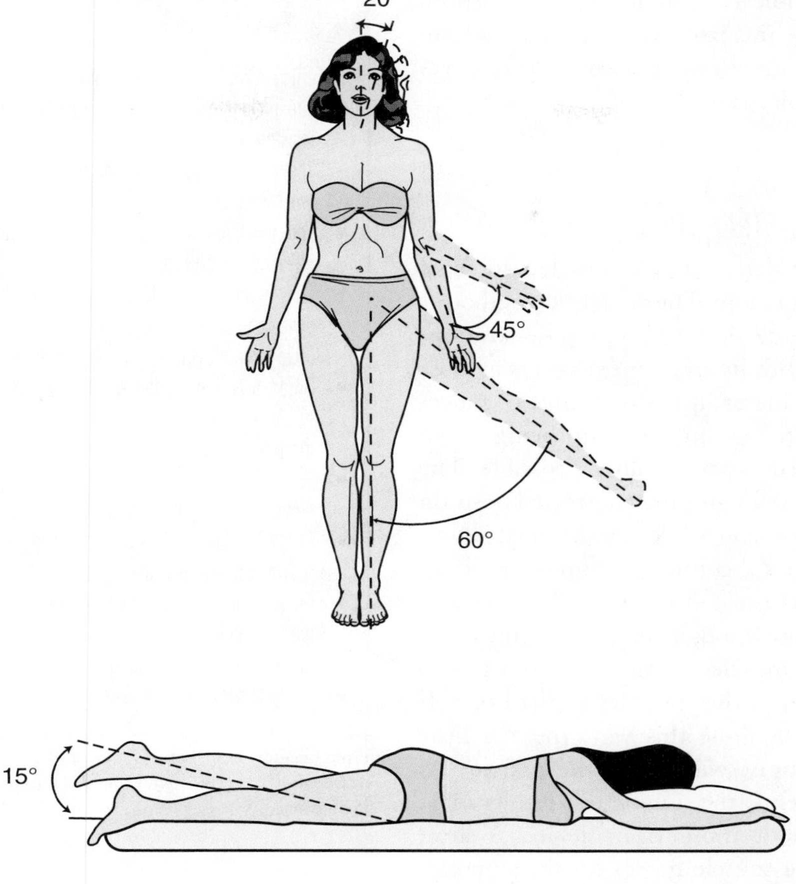

FIGURE 9-6 ■ Degrees of range of motion. (From Fritz S: *Mosby's essential sciences for therapeutic massage: anatomy, physiology, biomechanics, and pathology,* ed 2, St Louis, 2004, Mosby.)

- Subacute conditions cause pain at the end of the normal range.
- Chronic conditions may cause pain with slight overpressure at the end of active or passive motion.

Pain with passive motion at different ranges of the movement indicates a stage of healing that is the same as for active motion.

Interpreting the Assessment Findings

Range of Motion. Active and passive range of motion can identify limits of movement. If an empty, capsular, or hard end-feel is identified, the joint is damaged. Acute conditions are treated by the physician. Range of motion limited by muscle contraction may indicate an underlying problem with joint laxity, and caution is indicated before any muscle guarding present is reduced. Proceed slowly with massage until a balance is achieved between increased range of motion and maintaining joint stability. If joint stability is diminished by reducing muscle guarding too much, the patient usually has pain in the joint for a day or two after the massage. Simple edema around a joint is managed with lymphatic drainage. Any unexplained edema should be referred for diagnosis.

Range of motion should improve as the patient's tissues normalize with general massage. Progressive mobilization within the range of motion is an indication of improved function. Never force an increase in range of motion. Instead, allow it to be a natural outcome of effective massage application.

MUSCLE STRENGTH TESTING

Strength testing determines a muscle's force of concentric contraction. The preferred method is to isolate the muscle or muscle group by positioning the muscle with its attachment points as close together as possible or in the midrange of movement. The muscle or muscle group being tested should be isolated as specifically as possible. The patient holds or maintains the contracted position of the muscle isolation while the therapist slowly and evenly applies a counterpressure to pull the muscle out of its isolated position. The massage therapist must use enough force to recruit a full response by the muscles being tested, but not so much as to recruit other muscles in the body. If strength testing is done this way, there is little chance the therapist will injure the patient. As with all assessments, the muscle test results must be compared with those from a similar area, usually the same muscle group on the opposite side (Boxes 9-3 and 9-4).

In another testing method, a muscle group's strength is compared with its antagonist pattern. The body is designed so that the flexor, internal rotator, and adductor muscles are about 25% to 30% stronger than the extensor, external rotator, and abductor muscles. Also, the flexors and adductors usually work against gravity to move a joint. The main purposes of extensors and abductors are to restrain and control the flexor and adductor movement and to return the joint to a neutral position. Less strength is required because gravity assists the function.

Strength testing should reveal a difference in the pattern between the flexors, internal rotators, and adductors, and the extensors, external rotators, and abductors in an agonist-antagonist pattern. These groups should not be equally strong. Flexors, internal rotators, and adductors should show more muscle strength than extensors, external rotators, and abductors.

BOX 9-3 Muscle Strength Testing

For efficient muscle strength testing it is necessary to ensure that:

- The patient builds force slowly after engaging the barrier of resistance offered by the practitioner.
- The patient uses maximum controlled effort to move in the prescribed direction.
- The practitioner ensures that the point of muscle origin is efficiently stabilized.
- Care is taken to avoid use by the patient of "tricks" in which synergists are recruited.

Muscle strength is most usually graded as follows.

- Grade 5 is normal, demonstrating a complete (100%) range of movement against gravity, with firm resistance offered by the practitioner.
- Grade 4 is 75% efficiency in achieving range of motion against gravity with slight resistance.
- Grade 3 is 50% efficiency in achieving range of motion against gravity without resistance.
- Grade 2 is 25% efficiency in achieving range of motion with gravity eliminated.
- Grade 1 shows slight contractility without joint motion.
- Grade 0 shows no evidence of contractility.

From Chaitow L, DeLany JW: *Clinical applications of neuromuscular techniques-the upper body,* vol. 1. Edinburgh, 2001, Churchill Livingstone.

BOX 9-4 Two-Joint Muscle Testing

As a rule, good fixation is essential when testing a two-joint muscle. The same applies to all muscles in children and adults whose cooperation is poor and whose movements are uncoordinated and weak. The better the extremity is steadied, the less the stabilizers are activated and the better and more accurate are the results of the muscle function test (Janda, 1983).

From Chaitow L, DeLany JW: *Clinical applications of neuromuscular techniques-the upper body,* vol. 1, Edinburgh, 2001, Churchill Livingstone.

The following findings may be seen with muscle strength testing:

- A strong, painless contraction without muscle requietment indicates normal function.
- A strong but painful contraction usually indicates dysfunction in the tested muscle-tendon-periosteal unit.

- A weak, painless contraction may be the result of one or more of the following:
  - The muscle is inhibited because of a hypertonic antagonist pattern.
  - The muscle is inhibited because of dysfunction, illness, or injury to adjacent joint structures.
  - A spinal nerve condition is causing impingement upon or irritation of the motor nerve and weakness in the muscles innervated by that nerve.
  - The patient has a nerve illness or injury.
  - The muscle is deconditioned because of disuse caused by a previous illness, injury, or disease.
  - A long tension-length relationship is present.
  - A short tension-length relationship is present.

evolve 9-4

For specific muscle tests, see the Evolve website.

Postural and Phasic Muscles

Review this content on the Evolve website.

Postural, or stabilizer, muscles and phasic, or mover, muscles are made up of different kinds of muscle fibers. Postural muscles have a higher percentage of slow-twitch red fibers, which can hold a contraction for a long time before fatiguing. Phasic muscles have a higher percentage of fast-twitch white fibers, which contract quickly but tire easily. These two types of muscle are tested differently and develop different types of dysfunction.

Postural Muscles. **Postural (stabilizer) muscles** are relatively slow to respond compared with phasic muscles. They do not produce bursts of strength if asked to respond quickly, and they may cramp. They are the deliberate, slow, steady muscles that require time to respond. Using the analogy of the tortoise and the hare, these muscles are the tortoise. Inefficient neurologic patterns, muscle tension, reorganization of connective tissue with fibrotic changes, and trigger points are common in postural muscles.

If posture is not balanced, postural muscles must function more like ligaments and bones. When this happens, additional connective tissue develops in the muscle to give the body the ability to stabilize in gravity. The problem is that the connective tissue freezes the body in the position, because unlike muscle, which can actively contract and lengthen, connective tissue is a more static tissue.

Postural muscles tend to shorten and increase in tension in the strain-tension-length relationship. This information is important when the massage therapist is attempting to assess which muscles are tense and short, and therefore in need of lengthening, and which groups of muscle are apt to develop connective tissue changes and require stretching. Connective tissue shortening is dealt with mechanically through forms of stretching. Hypertension of concentric contracted muscles is dealt with through muscle energy methods and reflexive lengthening procedures.

Phasic Muscles. **Phasic (mover) muscles** jump into action quickly and tire quickly. Musculotendinous junction problems are more common in phasic muscles. The four most common problems are microtearing of the muscle fibers at the tendon, inflamed tendons (tendinitis), tendons adhering to underlying tissue, and bursitis.

Phasic muscles usually weaken in response to postural muscle shortening. Sometimes the weakened muscles also shorten. This shortening allows the weak muscle the same contraction power on the joint. It is important not to confuse this condition with hypertense muscles; these muscles are inhibited and weak.

Phasic muscles occasionally become overly tense and short. This almost always results from some sort of repetitive behavior and is a common problem in patients. Phasic muscles also become short in response to a sudden posture change that causes them to assist the postural muscles in maintaining balance. These common, inappropriate muscle patterns often result from an unexpected fall or near fall, an automobile accident, or some other trauma. Basic massage methods discussed in this text can be used to reset and retrain muscles that are out of sync.

KINETIC CHAIN ASSESSMENT

The body is a circular form divided into four quadrants: front, back, right side, and left side, with divisions on the sagittal and frontal planes. The body must be balanced in three dimensions to withstand the forces of gravity.

The body moves and is balanced in gravity in the following transverse plane areas, which easily allow movement: the atlas; the C6 and C7 vertebrae; the T12 and L1 vertebrae (the thoracolumbar junction); the L4, L5, and S1 vertebrae (the sacrolumbar junction); and at the hips, knees, and ankles (Figure 9-7). If a postural distortion exists in any of the four quadrants or within one of the jointed areas, the entire balance mechanism must be adjusted. This occurs as a pinball-like effect that jumps front to back and side to side in the soft tissue between the movement lines.

You can do a little demonstration for yourself to gain an understanding of postural balance. First, find a pole of some type (e.g., a broom handle without the broom portion will work). Tie a string around the pole. Now, try to balance the pole on its end using the string. Note that in trying to counter the fall pattern of the pole, you work *opposite* the fall pattern. If the pole tends to fall forward and to the left, you apply a counterforce back and to the right.

This is just what the body does if part of it moves off the balance line. The body is made up of many different poles stacked on top of one another. The poles stack at each of the movement segments. Muscles between the movement segments must be three dimensionally balanced in all four quadrants to support the pole in that area. Each area needs to be balanced. If one pole area tips a bit to the right, the body compensates by tipping the adjacent pole areas (above and/or below) to the left. If a pole area is tipped forward, adjacent poles are tipped back. A chain reaction

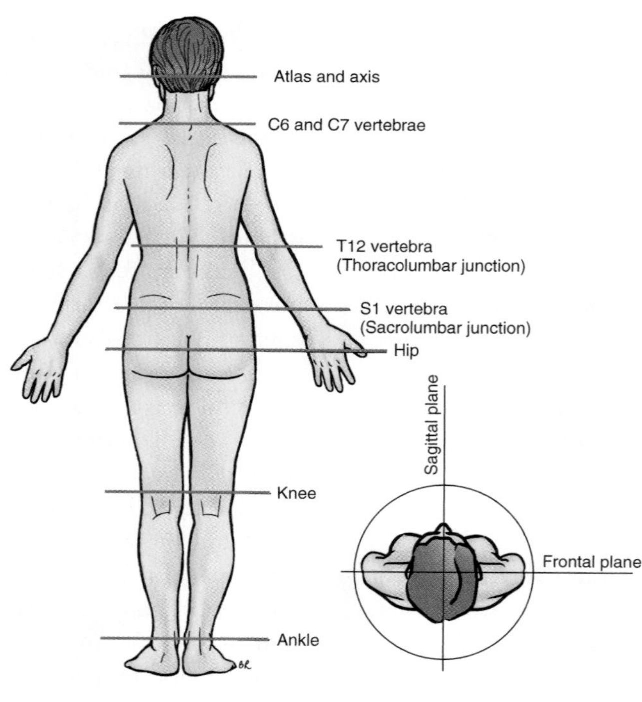

FIGURE 9-7 ■ Quadrants and movement segments. (From Fritz S: *Mosby's fundamentals of therapeutic massage,* ed 3, St Louis, 2004, Mosby.)

occurs, such that when compensating poles tip back, their adjacent areas must counterbalance the action by tipping forward. This is how the body-wide compensation pattern is set up.

Whether the pole areas sit nicely on top of each other with evenly distributed muscle action or whether they are tipped in various positions and counterbalanced by compensatory muscle actions, the body remains balanced in gravity. However, the "tippy pole" pattern is much more inefficient than the "balanced pole" pattern (Figure 9-8).

Intervention plans attempt to normalize the balance process by relaxing the tension pattern in overly tight and short areas (concentric caves), strengthening muscles in corresponding taut and long but weak areas (eccentric hills), and allowing the poles to straighten out. If a pole is permanently tippy, such as with scoliosis or kyphosis, intervention plans attempt to support the appropriate compensation patterns and prevent them from increasing beyond what is necessary for postural balance.

Muscle imbalance, discovered by observation, palpation, and through muscle testing procedures, often indicates how the body is compensating for postural and movement imbalances. Muscle testing also can locate the main muscle problems. When the primary dysfunctional group of muscles is concentrically contracted against resistance, the main compensatory patterns are activated, and the other body compensation patterns activate and exaggerate. The massage professional must then become a detective, looking for clues to unwind the pattern by concentrating on methods that restore symmetry of function.

A major muscle problem is overly short muscles. If these muscles can be relaxed, length-

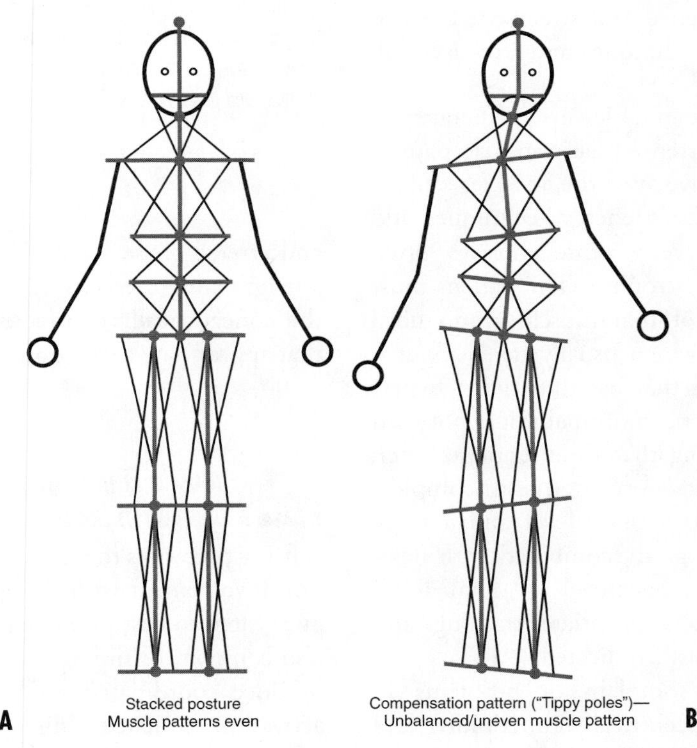

FIGURE 9-8 ■ Posture balance and imbalance. Stacked pole **(A)** versus tippy pole **(B)** postural influences on the body. (From Fritz S: *Mosby's fundamentals of therapeutic massage*, ed. 3, St. Louis, 2004, Mosby.)

ened and, if necessary, stretched to activate connective tissue changes, the rest of the dysfunctional pattern often resolves.

If the extensors and abductors are stronger than the flexors and adductors, major postural imbalance and postural distortion result. Similarly, if the extensors and abductors are too weak to balance the other movement patterns, the body curls into itself, and nothing works properly.

If gait and kinetic chain patterns are inefficient, more energy is required for movement, and fatigue and pain can result.

Shortened postural (stabilizer) muscles must be lengthened and then stretched. This takes time and uses all the massage therapist's technical skills. Because of the fiber configuration of the muscle tissue (red or white twitch fibers), techniques must be sufficiently intense and must be applied long enough to allow the muscle to respond.

Shortened and weak phasic (mover) muscles must first be lengthened and stretched. Eventually, strengthening techniques and exercises will be needed.

Long and weak muscles need therapeutic exercise. If the hypertense phasic muscle pattern is caused by repetitive use, the muscles can be normalized with muscle energy techniques and then lengthened. Overly tense muscles often increase in size (hypertrophy). The patient must reduce the activity of that muscle group until balance is restored, which usually takes about 4 weeks. Muscle tissue that has undergone hypertrophy begins to return to normal if it is not used for the activity during that time. Patients often display this pattern and very often resist complete inactivity. A reduced activity level and a more balanced exercise program, combined with flexibility training, can be beneficial for them. Refer these individuals to appropriate training and coaching professionals if indicated.

People usually complain of problems in the taut and long eccentrically functioning and inhibited muscle areas. Massage in these areas worsens the symptoms; the reason is, massage is excellent at increasing length and pliability, but these tissues already are too long. Instead, identify the short tissues and apply massage to lengthen and stretch these areas. The long muscles need strengthening exercises. Assessment must identify the concentrically contracted shortened areas so that appropriate correction can be applied (Figure 9-9).

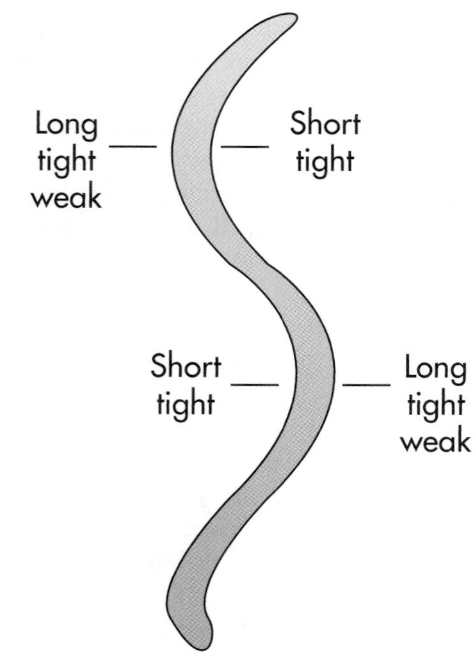

FIGURE 9-9 ■ First, massage application with stretching lengthens the short, tight areas. Coupled with therapeutic exercise, massage then stimulates the long, tight, and weak areas. (From Fritz S: *Mosby's essential sciences for therapeutic massage: anatomy, physiology, biomechanics, and pathology*, ed 2, St Louis, 2004, Mosby.)

Muscle Firing Patterns (Muscle Activation Sequences)

A firing pattern is the sequence of muscle contraction involvement with the agonist and the synergist geared to best produce joint motion. Muscles also contract, or fire, in a neurologic sequence to produce coordinated movement. If the muscle activation sequence is disrupted and muscles fire out of sequence or do not contract when they should, labored movement and postural strain result. Firing patterns can be assessed by initiating a particular sequence of joint movements and palpating for muscle activity to determine which muscles are responding first, second, and third to the movement.

The central nervous system recruits the appropriate muscles in specific firing patterns to generate the appropriate muscle function of acceleration, deceleration, or stability. If these firing patterns are abnormal, with the synergist becoming dominant, efficient movement is compromised and the joint position is strained. The general muscle activation sequence is prime movers, then stabilizers, then synergists. If the stabilizer also has to move the area (acceleration) or control movement (deceleration), it typically becomes short and tight. If the synergist fires before the prime mover, the movement is awkward and labored.

If one muscle is tight and short, it can cause reciprocal inhibition in the antagonist muscles. Reciprocal inhibition exists when a muscle with increased motor tone reduces nervous stimulation to its functional antagonist it causes reduced activity. For example, a short, tight psoas decreases the function of the gluteus maximus. The activation and force production of the prime mover (the gluteus maximus) are reduced, leading to compensation and substitution by the synergists (the hamstrings) and stabilizers (the erector spinae), creating an altered firing pattern.

The most common dysfunction of the muscle activation sequence is synergistic dominance, in which a synergist compensates for a prime mover to produce the movement. For example, if a patient has a weak gluteus medius, synergists (the tensor fasciae latae, adductor complex, and quadratus lumborum) become dominant to compensate for the weakness. This alters normal joint alignment, which further alters the normal length-tension relationships of the muscles around the joint. Box 9-5 presents the most commonly used assessment procedures and the intervention for altered firing patterns.

Each jointed area has an optimal muscle activation sequence pattern. The movement is a product of the entire mechanism, including bones; joints; ligaments; capsular components and design; tendons; muscle shapes and fiber types; interlinked fascial networks; nerve distribution; myotatic units of prime movers, antagonists, synergists, and fixators; neurologic kinetic chain interactions; the body-wide influence of reflexes, including the positional and righting reflexes of vision and the inner ear; circulatory distribution; general systemic balance; and nutritional influences. Assessment of a movement pattern as normal indicates that all parts are functioning in a well-orchestrated manner. When a dysfunction is identified, the causal factors can arise from any one or a combination of these elements. Often a multidisciplinary diagnosis is necessary to identify clearly the interconnected nature of the pathologic condition.

Inappropriate firing patterns can be addressed by inhibiting the muscles that are contracting out of sequence and stimulating the appropriate muscles to fire (contract). Tapotement is a good technique for stimulating muscles, as is pulsed muscle contraction. If the problem does not normalize easily, referral to an exercise professional may be indicated.

Gait Assessment

Understanding the basic body movements of walking helps the massage therapist recognize dysfunctional and inefficient gait patterns.

Disruption of the gait reflexes creates the potential for many problems. Common gait problems include a functional short leg caused by muscle shortening; tight neck and shoulder muscles; aching feet; weight distribution, such as during pregnancy or with obesity; and fatigue. The massage therapist must understand biomechanics, including posture, the interaction of joint functions, and gait. (A good text for learning about these biomechanical functions is *Kinesiology of the Musculoskeletal System* [Mosby, 2002] by Donald Neumann.) This is especially important in healing and rehabilitation regimens in which walking is either the goal or part of the program.

It is important to observe the patient from the front, the back, and both sides. To begin, the massage therapist should watch the patient walk, noticing the heel-to-toe foot placement. The toes should point forward with each step.

Observe the upper body. It should be relaxed and fairly symmetric. The head should face

Text continued on p. 290.

BOX 9-5 Common Muscle Firing Patterns

Trunk Flexion

Palpate either side of rectus abdominis to assess contraction of obliques and transverse abdomen.

1. Normal firing pattern
   a. Transverse abdominis
   b. Abdominal obliques
   c. Rectus abdominis
2. Assessment
   a. Client is supine with knees and hips approximately 90 degrees flexion.
   b. Client is instructed to perform a normal curl up.
   c. Massage practitioner assesses the ability of the abdominal muscles to functionally stabilize the lumbar-pelvic-hip complex by having the client draw the abdominal muscle in (as when bringing the umbilicus toward the back) and then do a curl just lifting the scapula off the table while keeping both feet flat. Inability to maintain the drawing-in position and/or to activate the rectus abdominis during the assessment demonstrates an altered firing pattern of the abdominal stabilization mechanism.
3. Altered firing pattern
   a. Weak agonist—abdominal complex
   b. Overactive antagonist—erector spinae
   c. Overactive synergist—psoas, rectus abdominis
4. Symptoms
   a. Low back pain
   b. Buttock pain
   c. Hamstring shortening

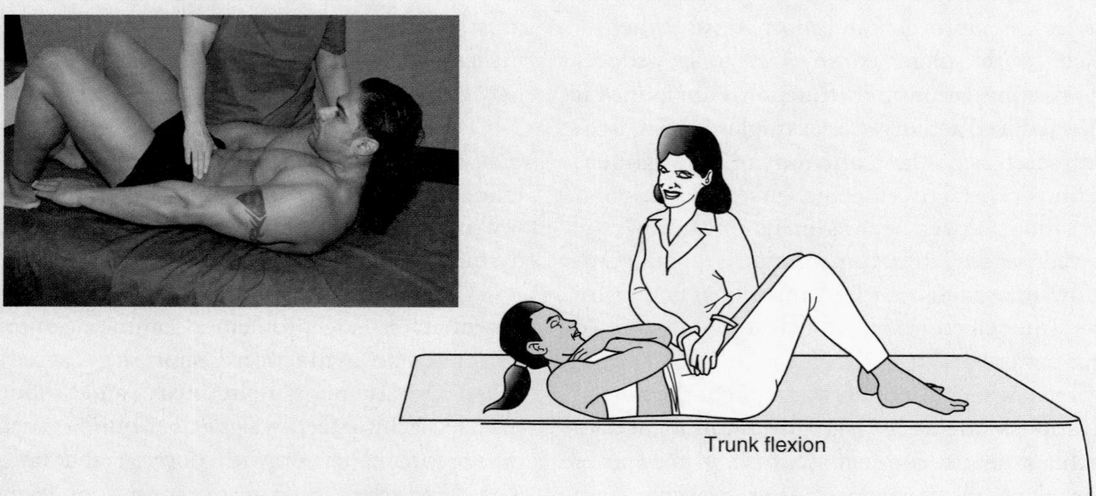

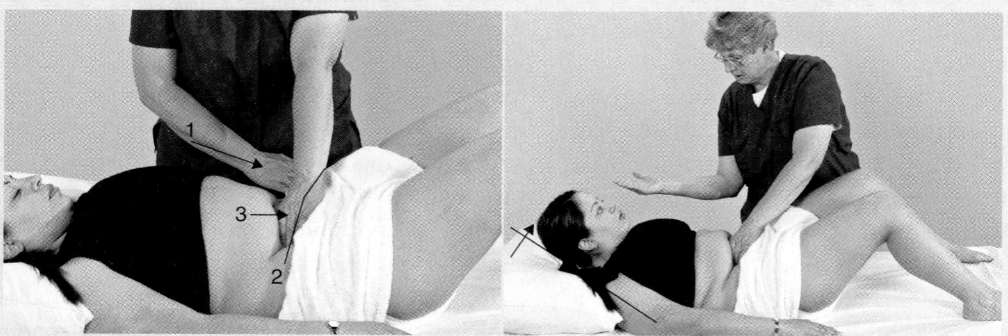

Palpate three positions lower. *1* and *2*: Lower abdominal obliques and transverse abdominis. *3*: Rectus abdominis.
Have patient lift head and shoulders. Instruct patient to perform draw-in maneuver. Pull belly button towards back.

BOX 9-5 Common Muscle Firing Patterns—cont'd

Hip Extension

1. Normal firing pattern
   a. Gluteus maximus
   b. Opposite erector spinae
   c. Same side erector spinae and hamstring
   OR
   a. Gluteus maximus
   b. Hamstring
   c. Opposite erector spinae
   d. Same side erector spinae
2. Assessment
   a. Client is prone.
   b. Massage practitioner palpates the erector spinae with the fingers of one hand while palpating the muscle belly of the opposite gluteus maximus and hamstring with the little finger and thumb of the other hand.
   c. Client is instructed to raise the hip more than 15 degrees off the table.
3. Altered firing pattern
   a. Weak agonist—gluteus maximus
   b. Overactive antagonist—psoas
   c. Overactive stabilizer—erector spinae
   d. Overactive synergist—hamstring
4. Symptoms
   a. Low back pain
   b. Buttock pain
   c. Recurrent hamstring strains

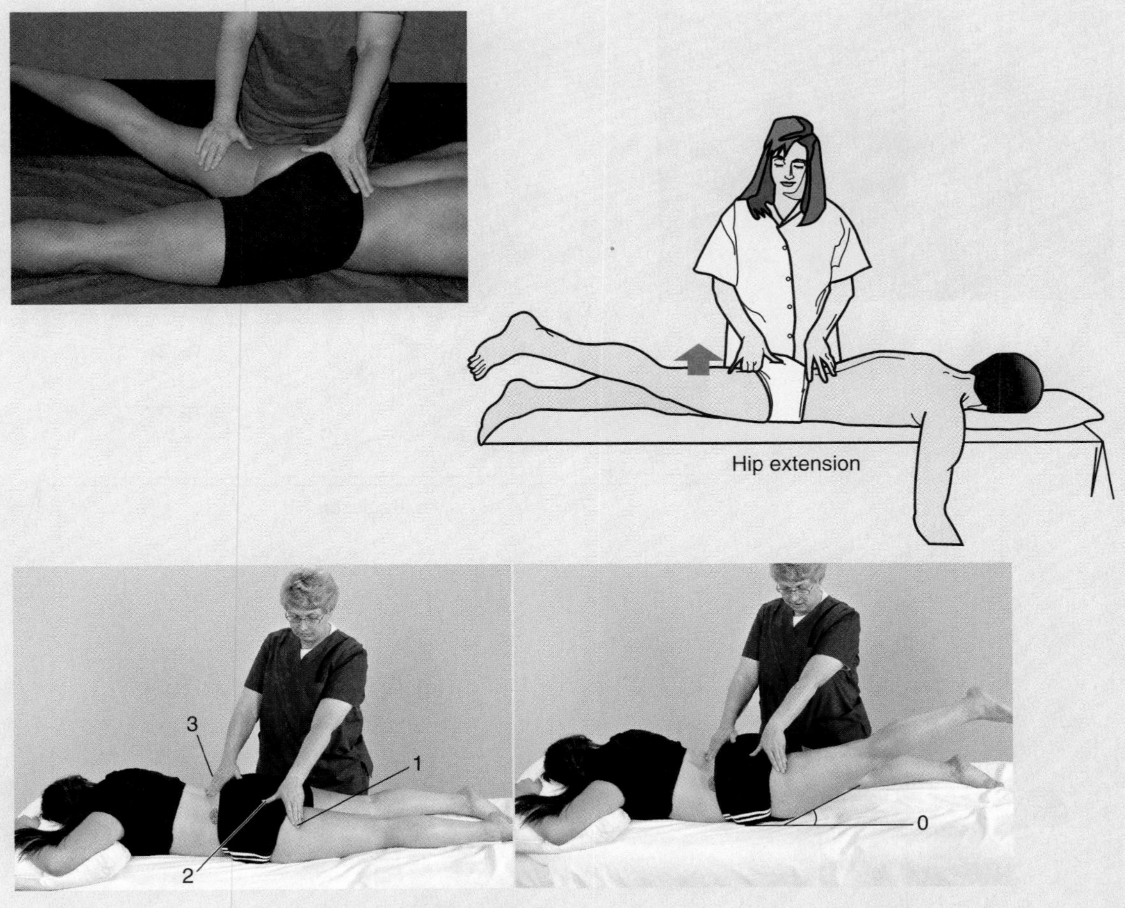

Palpate points 1 to 3. *1*, Upper hamstring. *2*, Gluteus maximus. *3*, Opposite lumbar.
Have patient extend hip at least 15 degrees.

Continued

BOX 9-5 Common Muscle Firing Patterns—cont'd

Hip Abduction

1. Normal firing pattern
   a. Gluteus medius
   b. Tensor fasciae latae
   c. Quadratus lumborum
2. Assessment
   a. Client is in side-lying position.
   b. Massage practitioner stands next to the client and palpates the quadratus lumborum with one hand and the tensor fasciae latae and gluteus medius with finger of the other hand.
   c. Client is instructed to abduct the leg from the table.
3. Altered firing pattern
   a. Weak agonist—gluteus medius
   b. Overactive antagonist—adductors
   c. Overactive synergist—tensor fasciae latae
   d. Overactive stabilizer—quadratus lumborum
4. Symptoms
   a. Low back pain
   b. Sacroiliac joint pain
   c. Buttock pain
   d. Lateral knee pain
   e. Anterior knee pain

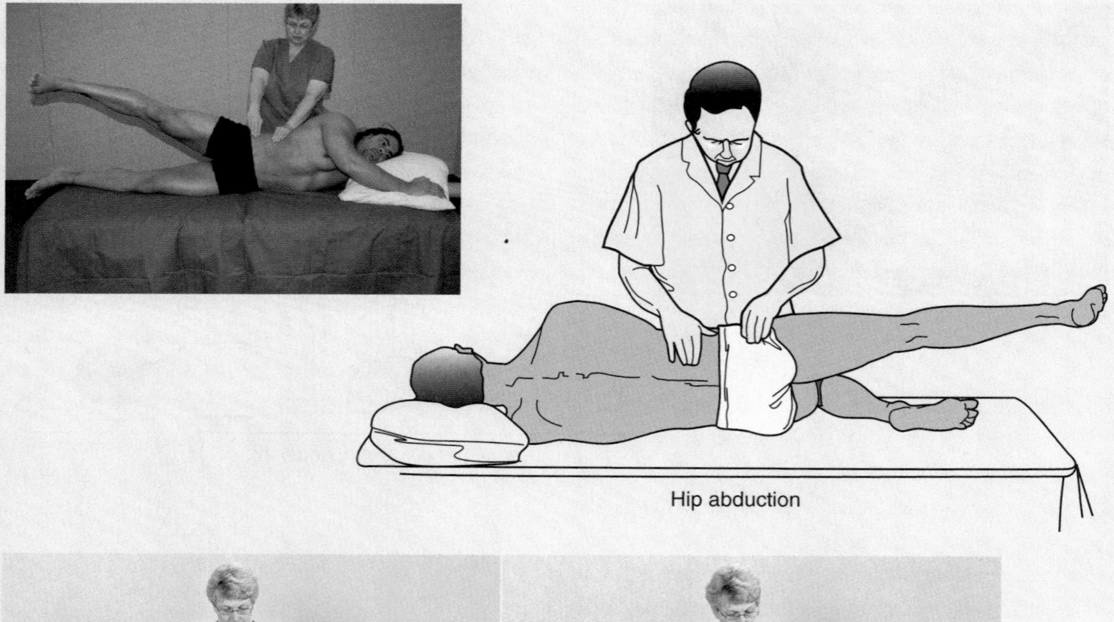

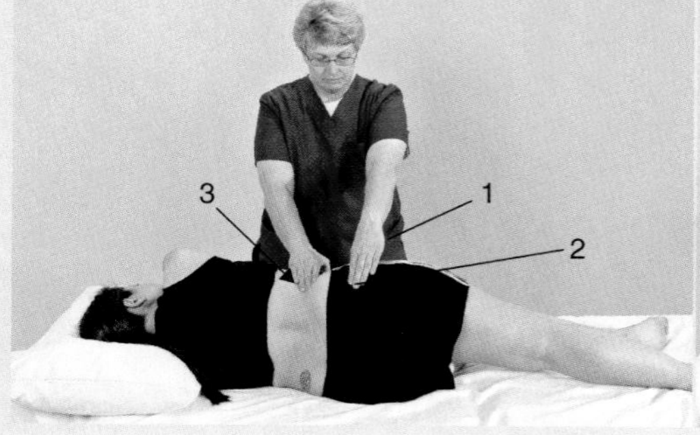

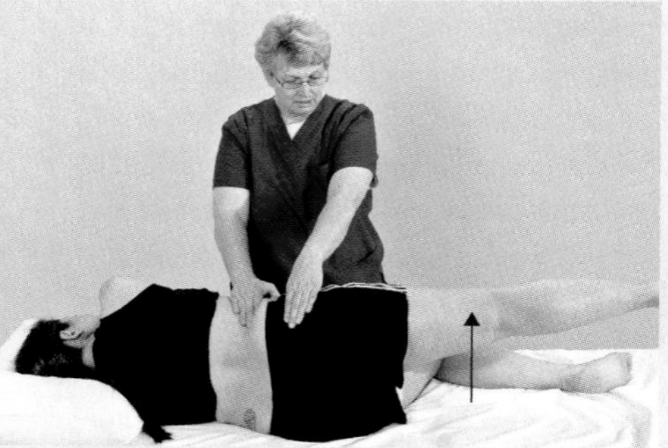

Begin palpation in three positions. *1*: Tensor fasciae latae. *2*: Gluteus medius. *3*: Quadratus lumborum. Have patient abduct leg.

BOX 9-5 Common Muscle Firing Patterns—cont'd

Knee Flexion

1. Normal firing pattern
   a. Hamstrings
   b. Gastrocnemius
2. Assessment
   a. Client is prone.
   b. Massage practitioner places fingers on the hamstring and gastrocnemius.
   c. Client flexes the knee.
3. Altered firing pattern
   a. Weak agonist—hamstrings
   b. Overactive synergist—gastrocnemius
4. Symptoms
   a. Pain behind the knee
   b. Achilles tendinitis

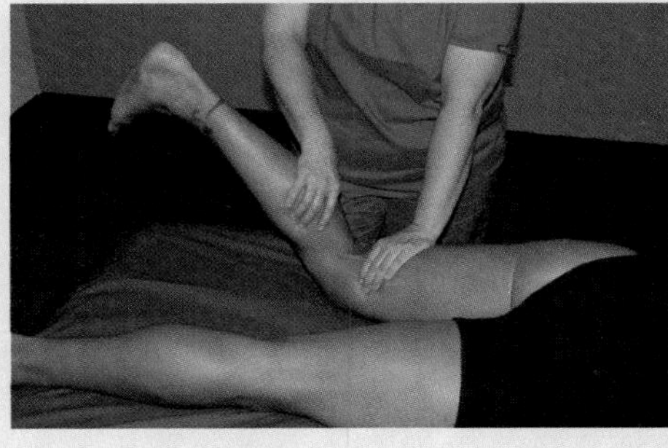

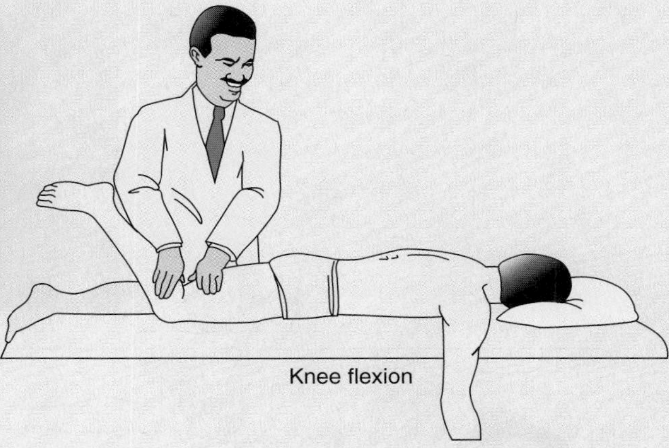

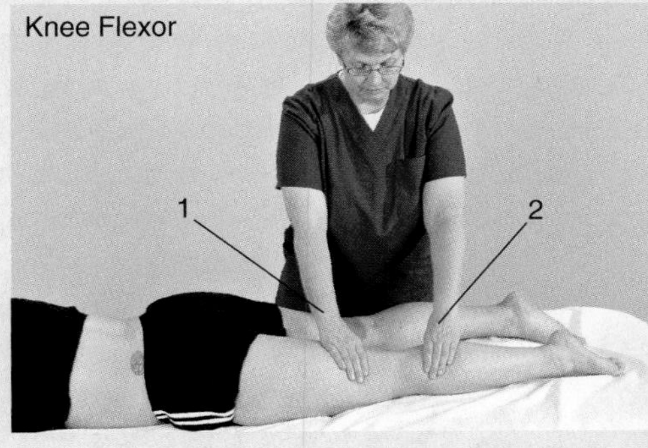

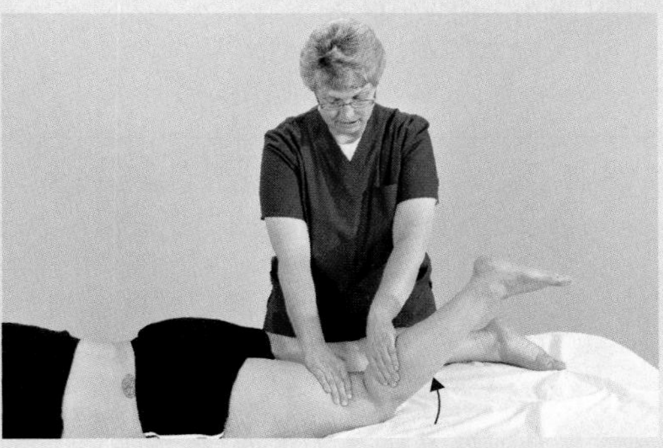

Begin palpation at two places. *1*: Hamstrings near knee. *2*: At calf near knee.
Have client flex knee.

Continued

BOX 9-5 Common Muscle Firing Patterns—cont'd

Knee Extension

1. Normal firing pattern
   a. Vastus medialis
   b. Vastus intermedius and vastus lateralis
   c. Rectus femoris
2. Assessment
   a. Client is supine with leg flat.
   b. Client is asked to pull the patella cranially (toward the head).
   c. Massage practitioner places finger on the vastus medialis oblique portion, vastus lateralis, and rectus femoris.
3. Altered firing pattern
   a. Weak agonist—vastus medialis, primarily oblique portion
   b. Overactive synergist—vastus lateralis
4. Symptoms
   a. Knee pain under patella
   b. Patellar tendinitis

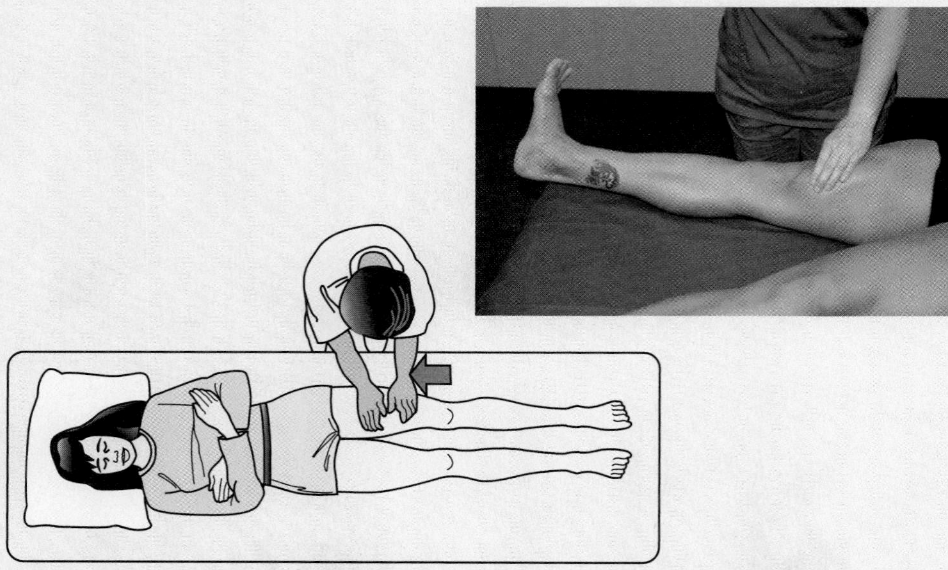

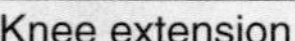

Knee extension

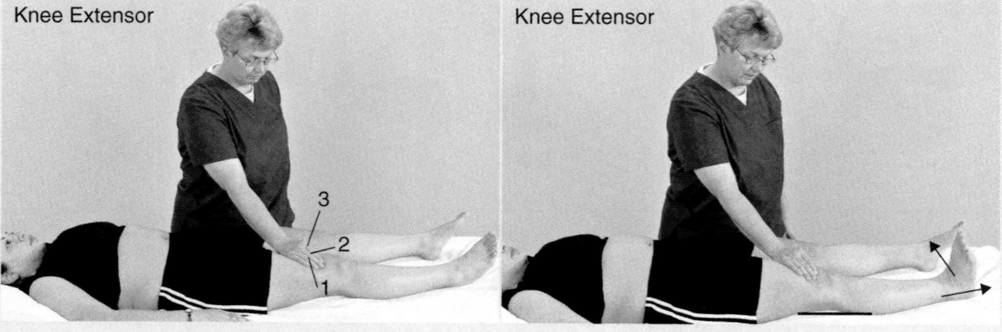

Begin with leg straight. Palpate three positions on quadriceps near knee. *1*: Vastus lateralis. *2*: Rectus femoris. *3*: Vastus medialis (oblique portion).

Have client extend knee by flattening leg—dorsiflexing and pushing heel out.

Box 9-5 Common Muscle Firing Patterns—cont'd

Shoulder Flexion

1. Normal firing pattern
   a. Supraspinatus
   b. Deltoid
   c. Infraspinatus
   d. Middle and lower trapezius
   e. Contralateral quadratus lumborum
2. Assessment
   a. Massage practitioner stands behind seated client with one hand on the client's shoulder and the other on the contralateral quadratus area.
   b. Client is asked to abduct the shoulder to 90 degrees.
3. Altered firing pattern
   a. Weak agonist—levator scapula
   b. Overactive agonist—upper trapezius
   c. Overactive stabilizer—ipsilateral quadratus lumborum
4. Symptoms
   a. Shoulder tension
   b. Headache at the base of the skull
   c. Upper chest breathing
   d. Low back pain

Intervention for Altered Firing Patterns

Use appropriate massage application to inhibit the dominant muscle. Then, strengthen the weak muscles.

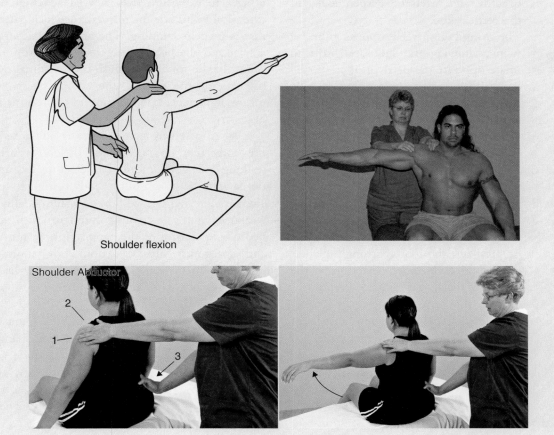

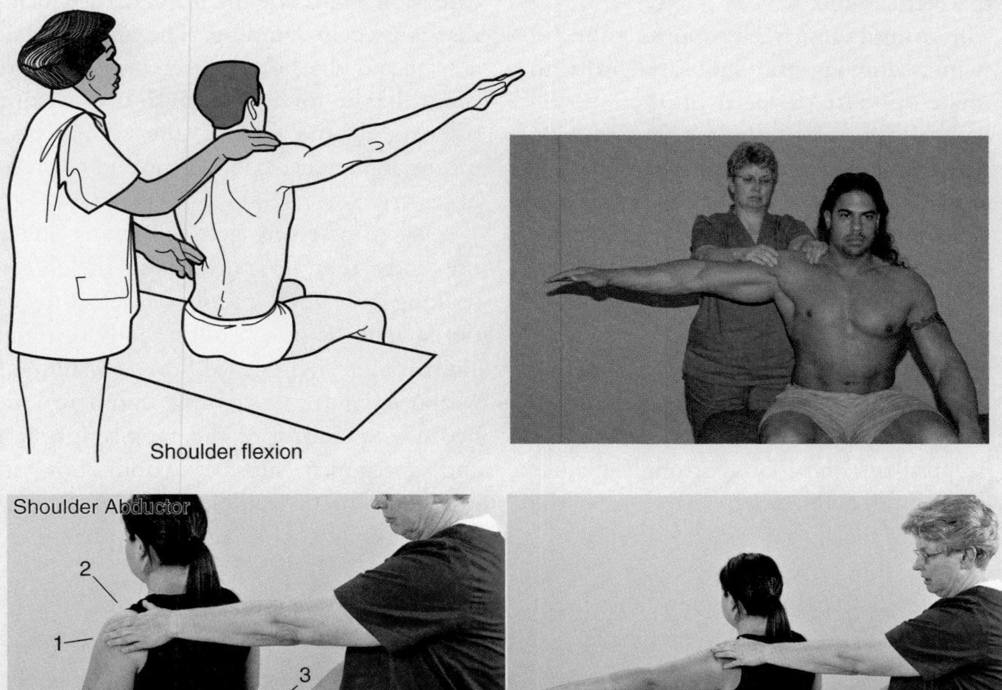

Begin palpation at three positions. *1*: Deltoid. *2*: Upper trapezius. *3*: Opposite quadratus lumborum. Have patient abduct shoulder.

forward with the eyes level with the horizontal plane. The natural arm swing is opposite to the leg swing. The arm swing begins at the shoulder joint. On each step the left arm moves forward as the right leg moves forward and then vice versa. This pattern provides balance. The rhythm and pace of the arm and leg swing should be similar. Walking speed increases the speed of the arm swing. The length of the stride determines the arc of the arm swing (Figures 9-10 and 9-11).

Observe the patient walking, and notice the person's general appearance. The optimum walking pattern is as follows:

1. The head and trunk are vertical, with the eyes easily maintaining forward position and level with the horizontal plane; the shoulders are level and perpendicular to the vertical line.
2. The arms swing freely opposite the leg swing, allowing the shoulder girdle to rotate opposite the pelvic girdle.
3. Step length and timing are even.
4. The body oscillates vertically with each step.
5. The entire body moves rhythmically with each step.
6. At the heel strike, the foot is approximately at a right angle to the leg.
7. The knee is extended but not locked.
8. The body weight is shifted forward into the stance phase.
9. At push-off, the foot is strongly plantar flexed, with defined hyperextension of the metatarsophalangeal joints of the toes.
10. During the leg swing, the foot easily clears the floor with good alignment and the rhythm of movement remains unchanged.
11. The heel contacts the floor first.
12. The weight then rolls to the outside of the arch.
13. The arch flattens slightly in response to the weight load.
14. The weight then is shifted to the ball of the foot in preparation for the spring-off from the toes and the shifting of the weight to the other foot.

During walking the pelvis moves slightly in a side-lying figure-eight pattern. The movements that make up this sequence are transverse, medial, and lateral rotation. The stability and mobility of the sacroiliac joints play very important roles in this alternating side figure-eight movement. If these joints are not functioning properly, the entire gait is disrupted. The sacroiliac (SI) joint is one of the few joints in the body that is not directly affected by muscles that cross the joint. It is a large joint, and the bony contact between the sacrum and ilium is broad. The rocking of this joint commonly is disrupted.

The hips rotate in a slightly oval pattern beginning with a medial rotation during the leg swing and heel strike, followed by a lateral rotation through the push-off. The knees move in a flexion and extension pattern opposite each other. The extension phase never reaches enough extension to initiate the normal knee lock pattern that is used in standing. The ankles rotate in an arc around the heel at heel strike and around a center in the forefoot at push-off. Maximal dorsiflexion at the end of the stance phase and maximal plantar flexion at the end of push-off are necessary.

When assessing gait, observing for areas of the body that do not move efficiently during walking is a good means of detecting dysfunctional areas. Pain causes the body to tighten and alters the normal relaxed flow of walking. Muscle weakness and shortening interfere with the neurologic control of the agonist (prime mover) and antagonist muscle action. Limitation of joint movement (hypomobility) and joint laxity (hypermobility) both result in protective muscle contraction.

If the situation becomes chronic, both muscle shortening and muscle weakness result. Changes in the soft tissue, including all the connective tissue elements of the tendons, ligaments, and fascial sheaths, restrict the normal action of the muscles. Connective tissue usually shortens and becomes less pliable.

Amputation disrupts the body's normal diagonal balance. Obviously, any amputation of the lower limb disturbs the walking pattern. What is not so obvious is that amputation of any part of the upper limb affects the counterbalance movement of the arm swing during walking. The rest of the body must compensate for the loss. Loss of

A

Heel strike = Initial contact

Hip	25° Flexion	Hip extensors eccentric
Knee	0°	Quadriceps concentric
Ankle	0°	Tibials concentric

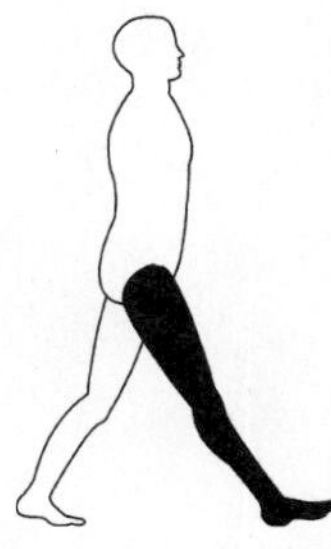

B

Foot Flat = Loading Response

Hip	26° Flexion	Hip extensors eccentric and hip abductors isometric
Knee	15° Flexion	Quadriceps eccentric
Ankle	10° Plantar flexion	Pretibials eccentric

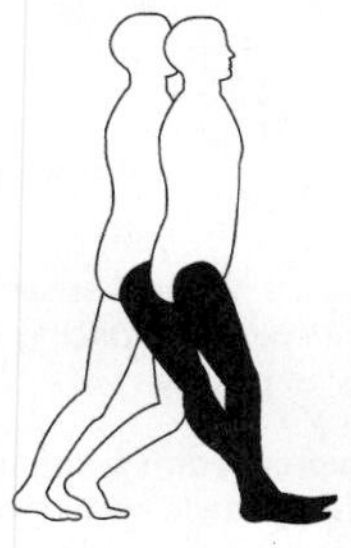

C

Midstance = Midstance

- The body (center of gravity) reaches its highest point in the gait cycle

Hip	0°	Hip abductors isometric
Knee	0°	Quadriceps concentric initially, then no muscle activity
Ankle	0°	Plantar flexors (calf) eccentric

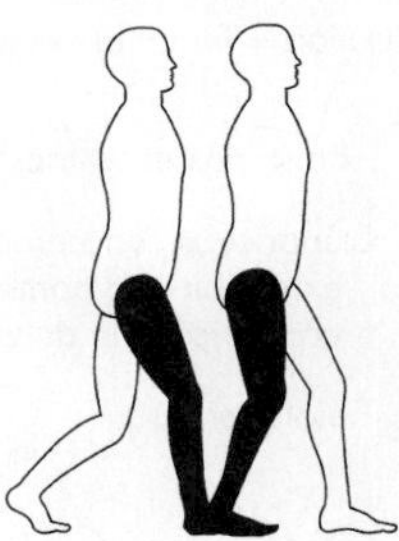

D

Heel-Off = Terminal Stance

Hip	20° Hip hyperextension	No muscle activity
Knee	0°	No muscle activity
Ankle	10° Dorsiflexion	Plantar flexors (calf) eccentric

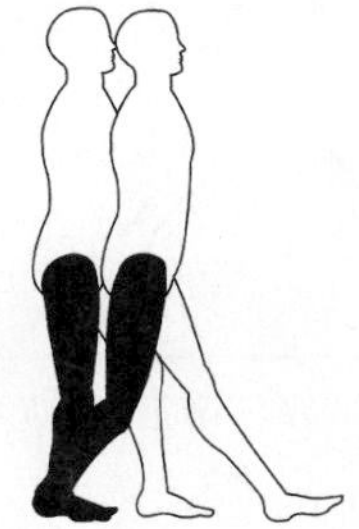

E

Toe-Off = Preswing

Hip	0°	Adductor longus
Knee	40° Knee flexion	No muscle activity
Ankle	20° Plantar flexion	Plantar flexors concentric initially, then no muscle activity

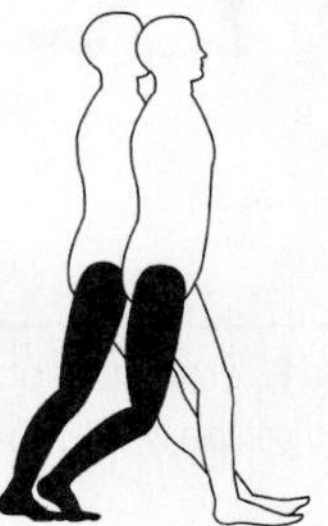

FIGURE 9-10 ■ **A** to **E,** Components of the stance phase. (Modified from Fritz S: *Mosby's essential sciences for therapeutic massage: anatomy, physiology, biomechanics, and pathology,* ed 2, St Louis, 2004, Mosby.)

A Acceleration = Initial swing

Hip	15° Hip flexion	Hip flexors concentric
Knee	60° Knee flexion	Knee flexors concentric
Ankle	10° Plantar flexion	Tibials concentric

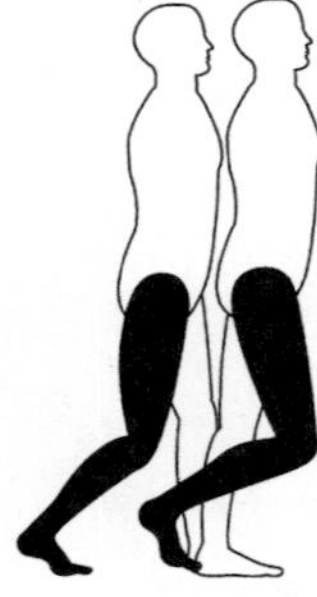

B Midswing = Midswing

Hip	25° Hip flexion	Hip flexors concentric initially, then hamstrings eccentric
Knee	25° Knee flexion	Knee extension is created by momentum and gravity and short head of biceps femoris control rate of knee extension through eccentric control
Ankle	0°	Tibials concentric

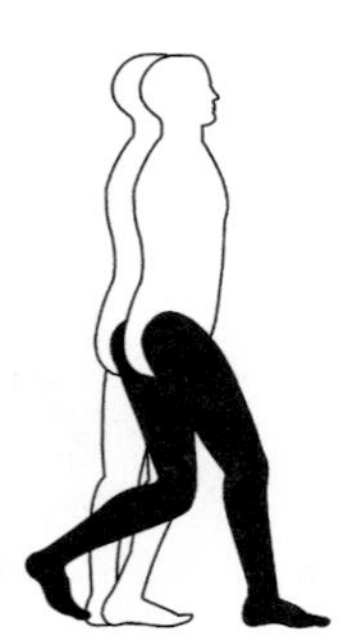

C Deceleration = Terminal swing

Hip	25° Flexion	Hamstrings eccentric
Knee	0°	Quadriceps concentric to insure knee extension and hamstrings are active eccentrically to decelerate the leg
Ankle	0°	Tibials concentric

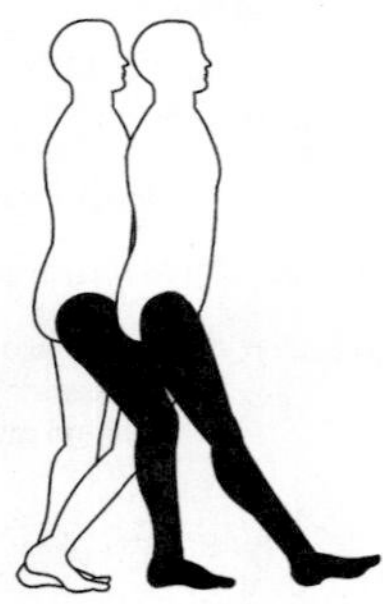

D Arm swing

- The upper extremities serve an important role in counterbalancing the shifts of the center of gravity.
- A reciprocal arm swing is seen in a mature gait (e.g., the left arm swings forward as the right leg swings forward and vice versa).
- As the shoulder girdle advances, the pelvis and limb trail behind. With each step, this is reversed.

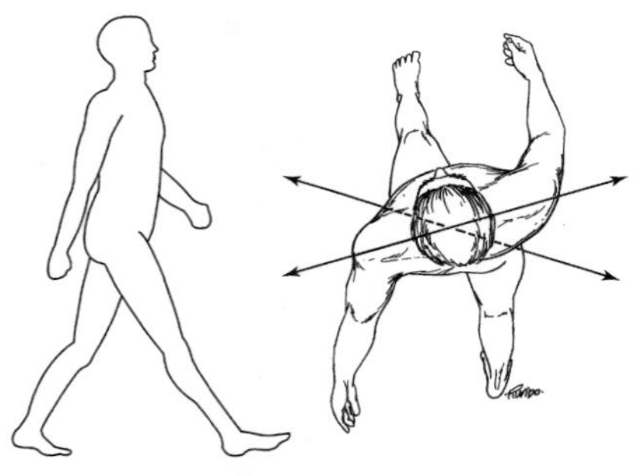

FIGURE 9-11 ■ **A** to **F,** Components of the swing phase. (Modified from Fritz S: *Mosby's essential sciences for therapeutic massage: anatomy, physiology, biomechanics, and pathology*, ed 2, St Louis, 2004, Mosby.)

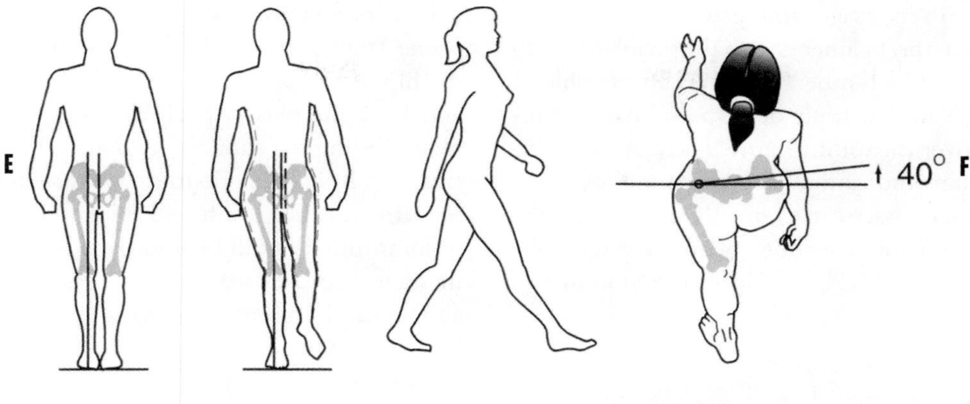

FIGURE 9-11, cont'd

any of the toes greatly affects the postural information sent to the brain from the feet.

Any disruption of the gait demands that the body compensate by shifting movement patterns and posture. Soft tissue dysfunction may exist without joint involvement. Any change in the tissue around a joint has a direct effect on the joint function. Changes in joint function eventually cause problems with the joint. Any dysfunction with the joint immediately involves the surrounding muscles and other soft tissue.

Because of this, all dysfunctional patterns are whole body phenomena. Working only on the symptomatic area is ineffective and offers limited relief. Therapeutic massage with a whole body focus is extremely valuable in dealing with gait dysfunction. Corrective measures also include normalizing muscle firing patterns and gait reflex patterns.

When interpreting the information gathered from gait assessment, the massage therapist should focus on areas that do not move easily when the patient walks and areas that move too much. Areas that do not move are restricted; areas that move too much are compensating for inefficient function. By releasing the restrictions through massage and re-educating the reflexes through neuromuscular work and exercise, the therapist can help the patient improve the gait pattern.

The techniques followed are similar to those for postural corrections. The shortened and restricted areas are softened with massage, then the neuromuscular mechanism is reset with muscle energy techniques, muscle lengthening, and stretches.

The patient should be taught slow lengthening and stretching procedures. After stimulating the muscles in weakened areas, the physical therapist can teach the patient strengthening exercises. The massage therapist must be sure the adaptation methods are built into the context of a complete massage rather than spot work on isolated parts of the body. Suggestions could be made to the patient to evaluate factors that may contribute to these adaptations, such as posture, footwear, chairs, tables, beds, clothing, work stations, physical tasks (e.g., shoveling), and repetitive exercise patterns.

Sacroiliac Joint Function

Proper functioning of the sacroiliac joint is an important factor in walking patterns. Because SI joint movement has no direct muscular component, the massage therapist will find it difficult to use any kind of muscle energy lengthening when working with this joint. The joint is embedded deep in supporting ligaments. To keep the surrounding ligaments pliable, direct and specific connective tissue techniques are indicated unless the joint is hypermobile. If that is the case, external bracing combined with rehabilitative movement may be indicated.

Sometimes the ligaments restabilize the area. Stabilization of the jointed area should be interspersed with massage and gentle stretching to ensure that the ligaments remain pliable and do not adhere to each other. To assess for possible SI joint involvement, apply deep, broad-based compression over the joint (Figure 9-12). An increase in symptoms indicates SI joint dysfunction.

Another assessment involves having the patient stand on one foot and then extend the trunk (Figure 9-13, *A*); this loads the SI joint and would increase symptoms. If the patient is lying prone (Figure 9-13, *B*), have the person extend the hip; then apply resistance to the opposite arm and have the person push against the resistance by extending the shoulder and arm. While doing this, also have the patient extend the contralateral hip; if it is easier to lift and if symptoms decline, SI joint function can be improved by exercise and massage, because force closure mechanisms can be addressed. If no improvement is seen, external bracing may help.

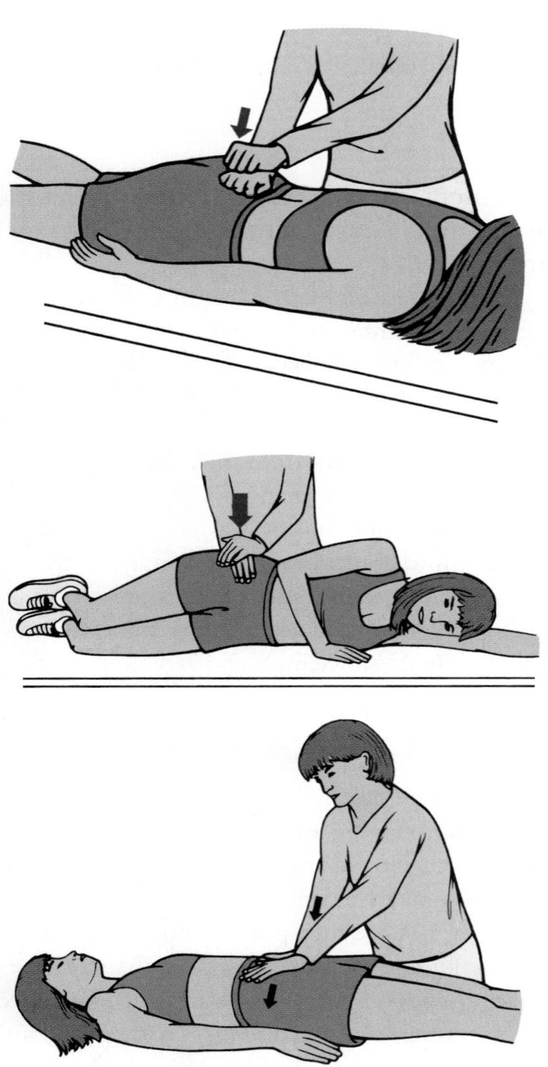

FIGURE 9-12 ■ Assessments for the sacroiliac (SI) joint. Pain in response to compression indicates SI joint dysfunction. (Modified from Saidoff DC, McDonough A: *Critical pathways in therapeutic intervention: extremities and spine,* St Louis, 2002, Mosby.)

Diagnosis of specific joint problems and fitting for external bracing are outside the scope of practice for therapeutic massage, and the patient must be referred to the appropriate professional.

Analysis of the Kinetic Chain

It is important to consider the pattern of muscle interactions that occurs with walking. Remember that gait has a certain pattern for efficient movement. For example, if the left leg is extended for the heel strike, the right arm also is extended. This results in activation of the flexors of both the arm and leg and inhibition of the extensors. A strength imbalance commonly is found in this gait pattern. One muscle out of sequence with the others can set up tense (too strong) or inhibited (weak) muscle imbalances. Whenever a muscle contracts with too much force, it overpowers the antagonist group, resulting in inhibited muscle function. The imbalances can occur anywhere in the pattern.

Muscle strength testing should reveal that the flexor and adductor muscles of the right arm should activate, facilitate, and coordinate with the flexors and adductors of the left leg. The opposite is also true; left arm flexors and adductors activate and facilitate with the right leg flexors and adductors. Extensors and abductors in the limbs coordinate in a similar fashion.

If the flexors of the left leg are activated, as occurs during strength testing, the flexors and adductors of the right arm should be facilitated and strength test strong. The flexors and adductors of the right leg and left arm should be inhibited and strength test weak. Also, the extensors and abductors in the right arm and left leg should be inhibited. All associated patterns follow suit

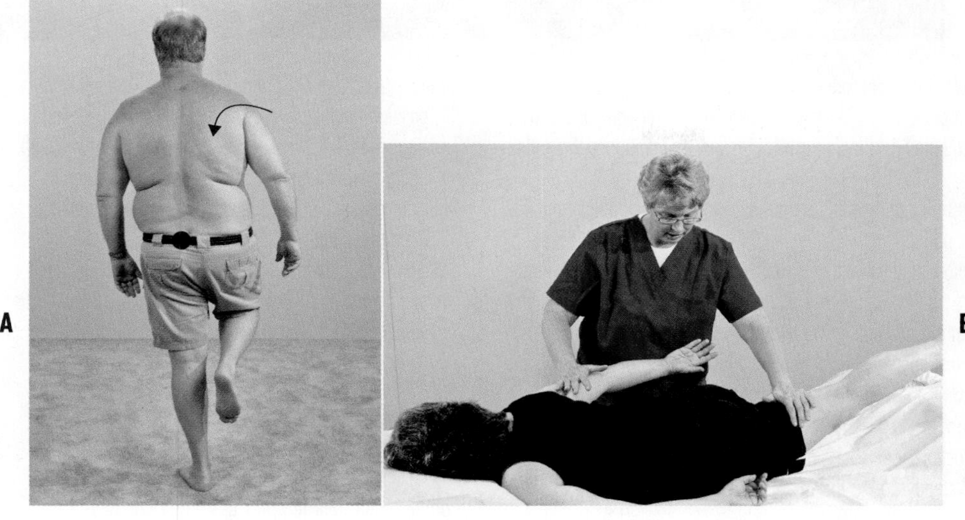

FIGURE 9-13 ■ **A,** Standing assessments for sacroiliac (SI) joint dysfunction. **B,** Prone assessment of SI joint function.

(i.e., activation of the right arm flexor pattern facilitates the left leg flexor pattern and inhibits left arm and right leg flexor muscles while facilitating extensors and abductors). In a similar way, activation of the adductors of the right leg facilitates the adductors of the left arm and inhibits the abductors of the left leg and right arm. The other adductor-abductor patterns follow the same interaction pattern.

All these patterns are associated with gait mechanisms and reflexes. If any pattern is out of sync, gait, posture, and efficient function are disrupted (Boxes 9-6 and 9-7).

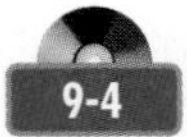

PALPATION ASSESSMENT

Palpation assessment can identify fibrotic changes in a muscle. Identifying changes in texture or tension, pliability, and signs of inflammation (heat, swelling, etc.) in the soft tissues during palpation assessment is a very important part of massage assessment. This requires the massage therapist to have a good understanding of the anatomy and physiology of the body–you simply cannot study anatomy and physiology enough.

Pain is an important indicator of dysfunction. If a client does not mention pain directly, look for nonverbal cues that include facial expressions (grimacing), flinching, and breathing changes. Pain upon palpation does not necessarily mean a problem exists as there are areas on the body that are naturally painful if pressed; these areas are often near surface nerves. Areas where the bone is prominent, such as the ribs, elbow, or patella, will be painful if the palpating pressure is too deep. If an area is painful when palpated, assess the same area on the other side of the body. If the sensation is similar, it is likely that the area is normal and the assessment process is flawed. However, if there is a difference, a problem may exist, and further assessment is indicated.

According to Dr. Leon Chaitow, during palpation varying depths of pressure should be used to reach all of the tissue types and layers. Almost all muscular dysfunctions, such as trigger points or microscarring from minute muscle tears, are found at the musculotendinous junction or in the belly of the muscle. Most acupressure points and motor points are also located in these areas.

Often three or more layers of muscle are present in an area. These layers are separated by deep fascia, and each muscle layer should slide over the one beneath it. Compressing systematically through each layer until the bone is felt is

Box 9-6 Kinetic Chain Protocol Testing

See the DVD for a demonstration

Control group: Serves as a standard or reference for comparison with a test group and is the group of muscles that initiates the reflex response.

Test group: The muscle group that responds to the stimulus from the control group.

Many gait-related kinetic chain patterns exist. We will concentrate on the main patterns involved in flexion, extension, abduction, and adduction at the shoulder and pelvic girdle. For testing the arm flexors/extensors, one should stabilize the humerus superior to the elbow joint and the femur above the knee.

The control group is activated first, the test group is next, and then both contractions are held simultaneously. Both groups should hold strong and steady during the test. One should chart the data to show any inhibitions.

The antagonist pattern should be initiated during the test. The antagonists should let go. If they do not let go, the contraction maintained is concentric instead of eccentric. One should chart the data.

Contralateral Patterns

Left Arm Flexor Test

Isolate and stabilize left arm and right leg in supine flexion.

Control group: Use right leg as control and have client hold right leg position against therapist's inferior/caudal pressure.

Test group: Test left arm flexors by having client hold left arm position against practitioner's inferior/caudal pressure.

Both groups should hold equally strong and steady. If test group is inhibited, chart the data.

Antagonist test: Test left arm extensors by having client hold against practitioner's superior/cranial pressure. These muscles should inhibit (let go). If test group remains concentrically contracted and holds, one should chart data.

Right Arm Flexor Test

Isolate and stabilize left leg and right arm in supine flexion.

Control group: Use left leg as control and have client hold left leg position against therapist's inferior/caudal pressure.

Test group: Test right arm flexors by having client hold right arm position against practitioner's inferior/caudal pressure.

Both groups should hold equally strong and steady. If test group is inhibited, chart data.

Antagonist test: Test right arm extensors by having client hold right arm position against practitioner's superior/cranial pressure. These muscles should inhibit (let go). If test group remains concentrically contracted and holds, one should chart data.

Left Leg Flexor Test

Isolate and support/stabilize left leg and right arm in supine flexion.

Control group: Use right arm as control and have client hold right arm position against therapist's inferior/caudal pressure.

Test group: Test left leg flexors by having client hold left leg position against practitioner's inferior/caudal pressure.

Both groups should hold equally strong and steady. If test group is inhibited, chart data.

Antagonist test: Test left leg extensors by having client hold against practitioner's superior/cranial pressure. These muscles should inhibit (let go). If test group remains concentrically contracted and holds, one should chart data.

Right Leg Flexor Test

Isolate and support/stabilize left arm and right leg in supine flexion.

Control group: Use left arm as control and have client hold left arm position against therapist's inferior/caudal pressure.

Test group: Test right leg flexors by having client hold right leg position against practitioner's inferior/caudal pressure.

Both groups should hold equally strong and steady. If test group is inhibited, chart data.

Antagonist test: Test right leg extensors by having client hold right leg position against practitioner's superior/cranial pressure. These muscles should inhibit (let go). If test group remains concentrically contracted and holds, chart data.

Contralateral Extensors

Left Arm Extensor Test

Isolate and stabilize left arm and right leg in supine flexion.

Control group: Right leg is control. Have client hold leg position against practitioner's superior/cephalad pressure.

Test group: Test left arm extensors by having client hold arm position against practitioner's superior/cephalad pressure.

Both groups should stay equally strong and steady. If test group is inhibited, chart data.

Antagonist test: Test left arm flexors by having client hold left arm position against practitioner's inferior/caudal pressure. These muscles should inhibit (let go). If test group remains concentrically contracted and holds, chart data.

Right Arm Extensor Test

Isolate and stabilize left leg and right arm in supine flexion.

Control group: Left leg is control. Have client hold left leg position against therapist's superior/cephalad pressure.

Test group: Test right arm extensors by having client hold arm position against practitioner's superior/cephalad pressure.

Both groups should hold equally strong and steady. If test group is inhibited, chart data.

Antagonist test: Test right arm flexors by having client hold against right arm position against practitioner's inferior/caudal pressure. These muscles should inhibit (let go). If test group remains concentrically contracted and holds, chart data.

BOX 9-6 Kinetic Chain Protocol Testing—cont'd

Left Leg Extensor Test

Isolate and stabilize left leg and right arm in supine flexion.

Control group: Right arm is control. Have client hold arm position against practitioner's superior/cephalad pressure.

Test group: Test left leg extensors by having client hold leg position against practitioner's superior/cephalad pressure.

Both groups should hold equally strong and steady. If test group is inhibited, chart data.

Antagonist test: Test left leg flexor by having client hold left leg position against practitioner's inferior/caudal pressure. These muscles should inhibit (let go). If test group remains concentrically contracted and holds, one should chart data.

Right Leg Extensor Test

Isolate and support/stabilize left arm and right leg in supine flexion.

Control group: Left arm is control. Have client hold arm position against practitioner's superior/cephalad pressure.

Test group: Test right leg extensors by having client hold leg position against practitioner's superior/cephalad pressure.

Both groups should hold equally strong and steady. If test group is inhibited, chart data.

Antagonist test: Test right leg flexors by having client hold right leg position against practitioner's inferior/caudal pressure. These muscles should inhibit (let go). If test group remains concentrically contracted pattern and holds, one should chart data.

BOX 9-7 Gait Muscle Testing as an Intervention Tool

An understanding of gait gives the massage therapist a powerful intervention tool: gait muscle testing. For example, a person trips and strains the left hip extensor muscles. Gait muscle testing reveals the imbalanced pattern by showing that the left hip extensor muscles are weak, whereas the flexors in the left hip and right arm/shoulder are overly tense. The hip and leg are sore and should not be massaged excessively, but the arm muscles are fine. By activating the extensors in the right shoulder and arm, the left hip extensor muscles can be facilitated. By activating the flexors of the left arm, the flexors of the left hip are inhibited. This process may restore balance in the gait pattern. Many combinations are possible based on the gait pattern and reflexes. Gait muscle testing provides the means of identifying these interactions.

important. Pressure used to reach and palpate the deeper layers of muscle must travel from the superficial layers down to the deeper layers. To accomplish this, the compressive force must be even, broad based, and slow. There should be no "poking" quality to the touch or abrupt pressure pushing through muscle layers, because the surface layers of muscle will tense up and guard, preventing access to the deeper layers.

Muscle tends to push up against palpating pressure when it is concentrically contracting. Having the client slowly move the joint that is affected can aid in the identification of the proper location of muscles being assessed.

Make sure to slide each layer of muscle back and forth over the underlying layer to detect any adherence between the muscle layers. The layers usually run cross-grain to each other. The best example of this is the abdominal muscle group. Even in the arm and leg, where all the muscles seem to run in the same direction, a diagonal crossing and spiraling of the muscle groups is evident. Muscles can feel tense and ropy in both concentric (short) and eccentric (long) patterns. Therefore, think of muscle functioning as short and tight and long and taut.

Applying compressive force into tissue and taking out all the slack puts the tissue in tension. Normally, pressing into the soft tissue does not cause pain, only a sense of pressure. If dysfunction is present, the following sensations may occur:

- Acute condition: The patient feels pain before the tissue is in tension.
- Subacute condition: The patient feels pain at tissue tension.
- Chronic condition: The patient may feel pain with overpressure.
- Inflammation: The patient feels an increase in pain as the pressure is maintained
- Increased motor tone: The patient feels a decrease in pain as pressure is maintained,

or reflexive guarding may occur. The patient feels pain and pressure both in the area and in tissue surrounding the point of compression.

Palpation assessment becomes part of the massage. In any given massage, about 90% of the touching is also assessment developed as part of gliding, kneading, compression, or joint movement. Palpation assessment meets tissue but does not override it or encourage it to change. This type of work generally relaxes or stimulates the patient, depending on the type of strokes used.

This text assumes that the therapist has been trained in the fundamentals of palpation. To review palpation skills, see *Mosby's Fundamentals of Therapeutic Massage* by Sandy Fritz or *Palpation and Skills* by Leon Chaitow.

Palpation findings of soft tissue include the following:

- Normal: The soft tissue feels resilient, homogeneous, relaxed, and pliable.
- Chronic condition: The soft tissue feels fibrous, thickened, stiff, and tight.
- Acute condition: The soft tissue feels taut or boggy, warm or hot.
- Atrophy: The soft tissue feels mushy and flaccid because of loss of motor tone or because it is dried out and fibrous.
- Fluid dynamics: Normal soft tissue is hydrated without feeling boggy or swollen. It is warm without feeling hot or sweaty. It blanches when compressed and then quickly returns to normal color.
- Temperature: Heat is an indication of inflammation. Cold often indicates a circulatory impairment.

It is important not to limit a palpation sense only to the hand. Body layers, differences in tissues, movement, heat, sensitivity, texture, and other sensations can be felt with the entire body. It is essential that the massage therapist's entire self become sensitive to subtle differences in the patient's body.

Levels and Types of Palpation

Near-Touch Palpation. The first application of palpation does not include touching the body. It detects hot and cold areas. This is best done just off the skin using the back of the hand, because the back of the hand is very sensitive to heat. The general temperature of the area and any variations should be noted. Very sensitive cutaneous (skin) sensory receptors also detect changes in air pressure and currents and the movement of the air. The ability to consciously detect subtle sensations is an invaluable assessment tool.

Hot areas may be caused by inflammation, muscle spasm, hyperactivity, or increased surface circulation. When the focus of intervention is to cool down the hot areas, one method to use is application of ice. Another way to cool an area is to reduce the muscle spasm and encourage more efficient blood flow in the surrounding areas.

Cold areas often are areas of diminished blood flow, increased connective tissue formation, or muscle flaccidity. Heat may be applied to cold areas. Stimulation massage techniques increase muscle activity, thereby heating up the area. Connective tissue approaches soften connective tissue, help restore space around the capillaries, and release histamine, a vasodilator, to increase circulation. These approaches can warm a cold area.

Palpation of the Skin Surface. The second application of palpation is very light surface stroking of the skin. First, determine whether the skin is dry or damp. Damp areas feel a little sticky, or the fingers drag. This light stroking also causes the root hair plexus that senses light touch to respond. It is important to notice whether an area gets more goose bumps (the pilomotor reflex) than other areas. This is a good time to observe for color, especially blue or yellow coloration. The therapist also should note and keep track of all moles and surface skin growths, pay attention to the quality and texture of the hair, and observe the shape and condition of the nails.

Skin should be contained, hydrated, resilient, and elastic, and have an even, rich coloring. Skin that does not spring back into original position after a slight pinch may be a sign of dehydration. The skin should have no blue, yellow, or red tinges. Blue coloration suggests lack of oxygen; yellow indicates liver problems, such as jaundice; and redness suggests fever, alcohol intake, trauma, or inflammation. Color changes are most noticeable in the lips, around the eyes, and under the nails.

Bruises must be noted and avoided during massage. Excessive bruising is an indication of a potentially serious condition. If a patient has any hot redness or red streaking, the individual should be referred to a physician immediately. This is especially important in the lower leg because of the possibility of deep vein thrombosis (the presence of a blood clot).

The skin should be watched carefully for changes in any moles or lumps. As massage professionals, we often spend more time touching and observing a person's skin than anyone else, including the person. If we keep a keen eye out for changes and refer patients to physicians early, many skin problems can be treated before they become serious.

Depending on the area, the skin may be thick or thin. The skin of the face is thinner than the skin of the lower back. The skin in each particular area, however, should be similar. The skin loses its resilience and elasticity over areas of dysfunction. It is important to know the visceral referred pain areas on the skin. If changes occur to the skin in these areas, refer the patient to the physician.

The skin is a blood reservoir. At any given time, it can hold 10% of the available blood in the body. The connective tissue in the skin must be soft to allow the capillary system to expand to hold the blood. Histamine, which is released from mast cells found in the connective tissue of the superficial fascial layer, dilates the blood vessels. Histamine is also responsible for the patient's reported sense of "warming and itching" in an area that has been massaged.

Damp areas on the skin are indications that the nervous system has been activated in that area. This small amount of perspiration is part of a sympathetic activation called a *facilitated segment.* Surface stroking with enough pressure to drag over the skin elicits a red response over the area of a hyperactive muscle. Deeper palpation of the area usually elicits a tender response. The small erector pili muscles attached to each hair also are under the control of the sympathetic autonomic nervous system. Light fingertip stroking produces goose bumps over areas of nerve hyperactivity. All of these responses can indicate potential activity, such as trigger points in the layers of muscle under the area.

The hair and nails are part of the integumentary system and can reflect health conditions. The hair should be resilient and secure; hair loss should not be excessive when the scalp is massaged. The nails should be smooth. Vertical ridges can indicate nutritional difficulties, and horizontal ridges can be signs of stress caused by changes in circulation that affect nail growth. Clubbed nails may also indicate circulation problems. The skin around the nails should be soft and free of hangnails. It is important to monitor the skin and associated structures continuously, because changes may be an early sign of a pathologic condition.

During times of stress, the epithelial tissues are affected first. Hangnails; split skin around the lips and nails; mouth sores; hair loss; dry, scaly skin; and excessively oily skin are all signs of prolonged stress, medication side effects, or pathologic conditions. These tissues offer one of the best means of assessing adaptive capacity. For example, slow wound healing indicates strain in the system.

A method such as kneading or skin rolling is used to further assess the texture of the skin by lifting it from the underlying fascial sheath and measuring the skin fold or comparing the two sides for symmetry. The skin should move evenly and glide on the underlying tissues. Areas that are stuck, restricted, or too loose should be noted, as should any areas of the skin that become redder than surrounding areas.

Palpation of Superficial Fascia. The third application of palpation is the superficial connective tissue/superficial fascia, which separates and connects the skin and muscle tissue. It allows the skin to glide over the muscles during movement. This layer of tissue is found by using compression until the fibers of the underlying muscle are felt. The pressure then should be lightened so that the muscle cannot be felt, but if the hand is moved, the skin also moves. This area feels a little like a very thin water balloon. The tissue should feel resilient and springy, like gelatin. The superficial fascia holds fluid and fat. If surface edema is

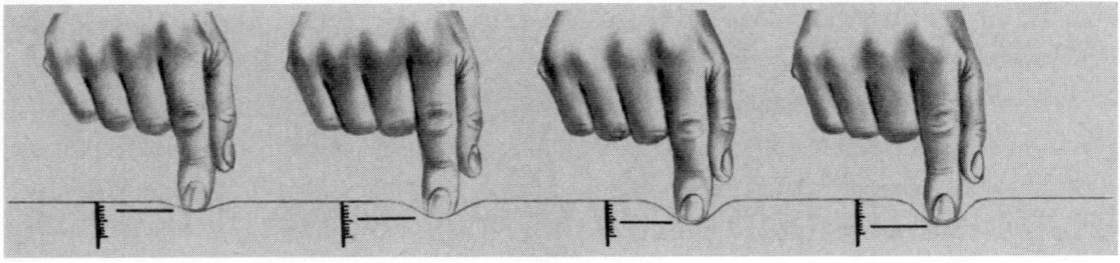
1+ Slight pitting, no visible distortion, disappears rapidly
2+ Somewhat deeper pit than in 1+, no readily detectable distortion, disappears in 10-15 sec
3+ Pit noticeably deep, may last more than a minute; the dependent extremity is swollen
4+ Pit very deep, lasts 2-5 min; dependent extremity is grossly distorted

FIGURE 9-14 ■ Assessment scale for pitting edema. (From *Mosby's nursing PDQ*, St Louis, 2004, Mosby.)

present, it is this tissue layer. This water-binding quality gives the area the feel of a water balloon, but it should not feel boggy or soggy or show pitting edema (i.e., the dent from the pressure stays in the skin) (Figure 9-14).

As mentioned previously, methods of palpation that lift the skin, such as kneading and skin rolling, provide much information. Depending on the area of the body and the concentration of underlying connective tissue, the skin should lift and roll easily. Loosening of these areas is very beneficial, and the therapist can achieve this by applying kneading and skin rolling methods slowly and deliberately, allowing for a shift in the tissues. A constant drag should be kept on the tissues, because both the skin and superficial connective tissue are affected.

Any areas that become redder than the surrounding tissue or that stay red longer than other areas are suspect for connective tissue changes. Usually, lifting and stretching of the reddened tissue (bend, shear, and torsion force) or use of the myofascial approaches can normalize these areas.

Palpation of Vessels and Lymph Nodes. The fourth application of palpation involves the circulatory vessels and lymph nodes. Just above the muscle and still in the superficial connective tissue lie the more superficial blood vessels. The vessels are distinct and feel like soft tubes. Pulses can be palpated, but if pressure is too intense, the feel of the pulse is lost. Feeling for pulses helps detect this layer of tissue.

In this same area are the more superficial lymph vessels and lymph nodes. Lymph nodes usually are located in joint areas and feel like small, soft gel caps. A patient with enlarged lymph nodes should be referred to a physician immediately. Enlarged lymph nodes may indicate local or systemic infection or more serious conditions.

Vessels should feel firm but pliable and supported. If any areas of bulging, mushiness, or constriction are noted, the therapist should refer the patient to a physician.

Pulses should be compared by feeling for a strong, even, full-pumping action on both sides of the body. If differences are perceived, the therapist should refer the patient to a physician. Sometimes the differences in the pulses can be attributed to soft tissue restriction of the artery or a more serious condition that can be diagnosed by the physician. Refill of capillaries in nail beds should be approximately 3 to 5 seconds and equal in all fingers.

Palpation of Skeletal Muscles. The fifth application of palpation is skeletal muscle. Muscle has a distinct fiber direction that can be felt. This texture feels somewhat like corded fabric or fine rope. Muscle is made up of contractile fibers embedded in connective tissue. The area of the muscle that becomes the largest when the muscle is concentrically contracted is in the belly of the muscle. Where the muscle fibers end and the connective tissue continues, the tendon develops; this is called the *musculotendinous junction*. It is a good practice activity to locate both of these areas for all surface muscles and as many underlying ones as possible. Almost all muscular dysfunctions, such as trigger points or microscarring from minute muscle tears, are found at the musculotendinous junction or in the belly of the muscle. Most acupressure points and/or motor points are also located in these areas.

Often three or more layers of muscle are present in an area. These layers are separated by fascia, and each muscle layer should slide over the one beneath it. It is important to compress systematically through each layer until the bone is felt. Pressure used to reach and palpate the deeper layers of muscle must travel from the superficial layers down to the deeper layers. To accomplish this, the compressive force must be even, broad based, and slow. The touch should not have a "poking" quality, and abrupt pressure should not be used to push through muscle layers, because the surface layers of muscle will tense up and guard, preventing access to the deeper layers. Muscle tends to push up against palpating pressure when it is concentrically contracting. Having the patient slowly move the affected joint can aid identification of the proper location of muscles being assessed.

Each layer of muscle must be slid back and forth over the underlying layer to make sure there is no adherence between the muscle layers. The layers usually run cross-grain to each other. The best example of this is the abdominal muscle group. Even in the arm and leg, where all the muscles seem to run in the same direction, a diagonal crossing and spiraling of the muscle groups is evident. Muscles can feel tense and ropy in both concentric (short) and eccentric (long) patterns. Therefore think of muscle functioning as short and tight and as long and taut (Figure 9-15).

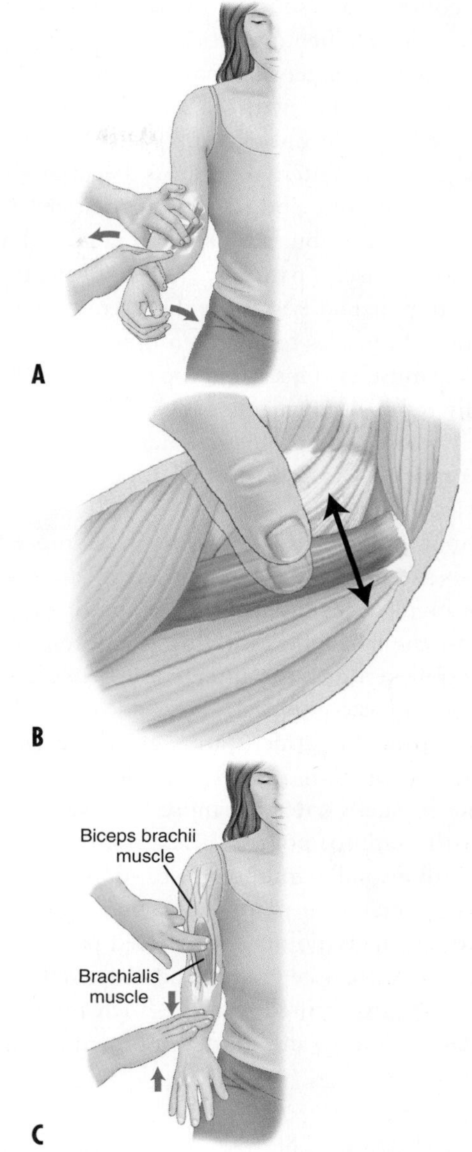

FIGURE 9-15 ■ Palpation. (From Muscolino JE: *Kinesiology: the skeletal system and muscle function,* enhanced edition, St Louis, 2006, Mosby.)

Skeletal muscle is assessed both for texture and for function. It should be firm and pliable. Soft, spongy muscle or hard, dense muscle indicates connective tissue dysfunction. Muscle atrophy results in a muscle that feels smaller than normal. Hypertrophy results in a muscle that feels larger than normal. Application of the appropriate techniques can normalize the connective tissue component of the muscle. Excessively strong or weak muscles can be caused by problems with neuromuscular control or imbalanced work or exercise demand. Weak muscle can be a result of wasting (atrophy) of the muscle fibers and neuroinhibition.

Tension can be felt in muscles that are either concentrically short or eccentrically long. Tension that manifests in short muscles that are concentrically contracted results in tissue that feels hard and bunched. When muscles are tense from being pulled into an extension pattern, they feel like long, taut bundles with some contraction and shortened muscle fiber groups. Usually, flexors, adductors, and internal rotators become short, whereas extensors, abductors, and external rotators palpate tense but are long and taut, and have eccentric muscle patterns. Massage treatment most often first addresses the short, concentrically contracted muscles to lengthen them rather than the long muscles. This is because massage methods usually result in longer tissues, which would ultimately worsen the problem. Therapeutic exercise is necessary to restore normal tone to the long muscles.

Spot work on isolated areas is seldom effective. Neurologic muscle imbalances are kinetic chain interactions linked by reflex patterns, most notably the gait reflexes, righting reflexes, oculopelvic reflexes, and the interaction between postural and phasic muscles.

Important treatment areas are the musculotendinous junction and the muscle belly, where the nerve usually enters the muscle. As was pointed out earlier, motor points cause a muscle contraction with a small stimulus. Disruption of sensory signals at the motor point causes many problems, including trigger points and referred pain, hypersensitive acupressure points, and restricted movement patterns caused by the increase in the physiologic barrier and the development of pathologic barriers.

Palpation of Tendons. The sixth application of palpation is the tendons. Tendons have a higher concentration of collagen fibers and feel more pliable and less ribbed than muscle. Tendons feel like duct tape. Under many tendons is a fluid-filled bursa cushion that assists the movement of the bone under the tendon.

Tendons should feel elastic and mobile. If a tendon has been torn, it may adhere to the underlying bone during the healing process. Some tendons, such as those of the fingers and toes, are enclosed in a sheath and must be able to glide within the sheath. If they cannot glide, inflammation builds, and the result is tenosynovitis. Overuse also can cause inflammation. Inflammation signals the formation of connective tissue, which can interfere with movement and cause the tendons to adhere to surrounding tissue. In tendons without a sheath, this condition is called *tendinitis.* Frictioning techniques help these conditions. Usually, tight tendon structures normalize when the muscle's resting length is normalized.

Palpation of Fascial Sheaths/Deep Fascia. The seventh application of palpation is the fascial sheaths. Fascial sheaths, which feel like sheets of plastic wrap, separate muscles and expand the connective tissue area of bone for muscular attachment. Some, such as the lumbodorsal fascia, the abdominal fascia, and the iliotibial band, run on the surface of the body and are thick, like a tarp. Others, such as the linea alba and the nuchal ligament, run perpendicular to the surface of the body and the bone like a rope. Still others run horizontally through the body. The horizontal pattern occurs at joints, the diaphragm muscle (which is mostly connective tissue), and the pelvic floor. Fascial sheaths separate muscle groups. They provide a continuous, interconnected framework for the body that follows the principles of tensegrity. Fascial sheaths are kept taut by the design of the cross-pattern and the action of muscles that lie between sheaths, such as the gluteus maximus, which lies between the iliotibial band and the lumbodorsal fascia and smooth muscle bundles embedded in the fascia.

The larger nerves and blood vessels lie in grooves created by the fascial separations. Careful comparison reveals that the location of the traditional acupuncture meridians corresponds to these nerve and blood vessel tracts. The fascial separations can be made more distinct and more pliable by palpating them with the fingers. With sufficient pressure, the fingers tend to fall into these grooves, which can then be followed. These areas need to be resilient but distinct, because they serve both as stabilizers and separators.

Fascial sheaths should be pliable, but because they are stabilizers, they may be denser than tendons in some areas. Problems arise if the fascial sheaths become stuck (adhere) to the adjacent tissue.

Myofascial approaches are best suited for dealing with fascial sheath dysfunction. Mechanical work, such as slow, sustained stretching, and methods that pull and drag on the tissue are used to soften the sheaths. Because this often is uncomfortable for the patient, causing a burning, stretching sensation, the work should not be done unless the patient is committed to regular appointments until the area is normalized. This may take 6 months to 1 year.

Chronic health conditions almost always show dysfunction in the connective tissue and fascial sheaths. Any techniques discussed as connective tissue approaches are effective as long as the therapist proceeds slowly and follows the tissue pattern. The massage therapist should not override the tissue or force the tissue into a corrective pattern. Instead, the tissue must be untangled or unwound gradually.

As mentioned, fascial separations between muscles create pathways for the nerves and blood vessels. When palpated, these pathways feel like grooves running between muscles. Narrowing or restriction of these areas may cause constriction of blood vessels and impingement upon the nerves. A slow, specific, stripping/gliding along these pathways can be beneficial. The nerves run in these fascial pathways, and the nerve trunks correlate with the traditional meridian system. Therefore most meridian and acupressure work takes place along these fascial grooves.

Muscle layers are also separated by fascia, and because muscles must be able to slide over each other, the massage therapist must make sure there is no adherence between muscles. This situation often occurs in the legs and anterior thorax. If assessment indicates that the muscles are stuck to each other, kneading and gliding can be used to slide one muscle layer over the other.

Water is an important element of connective tissue. To keep connective tissue soft, the patient must rehydrate.

Palpation of Ligaments. The eighth application of palpation is the ligaments. Most ligaments feel like bungee cords, and some are flat. Ligaments should be flexible enough to allow the joint to move, yet stable enough to restrict movement. It is important to be able to recognize a ligament and not mistake it for a tendon. With the joint in the midrange position, if muscles are isometrically contracted, the tendon moves but the ligament does not.

Palpation of Joints. The ninth application of palpation is the joints. Careful palpation should reveal the space between the synovial joint ends. Joints often feel like hinges. Most assessment is done with active and passive joint movements. An added source of information is palpation of the joint while it is in motion. The sense should be a stable, supported, resilient, and unrestricted range of motion.

As previously stated, with joint movements it is important to assess for end-feel. Simply, end-feel is the perception of the joint at the limit of its range of motion, and it is either soft or hard. In most joints it should feel soft. This means that the body is unable to move any more through muscular contraction, but a small additional move by the massage therapist still produces some give. A hard end-feel is what the bony stabilization of the elbow feels like on extension. No more active movement is possible, and passive movement is restricted by bone.

Movement of the joints through comfortable ranges of motion can be used as an evaluation method. Comparison of the symmetry of range of motion (e.g., comparing the circumduction pattern of one arm against that of the other) is effective for detecting limitations of a particular movement.

Muscle energy methods, as well as all massage manipulations, can be used to support symmetric range of motion functions. All these tissues and structures are supported by general massage applications, which result in increased circulation, increased pliability of soft tissue, and normalized neuromuscular patterns.

Massage can positively affect the normal limits of the physiologic barrier. When joints are traumatized, the surrounding tissue becomes "scared," almost as if saying, "This joint will never get in that position again." When this happens, all the proprioceptive mechanisms reset to limit the range of motion, setting up a pathologic barrier. Massage and appropriate muscle lengthening and general stretching, combined with muscle energy techniques and self-help, can have a beneficial effect on ligaments, joint function, and bone health. Ligaments are relatively slow to regenerate, and it takes time to notice prolonged improvement.

Palpation of Bones. The tenth application of palpation is the bones. Those who have developed their palpation skills find a firm but detectable pliability to bone. Bones feel like young sapling tree trunks and branches. For the massage therapist, it is important to be able to palpate the bony landmarks that indicate the tendinous attachment points for the muscles and to trace the bone's shape.

Palpation of the Abdominal Viscera. The eleventh application of palpation is the viscera. The abdomen contains the *viscera,* or internal organs of the body. It is important for the massage professional to know the positioning of the organs in the abdominal cavity and to be able to locate these organs. The massage therapist should be able to palpate the distinct firmness of the liver and the large intestine. The patient should be referred to a physician if any hard, rigid, stiff, painful, or tense areas are noted in the abdomen.

Close attention must be paid to the visceral referred pain areas. If tissue changes are noted, the therapist must refer the patient to a physician. The skin often is tighter in areas of visceral referred pain. Because cutaneous/visceral reflexes are a factor, stretching the skin in these areas may be beneficial. Some evidence indicates that normalizing the skin over these areas has a positive effect on the functioning of the organ. If nothing else, circulation is increased and peristalsis (intestinal movement) may be stimulated.

In accordance with the recommendations for colon massage, repetitive stroking in the proper directions may stimulate smooth muscle contraction and can improve elimination problems and intestinal gas (Figure 9-16). Also, psoas work often is done through the abdomen.

Palpation of Body Rhythms. The twelfth application of palpation is the body rhythms. Body rhythms are felt as even pulsations. Body rhythms, those mentioned and not mentioned, are designed to operate in a coordinated, balanced, and synchronized manner. In the body the rhythms all entrain. When palpating body rhythms, the therapist should get a sense of this harmony. Although the trained hand can pick out some of the individual rhythms, just as one can hear individual notes in a song, it is the whole connected effect that is important. When a person feels "off" or "out of sync," often the individual is speaking of disruption in the entrainment process of body rhythms.

Respiration. The breathing rhythm is easy to feel. It should be even and should follow good principles of inhalation and exhalation. Palpation of the breath is done by placing the hands over the ribs and allowing the body to go through three or more cycles as the therapist evaluates the evenness and fullness of the breath. Relaxed breathing should result in a slight rounding of the upper abdomen and lateral movement of the lower ribs during inhalation. Movement in the shoulders or upper chest indicates potential difficulties with the breathing mechanism.

Improved breathing function helps the entire body. The muscular mechanism for inhalation and exhalation of air is designed like a simple bellows system and depends on unrestricted movement of the musculoskeletal components of the thorax. The muscles of respiration include the scalenes, intercostals, anterior serratus, diaphragm, abdominals, and pelvic floor muscles. If a breathing pattern disorder is a factor and if the person is prone to anxiety, intervention softens and normalizes the upper body and supports the breathing mechanism.

Because of the whole body interplay between muscle groups in all actions, a not uncommon finding is tight lower leg and foot muscles that interfere with breathing.

Disruption of function in any of these muscle groups inhibits full and easy breathing.

General relaxation massage and stress reduction methods seem to help breathing the most. The patient can be taught slow lengthening and stretching methods and the breathing retraining pattern. More serious dysfunction should be referred to a respiratory therapist. The patient also can be advised not to wear restrictive clothing or hold in the stomach.

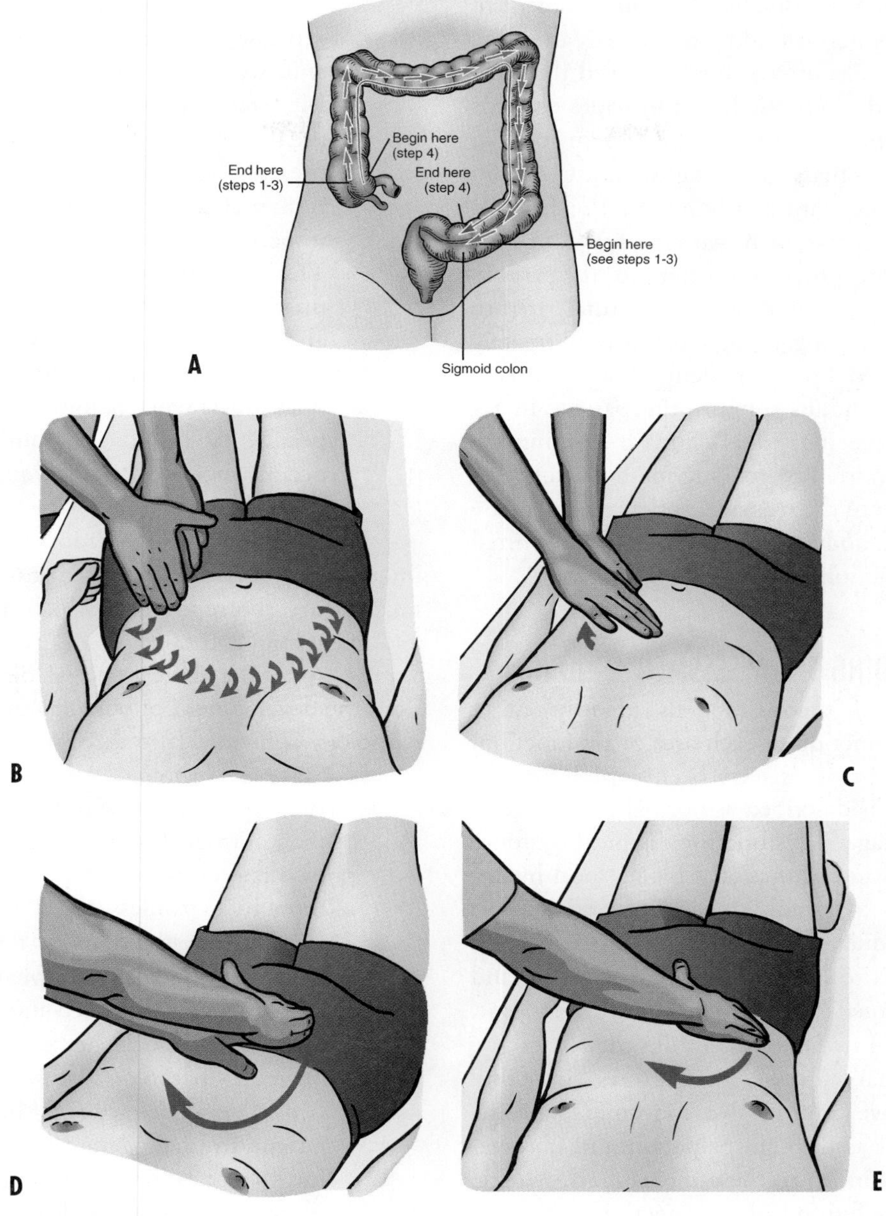

FIGURE 9-16 ■ Abdominal massage.

The circulation movement of the blood is felt at the major pulse points. The pulses should be balanced on both sides of the body. Basic palpation of the movement of the blood is done by placing the fingertips over pulse points on both sides of the body and comparing for evenness.

The vascular refill rate is another means of assessing the efficiency and rhythm of the circulation. To assess this rate, press the nail beds until they blanch (push blood out), then let go and count the seconds until color returns; normal is 3 to 5 seconds.

Many other biologic oscillators function in a rhythmic pattern. They are more difficult to palpate, but they contribute to the rhythmic pulsation of the body. The body rhythms are assessed before and after the massage. An improvement in rate and evenness should be noticed after the massage. Massage offered by a centered therapist with a focused, rhythmic intent provides patterns for the patient's body to use to entrain its own rhythms. The massage therapist must remain focused on the natural rhythm of the patient. Although the entrainment pattern of the therapist and the massage provides a pattern for the patient, it should not superimpose an unnatural rhythm on the patient. Any foreign patterns ultimately will be rejected by the patient's body. Instead, the therapist should support the patient in re-establishing the individual's innate entrainment rhythm. Supported by rocking methods, a rhythmic approach to the massage, and appropriate use of music, the body can re-establish synchronized rhythmic function (Figure 9-17).

UNDERSTANDING THE ASSESSMENT FINDINGS

The results of the assessment identify either appropriate function of each area or dysfunction. When all assessments have been completed, the overall result is described as normal or as stage 1, stage 2, or stage 3 dysfunction. Typical dysfunction includes local functional block, local hypermobility or hypomobility, an altered muscle activation sequence, and postural imbalance, all of which lead to changes in motor function and are accompanied by temporary or chronic joint, muscular, and nervous system disorders.

Functional assessment defines mobility through active and passive movements of the body, as well as through palpation and observation of a distortion in these movements. Muscle testing and definition of the functional relationships of muscles are also performed.

Often, distortions in functioning are measured and categorized in the following manner:

- First-degree dysfunction: Shortening or weakening of some muscles or the formation of local changes in tension or connective tissue in these muscles. For usual and simple movements, a person has to use additional muscles from different parts of the body. As a result, movement becomes uneconomical and labored.
- Second-degree dysfunction: Moderately expressed shortening of postural muscles and weakening of antagonist muscles. Moderately peculiar postures and movements of some parts of the body are present. Postural and movement distortion, such as altered firing patterns, begin to occur.
- Third-degree dysfunction: Clearly expressed shortening of postural muscles and weakening of antagonist muscles with the appearance of specific, nonoptimal movement. Significantly expressed peculiarity in postures and movement occurs. Increased postural and movement distortions result.

To determine the appropriate therapeutic intervention, it is very important to define which muscles are shortened and which are inhibited and likely long and taut.

Based on the three levels of distorted function, the development of postural and movement pathology is divided into three stages:

- Stage 1 pathology—functional tension: At this stage, a person tires more quickly than normal. This fatigue is accompanied by first- or second-degree limitation of mobility, painless local myodystonia (changes in the muscle tension/length relationship), postural imbalance in the first or second degree, and nonoptimal motor function of the first degree.
- Stage 2 pathology—functional stress: This stage is characterized by a feeling of fatigue from moderate activity, discomfort, slight pain, and the appearance of singular or multiple degrees of limited mobility that is painless or that results in first-degree pain. It may be accompanied by local hypermobility. Functional stress is also characterized by reflex vertebral-sensory dysfunction, fascial and connective tissue changes, and regional postural imbalance. It also is accompanied by first- or second-degree distortion of motor function in the muscle activation sequence and by pattern alterations.
- Stage 3 pathology—connective tissue changes in the musculoskeletal system:

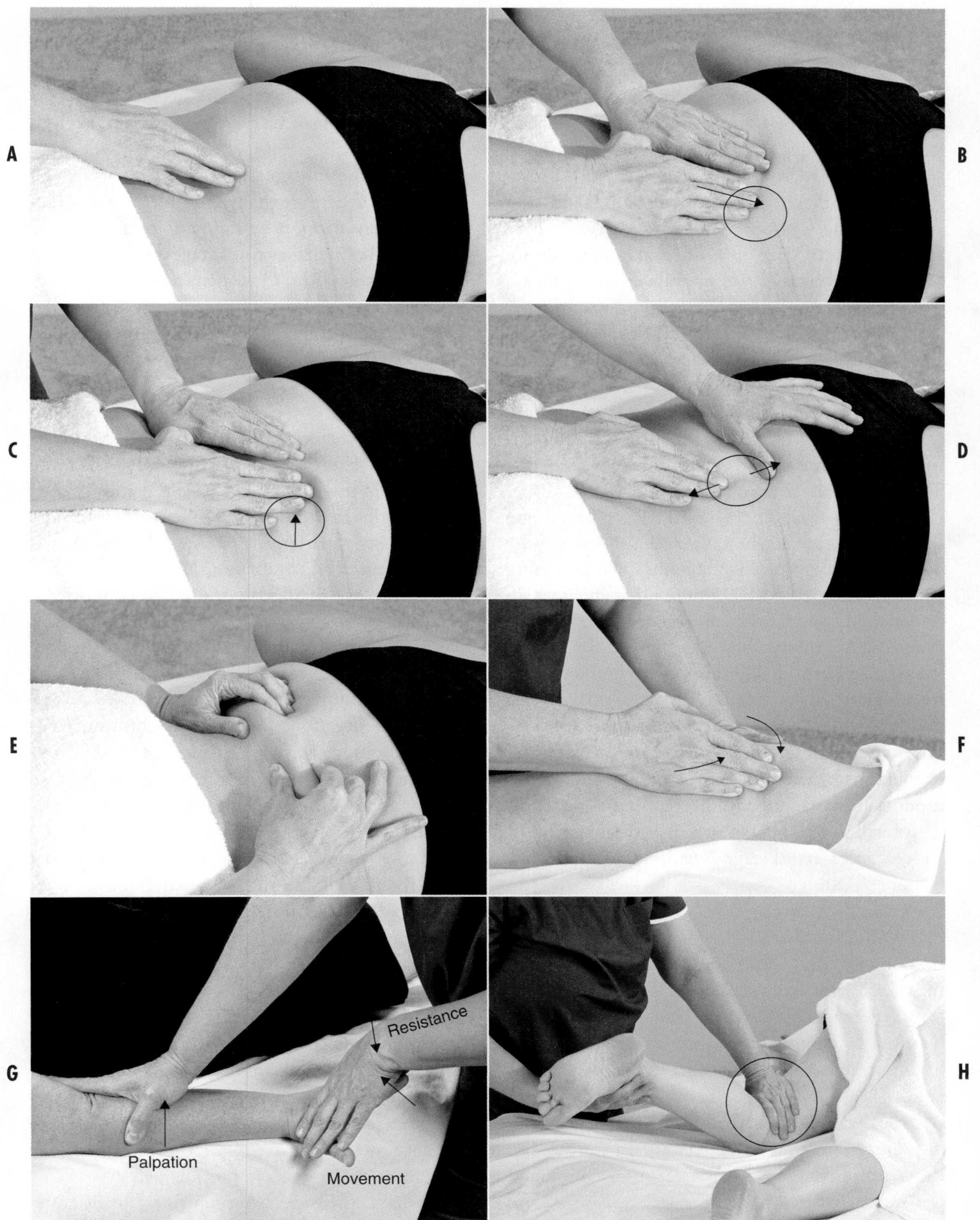

FIGURE 9-17 ■ Examples of palpation. **A,** Skin drag. **B,** Tissue movement, ease. **C,** Tissue movement, bind. **D,** Skin stretching. **E,** Skin fold. **F,** Sliding tissue layers. **G,** Palpating muscle. **H,** Palpating tendons and ligaments.

Connective tissue changes are caused by overloading, disturbances of tissue nutrition, microtrauma, microhemorrhage, unresolved edema, and other *endogenous* (inside the body) and *exogenous* (outside the body) factors. Hereditary predisposition is also a consideration. In a stage 3 pathologic condition, changes in the spine and weight-bearing joints may appear, with areas of local hypermobility and instability of several vertebral motion segments; hypomobility; widespread, painful muscle tension; fascial and connective tissue changes in the muscles; second- or third-degree regional postural imbalance in many joints; and temporary nonoptimal motor function with second- or third-degree distortion. Visceral disturbances may be present.

Stage 1 pathologic conditions (functional tension) often can be managed effectively by massage methods and by therapists with training equivalent to 500 to 1000 hours that includes an understanding of the information presented in entry level textbooks and technical training in the chosen method. This level of care often occurs in wellness environments and preventive care. Working with stage 2 and stage 3 pathologic conditions (functional stress and connective tissue changes) usually requires more training and proper supervision within a multidisciplinary approach. This textbook covers the information necessary to address stage 2 and stage 3 pathologic conditions (Figure 9-18).

Resourceful Compensation

Assessment also identifies areas of resourceful (i.e., successful) compensation. These compensation patterns occur when the body has been required to adapt to some sort of trauma or repetitive use pattern. Permanent adaptive changes, although not as efficient as optimal functioning, are the best pattern the body can develop in response to an irreversible change in the system. Resourceful compensation is not to be eliminated but supported.

Years of clinical experience have taught many therapists that most symptoms and dysfunctional patterns are compensatory patterns. Some problems are recent, and some qualify for archaeologic exploration, having developed in early life and compounded through time. Compensatory patterns often are complex, but the patient's body frequently can show us the way if we can listen to the story it tells.

The importance of compensation must be considered. There are many examples of **resourceful compensation,** a term used for the adjustments the body makes to manage a permanent or chronic dysfunction. One such example is protective muscle spasm (guarding) around a compressed disk. The splinting action of the spasms protects the nerves and provides additional stability in the area.

Decisions must be made about how and to what degree the compensatory pattern should be altered. It seems prudent to assume that the body knows what it is doing. The wise therapist spends time coming to understand the reasons for the compensatory patterns presented by the body. When resourceful compensation is present, therapeutic massage methods are used to support the altered pattern and prevent any more increase in postural distortion than is necessary to support the body change (compensation).

Some compensatory patterns are set up for short-term situations that do not require permanent adaptation. Having a leg in a cast and walking on crutches for a time is a classic example. The body catching itself during an "almost" fall is another classic set-up pattern. Unfortunately, the body often habituates these patterns and maintains them well beyond their usefulness. Over time, the body begins to show symptoms of pain, inefficient function, or both.

Many compensatory patterns develop to maintain a balanced posture, and even though the posture becomes distorted during compensation, the overall result is a balanced body in a gravitational line. It also is important to consider the pattern of muscle interactions, such as the ones that occur when walking, and to recognize that gait has a certain pattern for the most efficient movement that the body can manage.

No set system exists for figuring out the compensatory patterns. All these factors must be considered in devising a plan that best serves the patient.

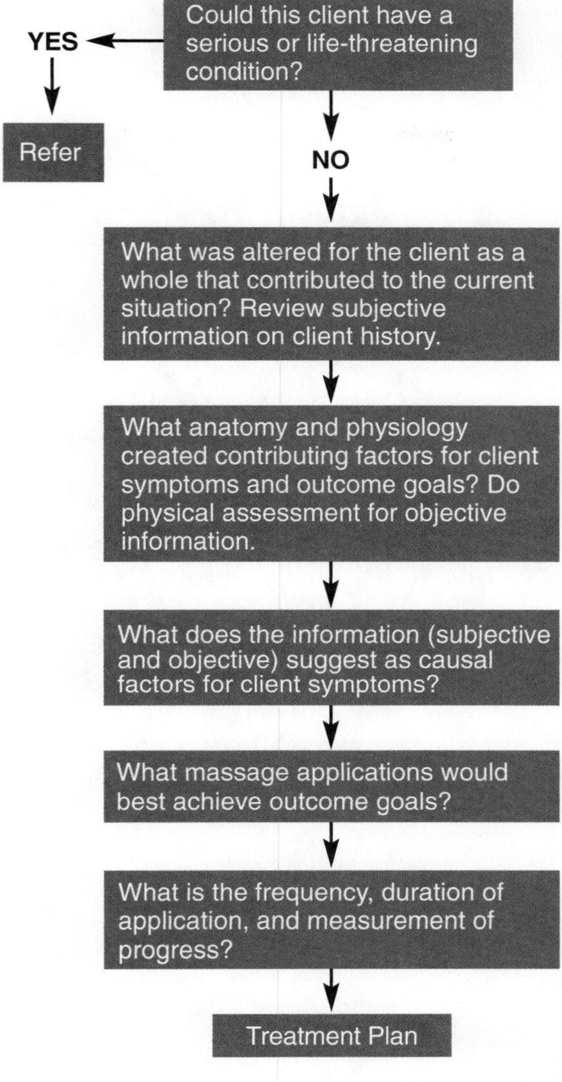

FIGURE 9-18 ■ Algorithm for development of a treatment plan.

ORGANIZING THE ASSESSMENT INFORMATION INTO TREATMENT STRATEGIES

If the massage therapist is working in a team environment, the physician does most of the assessment in conjunction with the physician assistant, nurse practitioner, physical therapist, or other health professionals. These team members also inform the massage therapist of the treatment plan and outcome goals. This does not mean that the massage therapist does not also do an assessment to identify the focus for massage application.

The body is an interrelated, relatively symmetric functional form. Both for assessment purposes and treatment approaches, it is helpful to consider these interrelationships. Science does not totally understand how our molecules stay together, let alone how the body constantly adapts, second by second, to internal and external environmental demands. Yet natural design is usually very simple and set up in repeating patterns that function together for efficiency.

The most recognized control of these interrelationships exists in the nervous system, especially various reflexes (i.e., oculopelvic, crossed extensor, withdrawal, gait, and other such patterns). Observation of the body reveals structural similarity in the design of the shoulder and pelvic girdles and the upper and lower limbs. It is logical to assume that similarly shaped areas function in similar ways.

The axial skeleton does not appear to show the similarity in design that the appendicular skeletal does; however, with a bit of imagination, it is there. Consider the rib cage as the central point: above it, you have the cervical vertebrae and the head; below it, the lumbar, sacrum, and coccyx (what is left of a tail). Most biologic forms have a head at one end and a tail at the other. Imagine if we could put a second head at the end of the coccyx, and there you go: symmetry.

The principles of postural balance and mobility factor in. The axial skeleton displays a mirror image as a top/bottom with the midpoint about the navel. Therefore, the imaginary head pairs with the real head, the coccyx pairs with the atlas, the axis with the sacrum, and the lumbar area with the cervical area. This mirror image can be considered functional for posture and stability. The muscles pair as follows: the occipital base and suprahyoids with the pelvic floor; the sternocleidomastoid and longus colli with the psoas and rectus abdominis; the scalenes with the quadratus lumborum; the internal and external intercostals with the internal and external obliques; and the transverse thoracis with the transverse abdominis. On the dorsal aspect of the thorax, you find the posterior serratus superior and inferior paired. Muscles that are oriented more vertically, such as the rectus abdominis and erector spinae group, pair on the dorsal and ventral aspects. If the pairs are also agonist/antagonists, either a reciprocal inhibition pattern can occur or a co-contraction situation can arise.

Therefore, if a patient has a short psoas, the sternocleidomastoid and longus colli may also be short. If the scalenes are short, the quadratus lumborum may show reflex shortening. Dysfunction in the occipital base may also involve pelvic floor dysfunction.

The girdles and limbs that attach to the axial skeleton move in contralateral patterns, the left lower with the right upper, and so forth. The scapula and clavicle pair with the pelvis. The SI joint pairs with both sternoclavicular joints. The humerus and femur, the tibia/fibula and radius/ulna, the carpals and tarsals, the metacarpals and metatarsals, the phalanges with the corresponding phalanges, the hip and shoulder joints, the elbow and knee, the ankle and wrist, and the foot and hand are all functional pairings.

This symmetry of the functional aspect of the axial soft tissue corresponds: the rotator cuff muscles with the deep lateral hip rotators; the deltoid with the gluteal group; the pectoralis minor and coracobrachialis with the pectineus; the pectoralis major and latissimus dorsi with the adductors; the quadriceps with the triceps and anconeus; the hamstrings with the biceps brachii; the brachialis with the popliteus; the wrist and finger flexors with the ankle plantar flexors; the wrist and finger extensors with the dorsiflexors; the supinators with the inverters and the pronators with the everters; and finally, the palm of the hand with the sole of the foot. These relationships should be easy to conceptualize (Figure 9-19).

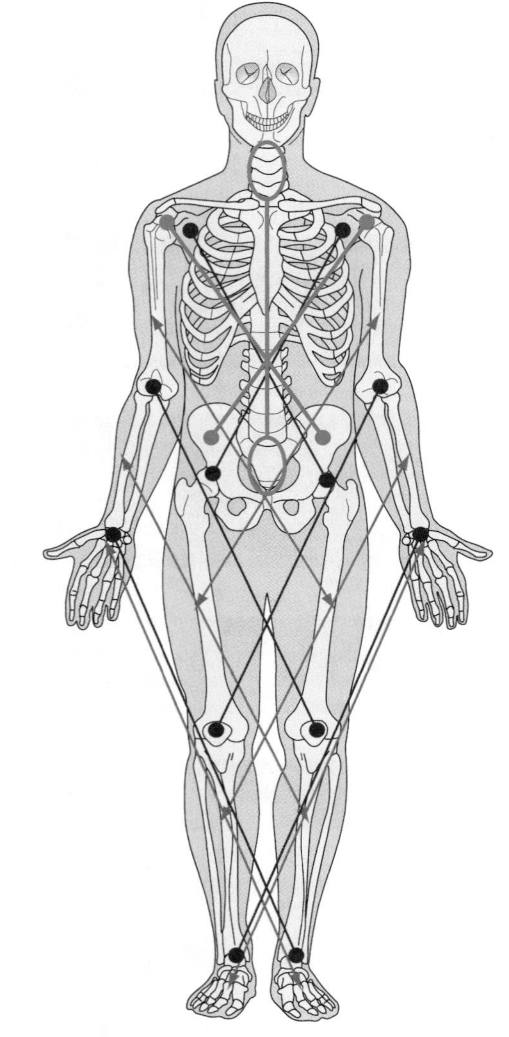

FIGURE 9-19 ■ Areas of symmetry. Arm/thigh, forearm/leg, hand/foot, shoulder/hip, elbow/knee, wrist/ankle, cervical spine/sacrum, and shoulder girdle/pelvic girdle. (From Fritz S: *Sports and exercise massage: comprehensive care in athletics, fitness, and rehabilitation,* St Louis, 2006, Mosby.)

Remember, a counterbalancing cross-pattern exists in the appendicular skeleton; therefore, again, the left arm pairs with the right leg and the right arm with the left leg. Consequently, a patient with a short hamstring on the left may also have a short biceps brachii on the right. A bruise on the right quadriceps may result in reflex guarding in the left triceps. A great toe sprain on the right may result in reflexive guarding in the left thumb. Bilateral short gastrocnemius muscles may reflexively include short wrist flexors bilaterally. Guarding patterns for a knee injury may occur reflexively around the opposite elbow. Right SI pain may be patterned with left sternoclavicular joint dysfunction. Short, deep lateral hip rotators on the left may involve reflexive guarding in the right rotator cuff, with changes in movement of the shoulder. Restricted shoulder/arm movement on the right may be a lingering response to a previous adductor/groin injury on the left. The possible interactions are numerous.

The simple way to use these potential patterns is in analysis of the assessment and in developing massage applications. For example, a patient has low back pain related to quadratus/psoas shortening. Ask if the person also is experiencing any symptoms in the neck. Assess the range of motion of the neck and palpate for especially tender areas. Before addressing the low back, make sure the scalenes and the sternocleidomastoid muscles are normal, and treat dysfunction with muscle energy methods or direct inhibition while the patient rotates the pelvis in various directions. Continue to assess for areas that overrespond to activation of the quadratus lumborum and psoas movement. Focus on those areas and reassess the low back function. Treat the remaining symptoms of the low back. While addressing the quadratus lumborum and the psoas, have the patient rotate the head in slow, large circles to activate the pattern and facilitate the release.

Another example: A patient was in an accident and has a thigh bruise that cannot be directly massaged other than with lymphatic drainage. To reduce reflexive guarding and pain, massage is applied to the opposite triceps group. The massage therapist may find a surprisingly sore area that corresponds to the location of the bruise.

When working with these patterns, remember the focus of the massage. If the goal of the massage is to increase the mobility of the left ankle, it may be helpful to have the patient slowly move the right wrist in circles; the intent is not to treat the wrist, but to influence the dysfunctional ankle. If the goal of the massage is to manage short hamstrings, the biceps muscle of the arm will be part of the treatment approach. The patient may notice changes in the arm when massage is applied, but he or she should be moving the knees back and forth so that the hamstrings are affected, because this is the goal of the massage.

The general protocol and many of the other specific recommendations for massage incorporate these concepts. Seemly unrelated symptoms are indeed part of the same process.

Additional guidelines for analyzing problems that can be found through the functional biomechanical assessment include the following:

- If an area is hypomobile, consider tension or shortening in the antagonist pattern as a possible cause.
- If an area is hypermobile, consider instability of the joint structure or muscle weakness in the fixation pattern or problems with antagonist/agonist co-contraction function.
- If an area cannot hold against resistance, consider weakness from reciprocal inhibition of the muscles of the prime mover and synergist pattern, as well as tension in the antagonist pattern, as possible causes.
- If pain or heaviness occurs on passive movement, consider joint capsule dysfunction and nerve entrapment syndromes as possible causes.
- If pain occurs on active movement, consider muscle firing patterns (activation sequences) and fascial involvement as a possible cause.
- Always consider body-wide reflexive patterns, as discussed in the sections on posture, gait, and the kinetic chain, as possible causes.

The following guidelines also are important:

- During muscle testing, the ability to easily resist the applied force should be the same or very similar bilaterally.
- Opposite movement patterns should be easy to assume.
- Bilateral asymmetry, pain, weakness, inability to assume the isolation position or to move into the opposite position, fatigue, or a heavy sensation may indicate dysfunction.
- Intervention or referral depends on the severity of the condition (stage 1, 2, or 3) and whether the dysfunction is joint related, neuromuscular related, or myofascial related.

JUST BETWEEN YOU AND ME

This is a lot of assessment. The doctor does assessment, other healthcare providers also assess, and then the massage therapist assesses. The patient can really get tired of assessment. Fortunately, most massage assessment is joint movement, muscle testing, and palpation, which can be structured to look and feel like a massage. The general protocol in Chapter 11 is set up that way. You just have to remember that the massage is assessment, and assessment is listening to what the body is telling you. Make sure to write down what you learn before you forget it. Remember, there is a lot to remember. Also, make sure patients realize that the first few massage sessions are assessment and information-gathering sessions, so that their expectations are realistic. Treatment does not begin until the information has been collected and analyzed; then the massage flows back and forth between assessment and treatment. At least the assessment-based massage does feel like a massage, and the patient will like that.

Whenever I write about or teach assessment, I think of one of my greatest teachers, Dr. David Gurevich. Dr. Gurevich was a Russian physician trained in the 1940s who immigrated to the United States in the early 1990s. He was meticulous about assessment and about understanding the body's story. He taught me many of my assessment skills. I remember once that Dr. Gurevich observed Dr. Leon Chaitow, another renowned expert in the bodywork field, giving a class. Dr. Gurevich later commented that Dr. Chaitow's skills were good, but improvement is always possible. He then drew himself up to his full 5 feet, 4 inches and stated that he would be happy to demonstrate some skills to Dr. Chaitow, since he (Dr. Gurevich) was older and therefore more experienced. Dr. Gurevich died in 1999, and I am thankful that I had the chance to learn from him for almost 8 years. More than anything he taught me to listen, observe, and seek to understand.

evolve 9-5

The following terms and expressions specific to Chapter 9 have already been used to search PubMed for the latest research literature available. The *Click Here for Massage* feature associated with this chapter on your textbook's Evolve website allows you to hyperlink to a continually updated PubMed search of research literature that corresponds to this subject.

Hyperlink Search Terms

Massage assessment
Massage assessment history
Massage care treatment plan
Massage clinical reasoning
Massage gait assessment
Massage healthcare assessment
Massage kinetic
Massage medical records
Massage objective assessment
Massage outcome goals
Massage palpation
Massage physician treatment order
Massage treatment order

SUMMARY

The main purpose of intervention is to help the body regain symmetry and ease of movement. Therefore, when observing gait or posture, the massage therapist should note areas that seem pulled, twisted, or dropped. The therapist's job is to use massage methods to lengthen shortened areas, untwist twisted areas, raise dropped areas, drop raised areas, soften hard areas, firm soft areas, warm cold areas, and cool hot areas.

During the assessment process, careful attention must be paid to the order of priority in which the patient relays the information. If the headache is mentioned first, the knee ache second, and the tight elbow last, the areas should be dealt with in that order, if possible, in the massage flow.

The importance of listening to understand is paramount. Many experienced professionals have learned that if we listen to our patients, they will tell us what is wrong and how to help them restore balance. Slow down, do not jump to conclusions, pay attention, and let the information unfold. Realize that each patient is the expert on himself or herself. Patients teach you about themselves, and in so doing they often begin to understand themselves better. In every session, approach each patient ready to be fascinated with what you will learn from the individual. No textbook, class, or instructor can equal the teaching provided by careful attention to the patient.

WORKBOOK

Because the information in this chapter is skill based, it does not conform well to the question–written response format. Therefore the following exercises are recommended. Using the checklists developed in questions 1 and 2, the student should complete 10 comprehensive assessments using all the methods covered in the chapter.

1. Develop a checklist of all history components covered.

2. Develop a checklist of all physical assessment components covered.

3. Develop a treatment plan based on each assessment.

4. Implement the treatment plan and reassess after 10 sessions. Chart each.

5. Write a postassessment narrative describing the outcomes achieved or not achieved by the patient.

CHAPTER 10 CONCEPT MAP

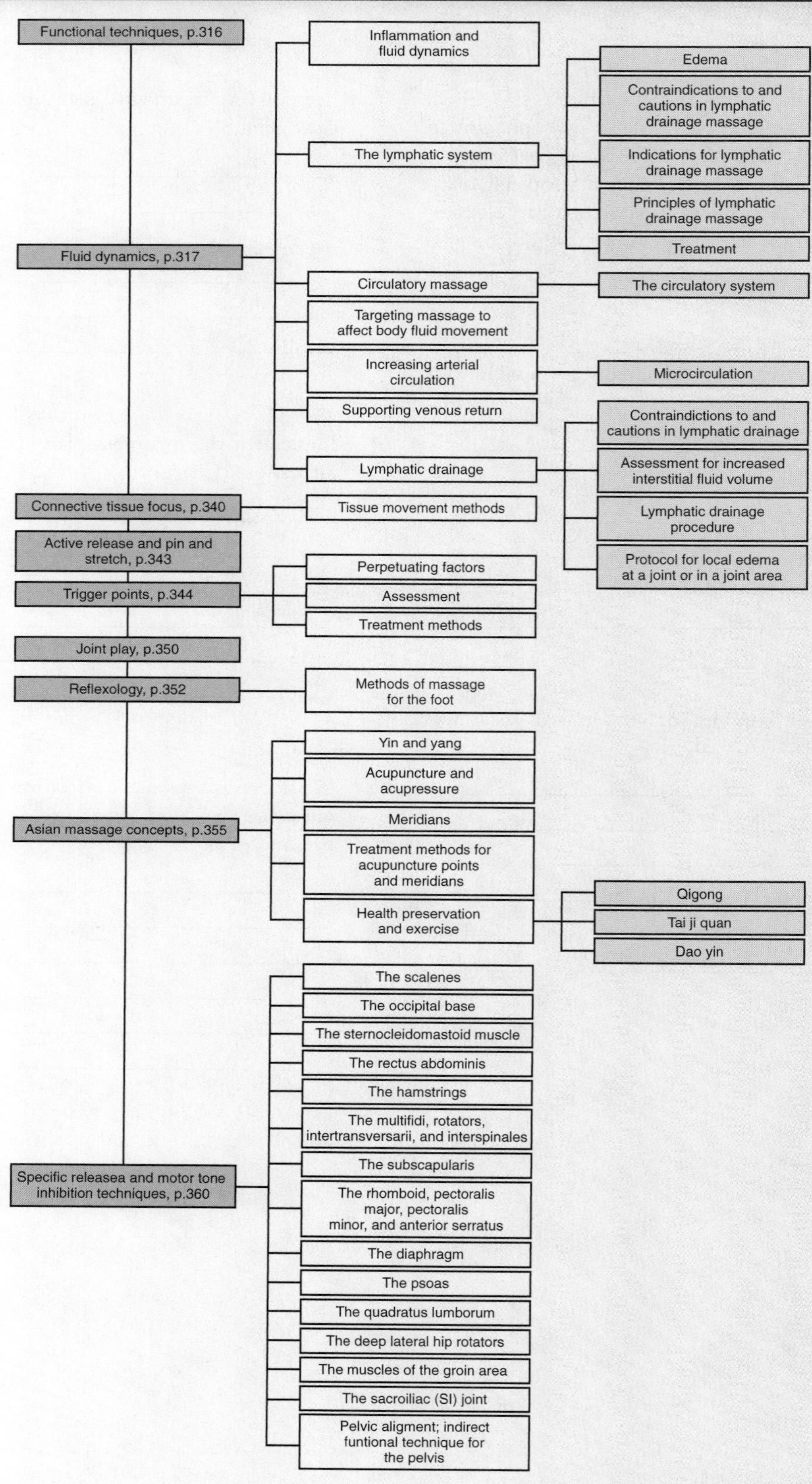

Functional techniques, p.316
Inflammation and fluid dynamics
Edema
Contraindications to and cautions in lymphatic drainage massage
The lymphatic system
Indications for lymphatic drainage massage
Principles of lymphatic drainage massage
Treatment
Fluid dynamics, p.317
Circulatory massage
The circulatory system
Targeting massage to affect body fluid movement
Increasing arterial circulation
Microcirculation
Supporting venous return
Contraindictions to and cautions in lymphatic drainage
Lymphatic drainage
Assessment for increased interstitial fluid volume
Connective tissue focus, p.340
Tissue movement methods
Lymphatic drainage procedure
Active release and pin and stretch, p.343
Perpetuating factors
Protocol for local edema at a joint or in a joint area
Trigger points, p.344
Assessment
Treatment methods
Joint play, p.350
Reflexology, p.352
Methods of massage for the foot
Yin and yang
Acupuncture and acupressure
Asian massage concepts, p.355
Meridians
Treatment methods for acupuncture points and meridians
Qigong
Health preservation and exercise
Tai ji quan
Dao yin
The scalenes
The occipital base
The sternocleidomastoid muscle
The rectus abdominis
The hamstrings
The multifidi, rotators, intertransversarii, and interspinales
The subscapularis
Specific releasea and motor tone inhibition techniques, p.360
The rhomboid, pectoralis major, pectoralis minor, and anterior serratus
The diaphragm
The psoas
The quadratus lumborum
The deep lateral hip rotators
The muscles of the groin area
The sacroiliac (SI) joint
Pelvic aligment; indirect funtional technique for the pelvis

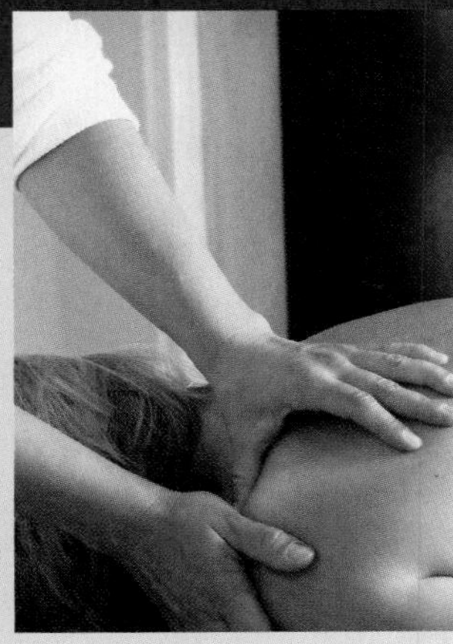

CHAPTER 10

FOCUSED MASSAGE APPLICATION

Key Terms

Active release technique
Acupressure
Acupuncture points
Anterior rotation
Bind
Connective tissue methods
Edema
Fluid dynamics
Indirect functional techniques
Inflare
Joint play
Lymph nodes
Lymphatic drainage massage
Meridians
Mobilization with movement (MWM)
Outflare
Pelvic alignment
Permeability
Pin and stretch technique
Posterior rotation
Reflexology
Sacroiliac (SI) joint
Trigger point
Yang
Yin

For definitions of key terms, refer to the Evolve website.

Objective

Upon completion of this chapter, the reader will have the information necessary to:

1. Correctly perform each of the following:
   - **Indirect functional technique**
   - **Circulation support and lymphatic drainage**
   - **Connective tissue applications**
   - **Trigger point treatment**
   - **Joint play methods**
   - **Reflexology**
   - **Simple acupressure and meridian massage**
   - **Specific releases**

This chapter discusses the use of various massage methods to target specific tissues or body functions. These methods include indirect functional techniques, fluid dynamics, connective tissue techniques, trigger point treatment, joint play methods, reflexology, acupressure, and specific releases. These methods are used as interventions to treat particular conditions. They should be used only if the application can be justified based on assessment findings and/or treatment orders. Some of these methods are intense, and all of them demand some degree of adaptation by the patient. If the patient's adaptive capacity is already strained, these techniques may not be beneficial until the person is in a healthier state and can respond appropriately. Remember, most massage in the medical setting involves generalized, nonspecific stress reduction, relaxation, pain management, and palliative care. None of these methods are nonspecific, and none of them target relaxation.

JUST BETWEEN YOU AND ME

Please don't confuse these specific treatment methods with the concept of medical massage. Most of the time, these methods are too intense and too aggressive to be used on sick or injured people. Clinical/medical massage is not a collection of methods, but rather an appropriate action in the setting of healthcare delivery. Another concept that creates confusion among massage professionals is the idea that orthopedic massage, which targets muscle, skeletal, and joint pathology, is medical massage. Orthopedic massage represents only one small, isolated element of massage therapy in healthcare. Hopefully one of these days the massage community will agree on this stuff.

FUNCTIONAL TECHNIQUES

INDIRECT TECHNIQUES

Functional techniques usually are referred to as *indirect techniques* or *indirect methods of treatment.* These methods are very gentle and safe to use on a fragile patient. Rather than specific modalities, functional indirect methods are concepts that need to be incorporated into the massage application regardless of whether the focus is soft tissue conditions or joint movement. Rather than engaging and attempting (by whatever means) to overcome resistance **(bind),** these methods do the exact opposite. The soft tissue or joint is taken in all directions of the point of maximum ease. The massage therapist simply maintains the joint or tissue in this ease position. No further treatment is done at this point, and after a period of time (a few seconds to a couple of minutes), the position is gently released.

A variation of this technique involves introducing a mild degree of overpressure at the point of maximum ease (the soft tissue actually is taken just into a bit of bind). This produces a reflex release of previously restricted tissues. It is essential that the therapist direct and control all movements. As a refinement of this application, gentle, focused oscillation can be added while the tissue or joint is in the ease position. Vibration, tiny shaking movements, and small, focused rocking are effective. In a further variation, the patient can produce the oscillation with tiny, pulsed movements against resistance provided by the massage therapist. Regardless of how the methods are performed, the underlying principles are the same: assessment of ease and bind and the natural tendency of the body to seek homeostasis.

Soft tissue or joint mobility is assessed for restriction of motion by palpation, range of motion, or both. Any problems then are treated by taking the dysfunctional tissue or joint in the direction of easier movement, which would be away from the restriction or bind and into the way the tissue or joint wants to go in all planes of movement (sagittal, frontal, and transverse). The ease position is held until a sense of softening is perceived. If the massage therapist cannot easily palpate or identify this sensation, the area is held for 30 to 60 seconds.

Breathing, which can increase the ease position, is assessed by inhalation and exhalation. The breath typically is held for a few seconds in the direction that further contributes to the ease of tissue tension. Because this is a noninvasive method, it should be the first approach attempted to normalize soft tissue and joint function.

DIRECT AND COMBINATION TECHNIQUES

Stretching is considered a *direct technique* because it engages the bind and moves through it. Stretching is more invasive than the indirect methods.

A variation of an indirect functional method involves moving back and forth between the ease position and the bind position; this could be described as an *indirect/direct functional technique.* First, the ease position is identified and held as previously described. Then the restrictive barrier of a joint or tissue is engaged in each plane of motion, and the tissue or joint is held taut at the barrier until softening occurs. The corrective activating force then moves slightly through the restrictive barrier, and again the area is held in this position for 30 to 60 seconds until the tissue changes. Various forms of oscillation can be added. Alternating two or three times between direct and indirect application is an effective approach. These methods are integrated into the general protocol in Chapter 11.

Indirect and direct functional methods also form the basis for **connective tissue methods.** An example of an indirect connective tissue technique would be placing a restricted area into the position of least resistance until relaxation occurs. An example of a direct connective tissue method would be placing the affected area against a restrictive barrier with constant force (i.e., stretching) until fascial release occurs.

Ease/indirect and bind/direct techniques can be combined with muscle energy methods. In muscle energy applications, muscle contractions are actively used to support the response. The muscles are placed in a specific direction, which can be either ease or bind, and the patient pushes slowly in a controlled manner against a counterforce that usually is supplied by the massage therapist.

FLUID DYNAMICS

The body is an interconnected network of fluid compartments that contain blood, interstitial fluid, lymph, synovial fluid, and cerebrospinal fluid. Normal flow within tissues and exchange of fluid between compartments are essential for homeostasis. Any impediment to normal flow leads to fluid stagnation, resulting in impaired tissue nutrition and repair. Stagnant tissue fluid becomes toxic and, as the protein content increases, can lead to fibrotic tissue changes.

Fluid tension in the body is called *hydrostatic pressure* (Figure 10-1). Body fluid is characterized as either *extracellular* (outside the cell) or *intracellular* (within the cell). About one third of the body's fluid is extracellular, and it is found in two compartments: (1) the blood circulatory system, including the arteries and veins, and (2) the interstitial anatomic space around cells and the lymphatic vessels.

Fluids also move across compartments, by means of diffusion, from areas of high salt concentration to areas of lower salt concentration. The rate and volume of fluid movement are determined by pumping mechanisms, such as the heart, muscle contraction and relaxation, rhythmic compression of fascial structures during movement, and respiration. The viscosity of a fluid also affects its movement, as do the permeability of the membranes and the size of the

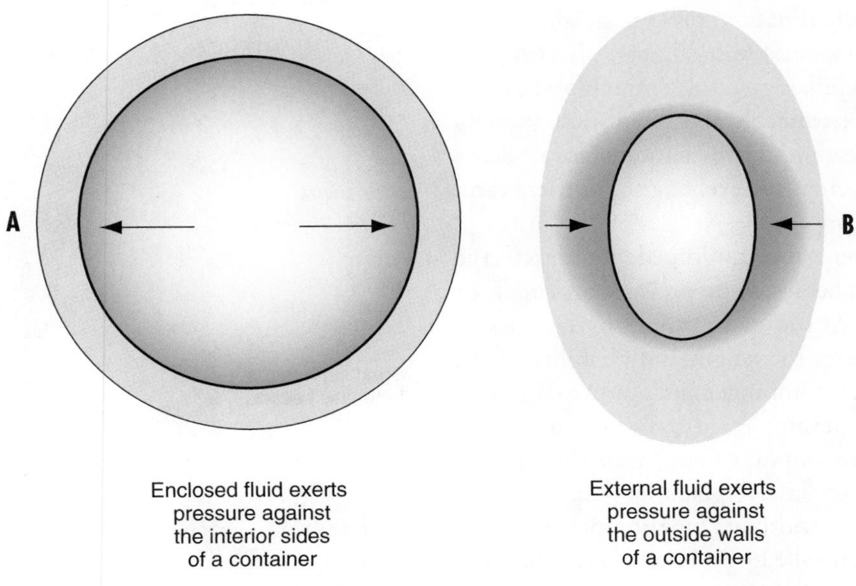
A
B
Enclosed fluid exerts pressure against the interior sides of a container
External fluid exerts pressure against the outside walls of a container

FIGURE 10-1 ■ The effect of hydrostatic pressure. **A,** Enclosed fluid exerts pressure against the interior walls of a container. **B,** External fluid exerts pressure against the outside walls of a container. (From Fritz S: *Sports and exercise massage: comprehensive care in athletics, fitness, and rehabilitation,* St Louis, 2006, Mosby.)

various vessels through which the fluid travels. Massage that addresses the extracellular fluid can mechanically support the movement of fluid within these compartments by stimulating *hydrokinetics* (the transport of fluid) along pressure gradients from high pressure to lower pressure.

Vasodilators and constrictors of the circulatory system affect the movement of body fluid. The mechanical pumping and oscillation applications of massage and the reflexive release of vasodilators (primarily histamine) produced during massage, coupled with the vasodilation or constriction response of hydrotherapy, interact in various ways to influence the outcome of the application.

INFLAMMATION AND FLUID DYNAMICS

Inflammation causes an increase in interstitial fluid, which raises hydrostatic pressure in the area. The tissue swelling causes pain by exerting pressure on pain receptors. This increase in tissue pressure can serve a protective function; it mechanically limits movement, and the pain serves as a warning sign of damage. This process is important during the first few days after an acute illness or injury, but it then needs to begin to reverse itself to allow normal healing to take place. The inflammatory process heightens the influence of chemical vasodilators, affecting the venules and capillaries. Locally, the blood vessels become more permeable and blood flow velocity declines; this leads to the formation of local edema and stasis, with reduced exchange of nutrients and waste products.

Other factors also can impede fluid exchange in the tissue. These include pressure on vessels or a reduction in tissue space caused by changes in muscle tone or in the length and pliability of the fascia or by bony impingement. In carpal tunnel syndrome, for example, fascial shortening and edema result in impingement upon the median nerve. Restoring fascial pliability and reducing edema supports normal functioning. Massage treatment uses tensile forces to elongate shortened connective tissue; compressive forces to support the body's pumping action, encouraging the movement of tissue fluid; and neuromuscular applications to reduce and normalize muscle tone.

THE LYMPHATIC SYSTEM

All massage stimulates the circulation and lymph movement. The lymphatic system drains fluid from around the cells through a system of filters. Interstitial fluid becomes lymph fluid once it enters the lymphatic capillaries.

The lymphatic system permeates the entire tissue structure of the body in a one-way drainage network of vessels, ducts, nodes, lacteals, and lymphoid organs. Segments of lymph capillaries are divided by one-way valves and a spiral set of smooth muscles called *lymphangions.* This system moves fluid against gravity in a peristalsis-type undulation.

The lymphatic tubes merge into one another until major channels and vessels are formed. These vessels run from the distal parts of the body toward the neck, usually alongside veins and arteries. Valves in the vessels prevent the back flow of lymph.

Lymph nodes are enlarged portions of the lymph vessels that generally cluster at the joints. This arrangement assists movement of the lymph through the nodes by means of the pumping action caused by joint movement (Figures 10-2 to 10-4).

All the body's lymph vessels converge into two main channels, the thoracic duct and the

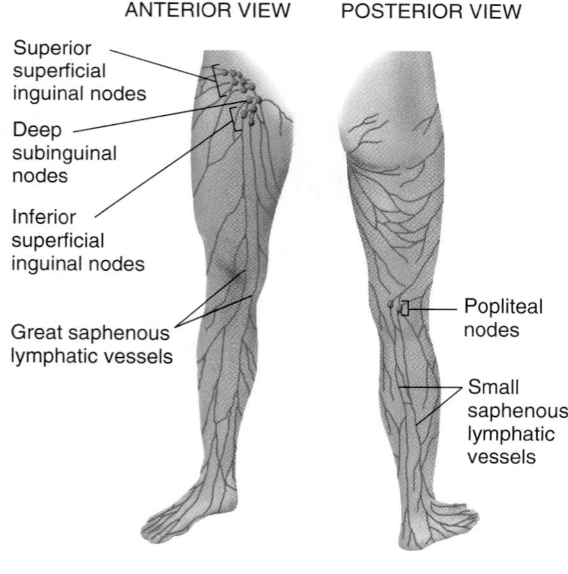

FIGURE 10-2 ■ Lymph vessels and node clusters—lower body. (From Seidel HM et al: *Mosby's guide to physical examination,* ed. 5, St. Louis, 2003, Mosby.)

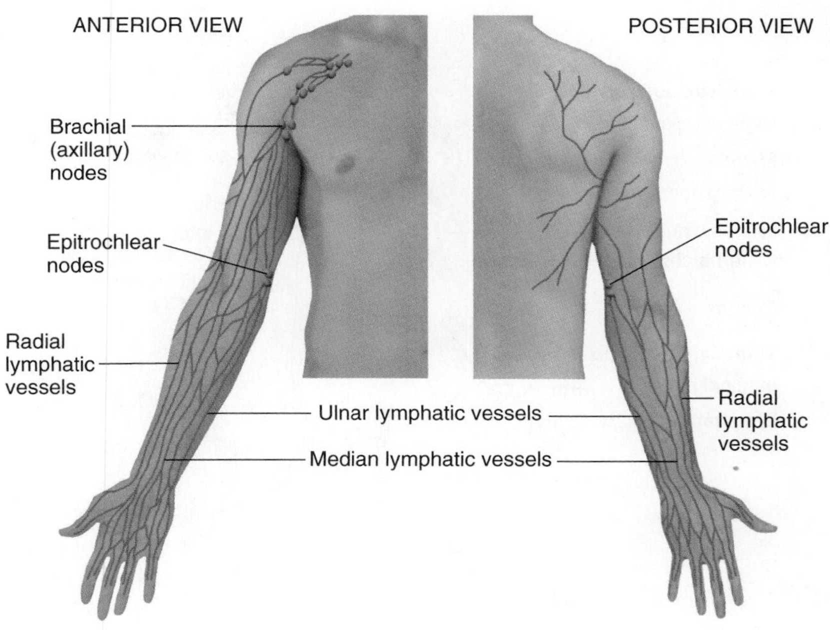

FIGURE 10-3 ■ Lymph vessels and node clusters—upper body. (From Seidel HM et al: *Mosby's guide to physical examination,* ed. 5, St. Louis, 2003, Mosby.)

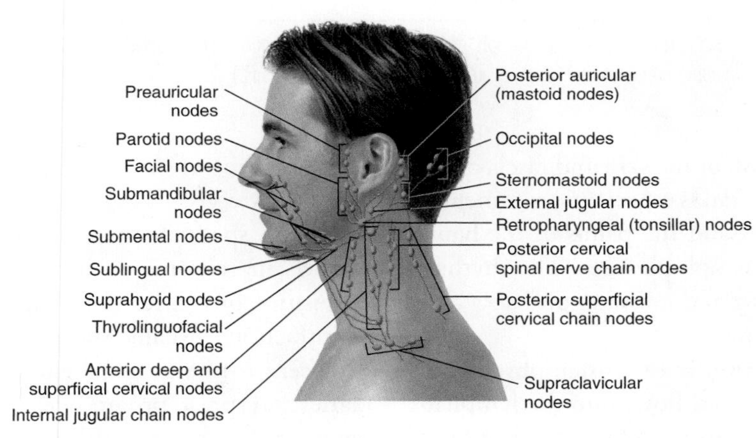

FIGURE 10-4 ■ Lymph vessels and node clusters—head and neck. (From Seidel HM et al: *Mosby's guide to physical examination,* ed. 5, St. Louis, 2003, Mosby.)

right lymphatic duct. Vessels from the entire left side of the body and from the right side of the body below the chest converge into the thoracic duct, which in turn empties into the left subclavian vein, situated beneath the left clavicle. The right lymphatic duct collects lymph from the vessels on the right side of the head, neck, upper chest, and right arm. It empties into the right subclavian vein beneath the right clavicle (Figures 10-5 and 10-6).

The movement of lymph occurs along a pressure gradient from areas of high pressure to areas of low pressure. Fluid moves from the interstitial space into the lymph capillaries by means of a pressure mechanism exerted by respiration, peristalsis of the large intestine, the compression of

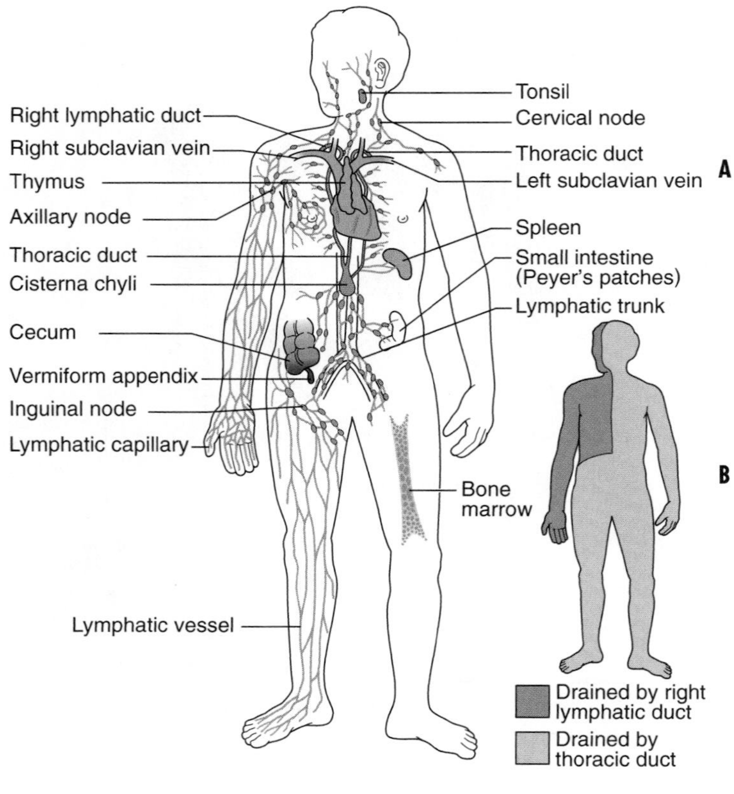

FIGURE 10-5 ■ Lymph organ vessels and drainage. (From Salvo S: *Massage therapy: principles and practice*, ed 2, St Louis, 2003, Saunders.)

muscles, and the pull of the skin and fascia during movement. This action is especially prominent on the soles of the feet and the palms of the hands, which have major lymph plexuses. The rhythmic pumping of walking and grasping probably facilitates lymphatic flow.

Lymph circulation is a two-step process:

1. Interstitial fluid flows into the lymphatic capillaries. Plasma is forced out of blood capillaries into the spaces around the cell walls (interstitial fluid). As fluid pressure increases between the cells, the cells move apart, pulling on the microfilaments that connect the endothelial cells of the lymph capillaries to tissue cells. The pull on the microfilaments causes the lymph capillaries to open like flaps, allowing tissue fluid to enter the lymph capillaries.
2. Lymph moves through the network of contractile lymphatic vessels. The lymphatic system does not have a central pump like the heart. Various factors assist the transport of lymph through the lymph vessels.

The spontaneous contraction of lymphatic vessels in response to increased lymphatic fluid pressure constitutes the lymphatic pump. These contractions usually start in the lymphangions adjacent to the terminal end of the lymph capillaries and spread progressively from one lymphangion to the next, toward the thoracic duct or the right lymphatic duct. The contractions are similar to abdominal peristalsis and are stimulated by increases in pressure inside lymphatic vessels. Contractions of the lymphatic vessels are not coordinated with the heart or breathing rate. If the pressure inside the lymphatic vessels exceeds or falls below certain levels, lymphatic contractions cease.

During inhalation, the thoracic duct is squeezed and fluid is pushed forward, creating a vacuum in the duct. During exhalation, fluid is pulled from the lymphatics into the thoracic duct to fill the partial vacuum.

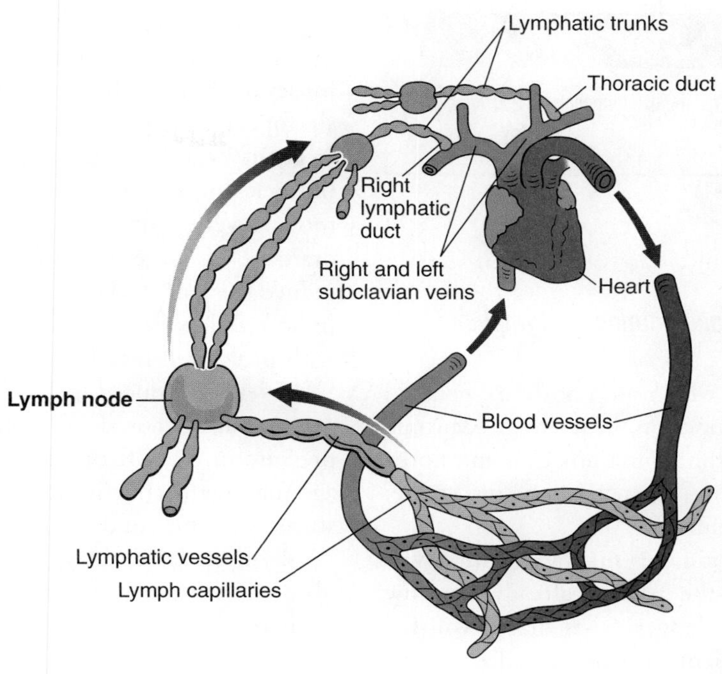

FIGURE 10-6 ■ Lymph circulation. (From Salvo S: *Massage therapy: principles and practice*, ed 2, St Louis, 2003, Saunders.)

Edema

Edema, which is an increase in interstitial fluid, can be caused by a variety of factors.

- *Lack of exercise.* Exercise, in which muscles alternately contract and relax, stimulates lymph circulation and cleans muscle tissue. If the muscles stay contracted or flaccid, lymph circulation decreases drastically inside the muscles, and edema can result.
- *Overexercising.* During exercise, blood pressure and capillary permeability both increase, allowing more fluid to seep into the interstitial spaces. If the movement of fluid exceeds the ability of the lymphatic capillaries to drain the areas, fluid accumulates. This seems to be a contributing factor to delayed onset muscle soreness.
- *Salt consumption.* The body maintains a specific ratio of salt to fluids. The more salt a person consumes, the more water is retained to balance it, resulting in edema.
- *Heart or kidney disease.* These diseases affect the blood and lymph circulations. Lymph massage stimulates the circulation of lymph. Caution is indicated, however, because the increase in fluid volume could overload an already weakened heart or kidneys.
- *Menstrual cycle.* Water retention and/or a swollen abdomen are common before or during the menstrual cycle.
- *Lymphedema.* Limbs affected by this condition become very swollen and painful, resulting in difficulty moving the affected limb and disfigurement. The cause is uncertain. Lymphedema can be life threatening. The interstitial fluid is contaminated, and even small wounds can become infected.
- *Inflammation.* Increased blood flow to an area of illness or injury and the release of vasodilators, which are part of the inflammatory response, can cause edema in the local area. This is a common response to injury and surgery.
- *Other causes.* Edema can be a side effect of medications such as steroids, hormones, and chemotherapeutic drugs used for cancer. Scar tissue and muscle tension can cause obstructive edema by restricting lymph vessels.

evolve 10-1

See the Evolve website for more information on the lymphatic system.

Contraindications to and Cautions in Lymphatic Drainage Massage

Edematous tissues, which are poorly oxygenated and have reduced function, heal slowly. Chronic edema results in chronic inflammation and fibrosis, which make the edematous tissue coarse, thicker, and less flexible.

Lymphatic drainage massage can lower blood pressure. If the patient already has low blood pressure, the danger exists that it will fall further and the patient may become dizzy when he or she stands up.

When a person is ill with a viral or bacterial infection and fever, circulation of lymph through the nodes slows, giving the lymphocytes more time to destroy the bacteria or virus. Because massage moves fluid through the lymphatic system more quickly, it can interfere with the body's efforts to defeat the attacking cells and can prolong the illness. During fever, white blood cells multiply more rapidly, whereas bacteria and viruses multiply more slowly; fever therefore is part of the body's healing process. Because lymph drainage massage may lower the body temperature, it should not be given to a patient with a fever.

Lymphatic drainage massage affects the circulation of fluid in the body and can overwhelm an already weak heart or kidneys. Do not give lymph drainage massage to anyone with congestive heart failure or kidney failure or anyone undergoing kidney dialysis unless it is specifically ordered by the patient's physician.

Indications for Lymphatic Drainage Massage

Simple edema (absent any contraindications) responds well to massage that focuses on the lymphatic system. This approach is helpful for soft tissue conditions, including postoperative conditions (with supervision), because it speeds healing and reduces swelling.

Traveler's edema is the result of enforced inactivity, such as sitting in an airplane or a car for several hours. The same is true for anyone who sits for extended periods. Interstitial fluid responds to gravity, causing swelling in the feet, hands, and buttocks of a person who has to sit without moving very much for a few hours. Lymphatic drainage massage can remove the edema and reduce the pain and stiffness it causes. Caution is indicated, however, because blood clots can form with prolonged inactivity.

Exercise-induced, delayed onset muscle soreness is partly caused by an increase in the fluid pressure in the soft tissues, and lymphatic drainage massage is effective at reducing the pain and stiffness of this condition.

Lymphatic drainage massage also softens fibrotic tissue and allows for improved circulation.

Principles of Lymphatic Drainage Massage

The pressure provided by massage mimics the drag and compressive forces of movement and respiration and can move the skin to open the lymph capillaries. The pressure gradient from high pressure to low pressure is supported by creating low-pressure areas in the vessels proximal to the area to be drained.

Depth of pressure, speed and frequency, direction, rhythm, duration, and drag are adjusted to support the lymphatic system.

Just enough pressure is applied to move the skin. The lymphatics are most affected by massage and are mostly located in superficial tissues (the outer 0.3 mm of the skin). Surface edema occurs in those superficial tissues, not in the deep tissue. Moving the skin moves the lymphatics. Stretching the lymphatics longitudinally, horizontally, and diagonally stimulates them to contract. Simple muscle tension puts pressure on the lymph vessels and may block them, interfering with efficient drainage. Massage can normalize this muscle tension. As the muscles relax, the lymph vessels open, and drainage is more efficient. The massage therapist should drain the surface areas and work on the areas of muscle tension using appropriate massage methods and pressure and then finish the area by repeating the surface lymphatic drainage.

Disagreement exists about the intensity of the pressure that should be used. Some schools of thought recommend very light pressure, such as that described by Vodder. Other methods, such as the technique described by Lederman, use a deeper pressure. Lederman holds that the stronger the compression, the greater the increase in the flow rate of lymph. Light pressure is used initially and then methodically increased as the area is drained and hydrostatic pressure decreases.

The more fluid present in the tissue, the slower the massage movements. Massage strokes are repeated slowly, at a rate of approximately 10 per minute in an area. This is approximately the rate at which the peripheral lymphatics contract.

Move lymph toward the closest cluster of lymph nodes, which are located in the neck, axilla, and groin for the most part. Massage near the nodes first and then move fluid toward them, working proximally from the swollen area toward the nodes. Massage the unaffected side first, then the obstructed side. For instance, if the right arm is swollen because of scar tissue from a mastectomy, massage the left arm first.

The approach is a rhythmic, slow repetition of the massage movements. Full body lymphatic drainage massage lasts about 45 minutes. Focus on local areas for about 5 to 15 minutes.

The methods of lymphatic massage are fairly simple, but lymphatic massage, when indicated, is a very powerful technique that elicits body-wide responses. Although disagreement exists about methodology, all approaches have some validity. Therefore the method described in this text combines the various techniques that support lymphatic movement in the body.

Treatment

See the photo sequence on p. 331.

The massage session begins with a pumping action on the thorax. Place both of your hands on the anterior surface of the thoracic cage. Have the patient exhale completely; your hands should passively follow the movements of the thorax. When the patient starts the inspiration, resist the movement of the thorax with counterpressure for 5 to 7 seconds. Repeat this procedure four or five times. Pumping action on the thorax increases the drainage of lymph through the lymphatic ducts by lowering intrapleural pressure and exaggerating the action of inhalation and exhalation.

Next, the massage application consists of a combination of short, light, pumping, gliding strokes that begin close to the torso at the node cluster and are directed toward the torso. The strokes methodically move distally. The phase of applying pressure and drag must be longer than the phase of release. However, the releasing phase cannot be too short because the lymph needs time to drain from the distal segment. Therefore the optimum duration of the pressure and drag phase is 6 to 7 seconds, and the optimum duration of the release phase is about 5 seconds. This pattern is followed by long, surface gliding strokes with a bit more pressure to influence deeper lymph vessels. The direction is toward the drainage points (Figure 10-7).

The focus of the initial pressure and finishing strokes is the dermis, which is just below the surface layer of the skin, and the superficial fascial layer, which is the tissue layer just beneath the skin and above the muscles. The superficial fascial layer contains 60% to 70% of the lymphatic circulation in the extremities. It does not take much pressure to contact the area. If too much pressure is applied, the capillaries are pressed closed, which nullifies any effect on the more superficial vessels. With lymphatic massage, generally light pressure is indicated initially; this increases to a moderate level (including kneading and compression as well as gliding) during repeated application to the area to reach the deep lymphatic vessels; the pressure then returns to a lighter level over the area. Drag is necessary to affect the microfilaments and open the flaps at the ends of the capillary vessels.

Pumping, rhythmic compression on the soles and the palms supports lymph movement. Rhythmic, gentle passive and active joint movement reproduces the body's normal means of pumping lymph. The patient helps the process by deep, slow breathing, which stimulates lymph flow in the deeper vessels. When possible, position the area being massaged above the heart so that gravity can assist the lymph flow.

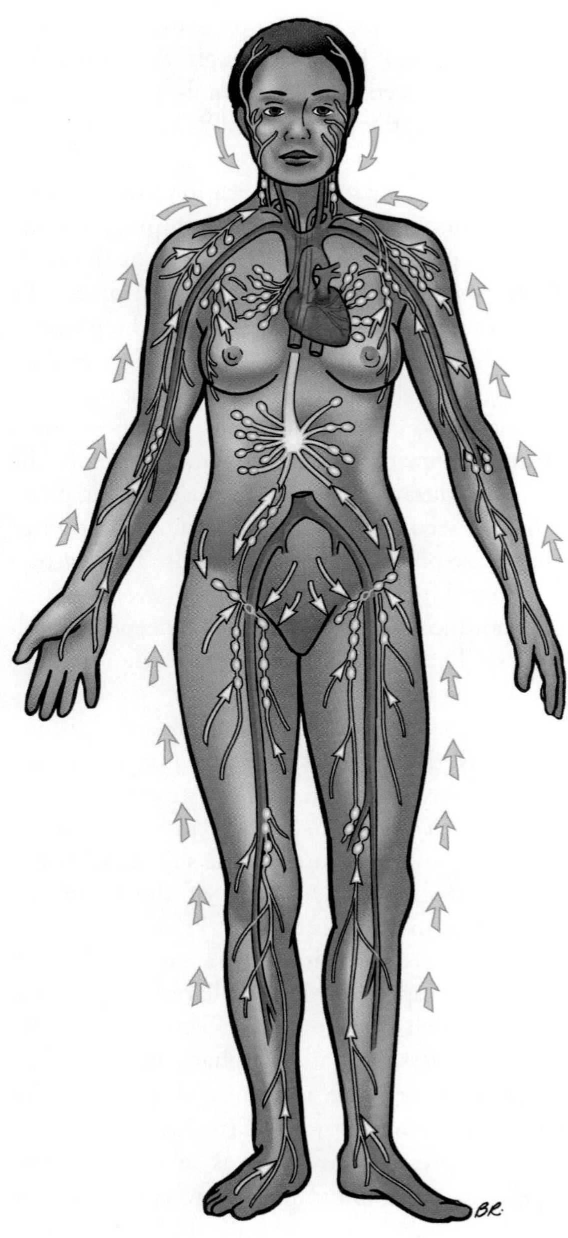

FIGURE 10-7 ■ Direction of strokes for facilitating lymphatic flow. (From Fritz S: *Mosby's fundamentals of therapeutic massage*, ed 3, St Louis, 2004, Mosby.)

CIRCULATORY MASSAGE

The purpose of circulatory massage is to stimulate the efficient flow of blood through the body. This type of massage tends to normalize blood pressure, tone the cardiovascular system, and undo the negative effects of occasional stress. It is an excellent massage approach to use after exercise. Circulatory massage also supports the inactive patient by increasing the blood movement mechanically; however, it in no way replaces exercise. Both the circulatory and lymphatic types of massage are very beneficial for a patient who is unable to walk or exercise aerobically.

The Circulatory System

The circulatory system is a closed system composed of a series of connected tubes and a pump. The heart (i.e., the pump) provides pressure for the blood to move through the body via the arteries and eventually into the small capillaries, where blood gas and nutrient exchange takes place. The blood returns to the heart by way of the veins. Venous blood flow is not under pressure from the heart. Rather, it relies on muscle compression against the veins to change the interior venous pressure. As in the lymphatic system, back flow of blood is prevented by a valve system (Figures 10-8 and 10-9).

Massage Methods for the Circulatory System

See the photo sequence on p. 328.

Massage to encourage blood flow to the tissues (arterial circulation) is different from massage to encourage blood flow from the tissues back to the heart (venous circulation). Because of the valve system of the veins and lymph vessels, deep, narrow-based stroking over these vessels from proximal to distal (from the heart out) is contraindicated. A small chance exists of breaking down the valves if this is done. However, compression (which does not slide, as does gliding or stripping) is appropriate for stimulating arterial circulation.

Treatment

Compression is applied over the main arteries (Figure 10-8). It begins close to the heart (proximal) and systematically moves distally to the tips of the fingers or toes. The manipulations are applied over the arteries, with a pumping action provided at a rhythm of approximately 60 beats per minute or whatever the patient's resting heart rate is. Compressive force changes the internal pressure in the arteries, stimulates the intrinsic contraction of arteries, and encourages the move-

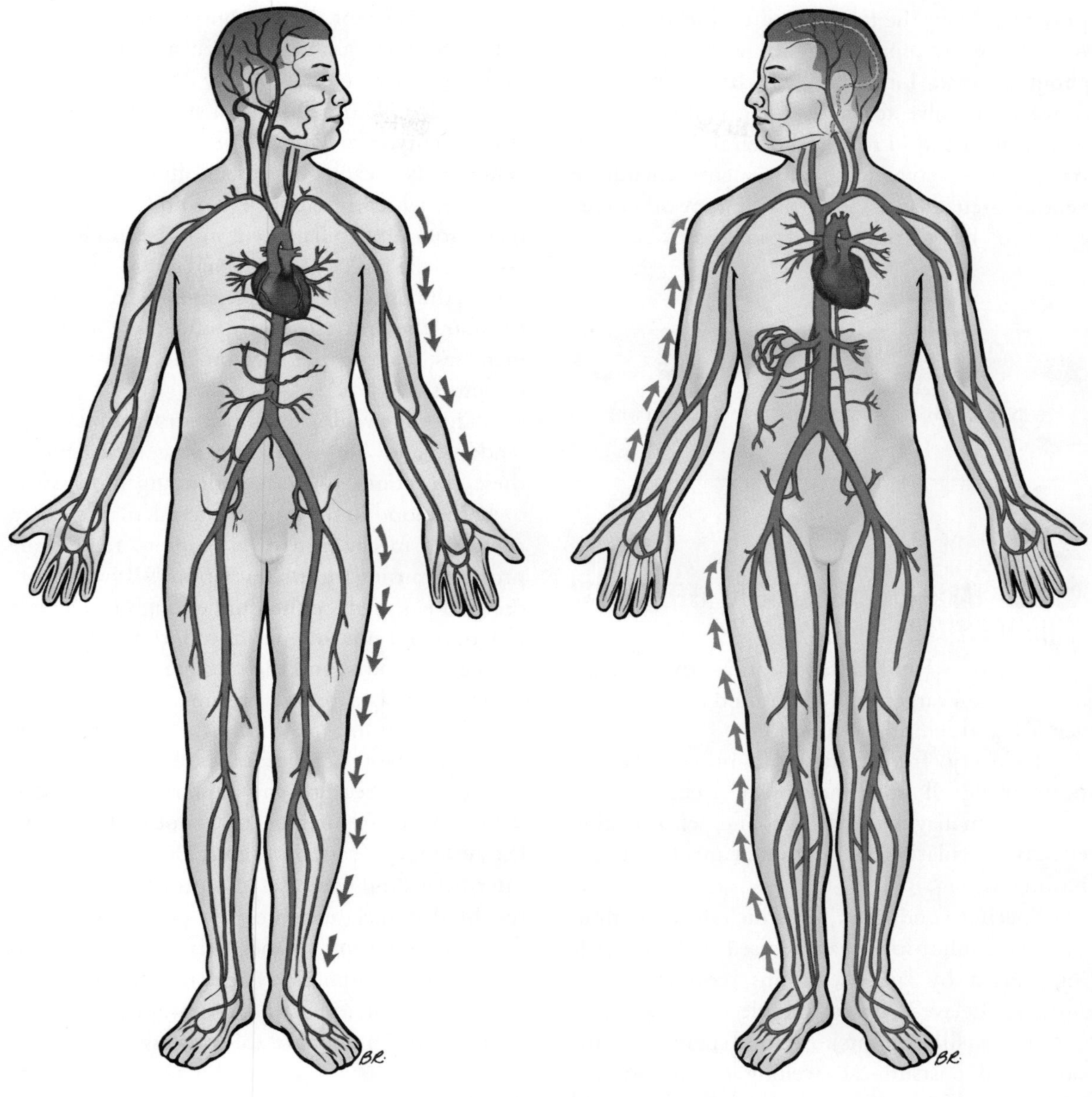

FIGURE 10-8 ■ Direction of compression over arteries to increase arterial flow. (From Fritz S: *Mosby's fundamentals of therapeutic massage*, ed 3, St Louis, 2004, Mosby.)

FIGURE 10-9 ■ Direction of gliding strokes to facilitate venous flow. (From Fritz S: *Mosby's fundamentals of therapeutic massage*, ed 3, St Louis, 2004, Mosby.)

ment of blood out to the distal areas of the body. Compression also begins to empty venous vessels and forms an arteriovenous pressure gradient, encouraging arterial blood flow.

Rhythmic, gentle contraction and relaxation of the muscles powerfully encourage arterial blood flow. Both active and passive joint movements support the transport of arterial blood.

The next step is to assist venous return flow. This process is similar to lymphatic massage in that a combination of short and long gliding strokes is used in conjunction with movement (Figure 10-9). The difference is that lymphatic massage is done over the entire body, and the movements usually are passive. With venous return flow, the gliding strokes move distal to proximal (from the fingers and toes to the heart) over the major veins. The gliding stroke is short, about 3 inches long. This enables the blood to move from valve to valve. Long gliding strokes carry the blood through the entire vein. Both passive and active joint movements encourage venous circulation. Placing the limb or other area above the heart brings gravity into assistance.

> **evolve 10-2**
>
> See the Evolve website for more information on the circulatory system.

10-1 TARGETING MASSAGE TO AFFECT BODY FLUID MOVEMENT

In terms of methodical application, the massage outcome can target each main fluid area: arterial, venous, and lymphatic function.

Recovery from illness or injury involves normalizing all fluid movement. Rehabilitation involves managing swelling and encouraging effective circulation to the injured area to support healing.

Specific conditions for which focused fluid massage applications may be used include swelling caused by sprains, strains, contusions, or surgery; delayed onset muscle soreness; and chronic swelling (joints). Strains, sprains, contusions, and postsurgical swelling require specific treatment. First- and second-degree (i.e., mild and moderate) levels of these local injuries benefit from both local and systemic lymphatic drainage. Decongesting the entire drainage region of the affected area is important; for example, a sprained ankle requires drainage of the entire leg into the trunk. For the first 24 hours after such injuries, treatment follows a regimen of protection, rest, ice, compression, and elevation (more commonly known by its acronym, PRICE). The movement of fluid from superficial tissues can begin after the acute stage starts to diminish; as always, proper medical care must be provided, and the medical team's orders must be followed.

Treatment for delayed onset muscle soreness (DOMS) can begin immediately after the activity as a preventive measure. Part of the process of DOMS is inflammation with increased capillary permeability. The sympathetic autonomic nervous system (ANS) exerts increased influence on blood pressure, which results in even more fluid movement from the capillary beds into the tissues. This increases the interstitial fluid and hydrostatic pressure in the tissue. The lymph capillaries are unable to drain the area effectively, and the congestion increases, putting pressure on the pain-sensitive receptors.

Chronic swelling usually occurs around joints, tendons, and bursae. Part of the treatment of these conditions involves addressing fluid issues of both blood and lymph. The edema acts as a protective mechanism to attempt to reduce the problem causing the inflammation. With massage, the goal is to reduce the fluid enough to increase function, but not so much as to interfere with the protective process and the increased stability provided by the hydrostatic pressure.

With contusions (bruises), the entire area around the contusion needs to be drained. Caution is necessary, because the capillaries have been damaged and the massage must not interfere with the healing process. However, the blood in the interstitial fluid increases the protein content of the fluid, which increases the potential for the formation of fibrotic tissue. This is why it is essential that the lymphatic system remove the interstitial fluid containing blood. Appropriate massage application can enhance this process.

Throughout its course, this textbook recommends the use of massage to increase arterial circulation, venous circulation, and lymphatic movement in order to aid patients involved in healing and rehabilitation programs. The following sections of this chapter provide precise descriptions first of the massage applications that affect arterial flow and then of those that support venous return. In both methods, the capillary beds are addressed, followed by a description of lymphatic drainage for interstitial fluid (extracapsular or tissue) and intracapsular fluid (inside the joint capsule).

Both mechanical and reflexive methods of fluid movement focus primarily on mechanical force. The massage therapist must understand both the structure and function of the vascular and lymphatic systems and appreciate the properties of a fluid, including the properties of water, colloids, and viscosity.

Some general rules about fluids include the following:

- Fluids naturally move from areas of high pressure to areas of low pressure with gravity.
- The more viscous the fluid, the slower it moves.
- Fluid moves against gravity only with the aid of a pump; the faster and stronger the pump, the more fluid is moved.
- Fluid that is enclosed exerts pressure against the interior sides of the container, and fluid outside the container can exert pressure against the outside walls.
- **Permeability** is the term used for how fast fluid (water) moves across a membrane. Fluid also moves by osmosis and diffusion.

The application of effective massage depends on all of these factors.

INCREASING ARTERIAL CIRCULATION

Various mechanisms can influence arterial circulation, and the massage application needs to address these factors. However, the most direct effect is produced by the mechanical influence of pressure in the vessels and the stimulation of vasodilation. These include:

- Increased sympathetic arousal, which increases both the stroke volume and heart rate
- Increased buildup of pressure within the vessels
- Vasodilation of the capillaries

The general massage is brisk and lasts 15 to 30 minutes. Active participation by the patient, such as various forms of range of motion and muscle energy methods, is effective both for increasing sympathetic arousal and for meeting the demand for blood caused by the muscle activity.

Deliberate, temporary pressure exerted by the massage therapist against the arteries results in a buildup of fluid pressure between the heart and the temporary blockage; consequently, the rate of blood flow increases when the pressure block is released. The result is compression of the arteries in a rhythmic fashion that moves the arterial blood faster toward the capillaries in order to supply the nutritional and oxygen requirements of the tissues. The target areas for this type of technique usually are the limbs, hands, and feet.

The main steps are as follows (Figure 10-10):

1. Position the target area below the heart, if possible; seated, standing, and semireclining positions are most desirable.
2. Use a broad-based compression force against the tissue over the arteries. Begin close to the torso.

   When the arms are the target, begin where the arms join the torso. The same applies for the leg. The compression must be deep enough to close off the arteries so that the pressure builds. The rate of the on/off compression of the arteries is timed to the patient's heart rate, which is determined by assessing the closest pulse rate in the area. For example, if the pulse rate is 60 beats per minute, the compression rate is approximately 1 second on, 1 second off. Counting can be helpful, such as "1 [compress] and 2 [release]."
3. Work systematically in a distal direction, toward the fingers and toes.
4. The patient can make a fist and release or curl the toes and release at the same rhythm.
5. Do 3 or 4 repetitions in the target area until the temperature of the distal area rises.
6. Rhythmically knead and compress the target area to increase blood flow and create hyperemia (histamine response and vasodilation). These methods squeeze out the capillary beds, allowing the movement of blood into the venous system and creating space for the arterial blood. They also facilitate the exchange of nutrients and gases, as well as the movement of plasma into the interstitial spaces.

Even passive pressure and squeezing techniques have a pumping effect on the circulation.

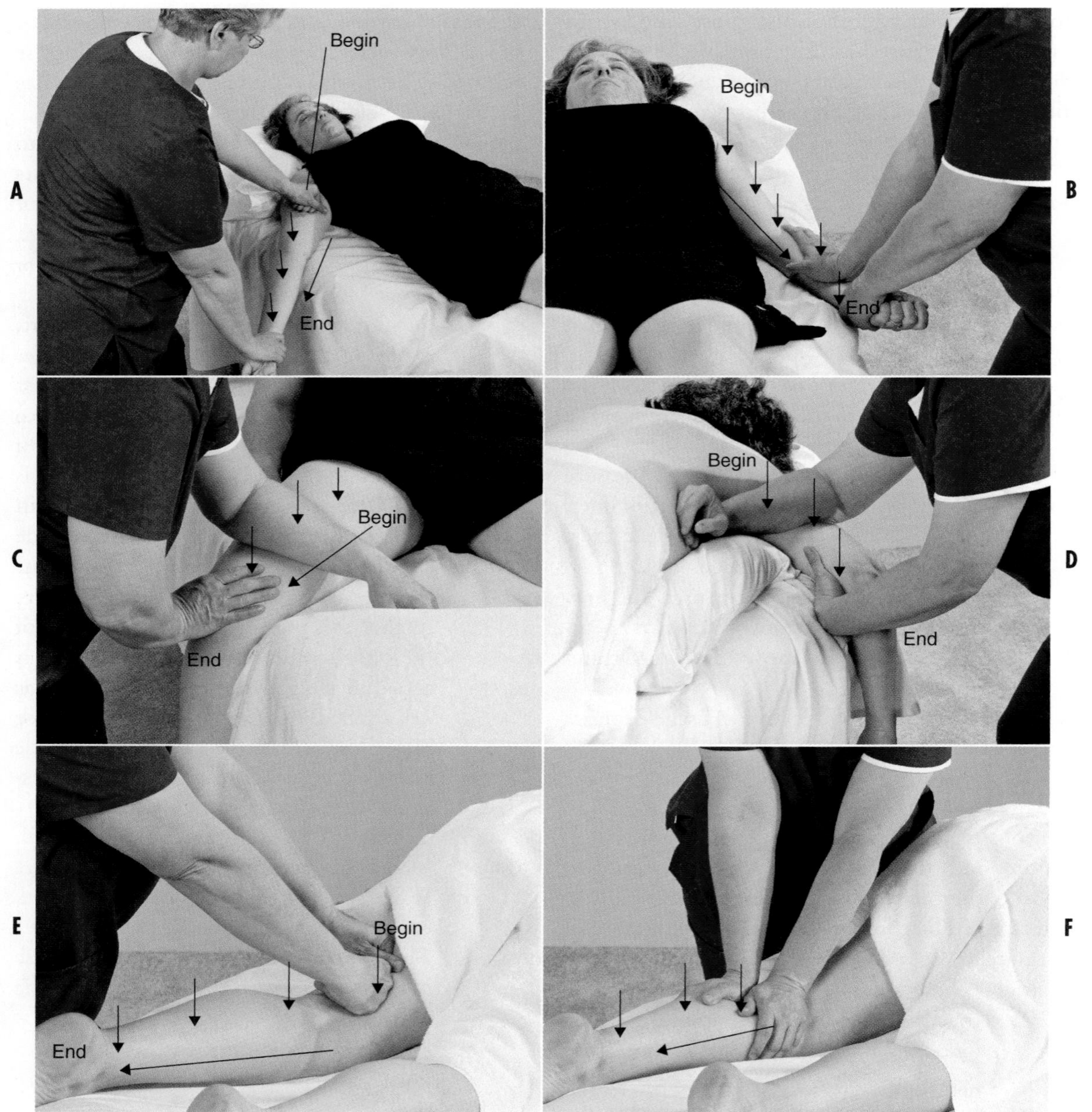

FIGURE 10-10 ■ The arterial circulation: examples of massage applications that support arterial flow to the extremities. **A,** Loose fist compression of major arteries on the upper limb to move blood toward the extremities. **B,** Compression of major arteries; the limb is positioned below the heart. **C,** Compression of the lower limb to support arterial flow to the extremities. **D,** Compression to support arterial blood flow with the limb positioned below the heart. **E,** Rhythmic compression to support arterial blood flow to the lower extremities. **F,** Rhythmic compression with the palms to support arterial blood flow.

Because the vessels have unidirectional valves, the pressure forces the blood out in one direction only, toward the heart. When the pressure is released, the vessels refill from the arterial supply.

Microcirculation

The walls of the blood vessels need to be soft and pliable so that they can assist the pumping action and allow filtration and absorption. As massage forces blood through the capillaries and arterioles, it has a stretching effect on the vessel walls, which can help increase their size, capacity, and function (Figure 10-11).

SUPPORTING VENOUS RETURN

As with all methods, the massage application supports the anatomy and physiology of normal function. To support normal venous circulation, the application mimics the venous pump. A combination of short and long gliding stokes is used over the veins. The depth of pressure is a bit more than that used for lymphatic drainage, because the intent is to actually pump the blood through a tube. Position the area, usually a limb, somewhat above the heart to allow gravity to assist the fluid movement. Then proceed as follows (Figure 10-12):

1. As with lymphatic drainage, begin close to the torso and glide no more than 3 inches in the direction toward the heart to take advantage of the valve system in the veins. Systematically move toward the distal end of the limb.
2. Use kneading to move the blood in the capillary beds, dispersing it through the soft tissue.
3. Have the patient actively contract and relax the muscles and move the joints in the area (think of the action as being a pump). Passive joint movement can be used if necessary. It is simple to move the joints in a circle through the entire range of motion.
4. Repeat the entire sequence and then shift the location a bit to address a different vein.
5. The calf muscles act as a secondary heart, especially influencing the venous return blood flow. The patient can move the ankle in slow circles to activate this pumping action (this also can be taught as a self-help method). This technique is especially effective if the patient is lying on a slant board with the head slightly lower than the heart, and the method is helpful even if the target area is not positioned above the heart.
6. The respiratory pump supports venous return by channeling thoracic pressure during breathing. This is primarily caused by the action of the diaphragm, therefore it is important for the breathing mechanism to be normal. See the protocol for breathing in Chapter 14.

LYMPHATIC DRAINAGE

The protocol presented in Figure 10-13 is meticulous and detailed. It covers all the current

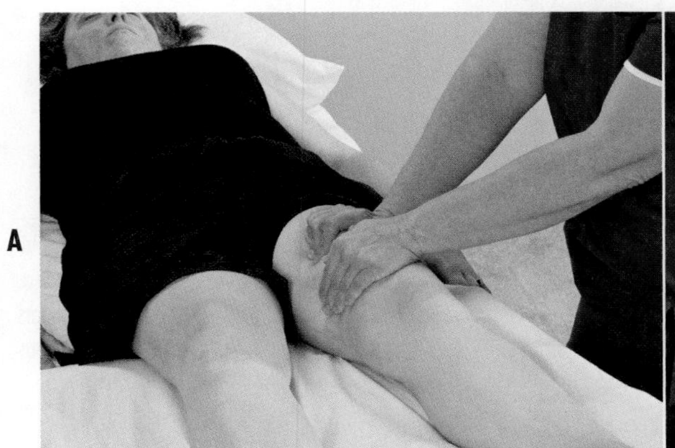

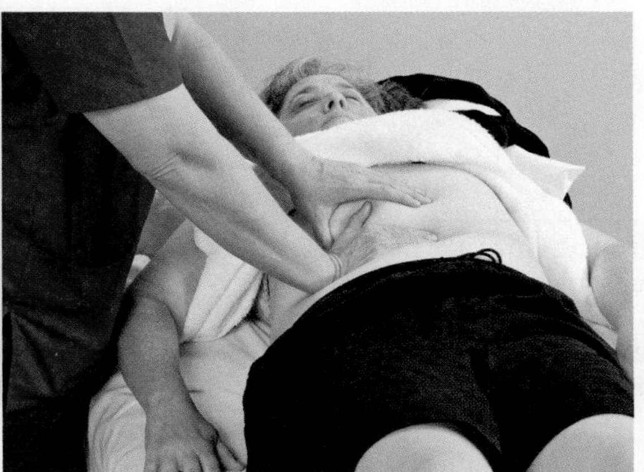

FIGURE 10-11 ■ The microcirculation and large vessels in the abdomen. **A,** Kneading the capillary beds supports the microcirculation; this should be done in all areas involved in the movement of blood, both arterial and venous. **B,** Abdominal kneading and compression support arterial and venous blood flow.

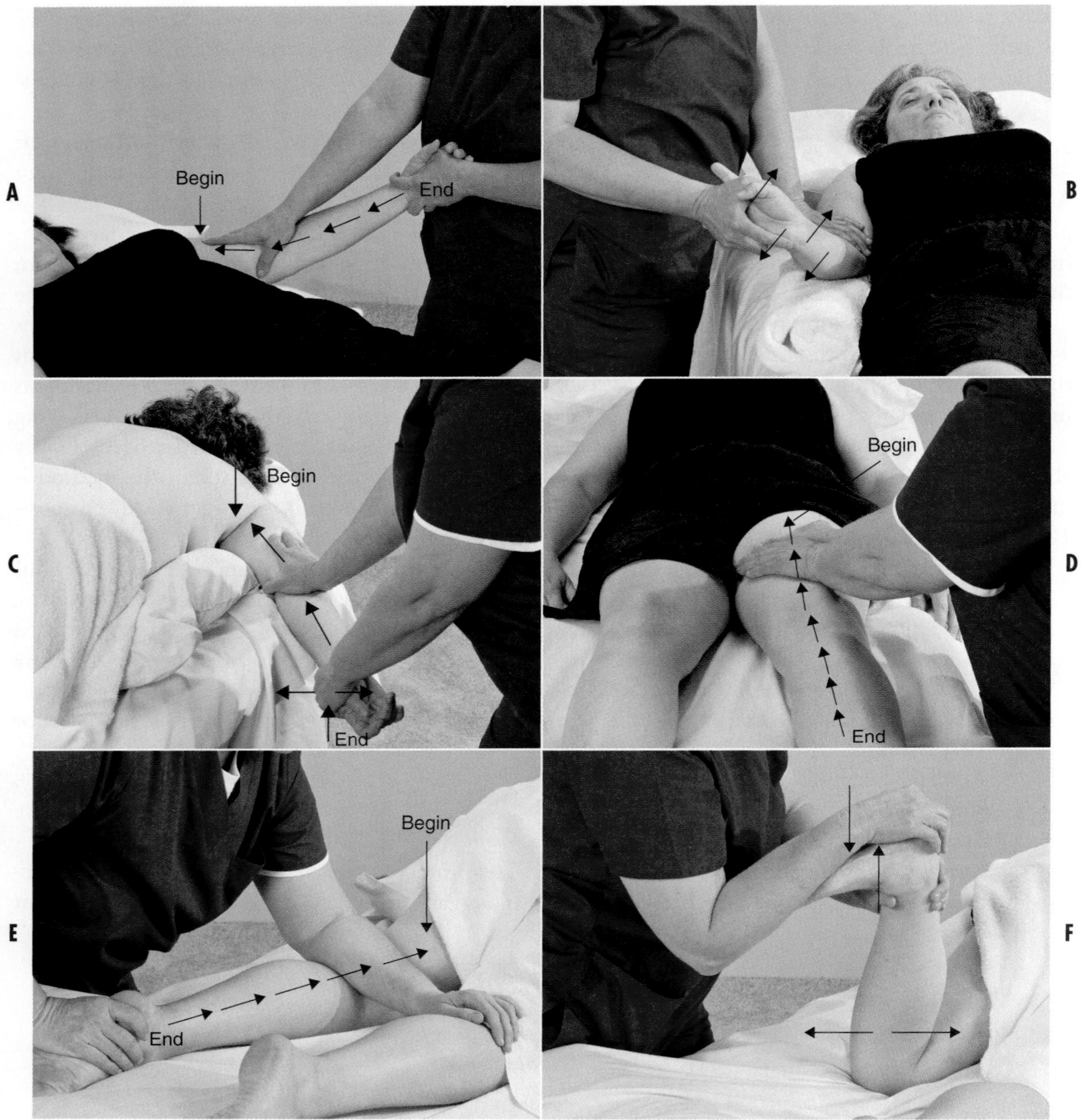

FIGURE 10-12 ■ The venous return circulation: examples of massage applications that support the return of venous blood from the extremities to the heart. **A,** Rhythmic gliding to support venous return; the arm is positioned above the heart. **B,** Rhythmic pumping to support venous return. **C,** Gliding with movement to support venous return (prone position). **D,** Gliding to support venous return (supine position); of wrist and elbow bolsters are positioned so the leg is above the heart. **E,** Gliding to support venous return (prone position). **F,** Rhythmic pumping of the calf to support venous return.

applications for lymphatic drainage that are based on physiologic mechanisms. It is presented in an effective order of application to target lymphatic fluid flow. (*Author's note:* I personally seldom perform the procedures as written here. Instead, I pick, choose, and modify. However, for learning purposes, I strongly suggest that you practice the protocols for both full body application and local application until you are comfortable with the concepts, procedures, and outcomes.) This

Text continued on p. 335.

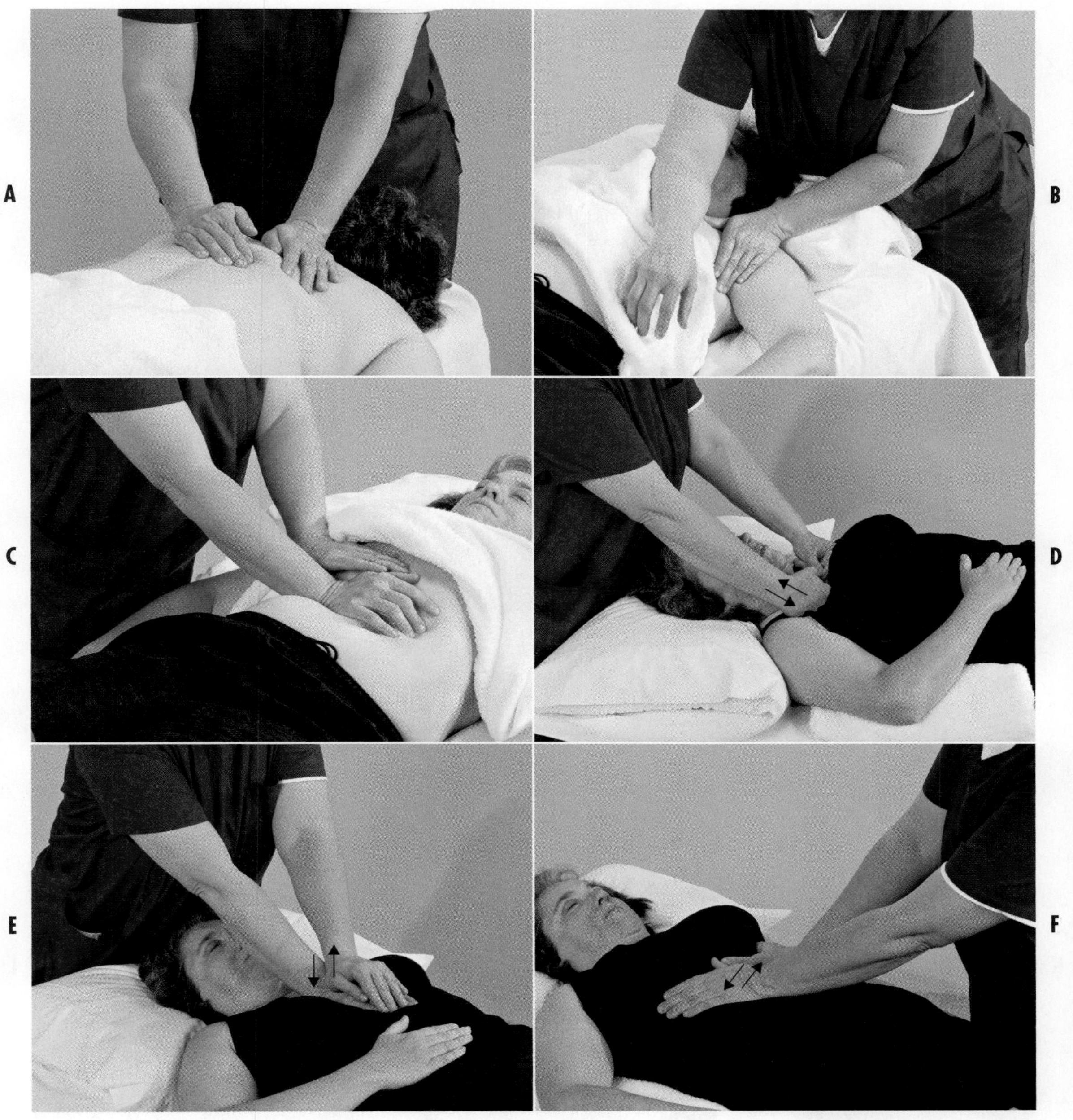

Figure 10-13 ■ Lymphatic drainage: examples of the various lymphatic drainage procedures described in the written protocol on pp. 323 and 336. (In addition, the DVD presents a demonstration of lymphatic drainage.) The general protocol photograph sequence in the Appendix presents examples of ways lymphatic drainage procedures can be incorporated into general massage application. **A,** Preparing the tissue position to prepare the thorax and neck for rhythmic pumping and drainage. **B,** Use of the forearm for chest compression and gliding to prepare the thorax for rhythmic pumping. **C,** Rhythmic rolling and pumping of the abdomen; these techniques are applied periodically during lymphatic drainage procedures. **D,** Position for lymphatic pumping: compression of the upper chest and neck. **E,** Position for lymphatic pumping: chest compression over the sternum. **F,** Position for lymphatic pumping: compression of the lower ribs.

Continued

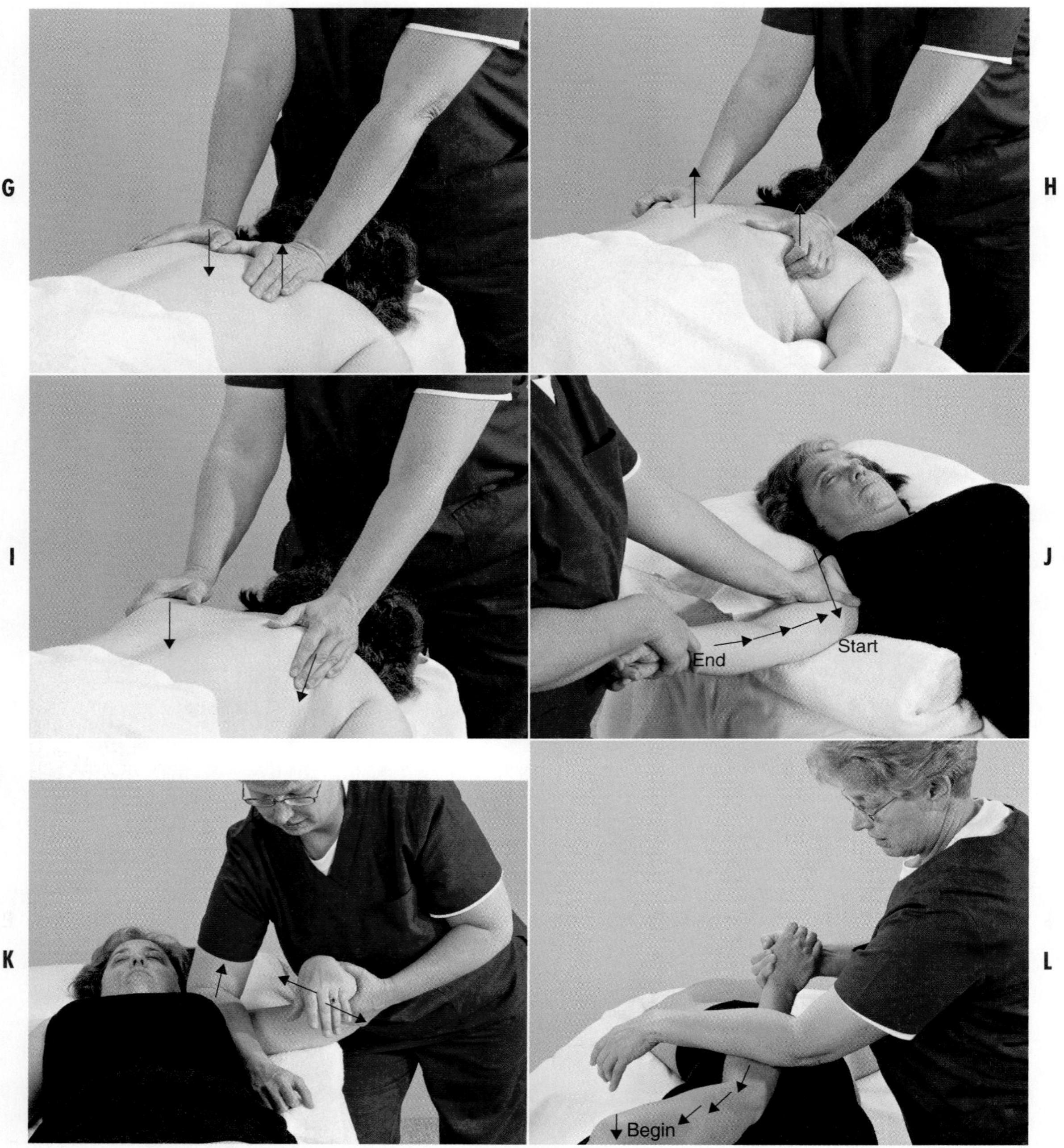

FIGURE 10-13, cont'd ■ **G,** Position of the thorax for lymphatic pumping. **H,** Lymphatic pumping: lower ribs. **I,** Lymphatic pumping: lower ribs. **J,** Position for lymphatic drainage of the arm (supine position). Notice the use of the bolster to support drainage. **K,** Rhythmic pumping with compression and joint movement. **L,** An example of the side-lying position and use of the forearm to create skin drag.

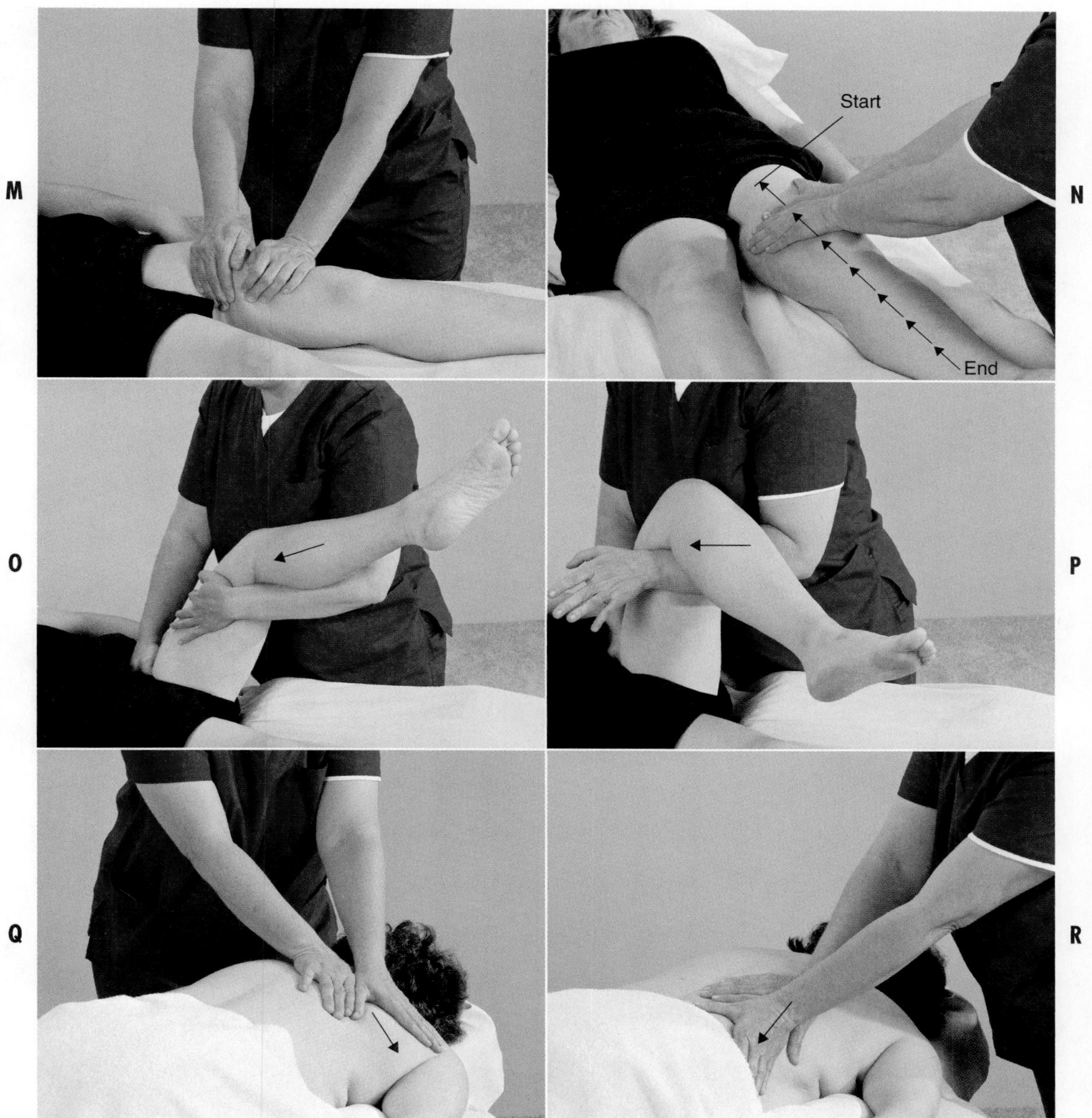

FIGURE 10-13, cont'd ■ **M,** Kneading of the deeper tissues during lymphatic drainage; this technique is applied to all body areas. **N,** Position for lymphatic drainage of the lower limb (supine position). Notice the use of the leg bolster. **O,** Rhythmic pumping of the lower limb (supine position). **P,** Rhythmic pumping of the lower limb. **Q,** Skin drag position for the cervical and upper torso (prone position). **R,** Skin drag for the lumbar area.

Continued

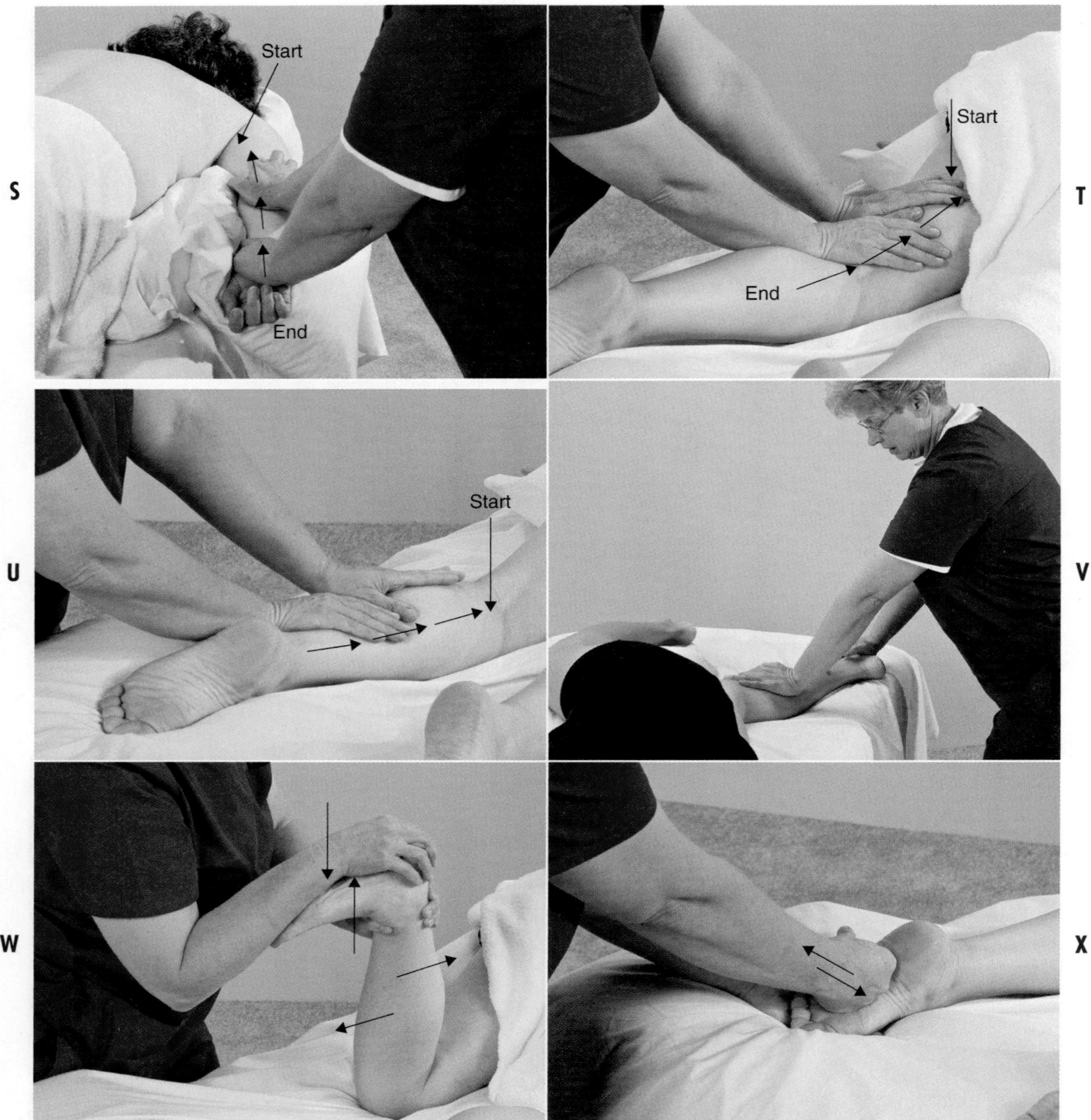

FIGURE 10-13, cont'd ■ **S,** Positioning of the arm for lymphatic drainage (prone position). Notice the use of the arm bolsters to support drainage. **T,** Skin drag of the thigh (prone position). **U,** Positioning of the leg for lymphatic drainage of the calf. **V,** An example of a side-lying skin drag technique or kneading and compression to prepare the tissues for rhythmic pumping. **W,** Lymphatic pumping using rhythmic joint movement. **X,** Rhythmic compression of the foot plexus.

protocol addresses increased movement of interstitial fluid into the lymphatic capillaries without fibrosis. The management of fibrotic tissue is covered on p. 340.

Contraindications to and Cautions in Lymphatic Drainage Massage

A number of factors may be contraindications to or cautions in lymphatic drainage massage, including the following:

- Compromised urinary or cardiovascular function, especially congestive heart or kidney failure, is a contraindication.
- Systemic illness (fever, diarrhea, vomiting, unexplained edema) requires caution.
- Edema in the acute phase of an illness or injury (i.e., the first 24 hours) is a contraindication.
- Edema that contributes to joint stability is a contraindication.

Surgery, abrasions, and puncture wounds break the protective skin barrier, therefore sanitation in the area of the wound is critical. Lymphatic drainage massage around such areas can be performed safely, but not within the first 24 to 48 hours. Extreme care must be taken not to disturb the tissue healing process. Direct work over a postsurgical area must wait until the incision sites have healed (usually 5 to 7 days, but possibly longer).

Lymphatic drainage targeted to a specific joint is most effective in the context of a general full body massage application.

Assessment for Increased Interstitial Fluid Volume

Common History Components

- Increased physical activity followed by 24 to 48 hours of relative inactivity
- Increased physical activity as above but with insufficient recovery time (common in training camp schedules)
- Increased salt intake
- Increased water intake without appropriate electrolyte balance
- Decreased fluid intake
- Water weight gain of 3 to 5 pounds

Common Complaints

- Delayed onset muscle soreness (sore all over, best described as "achy")
- Stiffness that does not stretch out and is not clearly confined to a particular area
- Sensation of the skin and muscles feeling fat or taut

Visual Assessment

- Loss of muscle and joint definition
- Swollen appearance
- Patient seems sluggish

Physical Assessment

- Skin and superficial fascia palpated as taut because of increased hydrostatic pressure
- Skin and superficial fascia palpated as boggy, spongy, or soggy (increased fluid but not enough to push against skin as just described)
- Difficulty palpating muscle fiber structure because of fluid accumulation overlay
- Decreased definition of joints
- Reduced range of motion of joints caused by edema
- Difficulty lifting the skin and fascia from the surface layer of muscles
- Pain caused by both deep, broad-based compression and narrow, superficial compression
- Pitting edema and prolonged blanching of the skin after compression
- Drag on the skin and superficial fascia produces pockets of fluid that feel like small water balloons

Other Observations

- Reflexive methods are ineffective at resolving complaints
- Connective tissue approach may make symptoms worse, at least temporarily

Supportive Measures

- Epsom salt soak. Use enough salt so that the water has a mineral taste; too much is better than not enough. The method works by means of diffusion of water from a lower mineral concentration to a higher concentration to equalize solutions on either side of a membrane (the skin). The edema close to the skin flows across the skin into the salty water.

- Increased fluid intake with proper electrolyte balance
- Early diuretic-type foods (e.g., pineapple, papaya, berries, cucumbers, radishes, celery, aloe vera juice, watermelon)

Lymphatic Drainage Procedure (Figure 10-13)

See the photo sequence on p. 331.

Full body lymphatic drainage takes 45 to 90 minutes, depending on the patient's size. Begin with the least affected areas and progress to the target area.

Step-by-Step Protocol for Full Body Lymphatic Drainage

Phase 1: Preparing the Torso

1. Position the patient on the back (supine) with the arms and legs bolstered above the heart but with no areas of joints in a close-packed position (typically, ends of range of motion).
2. Begin on the upper thorax and use gliding, kneading, and compression to prepare the tissue. The goals are to increase the pliability of the skin and connective tissue ground substance and to reduce any areas of muscle tension so that lymph capillaries and vessels are unobstructed. Continue into the abdomen, paying particular attention to the abdominal and diaphragm muscles.
3. Mobilize the ribs by applying gentle but firm, broad-based compression. Begin at the sternoclavicular joint and work down toward the lower ribs. Make two or three passes, working from the sternum out toward the lateral edge. If an area of restriction is found, various methods can be used to increase mobility in the area. Compressing the restricted area while the patient coughs usually is effective. Massage the intercostals.
4. Place the patient in the side-lying position and use gliding, kneading, and compression to continue to increase tissue pliability and rib mobility. Work from the iliac crests up toward the axilla. Pay particular attention to the anterior serratus. Repeat on the other side.
5. Place the patient prone (face down). Use gliding, kneading, and compression to increase tissue pliability and rib mobility. Begin at the iliac crest and systematically work toward the shoulder and neck. Do both the left and right sides.

OUTCOME: Pliability of the torso soft tissue and rib mobility allow effective deep breathing and movement of lymph into the torso.

Phase 2: Decongesting the Torso

1. Reposition the patient supine with the arms and legs bolstered above the heart.
2. Place the hands just below either clavicle and compress and release. Repeat 3 or 4 times. Compress with the exhale and release with the inhale. This begins to affect the thoracic duct by changing the thoracic pressure. NOTE: Repeat this procedure approximately every 15 minutes during the session.
3. Begin the surface drainage procedure. This consists of dragging and sliding the skin in various directions to pull on the microfilaments, opening the ends of the lymph capillaries, so that the interstitial fluid can move from around the cells into the lower pressure area of the lymph vessel. This needs to be done in a slow, rhythmic manner, like a pump. Drag the skin systematically in each area and then let it return to the original position. Drag the skin and let it return; drag it again, and so on. Each skin movement has a slightly different direction vertically, horizontally, diagonally, and circularly. The skin movement phase is a little longer than the release phase. Remember, the massage application is structured to mimic the pull of the skin and fascia that normally would affect the microfilaments attached to the lymphatic capillaries. Begin skin drag at the closest lymph node area and work in a distal direction. This decongests and lowers the pressure, allowing fluid to move from areas of high pressure to areas of low pressure.
4. Begin the skin movement at the thorax midline above the diaphragm and work toward the area under the clavicle. Do both sides. After this area has been thoroughly addressed, repeat the chest compressions.

5. Continue with skin movement below the diaphragm, and change direction to drain toward the groin.
6. Have the patient do deep breathing while you gently but firmly knead the abdomen, then repeat the chest compressions. Remember: compress on exhale, release on inhale.
7. Put the patient in the side-lying position and repeat the skin drag method. In the areas of the body from the waist up, drainage is directed toward the axilla; in the areas below the waist, drainage is directed toward the groin. Start proximal to the region where drainage occurs. Do both sides.
8. While the patient is in the side-lying position, rhythmically compress the ribs (compress on exhale, release on inhale).
9. Place the patient prone and perform drainage again (above the waist, toward the axilla; below the waist, toward the groin). Compress the ribs in rhythm with the breathing.

OUTCOME: The torso is decongested and able to receive fluid from the limbs.

Phase 3: The Limbs

1. Place the patient prone. Address the arms and legs systematically; the procedure is the same for both. Work the least congested area first. For example, if the arms have more fluid, begin with the legs. If the right arm is more congested, first work the legs, then the left arm, and then the right arm.
2. Begin with passive and active joint movement: hip/knee/ankle/foot, shoulder/elbow/wrist/hand.
3. Prepare the tissue in the limbs for drainage as was done for the torso. Use gliding, kneading, compression, and shaking to increase the pliability of the connective tissue and to reduce muscle tension. Restriction in these areas interferes with the fluid's ability to move into the lymphatic capillaries.
4. Passively and actively move the joints again.
5. Prop the limb above the heart as previously described. Begin the skin drag application close to the torso, in the groin, gluteal, or axillary area. Systematically, drag the skin slowly, rhythmically, and gently in multiple directions, ending in the direction of the closest set of lymph nodes. Work down toward the elbow (or knee).
6. Apply moderately deep gliding from the elbow (or knee) toward the axilla (or groin). The intent is to support the movement of the fluid once inside the vessels and to activate the lymphangions. Perform gliding with the twofold intent of moving the fluid from valve to valve and of increasing intravesicular pressure. Long, slow, moderately deep gliding from the knee or elbow to the groin or axilla also is appropriate.
7. Apply active and passive joint movement again. The intent is to pump fluid at the nodes located at the joints.
8. Knead and compress the soft tissue between the elbow and the axilla (or between the knee and the groin). The intent is to move the interstitial fluid in the deeper tissues to the more superficial lymphatic capillaries.
9. Repeat steps 3 through 5.
10. Apply active and passive joint movement.
11. Begin the skin drag application near the knee (or elbow) and work down to the ankle (or wrist). Move the skin in all directions and end in the direction toward the knee (or elbow).
12. Apply active and passive joint motion.
13. Redrain the limb as described in steps 3, 4, and 5.
14. Apply active and passive joint movement.
15. Knead and compress the soft tissue between the wrist and elbow (or the ankle and knee).
16. Repeat steps 8 through 12.
17. Apply moderately deep, short, and long gliding strokes from the wrist to the axilla (or the ankle to the groin).
18. Apply active and passive joint movement.
19. Apply broad-based, slow, rhythmic, moderately deep compression to the palms of the hands and the soles of the feet. Pump the plexuses located in these areas for about 60 seconds.
20. Repeat active and passive joint movement.
21. Turn the patient into the side-lying position.
22. Knead and compress the neck tissue to prepare it for drainage.
23. Begin skin drag methods close to the clavicle and work at the skull. The direction of the force is toward the clavicle.

24. Apply active and passive joint movement to the neck.
25. Use short and long gliding and moderately deep pressure to increase fluid movement in the vessels. Work from the skull toward the clavicles.
26. Repeat steps 24 and 25.
27. Apply broad-based compression to the thorax in a rhythmic pumping manner; have the patient do deep breathing to affect the thoracic duct pressure.
28. Repeat steps 23 through 27.
29. Position the patient supine and bolster the limbs above the heart.
30. Repeat steps 2 through 18 on each limb.
31. Repeat the rhythmic pumping compression of the ribs near the clavicles coupled with deep breathing. Remember to compress on the exhale and release on the inhale.

Protocol for Local Edema at a Joint or in a Joint Area

Swelling at joints occurs for many reasons. Rheumatoid arthritis is a cause of joint swelling that requires caution in the application of massage; any massage should be closely supervised by the medical team.

Osteoarthritis is another common cause of joint swelling. The fluid buildup usually is protective in nature. Intracapsular fluid can help keep pain-sensitive bone structures separated and can reduce rubbing and friction in the joint. Fluid around the capsule can provide stability for a joint and limit painful motion. In these cases, the goal is not to eliminate the fluid, but rather to keep it moving to reduce the tendency for stagnant, edematous tissue to become fibrotic and also to maintain appropriate levels of fluid. As just explained, some fluid buildup, both inside and outside the capsule, is beneficial. Too much is detrimental to effective healing and function.

Because it is essential in arthritic joint maintenance to maintain mobility, optimum **fluid dynamics** in the area is important. Traumas such as sprains, contusions, breaks, and surgery produce swelling as part of the acute inflammatory response. This tissue fluid must be managed because of its high protein content from tissue debris and blood. The fluid can quickly become fibrotic in the subacute healing phase. The key is to manage the accumulated fluid and keep it moving without increasing any inflammatory response or disrupting the healing process. In some cases skin drag is the only component of lymphatic drainage that can be used directly at the site of the trauma.

Treatment for Swelling of an Individual Joint Area or Contusion (Figure 10-14)

1. Identify the main areas of the trunk toward which the fluid will move. For the arm joints and tissues, these areas are the axillae and the area around the clavicles. For the joints and tissues in the leg, the destination areas are the groin and the lower abdomen. When targeting an isolated area, it may not be necessary to be as meticulous with full body lymphatic drainage as described previously. Using a shorter, less intense application to the whole body is helpful, even when a particular joint or area is the target. Passive and active range of motion and some skin dragging are appropriate as part of the general massage application, because increasing fluid movement anywhere in the body influences the movement of all the lymphatics.
2. Bolster the entire limb with the individual target areas in a relaxed position above the heart with the joints in the midrange, open position.
3. Prepare the tissue in the entire limb with gliding, kneading, compression, and shaking to increase the pliability of the connective tissue structures and to reduce any muscle tension on the lymphatic vessels.
4. Begin skin dragging close to the torso and meticulously drain to the next distal joint (either the elbow or the knee).
5. Apply passive and active movement, making sure the area of either the groin or the axilla is effectively compressed in a pumping fashion during the joint movement.
6. Knead and compress the soft tissue between the knee and the groin (or the elbow and the axilla) with the intent of affecting the deeper interstitial fluid movement.
7. Repeat active and passive joint movement.
8. Repeat steps 4 and 5.

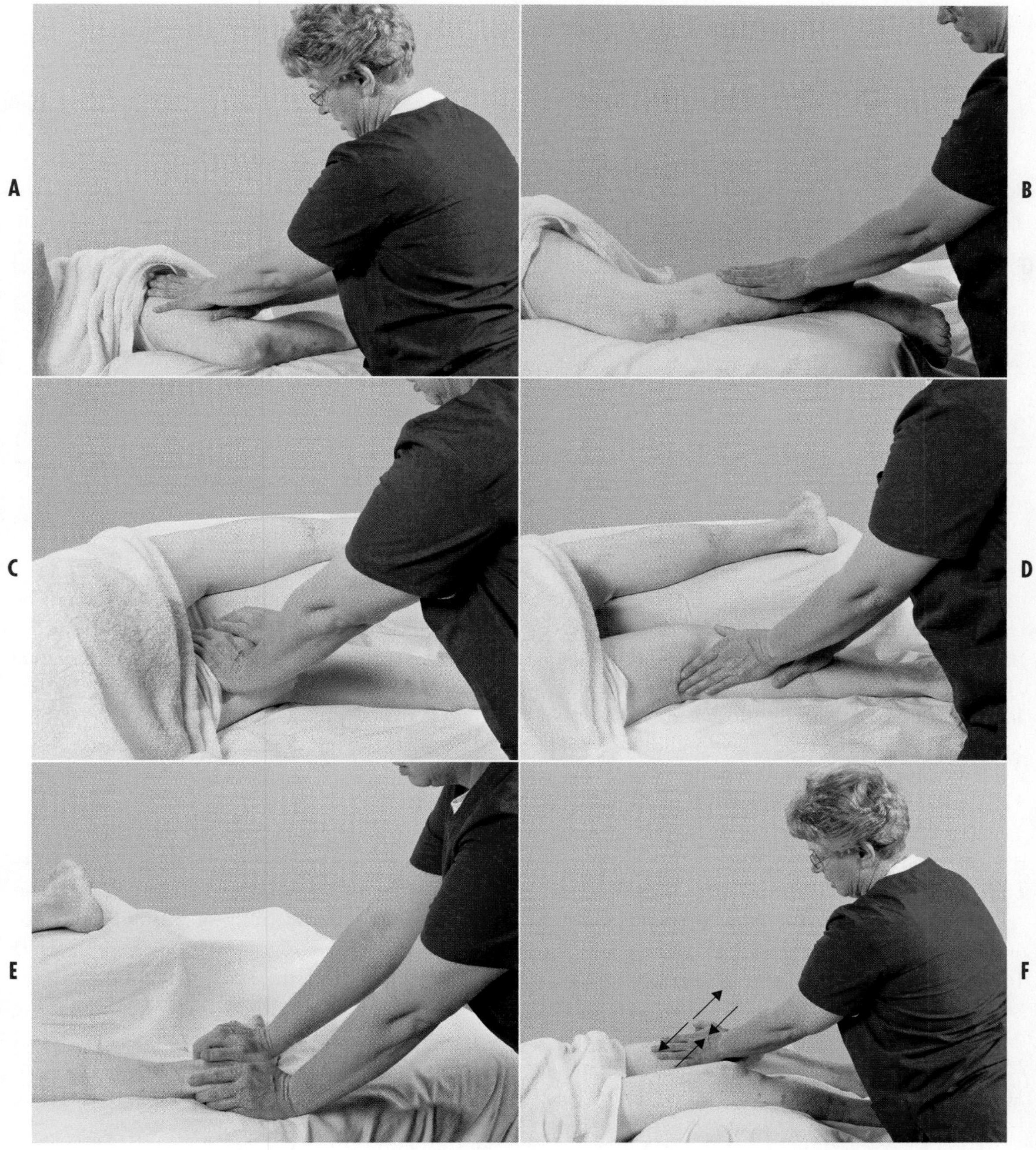

FIGURE 10-14 ■ Lymphatic drainage on an isolated area—the left knee joint—with bruises and edema on the thigh. **A,** Drainage of the entire limb. **B,** Drainage of the entire limb. **C,** Rhythmic compression and kneading. **D,** Target the area with skin drag. **E,** Rhythmic compression of the lymphatic plexus on the foot. **F,** Targeted rhythmic compression of the knee.

Continued

G 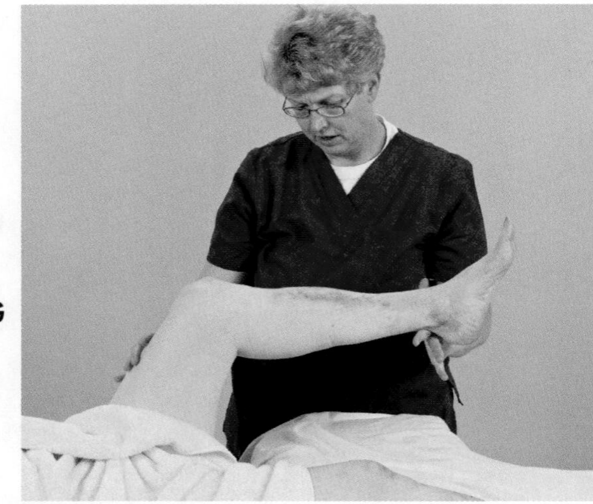 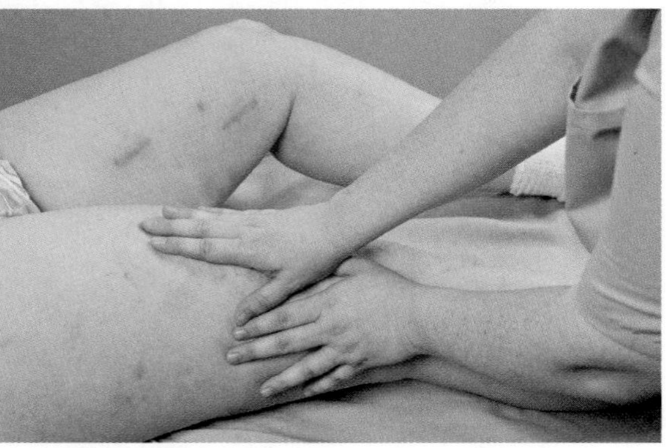 H

FIGURE 10-14, cont'd ■ **G,** Rhythmic and active joint movement. **H,** Only skin drag lymphatic drainage over bruised tissue.

9. Apply gliding strokes of moderate pressure toward the trunk. The intent is to increase fluid movement in the lymphatic vessels.
10. Repeat active and passive range of motion.
11. Prepare the tissue in the lower part of the limb (the arm or the leg) with gliding, kneading, compression, and shaking.
12. Repeat step 4, this time working all the way from the knee (or elbow) distally to the ankle (or wrist).
13. Repeat steps 5 through 10, including the entire limb from the wrist (or ankle) to the axilla (or groin).
14. Use compression to slowly and rhythmically pump the sole of the foot or the palm of the hand; continue for about 60 seconds.
15. Repeat active and passive joint movement.
16. Specifically address the swollen joint (i.e., hip, shoulder, knee, elbow, ankle, wrist, foot/hand, toes/fingers) or contusions by meticulously performing skin drag in all directions over the area unless the skin is damaged. If there is a breach in the skin, work near the area but not on it.
17. Apply active and passive joint movement.
18. Repeat steps 16 and 17.
19. If the target area is a joint, use a compressive action to slowly and rhythmically squeeze and release the tissue surrounding the joint. The smaller joints can be squeezed with one hand; the larger joints require the use of both hands to surround the joint and then squeeze together while maintaining the action.
20. Repeat the entire sequence if necessary.

10-3 CONNECTIVE TISSUE FOCUS

The quality of the connective tissue generally can be assessed by the pliability of the skin and subcutaneous layers. Thickened, adhered fascia is less mobile, and the skin glides only a short distance before feeling tight (bind). It is amazing how far healthy tissue can comfortably be stretched in all directions (Figure 10-15). In the treatment of musculoskeletal problems, the connective tissue of primary concern is the fascia that wraps the muscle fibers into bundles and compartments and then wraps all these together to form the whole muscle. The outer layer of fascia makes up the muscle's sheath, which maintains the overall shape and is smooth on the outside so that the muscle can move freely and independently of other structures. It is not contractile tissue, but it does (or should) have the same elasticity as the muscle.

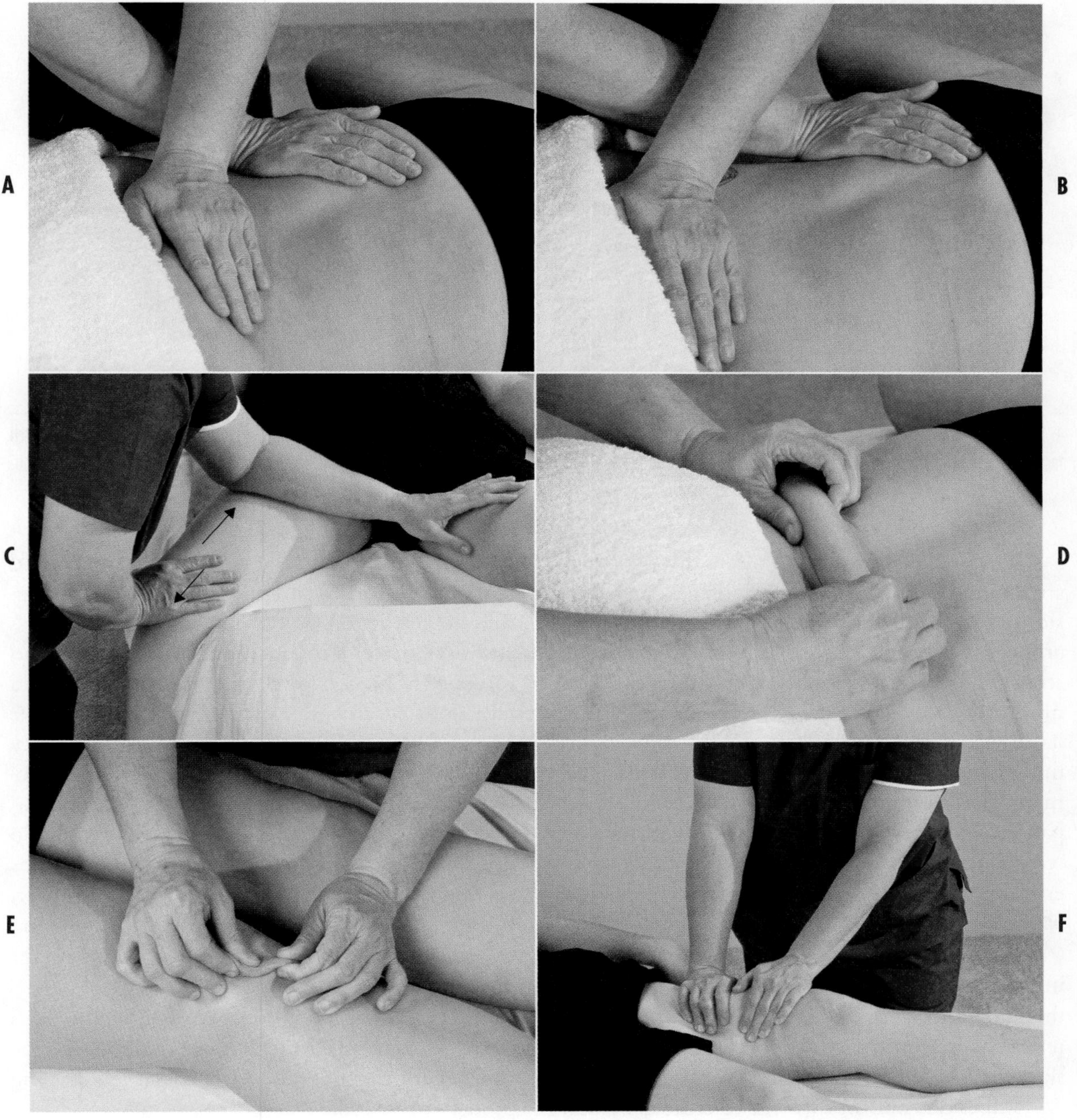

FIGURE 10-15 ■ Connective tissue methods. Typically, these approaches apply mechanical force to place and hold connective tissue structures at or slightly beyond tissue bind; then move tissue into and out of bind to increase pliability. **A,** Myofascial release, tension force: Begin at ease. **B,** Myofascial release: Move and hold tension at bind for 15 to 30 seconds. **C,** Tension force application with drag. **D,** Skin rolling: Bend force to bind. **E,** Shear force into and out of bind. **F,** Torsion force: Use an intensity sufficient to move the tissue into and out of bind.

Continued

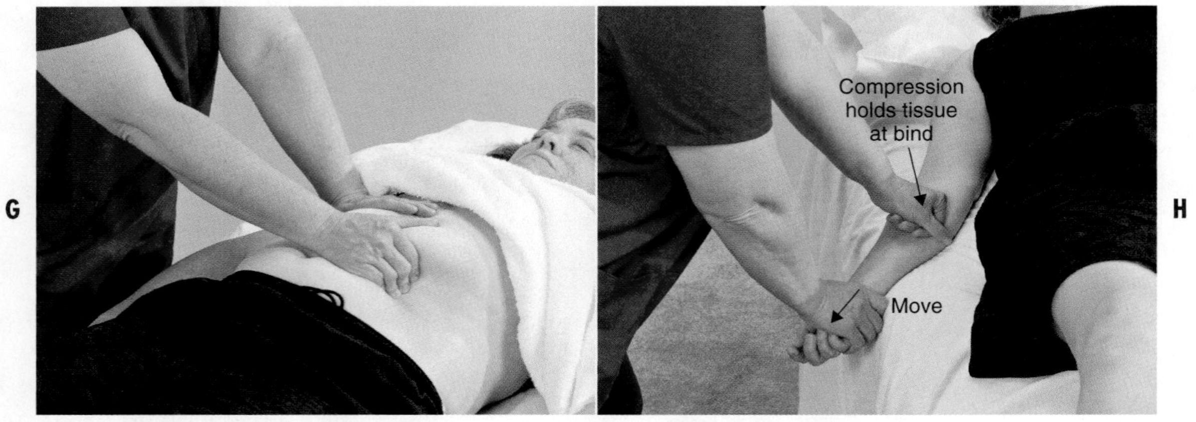

FIGURE 10-15, cont'd ■ **G,** Bend and tension force to bind; this is helpful for adhesions. **H,** Compression and tension: Pin and stretch technique uses passive joint movement. Active release uses active joint movement. Regardless of passive or active movement, maintain tissue at bind.

The fascia is subject to trauma through overstretching or impact, and scar tissue and adhesions can form. The main problem, however, arises from chronic changes caused by long-term stress. The fascia thickens and becomes more fibrous, which makes it less mobile and reduces its permeability. This affects the function of the underlying muscle and may restrict its free movement. Furthermore, if the interstitial fluid cannot pass freely through the fascia, the muscle may not receive an adequate supply of oxygen and nutrients and will be less able to eliminate metabolic waste.

Besides releasing excessive tension and relieving thickening in the fascia, connective tissue methods affect the ANS through a neurofascial reflex. This stimulates local blood flow, and the skin appears red and is warm.

Adhesions and fibrous tissue created by scar tissue cause the most dysfunction. In the early healing stages, scar tissue is quite sticky, and fibers can adhere together. For a muscle to function properly, the fibers must be able to glide smoothly alongside one another; when stuck together, they cannot do this, and the affected area does not function optimally. Over time, a local area of muscle fibers can mat together into a fibrous mass.

The noncontractile soft tissues also can be affected by fibrous adhesions, becoming less pliable. In addition, adhesions can form between different structures, such as between ligaments and tendons, muscles, and bone. This can lead to significant restriction of movement and function.

Transverse strokes using shear and bend forces can break down the fibrotic tissue and adhesions by literally tearing apart the adhesive bonds. Once the fibers have been separated, they are able to functionally slide again. Applied effectively, the massage methods should create a sensation of burning and localized pain, but they do not do any actual damage because the adhesions themselves have no blood vessels. However, further damage can result if these methods are applied too heavily or to tissue in an early stage of repair.

When a large, fibrous knot of compacted tissue has formed, little or no circulation may be running through it, therefore a natural healing process cannot take place. Massage increases tissue pliability and allows blood to flow more easily through the tissue, stimulating healing.

Massage methods are able to stretch specific localized areas of tissue in a way that may not be possible with other approaches. Longitudinal stroking (tension force) and kneading (bend and torsion force) can stretch the tissues by drawing them apart in all possible directions.

In most cases a lubricant is not used with connective tissue approaches because the drag quality on the tissue is necessary to produce results, and lubricant reduces drag.

Methods that affect primarily the ground substance require a quality of slow, sustained pressure, tension, and agitation. Most massage methods can soften the ground substance as long as the application is not abrupt. Tapotement and abrupt compression are less effective than slow gliding methods that have a drag quality. Kneading and skin rolling that incorporates a slow pulling action are effective as well. Appropriate application introduces one or a combination of the mechanical forces of tension, compression, bind, shear, and torsion.

Fiber components are affected by stretching methods (either longitudinal or cross-fiber) that elongate the fibers past their normal give and enter the plastic range past the bind. This creates either a freeing and unraveling of fibers or a small therapeutic (beneficial and controlled) inflammatory response that signals for change in the fibers.

TISSUE MOVEMENT METHODS

The more subtle connective tissue approaches rely on the skilled development of the following tissue movements.

1. Make firm but gentle contact with the skin. This is best accomplished with the tissue in the ease position.
2. Increase the downward, or vertical, pressure slowly until resistance/bind is felt; this barrier is soft and subtle.
3. Maintain the downward pressure at this point; now add horizontal drag (tension force) until the resistance barrier/bind is felt again.
4. Sustain the horizontal tension and wait.
5. The tissue will seem to creep, unravel, melt, slide, quiver, twist, or dip, or some other movement sensation will be apparent. Follow the movement, gently maintaining the tension on the tissues, encouraging the pattern as it undulates though various levels of release.
6. Slowly and gently release first the horizontal force and then the vertical force.

Twist-and-release kneading and compression applied in the direction of the restriction/bind can also release these fascial barriers.

The development of connective tissue patterns is highly individualized, and systems that follow a precise protocol and sequence often are less effective at dealing with these complex patterns. The important consideration in all connective tissue massage methods is that exerting pressure vertically and horizontally (compression and drag) actually moves the tissue to create tension, torsion, shear, or bend, generating forces and alteration of the ground substance long enough for energy to build up in it and soften it.

A good grip on the skin is essential, therefore no lotion or oil can be used. This grip can be achieved with the hands or forearms. The technique sometimes is even preformed with a towel, to provide stronger contact with the skin. The tissues are moved toward ease (i.e., the way they want to move) and are held for a few seconds to allow them to soften. The patient can add a neurologic component by contracting or relaxing the muscle as the massage therapist holds the tissues at ease. The entire procedure can be repeated while holding the tissues at bind (i.e., the way they do not want to move).

Some varieties of this process have been formalized into modality systems such as active release and pin and stretch.

ACTIVE RELEASE AND PIN AND STRETCH

With the **active release technique,** the massage therapist applies passive pressure and the patient provides the movement. In the **pin and stretch technique,** which is more passive, the therapist uses passive joint movement or direct tissue stretching. Assessment identifies a local area of fibrotic tissue and/or adhered fibers. Compression is applied to hold the area in a static position. The tissues then are stretched away from that point, either actively by the patient or passively by the massage therapist, or by the two together. The points where the pressure is applied often are the same as those used for typical trigger points.

The basic method starts with the muscle relaxed; it is held in a passive, shortened position by moving the associated joint. Focused compression is applied directly into the adhered fibers to fix them in position. The muscle then is stretched away from this fixed point in one of two ways: the therapist moves the joint (pin and stretch), or the patient provides the movement (active release). Pressure must be applied with sufficient force to prevent the target tissues from moving as the stretch takes place.

The use of active and resisted movements to stretch the muscle may be more effective than passive movements because the neuromuscular function is involved in addition to the focus on the connective tissue. The patient contracts the antagonist that reciprocally inhibits the muscle being treated and moves the area while the massage therapist maintains focused pressure. An easy way to do this is to have the patient move the associated joint areas in a slow circle (or back and forth if the joint is a hinge joint). The tissues also can be stretched away from the pressure point by using deep massage strokes done with the other hand or forearm. This is useful when moving the joint is not convenient, such as when treating the gluteal muscles with the patient in the prone position, and hip flexion to stretch the muscle would be impossible (Figure 10-16).

JUST BETWEEN YOU AND ME

Connective tissue methods sometimes are considered "deep tissue massage." This is very confusing, because connective tissue is found in both surface and deep tissue levels. I really don't know what "deep tissue massage" is. Massage should be applied with the appropriate depth and intensity to achieve outcomes. If third layer muscles are targeted, deeper pressure is required than for the first and second layer muscles. Deep tissue work is required if the connective tissues closest to the bone are the target, unless the connective tissue target is near a joint, where these tissues lie relatively close to the surface. Therefore, "deep tissue massage"—I just don't understand the concept.

A

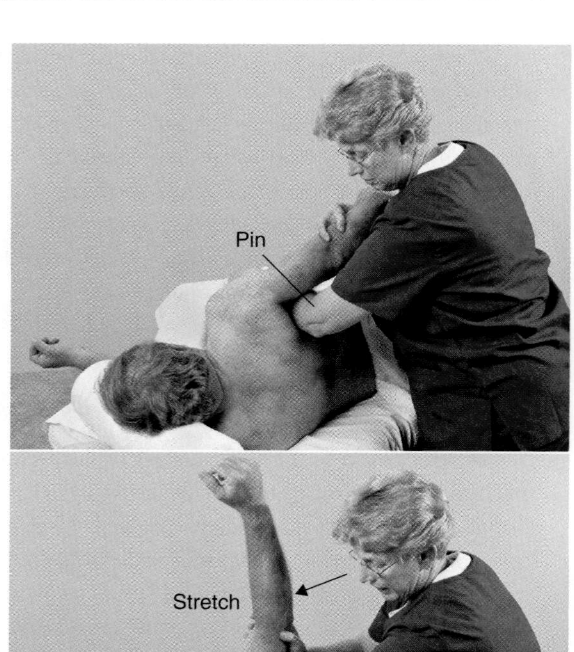

B

C

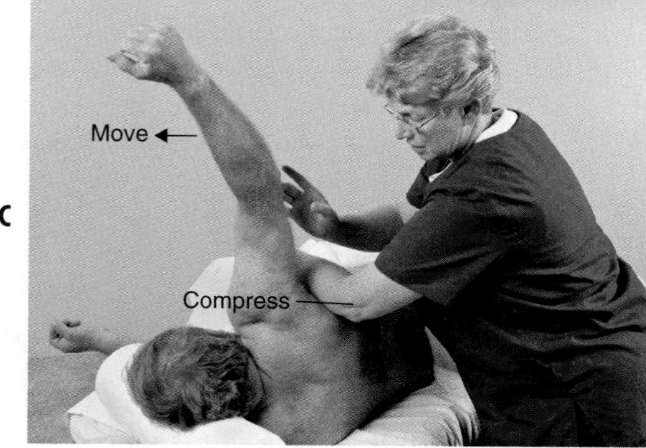

FIGURE 10-16 ■ Pin and stretch and active release techniques. **A,** Compression into the tissue, pin. **B,** The therapist moves the area: stretch. **C,** Active release: The therapist compresses the binding tissue and instructs the patient to move the area.

10-4 TRIGGER POINTS*

The terms *neuromuscular therapy* and *trigger point therapy* often are used interchangeably, which has created some confusion. *Neuromuscular therapy* is an umbrella term that encompasses a variety of treatment approaches, one of which is trigger point therapy. *Trigger point therapy* is one of many techniques useful in the treatment of neuromuscular and myofascial problems.

A **trigger point** is an area of local nerve facilitation and chemical imbalance of a muscle that is aggravated by stress of any sort affecting the

*For detailed information on trigger point therapy, see both volumes of the text by Leon Chaitow and Judith Delany, *Clinical application of neuromuscular techniques* (Edinburgh, 2002, Churchill Livingstone).

body or mind (Box 10-1). Trigger points are small areas of hyperirritability within soft tissues. They sometimes are located in the belly of the muscle, usually near the motor points where nerve stimulation initiates a contraction in a small, sensitive bundle of muscle fibers, which in turn activates the entire muscle at or near the tendon of a muscle attachment point. They also can be found in fascial tissues, especially scar tissue. If these areas are located near motor nerve points, the person may experience referred pain caused by nerve stimulation (Figure 10-17).

BOX 10-1 Common Physiologic Responses to Stress

Massage professionals recognize that the following physiologic signs of stress result from fluctuations in the autonomic nervous system and resulting shifts in endogenous chemicals.

- General irritability, hyperexcitation, or depression
- Pounding heart
- Dry throat and mouth
- Impulsive behavior and emotional instability
- Overpowering urge to cry, run, or hide
- Inability to concentrate
- Weakness or dizziness
- Fatigue
- Tension and extreme alertness
- Trembling and nervous tics
- Intermittent anxiety
- Tendency to be easily startled
- High-pitched, nervous laughter
- Stuttering and other speech difficulties
- Grinding of the teeth
- Insomnia
- Inability to sit still or physically relax
- Sweating
- Frequent need to urinate
- Diarrhea, indigestion, queasiness, and vomiting
- Migraine and other tension headaches
- Premenstrual tension or missed menstrual cycles
- Pain in the neck or lower back
- Loss of or excessive appetite
- Increased use of chemicals, including tobacco, caffeine, and alcohol
- Nightmares
- Neurotic behavior
- Psychosis
- Proneness to accidents

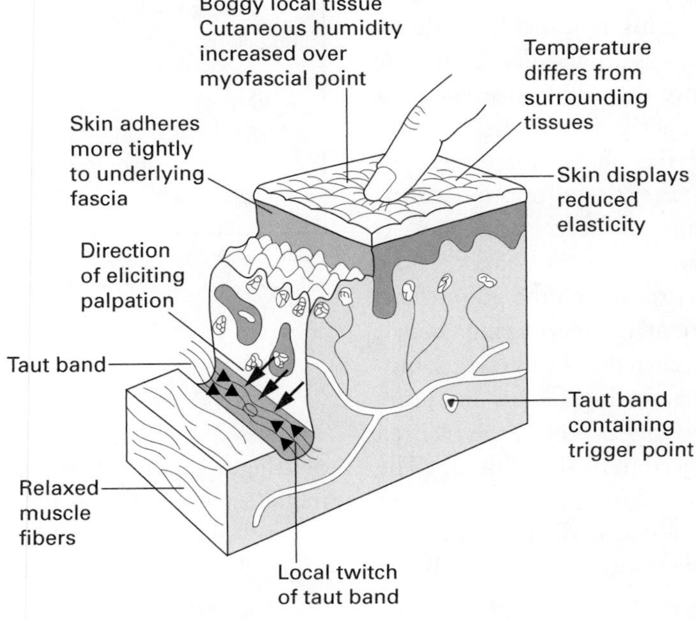

FIGURE 10-17 ■ Altered physiology of tissues in the region of a myofascial trigger point. (From Chaitow L, Delany J: *Clinical application of neuromuscular techniques, vol 1, The upper body,* Edinburgh, 2000, Churchill Livingstone.)

BOX 10-2 Active and Latent Trigger Points

- When pressure is applied to active trigger points, they refer a sensation pattern that is recognizable to the person (e.g., pain, tingling, numbness, burning, itching, or some other sensation).
- When pressure is applied to latent trigger points, they refer a pattern that is not familiar to the person or perhaps one that the person experienced in the past but has not recently.
- Activation may occur when the tissue is overused, strained by overload, chilled, stretched (particularly abruptly), shortened, or traumatized (as in a motor vehicle accident or a fall or blow) or when other perpetuating factors (e.g., poor nutrition, shallow breathing) result in less than optimal conditions of tissue health.
- Active trigger points may become latent trigger points, with their referral patterns subsiding for either brief or prolonged periods. They subsequently may be reactivated, with their referral patterns returning for no apparent reason, a condition that may confuse both practitioner and patient.

From Chaitow L, Delany J: *Clinical application of neuromuscular techniques, vol 1, The upper body,* London, 2000, Churchill Livingstone.

A trigger point area often is located in a tight band of muscle fibers. Palpation across the band may elicit a twitch response, which is a slight jump in the muscle fibers. This is difficult to detect when the trigger point is in the deeper muscle layers. Any of the more than 400 muscles in the body can develop trigger points. Trigger points are accompanied by the characteristic referred pain pattern and the restriction of motion associated with neuromuscular and myofascial pain.

Trigger points can be active or latent. If the trigger point is active, pressure on the point elicits the symptom the patient is experiencing. Latent trigger points are not currently producing symptoms but can be perpetuating factors in future problems. With classic trigger points, the referred pain pattern can be traced to its site of origin. The distribution of the referred trigger point pain does not usually follow an entire distribution of a peripheral nerve or dermatome segment (Boxes 10-2 and 10-3).

BOX 10-3 Theory of Trigger Point Formation

Some researchers have suggested that the formation of trigger points can be explained as follows:

1. Dysfunctional endplate activity occurs, commonly associated with a strain, overuse, or direct trauma.
2. Stored calcium is released at the site as a result of overuse or of tearing of the sarcoplasmic reticulum.
3. Acetylcholine (Ach) is released excessively at the synapse because of calcium-charged gates.
4. High calcium levels at the site keep the calcium-charged gates open, and Ach continues to be released.
5. Ischemia develops in the area, resulting in an oxygen and nutrient deficit.
6. A local energy crisis develops.
7. The tissue is unable to remove the calcium ions without available adenosine triphosphate (ATP), therefore Ach continues flowing.
8. Removal of the superfluous calcium requires more energy than sustaining a contracture, therefore the contracture remains.
9. The contracture is sustained not by action potentials from the cord but by the chemistry at the innervation site.
10. The actin/myosin filaments slide to a fully shortened position (a weakened state) in the immediate area around the motor endplate (at the center of the fiber).
11. As the sarcomeres shorten, a contracture knot forms.
12. The contracture knot is the *nodule,* which is a palpable characteristic of a trigger point.
13. The remainder of the sarcomeres of that fiber are stretched, creating the usually palpable taut band that also is a common trigger point characteristic.
14. Attachment trigger points may develop at the attachment sites of these shortened tissues (e.g., periosteal, myotendinous) where muscular tension provokes inflammation.

From Chaitow L, Delany J: *Clinical application of neuromuscular techniques, vol 1, The upper body,* London, 2000, Churchill Livingstone.

PERPETUATING FACTORS

Reflexive, mechanical, and systemic perpetuating factors are involved in the development of trigger points. Reflexive perpetuating factors include:

- Skin sensitivity in the area of the trigger point
- Scar tissue
- Joint dysfunction
- Visceral dysfunction in the viscerally referred pain pattern
- Vasoconstriction

Mechanical perpetuating factors include:

- Standing postural distortion
- Seated postural distortion
- Gait distortion
- Immobilization
- Vocational stress (this includes sport activity)
- Restrictive or ill-fitting clothing and shoes
- Poorly designed furniture

Systemic perpetuating factors include:

- Enzyme dysfunction
- Metabolic and endocrine dysfunction
- Chronic infection
- Dietary insufficiencies
- Psychological stress

ASSESSMENT

Often it is difficult to decide whether a tender spot is a trigger point, a point of fascial adhesion that requires frictioning, a motor point, or some other irritable reflex point, including an active acupuncture point. Stretching of trigger point areas is essential for effective treatment; therefore, if doubt exists about the nature of the point, it should be treated as a trigger point. The stretching can be longitudinal or direct.

The massage therapist usually finds trigger points during palpation or general massage using both light and deep palpation (Box 10-4). Remember, active trigger points produce pain familiar to the patient. Latent trigger points are painful only when stimulated by compression or stretching.

During assessment and treatment, the patient is aware of the trigger point but does not initiate protective mechanisms such as guarding (tightening up), breath holding, or flinching. The muscle must be relaxed to be assessed effectively. If the pressure is too great, severe local pain may overwhelm the referred pain sensation, making accurate evaluation impossible. In areas of deep inflammation, pain increases when pressure is sustained. In areas of increased motor tone, motor tone decreases when pressure is sustained. Trigger points refer pain into the massaged areas when pressure is sustained, and the pain sensation then diminishes. Trigger points that are so active that referred pain is already being produced do not require exaggerated pressure during assessment (Figure 10-18).

BOX 10-4 Palpation for Trigger Points

Light Palpation

In performing light palpation, the therapist may detect trigger points by the following responses:

- Skin changes: The skin may feel tense, with resistance to gliding strokes. The skin may be slightly damp as a result of perspiration caused by sympathetic facilitation, and the hand will stick or drag on the skin.
- Temperature changes: The temperature in a local area increases with acute dysfunction but decreases with ischemia, which indicates fibrotic changes within the tissues.
- Edema: Edema is an impression of fullness and congestion within the tissues. With chronic dysfunction, edema is replaced gradually by fibrotic (connective tissue) changes.

Deep Palpation

During deep palpation, the therapist establishes contact with the deeper fibers of the soft tissues and explores them for any of the following:

- Immobility
- Tenderness
- Edema
- Deep muscle tension
- Fibrotic changes
- Interosseous changes

From Fritz S: *Mosby's fundamentals of therapeutic massage,* ed 3, St Louis, 2004, Mosby.

TREATMENT METHODS

Only muscles that can actually be treated at the same visit should be examined. Palpation for trigger points can aggravate their referred pain activity, therefore only areas intended for treatment should be palpated.

Trigger point treatment should not be done for extended periods. It should be incorporated into a more general approach.

All the basic neuromuscular techniques, including the muscle energy techniques, deal effectively with trigger points if the hyperirritable area within a muscle is hyperstimulated and then lengthened and the connective tissue in the area is softened and stretched. After a trigger point has been identified, the massage therapist uses a

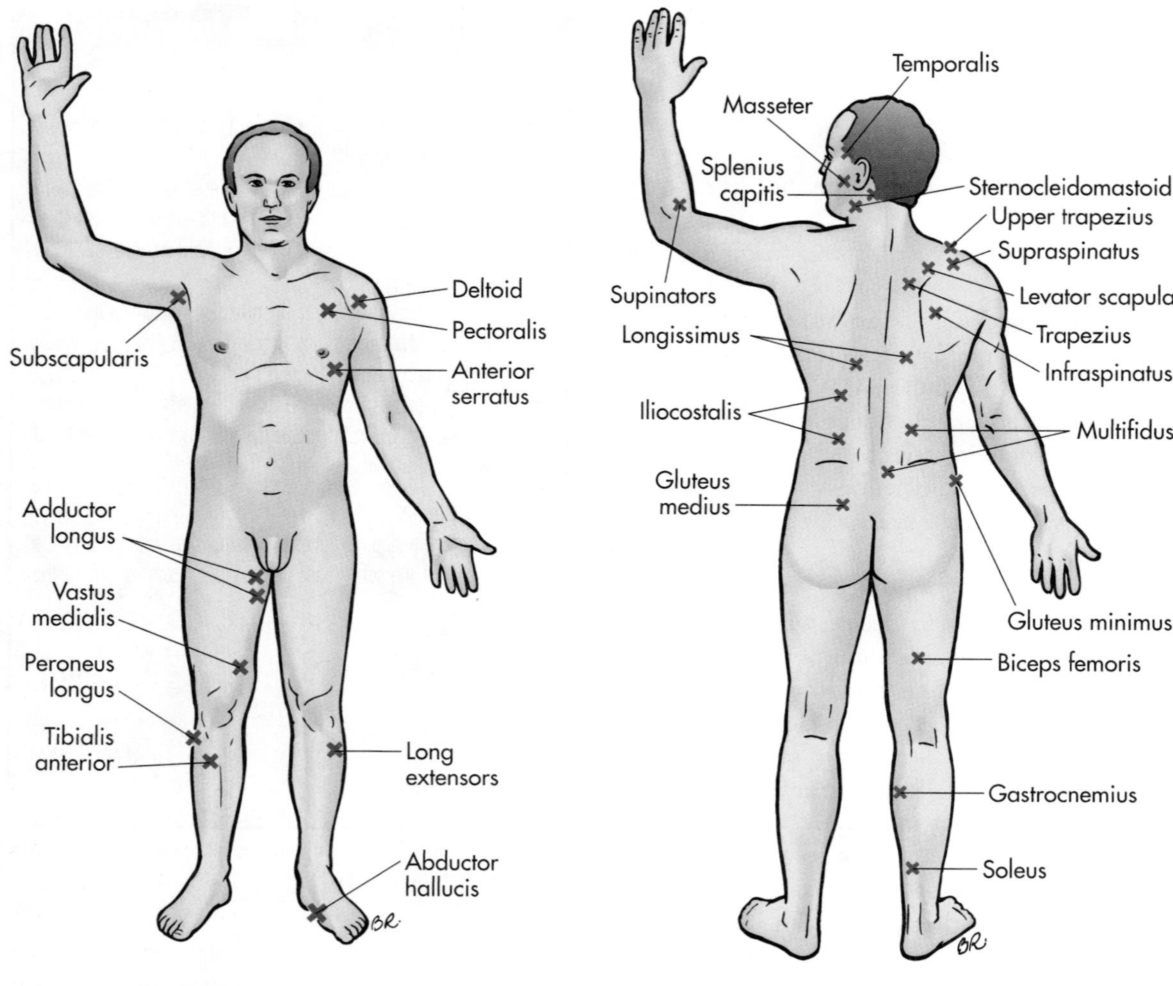

FIGURE 10-18 ■ Common trigger points. (From Fritz S: *Mosby's fundamentals of therapeutic massage,* ed 3, St Louis, 2004, Mosby.)

pressure technique, muscle energy, or a direct manipulation and stretch method to reduce hyperactivity in the point. Direct manipulation of proprioceptors by pushing or pulling on a muscle belly or its attachments is also effective. Intervention progresses from least aggressive to most aggressive. **Indirect functional techniques** in which the tissues over the trigger points and those containing the trigger points are moved into ease are beneficial. The tissues and proprioceptors in multiple areas of ease are held in ease for up to 60 seconds.

Positional release, with the appropriate stretching, is one of the most effective ways to treat trigger points. Positional release consists of identifying the painful point and positioning the body in the ease position that reduces the pain at the point. Positional release is the first step in the integrated muscle energy method, which introduces muscle contraction before lengthening.

Direct manipulation methods consist of pressing the belly of the muscle together to affect spindle cells and pushing the tendons apart to affect tendon receptors. If the belly of the muscle is pressed together and the desired effect is not achieved, the next step should be to separate the tissue from the middle of the muscle belly toward the tendons. Lengthening and direct manipulation are gentle methods and should be used next.

The integrated muscle energy method is more aggressive than positional release or direct manipulation but less aggressive than pressure or pinching methods and should be the next step. These methods often are effective and are worth trying before the more intense pressure or pinching techniques. The local area must be lengthened. This lengthening is performed either directly on the tissues or through movement of a joint.

If the trigger point remains after the less invasive methods have been attempted, pressure techniques can be tried. The pressure may take the form of direct pressure, in which the therapist presses the trigger point against an underlying hard structure (bone) or, when no bony tissue lies underneath, pinching pressure, as in the "squeezing" of the sternocleidomastoid muscle.

Pressure techniques can end the hyperirritability by mechanical disruption of the sensory nerve endings causing the trigger point activity. When using the direct pressure technique, the massage therapist must hold the compression long enough to stimulate the spindle cells.

When the trigger point has been located, the duration of applied pressure varies. Dr. Chaitow recommends gradually intensifying pressure, building up to 8 seconds. Pressure applied to the trigger point should be intense enough to bring about a physiologic change, but not so intense that the patient is in extreme pain. Acceptable discomfort is approximately how the patient grades pain sensation on a 0 to 10 pain scale, in which 10 is extreme pain. The pain intensity should be maintained at around 7. The process then is repeated for up to 30 seconds or as long as 2 minutes. The procedure should end when the patient reports that the referred pain has diminished or when the massage therapist feels a release in the trigger point tissue. The release sensation can be a softening of the tissues, a decrease in density, or lengthening.

Sufficient duration is determined by the fiber construction of the muscle. Muscles are made up of red (slow twitch) fibers and white (fast twitch) fibers. The type of fiber is determined by whether the muscle functions as a postural (stabilizer) muscle or a phasic (mover) muscle and by the demands exerted by the patient's lifestyle. Phasic muscle fibers are easier to fatigue than postural muscle fibers. After a muscle is fatigued, a period of recovery ensues in which the fibers will not contract, and the muscle can be lengthened effectively and stretched if necessary.

Dr. Chaitow also recommends variable pressure, rather than a uniform pressure from beginning to end, to prevent further irritation of the trigger area. This is a carefully changing pressure applied for a specific purpose, which reflects the therapist's sensitivity to what is happening as the tissue responds; the therapist applies more pressure as the tissue relaxes and accepts more pressure. When the massage therapist senses that the tissues are becoming tense, pressure is reduced.

As an alternative, deep cross-fiber friction over the trigger point can be effective, followed by lengthening and stretching. This method is beneficial if the massage therapist suspects that the connective tissue around the trigger point has become fibrotic and scar tissue is present.

Localized treatment of a muscle should always end with lengthening and stretching of the muscle, either passively or actively. Gradual, gentle lengthening to reset the normal resting length of the muscle's neuromuscular mechanism and stretching to elongate the muscle's shortened connective tissue must follow the positioning and/or pressure methods. Incomplete restoration of the full length of the muscle means incomplete relief of pain. Failure to lengthen and stretch the area results in the eventual return of the original symptoms. Muscle energy approaches are more effective than passive stretching at achieving the proper response. Trigger points in deep layers of muscle or in a muscle that is difficult to lengthen by moving the body are addressed with local bend, shear, and torsion forces to lengthen and stretch the area. This often is the most effective method with patients.

Trigger points in the belly of muscles usually are found in short, concentrically contracted muscles. Trigger points near the attachments usually are found in eccentric patterns and in long, inhibited muscles acting as antagonists to concentrically contracted muscles. Muscle shortening may serve as a response for compensation purposes. The best course of action is to address the trigger point activity in the short tissues first and wait to see whether the trigger points in the long muscles and at the attachments resolve as the posture of muscle interaction normalizes. Attachment points are treated only if tissue remains fibrotic.

Do not overtreat trigger points. Initially address only the trigger points that recreate symptoms the patient is experiencing. Remember, anything can feel like a trigger point if pressed on hard enough. Address only the trigger point that is most painful, most medial, and most proximal that recreates the patient's symptoms. Leave the rest alone. As the posture and function normalize with regular massage, many trigger points go away on their own. Continue to monitor latent trigger points to make sure they resolve over the treatment period for active trigger points. If the active points recur and if latent points do not go resolve within a reasonable period (10 treatments), begin to address them, starting with the closest active trigger point area.

Isometric contraction and concentric movements can be used to balance the long inhibited muscles. In an isometric contraction, the muscle is placed in a specific position within its range and the patient contracts against resistance, without any actual movement taking place. This is particularly useful for maintaining strength in a muscle that cannot be exercised normally because of dysfunction in the associated joint. The strengthening effect is greatest in the middle and inner range of movement.

Concentric movements are the most common type of muscle-strengthening activity. The muscle is contracted and shortened by taking it through its active range of movement with weighted resistance. For example, the biceps muscle concentrically contracts when lifting a weight by flexing the elbow.

A muscle produces its greatest force in the midrange. If a muscle is strengthened only in the midrange, it will function only in that range and may become chronically short. Therefore it is important always to include exercises with light resistance through the fullest range of both concentric and eccentric function, to develop length as well. The movements also should be done slowly to develop control throughout the contraction range. Sudden, quick contractions can lead to injury and are likely to increase muscle tension by overstimulating the nerve receptors (Figure 10-19).

JOINT PLAY

Synovial joints provide both stability and mobility. Synovial joints are constructed in such a way that there is an inherent movement of the bones inside the joint capsule; this is called **joint play.** Not uncommonly, this natural, small movement becomes reduced.

In general, all synovial joints have a concave bone end and a convex one. The position of the bone ends in the joint capsule is a factor in the efficiency of the joint function.

Working with specific joint function is beyond the scope of practice for therapeutic massage. It is best left in the care of the medical team, such as the chiropractor or physical therapist. However, an indirect functional technique that can be incorporated into the massage application to influence proper joint play is called **mobilization with movement (MWM).** This gentle method uses the ease position of a joint, combined with active movement by the patient, to settle the joint into a more functional position. MWM methodology typically involves translation or glide movement outside of voluntary control; the therapist holds this position while the patient moves the previously "stuck" or painful joint. Use of this method requires a thorough understanding of individual joint structure, the close-packed and least-packed position of each joint, and the normal range of motion of each joint (Table 10-1).

Before the MWM method is used, all soft tissues (muscle, tendons, and ligaments) must be relaxed and pliable. During assessment, the descriptive term the patient typically uses is "stuck." The patient usually can point to the stuck area and describes an event such as jamming the fingers when falling, being hit, stepping down hard, stepping into a hole, and so on.

Protocol for Mobilization with Movement

1. Normalize all tissues surrounding the joint.
2. Position the joint in least-packed position (typically the middle range of motion).

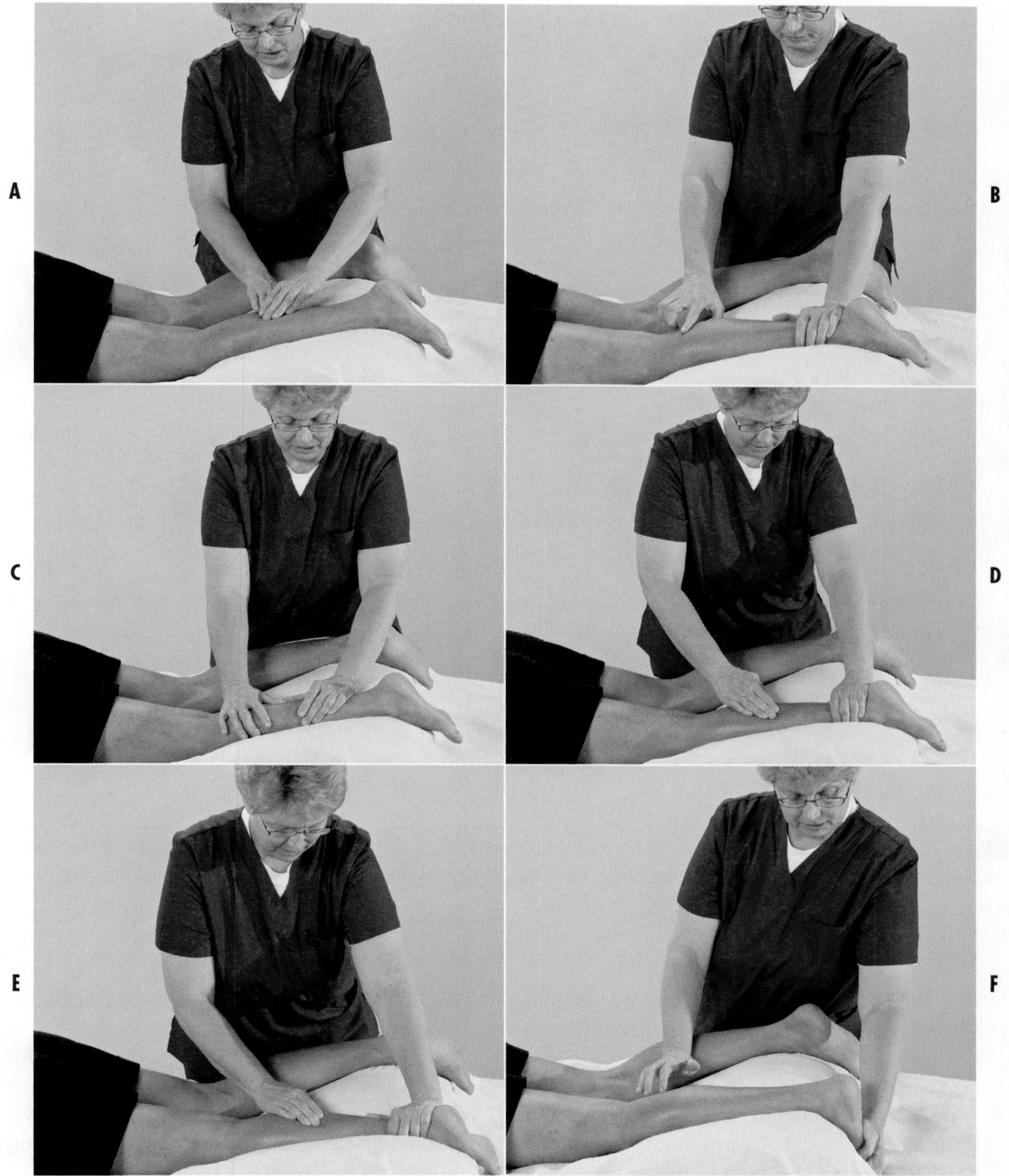

FIGURE 10-19 ■ Assessment and treatment of trigger points (least invasive techniques to most invasive). **A,** Assess using various forms of palpation. **B,** Identify the trigger point. **C,** Move the tissue containing the trigger point into ease; hold and then reassess. **D,** Move the tissue containing the trigger point into bind to treat and stretch. **E,** Use positional release. **F,** Stretch.

Continued

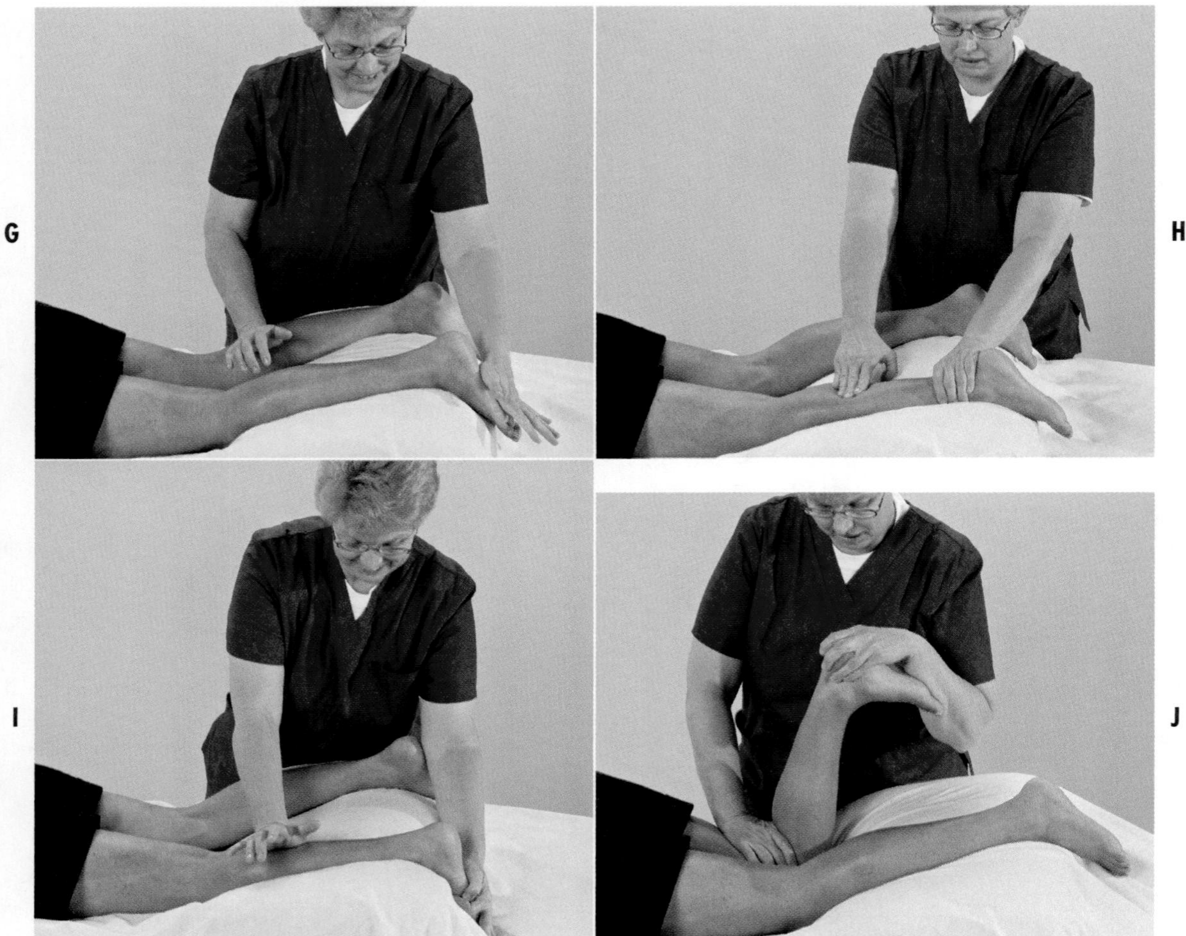

FIGURE 10-19 cont'd ■ **G,** Incorporate a muscle energy method with stretching. **H,** Apply direct inhibiting pressure and then stretch. **I,** Introduce combined loading in the form of pin and stretch, active release, and integrated muscle energy techniques. **J,** Know when to quit and move on with the massage.

3. Stabilize the most proximal end of the joint and gently pull in a straight line traction. Remember, no pain.
4. Translate/glide and twist/shunt one bone onto the other and have the patient introduce movement in the ease position.
5. Maintain the traction while introducing movement in a different direction (e.g., up, down; back, forth; rotation, diagonal). Identify the direction of the most ease.
6. Maintain the position of greatest ease, especially the traction, and instruct the patient to move the joint through the range of motion. The action of the muscles should pull the joint back into a more functional fit.

If the patient is unable to move the joint (including when sleeping), modify the technique by creating only traction and then passively move the joint through pain-free and normal range of motion (Figure 10-20).

REFLEXOLOGY

Reflexology is a bodywork method that applies the stimulus/response reflex principle to healing of the body (Figure 10-21). The foot has been

TABLE 10-1 Least-Packed Positions of Joints

Joints	Position
Spine	Midway between flexion and extension
Temporomandibular	Mouth slightly open
Glenohumeral	55 degrees abduction, 30 degrees horizontal adduction
Acromioclavicular	Arm resting by side in normal physiologic position
Sternoclavicular	Arm resting by side in normal physiologic position
Elbow	70 degrees flexion, 10 degrees supination
Radiohumeral	Full extension and full supination
Proximal radioulnar	70 degrees flexion, 35 degrees supination
Distal radioulnar	10 degrees supination
Wrist	Neutral with slight ulnar deviation
Carpometacarpal	Midway between abduction/adduction and flexion/extension
Thumb	Slight flexion
Interphalangeal	Slight flexion
Hip	30 degrees flexion, 30 degrees abduction and slight lateral rotation
Knee	25 degrees flexion
Ankle	10 degrees plantar flexion, midway between maximum inversion and eversion
Subtalar	Midway between extremes of range of motion
Midtarsal	Midway between extremes of range of motion
Tarsometatarsal	Midway between extremes of range of motion
Metatarsophalangeal	Neutral
Interphalangeal	Slight flexion

Modified from Magee DJ: *Orthopedic physical assessment,* ed 4, Philadelphia, 2002, WB Saunders.

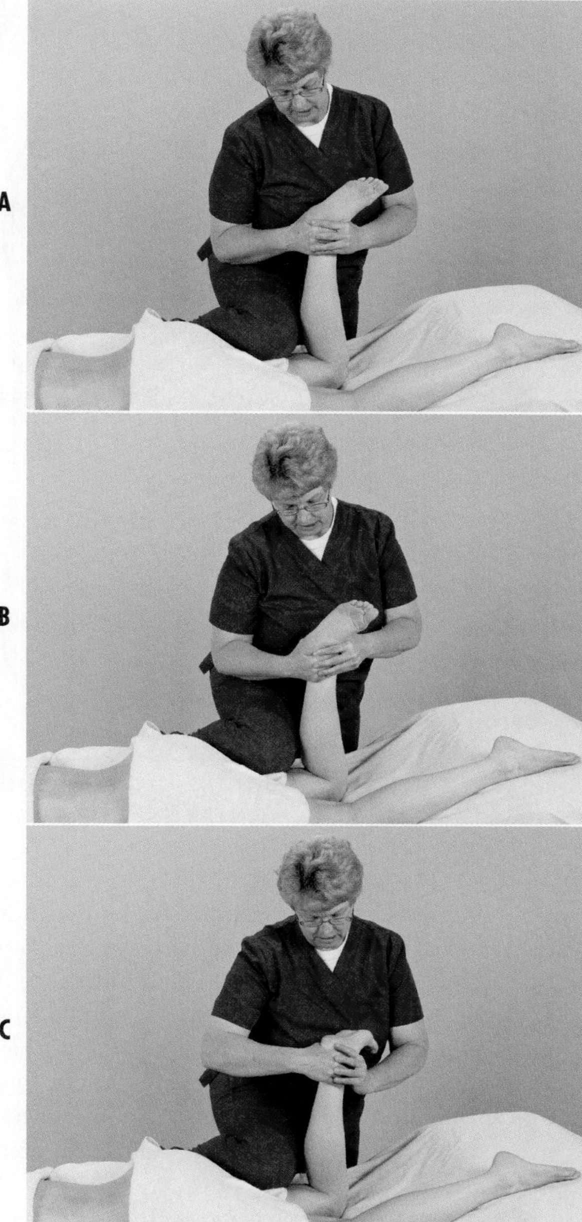

FIGURE 10-20 ■ Joint play. **A,** The therapist applies traction and maintains traction position. **B,** The therapist adds the second movement into ease. **C,** While the therapist maintains traction and the ease position, the patient moves the area.

mapped to show the areas to contact to affect different parts of the body. Charts mapping the foot and body relationship areas vary somewhat, but typically the large toe represents the head, and the junction of the large toe and the foot represents the neck. The other toes represent the eyes, ears, and sinuses. The waist is about midway on the arch of the foot, with various organs above and below the line. The reflex points for the spine are along the medial longitudinal arch.

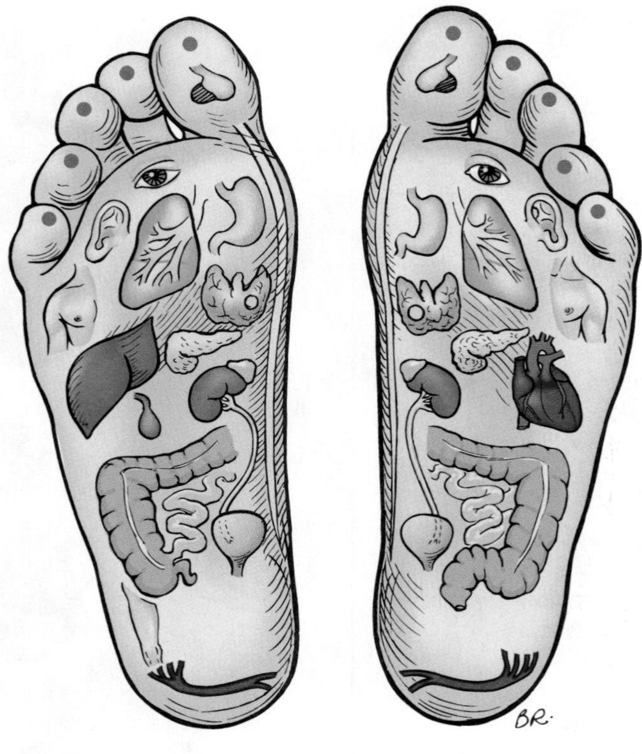

FIGURE 10-21 ■ A generalized reflexology chart. (From Fritz S: *Mosby's fundamentals of therapeutic massage,* ed 3, St Louis, 2004, Mosby.)

It is thought that this stimulus/response reflex is conducted through neural pathways in the body that activate the body's electrical and biochemical activities (see Figure 10-21). No scientific documentation exists for this method; however, it has shown up consistently in various forms in historical literature. The most thoroughly documented system is part of traditional Chinese medicine.

People usually appreciate having their feet massaged, and it does no harm to include these methods. The foot is a very complex structure. The ankle and foot consist of 34 joints, with many joint and reflex patterns and extensive nerve distribution to the feet and hands. The position of the foot sends considerable postural information from the joint mechanoreceptors through the central nervous system (CNS). The sensory and motor centers of the brain devote a large area to the foot and hand.

It seems logical to assume that stimulation of the feet activates the responses of the gate control mechanism and hyperstimulation analgesia, with activation of the parasympathetic ANS. Many nerve endings on the feet and hands correlate to acupressure points, which, when stimulated, trigger the release of endorphins and other endogenous chemicals. In addition, major plexuses for the lymph system are located in the hands and feet. Rhythmic compressive forces in these areas stimulate lymphatic movement, producing body-wide effects.

METHODS OF MASSAGE FOR THE FOOT

An excellent way to massage the foot is to apply pressure and movement systematically to the entire foot and ankle complex. The pressure stimulates the circulation, nerves, and reflexes. Moving all the joints stimulates large diameter nerve fibers and joint mechanoreceptors, initiating hyperstimulation analgesia. The result is a shift in proprioceptive and postural reflexes. The sheer volume of sensory information flooding the CNS has significant effects on the body that support parasympathetic dominance.

ASIAN MASSAGE CONCEPTS

According to Chinese theory, the meridians are internally associated with organs and externally associated with the surface of the head, trunk, and extremities. **Meridians** seem to be energy flows from nerve tracts in the tissue and are located in the fascial grooves.

YIN AND YANG

The Chinese perspective considers body functions in terms of balance between complementary forces. These complementary forces, often thought of as opposites, are actually part of a continuum. Physiologically the body is a closed system. Areas of "too much" energy cannot exist without reciprocal areas of "not enough" energy. Just as muscles work in pairs and facilitate and inhibit each other, so do meridians. The tool that helps to make sense of these complex interrelationships is the theory of yin and yang.

The **yin** and **yang** theory is a means of recognizing and defining patterns within highly complex, dynamic systems. It is a tool for perceiving order within supposed chaos and for allowing recognition of patterns of imbalance.

The body is described in terms of yin and yang (e.g., back and front, upper and lower, external and internal). Each part of the body can be subdivided into yin parts and yang parts. The internal organs are described as yin or yang characteristics according to their nature and function. Yin and yang manifest in all aspects of the body, interior and exterior interdependently related; therefore internal imbalances can be treated by working externally on the body.

ACUPUNCTURE AND ACUPRESSURE

Acupressure is a modified version of acupuncture that substitutes pressure for needle insertion. The results of acupressure are not as dramatic as those of acupuncture, but the technique is still effective, especially if it is repeated often and the pressure is held long enough.

Acupressure has a role in massage as an adjunct to the general protocol. It is especially helpful for systemic dysfunction, such as a cold or general fatigue.

Traditional Chinese medicine (TCM) methods are valued for sound physiologic reasons. Particular effects can be demonstrated after acupuncture treatment. Some of these effects involve alteration of the function of organs or systems. An analgesic effect and an anesthetic effect also occur, for those who find the physiology of these approaches difficult. It is not necessary to believe that disease is caused by an imbalance of yin and yang (the two equal and opposite forces of the universe, which act through qi). Instead, the benefits of acupuncture can be framed in terms of the body's homeostatic tendency, whereby a stable internal environment is maintained through the interaction of the various body processes and systems.

Some practitioners of Western medicine are integrating Chinese medicine techniques, including acupuncture, into their treatment regimens. The massage therapist needs to understand the basic concepts of Chinese medicine to support these healthcare professionals.

Stimulation of local points is the most basic use of acupressure and probably the most easily accessible for those accustomed to Western methods of treatment. However, this is only a small part of an ancient system of medical practice that includes needling, herbal therapy, manipulation, exercise, massage, and meditation. Many patients regularly use these methods.

MERIDIANS

The patterns that **acupuncture points** make on the body's surface have been charted for centuries by practitioners of acupuncture. They have been grouped together in lines called *channels,* or *meridians,* and have been allocated to the organs or functions upon which they appear to act (Figure 10-22). In addition to the 12 pairs of bilateral meridians, two meridians lie on the anterior and posterior midline of the trunk and head. Various extra meridians appear to relate to the body's organs and functions. Other points in the ear surfaces, hands, and face have specific reflex effects.

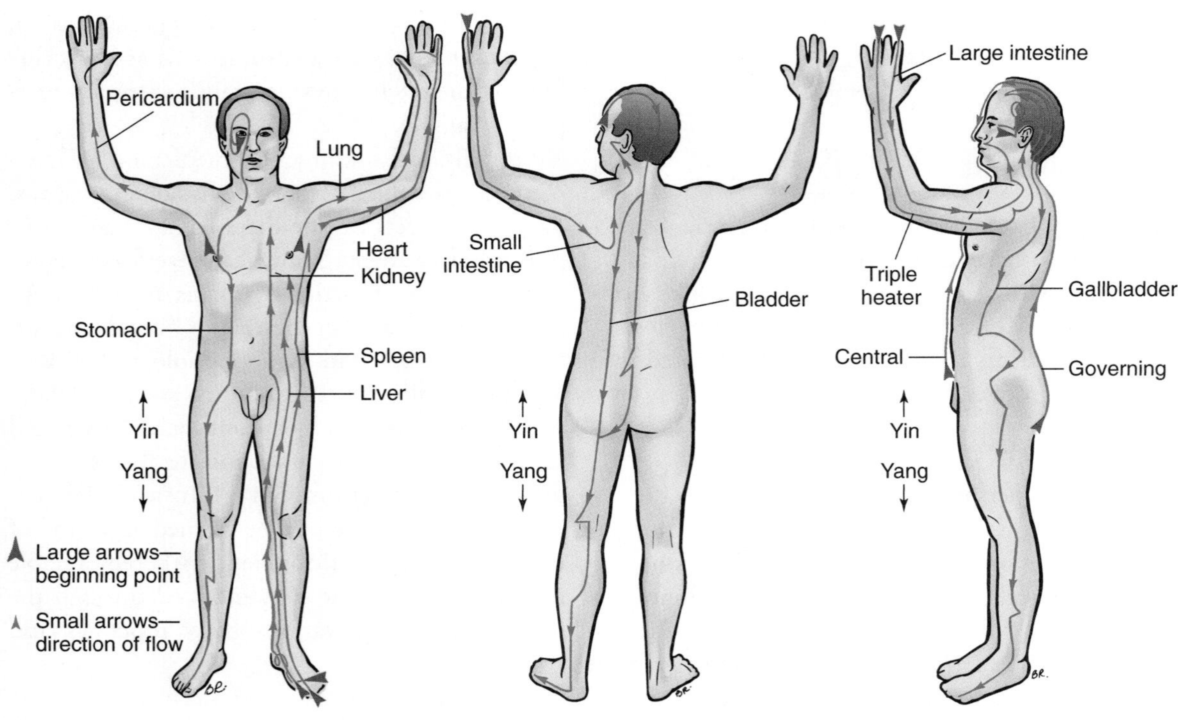

FIGURE 10-22 ■ Typical location of meridians. Meridians tend to follow nerves. (From Fritz S: *Mosby's fundamentals of therapeutic massage*, ed 3, St Louis, 2004, Mosby.)

According to Chinese theory, the meridians are internally associated with organs and externally associated with the surface of the head, trunk, and extremities. There are yin meridians and yang meridians. Yin meridians are associated with parasympathetic ANS responses and functions of the solid organs essential to life (e.g., the heart). Yin meridians are located on the inside soft areas of the body and flow from the feet up (Chinese anatomic position with the arms lifted into the air).

Yang meridians are associated with sympathetic ANS responses and hollow organs, the functions of which are supportive to life but not essential (e.g., the stomach). Chinese philosophy teaches that good health requires a balance between the forces of yin and yang. This balance changes according to the weather, seasons, and other rhythms of nature.

The 12 Main Meridians

The 12 main meridians are bilateral, symmetrically distributed lines of acupuncture points with an affinity for or effects upon the functions or organs for which they are named (Box 10-5).

Clinically, abundant evidence indicates the existence of reflex links between acupuncture points and specific organs and functions. In fact, no one really knows what an acupuncture point is. A large body of information is available about acupuncture points, their nature, structure, function, interrelationships, and interactions, as well as about the experience derived from thousands of years of the use of acupuncture points to treat illness.

The human body has hundreds of acupuncture points. Approximately 360 of the most used points are located on the 12 paired and the two unpaired centrally located meridians.

TREATMENT METHODS FOR ACUPUNCTURE POINTS AND MERIDIANS

Acupuncture meridians and points usually lie in a fascial division between muscles and near origins and insertions. A point feels like a small hole, and pressure elicits a "nervy" feeling. Unlike trigger

BOX 10-5 Meridians, Corresponding Number of Acupuncture Points, and Associated Pathologic Symptoms

The 12 Main Meridians

- **Lung (L) meridian** (yin): Begins on the lateral aspect of the chest, in the first intercostal space. It then passes up the anterolateral aspect of the arm to the root of the thumbnail. 11 acupuncture points.
  Pathologic symptoms: Fullness in the chest, cough, asthma, sore throat, colds, chills, and aching of the shoulders and back.
- **Large intestine (LI) meridian** (yang): Starts at the root of the fingernail of the first finger. It passes down the posterolateral aspect of the arm over the shoulder to the face. It ends at the side of the nostril. 20 acupuncture points.
  Pathologic symptoms: Abdominal pain, diarrhea, constipation, nasal discharge, and pain along the course of the meridian.
- **Stomach (ST) meridian** (yang): Starts below the orbital cavity and runs over the face and up to the forehead, then passes down the throat, thorax, and abdomen and continues down the anterior thigh and leg to end at the root of the second toenail (lateral side). 45 acupuncture points.
  Pathologic symptoms: Bloat, edema, vomiting, sore throat, and pain along the course of the meridian.
- **Spleen (SP) meridian** (yin): Originates at the medial aspect of the great toe. It travels up the internal aspect of the leg and thigh to the abdomen and thorax, where it finishes on the axillary line in the sixth intercostal space. 21 acupuncture points.
  Pathologic symptoms: Gastric discomfort, bloat, vomiting, weakness, heaviness of the body, and pain along the course of the meridian.
- **Heart (H) meridian** (yin): Begins in the axilla and runs up the anteromedial aspect of the arm, ending at the root of the little fingernail (medial aspect). 9 acupuncture points.
  Pathologic symptoms: Dry throat, thirst, pain in the cardiac area, and pain along the course of the meridian.
- **Small intestine (SI) meridian** (yang): Starts at the root of the small fingernail (lateral aspect) and travels down the posteromedial aspect of the arm and over the shoulder to the face, where it terminates in front of the ear. 19 acupuncture points.
  Pathologic symptoms: Pain in the lower abdomen, deafness, swelling in the face, sore throat, and pain along the course of the meridian.
- **Bladder (B) meridian** (yang): Starts at the inner canthus, then ascends and passes over the head and down the back and the leg to terminate at the root of the nail of the little toe (lateral aspect). 67 acupuncture points.
  Pathologic symptoms: Urinary problems, mania, headaches, eye problems, and pain along the course of the meridian.
- **Kidney (K) meridian** (yin): Starts on the sole of the foot. It ascends the medial aspect of the leg and runs up the front of the abdomen to finish on the thorax just below the clavicle. 27 acupuncture points.
  Pathologic symptoms: Dyspnea, dry tongue, sore throat, edema, constipation, diarrhea, motor impairment and atrophy of the lower extremities, and pain along the course of the meridian.
- **Circulation (C) meridian** (yin) (also known as heart constrictor or the pericardium): Begins on the thorax lateral to the nipple. It runs up the anterior surface of the arm and terminates at the root of the nail of the middle finger. 9 acupuncture points.
  Pathologic symptoms: Angina, chest pressure, heart palpitations, irritability, restlessness, and pain along the course of the meridian.
- **Triple-heater (TH) meridian** (yang): Begins at the nail root of the ring finger (ulnar side) and runs down the posterior aspect of the arm, over the back of the shoulder, and around the ear to finish at the outer aspect of the eyebrow. 23 acupuncture points.
  Pathologic symptoms: Abdominal distortion, edema, deafness, tinnitus, sweating, sore throat, and pain along the course of the meridian.
- **Gallbladder (GB) meridian** (yang): Starts at the outer canthus and runs backward and forward over the head, passing over the back of the shoulder and down the lateral aspect of the thorax and abdomen. It passes to the hip area and then down the lateral aspect of the leg to terminate on the fourth toe. 44 acupuncture points.
  Pathologic symptoms: Bitter taste in the mouth, dizziness, headache, ear problems, and pain along the course of the meridian.
- **Liver (LIV) meridian** (yin): Begins on the great toe, runs up the medial aspect of the leg, up the abdomen, and terminates on the costal margin (vertically below the nipple). 14 acupuncture points.
  Pathologic symptoms: Lumbago, digestive problems, retention of urine, pain in the lower abdomen, and pain along the course of the meridian.

The Midline Meridians

- **Conception (or Central) vessel (CV) meridian** (yin): Starts in the center of the perineum and runs up the midline of the anterior aspect of the body to terminate just below the lower lip; it is responsible for all yin meridians. 24 acupuncture points.
- **Governor vessel (GV) meridian** (yang): Starts at the coccyx and runs up the center of the spine and over the midline of the head, terminating on the front of the upper gum; it is responsible for all yang meridians. 28 acupuncture points.

Modified from Fritz S: *Mosby's fundamentals of therapeutic massage,* ed 3, St Louis, 2004, Mosby.

points, which may be found on only one side of the body, acupuncture points may be bilateral (i.e., found on both sides of the body), or they may be located on the central meridian (the anterior midline extending up to the mandibular gums) or the governing meridian (the posterior midline extending over the top of the head to the maxillary gums). To confirm the location of an acupuncture point, locate the point in the same place on the other side of the body.

The massage principles are (1) light massage of the meridian and (2) light or deep massage of a point.

To stimulate a hypoactive (not enough energy) acupuncture point, use a short vibrating or tapping action. This method is used if the area is sluggish or if a specific body function needs stimulation.

To sedate a hyperactive (too much energy) acupuncture point for pain reduction, elicit the pain response within the point itself. Use a sustained holding pressure until the painful excess energy dissipates and the body's own natural painkillers are released into the bloodstream. The pressure techniques are similar to those used for trigger points, but an acupuncture point need not be lengthened and stretched after treatment.

As with other reflex points, if the massage therapist is unsure of the nature of the hypoactive or hyperactive state of the acupuncture point, both techniques are applied in an alternating fashion and the body is allowed to adjust to the intervention. Often it can be difficult to determine whether the therapist is dealing with a trigger point or an acupressure point, because the two frequently overlap. The wisest course may be to lengthen and stretch the area gently after using direct pressure methods. This process does not interfere with the effect on the acupressure point, but without it, a trigger point cannot be treated effectively (Figure 10-23).

Massage Application

The physical aspects of meridians and points are addressed during the natural course of therapeutic massage. Trace the tract of the meridian path (these paths are found in the fascial grooves) and identify painful points; then treat as described.

HEALTH PRESERVATION AND EXERCISE

An important part of TCM is the discipline of preserving health and extending life. Foremost among the various methods that fall into this category are exercise and disciplines aimed at cultivating the inborn treasures of the body, mind, and spirit. Many can benefit by incorporating principles from these methods.

Qi Gong

Qi gong, or breathing exercise, refers to a variety of traditional practices consisting of physical, mental, and spiritual exercises. The regulation of the breath (qi) is a common feature of such exercise methods. The word *gong* means "achievement, result; skill; work; exercise." It is composed of two radicals. The radical on the left is also pronounced *gong* and means work. The radical on the right is the word *li* and means "strength" or "force." Qi gong can be understood as exercise designed to strengthen and harmonize the qi (life force), regulate the body and mind, and calm the spirit.

Tai Ji Quan

Tai ji quan (tai chi) is both a martial art and a meditative art. It therefore has complementary aspects that combine in a comprehensive discipline of physical culture and mental and spiritual discipline. The word *quan* means "fist; boxing; punch."

Dao Yin

Dao yin is a discipline involving meditation and breathing exercises that seeks to develop the ability to lead and guide the qi throughout the body for the benefit of the spirit, mind, and body. Dao yin exercises have a long history in China. They consist of bending, stretching, and otherwise mobilizing the extremities and the joints to free the flow of qi throughout the body. Like qi gong, dao yin emphasizes control of the breath (qi). It includes self-massage techniques that relieve fatigue and prolong life by activating and harmonizing the circulation of blood and qi. These techniques also stress the development of strength in the muscles and bones.

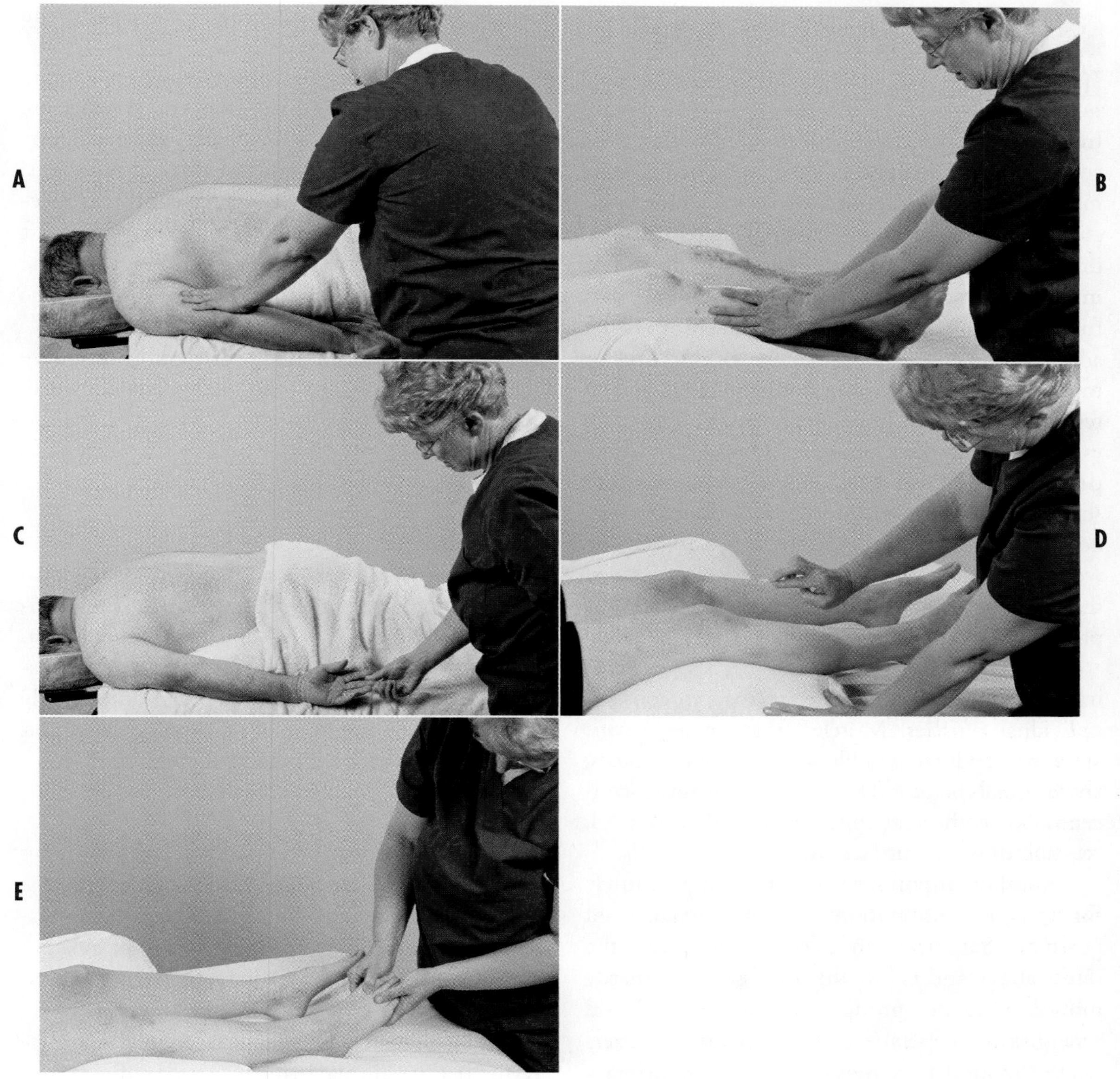

FIGURE 10-23 ■ An example of the incorporation of meridian flow and acupressure into general massage. **A,** Meridian sweeping. Follow the direction of meridian flow (yin flow: arms). **B,** Meridian sweeping (yang flow: legs). **C,** Squeeze the sides of each finger and toe near the nail. **D,** Tap points that are "under energy." **E,** Compress points that are "over energy."

The vastness of the TCM model and its elegance are far beyond the scope of this textbook, therefore no attempt is made to present scaled-down versions of these systems. The reference list at the end of this unit presents sources of further study. Massage therapists who are drawn to these concepts are encouraged to explore them in depth as they continue on their path of knowledge.

10-5 SPECIFIC RELEASE AND MOTOR TONE INHIBITION TECHNIQUES

Individual release and motor tone inhibition procedures should be done in the context of a general massage session with an awareness of whole body compensation patterns. No single muscle functions independently; all the muscles are linked in myotactic functional patterns. To restore optimal function, all muscles in the pattern must be addressed. Typically, when changes in one or more muscles result in hypertonicity and increased tension, corresponding antagonist patterns are inhibited, and those muscles weaken. To compensate, these same antagonist muscles may also shorten and become fibrotic. The opposite also occurs. Should one or more muscles become weakened, the antagonist patterns increase in tension and over time shorten and become less pliable.

It is more effective to think of muscle groups in terms of functioning patterns than to consider individual muscles. Muscles function as flexors, extensors, abductors, adductors, internal rotators, and external rotators. These actions are mostly concentrated in the extremities and at the occipital, cervical, thoracic, lumbar, and sacral junctions.

Another important consideration in muscle function is stabilization and maintenance of posture. Stabilizer muscles usually fix the joints above and below the joint being primarily moved. Muscle groups (prime mover and synergist or helpers) can function as stabilizers when the joint they move in is not the primary point of action. The massage therapist must consider all of this when working with isolated and localized procedures such as those described in the following sections. The question that needs to be addressed is, "Why is this muscle (or these muscles) dysfunctional?" Until the entire pattern is addressed, the symptoms will continue to return.

The main method for addressing dysfunctional areas is the application of inhibiting compressive force (direct pressure), either in the muscle belly or at the attachments, to reduce motor tone. These specific procedures address muscles that often are short and located in the deeper tissue layers, which makes access more difficult.

Remember, perform general massage before and after doing muscle releases.

Most inhibiting compressive force is applied to the muscle belly, unless the attachments are easier to access. Use a 45-degree angle to exert pressure on a "hill" instead of using a 90-degree angle in a valley unless 90-degree contact is specified. If you release or inhibit a muscle on the left side, make sure to release or inhibit the same muscle on the right side, even if tightness is assessed on only the one side.

These methods should be used only to achieve specific outcomes and should not be routinely incorporated into a massage.

THE SCALENES

Symptoms

Most symptoms relate to brachial or cervical plexus impingement, with symptoms of midthoracic pain near the midscapula and chest pain. Symptoms include arm pain that often is mistaken for carpal tunnel syndrome, an unreachable spot near the scapula, and occasionally pain that radiates into the head behind the eye.

Assessment

The best positions for assessment are side-lying and supine. Palpate to reproduce the symptoms. Systematically apply a flat, broad-based compression to the area between the upper trapezius and the sternocleidomastoid. Starting at the base of the skull, work down toward the clavicles, using sufficient pressure to reproduce referred pain patterns. If the pain pattern can be reproduced, the assessment result is positive.

The pain usually is caused by a contracted scalene muscle in conjunction with a chain pattern that often involves lumbar flexors or lateral flexion. The quadratus lumborum or psoas also is often involved.

Procedure

1. Use positional release if possible, relying on the position of the lower body to achieve the position of ease.
2. Apply compression at a 45-degree angle to recreate the symptoms. Have the patient activate antagonist patterns, either direct (e.g., the opposite scalene groups) or in the pattern

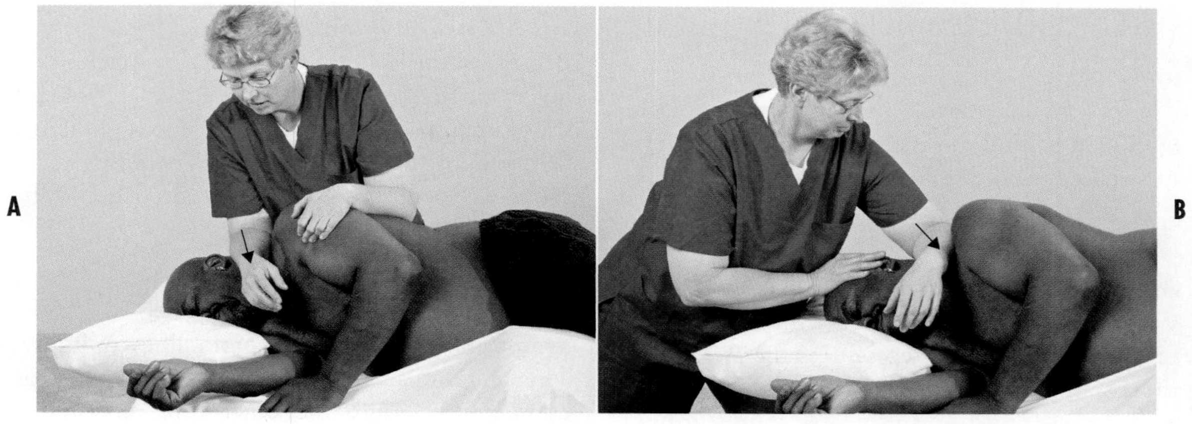

FIGURE 10-24 ■ Scalene release. **A,** Inhibitory pressure is applied to the belly of the muscle. **B,** Inhibitory pressure is applied to the distal attachments of the muscle.

(e.g., the quadratus lumborum), to initiate reciprocal inhibition. As the muscle softens, pinpoint the area of tension. This area will appear more taut than the surrounding tissue.

3. Have the patient use pulsed muscle energy, using both the muscle and the antagonist against the compression being held that recreates the symptoms.
4. Let the patient rest and lighten the pressure every 15 seconds or so. Resume until the tension diminishes, but no longer than 1 minute.
5. If the area does not release within 60 seconds, it is held by the chain compensation pattern, and work must focus on normalizing this pattern (Figure 10-24).

Once the muscle is inhibited, it must be lengthened gently (if the condition is acute) and then stretched (if the condition is chronic). The stretching will span several sessions. Keep the palpating hand in place and slowly move the head and rib cage until the palpating hand identifies the longest position of the muscle tissue. The tissue will feel taut in this position. Stabilize the head and lengthen and stretch from the thorax.

THE OCCIPITAL BASE

Symptoms

Symptoms include feeling the need to "crack" the neck (i.e., tension under the skull) and a headache from the occipital base to the forehead and typically involve the suboccipital muscles.

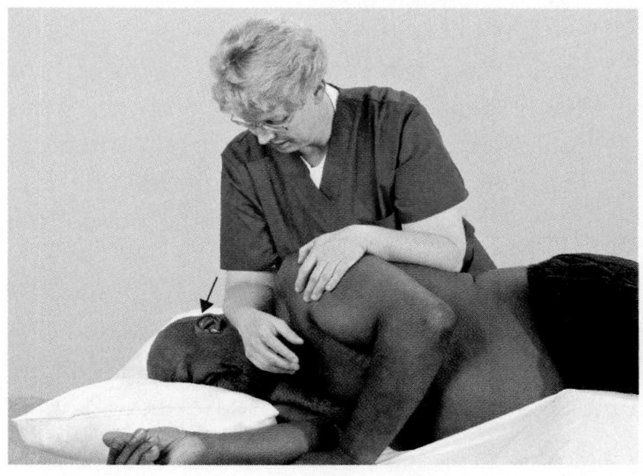

FIGURE 10-25 ■ Suboccipital release. Broad-based compression is applied to the suboccipital area.

Assessment

Apply compression into the area and determine whether the symptom is reproduced or increased. If so, the assessment result is positive.

Procedure

1. Place the patient in the side-lying position. Use the forearm or side of the hand to apply broad-based compression at a 45-degree angle into the occipital base under the occipital bone.
2. Have the patient roll the eyes in large circles; when the muscles activate, hold the position for up to 30 seconds. Repeat if necessary (Figure 10-25).

THE STERNOCLEIDOMASTOID MUSCLE

Symptoms

The patient may have a migraine-type headache with pain behind the eye and may find it painful to swallow. Also, the head position is altered.

Assessment

Compress the sternocleidomastoid using the pinch method; if this reproduces the symptoms, the assessment result is positive.

Procedure

1. Place the patient in the supine position with the head slightly turned. Stand above the patient's head.
2. Hold the target muscle in the palm of your hand between the thumb and fingertips and squeeze, starting superior and proceeding inferior. Have the patient roll the eyes in large circles and lift and depress the chin.
3. Bend and straighten the knees by sliding the heels onto the table to engage the psoas during release of the sternocleidomastoid (Figure 10-26).

THE RECTUS ABDOMINIS

Because of the location of the inferior attachments involved, first explain the procedure and obtain the patient's clear consent. Rule out a hernia before applying this method. When this technique is used, the hamstrings also should be addressed.

Symptoms

Symptoms mimic those of a groin illness or injury. This abdominal muscle tends to facilitate psoas tightening, because the other three abdominal muscles are inhibited when the rectus abdominis is tight.

Assessment

Palpation of the upper and lower attachments recreates symptoms.

Procedure

1. Use inhibiting compression at the superior attachments on the lower five ribs. Then use a shear force on the muscle belly to loosen the middle of the rectus abdominis. Caution is required if a female patient has had a cesarean section or hysterectomy because of the scar tissue in the muscle.

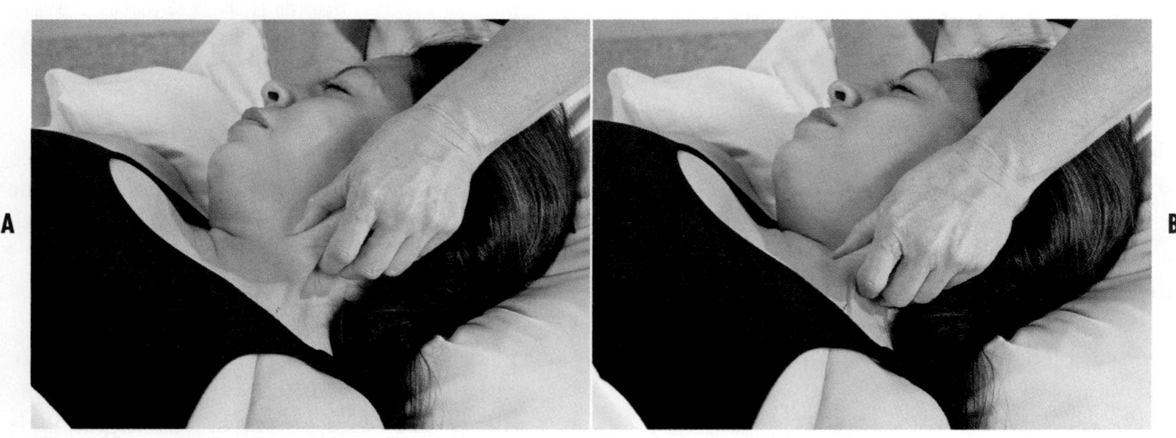

FIGURE 10-26 ■ Sternocleidomastoid release. **A,** Use pinch compression to apply inhibitory pressure, squeezing and lifting the muscle. Begin near the head. **B,** Systematically squeeze the muscle to the clavicular attachment. The patient can tip the chin toward the chest to introduce a muscle energy component into the release.

2. Apply inhibiting compression on the inferior attachments above and below the symphysis pubis for 30 seconds. Work over the patient's underwear, and hook your fingers under the symphysis pubis for 30 seconds while the patient raises the shoulder as if trying to do a situp. If you feel the tendons move while the patient is doing this, your fingers are in the right place (Figure 10-27).

THE HAMSTRINGS

Symptoms

Pain is felt at the proximal and/or distal attachments, accompanied by a sense of stiffness and aching. The patient hesitates to run and then stop quickly.

Assessments

Test to see whether the muscles are short: Can the patient bend at the waist and touch the toes while keeping the legs straight? Can the person flex the knees to touch the toes and then straighten the legs?

Procedure

1. Use a braced hand to apply inhibiting compression at the proximal and distal attachments. Attachments at the knee are most easily accessed when the knee is flexed.
2. Apply broad-based compression to the muscle belly while the patient flexes the knee (the side-lying position is the most effective for this). Alternately, with the patient prone, passively flex the knee on the target side by lifting the ankle and then apply inhibiting compression to the hamstrings, starting inferior, while moving the leg from side to side. Repeat while moving compression superiorly one step at a time (Figure 10-28).

THE MULTIFIDI, ROTATORS, INTERTRANSVERSARII, AND INTERSPINALES

As a group, the multifidi, rotators, intertransversarii, and interspinales produce small, refined movements of the vertebral column. They work in coordination, with each group of muscle fibers contributing to the entire action.

Symptoms

The patient often wants to have the back "cracked," yet manipulation does not provide relief. Stiffness is present upon initiation of movement, but once the movement begins, the stiffness diminishes. The patient is unable to stretch effectively to affect the muscle groups. Aching, as opposed to sharp pain, is felt.

Assessment

Palpation is the only effective assessment. These are small, deep muscles located between and along

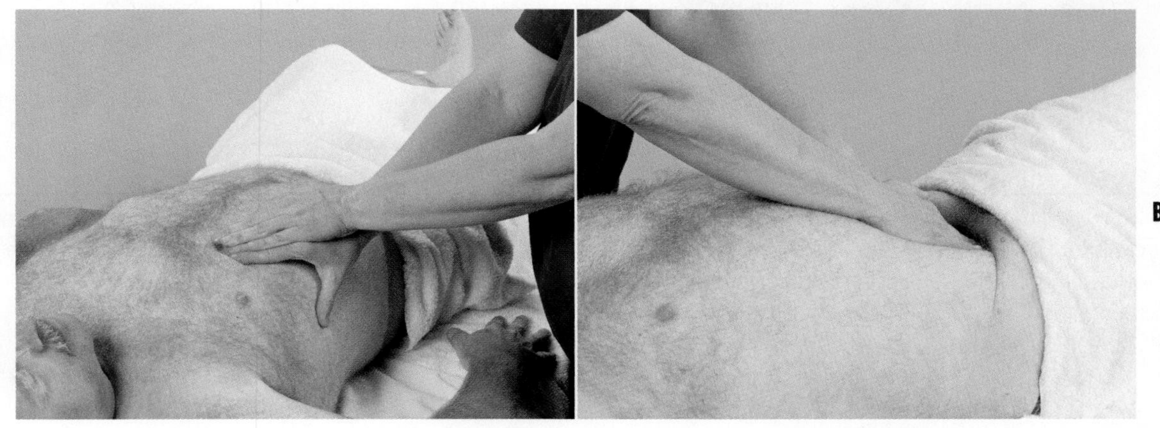

FIGURE 10-27 ■ Rectus abdominis release. **A,** Apply inhibitory pressure to the rib attachments. **B,** Apply inhibitory pressure to the symphysis pubis attachments, then massage the entire muscle.

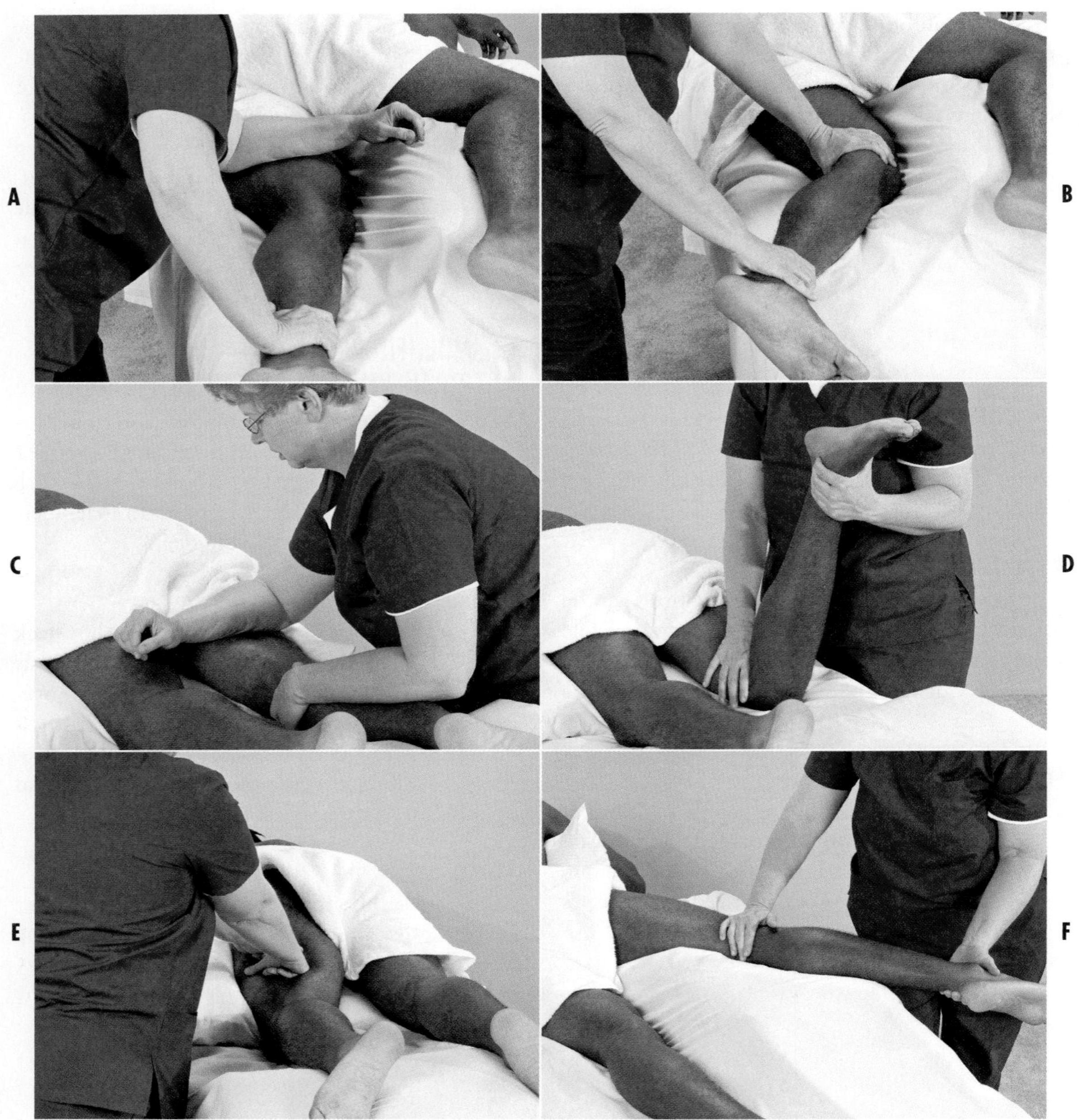

FIGURE 10-28 ■ Hamstring release. **A,** Use deep, broad-based gliding with compression force while moving the leg into knee flexion and extension. **B,** Apply inhibitory pressure at the distal attachments with movement. **C,** Apply compression at the proximal attachments to create inhibitory pressure. **D,** Apply inhibitory pressure at the distal attachments. **E,** Apply deep, slow compression to the belly of the muscle. **F,** Provide active assisted stretching; this also can be a position for muscle energy methods or active resisted movement.

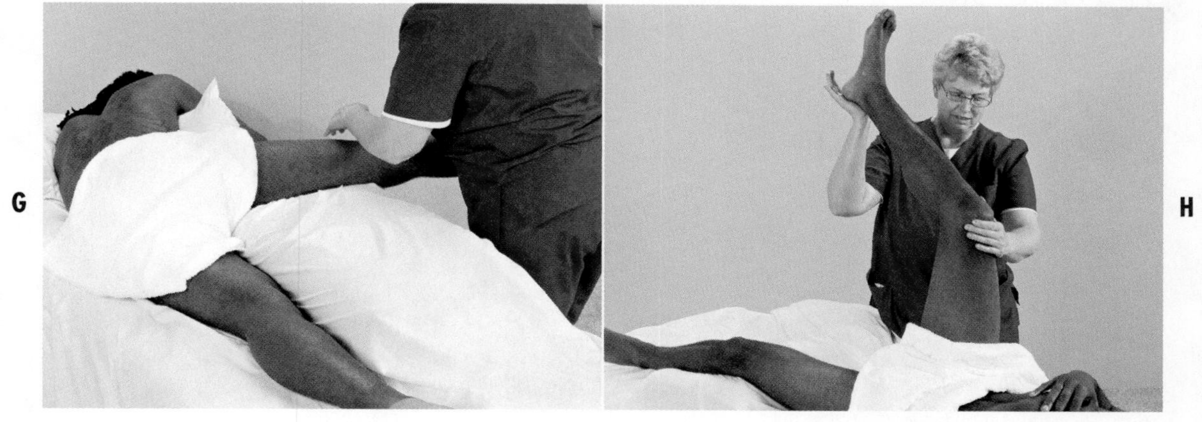

FIGURE 10-28, cont'd ■ **G,** An excellent side-lying position for stretching. **H,** Use muscle energy methods and lengthening specifically to target stretching at the knee.

the edge of the vertebrae. A history of being seated or of standing for extended periods is common. With the patient in both the prone and the side-lying positions, palpation deep into the spaces between the vertebrae reveals tough tissue bands that reproduce the symptoms. Effective palpation must go deep enough to contact the muscle group and get under the erector spinae muscles.

Procedure

Meticulous frictioning of the tight muscle bands combined with tissue stretching using compression is required. Softening and lengthening of the erector spinae and associated fascia are necessary before beginning this procedure.

1. Place the patient in the side-lying position with the affected side up and with a small amount of passive extension. The therapist may need to get on the table or use a stool or kneel to achieve an effective body mechanics position.
2. Angle in at 45 degrees against the groove next to the spinal column between the transverse and spinous processes, using a braced hand or a massage tool. Sink in until you can feel the spinous processes.
3. Hold the compression firmly against the affected tissue and have the patient slowly move the area back and forth from extension to flexion. Then have the patient remain in slight extension while you move down in a deep scooping action and then out, as if you were digging.
4. After the tissue has softened further, firmly hold the compression and have the patient move into spinal flexion very slowly until you feel the tissue become taut, so as to stretch the area. Hold this position until the tissue softens (Figure 10-29).

THE SUBSCAPULARIS

Symptoms

The patient complains of an aching or throbbing in the shoulder and upper arm. The wrist may also ache. The patient may have been told that he or she has a "frozen" shoulder or bursitis. Symptoms include pain or restriction in activities that require any form of external rotation.

Assessment

Visual assessment indicates an internally or medially rotated humerus. When the humerus is placed in external rotation and the patient is instructed to move it into internal rotation, pain is usually experienced but not always. This muscle usually is hypertonic if problems exist. It is part of the whole pattern of the body moving into a forward flexed protective and striking position. A history of overhead throwing (e.g., baseball or basketball) or of working in horizontal abduction and flexion or over the head with back and forth movements

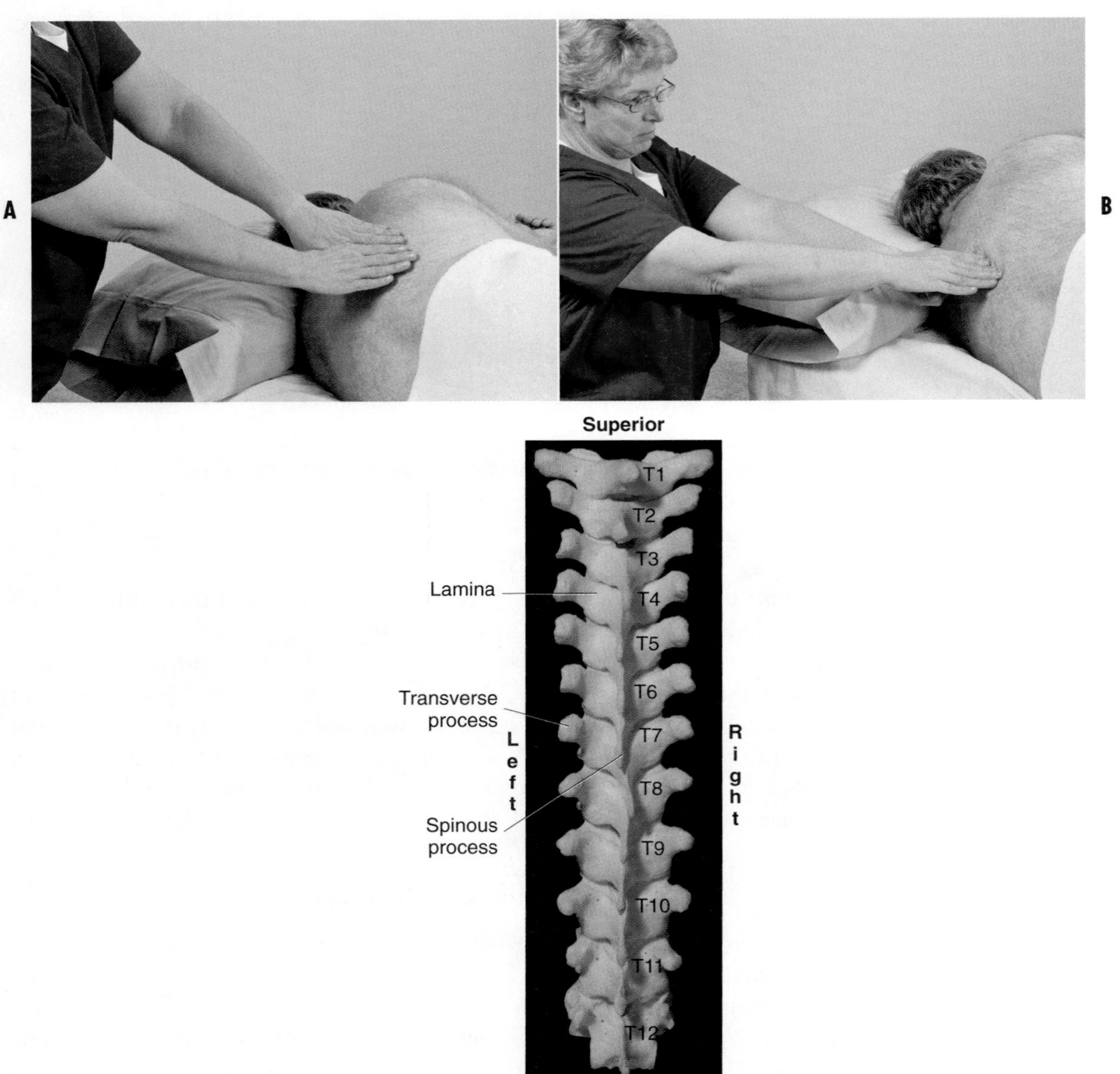

FIGURE 10-29 ■ Multifidi and rotator release. **A,** The position of the therapist's hand creates a broad but narrow contact that fits the area. **B,** Apply deep compression to the muscle, using small, gliding movements (friction), between the spinous and transverse processes. **C,** Posterior view of the thoracic spine. (**C** from Muscolino JE: *Kinesiology: the skeletal system and muscle function,* St Louis, 2006, Mosby.)

(e.g., painting) is common. This pattern of movement is stressed in activities such as driving and raking or shoveling for long periods, especially if the person is not used to the activity.

Palpation of the muscle reproduces symptoms. With the patient in the prone, supine, or side-lying position, the arm is horizontally abducted and externally rotated. Deep palpation is required in the groove between the latissimus to the back and the pectoralis to the front. Take care to avoid the vessels and nerves in this area; weave the supported four fingers in and down at a 45-degree angle until the scapula is felt. Probe in different areas by changing the angle of the hand until the symptoms are reproduced.

Procedure

1. Once the area of tissue that reproduces the symptoms has been located, continue to apply compression while the patient moves the arm back and forth from internal to external rotation.
2. Change the position of the humerus from 90 degrees to 130 degrees to access different aspects of the movement pattern as the patient moves the humerus into internal and external rotation. This movement can be active, active resisted, or passive, whichever is most effective for accessing the narrow band that constitutes the distal attachment of the subscapularis.
3. Maintain compression on the area and increase the movement at the end of each range to apply the stretch (Figure 10-30).

Because this procedure is painful, give the patient breaks but do not lose the position of the fingers. Avoid the brachial plexus.

THE RHOMBOID, PECTORALIS MAJOR, PECTORALIS MINOR, AND ANTERIOR SERRATUS

Symptoms

The patient generally complains of pain between the scapulae and reports that the back feels tight and fatigued. Sometimes a specific tender point or aching may exist in the upper rhomboid area.

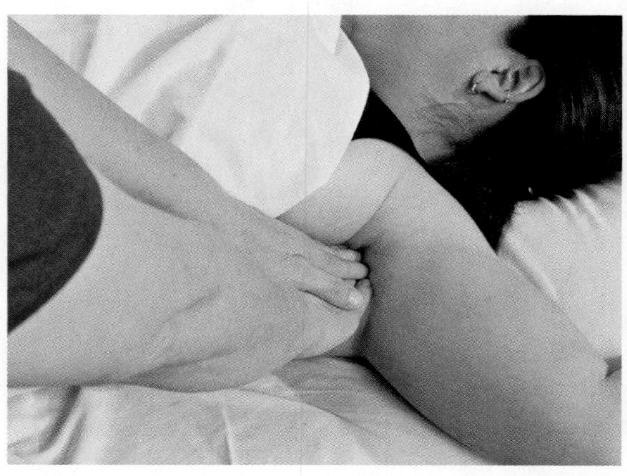

FIGURE 10-30 ■ Subscapularis release. Apply inhibitory pressure at a 45-degree angle to the belly of the subscapularis. Use caution around the nerves and vessels in this area.

Often the patient states that he or she is stretching the back, but when observed, the person is stretching the chest area. Breathing often is of the upper chest pattern and/or restricted.

Assessment

The most common problem is increased tension in the pectoralis major, pectoralis minor, and anterior serratus. Palpate these muscle areas for tender points. The patient usually is unaware that these points exist. The scapulae are difficult to wing, and the shoulders have a forward roll. The patient often has a history of static positioning of the arms forward and the use of small muscle action, such as with computer work. Any activity that requires pushing forward or pulling down sets up or aggravates the symptoms.

Procedure

Reducing tension and restoring length in the pectoralis muscles and the anterior serratus relieves tension on the rhomboids. Holding pressure on the tender points in the chest often is effective. If the pattern has become habitual or chronic, the fascia of the chest need to be stretched.

1. If possible, palpate for the tender points with the patient in either the side-lying or the supine position. Place one hand in the rhomboid region to feel for the interplay of the pressure applied into the chest involving the pectoralis major, the pectoralis minor, and the anterior serratus. These muscles pull the scapula forward. Compress or squeeze into the area to identify the tender points.
2. Once the tender points have been located, apply pressure against the rhomboid area, using various angles, to determine whether a position of release can be found. If not, have the patient move around slowly and repeat the application of pressure. Once the position of release has been located, follow the positional release or integrate the muscle energy procedure. It is important to stretch the area.
3. Stretching is accomplished manually by moving the scapula toward the spine while

the patient is in the side-lying position. This is facilitated either by having the patient pull the scapulae together or by applying firm tapotement to the rhomboid, reflexively creating a contraction reflex, while pushing the scapula toward the spine (Figure 10-31).

THE DIAPHRAGM

Symptoms

The patient complains of neck and shoulder tension and an aching or pulling at the area of the thoracolumbar junction. The symptoms get

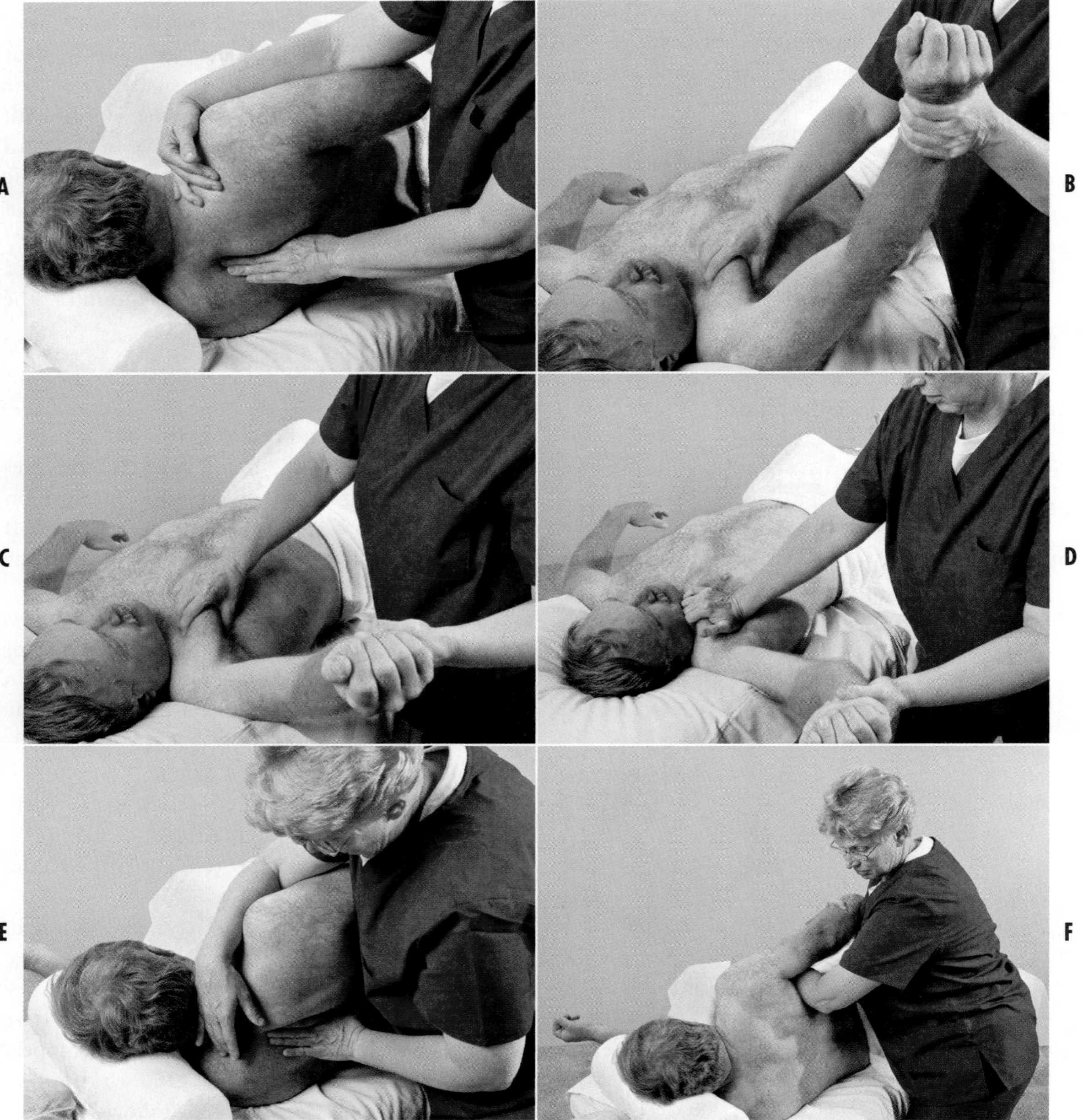

FIGURE 10-31 ■ Release of the rhomboids, pectoralis major and pectoralis minor, and anterior serratus. **A,** Rhomboids: Apply inhibitory pressure to the belly. **B,** Pectoralis major: Begin by grasping and lifting the muscle, then squeeze, lift, and move the arm away **(C). D,** Pectoralis minor: Apply compression to the muscle and externally rotate the arm to move the scapula. **E,** Anterior serratus, attachment on the scapula: Apply compression on the lateral aspect of the anterior serratus and pull the arm back to rotate the scapula. **F,** Anterior serratus belly: Use forearm to apply compression and move arm to activate muscles.

worse if anything restricts the abdomen, such as tight clothing or pulling in the stomach. Symptoms may also indicate a breathing pattern disorder.

Assessment

Perform all assessments for a breathing pattern disorder. In addition, palpate the area of the diaphragm along the edge of the rib cage for tenderness or rigidity.

Procedure

Release of the diaphragm should be performed in conjunction with procedures to address breathing pattern disorder and release of the psoas and quadratus lumborum.

1. Place the patient in the supine position with the knees slightly bent. Locate the edge of the rib cage and access it with either (1) an overlapping, double hand with braced finger contact or (2) the ulnar side of the hand, braced by the opposite hand.
2. While the patient exhales, slowly let the hand sink under the ribs. When resistance is felt, have the patient raise the arm up over the head, inhale, and then exhale deeply and slowly.
3. Follow the exhale, taking up any slack. The compressive force should be directed at an angle of about 25 degrees along and under the rib cage. Do not press directly down toward the spine, and avoid the liver. It may be helpful if the patient holds the breath to the end of the exhale and, while holding the breath, uses the muscles to try to push your hand out. Be aware of extended breath holding for anyone with high blood pressure.
4. Apply a broad-based, alternating, rhythmic compression to the lower rib attachments, gently but firmly pushing the rib cage in and out. Do not apply pressure on the xiphoid process. Then hook the fingers under the ribs and gently stretch up and out (Figure 10-32).

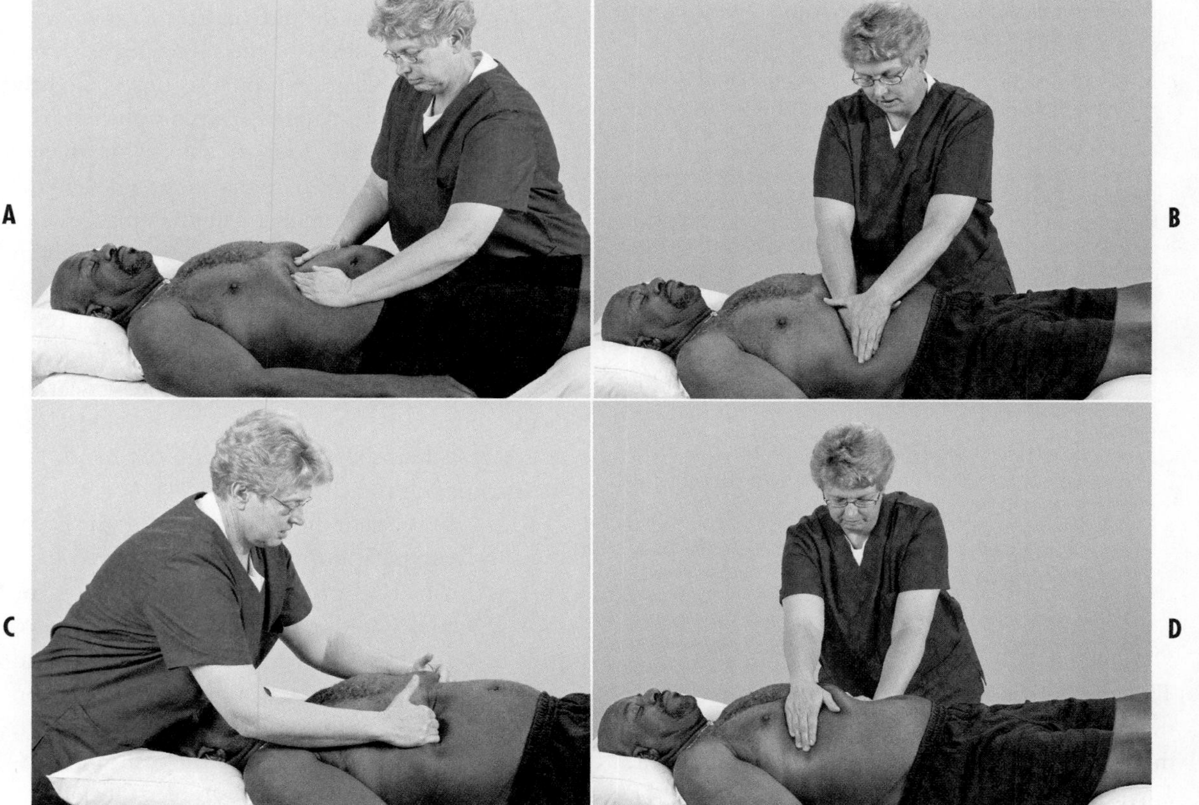

FIGURE 10-32 ■ Diaphragm release. **A,** Apply inhibitory pressure up and under the ribs. *Do not apply pressure to the liver.* **B,** This procedure can be performed on one side at a time. **C,** Stretch the area gently, lifting the lower ribs up and out. **D,** Mobilize the lower ribs.

THE PSOAS

Symptoms

The patient complains of generalized lumbar aching, aching into the tops of the thighs, low back pain when coughing or sneezing, and pain when lying on the stomach or flat on the back. The sensation can feel like menstrual cramps or labor pains, especially back labor.

Assessment

The gait stride is shortened, more so on the short side, and the leg on the short side is externally rotated. The patient often braces himself or herself with the hands against the thighs when sitting down or standing up. The leg is unable to fall into full extension (see the edge of the table test, below). The pelvis is rotated anteriorly on the short side.

NOTE: A shortened quadriceps group, quadratus lumborum, and tensor fasciae latae often are found with psoas dysfunction and should be addressed before the psoas muscles are treated. The sternocleidomastoid typically is also involved.

Two tests can help determine whether the psoas is short:

- *Edge of the table test:* The patient places the ischial tuberosity on the edge of the massage table, bringing one leg to the chest and rolling back to lie on the table. When the leg is held tightly to the chest, the other leg should lie horizontal on the table. If it is above the table, that psoas is short.
- *Sit-up test:* The patient lies supine on the table with the knees bent. The arms are extended at a slight angle toward the ceiling. The patient then lifts the torso off the table by reaching for the ceiling. The therapist holds or observes both feet. The foot on the side of the short psoas lifts off the table first.

Procedure

The procedures used include muscle energy lengthening and stretching in all positions: supine over the side of the table, supine, side-lying, and prone.

1. Position the patient.
   a. Supine over the side of the table: Make sure the pelvis is fixed firmly to the table and the knee on the opposite side is rolled as close to the chest as possible. The hands are placed above the knee for resistance force and lengthening.
   b. Supine: The patient lies close to the edge of the table and bends the knee not near the edge. The psoas being addressed is accessed by having the patient drop the leg over the edge of the table to achieve lengthening and stretching. The pelvis must be fixed and stabilized.
   c. Side-lying position: The bottom leg is drawn up toward the chest, and the therapist is positioned behind the patient. The torso remains fixed, and the lumbar area is stabilized. The patient bends the top knee, and the therapist cradles the thigh in his or her arm. The top leg then is slightly internally rotated, abducted, and extended.
   d. Prone: The pelvis is fixed to the table. The therapist is positioned opposite the side to be addressed. The leg remains straight on the side closest to the therapist. The knee of the target leg is flexed past 90 degrees, and the hip is slightly internally rotated (accomplished by allowing the foot to fall a bit to the outside) to prepare that side to be lengthened and stretched. The therapist reaches across and cradles the anterior thigh in his or her arm, lifts up, and leans back.

   NOTE: Decisions on which of these four positions is the most effective depend on the patient's statements and the size of the patient in relation to the therapist.
2. Access the psoas directly using the hand, the fist, or both.
   a. The patient lies supine or in the side-lying position with the knees flexed to at least 110 degrees. Both feet are flat on the table. The therapist stands on the side to be addressed. Either a flat, stabilized hand or a loose fist can be used; this decision is based on the patient's size and comfort. For the therapist, the fist position withstands a longer duration of treatment.
   b. With the patient side-lying and the knees flexed, the therapist kneels in front of the

patient and leans in, using a stabilized hand or loose fist. The leg can be used to pull the patient toward the pressure.

c. The muscle location is best accessed midline between the iliac crest and the navel and usually can be found by placing the metacarpophalangeal joint on the iliac crest. The fingers remain straight and the tips of the fingers identify the location of the muscle. This muscle is deep against the anterior aspect of the lumbar and lower thoracic spines. Slow, deliberate compression into the lower abdomen is required. The abdominal aorta, which can be palpated as pulsation, must not be compressed. The small and large intestines slide out of the way as a downward force is exerted. Identification of the proper location is confirmed if the patient flexes the leg against resistance and the therapist feels the psoas contract.

3. Apply a flat, sustained compression while the patient slowly moves the head in large, slow circles (these actions facilitate the psoas and serve as a contract-and-relax function for the muscle).
   a. The psoas can be inhibited by having the patient activate the neck extensor by slightly tipping the chin toward the ceiling and pushing the back of the head against the table. Alternating flexion and extension on the neck is valuable while maintaining a contraction against the psoas. All these neck actions can be supplemented with eye movement (i.e., the eyes look downward during forward flexion, sideways during lateral flexion, and upward during extension).
   b. In addition, the patient can slowly slide the heel of the foot out so that the leg becomes straight. If the patient contracts the buttocks when the leg is straight, the psoas is further inhibited. The patient then relaxes the gluteal muscles and slides the heel as close to the buttocks as possible to contract the psoas. This action is repeated while the compression is maintained.
4. Release at the distal attachment: If accessing the psoas through the abdomen is difficult, inhibiting compression can be applied where the muscle crosses over the pubic bone. Usually the leg is moved into an ease position to begin and into bind position while the inhibiting compression is maintained.

NOTE: The two techniques (abdominal access release and release at the distal attachment) can be used in coordination for a more intense interaction. The goal is to reduce motor tone in the psoas muscles. The release usually is palpated as a sinking in or a feeling of giving in of the tissues. The patient usually shifts the breathing by taking a deep breath and relaxing when the muscle lets go. This is a painful and intense procedure. Give the patient breaks during the process by reducing the pressure a bit, but do not lose contact with the muscle, because relocating it can cause discomfort.

5. When the treatment is complete, make sure the patient rolls first to the side and then rolls up to get off the table. Assist the person if necessary. Do not let the person sit straight up. It is best to perform the following sequence after applying inhibiting compression on the psoas.
6. Have the patient lie prone for a minute as a gentle lengthening position for the psoas. Then have the patient assume a four-point position by getting on the hands and knees.
   a. Have the patient assume the cat (swayback) position and then the camel (hunchback) position.
   b. The patient then slides the arms forward and brings the buttocks back against the hamstrings. Apply broad-based compression against the lumbar area while the patient is in this position.
   c. If the pain in the psoas is not acute and if disk involvement is a factor, have the patient drop gently into the yoga cobra position by lifting the head and chest, straightening the arms, and gently pushing the pelvis flat against the table.
   d. The patient then assumes the hands and knees position to get off the table. Each position can be sustained up to 3 minutes (Figure 10-33).

Healing and Rehabilitation Exercises

1. Teach the patient the sequence described in step 6, above:

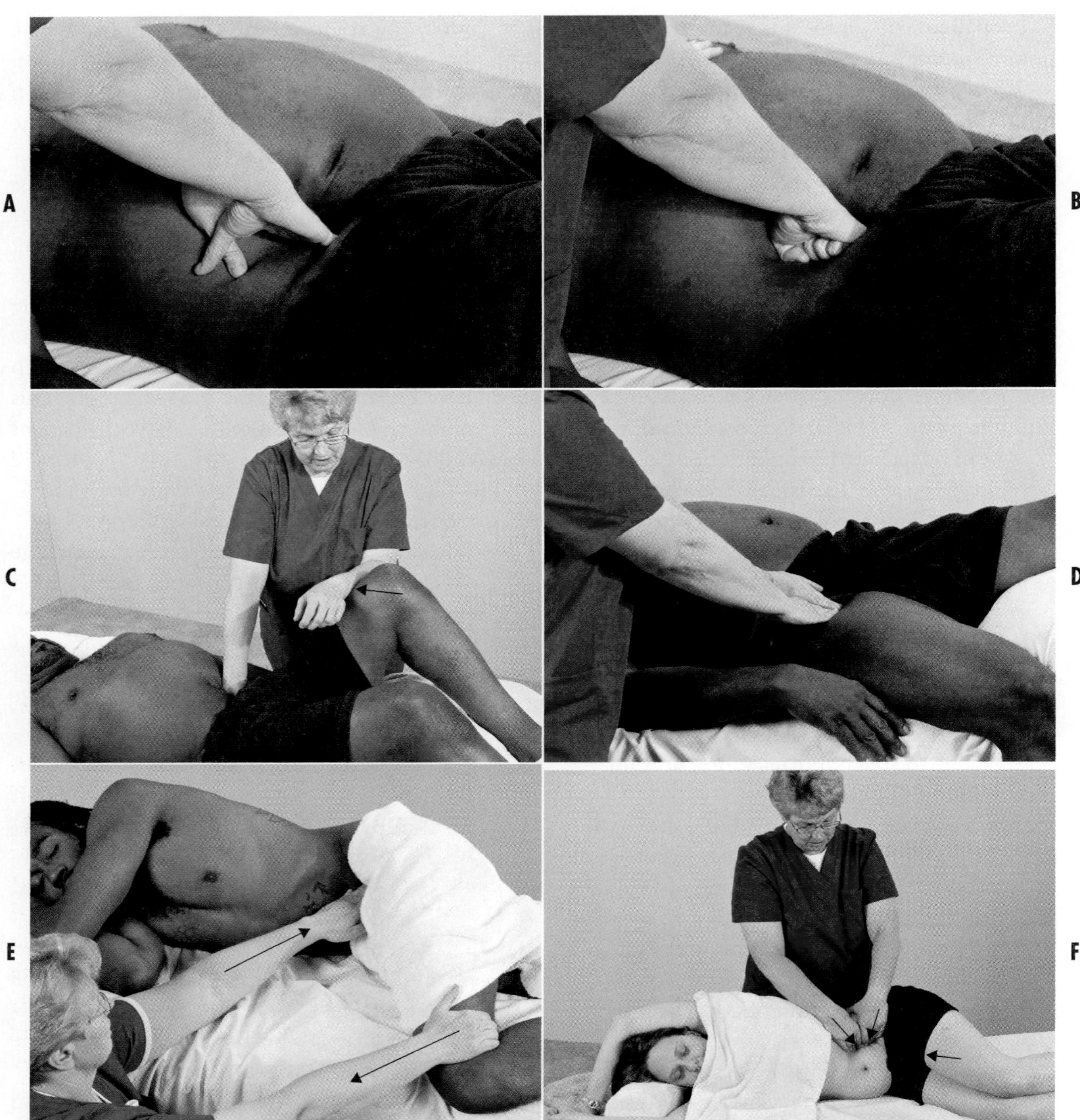

FIGURE 10-33 ■ Psoas release: Inhibiting pressure is applied at the belly of the muscle and in the distal attachment area where the muscle crosses over the pubic bone. **A,** With the patient supine, the therapist braces the fingers at a 45-degree angle toward the spine. **B,** Alternative position of the fist (patient supine); the therapist should use whichever position is most comfortable. **C,** The therapist should make sure the inhibiting pressure is exerted on the psoas by having the patient flex the hip against pressure; the therapist should feel the muscle contract. **D,** Inhibiting pressure is applied in the distal attachment area just where the muscle crosses the pubic bone. **E,** The side-lying position, with counterpressure used to apply inhibiting pressure. **F,** An alternative side-lying position for small patients. The therapist must make sure to access the psoas by moving the hip into flexion; care must be taken not to apply pressure to the iliacus by mistake.

- Lie on the stomach.
- Perform the cat and camel stretches.
- Perform the knee and arm stretches.
- Perform the yoga cobra.

2. Another beneficial activity involves using large gym balls for various low back exercises.

THE QUADRATUS LUMBORUM

Symptoms

Symptoms include deep, local low back pain that may be more intense on one side and pain radiating into the buttocks and down the side of the leg to the knee (nerve entrapment). The patient tends to wiggle or tries to stretch the lateral trunk and has restricted breathing. The leg may be shorter on the affected side (this may be functional or physical).

Assessment

1. Place the patient in the side-lying position. Palpate with either the forearms or the side of the hands in the space between the ribs and the iliac crest. Have the patient straighten and then lift the top leg. The palpated area should not be activated until the leg is raised more than 20 degrees. If it is activated sooner, the quadratus is tense and short.
2. Have the patient lie prone with the legs straight and assess leg length. A short leg may indicate a tight quadratus lumborum. If lateral flexion of the torso is restricted or asymmetric, the greatest restriction will be on the short/tense side (Figure 10-34).

Procedure

1. Place the patient in the side-lying position with the bottom leg bent slightly and the top leg straight with the hip slightly extended.
2. Stand behind the patient; apply compression into the space between the last rib and the top of the iliac crest. The angle of force is about 90 degrees (directed toward the table). When resistance is felt in the muscle, have the patient lift the top leg up and down. Make sure the hip stays in extension.
3. Alternately, have the patient move the neck and head back and forth in lateral flexion and extension. Both of these movements facilitate or inhibit the quadratus lumborum muscles. These neck movements can be supplemented with side-to-side eye movements.

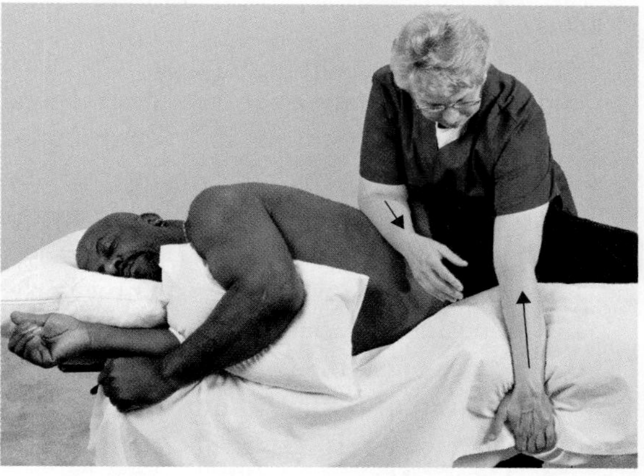

FIGURE 10-34 ■ Quadratus lumborum release. Apply inhibitory pressure with counterpressure. Do not apply pressure to the lower ribs.

4. After the muscle releases, it must be lengthened and stretched. Stabilize the thorax and lengthen by dropping the top leg even more into a lengthened and stretched position. Use a manual stretch by exerting force into the low back toward the table and side, bending the patient in extension with both the torso and the leg.
5. Self-help may include the following exercise: The patient is kneeling. The fingers are interlaced, the palms are turned up, and the arms are extended over the head. The pelvis is held stable and rolled forward. Side-bend and twist the patient into slight flexion to stretch the quadratus lumborum.

THE DEEP LATERAL HIP ROTATORS

Symptoms

The foot is externally rotated. The patient complains of pain deep in the gluteals, to which sciatic nerve impingement may be contributing.

Assessment

Perform physical assessment tests for the externally rotated foot. Palpate into the belly of the muscle to identify tender points that recreate symptoms. The patient may have difficulty standing on one foot on the affected side (Figure 10-34).

Procedure

1. Apply inhibiting compression with internal and external rotation of the deep lateral rotators. Use the forearms to apply compression while moving the hip into internal and external rotation. Incorporate muscle energy methods to facilitate release.
2. Perform stretching while the patient is in the supine position. Because of the placement of the attachments when the patient is in the supine position with the hip flexed to 90 degrees, the leg is externally rotated and pulled toward the chest (Figure 10-34).

THE MUSCLES OF THE GROIN AREA

NOTE: Special consent is required because of the location of muscle attachments. Perform over clothing or draping.

Symptoms

The patient reports a sensation of a high groin pull, but the therapist is unable to palpate tenderness in the adductor region. Symptoms include restricted breathing, shortened stride, and contralateral shoulder pain. An aching in the groin is similar to having to contract the sphincter muscles to retain urine or a sensation that feels like needing to urinate but being unable to do so.

Assessment

1. Assess by palpation. Place the patient in the side-lying position with the top leg bent and pulled up. Using the supported hand position with flat fingers, contact the ischial tuberosity from an inferior approach on the bottom and slide over it at a downward, 45-degree angle, moving superiorly and medially over the patient's body.
2. Shift the direction of force to identify tender areas that reproduce symptoms. Tell the patient to lift the bottom leg: if you feel the muscle move, you are on the right spot.

Procedure

1. Maintain contact with the tender points that create symptoms; increase the compressive force and have the patient slightly extend and gently adduct the bottom leg in a pulsating action.

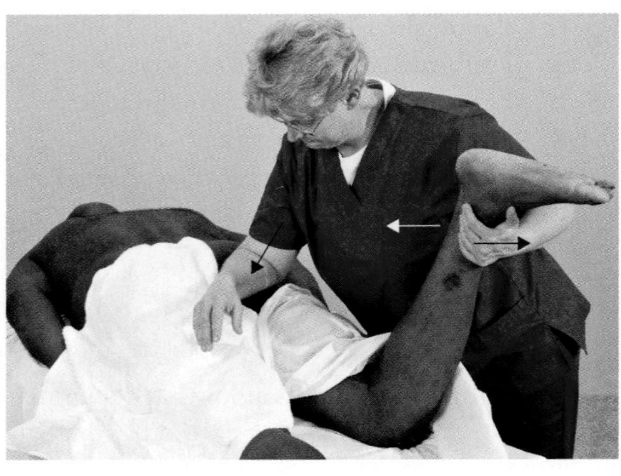

FIGURE 10-35 ■ Lateral hip release. Apply deep, broad-based compression to the deep hip muscles and add movement, both internal and external (lateral).

2. Continue the inhibiting compression until you feel the muscle relax and let you in deeper. Be sure to perform this procedure on both the right and left sides, or the patient will feel unbalanced when walking (Figure 10-35).

THE SACROILIAC (SI) JOINT

Symptoms

The patient reports pain over the **sacroiliac (SI) joint.** Symptoms increase when the patient stands on one leg or is sleeping at night. Pain also occurs when the individual is seated for long periods.

Assessment

Apply direct compression over the SI joint to determine whether symptoms increase. If they do, the assessment result is positive.

Procedure

1. Stabilize the sacrum with the hand, foot, or leg.
2. Place the patient in the prone position. Have the person extend the hips (knees straight), alternating as if walking backward.
3. Place the patient in the side-lying position. Move the joint by applying compression alternately at the iliac crest and ischial tuberosity to rock the joint back and forth. Also,

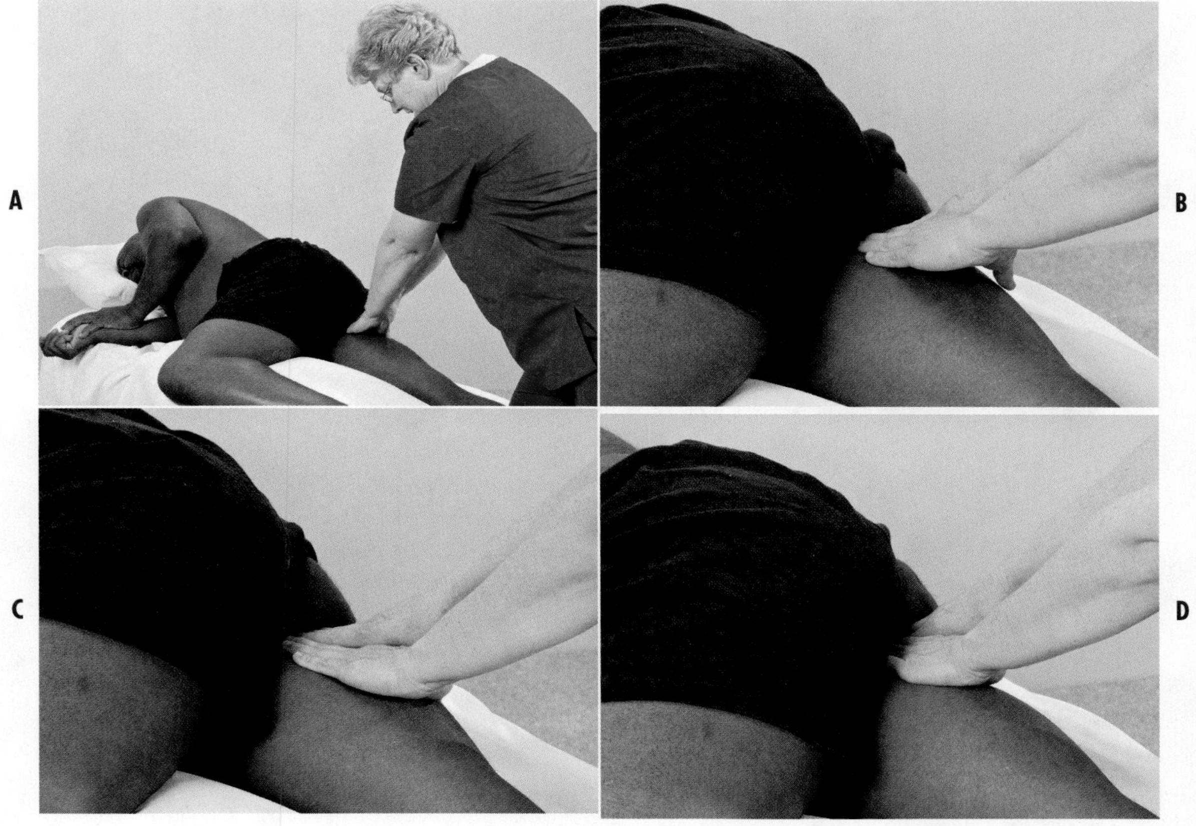

FIGURE 10-36 ■ **A,** The best body mechanics for applying inhibitory pressure (kneeling). This also can be done standing next to a table. **B,** Close-up of a stable hand position. **C,** Inhibitory pressure is exerted on the ischial tuberosity. **D,** Inhibitory pressure is applied proximal to the ischial tuberosity. The angle of contact is changed to allow the therapist to access various attachment structures.

compress the sacrum up and down and back and forth (Figures 10-36 and 10-37).

PELVIC ALIGNMENT: INDIRECT FUNCTIONAL TECHNIQUE FOR THE PELVIS

Symptoms

The patient reports having a "twisted" sensation and may have pain in the lower back, groin, or hip.

Assessment

First assess for asymmetry by comparing the two anterior superior iliac spines (ASISs) while the patient is in the supine position. Signs of dysfunction include the following:

- Bilateral anterior rotation: The ASIS palpates as forward and low.
- Bilateral posture rotation: The ASIS palpates as backward and high.
- Right or left anterior rotation: The ASISs palpate as one low and one high.
- Right or left posterior rotation: The ASISs palpate as one low and one high.
- Left, right, or bilateral inflare: The ASIS points toward the midline.
- Left, right, or bilateral outflare: The ASIS palpates away from the midline.

Procedure

1. **Anterior rotation:** Use the leg to bring the pelvis into increased anterior rotation by bringing the leg over the edge of the table. Have the patient pull the leg toward the shoulder. Apply moderate resistance and repeat 3 or 4 times. On the final move, stretch

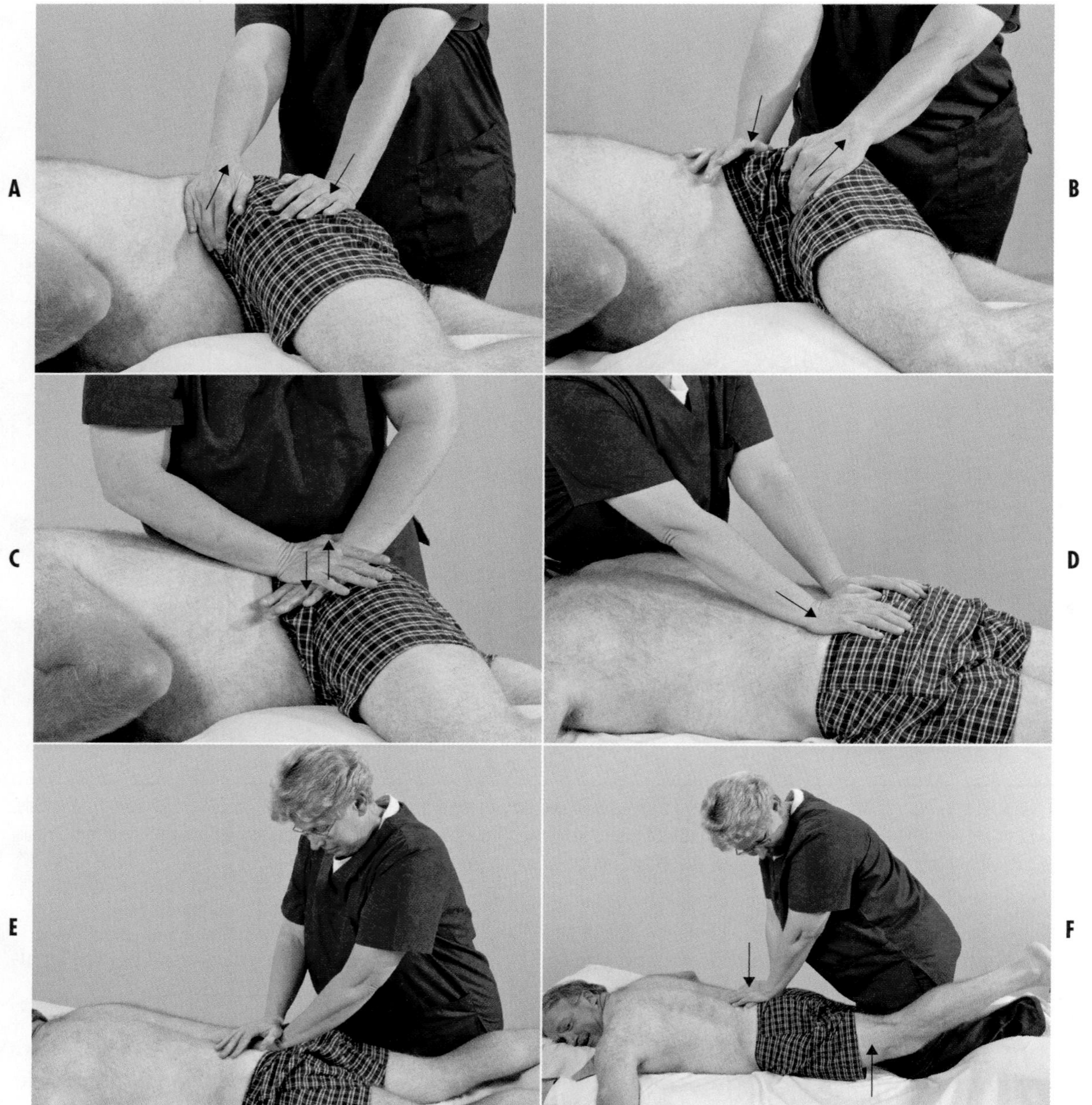

FIGURE 10-37 ■ Sacroiliac (SI) joint treatment. **A,** After massaging the area to increase tissue pliability, mobilize the SI joint with indirect and direct (ease and bind) movement. **B,** Move the joint back and forth from ease to bind. **C,** Apply rhythmic compression to the ilium just posterior to the iliac crest. **D,** Apply rhythmic compression to the ilium on either side of the SI joint. **E,** Apply rhythmic compression to the sacrum. **F,** Compress the sacrum while the patient alternately extends the hip, first right, then left, as if walking backward.

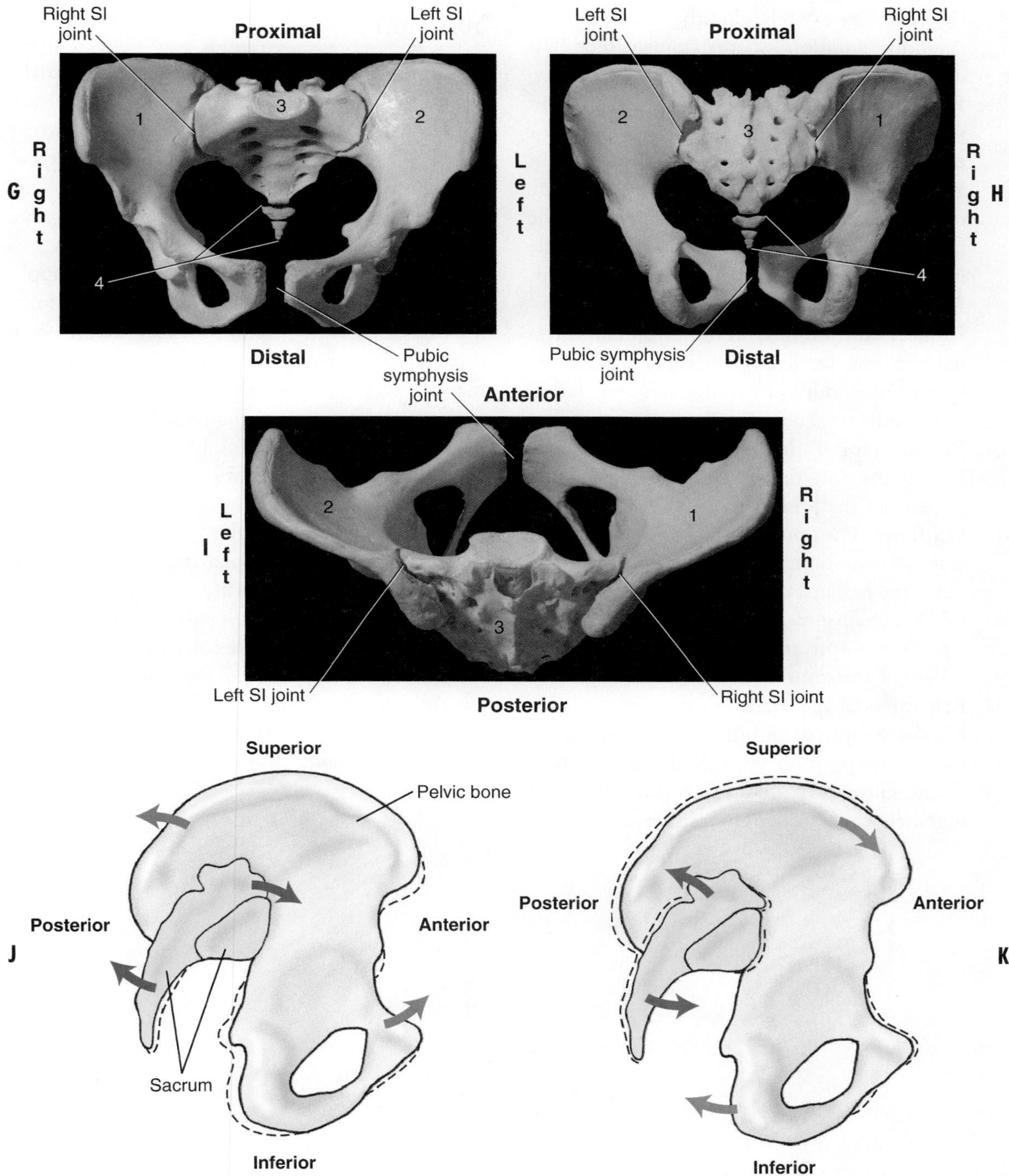

FIGURE 10-37, cont'd ■ **G,** Anterior view of the bones of the pelvis and the hip joint. **H,** Posterior view of the bones of the pelvis and the hip joint. **I,** Superior view of the bones of the pelvis and the hip joint. **J,** Intrapelvic motion of nutation (i.e., the sacrum can move within the pelvis relative to the two pelvic bones), in which the superior end of the sacrum moves anteriorly and inferiorly and the inferior end moves posteriorly and superiorly. The pelvic bone tilts relatively posteriorly. **K,** Intrapelvic motion of counternutation, in which the superior end of the sacrum moves posteriorly and superiorly and the inferior end moves anteriorly and inferiorly. The pelvic bone tilts relatively anteriorly. (**G** to **K** from Muscolino JE: *Kinesiology: the skeletal system and muscle function,* St Louis, 2006, Mosby.)

the soft tissue while slightly increasing the posterior rotation of the joint. Repeat if necessary

2. **Posterior rotation:** Begin with the leg bent toward the shoulder, increasing posterior rotation. Have the patient push the leg out and down over the table. Apply moderate resistance and repeat 3 or 4 times. On the final move, stretch the soft tissue while increasing the anterior rotation of the joint. Repeat if necessary.
3. **Inflare:** Position the hip in flexion and internal rotation, increasing the inflare. Have the patient push out against moderate resistance; the result is external rotation of the hip. Repeat 3 or 4 times. On the final move, stretch the soft tissues while increasing the outflare of the joint.
4. **Outflare:** Position the hip in flexion and external rotation, increasing the outflare. Have the patient move the full leg toward the midline against resistance. On the final move, stretch the soft tissue while increasing the inflare of the joint.
5. Regardless of the corrective procedure, stabilize the symphysis pubis. Place the patient in the supine position with the knees and hips flexed. Have the patient firmly push the knees together while you apply resistance.

SUMMARY

The applications discussed in this chapter usually are incorporated into the general massage protocol described in the Appendix and the Evolve website. These methods are interventions used to shift the patient's structure or function. As such, they can strain the person's adaptive capacity and should be used only as needed.

Metaphorically speaking, consider each application in this chapter as the seasoning in the main massage soup (the general protocol, described in the next chapter). In general, the biggest mistake massage therapists make is using either too much or too little seasoning. A massage that is too much of a strain or one that is too bland will not please the patient, and it will not be as therapeutic as it should be. A skilled therapist strives to get the flavor of the soup just right.

It cannot be overemphasized: these methods can strain adaptive capacity. Patients receiving healthcare typically are already stressed, and in some cases the methods are contraindicated. Clinical reasoning is essential for determining the patient's adaptive capacity, as well as the appropriate method that will produce a beneficial massage treatment.

WORKBOOK

1. For each of the following methods or structures, list at least three situations in which you feel you would use that method or work on that structure or structures. An example is provided in the first five methods.
   - Indirect function technique (Example: Tissue binds in the lumbar fascia)
   - Arterial circulation focus (Example: Cold feet)
   - Venous return focus (Example: Long plane ride)
   - General systemic lymphatic drainage (Example: Delayed onset muscle soreness)
   - Localized lymphatic drainage (Example: Ankle sprain)
   - Deep transverse friction
   - Connective tissue stretching (direct methods)
   - Trigger points
   - Joint play
   - Reflexology
   - Acupressure
   - Scalene/occipital/sternocleidomastoid release
   - Psoas release
   - Quadratus lumborum release
   - Subscapular release
   - Rectus abdominis release
   - Hamstring release
   - Groin attachments of hamstring and adductors
   - Multifidi, rotators, intertransversarii, and interspinales
   - SI joint
   - Lymphatic drainage
   - Mobilization with movement

Chapter 11 Concept Map

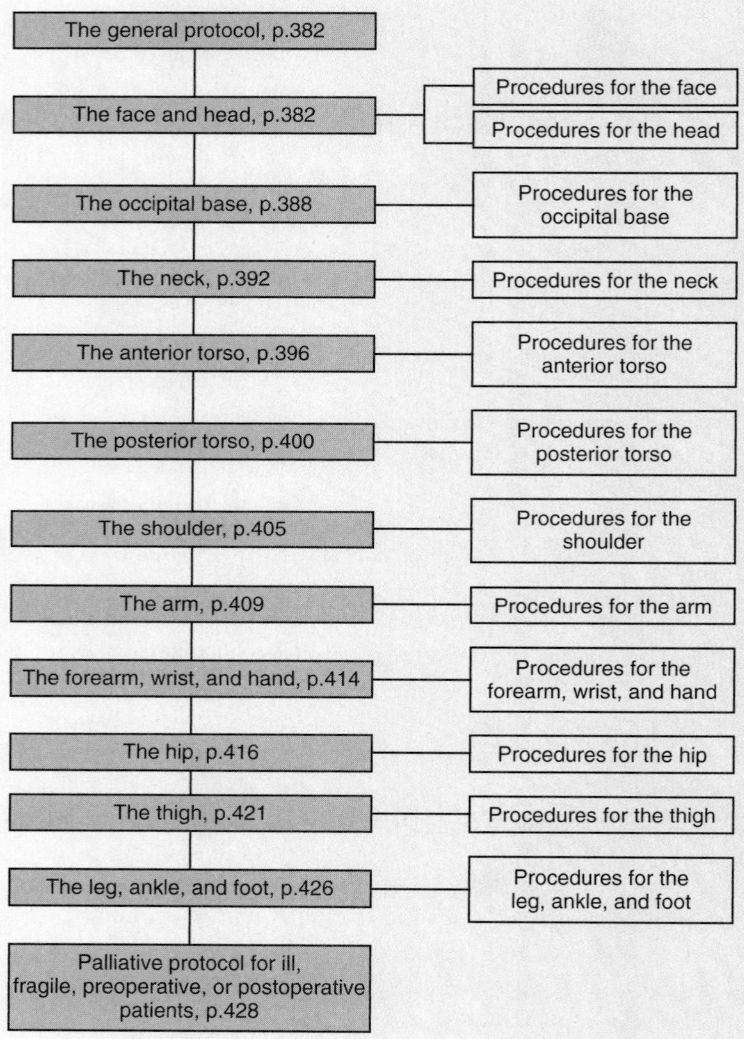

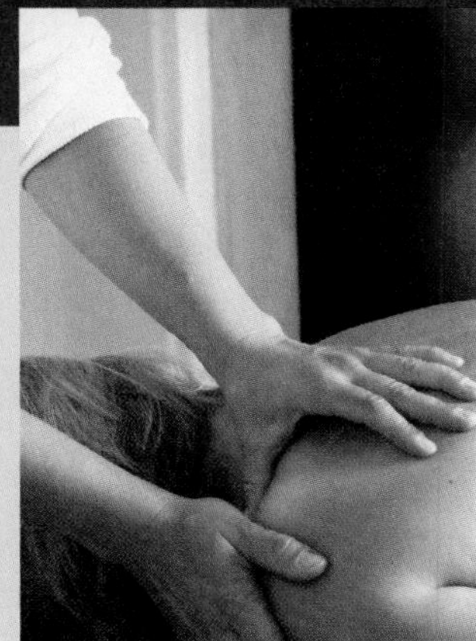

CHAPTER 11

GENERAL MASSAGE PROTOCOL AND PALLIATIVE VARIATION

OBJECTIVES

Upon completion of this chapter, the reader will have the information necessary to:

1. Complete a comprehensive, full body assessment and a general treatment massage application.
2. Modify the general protocol to achieve palliative outcomes.

NOTE: The appendix on p. 761 contains an example of the general massage protocol.

The protocol described in this chapter is used for general maintenance massage. Metaphorically, it can be considered a weekly or biweekly cleaning. Weekly sessions may provide enough intervention, especially if the person consistently follows an appropriate stretching program such as yoga. Any of the positions and method applications found throughout the textbook can be incorporated into the massage. Do not be limited by the illustrations in the sequence; the methods can be applied in many ways.

Massage application should have pleasurable aspects. It should both feel good and effectively produce results. The assessment and massage application should not produce a guarding response. During active treatment the sensations can be intense, and some forms of connective tissue applications can reproduce symptoms such as trigger point referral pain or a burning sensation when fascia is addressed. Depending on the desired patient outcomes, uncomfortable methods sometimes are necessary to achieve results. However, general massage application should be comfortable.

As long as the patient is able to respond to a full body massage, assessment and intervention should be provided for all of the areas discussed in the following sections. This need not be done in the order shown, but all these areas need to be addressed. Because of the interconnection of the fascial networks and neuromuscular reflex patterns, massage in one area influences the entire body, just as dysfunction or compensation in one area affects the whole body. The massage therapist must always be alert to and observe for the whole body effect.

In many cases this general protocol will be too intensive. For these patients, the modified palliative protocol presented at the end of the chapter is more appropriate.

The method of treatment is the same as with any general massage, minus the adaptive procedures described in Chapter 10. Remember, those methods are used only if necessary to achieve outcomes.

The protocol presented here is a comprehensive, sequential approach that can serve as the basis for massage in the clinical setting. Practitioners need not perform the protocol in this exact manner, and once they have learned it, they almost always need to alter it for the individual patient. However, this protocol provides a good foundation for learning, and you should practice it until you feel comfortable with the procedures. Then you should challenge yourself by modifying the patient's position and begin to practice ways to adapt the protocol.

JUST BETWEEN YOU AND ME

I always get nervous when I write a protocol. They never really work, but they are good formats for teaching and for gaining expertise. Therefore, practice, practice, practice—and then practice some more, and when you've gained experience and confidence in your abilities, you hopefully will never do this exact protocol again. Instead, you most likely will interweave bits and pieces of this protocol into the approaches you develop for yourself from what you have learned.

This protocol should not be used on a patient 48 hours before any medical procedure that requires any form of anesthesia, including local anesthesia. Do not use this protocol on postoperative patients or on patients who are fragile or fatigued. For those patients, use the modified palliative care protocol at the end of the chapter as a basis and modify it as needed.

THE GENERAL PROTOCOL

A general pattern approach is used during the massage session. The general approach consists of assessing each area (making the assessment part of the massage) and then addressing the outcome goals by applying the appropriate massage methods. See the Evolve website for more information about the general protocol.

The sequence is as follows:

- Skin, superficial fascia, and edema
- Deeper fascial structures, muscle layers, circulation, and edema
- Tissue density, ground substance, fluid contribution to muscle tone, and fascial tone
- Joint end-feel and intrinsic joint play
- Motor tone
- Reflex mechanisms
- Firing patterns (muscle activation sequences)
- Flexibility

This assessment and treatment protocol requires at least 60 minutes. This is an acceptable time frame if the patient is healthy; however, remember that most patients receiving healthcare (or should it be called "sick care"?) are not healthy. A session that lasts any longer than 60 minutes is too demanding for most patients. Sometimes 30 minutes is a better length for the massage. Instead of doing one long massage, break it up into shorter sessions.

The rehabilitative methods found in the previous chapter should be incorporated into this general approach as necessary to ensure full body normalization. Although some isolated spot work on specific target areas may be appropriate, a better response is achieved when such work is incorporated into a full body application (Figure 11-1). A comprehensive example of how the general protocol can be implemented can be found in the appendix and the Evolve website.

THE FACE AND HEAD (Figure 11-2)

Thorough massage of the face and head is very important. It is not uncommon to spend 15 minutes on the head and face. Many connective tissue structures are anchored and originate in this area. Because a fascial connection exists from the feet to the top of the head, connective tissue bind patterns can originate in the head area, or this area can manifest symptoms produced by various tension patterns in other parts of the body.

The muscles of the head and face are highly innervated, and some of them, such as the masseter, are very strong. Many pressure-sensitive structures (e.g., nerves, blood vessels, and lymph vessels) lie close to the muscles and connective tissue structures of the head and face. The sensitivity to pressure of these structures, combined with high sensation awareness, often results in pain in the head and face.

The skull bones must be able to move in very small increments to respond to normal fluctuations in intracranial fluid pressure. If the bones

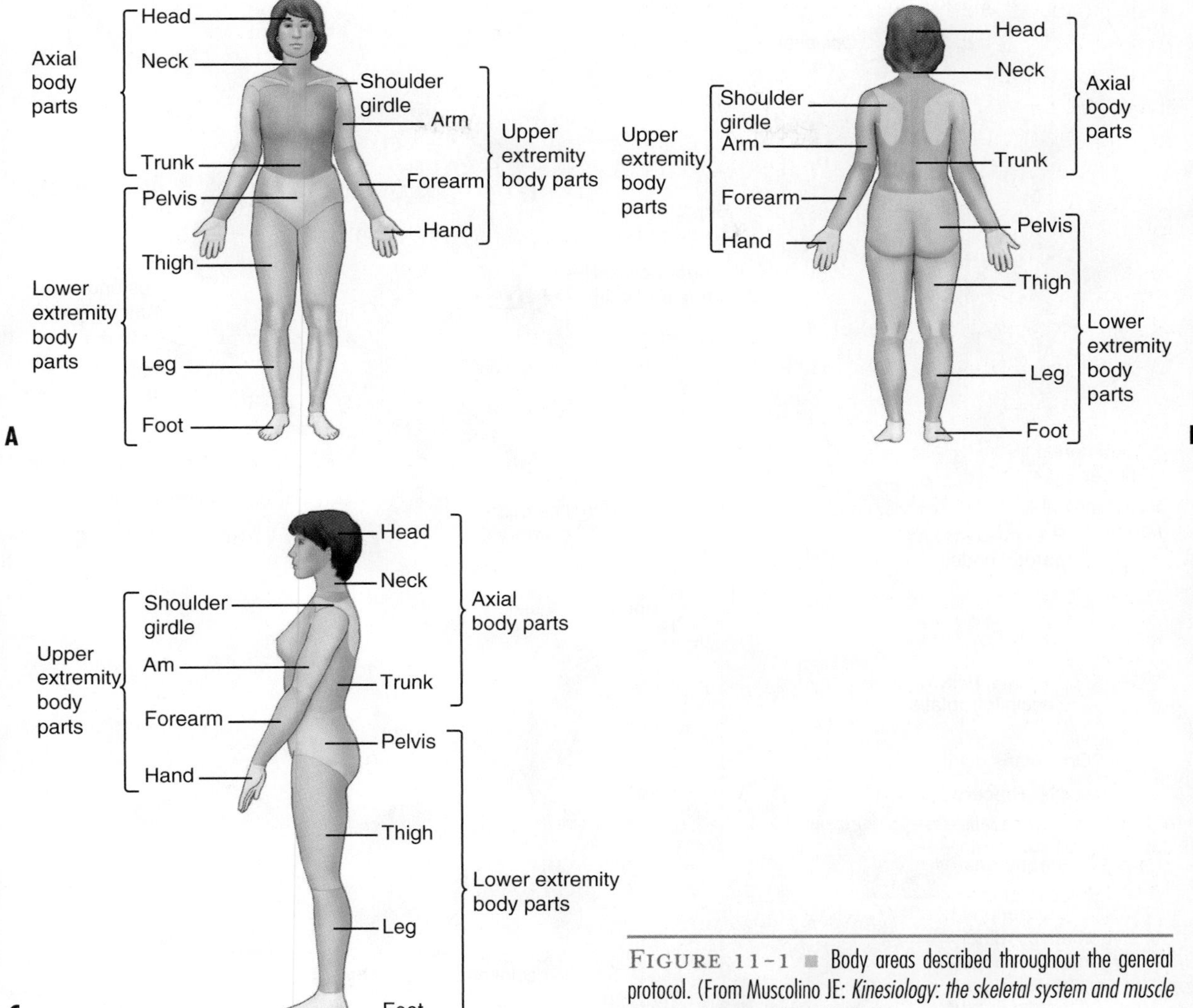

FIGURE 11-1 ■ Body areas described throughout the general protocol. (From Muscolino JE: *Kinesiology: the skeletal system and muscle function,* St Louis, 2006, Mosby.)

are fixed by tension patterns in the connective tissue, the muscles, or both, the person may feel pressure or an aching sensation.

Eyestrain and sun glare can cause tensing of the head and facial muscles; this is also common during physical activity.

The facial features should look symmetric, with little creasing of the skin from underlying increases in bind, tension, or tone in the myofascial structures.

The scalp should move easily on the skull in all directions. Fascial bands encircle the head, and these bands must be pliable or they restrict the movement of fluid and the cranial bones. The larger muscles (i.e., temporalis, occipital frontalis, and masseter) should feel resilient on palpation and should have no observable or palpable trigger point activity. If evidence of sinus congestion is noted, careful work on the small muscles of the face may allow better drainage.

The hair should not pull out during general massage of the scalp. If it does, the patient may have a systemic illness, fatigue, or nutritional deficiencies and should be referred for evaluation by the appropriate professional.

The skin should be resilient, soft, supple, and mostly free of blemishes. Changes in skin texture are indications of increased systemic strain. An increase in blemishes may indicate increased cortisol and androgen levels, also associated with the

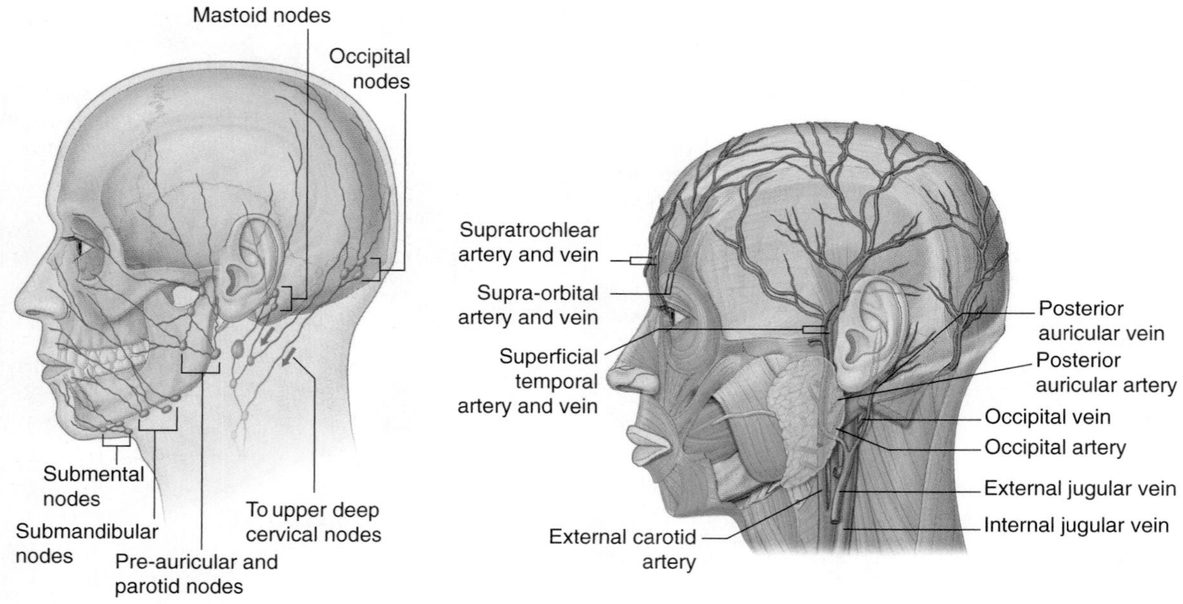

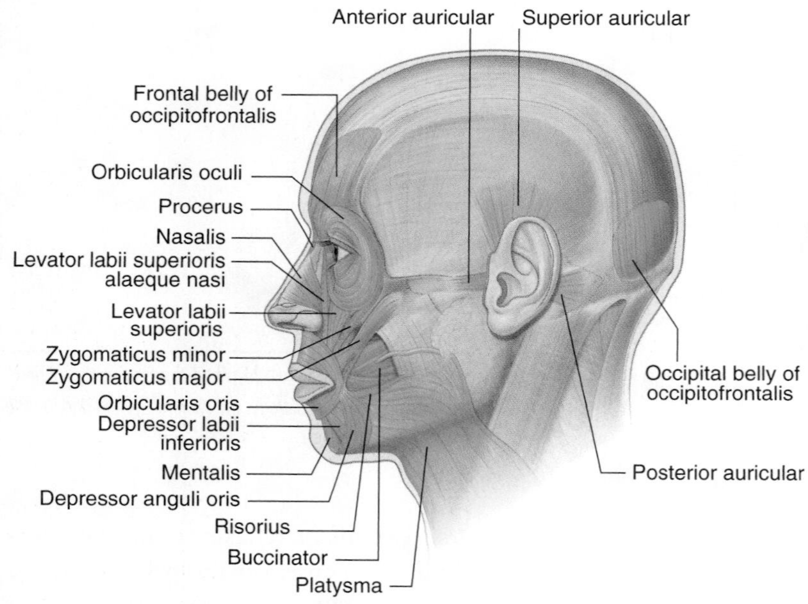

FIGURE 11-2 ■ Important structures in massage application to the face and head to assist the reader. **A,** Lymphatic drainage in the face and head. **B,** The arteries and veins of the scalp. **C,** The muscles of the face. (From Drake R, Vogl W, Mitchell A: *Gray's anatomy for students,* Edinburgh, 2005, Churchill Livingstone.)

stress response. If the skin is oily, be cautious about the type of lubricant you use, or work without it.

As for the eyes, four small but very sensitive eye muscles control eye movement. The proprioceptive feedback from these eye muscles contributes to postural reflexes.

It is appropriate to massage the head and facial muscles in all directions. Interestingly, when the facial muscles that create a smile are activated, the neurochemical response can shift. Therefore, when massaging the face, stroking in the direction that helps to create the shape of a smile may be beneficial.

PROCEDURES FOR THE FACE

Examples of treatment procedures for the face are shown in the Appendix.

The direction of lymphatic stroking should be toward the neck, and the strokes should have sufficient drag to pull the skin gently. Address this area with the patient in the supine or side-lying position.

- Lightly and systematically stroke the face to assess for temperature changes, tissue texture, and areas of dampness. If any such areas are identified, note them for further investigation.
- Use light compression to assess for bogginess or swelling. If an increase in interstitial fluid is suspected, use lymphatic drainage techniques to assist fluid flow.
- If you are in doubt about whether fluid stagnation is present, assume that it is and perform the methods. (Remember, when moving fluid, you cannot push a river. Moving fluid is deliberate work.)
- As mentioned previously, the direction of the lymphatic stroking should be toward the neck and have sufficient drag to gently pull the skin.
- After the area has been drained, remassage in the direction of the smile.
- Continuing with the face, carefully move the skin to identify any areas of bind in the superficial connective tissue. Be aware of any bind areas that correspond to the areas identified by the light stroking. Pay particular attention to any areas containing scars, because connective tissue bind is common in areas of scar tissue. Be aware that the soft tissues of the neck weave directly and indirectly into the soft tissues of the head and face. When palpating the soft tissue of the face, observe for tissue movement or bind in adjacent areas.
- Areas of bind can be addressed by slowly moving the tissue into ease, which is the way it most wants to go. Multiple load directions can be used. For example, if the skin and superficial fascia want to move up and to the right between the eyebrows, that is the direction of the forces introduced. Hold the tissue at ease for 30 to 60 seconds and reassess. Usually the pliability of the area will improve.
- Treat any remaining areas of superficial fascial bind with myofascial release methods that involve a slow, sustained drag on the binding tissues, introducing the lines of tension at each end of the binding tissue.
  - Place the finger pad(s) on one hand at one end of the bind and the finger pad(s) of the other hand at the other end of the bind.
  - Stretch the tissue gently but firmly and separate the hands, creating a tension force into the binding tissue. Bending force can also be introduced, but torsion force is too harsh for this tissue.
- Maintain the drag on the tissue until the thixotropic nature of the ground substance is affected and the ground substance becomes more pliable. Subtle changes in the lines of force serve to load and unload the tissue, resulting in hysteresis.

Next, address the muscle structures. The facial muscles are only one or two layers deep, therefore light to moderate compressive force is adequate to address the area.

- If muscle tone has increased as a result of sustained isometric contraction, use direct pressure to inhibit the spindle cells and the Golgi tendons. Apply this pressure in a broad-based compression with sufficient intensity to elicit tenderness or to reproduce the symptoms; however, do not make it so intense that a muscle tenses or breathing changes occur.
- Muscle energy methods can be used in combination with the compression by having the patient contract the muscle against the pressure applied by the therapist's hand. It may take a few experimental contractions before the right muscle pattern is discovered. When the correct muscle contracts, the area will tense or seem as if it is pushing against the therapist's pressure. Pulsed muscle energy, in which a repeated contract-relax, contract-relax pattern is used, is especially effective for the facial muscles.

Positional release can be achieved by working with eye positions until the pain is reduced in the compressed area.

- Apply pressure to the painful area until the patient can feel the tenderness or the reproduced symptoms. Maintain the pressure while the patient slowly moves the eyes into different positions until the pain, tenderness, or symptom sensation is reduced. When the tone begins to reduce, a bending or tension force can be applied to the muscle fibers. The intent is not to address connective tissue, but rather to pull the actin and myosin filaments apart mechanically to restore normal resting length.
- Address the muscles of the eyes by compressing the eyes gently and having the patient move the eyes in slow circles.
- Have the patient close the eyes, place the finger pads gently on the eyelids, and slowly press down just a bit. The patient should just feel the pressure.
- Use an on/off pumping action for a moment, then reapply sustained compression while the patient moves the eyes in circles.
- This method both stretches the eye muscles and resets their reflexes. As mentioned previously, four small but very sensitive eye muscles control eye movement. The proprioceptive feedback from these eye muscles contributes to postural reflexes.

Note: Increased fluid pressure in the eyes can produce a symptom of dull aching around the eyes, somewhat like a tension or pressure headache. If the patient has any trauma or history of trauma to the area around the eyes in addition to the symptoms described, the person should be immediately referred to a physician for further assessment.

Many patients chew gum or hold bite plates in the mouth. Pay particular attention to the masseter and other chewing muscles. The pterygoids are best reached from inside the mouth; make sure to use a latex or vinyl glove for this procedure. Inhibitory pressure on the belly of the muscle usually is sufficient to reduce tone, and it allows the muscle to be stretched.

- Apply a compression force to the chewing muscles by placing the thumb on the inside of the mouth near the temporomandibular joint (TMJ) and the finger pads on the outside on the cheek near the TMJ.
- Pinch the fingers and thumb together to apply inhibitory pressure to the belly of the muscles (to affect the spindle cell mechanisms) or close to the insertions (to inhibit the Golgi tendon receptors). Muscle energy methods can be used by having the patient clench the teeth.
- To lengthen the muscles, open the patient's mouth wide, but do not apply pressure against the lower jaw to try to stretch the muscles; this is too aggressive for the TMJ.
- Stretch, using the same method as that used when applying inhibitory pressure and introducing a bending force to the tissues. These are intense methods applied to areas with high levels of neurologic sensitivity. Although the application may be uncomfortable, the patient should not tense other body areas or change the breathing to endure the approach. Before you begin the application, tell the patient to wiggle the whole body to get comfortable, to take a deep breath, and to exhale slowly.

If the sinuses are problematic or as a preventive measure, a combination of compression on acupressure points and a light, rhythmic on/off pressure can be applied for about 10 repetitions against the sinus cavities; this encourages drainage.

To finish the face, return to the initial light stroking to reassess for temperature changes and other alterations. Normalization of areas that were hot, cold, damp, rough, or binding should have occurred.

Working with the face is relaxing. For this reason, doing this work first sets the stage for a calming whole body massage. Working with the face at the end of the session gently finishes the massage.

PROCEDURES FOR THE HEAD

Examples of treatment procedures for the face are shown in the Appendix.

Caution is necessary with any expensive hair design. Effective work on the head can be complicated by the patient's desire not to have the hair messed up. Various hairstyles that are tight to the head or that pull the scalp can be a problem.

Heavy hair also can pull on the scalp. Tight bands (e.g., sweat bands), restrictive elastic caps used to control or style hair, and protective sports headgear can interfere with the circulation of the scalp, restrict cranial bone movement, and put pressure on nerves and vessels in the head. This pulling or compression on the scalp can cause headaches, localized fascial restriction, and even body-wide binding and compensation. If these conditions are noted, a different hairstyle should be used, tight bands and head coverings should be avoided, and protective headgear should be properly fitted. Shaved heads can be irritated if the massage application rubs against the grain of the hair.

The scalp must be able to move freely in all directions on the skull to allow cranial bone movement and to reduce pressure on muscles, nerves, and vessels. As mentioned previously, distinct fascial bands encircle the head, and these bands must be pliable or they will restrict fluid and cranial bone movement.

Address this area with the patient in the prone, supine, and side-lying positions.

- Place your hands on either side of the patient's head by the ears. Turning the head to the side facilitates the application of pressure. Move the scalp in various directions to assess for bind.
- If an area binds, it can be addressed by slowly moving the tissue into ease, dragging it the way it most wants to go. Multiple load directions can be used. For example, if the skin and superficial fascia want to move up and to the right, that is the direction in which the forces are introduced.
- Once ease has been identified, introduce an increased force (i.e., tension or shear) and use the force rhythmically to load and unload the tissue to increase the pliability of the ground substance. Then move tissues into bind and repeat.
- Bend and shear forces are required to make the connective tissue bands less restrictive. Methodically move along the bands, assessing for bind, and address each area as it is found. The increase in the length and pliability of the connective tissue will be small but sufficient to allow for normal movement of the structures of the head.

Connective tissue structures in the neck that weave into the scalp can exert pressure into the scalp. In fact, the connective tissue plane that runs from the scalp superficially to the sacrum can create bind in the tissues of the head. Another pattern, from the scalp to the dorsolumbar fascia to the iliotibial (IT) band and then to the foot, can create bind in the scalp. The entire body must be addressed to ensure appropriate pliability in the fascial structures of the head.

- If superficial edema is present in the head, it should be drained after the connective tissue has been addressed. Drain patterns from the head run toward the neck.

The musculature of the head is very strong. The temporalis, which is part of the chewing mechanism, often has an increased tone as a result of gum chewing and gritting and clenching of the teeth. The suboccipital muscles weave into the posterior neck extensors via connective tissue attachments. The occipital muscles often become locked in isometric contraction patterns and eventually become fibrotic.

The frontalis and occipitalis are actually one muscle connected by connective tissues called the *galea aponeurotica.* This muscle attaches at the base of the skull and neck tissues and runs to the forehead. If the two portions of the muscle are not balanced, an uneven pull force, pain, or both can occur. If the occipitalis shortens, pain can be felt in the forehead and in some cases the eyebrows feel as if they are being pulled back. Squinting, scowling, and grimacing can increase tension in the frontalis and exert pull in the back of the head.

- If muscle tone has increased in any muscles of the head from sustained isometric contraction, use broad-based, direct pressure to inhibit the spindle cells and the Golgi tendons.
- Apply pressure using broad-based compression that is intense enough to elicit tenderness or to reproduce the symptoms but not so intense as to cause muscle tensing or breathing changes.
- Muscle energy methods can be used in combination with the compression by having the patient contract against the pressure applied by the massage therapist's hand or forearm. It may take a few experimental contractions

before the right muscle pattern is discovered. When the correct muscle contracts, the area will tense or seem as if it is pushing against the therapist's pressure.

- Pulsed muscle energy methods in which a contract-relax, contract-relax pattern is used are especially effective for the muscles of the head. When the tone begins to reduce, bend or tension force can be applied to the muscle fibers. The intent is not to address connective tissue, but rather to pull the actin and myosin filaments apart mechanically to restore normal resting length.

Eye fatigue is common. Applying systematic pressure on the muscles of the head while the patient slowly moves the eyes in circles seems to help and certainly does no harm.

- Some patients enjoy having their hair gently pulled. The hair can be used as a handle to pull the scalp away from the skull. Make sure you grasp a large bunch of hair; then, introduce a gentle pull to bind, hold, and then release. Done systematically this application addresses the entire scalp.
- Compression to the sides of the head and to the front and back of the head, coupled with a scratching motion to the scalp, can be very pleasant. The compression aspect of this technique can be a typical craniosacral sequence if the massage professional is trained in this bodywork method.

THE OCCIPITAL BASE (Figure 11-3)

The occipital base is the transition point between the head and the neck. Transition areas usually involve fairly mobile, jointed areas. The joints in this area are the atlas and the axis. Local muscles are involved in the stability of this area and consist primarily of the suboccipital group. These muscles also act as proprioceptive feedback stations on the position of the head in relation to the rest of the body and work with the ocular, tonic neck, and pelvic reflexes to maintain posture and balance. In some cases the suprahyoid may also work to balance the head, exerting a small counterforce to the suboccipitals. The global muscles that can influence the occipital base are the sternocleidomastoid, platysma, semispinalis, splenius capitis, and trapezius. Listing individual muscles that can influence any particular area is difficult, because the body is such an interconnected structure; however, these are the main muscles that affect the local joint stability, proprioceptive information, and global movement of this area. The local muscles are deep; the global muscles, which are more superficial, comprise the first and second layers of tissue.

The cervical plexus and the vessels supplying the head are located in the area of the occipital base, and impingement is common. It is essential that this area function normally, to ensure the proper positional reflexes necessary for agility and precise movement. Sympathetic dominance increases muscle tone in the area, and decreased connective tissue pliability is often a factor.

PROCEDURES FOR THE OCCIPITAL BASE

Examples of treatment procedures for the occipital base area are shown in the Appendix.

Address this area with the patient in the prone and side-lying positions.

- Systematically lightly stroke the area to assess for temperature changes, skin texture, and damp areas. Observe for skin reddening (histamine response) and goose bumps (pilomotor response). These signs indicate possible changes in skin pliability. The accumulation of interstitial fluid may be indicated by the presence of edematous tissue and/or increased skin pressure (the sensation is much like pressing on a water balloon).
- If increased fluid pressure is evident, drain the area; use a combination of light pressure to drag the skin and deeper, rhythmic, broad-based compression and kneading to stimulate the deeper vessels.
    - Begin with lighter pressure directed toward the collarbone and cover the entire area.
    - Then introduce pumping, broad-based compression and combine it with active movement (i.e., have the patient slowly rotate the head in circles, first one way and then the other) and passive movement.
    - Return to dragging the skin. Alternate between dragging and compression until the area has been drained (about 5

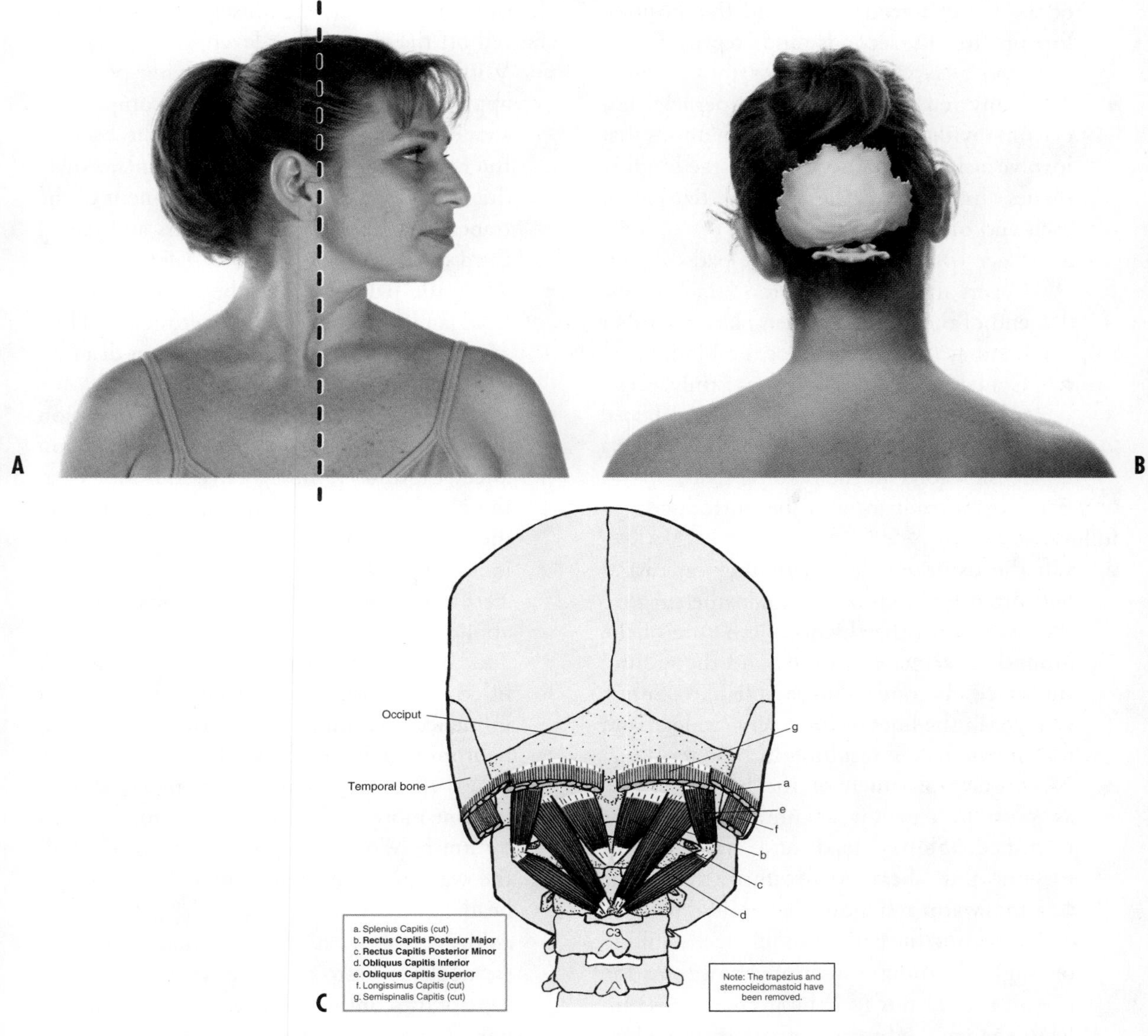

FIGURE 11-3 ■ Important structures in massage application to the occipital base to assist the reader. The bones of the occipital base are shown in a side view **(A)** and a posterior view **(B)**. **C,** The muscles of the occipital base. (**A** and **B** from Muscolino JE: *Kinesiology: the skeletal system and muscle function,* St Louis, 2006, Mosby; **C** from Muscolino JE: *The muscular system manual: the skeletal muscles of the human body,* ed 2, St Louis, 2005, Mosby.)

minutes). (Remember, when moving fluid, you can't push a river.)

- If you are in doubt about whether fluid retention is present, assume that it is and drain the area.

Next, address the superficial fascia by assessing for tissue bind. Always observe for involvement in adjacent areas such as the upper back, chest, head, and face.

- Move the skin to identify any areas of bind in the superficial connective tissue. Notice whether any bind areas correspond to the areas of skin reddening or goose bumps identified by the light stroking. Pay particular attention to any scars, because connective tissue bind is common at these sites.
- Address areas of bind by slowly moving the tissue into ease, dragging it the way it most wants to go. Multiple load directions can be used. For example, if the skin and superficial fascia want to move down and to the left at the base of the skull, that is the direction

of the forces introduced. Hold this position for up to 30 seconds and repeat. Then reassess.

- Treat any remaining areas of superficial fascial bind with myofascial release methods that involve a slow, sustained drag on the binding tissues, introducing the lines of tension at each end of the binding tissue.
    - Place your flat hand (or the pads of your fingers if your hand is too large) at one end of the bind, and then place the other hand at the other end of the bind.
    - Contact the tissue gently but firmly, pressing only as deep as the superficial fascial layer; then separate your hands, creating a tension force in the binding tissue.

Bending force can also be introduced as follows:

- Lift the tissue much as a mother cat carries her kitten by its neck; maintain the drag on the tissue until the thixotropic nature of the ground substance is affected and the ground substance becomes more pliable. Subtle changes in the lines of force serve to load and unload the tissue, resulting in hysteresis.
- Next, grasp as much of the binding tissue as possible and lift it until the bind is identified. Slowly load and unload with torsion and shear force until the tissue becomes warm and more pliable. This method is intense, and the patient should feel a pulling or slight burning sensation; however, the person should not feel the need to tense up or to change the breathing pattern to endure the application.
- Work slowly and deliberately, interspersing the process with lymphatic drainage–type stroking every minute or so.

The posterior tissue is very thick, and work in this area can be relatively aggressive. The anterior tissue between the chin and hyoid, on the other hand, is more delicate, and gentler methods need to be used in this area.

The musculature in the posterior region is addressed in layers by moving systematically from superficial to deep. Depending on the size of the neck, the depth to the suboccipitals can be more than 2 inches. It is important to make sure that the muscle layers are not adhering to each other. If adhesion is present, the muscle layer should be sheared off the next deeper layer.

- With the patient in the side-lying position, apply gliding strokes with a compressive element. Begin at the middle of the back of the head at the trapezius attachments; slowly drag the tissue to the distal attachment of the trapezius at the acromion process and lateral third of the clavicle.
- With the patient prone, begin again at the head and glide toward the acromion. Then reverse the direction and work from distal to proximal.
- Next, glide slowly across the fiber direction using enough pressure to ensure that you affect the muscle fiber. This addresses both the connective tissue and neuromuscular elements of the muscle. Repeat 3 or 4 times, increasing the depth and drag each time. Be alert to the movement of the muscle with the application.
- The upper trapezius area can be grasped, lifted, kneaded, and shaken, all of which influence the fluid, connective tissue, and neuromuscular elements. Fluid should move more effectively, connective tissue should become more pliable, and muscle tone should diminish. Work the upper trapezius tissue all the way to the proximal attachments at the head.
- Address the sternocleidomastoid using the sternocleidomastoid release (see Chapter 10). Do not use compression because of the underlying pressure-sensitive vessels and nerves. Instead, place the head so that one of the sternocleidomastoids is slackened, then grasp the muscle, lift it slightly, and systematically work with a squeezing motion from the belly to both attachments.
- Repeat slowly while introducing a shear and bend; move just past bind to lengthen the fibers and increase the pliability of the connective tissue.
- Gently lift the tissue that includes the platysma and bend it to normalize both the neuromuscular and connective tissue elements.

Narrow the focus to address the next layer of muscle, the splenius and semispinalis capitis group. Make sure the more superficial muscles slide over these muscles.

- Use a wavelike motion over the area to assess for sliding. If the tissues are adherent, reintroduce connective tissue methods by grasping the surface layer, lifting it off the underlying tissue, and systematically shearing the tissue until it is freed from the underlying area. If the area is very adherent, many sessions may be required to separate the layers enough to allow proper muscle action.
- Work for up to 3 minutes on an area or until it gets warm.
- Maintaining a broad-based contact, increase the compressive force and contact the next layer of tissue. Again, glide and drag the tissue from proximal attachment to distal attachment and then reverse. Repeat 3 or 4 times.
- Knead, glide, and use friction across the muscle fibers, making sure that bend, shear, and torsion forces are sufficient to move the muscles and that they do not adhere to the deeper layer of tissue.

Narrow the focus again to address the suboccipitals. These muscles are too small for gliding strokes. However, they respond to compression of the muscle belly; this serves to bend the muscle and to exert a tension force at the attachment, affecting the proprioceptors in these locations. When addressing deeper tissue layers, always remember to protect the more superficial muscles by applying pressure gradually and with as broad a base of contact as the area allows.

The side-lying position is best for applying the compression. The supine position is too hard on the massage therapist's hands, and in the prone position, the patient's head has just enough extension to make the muscles difficult to reach and address. The muscles can be accessed if the head is dropped off the table edge into forward flexion, but the pressure must be applied through the taut, more superficial tissue. With the patient in the side-lying position, the more superficial tissue is more passive and the muscle can be addressed using the forearm (if the area is very small, use the supported fingers). Use the suboccipital release described in Chapter 10.

- Because this area is extremely active in proprioceptive functions, muscle energy methods are effective, especially the use of motion and positioning of the eyes. Depending on the situation, use varying degrees of intensity. The gentlest method involves using the eye position to locate the position of release.
  - Locate the tender point.
  - While maintaining pressure on the area, have the patient slowly move the eyes in circles until the tenderness dissipates.
  - Hold for up to 30 seconds.
  - Next, if the area is not acutely painful, maintain the same pressure contact with the tender area and have the patient look hard, moving only the eyes toward the pain. This initiates a tensing of the muscles.
  - Have the patient hold this position for a few seconds and then look in the opposite direction; this activates opposing antagonist patterns and initiates reciprocal inhibition. Have the patient hold this position for a few seconds and then slowly turn the head in the direction of the eyes, as far as possible from the pain. When the end of range is reached, apply a small overpressure to lengthen the muscles. After a few seconds, apply a bit more tension to the bind and stretch the connective tissue.

The most aggressive muscle energy pattern used in this area involves appropriate facilitation and inhibition of muscle contraction.

- Place the patient's head in a neutral position (the patient may be in the supine, prone, side-lying, or seated position).
- Place your hands on either side of the patient's head just above the ears and stabilize the head. Instruct the patient to push against one of your hands and to look hard in that direction. Apply sufficient resistance so that the contraction remains isometric.
- Next, have the patient continue to push, but instruct him or her to turn only the eyes in the opposite direction, to inhibit the contacting muscles. Apply a slightly increased pressure to determine whether the area is inhibited. The patient should not be able to hold against the increased pressure unless using other muscles or holding the breath.

- If the area does not inhibit, apply sufficient overpressure to move the head 1 inch. Slowly let go and repeat until the area inhibits easily.
- If a change is not noted in 2 or 3 attempts, the problem likely is more global and connected to some other reflex or proprioceptive pattern. Leave it alone.
- Repeat on the other side, then go front to back and on each diagonal. During the treatment, do not let the patient recruit other muscles or hold the breath.

This series of moves can substantially reduce the sensation of tightness in the neck, especially the need to "crack" the neck.

Gentle, rocking, rhythmic range-of-motion movements (oscillation) may be used to continue to relax the area. The more global muscles can be remassaged gently, or lymphatic drainage massage can complete the procedure.

THE NECK (Figure 11-4)

The neck area includes the cervical vertebrae, particularly from C2 to T1. This is an area of many joints that permit flexion, extension, and rotation, as well as many combinations of these movements, to allow orientation of the head and ultimately the eyes, ears, and nose in many different directions. The tissues in this area have to supply both stability to maintain the position of the head and mobility for both large and small precise movements. The neck has both local and global muscle patterns, and the connective tissue of the area is a major factor. The more global muscles were addressed in massage of the occipital area but are described again in relation to cervical movement and stability. The local muscles stabilize the cervical vertebrae and guide movement, making it more precise. This deeper layer of muscle often creates the sensation of a tight neck.

The neck region consists of either three or four tissue layers, depending on how the anatomy is interpreted. In addition to the muscles that attach to the cervical area, several muscles that do not attach to the head are discussed, including the scalenes, levator scapula, longissimus cervicis, semispinalis cervicis, iliocostalis cervicis, spinalis, longus colli, and infrahyoids, as well as the multifidi, rotators, interspinales, and intertransversarii at each vertebra.

The neck area has many vessels and nerves, including the brachial plexus. Impingement is common, with referral patterns in the neck, down to the chest, and to the arms. This is the area where thoracic outlet syndrome occurs. Preventive care is needed for this condition. Also, if a person suffers impact trauma to the head, the neck absorbs the force and restrains the motion.

The neck is involved in many reflex patterns, including the tonic neck reflex. The muscles that insert on the ribs often become short with upper chest breathing patterns. The outcome of this may be symptoms of chronic overbreathing and breathing pattern syndrome.

PROCEDURES FOR THE NECK

Examples of treatment procedures for the neck are shown in the Appendix.

This area is effectively addressed with the patient in the supine, prone, side-lying, and seated positions.

- Systematically lightly stroke the area to assess for temperature changes, skin texture, and damp areas. Observe for skin reddening (histamine response) and goose bumps (pilomotor response). These signs indicate possible changes in the connective tissue, muscle tone, or circulation patterns.
- Increase the pressure slightly and assess for superficial fascial bind, changes in skin pliability, and the accumulation of interstitial fluid, as indicated by boggy or edematous tissue and/or increased skin pressure (the sensation is much like pressing on a water balloon).
- If increased fluid pressure is evident, drain the area; use a combination of light pressure to drag the skin and deeper, rhythmic, broad-based compression and kneading to stimulate the deeper vessels.
  - Begin with lighter pressure directed toward the collarbone and cover the entire area.
  - Then introduce pumping, broad-based compression, and kneading, and com-

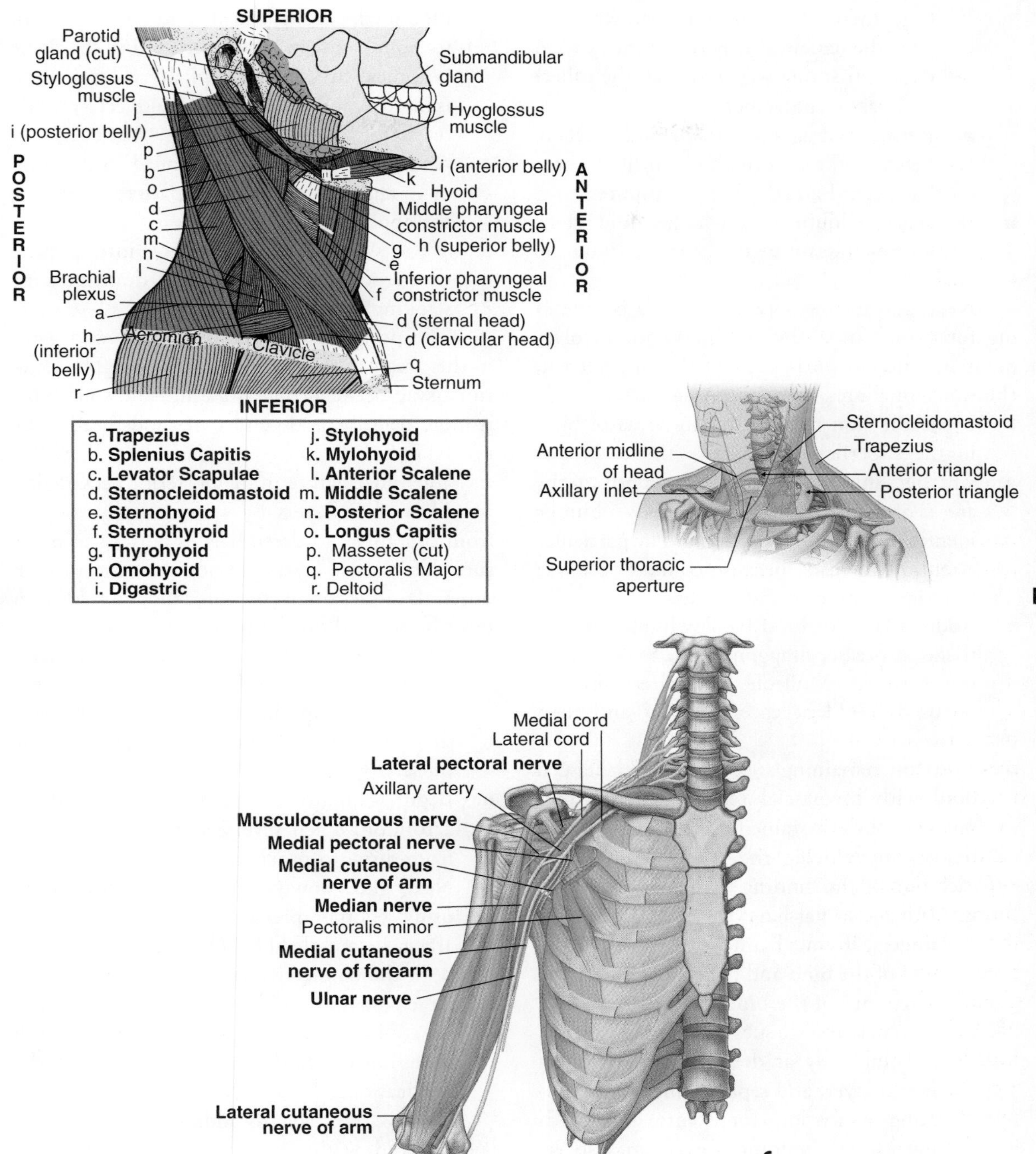

FIGURE 11-4 ■ Important structures in massage application to the neck to assist the reader. **A,** The muscles of the neck. **B,** The anterior and posterior triangles of the neck. **C,** The brachial plexus. (**A** from Muscolino JE: *The muscular system manual: the skeletal muscles of the human body,* ed 2, St Louis, 2005, Mosby; **B** and **C** from Drake R, Vogl W, Mitchell A: *Gray's anatomy for students,* Edinburgh, 2005, Churchill Livingstone.)

bine them with active movement (i.e., have the patient slowly rotate the head in circles, first one way and then the other) and passive movement.
    - Return to dragging the skin and alternate between the two methods until the area has been drained (about 5 minutes).
- If you are in doubt about whether fluid retention is present, assume that it is and drain the area.

Next, address the superficial fascia by assessing for tissue bind. Always observe for involvement in adjacent areas such as the upper back, chest, occipital area, face, and head.

- Move the skin to identify any areas of bind in the superficial connective tissue. Notice whether any bind areas correspond to the areas of skin reddening or goose bumps identified by the light stroking. Pay particular attention to scars, because connective tissue bind is common in these areas.
- Address areas of bind by slowly moving the tissue into ease, dragging it the way it most wants to go. Multiple load directions can be used. Hold at each position and then reassess.
- Treat any remaining areas of superficial fascial bind with myofascial release methods that involve a slow, sustained drag on the binding tissues, introducing the lines of tension at each end of the binding tissue.
    - Place your flat hand (or the pads of your fingers, if your hand is too large) at one end of the bind and the other hand at the other end of the bind.
    - Contact the tissue gently but firmly, pressing only as deep as the superficial fascial layer, and separate the hands, creating a tension force into the binding tissue. Bending force can also be introduced.
- Maintain the drag on the tissue until the thixotropic nature of the ground substance is affected and the ground substance becomes more pliable. Subtle changes in the lines of force serve to load and unload the tissue, resulting in hysteresis.
- Next, grasp as much of the binding tissue as possible and lift it until the resistance is identified. Slowly load and unload with torsion, bend, and shear forces until the tissue becomes warm and more pliable. This method is intense, and the patient should feel a pulling or slight burning sensation; however, the person should not feel the need to tense up or to change the breathing pattern to endure the application.
- Work slowly and deliberately, interspersing the process with lymphatic drainage–type stroking every minute or so.

The posterior tissue is very thick, and work in this area can be relatively aggressive. The anterior tissue between the hyoid and the collarbone is more delicate, and gentler methods need to be used there.

The musculature in the posterior neck region is addressed in layers by systematically moving from superficial to deep. It is important to make sure that muscle layers are not adhering to each other. If adhesion is present, the muscle layer must be sheared off the next deeper layer.

- Use gliding with a compressive element, beginning at the middle of the back of the head at the trapezius attachments, and slowly drag the tissue to the distal attachment of the muscle.
- Begin again at the head and glide toward the acromion. Then reverse direction and work from distal to proximal.
- Next, glide slowly across the fiber direction, using enough pressure to ensure that you affect the muscle fiber. This method addresses both the connective tissue and neuromuscular elements of the muscle. Repeat 3 or 4 times, increasing the depth and drag each time. Be alert to the muscle moving with the application.

Narrow the focus to address the next tissue layer, including the levator scapula and scalenes. Make sure the surface muscles slide over these muscles.

- Use a wavelike motion over the area to assess for sliding. If sliding does not occur, reintroduce connective tissue methods by grasping the surface layer, lifting it off the underlying tissue, and systematically shearing the tissue until it is freed from the underlying area. If the area is very adherent, many sessions may be needed before the layers separate sufficiently to allow proper muscle action.

- Work for 2 minutes or longer or until that particular area gets warm, and then continue with the rest of the area.
- While maintaining a broad-based contact, increase the compressive force. Glide and drag the tissue from the proximal attachment to the distal attachment and then reverse. Repeat 3 or 4 times.
- Knead and glide across the muscle fibers, making sure that bending, shear, and torsion forces are sufficient to move the muscles accurately and to make sure they do not adhere to the deeper layer of tissue.
- Compression is best applied with the patient in the side-lying position and with the massage therapist using the forearm in the valley of the neck. By changing the angle of the contact, the therapist can use compression to identify any areas where short muscle structures are impinging on the nerves. When such an area has been located, the symptoms that have troubled the patient will be reproduced.
- First apply compression and then combine it with muscle energy methods. Start from the least invasive positional release using movement of the eyes.
- If the target muscle is not released, progress to positional release using movement of the head, neck, arms, and pelvis and finally to pulsed muscle energy methods.
- If necessary, use the more aggressive reciprocal inhibition and tense and relax methods. The goal is to temporarily inhibit the motor tone of the muscle bundle that is problematic so that it can be lengthened to the appropriate resting length that results in reduced pressure on the nerves or vessels.

Narrow the focus to the third layer of tissue. These muscles are too small for gliding techniques, but they respond to compression of the belly of the muscles. This serves to bend the muscle and exert a tension force at the insertion to affect the proprioceptors in these locations. The side-lying position is best for applying the compression. The supine position is too hard on the massage therapist's hands.

The patient also can be positioned prone with the head dropped slightly into forward flexion. If the superficial tissue is not too taut, the deeper muscle and connective tissue can be addressed. With the patient in the side-lying position, the more superficial tissue is relatively passive, and the muscle can be addressed using the forearm (or, if the area is very small, the supported fingers). When addressing deeper tissue layers, always remember to protect the more superficial muscles by applying pressure gradually, with as broad a base of contact as the area allows.

Neuromuscular reflex patterns can be addressed as follows:

- Place the patient's head in neutral position (the patient may be in the supine, prone, side-lying, or seated position).
- Place your hands on either side of the head just below the ears and stabilize the head. Instruct the patient to push against one of your hands and look hard in that direction. Apply sufficient resistance so that the contraction remains isometric.
- Next, have the patient continue to push, but have the person turn the eyes and look in the opposite direction; this should inhibit the contacting muscles. Apply slightly increased pressure to determine whether the area is inhibited. If it is, the patient will not be able to hold against the increased pressure unless other muscles are used or the person holds the breath.
- If the area does not inhibit, apply sufficient overpressure to move the head about 2 inches. Let go and repeat until the area inhibits. If a change is not noted in 2 or 3 attempts, the problem probably has a more global connection involving some other reflex or proprioceptive pattern. Leave it alone.
- Repeat the process on the other side, then go from front to back and on each diagonal and in both rotational patterns. Do not let the patient recruit other muscles or hold the breath.
- Have the patient flex the head and neck by looking toward the navel and rolling the pelvis toward the navel. Tell the patient to hold this position (without using other muscles or holding the breath).

- Apply a gentle but firm pressure to the forehead to push the neck into extension. It should hold the contraction easily.
- If it does not hold the contraction, have the patient maintain the pelvic position while gently performing pulsing contractions against the therapist's hand on the patient's forehead; this stimulates the neck flexors. Flexion should normalize with 10 to 15 pulses.
- Next, have the patient look toward the navel and roll the pelvis in the opposite direction (which will slightly arch the low back) and hold again while continuing to breathe normally. Apply a gentle but firm pressure to the patient's forehead to push the neck into extension. The neck flexors should have difficulty holding the contraction and should let go. If they do not inhibit, apply a gentle but firm pressure to the forehead to move the neck into extension while the patient rocks the pelvis back and forth. Three or four repetitions should reset the reflex.

This series of moves can substantially reduce the sensation of tightness in the neck, especially the need to "crack" the neck.

Use a gentle, rocking, rhythmic range of motion to continue to relax the area. The more global muscles can be remassaged gently, or a lymphatic drainage application can be used to complete the massage of the area.

THE ANTERIOR TORSO (Figure 11-5)

The anterior torso is best addressed before the posterior torso because it is the location of the structures that cause most of the aching and dysfunction in the posterior torso.

The anterior torso consists of the rib cage, which protects the vital organs, and the abdominal contents. The muscles in the anterior torso area are primarily responsible for breathing. The pectoralis major and pectoralis minor provide the arm and scapula with both movement and stability. The abdominal muscles are layered and quite intricate in design and are extensively encased and supported by fascial structures. This is an important area of core stability, and the massage therapist must understand how the abdominal group functions in posture.

Attachments of the muscles from the neck (platysma, sternocleidomastoid, scalenes) and the connective tissue connections that unify the body are situated in the upper chest. The muscles of the anterior torso are in functional units with the head and neck flexors. The muscles of this area are involved in flexion and adduction movements in the frontal and sagittal planes. The fiber orientation of the muscles and fascia is multidirectional, with a strong diagonal and perpendicular focus.

Three major cross sections of tissue in the transverse plane define this area. First, the muscles of the neck overlap with the muscles of the upper thorax and the back of the neck and torso to form the thoracic diaphragm. Second, the diaphragm muscle itself separates the upper and lower torso, and third, the pelvic floor is closed by the crisscross design of the pelvic floor muscles. These transverse layers of tissue provide stability and are involved in respiration.

PROCEDURES FOR THE ANTERIOR TORSO

Examples of treatment procedures for the anterior torso are shown in the Appendix.

Address this area with the patient in the side-lying or supine position; the use of both is most desirable. The massage begins with superficial work, progresses to deeper tissue layers, and finishes off with superficial work. Initial applications involve palpation assessment to identify temperature and superficial tissue changes.

- Systematically lightly stroke the area to assess for temperature changes, skin texture, and damp areas. Observe for skin reddening (histamine response) and goose bumps (pilomotor response). These signs indicate possible changes in the connective tissue, muscle tone, or circulation patterns.
- Increase the pressure slightly and assess for superficial fascial bind, changes in skin pliability, and the accumulation of interstitial fluid, as indicated by boggy or edematous tissue and/or increased skin pressure (the sensation is much like pressing on a water balloon).

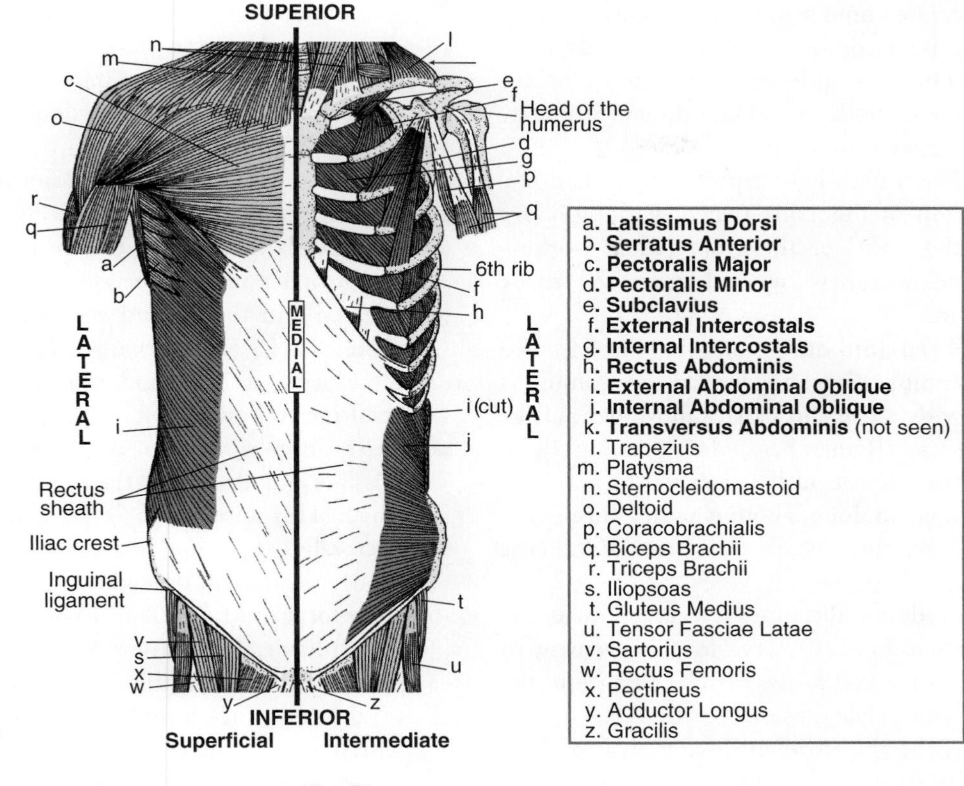

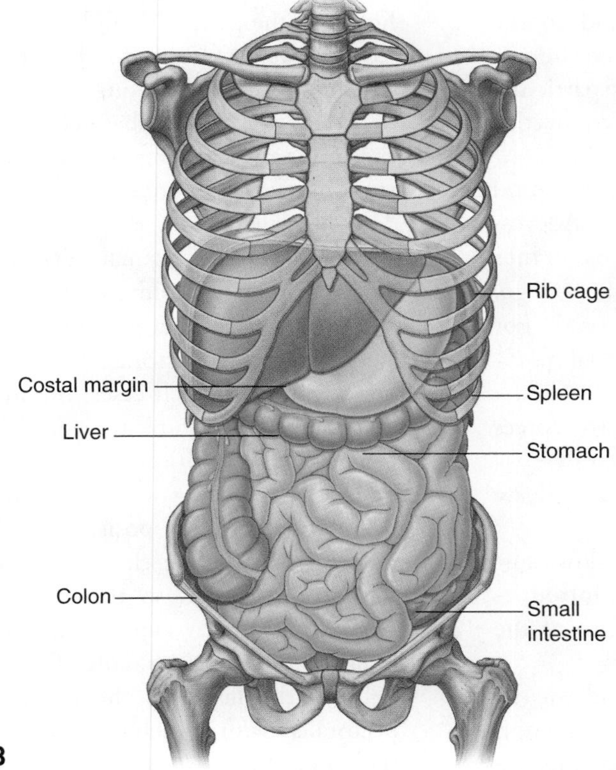

FIGURE 11-5 ■ Important structures in massage application to the anterior torso to assist the reader. **A,** The muscles of the anterior torso. **B,** The abdomen contains and protects the abdominal viscera. (**A** from Muscolino JE: *The muscular system manual: the skeletal muscles of the human body,* ed 2, St Louis, 2005, Mosby; **B** from Drake R, Vogl W, Mitchell A: *Gray's anatomy for students,* Edinburgh, 2005, Churchill Livingstone.)

- If increased fluid pressure is evident, drain the area; use a combination of light pressure to drag the skin and deeper, rhythmic, broad-based compression and kneading to stimulate the deeper vessels.
  - Begin with lighter pressure in the direction of the axilla (when working above the waist) or the groin (when working below the waist) and cover the entire area.
  - Then introduce pumping, broad-based compression, which can be combined with active and passive movement of the area. (Remember, when moving fluid, you cannot push a river.)
- If you are in doubt about whether fluid retention is present, assume that it is and drain the area.

Next, address the superficial fascia by assessing for tissue bind. Observe for involvement of adjacent areas, such as the tissue leading into the shoulder and pelvic girdles.

- Move the skin to identify any areas of bind in the superficial connective tissue. Notice whether any bind areas correspond to the areas of skin reddening or goose bumps identified by the light stroking. Pay particular attention to any scars, because connective tissue bind is common at these sites.
- Treat areas of superficial fascial bind with myofascial release methods. Address these areas by slowly moving the tissue into ease, dragging it the way it most wants to go. Multiple load directions can be used. For example, if the skin and superficial fascia want to move up and to the right at the sternum, that is the direction of the forces introduced.
- Hold the tissue in ease position until release is felt or for 30 to 60 seconds.
- Next, work into the bind. Use a slow, sustained drag on the binding tissues, introducing the lines of tension at each end of the binding tissue.
  - Place your forearm or flat hand (or the pads of your fingers if your hand is too large) at one end of the bind and the other forearm or hand at the other end of the bind.
  - Contact the tissue gently but firmly, pressing only as deep as the superficial fascial layer, and separate your forearms or hands, creating a tension force in the binding tissue.

Bend and torsion forces and joint movement can be introduced as well.

- Maintain the drag on the tissue until the thixotropic nature of the ground substance is affected and the ground substance becomes more pliable. Subtle changes in the lines of force serve to load and unload the tissue, resulting in hysteresis.
- Next, grasp as much of the binding tissue as possible and lift it until the resistance is identified. This application is possible with the pectoralis major and the rectus abdominis. Slowly load and unload with torsion and shear force until the tissue becomes warm and more pliable. The arm movements previously described can be combined with direct lifting of the tissue to introduce multiple forces. This method is intense, and the patient should feel a pulling or slight burning sensation; however, the patient should not feel the need to tense up or change the breathing pattern to endure the application.
- Work slowly and deliberately, interspersing the process with lymphatic drainage–type stroking every minute or so.

The musculature in the anterior thorax is addressed in layers by systematically moving from superficial to deep. It is important to make sure that muscle layers are not adhering to each other. Most commonly, the pectoralis major sticks to the pectoralis minor. In such cases, the muscle layer must be sheared off the next deeper layer.

- It is helpful to position the patient so that the surface layer is in a slack position. This can be accomplished by positioning the attachments of the muscle close together and bolstering the patient so that the person can remain relaxed. In some situations, the side-lying position may be more efficient.
- Because the fascia in the chest covers the pectoralis major, which extends into the arm, the arm can be used to increase or release the tension force on the tissue. When the arm is passively internally rotated and horizontally

adducted, the fascia is slack. With the torso stabilized and the arm externally rotated, abducted, and extended, the fascia is taut. Moving back and forth between these two positions loads and unloads the tissue.

- Whether using the more direct methods or the movements of the arms, maintain the drag on the tissue until the thixotropic nature of the ground substance is affected and the ground substance becomes more pliable. Subtle changes in the lines of force serve to load and unload the tissue in various orientations.
- Beginning at the shoulder, use gliding with a compressive element and work from the distal attachment of the pectoralis major at the arm toward the sternum, following the fiber direction. This can be done in the supine or side-lying position with the patient rolled. Repeat 3 or 4 times, each time increasing the drag and moving slower.
- Move to the abdomen to address the rectus abdominis. If any area binds against the drag, working across the grain of the muscle and in the opposite direction may be beneficial.
- Any areas that redden may be sites of trigger point activity. Latent trigger points can cause muscles to fire out of sequence, therefore it is important to restore as much normalcy to the tissue as possible.
- To increase circulation to the area and shift the neuroresponses of latent trigger points, move the skin over the point into multiple directions of ease and hold the ease position for 30 to 60 seconds.
- If the tenderness is not relieved, the next option is positional release, followed by muscle energy methods if necessary.
- Local lengthening of the tissue containing the trigger points is effective, and authorities have found that it is needed to complete the release of trigger points. Local lengthening is accomplished by using tension, bend, or torsion force on the tissue with the trigger point and taut band. Do not use direct pressure or transverse friction, because they may cause tissue damage.
- If the trigger point does not release with the methods described, it is part of a compensation pattern that must be dealt with, and it probably serves a useful function. Leave it alone.

Once the surface tissue has been addressed, the second layer of muscle is massaged. It is important to make sure the surface tissue and the fascial separation between muscle layers are not adhering to each other in any way. Assess by lifting the surface tissue and moving it back and forth in a wavelike movement. The main muscles addressed in this group are the pectoralis minor, anterior serratus, and external and internal abdominal obliques.

- Use compression with gliding; apply it deeply enough to address this layer of tissue.
- Broaden the base of contact so that the surface tissue does not tighten to guard against poking.
- Glide in various directions, both with and against the grain of the muscle fibers.
- Repeat 3 or 4 times. Provide each application more slowly and at a slightly different angle to access the multiple fiber directions of these muscles.
- Next, knead slowly across the fiber direction, using enough pressure and lift to ensure that you affect the muscle fiber in this layer. These methods address both the connective tissue and neuromuscular elements of the muscle.
- Repeat 3 or 4 times, increasing the depth and drag each time. Be alert to the muscle moving with the application. Work the entire length of the area and repeat.

Narrow the focus to address the third tissue layer, including the intercostals. Make sure the surface muscles slide over these muscles.

- Use a wavelike motion over the area to assess for sliding. If adhesion is identified, reintroduce connective tissue methods by grasping the surface layer, lifting it off the underlying tissue, and systematically shearing or bending the tissue until it is freed from the underlying area. If the area is very adherent, many sessions may be needed before the layers separate enough to allow proper muscle action. Work for up to 2 to 3 minutes or until the area becomes warm.
- The side-lying position is best. Use the braced finger to contact the tissue between the ribs.

Gently and confidently increase the compressive force and contact this layer of tissue. This is commonly a ticklish area, so do not use a hesitant touch.

- Glide and drag the tissue using the fingers; these are not long moves, because the span of these muscles is between the ribs.
- Repeat 3 or 4 times.
- Tender points are treated with positional release. Often the position of release can be reached by using different compressive forces on the ribs to change the shape of the rib cage. If bones are brittle in this area, be cautious. If direct movement of the rib cage is not possible, moving the hips or shoulders also changes the position of the ribs. It is very important to address these tender points, because they can interfere with effective movement of the ribs during breathing.
- When addressing deeper tissue layers, always remember to protect the more superficial muscles by applying pressure gradually, using as broad a base of contact as the area allows.

Accessing the Diaphragm Muscle, Psoas, and Colon

The proprioceptors in the diaphragm muscle's attachments on the anterior ribs can be stimulated with careful direct pressure by applying compression up and under the rib cage. Care must be taken to protect the liver, stomach, and spleen. (See Chapter 10 to review the procedure for diaphragm release.)

- Muscle energy methods are introduced by having the patient inhale and exhale. Be aware that the pelvic floor muscles and diaphragm may interact in an antagonist pattern. Recall that these are like sheets of muscle that divide the thorax into separate cavities. Even though this muscle interaction has not been verified, contracting and relaxing the pelvic floor may affect the tone pattern of the diaphragm. Introduce this pelvic floor contraction and relaxation while applying compression to the diaphragm's rib attachments.
- The diaphragm can also be addressed by applying a compressive or lifting force to the bottom ribs to change the shape of the rib cage. Rib contraindications apply.
- Systematic compression into the linea alba also has been used to release the diaphragm. The inferior attachment of the rectus abdominis to the pubic bone is addressed at this time if assessment indicates involvement. Shortening of the rectus abdominis can mimic a groin pull. This area should be addressed only if necessary, based on assessment and patient goals, with specific informed consent and other prudent cautions, such as having an additional person present.
- Likewise, the proximal attachments of the hamstrings and adductors on the ischial tuberosity and pubic bone can be addressed if assessment indicates involvement. This area should be addressed only if necessary, based on assessment and patient goals, with specific informed consent and other prudent cautions, such as having an additional person present (see the section on specific releases). The area tends to shorten in the patient.
- When working the anterior torso, the quadratus lumborum is addressed when the patient is in the side-lying position.
- The abdominal organs can be rolled to encourage peristalsis. Specific massage to the large intestine can support normal bowel elimination.
- If assessment identifies psoas symptoms, the psoas muscles can be addressed at this time.
- The following can be used to complete treatment of the anterior torso:
  - Apply rhythmic compression to the entire area of the anterior torso to simulate lymph flow.
  - Assess and correct firing patterns for the abdomen if possible. Usually the area requires therapeutic exercise.

THE POSTERIOR TORSO (Figure 11-6)

The posterior torso consists of the thoracic vertebrae, ribs, lumbar vertebrae, sacrum, and coccyx and the structures that attach to these bones. The most superficial layer of muscle serves to connect, stabilize in force couples, and move the limbs. These soft tissue structures are relatively global. The second, third, and fourth layers of muscle attach intrinsically on the vertebral column and ribs. These muscles and soft tissue structures

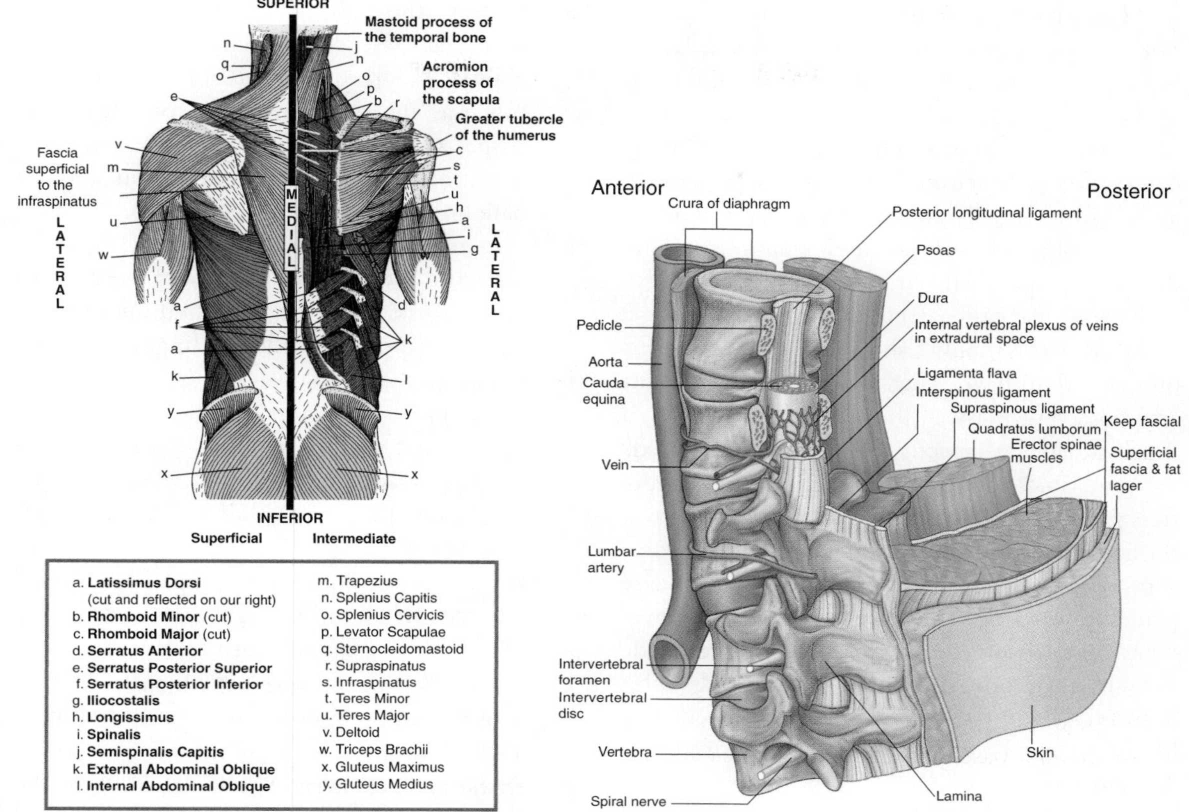

FIGURE 11-6 ■ Important structures in massage application to the posterior torso to assist the reader. **A,** The muscles of the posterior torso. **B,** The structures of the vertebral canal and the back. (**A** from Muscolino JE: *The muscular system manual: the skeletal muscles of the human body,* ed 2, St Louis, 2005, Mosby; **B** from Drake R, Vogl W, Mitchell A: *Gray's anatomy for students,* Edinburgh, 2005, Churchill Livingstone.)

become progressively more local the deeper they are oriented.

The middle layer of muscles has multiple attachments on the vertebrae and ribs that orient in a direction parallel to the spine. These muscles, collectively called the *sacrospinal* or *erector spinae,* function to extend and stabilize the back. Because the degree of movement for these muscles is limited, the stabilization of posture becomes their primary function. Stabilization involves smaller concentric and eccentric muscle function with sustaining isometric contraction. Therefore these muscles often will feel tense to the patient.

Major connective tissue structures begin at the head and cover the entire posterior trunk. These structures spread into the shoulder and pelvis as part of the supporting structures of limbs. Think of a traditional ground-based television or radio broadcast antenna (the spine) supported by its guy wires (connective tissue, including fascia).

The deeper layer of muscles (the multifidi, rotators, intertransversarii, and interspinales) are primarily stabilizers with important proprioceptive functions for the position of the spine. The deep muscles, which attach from one vertebra to the next, shorten and become hypersensitive to movement. They are difficult to stretch and tense, and often the patient feels as if he or she wants to "crack" the back.

Many nerves exit the spine, and the potential for entrapment exists. The most common locations where this may occur in the lumbar area are the lumbar and sacral plexuses.

The quadratus lumborum is a deep muscle that often has trigger point activity, with referred pain to the low back, which causes difficulty during the firing patterns of leg abduction.

The functions of the soft tissue in the posterior torso include extension, rotation, and lateral flexion, but the main function is maintaining an upright posture.

The posterior torso often is the cause of many complaints. The tension, binding, trigger points, and so forth usually are compensatory and adaptive to some sort of postural strain. Applying direct massage work in the area without also addressing the causal factors is purely palliative, and its effects last only a short time. However, this outcome does have value, especially in pre-event and postevent massage for athletes. Otherwise, a much broader perspective for massage is desired.

Anterior flexion, internal rotation, and adduction patterns usually are more likely to be part of the actual cause of backaches because they involve a pulling forward in the sagittal and transverse planes toward the midline. When these movement patterns are too strong, posterior thoracic structures become inhibited, long, and tight; however, there are exceptions, usually in the lumbar area, where muscles and connective tissue can shorten.

Be cautious in addressing trigger points and connective tissue bind in inhibited and long muscles of the posterior torso, because these conditions may be part of a resourceful compensation pattern. Instead, focus treatment on the anterior thorax and then reassess the posterior structures. Use hyperstimulation and counterirritation methods in the inhibited and long areas to reduce symptoms.

PROCEDURES FOR THE POSTERIOR TORSO

Examples of treatment procedures for the posterior torso are shown in the Appendix.

As described previously, massage begins with superficial work, progresses to the deeper tissue layers, and finishes off with superficial work. Initial applications are palpation assessments to identify temperature and surface tissue changes.

- Systematically lightly stroke the area to assess for temperature changes, skin texture, and damp areas. Observe for skin reddening (histamine response) and goose bumps (pilomotor response). These signs indicate possible changes in the connective tissue, muscle tone, or circulation patterns.
- Increase the pressure slightly and assess for superficial fascial bind, changes in skin pliability, and the accumulation of interstitial fluid, as indicated by boggy or edematous tissue and/or increased skin pressure (the sensation is much like pressing on a water balloon).
- If increased fluid pressure is evident, drain the area; use a combination of light pressure to drag the skin and deeper, rhythmic, broad-based compression and kneading to stimulate the deeper vessels.
    - Begin with lighter pressure in the direction of the axilla (when working above the waist) or the groin (when working below the waist) and cover the entire area.
    - Then introduce pumping, broad-based compression. (Remember, when moving fluid, you cannot push a river.)
- If you are in doubt about whether fluid retention is present, assume that it is and drain the area.

Next, address the superficial fascia by assessing the tissue bind. Always observe for involvement in adjacent areas, such as the tissue leading into the shoulder and pelvic girdles.

- Move the skin to identify any areas of bind in the superficial connective tissue. Notice whether any bind areas correspond to the areas of skin reddening or goose bumps identified by the light stroking. Pay particular attention to any scars, because connective tissue bind is common at these sites.
- Treat areas of superficial fascial bind with myofascial release methods. Address these areas by slowly moving the tissue into ease, dragging it the way it most wants to go. Multiple load directions can be used. For example, if the skin and superficial fascia want to move up and to the right between the scapulae, that is the direction of the forces introduced.
- Hold the tissue in the ease position for up to 30 to 60 seconds.
- Next, work into the bind with a slow, sustained drag on the binding tissues, introducing the lines of tension at each end of the binding tissue.

- Place your flat hand (or the pads of your fingers if your hand is too large) at one end of the bind and the other hand at the other end of the bind.
- Contact the tissue gently but firmly, pressing only as deep as the superficial fascial layer, and separate the hands, creating a tension force in the binding tissue. Bending force can also be introduced.

- Maintain the drag on the tissue until the thixotropic nature of the ground substance is affected and the ground substance becomes more pliable. Subtle changes in the lines of force serve to load and unload the tissue, resulting in hysteresis.
- Next, grasp as much of the binding tissue as possible and lift it until the resistance is identified. Slowly load and unload with torsion and shear force until the tissue becomes warm and more pliable. This method is intense, and the patient should feel a pulling or slight burning sensation; however, the person should not feel the need to tense up or change the breathing pattern to endure the application.
- Work slowly, interspersing the process with lymphatic drainage–type stroking every minute or so.

The fascial tissue of the posterior torso is very thick, especially at the thoracolumbar aponeurosis, and work in this area can be more intense than in other areas of the body.

The musculature in the posterior thoracic region is addressed in layers by systematically moving from superficial to deep. It is important to make sure that muscle layers are not adhering to each other. If they are, the layer of muscle should be sheared off the next deeper layer.

- It is helpful to position the patient so that the surface layer is in a slack position. This can be accomplished by positioning the attachments of the muscle close together and propping the patient so that the person stays relaxed. In some situations, the side-lying position may be better for this.
- Using gliding with a compressive element, begin at the iliac crest and work diagonally along the fibers of the latissimus dorsi, ending at the axilla. Repeat 3 or 4 times, each time increasing the drag and moving slower.
- Move up to the thoracolumbar junction and repeat the same sequence on the lower trapezius.
- Then, begin near the tip of the shoulder and glide toward the middle thoracic area to address the middle trapezius. Repeat 3 or 4 times, increasing drag and decreasing speed.
- Begin again near the acromion and address the upper trapezius with one or two gliding stokes to complete the surface area.
- If any area binds against the drag, working across the grain of the muscle and in the opposite direction may be beneficial.
- Any areas that redden may be sites of trigger point activity. Latent trigger points can cause muscles to fire out of sequence, therefore it is important to restore as much normalcy to the tissue as possible.
- To increase circulation to the area and shift the neuroresponses of latent trigger points, move the skin over the latent trigger point into multiple directions of ease and hold the ease position for 30 to 60 seconds.
- If the tenderness is not relieved, positional release is the next option, followed by muscle energy methods if necessary.
- Local lengthening of the tissue containing the trigger points is effective, and leading authorities have found that it is necessary to complete the release of trigger points. Local lengthening is accomplished by using tension, bend, or torsion force on the tissue with the trigger point and taut band. Do not use direct pressure or transverse friction, because they may cause tissue damage.
- If the trigger point does not release with the methods described, it is part of a compensation pattern. In this situation, the trigger point probably serves a useful function, especially in the posterior muscles, which often are in a long, taut state. In these cases, the trigger point areas shorten the tissue and add some counterforce to the areas that are short and pulling.
- Finish the area with kneading, making sure that the muscle tissue easily lifts off the layer underneath it.
- If adhesion is identified, introduce a bend, shear, or torsion force until the tissue becomes

more pliable. This method can be intense and can create a burning sensation; however, the patient should not guard, display pain behaviors, or hold the breath during application.

- Repeat this sequence bilaterally.

Once the surface tissue has been addressed, target the second layer of muscle. It is important to assess to make sure the surface tissue and the fascial separation between muscle layers are not adhering to each other in any way. The main muscles addressed at this point are the erector spinae, serratus posterior inferior and superior (especially if the patient is coughing, sniffling, or has any other breathing dysfunction), and rhomboids.

- Begin at the iliac crest. Use gliding strokes deep enough to address this layer of tissue and follow the direction of the tissue fiber. Maintain a broad base of contact so that the surface tissue does not tighten to guard against poking. Glide toward the scapula, ending just past the rhomboids.
- Repeat 3 or 4 times, slowing each stroke and delivering them at slightly different angles to access the multiple fiber directions of these muscles. Then reverse the direction and work from superior to inferior.
- Next, knead slowly across the fiber direction using enough pressure and lift to ensure that you affect the muscle fiber in this layer. These methods address both the connective tissue and neuromuscular elements of the muscle.
- Repeat 3 or 4 times, increasing the depth and drag each time. Be alert to the muscle moving with the application.
- Work the entire length of the area and repeat.

Narrow the focus to address the next layer, which includes the multifidi, rotators, intertransversarii, and interspinales. Make sure the more superficial muscles slide over these muscles.

- Use a wavelike motion over the area to assess for sliding. If the tissues do not slide, reintroduce connective tissue methods by grasping the surface layer, lifting it off the underlying tissue, and systematically shearing or bending the tissue until it is freed from the underlying area. If the area is substantially adherent, many sessions may be needed before the layers separate sufficiently to allow proper muscle action.
- Work for up to 2 or 3 minutes on a specific area, or until it gets warm, and then continue with the rest of the area.
- Maintain broad-based contact, increase the compressive force, and contact this layer of tissue.
- Glide and drag the tissue, using the forearm and fingers, from the proximal attachment to the distal attachment, and then reverse. These are not long moves, because the span of these muscles is between one and three vertebrae.
- Repeat 3 or 4 times. The prone or side-lying position can be used successfully.
- By changing the angle of contact, the therapist can use compression to identify any area where short muscle structures are impinging upon the nerves. When the area is located, the symptoms that have been troubling the patient will be reproduced.
- Apply compression combined with muscle energy methods, starting from the least invasive method (i.e., positional release using the eyes) and progressing to the more invasive contract-relax and antagonist-contract methods. Rotary movements of the torso while the patient is in the side-lying position work well in this area to isolate muscles for muscle energy methods. The goal is to inhibit temporally the motor tone of the problematic muscle bundle so that it can be lengthened to the appropriate resting length and reduce pressure on the nerves or vessels.
- After the muscle energy application, lengthen and stretch the area by using rotation as demonstrated. These small muscles respond to compression in the muscle belly; this serves both to bend the belly and to exert tension force at the insertion to affect the proprioceptors in these locations. (When needed, use the specific releases discussed in Chapter 10.)

In addressing deeper tissue layers, always remember to protect the more superficial tissues by applying pressure gradually and with as broad a base of contact as the area allows.

- Address the quadratus lumborum if symptoms indicate (see specific releases in Chapter 10).

- Address muscle firing patterns for hip extension at this point. (See the discussion of hip extension firing patterns in Chapter 9.)

Using a myofascial release method, massage the back with the patient in the seated position. Finish the area with superficial work.

THE SHOULDER (Figure 11-7)

The shoulder is a complex musculoskeletal unit. The joint structure is so mobile that it relies more than other major joints on muscles and fascia to provide stability. The scapula and the acromiocla-

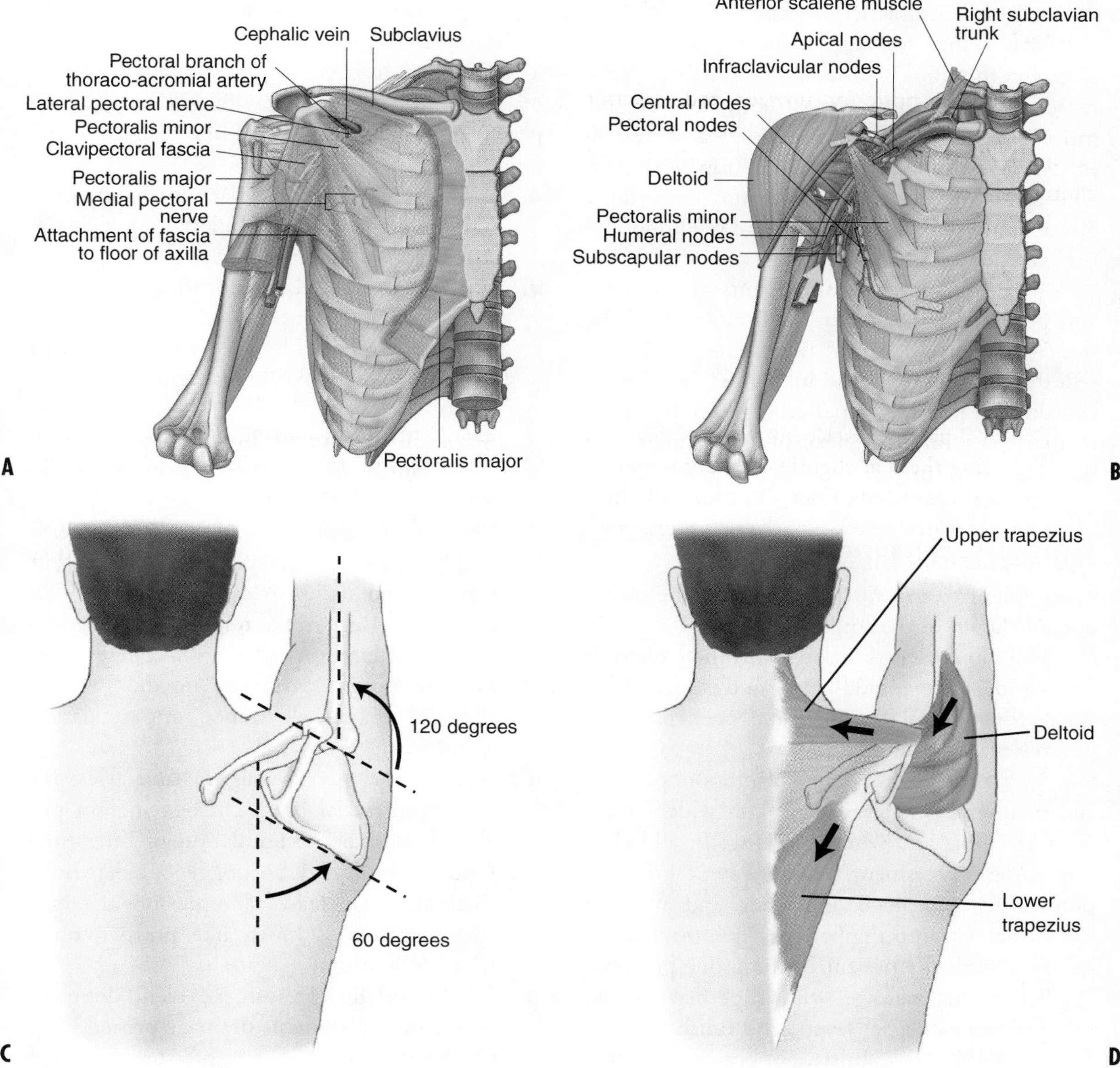

FIGURE 11-7 ■ Important structures in massage application to the shoulder to assist the reader. **A,** Structures that influence shoulder movement. **B,** The lymph nodes and musculature in the shoulder area. **C,** Coupled actions for shoulder and arm movement: humeral motion at the shoulder joint and scapular motion at the scapulocostal (ScC) joint. **D,** The deltoid is the mover of abduction of the arm at the shoulder joint, and the upper trapezius and lower trapezius are the movers of upward rotation of the scapula at the ScC joint. (**A** and **B** from Drake R, Vogl W, Mitchell A: *Gray's anatomy for students,* Edinburgh, 2005, Churchill Livingstone; **C** and **D** from Muscolino JE: *Kinesiology: the skeletal system and muscle function,* St Louis, 2006, Mosby.)

vicular (AC), sternoclavicular (SC), and glenohumeral joints must move in a coordinated fashion for both maximal mobility and stability of the area. The inner (local) muscle unit, rotator cuff muscles, and coracobrachialis hold and guide the humerus in the glenoid fossa, using the scapula as a broad-based attachment. The deltoid muscle is expansive and actually functions as three separate units. It also acts as a protective cover for the shoulder. Other muscles of the torso and arm (e.g., the rhomboids, anterior serratus, pectoralis minor, trapezius, and triceps) both stabilize and move the scapula, performing a series of muscle actions and working together in force couples. The pectoralis major and latissimus dorsi form global units that extend the range of motion of the arm.

Muscle and fascial components of the torso and neck affect the stability and mobility of the shoulder. Because of the involvement of gate reflexes, the shoulders and hips must function in coordinated movement patterns. Nerve impingement of the brachial plexus refers pain to the shoulder and arm.

PROCEDURES FOR THE SHOULDER

Examples of treatment procedures for the shoulder are shown in the Appendix.

The shoulder is massaged with the patient in the supine, prone, side-lying, and seated positions. Massage of the torso and neck naturally progresses to the shoulder.

Assessment of all range-of-motion patterns and of muscle strength determines which structures are short and which are long. In addition, gate pattern assessment should provide information about neurologic efficiency and whether muscle activation firing patterns are optimal.

- Start with the patient in the prone position. Begin the massage with superficial work, progress to deeper layers, and finish off with superficial work. Initial applications are palpation assessment, range of motion, strength, and neurologic assessment, including firing patterns, gait assessment, and all kinetic chain relationships (see Chapter 9).
- Move the shoulder actively and passively through flexion, extension, internal and external adduction and abduction, and full circumduction (i.e., in a circle). Compare active and passive movements.
- Gently compress the joint to make sure there is no intercapsular involvement. If pain occurs, refer the patient to an appropriate specialist. Massage can still be performed, but be aware that muscle tension patterns may be a guarding response to create appropriate compensation.

Take care to make sure the scapula is mobile on the scapulothoracic junction and that appropriate movement occurs at the AC and SC joints.

- With the patient prone, place one hand under the top of the scapula and the other at the lateral border near the apex.
- With the patient relaxed, lift the scapula away from the ribs and move in various directions. The scapula should move easily but with stability and without any winging off the rib cage.

Any areas that are not functioning optimally should be noted and reassessed after they have been massaged.

- Resume by lightly stroking the area systematically to assess for temperature changes, skin texture, and damp areas. Observe for skin reddening (histamine response) and goose bumps (pilomotor response). These signs indicate possible changes in the connective tissue, muscle tone, or circulation patterns.
- Increase the pressure slightly and assess for superficial fascial bind, changes in skin pliability, and the accumulation of interstitial fluid, as indicated by boggy or edematous tissue and/or increased skin pressure or turgor (the sensation is much like pressing on a water balloon).
- If increased fluid pressure is evident, drain the area using a lymphatic drainage procedure.
    - Begin with lighter pressure directed toward the axilla and cover the entire area.
    - Then introduce pumping, broad-based compression, which works more efficiently if followed by or combined with active and passive movements.

- If you are in doubt about whether fluid retention is present, assume that it is and drain the area.

Next, address the superficial fascia by assessing for tissue bind. Always observe for involvement of the superficial fascia in adjacent areas, such as the tissue leading into the torso and neck.

- Move the skin to identify any areas of bind in the superficial connective tissue. Notice whether any bind areas correspond to the areas of skin reddening or goose bumps identified by the light stroking. Pay particular attention to any scars, because connective tissue bind is common at these sites.
- Treat any areas of superficial fascial bind with myofascial release methods. Address these areas by slowly moving the tissue into ease, applying drag to move it the direction it most easily wants to go. Multiple load directions can be used. For example, if the skin and superficial fascia want to move up and to the left on the deltoid, that is the direction of the forces introduced.
- Hold the ease position up to 30 to 60 seconds and then reassess.

Any remaining areas of bind can be treated with the following myofascial release methods:

- Work into the bind using a slow, sustained drag on the binding tissues, introducing the lines of tension at each end of the binding tissue.
  - Place your flat hand (or the pads of your fingers if your hand is too large) at one end of the bind and the other hand at the other end of the bind.
  - Contact the tissue gently but firmly, pressing only as deep as the superficial fascial layer, and separate your hands, creating a tension force in the binding tissue.
  - Maintain the drag and introduce subtle changes in the lines of force, loading and unloading the tissue until it becomes more pliable.
- Next, grasp as much of the binding tissue as possible and lift it until the resistance is identified. Slowly load and unload with torsion and shear force until the tissue becomes warm and more pliable. This method is intense, and the patient should feel a pulling or slight burning sensation; however, the patient should not feel the need to tense up or change the breathing pattern to endure the application.
- Work slowly and deliberately, interspersing the process with lymphatic drainage–type stroking every minute or so.

The musculature is addressed in layers by systematically moving from superficial to deep. It is important to make sure the muscle layers are not adhering to each other. If any are, superficial tissue should be sheared off the next deeper layer.

- It is helpful to place the patient so that the surface layer is in a slack position; this is achieved by positioning the attachments of the muscle close together and propping the patient with bolsters so that the person stays relaxed. In some cases the side-lying position may be better for this.
- Begin on the posterior aspect and address the midthoracic region that connects with the shoulder. This area is covered by the trapezius (the first layer of the muscle). The area was addressed during massage of the torso, but it now is massaged again in relation to the shoulder. Carry the strokes into the posterior deltoid.
- Use gliding with a compressive element from the upper, middle, and lower aspects of the trapezius, slowly dragging tissue toward its distal attachment at the shoulder. Repeat with the latissimus dorsi, again in relation to shoulder function, and carry the stroke into the posterior deltoid. If any area binds against the drag, working across the grain of the muscle and in the opposite direction may be beneficial.
- Any areas that redden may be sites of trigger point activity. Trigger points can cause muscles to fire out of sequence, therefore as much normalcy as possible must be restored.
- To increase circulation to the area and shift the neuroresponses of trigger points, move the skin over the trigger points into multiple directions of ease and hold the ease position for up to 30 to 60 seconds.

- If this does not relieve the tenderness, positional release is the next option, followed by more aggressive muscle energy methods if necessary.
- Local lengthening of the tissue containing trigger points is effective. Local lengthening is accomplished by using tension, bend, or torsion force on the tissues with the trigger points and taut band. Do not use direct pressure or transverse friction, because they may cause tissue damage.
- If a trigger point does not release using these methods, it is part of a compensation pattern that must be dealt with. The trigger point likely serves a useful function, especially because the posterior muscles often are in a long, taut state. In this situation, the trigger point areas create stability in the tissues and exert some counterforce to the pulling areas that are short in the anterior.
- Finish the area with kneading, making sure the muscle tissue easily lifts off the layer beneath it.
- If adhesions are identified, introduce a bend, shear, or torsion force until the tissue becomes more pliable. This method can be intense, and the patient may feel a burning sensation; however, it should not cause the patient to show guarding or pain behaviors or hold the breath during application.
- Repeat the sequence bilaterally.

Once you have addressed the surface tissue, massage the second layer of muscle. It is important to assess to make sure the surface tissue and the fascial separation between muscle layers are not adhering to each other in any way. The main muscles addressed in this sequence are the rhomboids, infraspinatus, teres major and teres minor, and subscapularis, as well as the deeper layers of the deltoid muscle.

- Begin at the vertebral attachments of the rhomboids. Use a compressive gliding parallel to the muscle fibers that is deep enough to address this layer of tissue. Maintain a broad base of contact so that the surface tissue does not tighten to guard against poking.
- Glide toward the scapula. Repeat 3 or 4 times, each time slowing the strokes and providing them at a slightly different angle.
- Knead slowly across the fiber direction, using enough pressure and lift to ensure that you affect the muscle fibers in this layer. These methods address both the connective tissue and neuromuscular elements of the muscle. Repeat 3 or 4 times, increasing depth and drag each time. Be alert to the muscle moving with the application.
- Next, address the supraspinatus. Glide from the medial border of the scapula toward the acromion. Work above the spine of the scapula to access the supraspinatus. The soft heel of the palm may fit better in these areas than the forearm. Reverse direction and then knead the area slowly and deeply. Make sure the upper trapezius is not binding on the supraspinatus.
- Repeat the sequence from the medial and lower medial border to address the infraspinatus and the teres major and teres minor.
- Using gliding and kneading, massage the triceps toward the attachment on the lateral border of the scapula.
- Next, slowly and deeply knead the posterior and medial deltoid.
- Place the patient in the side-lying position (this is a good position for addressing the latissimus and the teres major and teres minor attachments on the arm).
- Repeat the sequences described and add placement of the arm over the head. Perform active and passive movements while the area is massaged. Positioning the arm over the head allows the medial border of the scapula to be lifted and mobilized in rotary movements.
- Massage and compress the attachments of the rhomboids and anterior serratus on both sides.
- The pectoralis minor also can be addressed with the patient in the side-lying position. Use a diagonal compression to move under the pectoralis major from the axilla.
- Place the arm in a passive flexed and adducted position to create slack in the tissues; then, slowly follow the contour of the ribs to contact the pectoralis minor. This method can be intense, and a confident touch is necessary.

When addressing deeper tissue layers, always remember to protect the more superficial muscles by applying pressure gradually and with as broad a base of contact as the area allows.

The subscapularis tendon and the belly of the muscle can be accessed with the patient in either the side-lying or the supine position.

- With the fingers placed at a 45-degreee angle, glide posteriorly to access the anterior surface of the scapula. Be careful of the nerves and vessels in the area. The belly of the muscle can be reached near the shoulder attachment (see the description of subscapularis release in Chapter 10). When symptoms are recreated or when bind is felt, use compression against the scapula with internal and external rotation of the arm, either passively or actively, to release the area.

The attachments of the latissimus dorsi and both teres muscles at the axilla also can be reached with the patient in the side-lying, prone, or supine position.

- Combine compression with active or passive movements (or both) of the arm.
- Slow circumduction of the shoulder tends to access all areas.

The coracobrachialis can be accessed with the patient in either the side-lying or supine position. Address this muscle if extension and abduction are limited.

- Place your fingers on the muscle belly and have the patient flex and adduct the arm.
- Reverse the movement.
- If tender points are found, use positional release if possible.

Reassess for firing patterns and gait pattern dysfunction of the shoulder and correct any imbalance that remains.

- Palpate at the AC joint while the patient moves the arm through circumduction. (I tell the patient to swim using an overhand stroke.) The AC joint should easily hinge back and forth. If it does not move easily, increase compression on the joint slightly and have the patient repeat the arm movements 2 or 3 times.
- Palpation of the SC joint bilaterally should indicate that the clavicles are spinning evenly on the manubrium when the patient lifts the arm over the head. If the joint does not move easily, increase compression on it slightly and have the patient repeat the arm movements 2 or 3 times.
- Finish by gliding and kneading the entire area. Add oscillation (shaking and rocking) in various positions. In addition, you might drain the area.

THE ARM (Figure 11-8)

The arm functions as an open chain most of the time; this means that the wrist, elbow, and shoulder joints can function independently of each other. However, even in open chain function, the joints and tissues influence each other. When the hands are fixed, as when doing a pushup or some sort of handspring, the chain is closed, meaning that the wrist, elbow, and shoulder function in a coordinated movement.

The muscles of the arm work primarily at the elbow. The triceps and biceps cross two joints and also function at the shoulder. Some of the muscles of the forearm also cross the elbow.

The gait reflexes coordinate the interaction of the arms and legs. For example, flexor, adductor, and internal rotation patterns on the left arm and right leg work together during forward motion (concentric contraction). The antagonists function eccentrically, decelerating the movement with some inhibition to allow stability and agility during movement. Movement then reverses to the right arm and left leg, and the opposite pattern is activated. At the same time, the extensor, abductor, and external rotation pattern facilitates in concentric contraction in the opposite pattern while the antagonist pattern functions eccentrically. This back and forth gait movement is necessary for agility and postural balance. It can be disrupted by illness, injury, or repetitive training activities, especially if the movement patterns are altered. A prime example of this is bilateral weight training (e.g., biceps curls) in which both muscles concentrically contract during flexion and then eccentrically function during extension, without contralateral balancing by leg movement and instead of the normal opposite swing pattern. Although this may increase strength in the arms, it has a tendency to disrupt gait patterns and can cause an increase in the motor tone of the hamstrings.

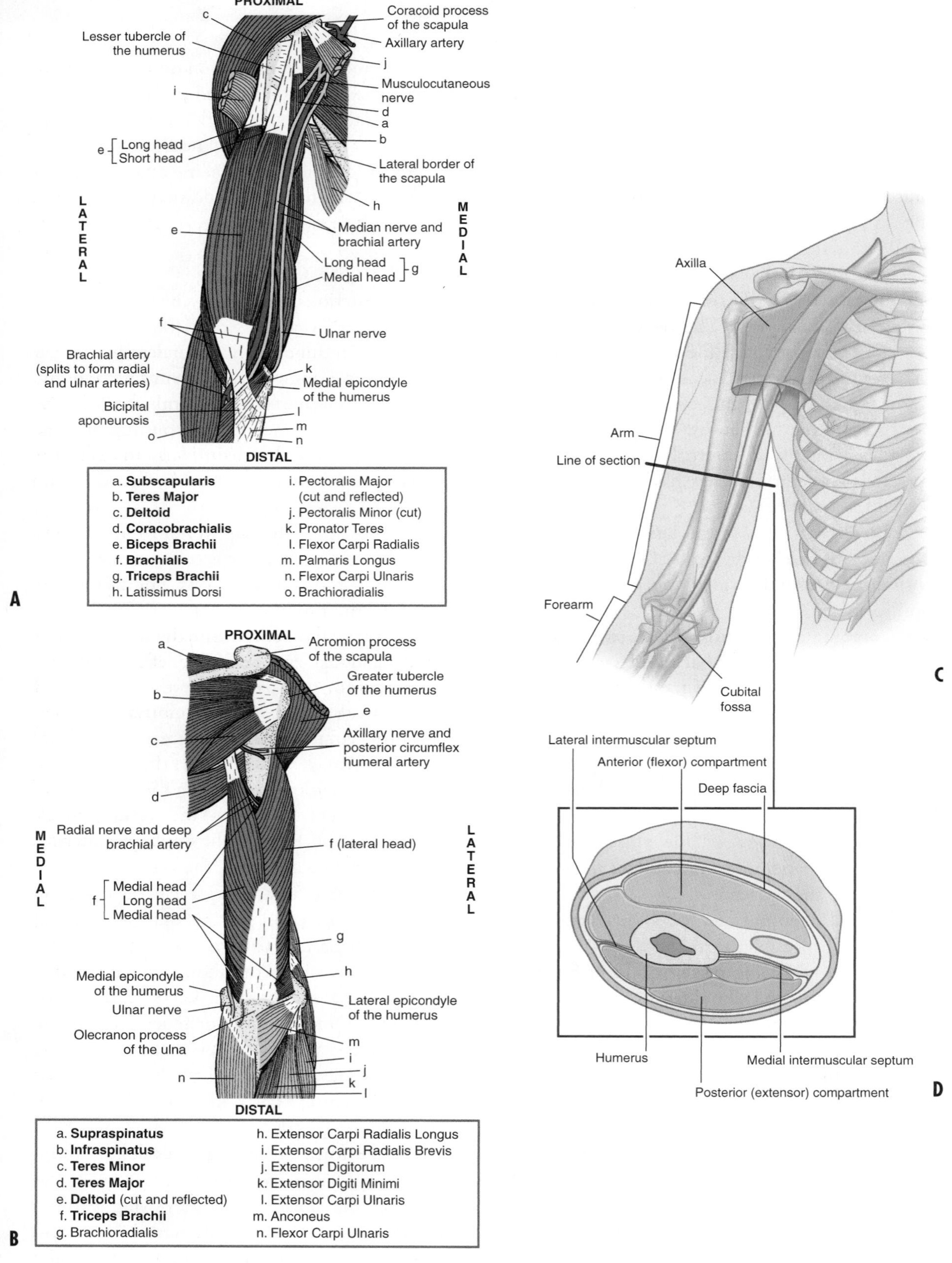

FIGURE 11-8 ■ Important structures in massage application to the arm to assist the reader. **A,** Anterior view of the right arm (superficial). **B,** Posterior view of the right arm. **C,** Proximal and distal relationships in the arm. **D,** Transverse section through the middle of the arm. (**A** and **B** from Muscolino JE: *Kinesiology: the skeletal system and muscle function,* St Louis, 2006, Mosby; **C** and **D** from Drake R, Vogl W, Mitchell A: *Gray's anatomy for students,* Edinburgh, 2005, Churchill Livingstone.)

Often the massage therapist must work with the arms and legs in some sort of coordinated pattern to increase the effectiveness of the massage. For example, the patient can actively swing the knee back and forth in an open chain position while massage is applied to the opposite arm. The flow of the massage application can proceed from the left arm to the right leg and then from the right arm to the left leg. Also, the therapist can work with the right biceps and the left hamstring, then work with the right triceps and the left quadriceps, and vice versa. The side-lying position gives the best access for optimal body mechanics, but the supine or prone position also can be used.

The muscles of the arm are arranged in two layers. The two heads of the biceps and the three heads of the triceps are thick muscles, each with attachments on the shaft of the humerus that can bind. The brachialis and anconeus constitute the second layer of muscles.

The arm can be massaged in all basic positions and often is addressed more than once during the massage. The back of the arm is accessible when the patient is in the prone position. The lateral and medial aspects can be reached when the patient is in the side-lying position. With the patient in the supine position, the anterior arm is easily reached, and the lateral, medial, and posterior regions also can be massaged. These muscles need to glide over the bone, therefore it is important to make sure the tissues roll over the humerus.

Some patients have arms that are highly developed and bulky. To obtain adequate pressure without poking, the massage therapist sometimes must use the knees and feet to apply compression while the patient is lying on the floor.

PROCEDURES FOR THE ARM

Examples of treatment procedures for the arm are shown in the Appendix.

Massage of the arm naturally progresses from the shoulder to the forearm and then to the hand. Assessment of all range-of-motion patterns and of muscle strength determines which structures are short and which are long. In addition, gate pattern and firing pattern assessment should provide information about neurologic efficiency or demonstrate whether patterns are optimal.

The arm can be massaged with the patient in the supine, side-lying, or prone position. The massage begins with superficial work, progresses to deeper layers, and finishes with superficial work. The initial applications are palpation, range of motion, strength, and neurologic assessment. This sequence focuses on massage of the arm with the patient in the prone and side-lying positions.

- Move the arm actively and passively through all joint motion patterns. Compare active and passive movements of the arms for balanced function.
- Gently compress the elbow joint to make sure there is no intracapsular involvement. If pain occurs, refer the patient to the appropriate professional. Massage can be performed, but be aware that muscle tension patterns may be a guarding response to create appropriate compensation.

Any areas that are not functioning optimally should be noted and reassessed after they have been massaged.

- Lightly stroke the area systematically to assess for temperature changes, skin texture, and damp areas. Observe for skin reddening (histamine response) and goose bumps (pilomotor response). These signs indicate possible changes in the connective tissue, muscle tone, or circulation patterns.
- Increase the pressure slightly and assess for superficial fascial bind, changes in skin pliability, and the accumulation of interstitial fluid, as indicated by boggy or edematous tissue and/or increased skin pressure (the sensation is much like pressing on a water balloon).
- If increased fluid pressure is evident, drain the area using a lymphatic drainage technique.
- If you are in doubt about whether fluid retention is present, assume that it is and drain the area.

Next, address the superficial fascia by assessing for tissue bind. Always observe for involvement in adjacent areas, such as the tissue leading into the shoulder.

- Move the skin to identify any areas of bind in the superficial connective tissue. Notice whether any bind areas correspond to the areas of skin reddening or goose bumps identified by the light stroking. Pay particular attention to any potential connective tissue bind in areas of scar tissue.
- Treat any areas of superficial fascial bind with myofascial release methods. Address these areas by slowly moving the tissue into ease, dragging it the way it most wants to go. Multiple load directions can be used. For example, if the skin and superficial fascia want to move down and to the right, that would be the direction of the forces introduced.
- Hold each position for about 30 to 60 seconds.
- Then, work into the bind with a slow, sustained drag on the binding tissues, introducing the lines of tension at each end of the binding tissue.
    - Place your flat hand (or the pads of your fingers if your hand is too large) at one end of the bind and the other hand at the other end of the bind.
    - Contact the tissue gently but firmly, pressing only as deep as the superficial fascial layer, and separate the hands, creating a tension force in the binding tissue.

Bend and torsion forces using compression and kneading can also be introduced.

- Maintain the drag on the tissue until the thixotropic nature of the ground substance is affected, and the ground substance becomes more pliable. Subtle changes in the lines of force serve to load and unload the tissue, resulting in hysteresis.
- Next, grasp as much of the binding tissue as possible and lift it until the resistance is identified. Slowly load and unload with bend, torsion, and shear forces until the tissue becomes warm and more pliable.
- Finally, if the arm is small enough, grasp the tissue and twist it around the arm. If the arm is large (or as an alternative), apply broad-based compression (the foot works well) and have the patient roll the arm back and forth. These methods are intense, and the patient should feel a pulling or slight burning sensation; however, the patient should not need to tense up or change the breathing pattern to endure the application.
- Work slowly and deliberately, interspersing the process with lymphatic drainage–type stroking every minute or so.

The musculature is addressed in layers by systematically moving from superficial to deep. It is important to make sure the muscle layers are not adhering to each other. With the biceps and triceps, make sure the heads of the muscles are not stuck together, because each part of the muscle has a somewhat different angle of pull. If any are adhering, each muscle layer should be sheared off the next deeper layer.

- It is helpful to place the patient so that the surface layer is in a slack position; this can be accomplished by positioning the attachments of the muscle close together and bolstering the patient so that the person stays relaxed. With the patient prone, the arm should be in passive extension so that the tissues are on a slack (i.e., loose).
- Place the patient in the prone position. Begin at the elbow and carry the strokes into the posterior deltoid and the scapular attachment.
- Reverse direction; use compression that ends at the elbow and then glide again toward the shoulder. Repeat 3 or 4 times, each time working slower and deeper while maintaining broad-based contact to protect the more superficial tissue and reduce the potential for guarding.
- If any area binds against the drag, working across the grain of the muscle and in the opposite direction may be beneficial.

Any areas that redden may be sites of trigger point activity. Because trigger points can cause muscles to fire out of sequence, it is important to restore as much normalcy as possible to the tissue.

- To increase circulation to the area and shift the neuroresponses of trigger points, move the skin over the points into multiple directions of ease and hold the ease position for up to 30 to 60 seconds.
- If the tenderness is not relieved, positional release is the next option, followed by

more aggressive muscle energy methods if necessary.

- Local lengthening of the tissue containing the trigger points is effective, and authorities have found that it is needed to complete the release of trigger points. Local lengthening is accomplished by using a tension, bend, or torsion force on the tissue with the trigger point and taut band. Do not use direct pressure or transverse friction, because they may cause tissue damage.
- If the trigger point does not release with the methods described, it is part of a compensation pattern that must be dealt with, and the trigger point likely serves a useful function. Leave it alone.
- Finish the area with kneading. Make sure the muscle tissue easily lifts off the layer beneath it and rolls around the bone structure.
- If adhesions are identified, apply a bend, shear, or torsion force until the tissue becomes more pliable. This method can be intense and can cause a burning sensation; however, the patient should not show guarding or pain behaviors or hold the breath during application.
- Repeat this sequence bilaterally.

Once the surface tissue has been addressed, the deep surface of the triceps muscle is massaged. It is important to make sure that the surface tissue and the fascial separation between muscle segments are not adhering to each other in any way.

- Apply compressive gliding parallel to the fibers that is deep enough to address this layer of tissue. Broaden the base of contact so that the surface tissue does not tighten to guard against poking. Adding passive movement to the compression serves to move the bone a bit against the deep tissue, creating combined loading. Repeat 3 or 4 times, each time working slower and at a slightly different angle.
- Next, glide and knead slowly across the fiber direction, using enough pressure and lift to ensure that you affect the muscle fiber and that the tissue can slide around the bone. These methods address both the connective tissue and the neuromuscular elements of the muscle. Repeat 3 or 4 times, increasing depth and drag each time. Be alert to the muscle moving with the application.

With the patient in the side-lying position, place the patient's arm on the torso. This makes it easier for the massage therapist to use the forearm to massage the patient's arm.

- Systematically lightly stroke the area to assess for temperature changes, skin texture, and damp areas. Observe for skin reddening (histamine response) and goose bumps (pilomotor response). These signs indicate possible changes in the connective tissue, muscle tone, or circulation patterns.
- Increase the pressure slightly and assess for superficial fascial bind, changes in skin pliability, and the accumulation of interstitial fluid, as indicated by boggy or edematous tissue and/or increased skin pressure (the sensation is much like pressing on a water balloon).
- If increased fluid pressure is evident, drain the area; use a combination of light pressure to drag the skin and deeper, rhythmic, broad-based compression and kneading.
  - Begin with lighter pressure directed toward the shoulder and cover the entire area.
  - Then introduce pumping, broad-based compression; combine this with active movement (i.e., have the patient flex and extend the elbow and shoulder) and then perform passive movement. (Remember, when moving fluid, you cannot push a river.)
- If you are in doubt about whether fluid retention is present, assume that it is and drain the area (the direction of drainage is toward the axilla).

Next, address the superficial fascia by assessing for tissue bind. Always observe for involvement in adjacent areas, such as the tissue leading into the shoulder, neck, and forearm.

- Move the skin to identify any areas of bind in the superficial connective tissue. Notice whether any bind areas correspond to the areas identified by the light stroking. Pay particular attention to any scars, because connective tissue bind is common at those sites.

- Treat any areas of superficial fascial bind with myofascial release methods. Address these areas by slowly moving the tissue into ease (i.e., dragging it the way it most wants to go). Multiple load directions can be used. Hold each position up to 30 to 60 seconds.
- Next, work into the bind with a slow, sustained drag on the binding tissues, introducing the lines of tension at each end of the binding tissue.
  - Place your forearm (or your flat hand if your forearm is too large) at one end of the bind and the other forearm at the other end of the bind.
  - Contact the tissue gently but firmly, pressing only as deep as the superficial fascial layer, and separate the forearms, creating a tension force in the binding tissue.

A bend force also can be introduced through kneading, and tension force can be added.

- Have the patient actively or passively move the arm into slight flexion and extension and then back into the original position while the massage is applied. Repeat the movement back and forth until a change is noted.
- Maintain the drag on the tissue until the thixotropic nature of the ground substance is affected, and the ground substance becomes more pliable. Subtle changes in the lines of force serve to load and unload the tissue, resulting in hysteresis.
- Grasp as much of the binding tissue as possible and lift it until the resistance is identified. Slowly load and unload with torsion and shear force (or by having the patient move the arm) until the tissue becomes warm and more pliable. This method is intense, and the patient should feel a pulling or slight burning sensation; however, the patient should not feel the need to tense up or to change the breathing pattern to endure the application.
- Work slowly and deliberately, interspersing the process with lymphatic drainage–type stroking every minute or so.
- When you locate an area that is bothering the patient, familiar symptoms will be reproduced. Compression combined with muscle energy methods, from the least invasive (i.e., positional release) to the more aggressive integrated methods, can be used to create a shift in function. The goal is to inhibit temporally the motor tone of the muscle bundle that is problematic so that it can be lengthened to the appropriate resting length and the patient feels reduced pressure on the nerves or vessels.

With the patient in the side-lying position, the lateral, posterior, and anterior areas can be massaged simply by changing the arm position, and range of motion is not limited by the table. When addressing deeper tissue layers, always remember to protect the more superficial muscles, applying pressure gradually and with as broad a base of contact as the area allows.

The triceps belly and tendon at the scapula are best accessed with the patient in the side-lying position.

- Have the patient flex and extend the elbow and circumduct the shoulder.
- Combine compression with active or passive movements (or both) of the arm. Slow circumduction tends to access all areas.
- Assess firing patterns for the arm.
- Finish by gliding and kneading the entire area with the patient in the supine position. Add oscillation (rocking and shaking) in various positions. In addition, you might drain the area.

THE FOREARM, WRIST, AND HAND (Figure 11-9)

The forearm muscles function to work the wrist and fingers. They also weakly assist elbow movements. This can be an issue when the elbow, wrist, and fingers must function as a unit, such as in throwing a ball; the fingers must grasp (isometric), but the wrist and elbow have to move (concentric and eccentric). This situation creates the potential for rubbing at the attachments. The end result of repetitive movements such as this can be tendinitis and bursitis. Muscles near the elbow and wrist allow supination and pronation of the hand.

Repetitive movement is common for the forearm, wrist, and hand tissues, as are repetitive

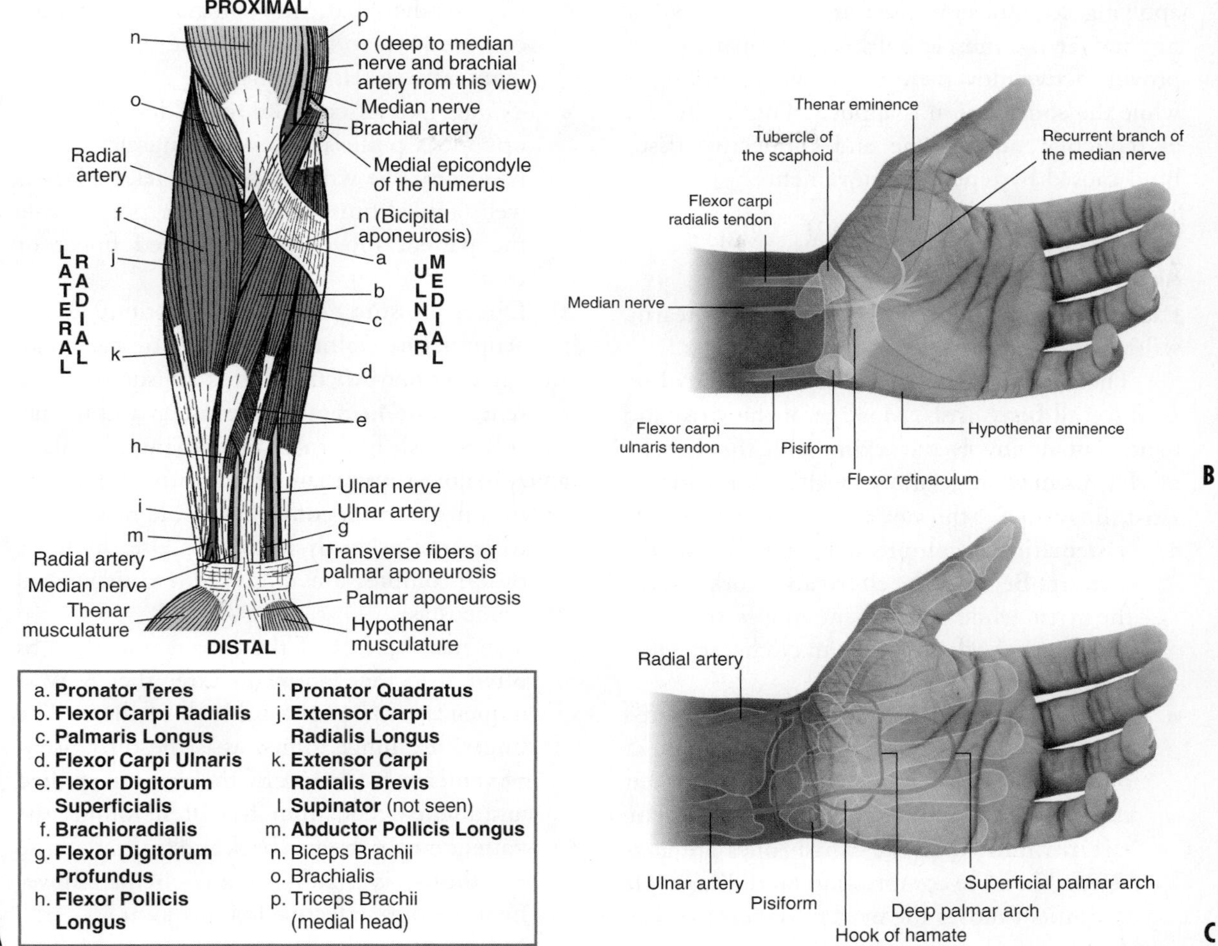

FIGURE 11-9 ■ Important structures in massage application to the forearm, wrist, and hand to assist the reader. **A,** The muscles of the forearm, wrist, and hand. **B,** The wrist. **C,** The structures of the hand. (**A** from Muscolino JE: *The muscular system manual: the skeletal muscles of the human body,* ed 2, St Louis, 2005, Mosby; **B** and **C** from Drake R, Vogl W, Mitchell A: *Gray's anatomy for students,* Edinburgh, 2005, Churchill Livingstone.)

strain illness and injury. The goal of the massage is to maintain normal tissue function so that repetitive movement does not become repetitive strain.

The muscles of the forearm are categorized as superficial, intermediate, and deep. They are best addressed as three layers, which include the supinator, pronator teres, and pronator quadratus. These muscles can adhere to each other, both on top of one other and in the side-by-side position. Because the range of the movements of the fingers is slightly different from that of the wrist, it is essential that these muscles glide easily over one another. The superficial muscle layer functions primarily at the wrist with some activity at the elbow. The deep layers work the fingers with some activity at the wrist.

The bellies of these muscles are closer to the elbow, and they taper to the tendons in the wrist and fingers. It is important to gauge the pressure of the massage, which is more intense along the proximal half of the forearm where the muscle bulk is located. Connective tissue bind often shows up in the distal half of the forearm and into the hand.

The massage therapist typically uses the forearm or the flat, soft palm to massage the forearm, but the foot also works very well for applying compression. The arch of the foot fits nicely over the muscle bulk, and the patient can provide active movement of the wrist and fingers while the compression is applied. This is effective at reducing muscle tone and connective tissue bind caused by repetitive movements.

PROCEDURES FOR THE FOREARM, WRIST, AND HAND

Examples of treatment procedures for the forearm, wrist, and hand are shown in the Appendix.

The massage pattern is very similar to that used for all body areas. Massage of the wrist and hand initially involves working with the muscles of the forearm in relation to the action of the wrist, fingers, and thumb.

- Systematically compress the muscles of the forearm. Begin at the elbow and work toward the wrist while the patient moves the wrist and fingers back and forth in circles or makes and releases a fist.
- To isolate a particular muscle function related to a wrist or finger action, have the patient move the wrist or finger in the way that creates the symptom and then palpate the forearm muscles to see which ones are activated. Then use compression or gliding while the patient moves the wrist or fingers to affect the identified area. Occasionally, trigger point type application is necessary.

Next, address the range of motion of the wrist. The wrist is often jammed, which reduces joint play. A general method for restoring joint play is the mobilization with movement (MWM) sequence.

- Apply traction to the joint and then move it into the ease and pain-free position. The patient is passive while the position is found. The therapist then maintains the position while the patient actively moves the joint through a range of motions. For the wrist, having the patient move the wrist in a circle is effective.

Next, address the intrinsic muscles of the hand.

- Systematically work the area, using compression and gliding of the soft tissues between the fingers and the web of the thumb and on the palm.
- To assist lymphatic movement, use rhythmic compression to stimulate the network of lymphatic vessels in the palm.
- Trigger points commonly are found in the opponens pollicis and other muscles of the palm near the wrist. Positional release works well; apply compression on the point while the patient moves the associated finger or thumb.
- Direct pressure or tapping can stimulate the acupuncture points at the side of each nail. An easy way to do this is to squeeze and release 3 or 4 times on the lateral and medial side of each fingernail and the thumbnail.
- A major acupuncture point in the web of the thumb is used to control pain and nausea and to address other dysfunctions. Use rhythmic on-off compression of this point to aid general homeostasis.
- The many joints of the fingers and thumbs often become jammed, and the MWM sequence can be used on each of them. The fingers are hinge joints, as is the distal joint of the thumb. Once traction has been applied and the ease position has been found, the patient moves the area back and forth. Because the thumb is a saddle joint, circular movement is more effective for this joint.
- Next, address the metacarpal joints. Moving the carpal bones back and forth is effective.
- To finish off, use oscillation (rocking and shaking) and lymphatic drainage.

THE HIP (Figure 11-10)

The hip is a complex musculoskeletal unit. The joint structure is mobile, relying on a deep joint capsule, ligaments, muscles, and fascia to provide stability. However, it is less mobile than the shoulder. The sacroiliac (SI) and femoral joints must move in a coordinated fashion for maximum mobility and stability of the area.

The inner (local muscle) unit (i.e., deep lateral rotator muscles) and an extensive ligament structure hold and guide the femur in the acetabulum, using the bones of the pelvis as a broad-based attachment point. The gluteus maximus is an expansive outer unit (global muscles) that inter-

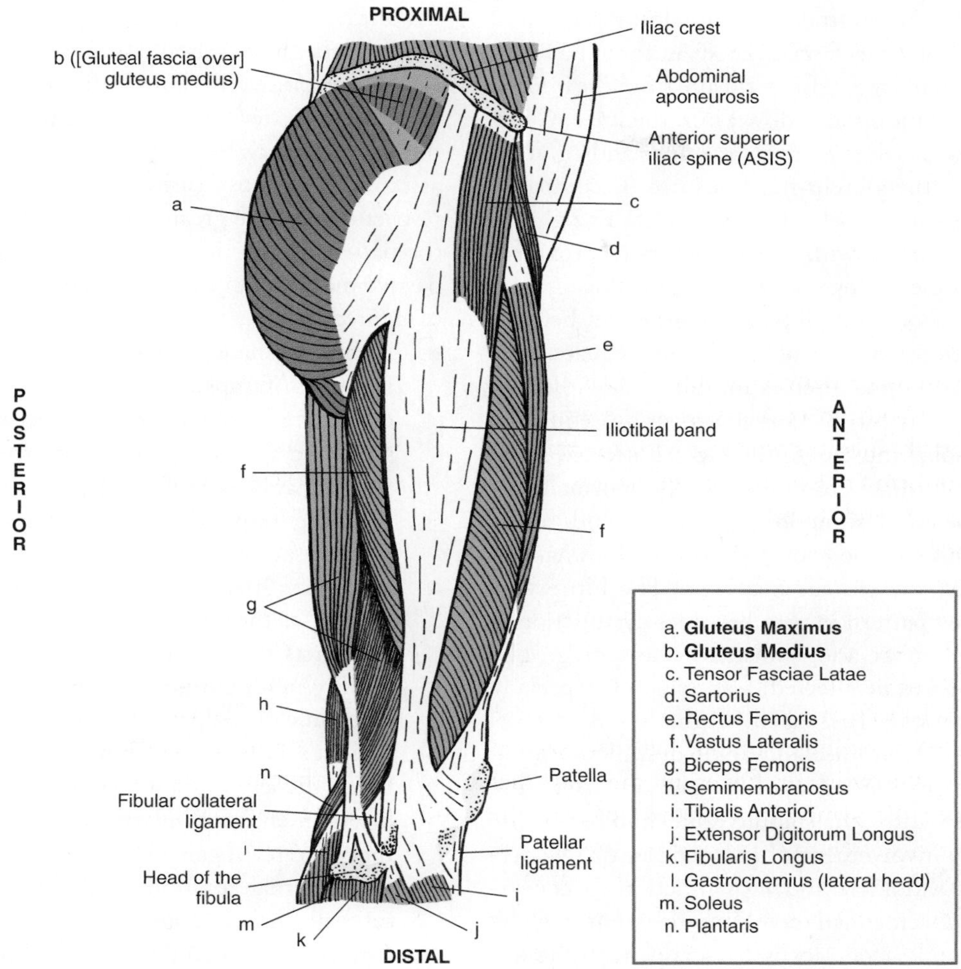

PROXIMAL
Iliac crest
b ([Gluteal fascia over] gluteus medius)
Abdominal aponeurosis
Anterior superior iliac spine (ASIS)
a
c
d
e
POSTERIOR
ANTERIOR
Iliotibial band
f
f
g
h
n
Fibular collateral ligament
l
Head of the fibula
m
k
Patella
Patellar ligament
i
j
DISTAL
a. Gluteus Maximus
b. Gluteus Medius
c. Tensor Fasciae Latae
d. Sartorius
e. Rectus Femoris
f. Vastus Lateralis
g. Biceps Femoris
h. Semimembranosus
i. Tibialis Anterior
j. Extensor Digitorum Longus
k. Fibularis Longus
l. Gastrocnemius (lateral head)
m. Soleus
n. Plantaris

A

Greater trochanter
Sciatic nerve
Ischial tuberosity
Gluteal fold

B

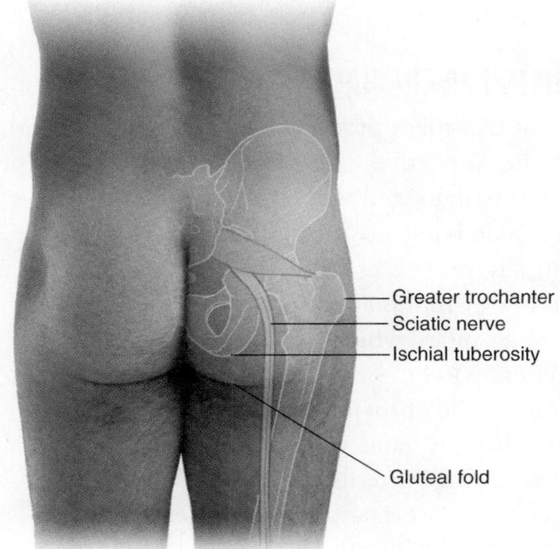

FIGURE 11-10 ■ Important structures in massage application to the hip to assist the reader. **A,** The muscles of the hip. **B,** Posterior view of the gluteal region of a man, showing the position of the sciatic nerve. (**A** from Muscolino JE: *The muscular system manual: the skeletal muscles of the human body,* ed 2, St Louis, 2005, Mosby; **B** from Drake R, Vogl W, Mitchell A: *Gray's anatomy for students,* Edinburgh, 2005, Churchill Livingstone.)

acts with the contralateral latissimus dorsi and ipsilateral tensor fasciae latae and IT band to provide stability and force closure from the lumbar back and SI joint area down into the knee. Combined with the gluteus medius and gluteus minimus, the gluteus maximus can be compared to the deltoid muscle of the shoulder. The gluteal muscles interact with the adductors to provide a force couple arrangement during gait.

The psoas and gluteus maximus can become dysfunctional if core stability is inadequate. The gluteus maximus often is inhibited as a result of a short, tight psoas. Muscle activation sequences of the global muscles of the hip are affected if the lower abdominal group does not fire normally. In this type of dysfunction, the psoas and rectus abdominis fire too soon (synergistic dominance), inhibiting the gluteus maximus. The hip extension firing pattern in turn becomes dysfunctional, causing lumbar and hamstring shortening. The knee also can be affected. Calf muscles, especially the gastrocnemius, then begin to dominate, leading to both knee and ankle dysfunction.

The muscle and fascial components of the torso also affect the stability and mobility of the hip. The involvement of gait reflexes necessitates that the shoulders and hips function in coordinated movement. Nerve impingement by the lumbar and sacral plexuses refers pain to the hip and leg.

PROCEDURES FOR THE HIP

Examples of treatment procedures for the hip are shown in the Appendix.

The hip is massaged with the patient in the prone and side-lying positions. Massage of the torso naturally progresses to the hip. Assessment of all range-of-motion patterns and muscle strength determines which structures are short and which are long. In addition, gait pattern assessment should provide information about neurologic efficiency and whether firing patterns are optimal. Firing patterns in this area are especially important. Assess patterns for hip extension and abduction (see Chapter 9).

The massage begins with superficial work, progresses to deeper layers, and finishes off with superficial work. The initial applications are palpation, range of motion, strength, and neurologic assessment. The hip should be moved first actively and then passively though flexion, extension, internal and external rotation, adduction, abduction, and full circumduction. This part of the assessment is most easily done, with the least restriction and the greatest range of motion, with the patient in the side-lying position. Active and passive movement of left and right hips should be compared.

- Compress the joint gently to make sure there is no intracapsular involvement. If pain occurs, refer the patient to the appropriate specialist. Massage can be performed, but be aware that muscle tension patterns may be a guarding response to create an appropriate compensation.
- With the patient in the prone position, palpate at the SI joint while the patient circumducts the hip; the SI joint should move slightly in a figure-eight pattern.
- Continue to palpate the SI joint. Bend the patient's knee and internally and externally rotate the leg. Initial movement occurs in the hip joint, and secondary movement occurs at the SI joint. In general, 45 degrees of internal and external rotation in this position indicates normal function. Any alteration in this pattern indicates a potential for both SI joint and hip joint dysfunction.

Any areas that do not function optimally should be noted and reassessed after the area has been massaged. If the pattern does not normalize, the patient must be referred to appropriate medical personnel.

- Systematically lightly stroke the area to assess for temperature changes, skin texture, and damp areas. Observe for skin reddening (histamine response) and goose bumps (pilomotor response). These signs indicate possible changes in the connective tissue, muscle tone, or circulation patterns.
- Increase the pressure slightly and assess for superficial fascial bind, changes in skin pliability, and the accumulation of interstitial fluid, as indicated by boggy or edematous tissue and/or increased skin pressure (the sensation is much like pressing on a water balloon).

- If increased fluid pressure is evident, drain the area.
- If you are in doubt about whether fluid retention is present, assume that it is and drain the area.

Next, address the superficial fascia by assessing for tissue bind. Always observe for involvement in adjacent areas, such as the tissue leading into the torso and leg.

- Move the skin to identify any areas of bind in the superficial connective tissue. Notice whether any bind areas correspond to the areas of skin reddening or goose bumps identified by the light stroking. Pay particular attention to any scars, because connective tissue bind is common at these sites.
- Treat areas of superficial fascial bind with myofascial release methods. Address these areas by slowly moving the tissue into ease, dragging it the way it wants to go. Multiple load directions can be used. For example, if the skin and superficial fascia want to move up and to the right near the sacrum, that is the direction of the forces introduced.
- Hold the ease position for up to 30 to 60 seconds
- Next, work into the bind with a slow, sustained drag on the binding tissues, introducing the lines of tension at each end of the binding tissue.
  - Place your flat forearm or hand at one end of the bind and the other forearm or hand at the other end of the bind.
  - Contact the tissue gently but firmly, pressing only as deep as the superficial fascial layer, and separate the forearms or hands, creating a tension force in the binding tissue.
- Maintain the drag on the tissue until the thixotropic nature of the ground substance is affected, and the ground substance becomes more pliable. Subtle changes in the lines of force serve to load and unload the tissue, resulting in hysteresis. Active and passive range of motion can serve to load and unload tissues.
- Next, grasp as much of the binding tissue as possible and lift it until the resistance is identified. Slowly load and unload with torsion and shear force until the tissue becomes warm and more pliable. This method is intense, and the patient should feel a pulling or slight burning sensation; however, the patient should not feel the need to tense up or to change the breathing pattern to endure the application.
- Work slowly and deliberately, interspersing the process with lymphatic drainage–type stroking every minute or so.

The musculature is addressed in layers by moving from superficial to deep. It is important to make sure the muscle layers are not adhering to each other. If adhesions exist, the muscle layer should be sheared off the next deeper layer. Layers tend to stick where the gluteus maximus weaves into the IT band at a lengthy musculotendinous junction. Use a wavelike motion to assess the tissue.

- It is helpful to place the patient so that the surface layer is in a slack position; this is achieved by positioning the attachments of the muscle close together and propping the patient with bolsters so that the person stays relaxed. In some situations the side-lying position may be better for this.
- Begin on the posterior side, addressing the lumbar region that connects with the hip. This area was addressed during massage of the torso, but it now is massaged in relation to the hip.
- Carry the strokes into the gluteus maximus. Use gliding with a compressive element and drag toward the hip.
- Repeat with the latissimus dorsi in relation to hip function. Begin at the shoulder and carry the stroke all the way into the opposite gluteus maximus. If any area binds against the drag, working across the grain of the muscle and in the opposite direction may be beneficial.

Any areas that redden may be sites of trigger point activity. Because trigger points can cause muscles to fire out of sequence, it is important to restore as much normalcy as possible to the tissue.

- To increase circulation to the area and shift the neuroresponses of the trigger points, move the skin into multiple directions of ease over the suspected trigger point area and hold the ease position for 30 to 60 seconds.

- If the tenderness is not relieved, positional release is the next option, followed by muscle energy methods if necessary.
- Local lengthening of the tissue containing the trigger points is effective. Local lengthening is accomplished by using tension, bend, or torsion force on the tissue with the trigger point and taut band. Do not use direct pressure or transverse friction, because they may cause tissue damage.
- If the trigger point does not release with the methods described, it likely is part of a compensation pattern that must be dealt with, and the trigger point serves a useful function. Leave it alone.
- Finish the area with kneading, making sure the muscle tissue lifts easily off the layer beneath it.
- If adhesions are identified, introduce a bend, shear, or torsion force until the tissue becomes more pliable. This can be intense and can cause a burning sensation; however, the patient should not need to show any guarding or pain behaviors or hold the breath during application.
- Repeat this sequence bilaterally.

Once the surface tissue has been addressed, the second layer of muscle is massaged. It is important to make sure that the surface tissue and the fascial separation between muscle layers are not adhering to each other in any way. To assess for adhesion, use a wavelike motion on the surface muscle to slide it back and forth or lift the muscle tissue up and move it back and forth.

The main muscles addressed are portions of the gluteus medius, gluteus minimus, and deep lateral hip rotators.

- It is helpful to place the surface layer of tissue in a slack position; this is achieved by passively supporting the hip in extension with the patient in either the prone or side-lying position.
- Begin at the iliac crest attachments. Use a compressive gliding technique, working deep enough to address this layer of tissue. Broaden the base of contact so that the surface tissue does not tighten to guard against poking.
- Glide toward the greater trochanter. Repeat 3 or 4 times, each time working slower and at a slightly different angle.
- Glide and knead slowly across the fiber direction, using enough pressure and lift to ensure that you affect the muscle fiber in this layer. These methods address both the connective tissue and the neuromuscular elements of the muscles. Repeat 3 or 4 times, increasing the depth and drag each time. Be alert to the muscle moving with the application.

  Next, address the deep lateral hip rotators.
- With the surface layer still in a slack position, use the forearm to apply broad-based compression into the space between the sacrum and the greater trochanter. This is best accomplished with the patient in the prone position.
- Bend the patient's knee and move the hip back and forth from medial to lateral rotation. This can be thought of as moving "into the 4 and out of the 4." The action can be active or passive.
- Repeat 3 or 4 times, slightly changing the angle. Do not apply constant compression on the sciatic nerve. Lighten the compressive force at least every 30 seconds to allow for proper circulation to the area.

The side-lying position is effective for addressing the gluteus medius and tensor fasciae latae on the upper side and the quadratus femoris on the opposite (closer to the table) side. Broad-based compression with the forearm on the gluteus and a stabilized hand position are best for working on the quadratus femoris. Because the quadratus femoris muscle is in the groin area, ask permission before working in this area.

The quadratus femoris is a deep lateral rotator; however, unlike the others, which are abductors, it is an adductor and often is short. Active and passive movement can be added while the area is compressed.

- Assess the SI joint by palpating it and by internally and externally rotating the hip. The hip should be able to move 45 degrees in either direction without producing a feel of bind at the joint.
- Perform passive and active mobilization of the SI joint and symphysis pubis (see specific release procedures in Chapter 10).

- Assess firing patterns (see Chapter 9).
- Finish by gliding and kneading the entire area. Add oscillation (rocking and shaking) in various positions. In addition, you might drain the area.

THE THIGH (Figure 11-11)

Lumbar and sacral plexus impingement can cause radiating pain in the legs. The muscles that most often cause impingement are the quadratus lumborum and the multifidi. Lumbar plexus impingement causes radiating pain in the thigh, whereas sacral plexus impingement causes radiating pain in the back of the thigh and the calf.

The thigh and leg are in closed chain function most of the time, meaning that the hip, knee, and ankle do not function independently of each other. Even in open chain function, these joints and tissues influence each other.

The muscles of the thigh work primarily at the knee. The rectus femoris, hamstring group, and sartorius cross two joints and function both at the hip and the knee. Some of the muscles of the leg (e.g., the gastrocnemius) also cross the knee.

The gait reflexes coordinate the interaction of the arms and legs. A flexor, adductor, and internal rotation pattern on the left arm and right leg is seen during forward motion (concentric contraction), facilitating with antagonists that function eccentrically for deceleration. Then, concentric contraction transfers into the right arm and left leg, and the opposite pattern is activated. At the same time, the extensor, abductor, and external rotation pattern facilitates concentric contraction on the contralateral side of the body, and the antagonist pattern functions eccentrically. This back and forth movement of gait is necessary for postural stability, fluid motion, and agility.

Gait function can be disrupted by illness or injury, by repetitive training activities, or by competing when fatigued, especially if the movement patterns are altered. A prime example of this is bilateral weight training (e.g., hamstring strengthening) in which both left and right hamstring muscles are concentrically contracted and then eccentrically contracted at the same time instead of in the opposite swing pattern. Although this may increase strength in the legs, it has a tendency to disrupt gait patterns, with a corresponding increase in muscle tone in both biceps brachii.

Often the massage therapist must work with the arms and legs in some sort of coordinated pattern to increase the effectiveness of the massage. For example, the patient can actively bend the elbow back and forth in an open chain position while the therapist massages the opposite leg, or the flow of the massage application can proceed from the left arm to the right leg and then from the right arm to the left leg. Put another way, the therapist could work with the right biceps and the left hamstring, then the right quadriceps and the left triceps, and vice versa. The side-lying position gives access for optimum body mechanics, but the supine or prone position also can be used.

The thigh muscles are basically arranged in two layers. In the superficial layer, the three heads of the hamstrings are thick muscles that superiorly attach near each other on the ischial tuberosity; these muscles can bind or get stuck together. The four heads of the quadriceps are also thick muscles, three of which have proximal attachments on the shaft of the femur, and all four have distal attachments on the tibia, which can become a source of bind if layers are stuck together. The vastus intermedius is the main second layer muscle.

The thigh also has a large group of adductor muscles that is very involved in core stability and antigravity function.

The thigh can be massaged in all basic positions and often is addressed more than once during a massage. When the patient is in the prone position, the back of the thigh is accessible. With the patient in the side-lying position, the adductors and IT band are accessible. With the patient supine, the anterior thigh is easily reached, and the lateral, medial, and posterior regions can be assessed. The quadriceps muscles are effectively massaged with the patient seated.

The thigh muscles must be able to glide over the bone, therefore rolling tissues over the femur is important. For patients with highly developed, bulky thighs, it often is advisable to have the patient lie on the floor while the therapist uses the knees and feet to apply compression.

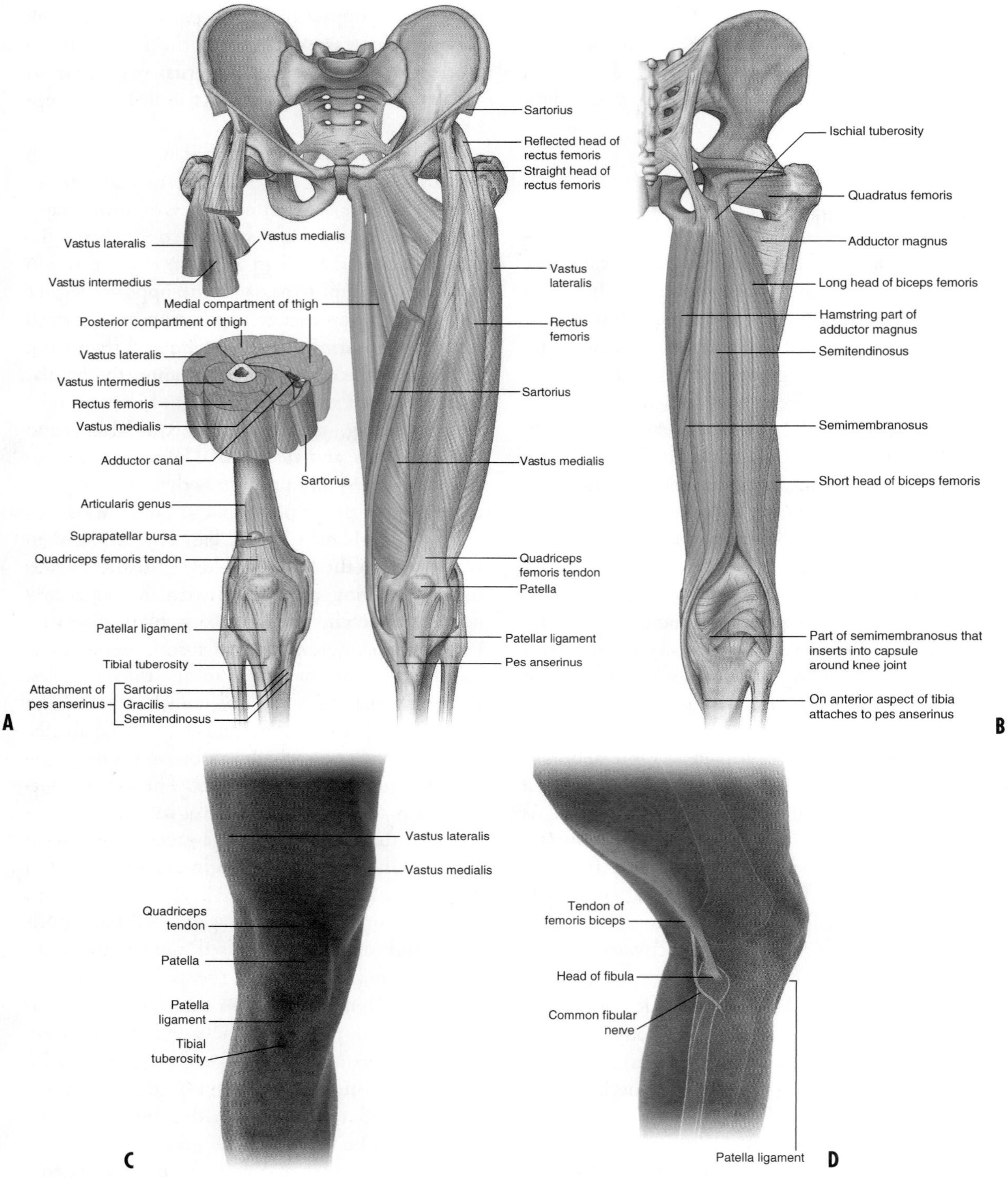

FIGURE 11-11 ■ Important structures in massage application to the thigh to assist the reader. **A,** The anterior compartment of the thigh. **B,** The posterior compartment of the thigh. **C,** Anterior view of the right knee. **D,** Lateral view of the right knee. (From Drake R, Vogl W, Mitchell A: *Gray's anatomy for students,* Edinburgh, 2005, Churchill Livingstone.)

PROCEDURES FOR THE THIGH

Examples of treatment procedures for the thigh are shown in the Appendix.

Massage of the thigh naturally progresses from the hip and calf. Assessment of all range-of-motion patterns and muscle strength determines which structures are short and which are long. In addition, gait pattern and firing pattern assessment should provide information about neurologic efficiency or whether tone patterns are affected.

As with other body regions, the massage begins with superficial work, progresses to deeper layers, and finishes off with superficial work. The initial applications are palpation assessment, range of motion, strength, and neurologic assessment. The massage should begin with the patient in the prone position.

- Move the thigh and knee both actively and passively through flexion, extension, and internal and external rotation. Compare active and passive movement of the right and left limbs.
- Gently compress the knee joints to make sure there is no intracapsular involvement. If pain occurs, refer the patient to the appropriate specialist. Massage can still be performed, but be aware that muscle tension patterns may be a guarding response to create appropriate compensation.

Any areas that do not function optimally should be noted and reassessed after the area is massaged.

- Systematically lightly stroke the area to assess for temperature changes, skin texture, and damp areas. Observe for skin reddening (histamine response) and goose bumps (pilomotor response). These signs indicate possible changes in the connective tissue, muscle tone, or circulation patterns.
- Increase the pressure slightly and assess for superficial fascial bind, changes in skin pliability, and the accumulation of interstitial fluid, as indicated by boggy or edematous tissue and/or increased skin pressure (the sensation is much like pressing on a water balloon).
- If increased fluid pressure is evident, drain the area; use a combination of light pressure to drag the skin and deeper, rhythmic, broad-based compression and kneading to stimulate the deeper vessels.
  - Begin with lighter pressure directed toward the groin and cover the entire area.
  - Then introduce pumping, broad-based compression, combined first with active movement (i.e., have the patient slowly flex and relax the hip) and then with passive movement.
  - Return to dragging the skin, and alternate between the two methods until the area is drained (about 5 minutes). (Remember, when moving fluid, you can't push a river.)
- If you are in doubt about whether fluid retention is present, assume that it is and drain the area.

Next, address the superficial fascia by assessing for tissue bind. Always observe for involvement in adjacent areas, such as the tissue leading into the hip and knee. Pay particular attention to the IT band and the junctions of the hamstring and quadriceps with this connective tissue structure.

- Move the skin to identify any areas of bind in the superficial connective tissue. Notice whether any bind areas correspond to the areas of skin reddening or goose bumps identified by the light stroking. Pay particular attention to any scars, because connective tissue bind is common at these sites.
- Treat areas of superficial fascial bind with myofascial release methods. Address these areas by slowly moving the tissue into ease, dragging it the way it most wants to go. Multiple load directions may be used. For example, if the skin and superficial fascia want to move up and to the right on the IT band, that is the direction of the forces introduced. Hold the ease position for up to 30 to 60 seconds.
- Then, work into the bind; use a slow, sustained drag on the binding tissues, introducing the lines of tension at each end of the binding tissue.
  - Place your flat hand at one end of the bind and the other hand at the other end of the bind.

- Contact the tissue gently but firmly, pressing only as deep as the superficial fascial layer; then separate your hands, creating a tension force in the binding tissue.

Kneading can be used to introduce bend and torsion forces; these methods are especially effective on the IT band. Subtle changes in the lines of force serve to load and unload the tissue.

- Grasp as much of the binding tissue as possible and lift it until the resistance is identified. Slowly load and unload with bend, torsion, and shear forces until the tissue becomes warm and more pliable. This method is intense, and the patient should feel a pulling or slight burning sensation; however, the patient should not feel the need to tense up or to change the breathing pattern to endure the method. Work slowly and deliberately.
- Do not use a tension force application (gliding) with deep pressure over the IT band, because this may cause compression of the nerve structures. Use a kneading technique instead.

The muscle layers are addressed systematically by moving from superficial to deep. It is important to make sure the muscle layers are not adhering to each other, particularly in the thigh. The most common points of adherence are (1) at the rectus femoris on the vastus intermedius; (2) at the edges of the two medial hamstrings (semimembranosus and semitendinosus) where they meet in the middle of the posterior thigh; and (3) where the vastus lateralis and lateral hamstring (biceps femoris) weave into the IT band near their distal insertions. In both the quadriceps and hamstring groups, make sure the heads of the muscles are not stuck together, because each part of the muscles has a somewhat different angle of pull. If adhesions are found, the affected muscle layer should be sheared off the next deeper layer and off the structures next to it.

- It is helpful to place the patient so that the surface layer is in a slack position. This can be accomplished by positioning the attachments of the muscle close together and bolstering the patient so that the person stays relaxed.
- Begin at the knee and carry the strokes into the posterior hip. Then, reverse direction; use compression toward the knee and then gliding again toward the hip. Repeat 3 or 4 times, each time working slower and deeper and maintaining broad-based contact to protect the more superficial tissue and reduce the potential for guarding.
- If any area binds against the drag, working across the grain of the muscle and in the opposite direction may be beneficial.
- Glide slowly across the fiber direction, using enough pressure to make sure you affect the muscle fiber. This method addresses both the connective tissue and the neuromuscular elements of the muscle. Repeat 3 or 4 times, increasing the depth and drag each time. Be alert to the muscle moving with the application.

Any areas that redden may be sites of trigger point activity. Trigger points can cause muscles to fire out of sequence, therefore it is important to restore as much normalcy as possible to the tissue.

- To increase circulation to the area and shift the neuroresponses of the trigger points, move the skin into multiple directions of ease over the area and hold the ease position for 30 to 60 seconds.
- If the tenderness is not relieved, positional release is the next option, followed by muscle energy methods if necessary.
- Local lengthening of the tissue containing the trigger points is effective. This is accomplished by using tension, bend, or torsion force on the tissue with the trigger point and taut band. Do not use direct pressure or transverse friction, because they may cause tissue damage.
- If the trigger point does not release with these methods, it is part of a compensation pattern that must be dealt with, and the trigger point likely serves a useful function. Leave it alone.
- Assess for firing patterns for hip extension and knee flexion and correct if necessary.
- Finish the area with kneading, making sure the muscle tissue easily lifts off the layer beneath it.

- If adhesions are identified, introduce a bend, shear, or torsion force until the tissue becomes more pliable. This method can be intense and can cause a burning sensation; however, the patient should not show guarding or pain behaviors or hold the breath during application.
- Repeat this sequence bilaterally.

With the patient in the side-lying position, the medial, lateral, posterior, and anterior thigh can be massaged, and range of motion is not limited by the table. This is the best position for massage of the medial and lateral thigh. The supine position is most effective for massage of the anterior thigh.

- Systematically lightly stroke the area to assess for temperature changes, skin texture, and damp areas. Observe for skin reddening (histamine response) and goose bumps (pilomotor response). These signs indicate possible changes in the connective tissue, muscle tone, or circulation pattern.
- Increase the pressure slightly and assess for superficial fascial bind, changes in skin pliability, and the accumulation of interstitial fluid, as indicated by boggy or edematous tissue and/or increased skin pressure (the sensation is much like pressing on a water balloon).
- If increased fluid pressure is evident, drain the area. (Remember, when moving fluid, you can't push a river.)
- If you are in doubt about whether fluid retention is present, assume that it is and drain the area.

Next, address the superficial fascia by assessing for tissue bind. Always observe for involvement in adjacent areas, such as the tissue leading into the hip and knee.

- Move the skin to identify any areas of bind in the superficial connective tissue. Notice whether any bind areas correspond to the areas of skin reddening or goose bumps identified by the light stroking. Pay particular attention to any scars, because connective tissue bind is common at these sites.
- Treat areas of superficial fascial bind with myofascial release methods. Address these areas by slowly moving the tissue into ease with multiple load directions.
- Next, work into the bind, using a slow, sustained drag on the binding tissues and introducing the lines of tension at each end of the binding tissue.
  - Place your forearm (or your flat hand if your forearm is too large) at one end of the bind and the other forearm at the other end of the bind.
  - Contact the tissue gently but firmly, pressing only as deep as the superficial fascial layer, and then separate your forearms, creating a tension force in the binding tissue.
- Bend force can also be introduced through kneading. Tension force can be added by having the patient actively or passively move the knee into slight flexion and then back into the original position. For passive motion, use of the foot and leg to do this is very effective.
- Repeat the movement back and forth until a change is noted. Maintain the drag on the tissue until the ground substance becomes more pliable. Subtle changes in the lines of force serve to load and unload the tissue, resulting in hysteresis.
- Next, grasp as much of the binding tissue as possible and lift until you feel the bind. Slowly load and unload with torsion and shear force, or by having the patient move the knee, until the tissue becomes warm and more pliable. This method is intense, and the patient should feel a pulling or slight burning sensation; however, the patient should not feel the need to tense up or to change the breathing pattern to endure the method.
- Work slowly and deliberately, interspersing the process with lymphatic drainage–type stroking every minute or so.

When an area is found that produces the symptoms that are bothering the patient, compression combined with muscle energy methods, from the least invasive positional release to integrated methods, can be used. The goal is to inhibit temporally the motor tone of the muscle bundle that is problematic so that it can be lengthened to the appropriate resting length, reducing the pressure on the nerves or vessels.

When addressing deeper tissue layers, always remember to protect the more superficial muscles by applying pressure gradually and with as broad a base of contact as the area allows.

The side-lying position allows access to the attachments of the hamstrings and adductors in the groin. Because groin problems often occur, this is an important but difficult area to massage. Compression applied at the attachments is effective and can be done through thin clothing if necessary.

- With the fingers placed on muscle attachments, combine compression with active or passive movement (or both) of the hip and knee. A slow circumduction tends to access all areas.
- Finish by gliding and kneading the entire area. Add oscillation, (rocking and shaking) in various positions. In addition, you might drain the area.

THE LEG, ANKLE, AND FOOT (Figure 11-12)

The leg muscles function at the knee, ankle, and foot. Repetitive movement is common for these muscles, as is repetitive strain illness and injury. The goal of the massage is to maintain normal tissue function so that repetitive movement does not become repetitive strain.

The muscles of the leg are categorized as superficial, intermediate, and deep. The muscles can adhere to each other in their side-by-side positions and between layers. It is especially important to make sure the popliteus, soleus, and gastrocnemius are not stuck together. The superficial muscle layer primarily functions at the ankle, with some activity at the knee. The intermediate layer functions at the ankle, and the deep layer works the toes, with some activity at the ankle.

The bellies of these muscles lie closer to the knee, and they taper to the tendons in the ankle and foot. It is important to gauge the pressure you use in the massage. Deeper pressure is used in the proximal half of the lower leg, where the muscle bulk is located. Connective tissue binding often occurs in the distal half of the lower leg into the foot and is common at the Achilles tendon and plantar fascia.

Typically, the forearm or flat hand is used to massage the leg, but the foot works very well for applying compression. The arch of the foot fits nicely over the muscle bulk, and the patient can provide active movement of the ankle and toes while the compression is applied. This is effective at reducing muscle tone and connective tissue binding in the tissues.

PROCEDURES FOR THE LEG, ANKLE, AND FOOT

Examples of treatment procedures for the ankle and foot are shown in the Appendix.

The knee joint is complex and should be addressed by massage of the thigh and lower leg. In addition, move the patella gently to make sure it moves freely.

The pes anserinus tendon on the medial aspect of the tibia is where the distal attachments of the sartorius, gracilis, and semitendinosus blend into one structure just below the knee. Bending can interfere with knee function. A connective tissue application is effective for this.

The massage pattern is very similar to that presented in other areas. All three basic positions can be used. Massage of the ankle and foot first involves working with the muscles of the lower leg in relation to the actions of the ankle, foot, and toes.

- Apply systematic compression to the muscles of the lower leg, beginning at the knee and working toward the ankle, while the patient moves the ankle and toes in circles.
- To isolate a particular muscle pain caused by ankle or foot action, have the patient move the ankle or foot in the way that creates the symptom; palpate the muscles to see which ones are activated and then address those muscles.

Next, address the range of motion of the ankle. Proper ankle mobility is necessary for knee and hip function. Often knee pain is related to disruption of ankle function. The ankle may be jammed, with a reduction in joint play. A general method for restoring joint play is the MWM sequence.

Apply traction to the joint and then move it into the ease and pain-free position. The patient is passive while the position is found. The therapist then maintains the position while the patient actively moves the joint through a range of

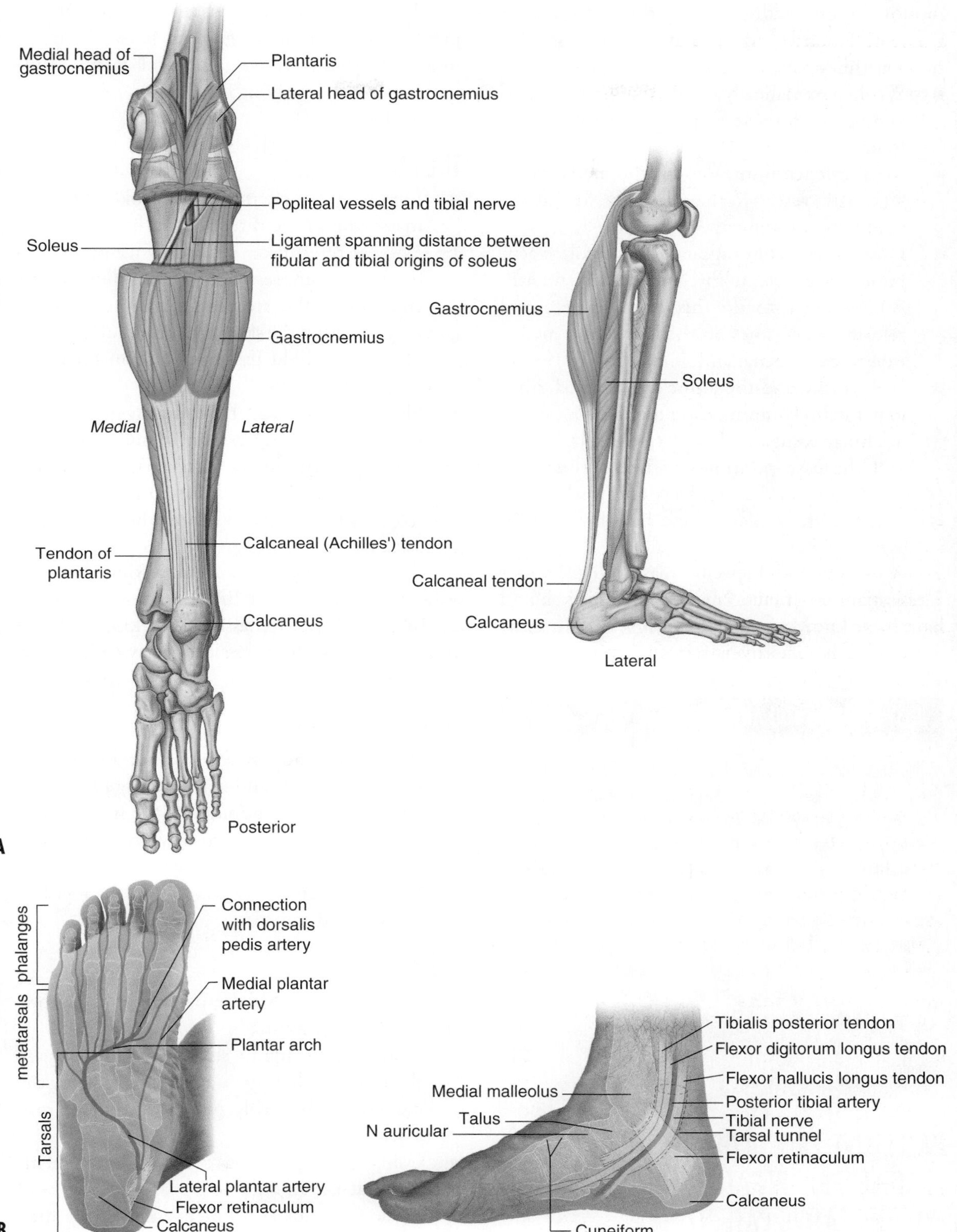

FIGURE 11-12 ■ Important structures in massage application to the leg, ankle, and foot to assist the reader. **A,** Superficial muscles in the posterior compartment of the leg (posterior and lateral views). **B,** The tarsal tunnel of the foot. **C,** The plantar arch. (From Drake R, Vogl W, Mitchell A: *Gray's anatomy for students,* Edinburgh, 2005, Churchill Livingstone.)

motions. Next, address the intrinsic muscles of the foot. The side-lying position is the best position for this work.

- Work systematically, using compression and gliding of the soft tissue of the sole of the foot.
- Rhythmic compression of the network of lymphatic vessels in the sole of the foot assists lymphatic movement.
- Direct pressure or tapping can stimulate acupuncture points at the side of each toenail. An easy way to do this is to squeeze and release 3 or 4 times on the lateral and medial side of each toenail.
- If the tarsal and toe joints are jammed, joint play methods can increase mobility. The toes are hinge joints, and once traction is applied and the ease position has been found, the patient moves the toes back and forth.
- Finish with oscillation and lymphatic drainage.

A thorough and specific massage of the foot is essential for patients. Massage therapists should have some knowledge of reflexology, and integrating it into the massage is appropriate.

JUST BETWEEN YOU AND ME

This whole body general protocol, in all its variations, is what I call my "weekly house-cleaning" massage. I have performed some version of it at least 25,000 times over my 25+ years of practice. It really is the same thing over and over, moving from one region of the body to another, with only the names of the bones, joints, and muscles changing. However, specific cautions and suggestions apply for particular regions, and this textbook plays a vital role as a reference source for those. I believe that many massage therapists will use specific sections of this protocol during massage, either as students, while learning, or later on, as practitioners, to recall details. Therefore this is a deliberate strategy; you can find what you need about any particular region of the body in this resource material.

PALLIATIVE PROTOCOL FOR ILL, FRAGILE, PREOPERATIVE, OR POSTOPERATIVE PATIENTS

For an example of this protocol, refer to the appendix on p. 759.

This palliative massage is a general inhibition, pleasure-based application that lasts 30 to 45 minutes. Assessment is basic and targets contraindications involving alteration of massage application.

THE FACE

- Lightly and systematically stroke the face, massaging in the direction of the smile.
- Address the muscle structures using light to moderate compressive force. To increase circulation to the area and shift the neuroresponses, move the skin into multiple directions of ease and hold the ease position for up to 30 to 60 seconds.
- Sinus drainage can be encouraged by compression on acupressure points combined with light, rhythmic, on-off pressure against the sinus cavities for about 10 repetitions.
- To finish the face, return to the initial light stroking.

Working with the face is relaxing. For this reason, doing this work first sets the stage for a calming whole body massage. Working with the face at the end of the session gently finishes the massage.

THE HEAD

- Place your hands on either side of the patient's head by the ears and gently apply pressure.
- Compression to the sides of the head and to the front and back, coupled with a scratching motion to the scalp, can be very pleasant.
- Some patients enjoy having the hair gently stroked and pulled.

THE NECK

Address this area with the patient in the prone and side-lying positions.

- Systematically lightly stroke the skin. Increase the pressure slightly, as is comfortable for the patient, while slowly moving the tissue into ease.
- Using gliding with a compressive element, begin at the middle of the back of the head at the trapezius attachments and slowly drag the tissue to the distal attachment of the trapezius at the acromion process and lateral third of the clavicle.

- With the patient prone, begin again at the head and glide toward the acromion. Then, reverse direction and work from distal to proximal.
- Then knead and glide across the muscle fibers, making sure that bend, shear, and torsion forces are only sufficient to create a pleasurable sensation.
- Gentle rocking, rhythmic ranges of motion (oscillation) may be used to continue to relax the area.

THE ANTERIOR TORSO

- Begin the massage superficially, progress to deeper tissue layers, and finish off by returning to superficial work. In general, as the massage progresses, hold the tissue in the ease position until you feel it release (up to 30 to 60 seconds).
- Using gliding with a compressive element, begin at the shoulder and work from the distal attachment of the pectoralis major at the arm toward the sternum, following the fiber direction. This can be done with the patient rolled in the supine or side-lying position. Repeat 3 or 4 times, each time increasing the drag and moving more slowly.
- Move to the abdomen and knead slowly across the fiber direction. The abdominal organs can be rolled to encourage peristalsis.
- Rhythmic compression of the entire anterior torso stimulates lymphatic flow, blood circulation, and relaxed breathing.

THE POSTERIOR TORSO

- As described previously, begin the massage superficially, progress to deeper layers, and finish off by returning to superficial work. It is helpful to place the patient so that the surface layer is in a slack position; this is accomplished by positioning the attachments of the muscle close together and propping the patient so that the person remains relaxed. In some situations the side-lying position may be better for this.
- Using gliding with a compressive element, begin at the iliac crest and work diagonally along the fibers of the latissimus dorsi, ending at the axilla. Repeat 3 or 4 times, each time increasing the drag and moving more slowly.
- Move up to the thoracolumbar junction and repeat the same sequence on the lower trapezius.
- Then, begin near the tip of the shoulder and glide toward the middle thoracic area to address the middle trapezius. Repeat 3 or 4 times, increasing drag and decreasing speed.
- Begin again near the acromion and address the upper trapezius with one or two gliding strokes to complete the surface area.
- Kneading of the area is pleasurable for the patient. To increase circulation to the area and shift the neuroresponses, move the skin into multiple directions of ease and hold the ease position for up to 30 to 60 seconds.
- Rhythmic compression to the area stimulates various aspects of fluid movement and supports relaxed breathing.

THE SHOULDER, ARM, AND HAND

The area is massaged with the patient in the supine, prone, side-lying, and seated positions. Massage of the torso and neck naturally progresses to the shoulder, arm, and hand.

- Place the patient in the prone position. Begin the massage superficially, progress to deeper layers, and complete the process by returning to superficial work. Finish the area with kneading, compression, and gliding.
- To increase circulation to the area and shift the neuroresponses, move the skin into multiple directions of ease and hold the ease position for up to 30 to 60 seconds.
- Combine compression with passive movements of the arm. A slow circumduction tends to access all areas.
- Next address the intrinsic muscles of the hand. Systematically work the area, using compression and gliding of the soft tissue between the fingers, the web of the thumb, and on the palm.
- Rhythmic compression of the network of lymphatic vessels in the palm assists lymphatic movement.

THE HIP

The hip is massaged with the patient in the prone and side-lying positions. Massage of the torso naturally progresses to the hip

- Begin the massage superficially, progress to deeper layers, and finish off by returning to superficial work.
- Systematically lightly stroke the area. To increase circulation to the area and shift the neuroresponses, move the skin into multiple directions of ease and hold the ease position for up to 30 to 60 seconds.
- Increase the pressure slightly. Begin on the posterior to address the lumbar region that connects with the hip. This area was addressed during massage of the torso but now is massaged in relation to the hip. Carry the strokes into the gluteus maximus.
- Using gliding with a compressive element, glide toward the hip. Repeat with the latissimus dorsi, again in relation to hip function. Begin at the shoulder and carry the stroke all the way into the opposite gluteus maximus.
- Finish by gliding and kneading the entire area. Add oscillation (rocking and shaking) in various positions. In addition, you might drain the area.

THE THIGH, LEG, AND FOOT

These areas can be massaged in all the basic positions. The massage naturally progresses from the hip.

- As with other body regions, begin the massage superficially, progress to deeper layers, and finish by returning to superficial work.
- To increase circulation to the area and shift the neuroresponses, move the skin into multiple directions of ease and hold the ease position for up to 30 to 60 seconds. Move the hip and knee passively through flexion, extension, and internal and external rotation *if comfortable.*
- Increase the pressure slightly and again use gliding and kneading to the entire area. Add gentle shaking and oscillation in various positions.
- Next, address the intrinsic muscles of the foot (the side-lying position is best for this). Work systematically, using compression and gliding of the soft tissue of the sole of the foot.
- Rhythmic compression of the network of lymphatic vessels in the sole assists lymphatic movement.
- Direct pressure or tapping on acupuncture points at the side of each toenail can stimulate these points. An easy way to do this is to squeeze and release 3 or 4 times on the lateral and medial sides of each toenail.
- Finish by using gentle shaking and oscillation, compression, and passive movement.

evolve 11-2

The following terms and expressions specific to Chapter 11 have already been used to search PubMed for the latest research literature available. The *Click Here for Massage* feature associated with this chapter on your textbook's Evolve website allows you to hyperlink to a continually updated PubMed search of research literature that corresponds to this subject.

Hyperlink Search Terms

Massage fragile
Massage general protocol
Massage palliative
Massage protocol
Massage protocol ill
Massage surgery patient

SUMMARY

This chapter provided a detailed, comprehensive, and repetitive approach to massage, as well as a modified version for palliative care. Hopefully, at this point the reader realizes that regardless of the body area worked, the general sequence of the massage is the same. The protocol need not be used exactly as presented; applications can be incorporated or deleted. More often, this protocol will be modified based on the patient's goals, initial patient positioning, and other contributing factors. As described, specific areas are addressed as needed. This protocol is the basic, general maintenance massage approach used for performance and recovery massage. Healing and rehabilitation massage procedures are presented in Unit Three. The general and palliative protocols are shown on video on the Evolve website.

WORKBOOK

1. Review the protocol and identify the repeating sequences, then write down the sequence.

___

___

___

___

2. Rewrite the protocol in a way that makes the best sense to you.

___

___

___

___

3. Review the chapter text and the corresponding Evolve material, then list all the figures that demonstrate ways to massage the following:

   Face

   Head

   Occipital area

   Neck

   Anterior torso

   Posterior torso

   Shoulder

   Arm, wrist, and hand

   Hip

   Leg, ankle, and foot

___

___

___

___

4. Using the photographs and DVD material from question 3, write an entirely different massage protocol; include a variation that targets palliative care.

___

___

___

___

Chapter 12 Concept Map

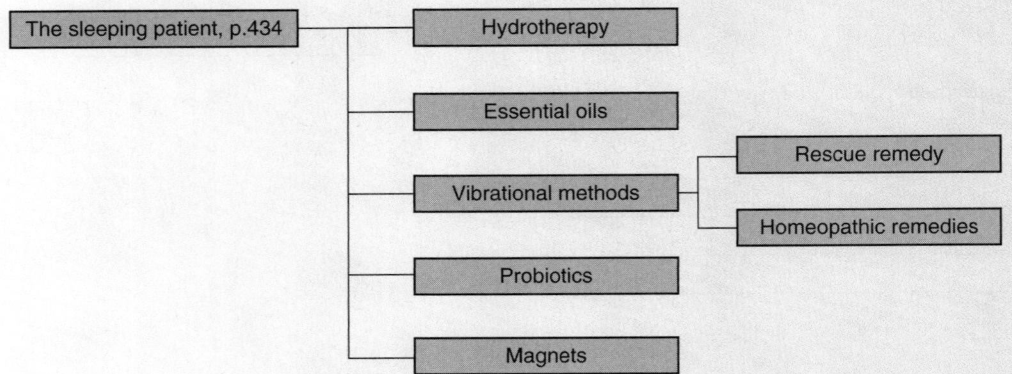

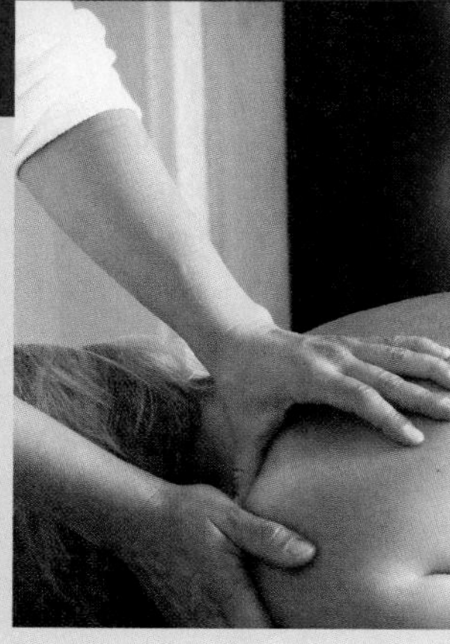

CHAPTER 12

UNIQUE CIRCUMSTANCES AND ADJUNCT THERAPIES

Key Terms

Aromatherapy
Diffusion
Essential oils
Homeopathy
Magnets
Probiotics

For definitions of key terms, refer to the Evolve website.

OBJECTIVES

Upon completion of this chapter, the reader will have the information necessary to:

1. Alter the massage application to work effectively with a sleeping patient.
2. Alter the massage application to adjust to unique draping concerns and medical equipment.
3. Provide massage in various environments.
4. Use simple, safe applications of adjunct therapies to support the massage outcome.

This final chapter of Unit Two discusses some of the specific situations that massage therapists often encounter. The information is based on years of professional experience. Because each person comes with his or her own unique set of circumstances, the massage therapist needs ingenuity, flexibility, creativity, and a sense of humor. As mentioned at the beginning of this textbook, many different situations arise that can stretch the massage therapist's ability to perform an effective massage. The main challenges are a sleeping patient, draping considerations, and dealing with medical devices.

Patients often are open to the use of essential oils, homeopathy, and magnet treatments. The massage therapist needs to be ethical and informed about such approaches. Many of these products are expensive and may have little value beyond a placebo effect. The methods may offer possibilities as self-help treatments or as a means to support or extend the effects of massage. However, the therapist must always obtain the doctor's approval before recommending any adjunct method.

This chapter provides information on adjunct therapies such as aromatherapy, hydrotherapy, homeopathy, and magnet therapy. Hydrotherapy is well researched and is used extensively by those involved in sports fitness and in healing and rehabilitation. **Aromatherapy** (the use of essential oils) is also a useful method, and valid research is providing insight into its mechanisms and effects. This chapter describes the oils that are generally safe and that I have found most useful.

Magnet therapy and other energy methods, such as homeopathy, have a less solid research base. However, some patients use magnets, therefore it is important to understand the current theories. My personal experience indicates that a couple of homeopathic remedies are helpful, especially arnica for preoperative and postoperative uses. Rescue Remedy, a flower essence preparation made by Bach, also seems to help with the ongoing trauma and shock these patients experience.

As mentioned earlier, always obtain permission before combining an adjunct therapy with massage. The doctor or other supervising healthcare professional may want to discuss the methods with the patient and then decide whether to recommend them. Aromatherapy best works directly with massage, but essential oils should not be used without specific permission, because they may interact with other treatments.

THE SLEEPING PATIENT

Patients commonly fall asleep during a massage. Because restorative sleep is so important, the massage therapist must be able to adapt a massage application so as to accommodate sleep and continue to achieve outcomes. The most obvious challenges are active assessment and the use of methods that require active participation. Altering the flow of the application so that these methods are used at the beginning of the massage and afterward usually solves such problems.

Extra blankets and pillows, as well as bolsters, usually are required. The circulation changes during both sleep and massage, and patients become cool. The patient's position must be changed gently and smoothly so that the person is disturbed as little as possible.

Use rhythmic rocking to settle the patient if the person rouses a bit from sleep; this usually allows the individual to go back to sleep. Patients can be roused by position changes, the use of passive range of motion and stretching methods, and application of an unexpectedly painful method.

Try to do most of the massage with the person in the side-lying and supine positions. The prone position can cause the sinuses to clog up and strains the lower back; use it when the patient is most wakeful and bolster the lower leg to reduce lumbar strain.

The massage needs to be given in a confident, rhythmic manner. All movement should be secure and stabilized appropriately. The massage therapist needs to be focused, observant of the patient's responses, and quiet. Passive methods, such as lymphatic drainage and other fluid dynamics techniques, are easy to apply during sleep. A skilled therapist can alter some of the more active applications and assessment procedures and apply them passively.

In general, assessment is accomplished primarily through observation and palpation. For more active assessment methods, such as evaluating muscle firing patterns, a rule of thumb is that heat and muscle tension can indicate a synergistic dominance pattern. If you are in doubt, assume that the firing pattern indicates synergistic dominance. Some massage methods can be focused to reduce tone in the misfiring muscles, and more stimulating methods can be applied to the inhibited muscles.

To address gait patterns, work the arm and leg on opposite sides of the body in sequence as follows:

1. Left biceps with left quadriceps and right hamstring
2. Left triceps with left hamstring and right quadricep
3. Right biceps with right quadriceps and left hamstring
4. Right triceps with right hamstring and left quadriceps
5. Left wrist and finger flexors with left foot dorsiflexors and evertors and right plantar flexors and invertors
6. Left wrist and finger extensors with left foot plantar flexors and invertors and right foot dorsiflexors and evertors
7. Right wrist and finger flexors with right foot dorsiflexors and evertors and left plantar flexors and invertors

8. Right wrist and finger extensors with right foot plantar flexors and invertors and left foot dorsiflexors and evertors
9. Left hand with right foot
10. Right hand with left foot

Joint play is restored by tractioning the joint and moving it passively within the normal range of motion.

Passive massage application usually is less effective than applications that incorporate the patient's active participation; however, benefits are still achieved when sleep is also an important goal. Indirect functional techniques become a primary treatment method. They replace the more invasive connective tissue methods and trigger point applications. Pay attention to the sleep cycle, which naturally fluctuates about every 45 minutes, and time the massage to end about when the patient would begin to wake up.

HYDROTHERAPY

Hydrotherapy is a distinct form of therapy that combines well with massage. Water is a near-perfect natural body balancer and is necessary for life. It accounts for the largest percentage of our body weight.

The effects of water are primarily reflexive and focus on the autonomic nervous system. The addition of heat energy or the dissipation of heat energy from tissues can be classified as a mechanical effect. In general, cold stimulates sympathetic responses, and warmth activates parasympathetic responses. Short- and long-term applications of hot or cold differ in effect. For the most part, short cold applications stimulate and cause vasoconstriction, with a secondary effect of increased circulation as blood is channeled to the area to warm it. Long cold applications depress and decrease circulation. Short applications of heat cause vasodilation of vessels and depress and deplete tone, whereas long heat applications result in a combined depressant and stimulant reaction.

Different water pressures can exert a powerful mechanical effect on the nerves and blood supply of the skin. Techniques include a friction rub with a sponge or wet mitt and directing pressurized streams of hot and cold water at various parts of the body (Box 12-1).

Diffusion is a principle of hydrotherapy by which water moves across a permeable or semipermeable membrane from a low mineral salt concentration to a high concentration to equalize the solution's consistency. If the salt content of the water used for hydrotherapy is lower than that of the body fluids, water moves from the outside of the body to the inside through the semipermeable superficial tissue of the skin and superficial fascia. If the salt content of the water external to the skin is higher (e.g., as in mineral salt baths), water from the body moves into the external soak water. This reduces surface edema.

In the medical and physical therapy settings, the physician assistant, medical technician, or physical therapist applies hydrotherapy. The massage therapist must make sure that massage techniques do not interfere with the outcomes of these treatments. Primarily, do not massage an area that has been iced. Let the body restore circulation to the area to warm it. Hot and cold contrast hydrotherapy is effective at supporting fluid movement. Epsom salts and salves can help manage surface edema.

Cold is most effective for just about everything, and the application of ice is a component of acute care for many injuries (i.e., *p*rotection, *r*est, *i*ce, *c*ompression, and *e*levation [PRICE]). When in doubt, put ice on it. Real ice is safer than chemical ice packs. Immersing an area in ice water is extremely effective, especially for sprains, strains, and similar injuries. Heat is more effective for palliative care and as a surface muscle relaxer.

If neither illness nor injury is a factor, a general rule can be: ice joints and heat muscles. Warm applications (e.g., rice or seed bags that can be heated in the microwave) are pleasant during a massage, especially on the feet. You can easily make such a bag by filling tube socks (I like hunting socks) with rice and tying them off. I put one sock inside another and tie each one so that the outer sock can be removed and laundered. Warm the rice bag in the microwave for 1 to 3 minutes.

ESSENTIAL OILS

Essential oils are the highly concentrated oils of aromatic plants, and aromatherapy is the art of using these oils to promote healing of the body

Box 12-1 Effects of Hydrotherapy Using Heat, Cold, and Ice Applications

Heat Applications

Effects

- Increased circulation
- Increased metabolism
- Increased inflammation
- Increased respiration
- Increased perspiration
- Decreased pain
- Decreased muscle spasm
- Decreased tissue stiffness
- Decreased white blood cell production

Hydrotherapy Uses

- *Sedation:* Water is a very efficient, nontoxic, calming substance. It soothes the body and promotes sleep.
  - *Techniques:* Use hot and warm baths to quiet and relax the entire body. Salt baths, neutral showers, or damp sheet packs can be used to relax certain areas.
- *Elimination:* The skin is the largest organ, and simple immersion in a long, hot bath or a session in a sauna or steam room can stimulate the excretion of toxins from the body through the skin. Inducing perspiration is useful in treating acute diseases and many chronic health problems.
  - *Techniques*: Use hot baths, Epsom salt or common salt baths, hot packs, dry blanket packs, and hot herbal drinks.
- *Antispasmodic:* Water effectively reduces cramps and muscle spasms.
  - *Techniques:* Use hot compresses (depending on the problem), herbal teas, and abdominal compresses.

Cold and Ice Applications

Effects

Cold

- Increased stimulation
- Increased muscle tone
- Increased tissue stiffness
- Increased white blood cell production
- Increased red blood cell production
- Decreased circulation (primary effect); increased circulation (secondary effect)
- Decreased inflammation
- Decreased pain
- Decreased respiration
- Decreased digestive processes

Ice

- Increased tissue stiffness
- Decreased circulation
- Decreased metabolism
- Decreased inflammation
- Decreased pain
- Decreased muscle spasm

Types of Applications

- Ice packs
- Ice immersion (ice water)
- Ice massage
- Cold whirlpool
- Chemical cold packs
- Cold gel packs (use with caution)

Contraindications to Ice

- Vasospastic disease (spasm of blood vessels)
- Cold hypersensitivity; signs include:
  - *Skin:* Itching, sweating
  - *Respiratory:* Hoarseness, sneezing, chest pain
  - *Gastrointestinal:* Abdominal pain, diarrhea, vomiting
  - *Eyes:* Puffy eyelids
  - *General:* Headache, discomfort, uneasiness
- Cardiac disorder
- Compromised local circulation

Precautions for Ice

- Do not apply frozen gel packs directly to the skin.
- Do not use ice applications (cryotherapy) for longer than 30 minutes continuously.
- Do not do exercises that cause pain after cold applications.
- Do not use cryotherapy on individuals with certain rheumatoid conditions or on those who are paralyzed or have coronary artery disease.

Hydrotherapy Uses

Ice is a primary therapy for strains, sprains, contusions, hematomas, and fractures. It has a numbing, anesthetic effect and helps control internal hemorrhage by reducing circulation to and metabolic processes within the area.

- *To restore and increase muscle strength and increase the body's resistance to disease:* Cold water boosts vigor, adds energy and tone, and aids digestion.
  - *Techniques:* Use cold water treading (standing or walking in cold water), whirlpool baths, cold sprays, alternate hot and cold contrast baths, showers and compresses, salt rubs, apple cider vinegar baths, and partial packs.
- *For injuries:* Application of an ice pack controls the flow of blood and reduces tissue swelling.
  - *Technique:* Use an ice bag in addition to compression and elevation.
- *For anesthesia:* Ice can dull the sense of pain or sensation.
  - *Technique:* Use ice to chill the tissue.
- For *minor burns:* Water, particularly cold water and ice water, has been rediscovered as a primary healing agent.
  - *Technique:* Use ice water immersion or saline water immersion.
- *To reduce fever:* Water is nature's best cooling agent. Unlike medications, which usually only diminish internal heat, water both lowers the temperature and removes heat by conduction.
  - *Technique:* Use ice bag applications at the base of the neck and on the forehead and feet; cold water sponge baths; and drinking cold water.

Modified from Fritz S: *Mosby's fundamentals of therapeutic massage,* ed 3, St Louis, 2004, Mosby.

and the mind. Aromatherapy combines well with massage.

The oils are found in different parts of the plant (e.g., the flowers, twigs, leaves, and bark) or in the rind of fruit. Because a large amount of plant material is required to produce an essential oil, pure essential oils are expensive. However, they also are highly effective; only a few drops at a time are required to achieve the desired effect. Essential oils are chemicals that interact with the body's physiology. Although their influence generally is subtle, care must be taken when using them. Specific therapeutic treatment should be provided only by a qualified aromatherapist.

Most essential oils are *volatile* (i.e., they evaporate quickly), and the molecules pass readily into the bloodstream. Essential oils have an immediate impact on the sense of smell. When they are inhaled, first the olfactory receptor cells and then the hypothalamus are stimulated, and the impulse is transmitted to the emotional center of the brain, the limbic system. Recent research has shown that the hypothalamus has both neurotransmitter and neuroendocrine activity. The hypothalamus, therefore, accesses both the nervous and endocrine systems. Researchers currently are tracing the hormones found in the hypothalamus to try to determine where they go in the body and what effects they have.

The limbic system is connected to areas of the brain linked to memory, breathing, and blood circulation, as well as to the endocrine glands, which regulate hormone levels in the body. The properties of each oil, its fragrance and effects, determine the stimulation of these systems. Also, the active chemicals in the oil are directly absorbed by the mucous membranes in the nose.

When used in massage, essential oils are not only inhaled but also absorbed through the skin. Upon absorption, they enter the bloodstream, where they are transported to the body's organs and systems. Essential oils have differing rates of absorption (generally 20 minutes to 2 hours). Therefore, to ensure maximum effectiveness, the patient should be advised not to bathe or shower directly after a session in which essential oils were applied.

Essential oils work in the body in a number of ways. They can influence fluid dynamics. They also can have antibacterial, antiviral, antifungal, antiinflammatory, analgesic (pain reducing), stimulating, or sedative effects. Just a few of the more common uses are as follows:

- If a patient has just added an exercise program or has increased the physical intensity of exercise and has delayed onset muscle soreness (a combination of inflammation and fluid retention), use German chamomile and juniper berry.
- If a patient has a bruise, use helichrysum.
- If a patient is fatigued but having trouble sleeping, use balsam fir and lavender.
- If a patient is getting a cold, use eucalyptus, tea tree, and thyme.
- If a patient feels achy and stiff, use black pepper and lemon grass.
- If a patient has a mild ankle sprain, use helichrysum, German chamomile, and rosemary.
- If a patient has aching joints (e.g., arthritis), use eucalyptus, lemongrass, and peppermint.
- If a patient has a headache, use peppermint and lavender.

If you do not know what to use, have the patient smell the oils and pick two or three favorites; then, mix those oils together. It is interesting to do this and then compare the properties of the oils with the patient's symptoms and outcome goals.

The essential oils presented in Table 12-1 have focused benefits for patients. They are reasonably safe when used in small amounts mixed into a carrier oil. Good carrier oils include high-quality olive oil and almond oil. The essential oil also can be mixed into melted food grade coconut oil. When the coconut oil solidifies, the result is somewhat like an ointment.

When purchasing essential oils, buy only pure, high-quality, therapeutic-grade products from well-known suppliers.

Typically, 10 drops of essential oil in 1 ounce of carrier oil is all that is necessary (some essential oils are used in even smaller amounts). It is best to blend no more than three essential oils together. Each ounce of carrier oil should have no more than 15 drops total of essential oil. Or mixed oil lasts for some time, because c amount is used at a time.

TABLE 12-1 Examples of Essential Oils and Their Uses

Essential Oil	Characteristics	Uses
Balsam fir	Fresh, balsamic aroma	Used to relieve muscle aches and pains; relieve anxiety and stress-related conditions; fight colds, flu, and infections; and relieve bronchitis and coughs.
Black pepper	Warm, peppery aroma	Used to energize; increase circulation; warm and relieve muscle aches and stiffness; and fight colds, flu, and infections. Use with care; only a small amount is required (3 to 5 drops in 1 ounce of carrier oil).
Eucalyptus	Strong camphoraceous aroma	Used for colds; as a decongestant to relieve asthma and fevers; for its bactericidal and antiviral actions; and to ease aching joints. Do not use if you or your patient have high blood pressure or epilepsy.
Geranium	Leafy, roselike scent	Used to reduce stress and tension; ease pain; balance emotions and hormones; ease premenstrual syndrome (PMS); relieve fatigue and nervous exhaustion; lift depression; and lessen fluid retention.
German chamomile	Strong, sweet, warm herbaceous aroma; blue in color; has many of the same properties as Roman chamomile, but its much higher azulene content gives it greater antiinflammatory activity	Used to relieve muscle pain; heal skin inflammation, acne, and wounds; also used as a sedative to ease anxiety and nervous tension and help with sleeplessness. It should not be used during early pregnancy and may cause skin reactions in some people. Before using, test a small area of skin (e.g., the medial ankle) for a reaction.
Helichrysum	Intense aroma resembling honey and tea	Used to heal bruises (internal and external), wounds, and scars; to detoxify the body, cleanse the blood, and increase lymphatic drainage; heal colds, flu, sinusitis, and bronchitis; relieve melancholy, migraines, stress, and tension.
Juniper berry	Fresh, pine needle aroma	Used to energize and relieve exhaustion; ease inflammation and spasms; improve mental clarity and memory; purify the body; lessen fluid retention; and disinfect. It should not be used in pregnant patients or those with kidney disease.
Lavender	Fresh, sweet scent	Used to balance emotions; relieve stress, tension, and headache; promote restful sleep; heal the skin; lower high blood pressure; help breathing; and disinfect.
Lemongrass	Powerful lemonlike aroma	Used to relieve muscle pain; ease headaches, nervous exhaustion, and other stress-related problems; and to increase circulation. Use with care; only a small amount is required (3 to 5 drops in 1 ounce of carrier oil). Do not use during pregnancy.
Peppermint	Sweet, minty aroma	Used to boost energy; brighten mood; reduce pain; help breathing; and improve mental clarity and memory. Skin test required, because it may irritate sensitive skin. Do not use during pregnancy.
Pine	Strong, coniferous, woodsy aroma	Used to ease breathing; as an immune system stimulant; to increase energy; and to relieve muscle and joint aches.
Rosemary	Camphoraceous aroma	Used to energize; relieve muscle pains, cramps, or sprains; brighten mood and improve mental clarity and memory; ease pain; relieve headaches; and disinfect. Do not use if you or your patient are pregnant, epileptic, or have high blood pressure.
Tea tree	Spicy, medicinal aroma; scientifically, one of the most extensively researched oils	Used as an immunostimulant, particularly against bacteria, viruses, and fungi; also used to relieve inflammation and to disinfect.
Thyme	Sweet, intense, medicinal herb aroma	Used to inhibit infectious diseases; treat colds and bronchitis; relieve muscle aches and pains; aid concentration and memory; and relieve fatigue.

Target the essential oil to the goals of the massage. The patient can use the mixed oil as a self-help measure. If you are in doubt about whether the patient's skin is sensitive to a particular oil, do a skin test on a small area (e.g., the medial ankle) to check for reactions.

Some essential oils are not safe for use in massage.

- *Oils that are not suitable for massage:* Cinnamon, clove, hyssop, and sage (and others).
- *Oils that should not be used during pregnancy:* Basil, clove, cinnamon, fennel, hyssop, juniper, lemongrass, marjoram, myrrh, peppermint, rosemary, sage, and white thyme (and others).
- *Oils that should not be used with steam:* Bay, clary sage, ginger, juniper, pine, and tea tree (and others).
- *Oils that are photosynthesizing:* Lemon, bergamot, lime, and orange (and others). The patient should be instructed to stay out of the sun for at least 2 hours after application of these oils to the skin.

These cautions apply to both the patient and therapist, because oils are absorbed not only through the skin, but also through the olfactory bulb and hypothalamus. If you use multiple oils during your massage work, be sure to ground and center yourself by going outside for fresh air, stretching, or drinking water before and after using the oils. Otherwise, the aromatic effects can distort your thinking, judgment, and sensations as a therapist.

VIBRATIONAL METHODS

Rescue Remedy

As mentioned previously, Rescue Remedy is a premixed flower essence combination that is specifically used for trauma. It is obvious why this preparation is appropriate for patients. Rescue Remedy can be applied as a first aid measure in emergencies of all kinds. The solution consists of the following flower essences:

- Star of Bethlehem (for shock)
- Rock rose (for acute fear and panic)
- Impatiens (for inner tension and stress)
- Cherry plum (for fear of breaking down and despair)
- Clematis (for the feeling of being "not completely here")

Rescue Remedy is appropriate for use in situations that appear threatening to an individual or that indeed might be life threatening. The proposed basis for this therapy is that a state of shock paralyzes the body's energy system, and as a result the conscious mind has a tendency to withdraw itself from the body or in extreme cases even to leave it. In such cases the body is left completely on its own and therefore is unable to activate self-healing energy. Rescue Remedy is said to remove the energy block very quickly, enabling the body's regulatory system to initiate the necessary measures for emergencies.

Rescue Remedy is very safe, because it is an energy interaction that is being held in the water molecules. One to four drops in a glass of water or water bottle cannot hurt and may help. If the patient does not want to take the remedy internally, it can be rubbed on the skin.

Homeopathic Remedies

Homeopathic remedies usually are prepared as small, sweet-tasting pellets that dissolve easily or as liquids or tablets. They are derived from natural substances (animal, vegetable, or mineral) that are listed in the homeopathic *Pharmacopoeia of the United States.*

Homeopathic remedies are created by obtaining the source in its most concentrated form and then, through a long process of dilution, preparing a remedy with a potency sufficient to effect a physiologic change by vibrational or energy means. The potency describes the measure of the dilution of the remedy and is denoted by the number that follows the name of the medicine itself. The higher the number, the greater the dilution (up to 1 part source to 1 trillion parts diluent) and the stronger the effect.

Because of the very, very small doses used, homeopathic remedies are safe and nonaddictive, and have no unwanted side effects.

These remedies cannot harm the patient and have the potential to be beneficial. They may do nothing, but they also could help. They are especially useful in the acute stages of illness and injury and before and after surgery. Combination homeopathic remedies for specific conditions also can be helpful. These can be found at health food stores and generally cost about $5 to $10 a bottle. Homeopathic treatment for specific conditions is a complex discipline, and referral to a qualified professional is necessary.

Arnica montana. Arnica montana is a natural homeopathic remedy that frequently is taken in oral pellet form to help reduce bruising and swelling. In addition to those effects, this homeopathic herb, which is grown in mountain regions, is said to help promote healing and reduce postoperative pain and discomfort. Arnica montana may also help prevent bruising and muscle fatigue.

PROBIOTICS

Many microbiologists and scientists are studying the effects of healthy living, which includes components such as organic foods, unrefined grains and sugar, and vitamin and mineral supplements. Gastrointestinal conditions are on the rise, as is the use of drugs to treat their symptoms. Probiotics can be found naturally in some foods such as yogurt and other milk products. Supplements are also available that carry a much larger amount in a smaller portion. When choosing a supplement, it is important to make sure the product contains live strains of bacteria.

MAGNETS

In general, magnets seem to help manage pain, especially acute pain. They also may support tissue healing. The results may simply be due to a placebo effect. However, if appropriate cautions are followed, these therapies are safe and noninvasive. The following information is presented to help the massage therapist educate the patient. No research is available indicating that expensive specialty magnets work any better than inexpensive ones. However, care must be taken not to drop them, which can demagnetize them.

Magnet applications are similar to those for ice or heat; that is, they are applied for about 20 minutes 2 or 3 times a day. They also can be strapped, taped, or wrapped on the body for extended use.

Magnet power is measured in *gauss* (g), the line of force per unit area of the pole. A magnet's gauss rating determines the speed at which it works, and the thickness determines the depth of penetration. The earth's surface is approximately 0.5 gauss. Many manufacturers rate their products using internal gauss and external gauss to indicate strength. Typical classifications of magnetic strength are as follows:

Low gauss: 300 to 700 g
Medium gauss: 1000 to 2500 g
High gauss: 3000 to 6000 g
Super gauss: 7000 to 12,000 g

The *surface gauss rating* refers to the external strength of the magnet. This value depends on the size, shape, polarity, and grade of the magnetic material. Some experts in magnet therapy begin treatment at low gauss and gradually increase strength as necessary.

Some companies list their products by internal gauss and others use the external gauss rating. To determine the proper gauss strength, a quick rule of thumb can be stated in equation form as follows:

$$\text{External gauss rating} \times 3.9 \text{ (approximate)} = \text{Internal gauss rating}$$

For example, an external gauss rating of 800 g is appropriate. Thus:

$$800 \times 3.9 = 3120 \text{ (approximate)}$$

Therefore a magnet with an external gauss rating of 800 g has an approximate internal gauss rating of 3120 g. If the internal gauss rating is used, do not be misled into believing you are getting a higher strength product; both ratings are correct for the same magnet.

There are about as many types of magnets as there are body parts. Magnetic mattresses and pads are designed to be slept on; magnetic insoles fit inside shoes; block magnets can be placed under mattresses, pillows, or seat cushions; and some types of back supports have slots for inserting magnets. Magnets are also available as body wraps with Velcro-type closures, jewelry, and magnetic foil.

Most magnets are made of ferrites, which are iron oxides combined with cobalt, nickel, barium, and other metals to make a ceramic-like material. Flexible magnets are combined with plastic, rubber, or other pliable materials. The strongest magnets are made of neodymium, a rare earth element.

Claims of magnets' therapeutic effects should still be regarded with considerable skepticism. Most of the testimonials to the effectiveness of magnetic therapy can be attributed to the placebo effect and to other effects that derive secondarily from the use of magnets. For example, magnetic back braces may help ease back pain by providing mechanical support, warmth, and a constant reminder not to overexert the muscles. All these effects are helpful, with or without magnets.

Most valid research has not found the use of magnets to be beneficial. One highly publicized exception is a double-blind study done at Baylor College of Medicine, which compared the effects of magnets and sham magnets on the knee pain of 50 postpolio patients. The experimental group reported a significantly greater reduction in pain than the control group. No replication of these results has been done, but the Baylor study raises the possibility that at least in some cases, topical application of magnets may indeed be useful for pain relief. A controversial theory, which has not been proven scientifically, suggests that magnets do not heal, but rather stimulate the body to heal naturally.

An important aspect of magnetic therapy is magnet polarity and its influences (Box 12-2). This relates to the direction in which the magnet is placed. The north pole corresponds to yin, or negative polarity. The south pole corresponds to yang, or positive polarity.

If the body appears to lack both positive and negative energies to heal, two magnets can be used to apply the north and south poles simultaneously (i.e., bipolar magnet therapy). Bipolar magnet therapy may be used to heal fractures or to treat chronic pain. Unipolar magnets also are available for cases in which use of a particular pole is not required. However, these types of magnets tend to be more expensive. When in doubt, use the north pole.

As with any treatment, cautionary measures must be followed in magnetic therapy. Magnets should not be used during pregnancy; on patients who have internal bleeding, a history of epilepsy, or who are taking blood-thinning medications; or on bleeding wounds. Magnets should *never* be used on a patient who has a pacemaker or metal implants that could be dislodged by the magnet. Also, many patients have had broken bones that are pinned or screwed together. Do not use magnets on these areas.

BOX 12-2 Use of the North and South Poles in Magnetic Therapy

Important Factors	North Pole	South Pole
Characteristics	Sedating, cooling, negative polarity (yin)	Stimulating, heating, positive polarity (yang)
Conditions treated	Acute headaches, arthritis, bursitis, fractures, inflammation, low back pain, sharp pain, tendinitis	Fibrosis, numbness, paralysis, scars, tingling, weak muscles

evolve 12-1

The following terms and expressions specific to Chapter 12 have already been used to search PubMed for the latest research literature available. The *Click Here for Massage* feature associated with this chapter on your textbook's Evolve website allows you to hyperlink to a continually updated PubMed search of research literature that corresponds to this subject.

Hyperlink Search Terms
Massage and magnets
Massage and aromatherapy
Massage and essential oils
Massage and probiotics

SUMMARY

Massage therapists need to remain open minded and supportive of each patient's unique path to health, while at the same time exercising caution with regard to products that are harmful or that could interfere with other medical treatments. It is also necessary to be flexible when addressing unique circumstances.

From an ethical standpoint, it probably is not the best professional practice to sell these products to patients, because the potential for conflict and dual roles is too great. The products are easily obtained, and patients can find and purchase them on their own.

Essential oils can be mixed and given to a patient as a self-help measure. Massage therapists should never sell these to the patient; rather, they should be incorporated into the therapeutic massage application.

WORKBOOK

1. Describe a situation in which you might use or recommend each of the following:

 a. Cold hydrotherapy

 b. Warm hydrotherapy

 c. Hot and cold contrast hydrotherapy

 d. Epsom salts soak

 e. Aromatherapy

 f. Rescue Remedy

 g. Arnica montana

 h. North pole magnetic therapy

 i. South pole magnetic therapy

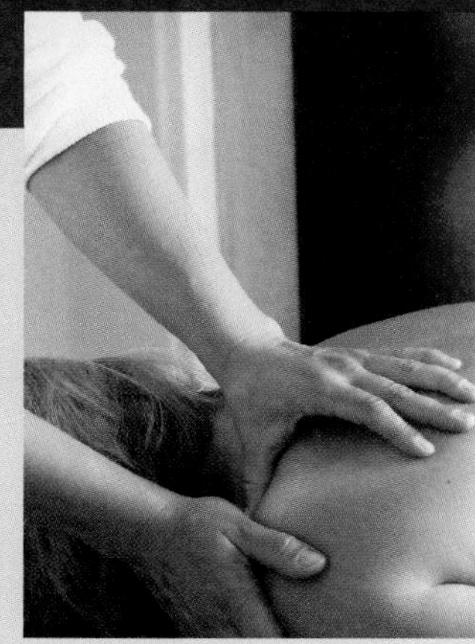

UNIT TWO REFERENCES

Academy of Traditional Chinese Medicine: *An outline of Chinese acupuncture,* Beijing, 1975, Foreign Languages Press.

Adams KE, Cohen MH, Eisenberg D et al: Ethical considerations of complementary and alternative medical therapies in conventional medical settings, *Ann Intern Med* 137: 660-664, 2002.

Ahluwalia S: Distribution of smooth muscle acting-containing cells in the human meniscus, *J Orthopaed Res* 19:659-664, 2001.

American Association of Naturopathic Physicians: *Naturopathic medicine: What it is. What it can do for you!* Seattle, Washington, 1998, The Association.

American Massage Therapy Association: *Demand for massage therapy,* Evanston, Ill, 2002, The Association.

American Psychiatric Association: *Diagnostic and statistical manual of mental disorders,* ed 4, DSM-IV, Washington, DC, 1994, The Association.

Aourell M, Skoog M, Carleson J: Effects of Swedish massage on blood pressure, School of Physiotherapy, Karolinska Institutet, Novum, S-171 76, Stockholm, Sweden, *Complement Ther Clin Pract* 11:242-246, 2005.

Associated Bodywork and Massage Professionals: *Thinking about career options,* Evergreen, Colo, 1999, Associated Bodywork and Massage Professionals.

Astin JA: Why patients use alternative medicine: results of a national study, *JAMA* 279: 1548-1553, 1998.

Baechle TR, Roger WE: *Essentials of strength and conditioning,* ed 2, Champaign, Ill, 2000, Human Kinetics.

Bandy WD, Irion JM, Briggler M: The effect of time and frequency of static stretching on flexibility of the hamstring muscles, *Phys Ther* 77:1090-1096, 1997.

Barnes P, Powell-Griner E, McFann K, Nahin R: Complementary and alternative medicine use among adults: United States, 2002, *CDC Advance Data Report #343,* 2004.

Benford MS: Radiogenic metabolism: an alternative cellular energy source, *Med Hypotheses* 56:33-39, 2001.

Bensky D, Gamble A: *Chinese herbal medicine: materia medica,* Seattle, 1993, Eastland Press.

Brostoff J: *Complete guide to food allergy,* Bloomsbury, London, 1992.

Brucini M, et al: Pain thresholds and EMG features of periarticular muscles in patients with osteoarthritis of the knee, *Pain* 10: 57-66, 1982.

Cafarelli E, Flint F: The role of massage in preparation for and recovery from exercise, *Sports Med* 14:1-9, 1992.

Cambron JA, Dexheimer J, Coe P: Changes in blood pressure after various forms of therapeutic massage: a preliminary study, *J Altern Complement Med* 12:65-70, 2006.

Cantu RI, Grodin AJ: *Myofascial manipulation: theory and clinical application,* New York, 2001, Aspen.

Cash M: *Sport and remedial massage therapy*, New York, 1996, Random House.

Chaitow L: *Cranial manipulation theory and practice: osseous and soft tissue approaches,* London, 1999, Churchill Livingstone.

Chaitow L: *Fibromyalgia syndrome: a practitioner's guide to treatment,* London, 2000, Churchill Livingstone.

Chaitow L: *Muscle energy techniques,* ed 2, New York, 2001, Churchill Livingstone.

Chaitow L: *Modern neuromuscular technique,* ed 2, Edinburgh, 2003, Churchill Livingstone.

Chaitow L, Bradley D, Gilbert C: *Multidisciplinary approaches to breathing pattern disorders,* Edinburgh, 2002, Churchill Livingstone.

Cherkin DC, Deyo RA, Sherman KJ et al: Characteristics of visits to licensed acupuncturists, chiropractors, massage therapists, and naturopathic physicians, *J Am Board Fam Pract* 15:463-472, 2002.

Cherkin D, Sherman K, Deyo R et al: A review of the evidence for the effectiveness, safety, and cost of acupuncture, massage therapy, and spinal manipulation for back pain, *Ann Intern Med* 138:898-906, 2003.

Chikly B: *Silent waves: theory and practice of lymph drainage therapy, with applications,* Scottsdale, Ariz, 2001, IHH Publishing.

Chlan L: Music intervention. In Snyder M, Lindquist R, editors: *Complementary/alternative therapies in nursing,* ed 4, New York, 2001, Springer.

Clews W: Making muscles malleable, *Sport Health* 14:32-33, 1996a.

Clews W: Where does massage draw the line? *Sport Health* 11:20-21, 1996b.

Cohen MH: *Complementary and alternative medicine: legal boundaries and regulatory perspectives,* Baltimore, 1998, Johns Hopkins University Press.

Cohen MH: *Beyond complementary medicine: legal and ethical perspectives on health care and human evolution,* Ann Arbor, Mich, 2000, University of Michigan Press.

Cohen MH, Eisenberg DM: Potential physician malpractice liability associated with complementary and integrative medical therapies, *Ann Intern Med* 136:596-603, 2002.

Colby LA, Kisner C: *Therapeutic exercise: foundations and techniques,* ed 4, Philadelphia, 2002, FA Davis.

Commerford M, Mottram S: Movement and stability dysfunction: contemporary developments, *Man Ther* 6:15-26, 2001.

Commerford M, Mottram S: Functional stability retraining: principles and strategies for managing mechanical dysfunction, *Man Ther* 6: 3-14, 2001.

Coombes J, Powers S, Hamilton K et al: Exercise intensity and longevity in men: the Harvard Alumni Health Study, *JAMA* 273: 1179-1184, 1995.

Cooper RA, Stoflet SJ: Trends in the education and practice of alternative medicine clinicians, *Health Aff (Millwood)* 15:226-238, 1996.

Cucherat M, Haugh MC, Gooch M et al: Evidence of clinical efficacy of homeopathy: a meta-analysis of clinical trials, Homeopathic Medicines Research Advisory Group, *Eur J Clin Pharmacol* 56:27-33, 2000.

Drug Facts and Comparisons, St Louis, 1999, Mosby.

Druss BG, Rosenheck RA: Association between use of unconventional therapies and conventional medical services, *JAMA* 282:651-656, 1999.

Eisenberg DM, Davis RB, Ettner SL et al: Trends in alternative medicine use in the United States, 1990-1997: results of a follow-up national survey, *JAMA* 280:1569-1575, 1998.

Emoto M: Healing with water, *J Altern Complement Med* 10:19-21, 2004.

Ernst E: Complementary and alternative medicine in rheumatology, *Baillieres Best Pract Res Clin Rheumatol* 14:731-749, 2000.

Field T, Hernandez-Reif M, Diego M et al: Cortisol decreases and serotonin and dopamine increase following massage therapy, *Int J Neurosci* 115:1397-1413, 2005.

Fritz S: *Fundamentals of therapeutic massage,* ed 3, St Louis, 2004, Mosby.

Fryer G, Hodgson L: The effect of manual pressure release on myofascial trigger points in the upper trapezius muscle, *J Bodywork Move Ther* (in press).

Goertz CH, Grimm RH, Svendsen K et al: Treatment of Hypertension with Alternative Therapies (THAT) Study: a randomized clinical trial, *J Hypertens* 20:2063-2068, 2002.

Greenman P: *Principles of manual medicine,* ed 3, Baltimore, 2003, Williams & Wilkins.

Greenman TW, Flynn PE: *Thoracic spine and rib cage: musculoskeletal evaluation and treatment,* Oxford, 1996, Butterworth-Heinemann.

Gunn C: *Bones and joints,* ed 4, New York, 2002, Churchill Livingstone.

Hardy ML: Research in Ayurveda: where do we go from here? *Altern Ther Health Med* 7: 34-35, 2001.

Hastreiter D, Ozuna RM, Spector M: Regional variations in certain cellular characteristics in human lumbar intervertebral discs, including the presence of smooth muscle actin, *J Orthop Res* 19:597-604, 2001.

Hendrickson T: *Massage for orthopedic conditions,* Philadelphia, 2002, Lippincott Williams & Wilkins.

Hondras MA, Linde K, Jones AP: Manual therapy for asthma. Cochrane Database of Systematic Reviews, CD001002. Accessed April 30, 2004, at www.cochrane.org

Janda V: Muscles, central nervous motor regulation, and back problems. In Korr IM, editor: Neurobiologic mechanisms in manipulative therapy, New York, 1978, Plenum Press.

Keen J, et al: *Mosby's critical care and emergency medication reference,* ed 2, St Louis, 1996, Mosby.

Keer R, Grahame R: *Hypermobility syndrome,* Edinburgh, 2003, Butterworth-Heinemann.

Kemper KJ, Kelly EA: Treating children with therapeutic and healing touch, *Pediatr Ann* 33:248-252, 2004.

Kleijnen J, Knipschild P, ter Riet G: Clinical trials of homeopathy, *Br Med J* 302:316-323, 1991.

Kshettry VR, Carole LF, Henly SJ et al: Abbott Northwestern Hospital, Minneapolis Heart Institute Foundation, Minneapolis, Minnesota, USA.

Leake R, Broderick JE: Current licensure for acupuncture in the United States, *Altern Ther Health Med* 5:94-96, 1999.

Lederman E: *Fundamentals of manual therapy physiology, neurology, and psychology,* New York, 1997, Churchill Livingstone.

Lee BY, LaRiccia PJ, Newberg AB: Acupuncture in theory and practice, *Hosp Physician* 40: 11-18, 2004.

Lin YC, Lee AC, Kemper KJ, Berde CB: Use of complementary and alternative medicine in pediatric pain management service: a survey, *Pain Med* 6:452-458, 2005.

Linde K, Clausius N, Ramirez G et al: Are the clinical effects of homeopathy placebo effects? A meta-analysis of placebo-controlled trials, *Lancet* 350:834-843, 1997.

Linde K, Hondras M, Vickers A et al: Systematic reviews of complementary therapies: an annotated bibliography. Part 3. Homeopathy, *BMC Complement Altern Med* 1:4, 2001.

Logani MK, Bhanushali A, Anga A et al: Combined millimeter wave and cyclophosphamide therapy of an experimental murine melanoma, *Bioelectromagnetics* 25:516, 2004.

Lund I, Yu LC, Uvnas-Moberg K et al: Repeated massage-like stimulation induces long-term effects on nociception: contribution of oxytocinergic mechanisms, *Eur J Neurosci* 16: 330-338, 2002.

Luskin FM, Newell KA, Griffith M et al: A review of mind/body therapies in the treatment of musculoskeletal disorders with implications for the elderly, *Altern Ther Health Med* 6: 46-56, 2000.

Maitland G: *Maitland's vertebral manipulation,* ed 6, Oxford, 2001, Butterworth-Heinemann.

Martiny K, Simonsen C, Lunde M et al: Decreasing TSH levels in patients with seasonal affective disorder (SAD) responding to 1 week of bright light therapy, *J Affect Dis* 79:253-257, 2004.

Mathie RT: The research evidence base for homeopathy: a fresh assessment of the literature, *Homeopathy* 92:84-91, 2003.

McCaffery M, Pasero C: *Pain: a clinical manual,* ed 2, St Louis, 1999, Mosby.

Meeker WC, Haldeman S: Chiropractic: a profession at the crossroads of mainstream and alternative medicine, *Ann Intern Med* 136:216-227, 2002.

Miles R, Traub RD, Wong RKS: Spread of synchronous firing in longitudinal slices from the CA3 region of the hippocampus, *J Neurophysiol* 60:1481-1496, 1995.

Milgrom LR: Vitalism, complexity and the concept of spin, *Homeopathy* 91:26-31, 2002.

Mitchell BB: *Acupuncture and Oriental medicine laws,* Gig Harbor, Wash, 1999, National Acupuncture Foundation.

National Center for Complementary and Alternative Medicine (NCCAM): Manipulative and body-based practices: an overview. Publication No. D238. Accessed August, 2005, at nccam.nih.gov

National Certification Commission for Acupuncture and Oriental Medicine (NCCAOM): NCCAOM certification programs. Accessed October 28, 2002, at www.nccaom.org

National Institutes of Health Consensus Panel: Acupuncture: National Institutes of Health consensus development statement. Accessed April 30, 2004, at odp.od.nih.gov/consensus/cons/107/107_statement.htm

Ni H, Simile C, Hardy AM: Utilization of complementary and alternative medicine by United States adults: results from the 1999 National Health Interview Survey, *Med Care* 40:353-358, 2002.

Olney CM: The effect of therapeutic back massage in hypertensive persons: a preliminary study, *Biol Res Nurs* 7:98-105, 2005.

Oschman JL: *Energy medicine: the scientific basis of bioenergy therapies,* Philadelphia, 2000, Churchill Livingstone.

Palinkas LA, Kabongo ML: The use of complementary and alternative medicine by primary care patients: a SURF*NET study, *J Fam Pract* 49:1121-1130, 2000.

Polgar S, Thomas SA: *Introduction to research in the health sciences,* ed 4, London, 2001, Churchill Livingstone.

Reddy GK: Photobiological basis and clinical role of low-intensity lasers in biology and medicine, *J Clin Laser Med Surg* 22:141-150, 2004.

Rojavin MA, Ziskin MC: Medical application of millimetre waves, *QJM* 91:57-66, 1998.

Russek L, Schwartz G: Energy cardiology: a dynamical energy systems approach for integrating conventional and alternative medicine, *Adv J Mind-Body Health* 12:4-24, 1996.

Sancier KM, Holman D: Commentary: multifaceted health benefits of medical qigong, *J Altern Complement Med* 10:163-165, 2004.

Sisken BF, Walder J: Therapeutic aspects of electromagnetic fields for soft tissue healing. In Blank M editor: *Electromagnetic fields: biological interactions and mechanisms,* Washington, DC, 1995, American Chemical Society.

Smith MJ, Logan AC: Naturopathy, *Med Clin N Am* 86:173-184, 2002.

Szabo I, Manning MR, Radzievsky AA et al: Low power millimeter wave irradiation exerts no harmful effect on human keratinocytes in vitro, *Bioelectromagnetics* 24:165-173, 2003.

Tiller WA, Dibble WE Jr, Nunley R et al: Toward general experimentation and discovery in conditioned laboratory spaces. I. Experimental pH change findings at some remote sites, *J Altern Complement Med* 10:145-157, 2004.

United Kingdom Parliament, House of Lords Select Committee on Science and Technology: Sixth report: complementary and alternative medicine. Accessed October 28, 2002, at www.parliament.the-stationery-office.co.uk/pa/Id199900/Idselect/Idsctech/123/12301/htm

Vibhu A: Complementary alternative medical therapies for heart surgery patients: feasibility, safety, and impact, *Thoracic Surg* 81: 201-205, 2006.

Wieting JM, Cugalj AP, Kaplan RJ et al: Massage, traction, and manipulation. Accessed August, 2005, at www.eMedicine.com

Williams AL, Selwyn PA, Liberti L et al: A randomized controlled trial of meditation and massage effects on quality of life in people with late-stage disease: a pilot study, *J Palliat Med* 8:939-952, 2005.

Winstead-Fry P, Kijek J: An integrative review and meta-analysis of therapeutic touch research, *Altern Ther Health Med* 5:58-67, 1999.

Yahia LH, Pigeon P, DesRosiers EA: Viscoelastic properties of the human lumbodorsal fascia, *J Biomed Eng* 15:425-429, 1993.

Yates J: *A physician's guide to therapeutic massage,* ed 3, Toronto, 2004, Curties-Overzet.

Zimmerman J: Laying-on-of-hands healing and therapeutic touch: a testable theory, *BEMI Currents* 2:8-17, 1990.

Additional Resources

Agency for Health Care Policy and Research (AHCPR)
http://www.ahcpr.gov

American Academy of Orthopedic Surgeons
6300 North River Road
Rosemont, Illinois 60018-4262
www.aaos.org
Telephone: 847-823-7186; 800-346-2267
Fax: 847-823-8026
e-mail: julitz@mac.aaos.org

American Academy of Physical Medicine and Rehabilitation*
One IBM Plaza, Suite 2500
Chicago, Illinois 60611-3604
www.aapmr.org
Telephone: 312-464-9700
Fax: 312-464-0227
e-mail: info@aapmr.org

American Heart Association Biostatistical Fact Sheets http://americanheart.org/statistics/biostats/index.html

American Physical Therapy Association
1111 North Fairfax Street
Alexandria, Virginia 22314-1488
www.apta.org
Telephone: 703-684-2782; 800-999-2782 ext 3395 Service Center

Arthritis Foundation
P.O. Box 7669
Atlanta, Georgia 30357-0669
Telephone: 404-872-7100 (or call your local chapter)
www.arthritis.org

Congenital Heart Information Network
www.tchin.org/

CPR You can do it!
http://depts.washington.edu/learncpr/pocket.html

Heart Failure Online
www.heartfailure.org

Life and Health Insurance Foundation for Education
http://www.life-line.org

Mayo Clinic
www.mayoclinic.org/healthinfo

National Center for Complementary and Alternative Medicine (NCCAM) Clearinghouse
NCCAM Clearinghouse provides information on complementary and alternative medicine and NCCAM, including publications and searches of federal databases of scientific and medical literature. It does not provide medical advice, treatment recommendations, or referrals to practitioners.
nccam.nih.gov
e-mail: info@nccam.nih.gov

Occupational Safety and Health Administration
www.OSHA.gov

Open the Door to a Healthy Heart
www.healthyfridge.org

The Heart: Online Exploration
http://www.fi.edu/learn/heart/index.html

Touch Research Institute
University of Miami School of Medicine
Miami, Florida 33101

Universal College of Reflexology
www.universalreflex.com

WebMD
www.webmd.com

Wikipedia
en.wikipedia.org/wiki/Medication
You've had a heart attack—what now? http://staff.washington.edu/bmperra/heart-help.html

http://www.healthtouch.com

www.medicationwizard.com
http:www.revolutionhealth.com

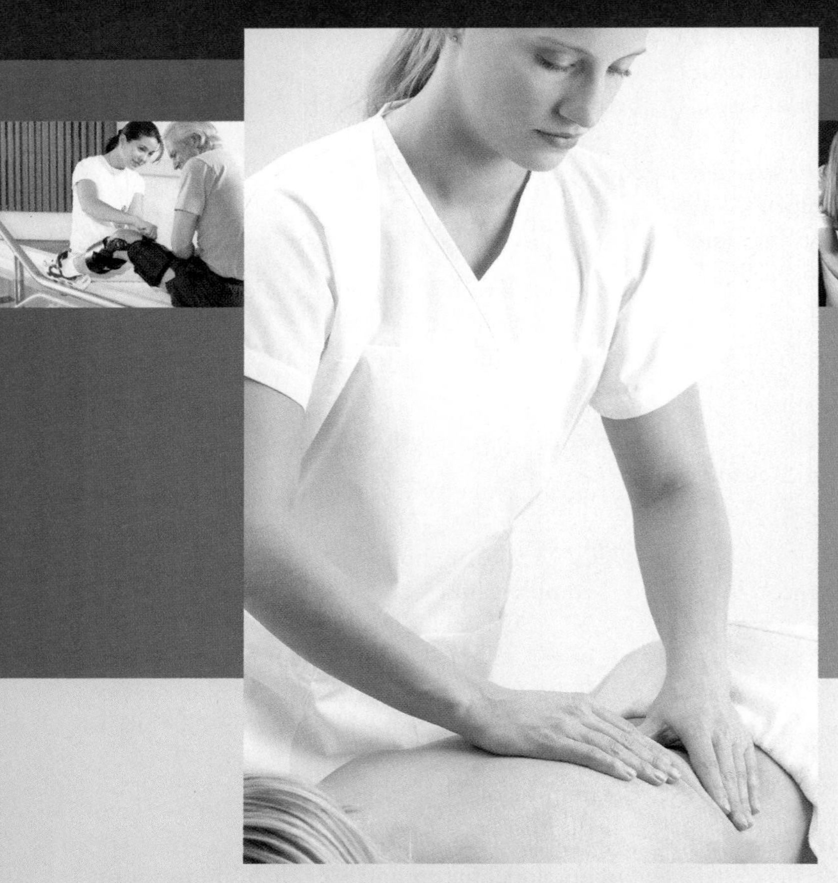

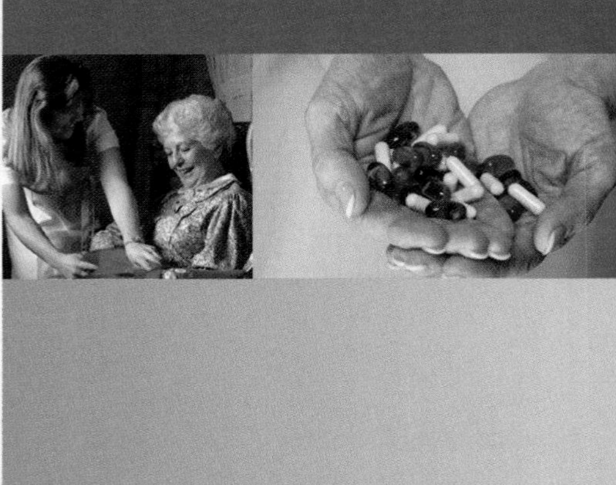

13 *Overview of the Illness and Injury Processes, 452*

14 *General Massage Treatment for Predisposing and Perpetuating Factors and Symptom Management, 472*

15 *Medical Treatment for Illness and Injury, 514*

16 *Population Similarities in Healthcare, 534*

17 *Common Categories of Illness and Injury and the Clinical Reasoning Process, 594*

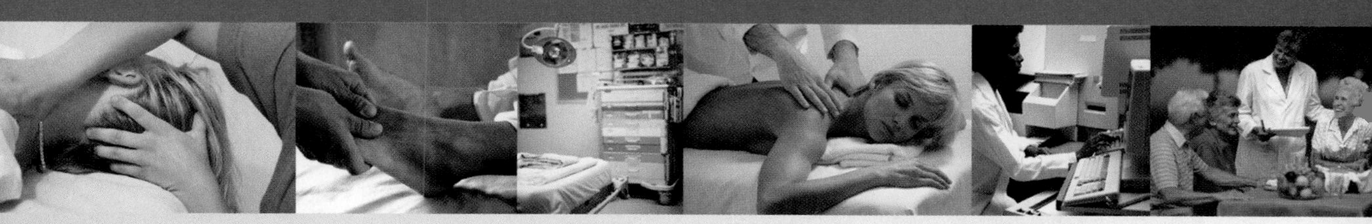

Unit Three

MASSAGE APPLICATION FOR SPECIFIC HEALTHCARE OUTCOMES

This unit describes massage application to address specific healthcare outcomes. This task is difficult both to write and to learn. The material in Unit One is relatively concrete; that is, how the healthcare system is organized and how massage therapy is integrated into it. Because of the ever-changing nature of healthcare, the information in Unit One will evolve; however, current trends seem predictable enough to allow the information to be presented with confidence. Unit Two is all about massage, and this information also is relatively uniform these days. Some controversy and differences in opinion remain, especially about terminology and body mechanics, but the Unit Two content is relatively standardized. This third unit is much more abstract and has elements of the author's experiences integrated with the more factual data about the various health conditions.

The content of this unit is presented in four ways:

- By outcomes (e.g., pain management, increased mobility, scar tissue management, and support of restorative sleep)
- By client population (e.g., mental health, pediatrics, geriatrics, obstetrics, end-of-life care, and hospice)
- By general classification of disease categories (e.g., infection; musculoskeletal, autoimmune, and cardiovascular diseases; and cancer)
- By pathologic conditions of each body system

The Evolve site expands on much of the material covered in this unit and should be used in conjunction with the textbook. The intent of this unit is to teach the student how to sort through information to make justifiable clinical decisions. This is sometimes a messy process, which eventually leads to a concise plan. Therefore although the unit's organization may seem a bit disjointed, it ultimately will help lead you to effective thinking.

The process of research for factual data for this book was extensive, and many resources have been consulted and compiled. Many of the resources consulted provided the same information in a number of ways. At least five sources were consulted and the data compared. The data that emerged consistently in these sources were compiled for this text. Only information that was found in multiple sources was included in this text, to ensure that the information is valid.

Chapter 13 Concept Map

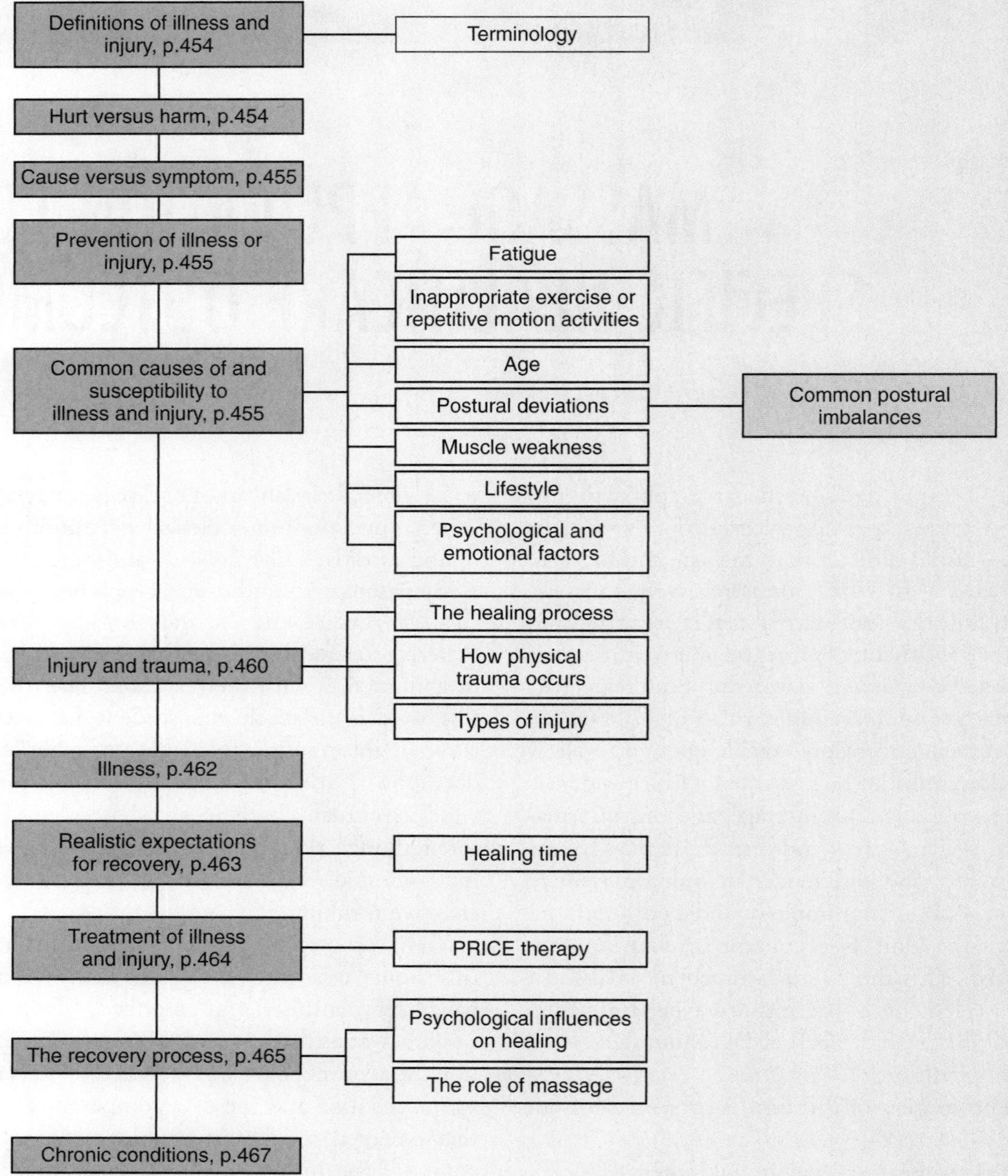

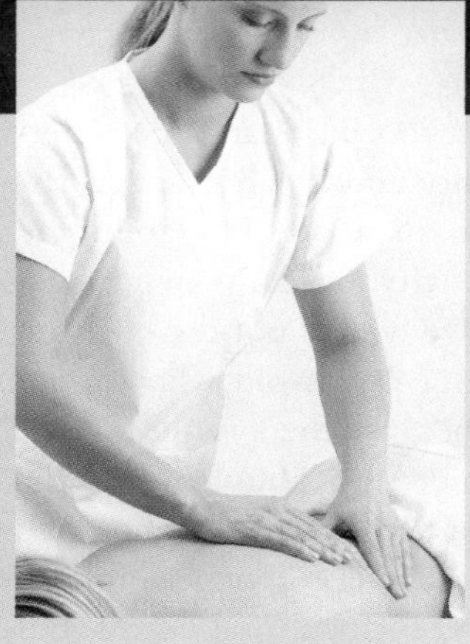

CHAPTER 13

OVERVIEW OF THE ILLNESS AND INJURY PROCESSES

Key Terms

Acute illness
Acute injury
Acute reinjury of a chronic condition or earlier trauma
Cause
Chronic condition
Chronic or overuse trauma
Disability
Deformation
Direct trauma
Force
Handicap
Hardiness
Harm
Hurt
Illness
Indirect trauma
Injury
Internal response
Load
Mechanical stress
Mental/emotional trauma
Nonsteroidal antiinflammatory drugs (NSAIDs)
Pathomechanics
Physical trauma
Protection, rest, ice, compression, and elevation (PRICE)
Repetitive injury
Resistance
Risk factors
Secondary gain
Symptom
Trauma
Traumatic injury
Yield point

For definitions of key terms, refer to the Evolve website.

OBJECTIVES

Upon completion of this chapter, the reader will have the information necessary to:

1. Identify the risk factors for illness and injury.
2. List the common causes of physical activity injuries.
3. List strategies for preventing illness and injury.
4. Define trauma.
5. List the three phases of healing and relate them to massage application.
6. Describe acute and chronic inflammation and relate the inflammation process to the three stages of healing.
7. Define illness.
8. Estimate the general healing time for various injuries and illnesses.
9. Explain and perform PRICE therapy.
10. Devise effective massage strategies to support the recovery process during the acute, subacute, and remodeling phases of healing.
11. Explain the basic etiology of chronic illness.
12. Explain the difference between acute and chronic illness.
13. Develop realistic expectations for working with people who have a chronic illness.

This first chapter in Unit Three presents an overview of the processes of illness and injury. It discusses a number of factors, including common causes of and susceptibility to illness and injury, trauma, assessment of illness and injury, types of illness, general categories of treatment, the phases of healing, realistic expectations for recovery, the recovery process, and chronic illness and pain. As a massage therapist, you need to understand why some people are susceptible to the development of a pathologic condition. You also must have some knowledge of the nature of healing and recovery, and of maintenance in chronic conditions. Armed with this knowledge, you will be better able to anticipate the course of an illness or injury and to identify realistic outcomes and time frames for massage intervention.

DEFINITIONS OF ILLNESS AND INJURY

Illness is different from injury. In general, **illness** involves the whole body, whereas **injury** is a more localized condition. Various illnesses can target a body system. For example, a cold is an upper respiratory inflection. This is different from a localized bruise on the quadriceps, which is an injury. Illness occurs as a dysfunction of the immune response. It can be caused by infectious organisms (bacteria, viruses, or fungi); illness results because the immune system is unable to stop the progression of invasion. Illness often is the result of a flawed autoimmune response or an overreaction of the immune response (e.g., allergies, multiple sclerosis). Illness also can be caused by failure of a body system (e.g., cardiovascular disease, kidney failure, diabetes).

TERMINOLOGY

For purposes of describing a person who has an illness or injury, the current terminology stresses the individual and then mentions the condition (e.g., an individual with chronic fatigue syndrome [CSF], a person who has hepatitis). This language clearly acknowledges that the person is much more than simply the illness or injury.

It also is important to understand the difference between a disability and a handicap. A **disability** is a restriction in a person's ability to perform a normal activity of daily living that someone of the same age who is not disabled can perform. For example, a 3-year-old who cannot walk has a disability, because the average 3-year-old can walk independently. **Handicap** is the term used to describe a person who, because of a disability, is unable to achieve a typical role in society based on age and sociocultural norms. For example, a 16-year-old who cannot prepare meals or perform personal toileting or hygiene routines is handicapped. On the other hand, a 16-year-old who can walk only with the assistance of crutches but who attends a regular school and is fully independent in activities of daily living is disabled, not handicapped.

All disabled individuals are impaired, and all handicapped people are disabled. However, a person can be impaired but not disabled, and an individual can be disabled without being handicapped. In the past, the general public and even literature have shown a disturbing lack of awareness and sensitivity about the terminology used to discuss people with disabilities. Fortunately, increasing attention is being paid to the use of respectful language for these members of our society.

HURT VERSUS HARM

People should listen to their bodies. Pain is a warning sign of illness or injury. The difference between hurt and harm is important. Lots of things can cause pain **(hurt),** but they do not **harm** (i.e., cause damage). Although pain is a very important warning sign of harm, pain itself does not cause harm. Dealing with pain is stressful, which can be harmful. However, it is the stress response and not the pain sensation (hurt) that harms. An awareness of this distinction is extremely important for patients with chronic pain. It also is important for those who are in rehabilitation or who require medical treatment, in which the process may very well be painful but is targeted to help, not harm.

CAUSE VERSUS SYMPTOM

The **cause** of an illness or injury may be any of a number of factors, such as a person's lifestyle, an event or activity, organ system dysfunction, immune disruption, or pathogenic invasion. A **symptom** is the effect the person experiences in response to the cause (e.g., pain, fatigue, bruising, stiffness, anxiety).

Healthcare intervention is most effective when the cause can be altered, eliminating the reason for the symptoms, and symptoms can be treated effectively until the person is cured (i.e., the cause is eliminated). Causes can harm. Symptoms can be distressing, painful, and a cause of suffering, but they tend not to be a direct cause of harm. However, symptoms drive people to seek treatment. Many health conditions cannot be cured; instead, they are managed. Management involves slowing the degenerative progression, supporting self-regulating mechanisms, and managing symptoms.

Massage therapy is best at managing symptoms and supporting self-regulating and healing mechanisms. Unlike surgery and some medications, massage seldom is curative. But that's okay. The massage profession is uniquely positioned to alleviate suffering by managing symptoms. It is a wonderful gift we give.

PREVENTION OF ILLNESS OR INJURY

Prevention is important. A person who is not fit is more likely to develop an illness or sustain an injury. Being fit really means choosing a healthy lifestyle, in which a person can express emotions effectively, maintain good relationships with others, and be confident about decision-making abilities, ethics, values, and spirituality. Paying attention to the elements of a healthy lifestyle (e.g., physical fitness, good nutrition, stress management, control of alcohol consumption, avoidance of drug abuse, smoking cessation, and weight management) helps prevent illness and injury (Figure 13-1).

COMMON CAUSES OF AND SUSCEPTIBILITY TO ILLNESS AND INJURY

A massage therapist who wants to work with ill or injured patients or those in rehabilitation first must understand the different **risk factors** that can lead to illness or injury.

FATIGUE

A person who is tired is less attentive to his or her surroundings and more apt to have an accident. Fatigue also strains the adaptive responses and suppresses the immune system.

INAPPROPRIATE EXERCISE OR REPETITIVE MOTION ACTIVITIES

Common causes of musculoskeletal injury are nonoptimal movement strategies, excessive exercise or lack of fitness-based exercise, and repetitive movement. Repetitive movement injury is a common cause of employment-related disability.

AGE

Those most vulnerable to illness and injury are the very young and the very old. These extremes of age are marked by less efficient homeostatic and immune function. Adolescents and the middle aged are also vulnerable, but illness or injury in these individuals more often is the result of strain on the body caused by hormonal changes and the pressure of daily life.

The aging process alters the metabolic processes involved in recovery after activity. Tendons become less well lubricated and therefore are more prone to damage. Repetitive movement over time can cause wear and tear on the joints. Older patients basically need to put more effort into helping the natural recovery processes work better; this usually means a longer recovery time in general. Massage is especially beneficial for the older patient.

POSTURAL DEVIATIONS

Postural deviations often are a major underlying cause of injuries and chronic musculoskeletal dysfunction. Postural misalignment may be the result of muscle and soft tissue asymmetries or

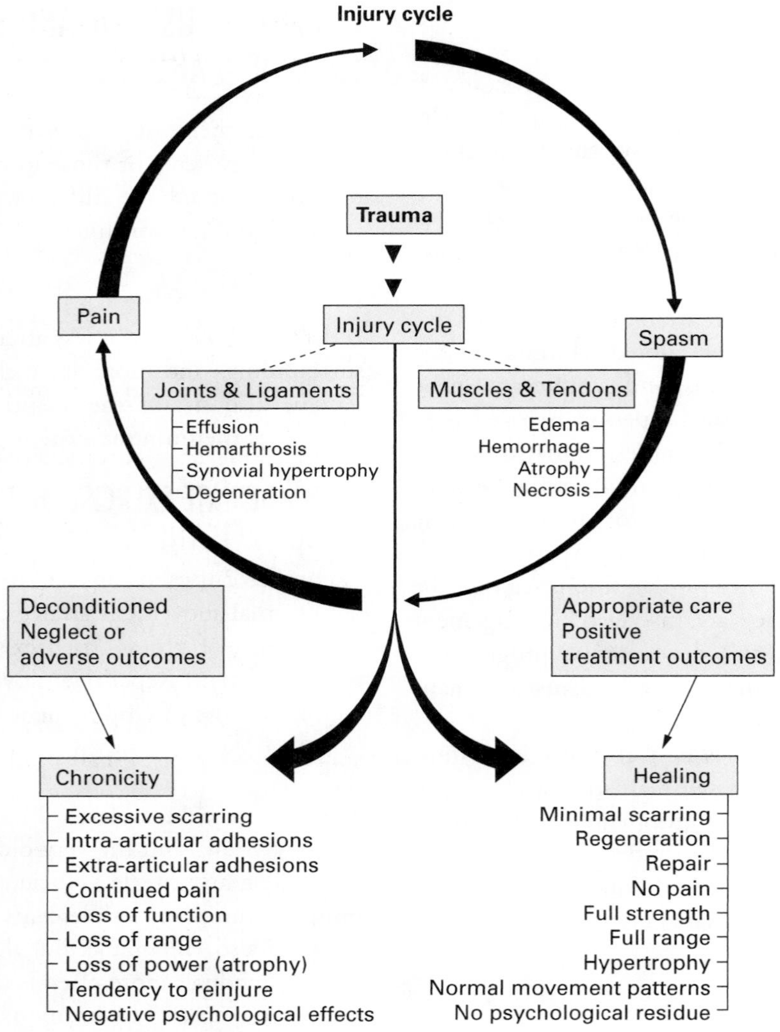

FIGURE 13-1 ■ Schematic representation of the injury cycle. (From Chaitow L, Delany J: *Clinical application of neuromuscular techniques, vol 1, The upper body,* London, 2000, Churchill Livingstone.)

bony asymmetries. As a result, the individual engages in poor mechanics of movement (**pathomechanics**).

Common Postural Imbalances

Some of the common postural imbalances are:

- Cervical lordosis: Short upper erector spinae. This usually is a postural compensation for a thoracic curvature. The sternocleidomastoid muscles may not be weak, although they may shorten and become tense.
- Thoracic kyphosis: Weak erector spinae, short abdominals and sternocleidomastoids.
- Lumbar lordosis: Short lower erector spinae, weak abdominals.
- Forward-tilting (anterior) pelvis: Short gluteus maximus and rectus femoris; weak abdominals, hamstrings, and iliopsoas.
- Backward-tilting (posterior) pelvis: Short hip extensors, abdominals, iliopsoas, and hamstrings; weak rectus femoris.

- Rotated (left or right pelvis): Short, tight structures in the concave areas; long, taut, inhibited muscles and structures in the convex areas.
- Swayback (hyperextended) knees: Short calf muscles and rectus femoris; weak hamstrings.

Distortions can occur in many lateral and rotational directions. These involve imbalances between the postural muscles on either side of the body and reciprocal imbalances in some of the voluntary muscles of the torso. None of these postural imbalances occurs in isolation. An imbalance in one area generally leads to a compensatory imbalance in adjacent areas. The combined postural distortion patterns are the upper crossed, lower crossed, and pronation distortion patterns. These can occur singularly or in combination.

Muscle imbalance can lead to problems in the bone structure, and structural bone problems lead to muscle imbalance; both require attention. Although massage therapists do not directly treat the bone structures, working with the soft tissue can be beneficial and can support methods such as physical therapy or chiropractic in targeting bony structures.

No single answer covers all these postural problems. For significant improvement, a variety of specialized skills usually is needed to rectify muscle balance, structural alignment, and joint function.

MUSCLE WEAKNESS

Muscles may become weak because of a combination of illness, injury, lack of use, and nerve inhibition. Once the cause of the problem has been resolved, normal use or exercise should restore muscle strength. However, the body learns to adapt and compensate for small areas of weakness. The complexity of the muscular system permits altered movement patterns that avoid using weak muscles but still allow performance of daily activities. The weak muscle does not get the exercise it needs and does not improve.

Whether it is the cause or the consequence, nerve stimulation to a weak muscle declines, and eventually nerve function becomes poor. Nerve conductivity improves very quickly when stimulated. This is the reason a person initially notes improvement in apparent strength when starting an exercise program; the increased nerve stimulation, rather than true strength, is responsible. Isolating the specific muscle that is weak and making it work stimulates the nerves, rapidly improving the muscle's function. In fact, a real improvement usually can be felt after only four or five contractions, and the functional effect sometimes can be remarkable. The person immediately feels that movement is better and therefore uses the muscle more normally. Correcting gait reflexes and muscle activation sequence firing patterns, as described in Unit Two, are examples of neural stimulation.

In a long-term chronic situation, nerve conductivity may have become so poor that the person has real difficulty creating any movement and feels that he or she does not even know how to move the area. In such cases, the condition must be addressed with passive movement, which allows the person to see, feel, and experience the movement. Next, the area is moved as the person assists and watches the movement (active assisted movement). Finally, full active movement methods are used.

LIFESTYLE

The general environment in which a person lives, works, and plays can involve high levels of stress, which can have a direct effect on the structure and function of the body and lead to health problems. Increased mental demand and worry can drain energy and lead to muscle fatigue and tension. Poor environmental conditions (i.e., cold, damp, polluted, or noisy) can add to the physical stress. The prior health history may hold the potential for future health concerns. The potential for illness and injury is increased by factors such as lack of sleep; being distracted and having unrealistic expectations, which create stress responses; poor nutrition; and using dangerous substances such as alcohol and tobacco. Any and all aspects of life may contribute to a decline in overall health. On the positive side, lifestyle changes can help increase a person's likelihood of enjoying good health.

PSYCHOLOGICAL AND EMOTIONAL FACTORS

Psychology and emotion play a part in all aspects of life, and health issues are no exception. In some clinical situations, despite good and apparently effective treatment, the patient continues to suffer painful or distressful symptoms. Some people seem to suffer continually from one illness or injury or another.

A person may hold on to a condition because it satisfies other needs; this is called **secondary gain.** The health condition may obtain for the individual the support and sympathy of the people around him or her. It also may provide an excuse to avoid activities, responsibility, and possible failure. It makes a good excuse for poor work performance. Continuing to function despite the pain makes the person appear to be a martyr.

Because the individual benefits in some way from the condition (often on a subconscious level), he or she often has had health problems for a long time and probably has sought out many different types of healthcare. The person's symptoms may have a physical or medical basis, but underlying psychological factors also may be influencing the situation. Although this is not an area in which the massage therapist should attempt to work directly, therapists must be aware of the possibility of these emotional influences. It is important to accept that the pain the person feels usually is quite real, and it is wrong to tell the individual that there is no problem. Massage therapists should not try to deal with the psychological aspects of an illness or injury without proper training. However, serving as an empathetic listener can sometimes help the patient see the problem for himself or herself.

The assessment process described in Unit Two should identify the underlying causes of illness and injury. Ultimately, healthcare intervention at this fundamental level is necessary for a reasonable expectation of successful treatment. This is treating the cause as well as the symptoms (Box 13-1 and Figure 13-2).

BOX 13-1 Biochemistry, the Mind, and Neurosomatic Disorders

Goldstein (1996) has described many chronic health conditions, including chronic fatigue syndrome (CFS) and fibromyalgia syndrome (FMS), as neurosomatic disorders. In doing so, he quoted Yunus (1994), who stated that these disorders are "the commonest group of illnesses for which patients consult physicians."

Neurosomatic disorders, Goldstein says, are illnesses that are caused by "a complex interaction of genetic, developmental, and environmental factors." According to Fry (1993), these factors often include the possibility of early physical, sexual, or psychological abuse. Symptoms emerge as a result of impaired processing of sensory information by the neural network, including the brain. For example, a light touch may be painful; mild odors may cause nausea; walking a short distance may be exhausting; climbing stairs may seem like going up a mountain; and reading light material may cause cognitive impairment. All of these examples are true for many people with CFS or FMS.

Goldstein is critical of psychological approaches to the treatment of such conditions, apart from cognitive behavior therapy, which he suggests "may be more appropriate, since coping with the vicissitudes of these illnesses, which wax and wane unpredictably, is a major problem for most of those afflicted." He claims that most major medical journals, concerned with psychosomatic medicine, rarely discuss neurobiology and "apply the concept of somatization to virtually every topic between their covers" (Hudson, 1992; Yunus, 1994).

According to Goldstein, the four basic influences on neurosomatic illness are as follows:

1. Genetic susceptibility, which can be strong or weak. If only a weak tendency exists, other factors are needed to influence the trait.
2. A feeling of being unsafe between birth and puberty. If a child has such a feeling, hypervigilance may develop, altering interpretation of sensory input.
3. Genetically predetermined susceptibility to viral infections affecting the neurons and glia. Persistent viral infections that affect the central nervous system could alter both the production of transmitters and cellular mechanisms.
4. Increased susceptibility to environmental stressors as a result of a reduction in neural plasticity (caused by any or all of the factors already listed). This might include a deficiency of glutamate or nitric oxide (NO) secretion, which are crucial to the encoding of new memory. The neural plasticity capacity may easily be overtaxed in such individuals, which is why neurosomatic patients often develop problems after a degree of increased exposure to environmental stressors such as acute infection, sustained attention, exercise, immunization, emergence from anesthesia, or trauma.

The brain's involvement in the neurosomatic disorders centers on alterations in the limbic system. Goldstein described the limbic system and its dysregulation as follows:

1. Because the limbic system acts as a regulator (integrative processing) in the brain, it affects fatigue, pain, sleep, memory, attention, weight, appetite, libido, respiration, temperature, blood pressure, mood, and immune and endocrine functions.
2. Dysregulation of the limbic system can affect any or all of these functions and systems.
3. Regulation of autonomic control of respiration derives from the limbic system, and major abnormalities in breathing function (e.g., hyper-

BOX 13-1 Biochemistry, the Mind, and Neurosomatic Disorders—cont'd

ventilation tendencies, irregularity in tidal volume) are noted in people with CFS, along with abnormal responses to exercise (e.g., failure to find expected levels of cortisololamines, growth hormone, somatostatin; and increased core temperature) (Gerra, 1993; Goldstein and Daly, 1993; Griep, 1993; Munschauer, 1991).

4. Dysfunction of the limbic system can result from central or peripheral influences (e.g., stress).
5. Sensory gating (the weight given to sensory inputs) has been shown to be less effectively inhibited in women than in men (Swerdlow, 1993).

Many biochemical imbalances are involved in limbic dysfunction, and no attempt is made in this summary to detail them all. Some of the more important ones, according to Goldstein, are as follows:

- The trigeminal nerve modulates limbic regulation. "The trigeminal nerve may produce expansion of the receptive field zones of wide dynamic-range neurons and nociceptive-specific neurons under certain conditions, perhaps involving increased secretion of substance P, so that a greater number of neurons will be activated by stimulation of a receptive zone, causing innocuous stimuli to be perceived as painful" (Dubner, 1992).
- NO, a primary vasodilator in the brain, has profound influences on glutamate secretion and the neurotransmitters that influence short-term memory (Sandman, 1993), anxiety (Jones, 1994), dopamine release (thereby affecting fatigue) (Hanabauer, 1992), descending pain inhibition processes, sleep induction, and even menstrual problems. "Female patients with CFS/FMS usually have premenstrual exacerbations of their symptoms. Most of the symptoms of late luteal phase dysphoric disorder are similar to those of CFS, and it is likely that this disorder has a limbic etiology similar to CFS/FMS" (Iadecola, 1993).

Allostasis is a primary feature of Goldstein's model. Allostasis is the regulation of the internal milieu through dynamic changes in a number of hormonal and physical variables that are not in a steady-state condition. In this regard, Goldstein reported the following:

1. Approximately 40% of FMS or CFS patients screened had been physically, psychologically, or sexually abused in childhood. Brain electricity activity mapping (BEAM) demonstrated abnormalities in the left temporal area, a feature of people who have been physically, psychologically, or sexually abused in childhood (compared with nonabused controls) (Teicher, 1993).
2. Major childhood stress increases cortisol levels, which can affect the structure and function of the hippocampus (McEwan, 1004; Sapolsky, 1990). Early experience and environmental stimuli, interacting with undeveloped biologic systems, lead to altered homeostatic responses. For example, exaggerated or insufficient HPA [hypothalamus-pituitary axis] responses to defend a homeostatic state in a stressful situation could result in behavioral and neuroimmunoendocrine disorders in adulthood, particularly if stimuli that should be nonstressful were evaluated inappropriately by the prefrontal cortex (Meany, 1994).
3. Sapolsky (1990) identified a sense of lack of control as a primary feature of disrupted allostasis. This researcher also noted a sense of lack of predictability and various other stressors that influence the HPA and that are less balanced in individuals with CFS or FMS. Sapolsky found that all of these stressors involve a "marked absence of control, predictability, or outlets for frustration."
4. Patients with CFS or FMS predominantly attribute their symptoms to external factors, such as a virus, whereas control subjects (depressives) usually show inward attribution (Powell, 1990).
5. In contrast to homeostatic mechanisms, which stabilize deviations in normal variables, allostatic load is the price the body pays for containing the effects of arousing stimuli and expectation of negative consequences (Schulkin, 1994).
6. Chronic negative expectations and subsequent arousal seem to increase allostatic load. This state is characterized by anxiety and anticipation of adversity, leading to elevated levels of stress hormones (Sterling and Eyer, 1981).

Goldstein attempts to explain the immensely complex biochemical and neural interactions that mark the disruptive scenario. These interactions involve areas of the brain such as the amygdala, prefrontal cortex, lower brainstem, and other sites, as well as myriad secretions, including hormones (e.g., glucocorticoids), neurotransmitters, substance P, dopamine, and NO.

Functioning of the prefrontal cortex, Goldstein states, can be altered by numerous triggering agents in an individual who is predisposed (e.g., through genetic factors or early trauma). These agents include the following:

- Viral infections that alter neuronal function
- Immunizations that deplete amines (Gardier, 1994)
- Organophosphate or hydrocarbon exposure
- Head injury
- Childbirth
- Exposure to electromagnetic fields
- Sleep deprivation
- General anesthesia
- Stress (physical, mental, or emotional)

Goldstein's theory describes an altered neurohumoral response in individuals whose defense and repair systems are predisposed to this condition, either because of inherited tendencies or because of early developmental (physical or psychological) insults, to which multiple stressors have been added. His solution is a biochemical (drug) modification of the imbalances he identifies as the key features of this condition. Alternate approaches might attempt to modify behavior or alter other aspects of neurosomatic disturbances, possibly using nutritional approaches.

Goldstein offers his own insights and solutions for these complex conditions. They will not necessarily be accepted by everyone, but the illumination he has shed on the highly complicated mechanisms involved is to be commended.

Modified from Chaitow L, Delany J: *Clinical application of neuromuscular techniques, vol 1, The upper body,* London, 2000, Churchill Livingstone.

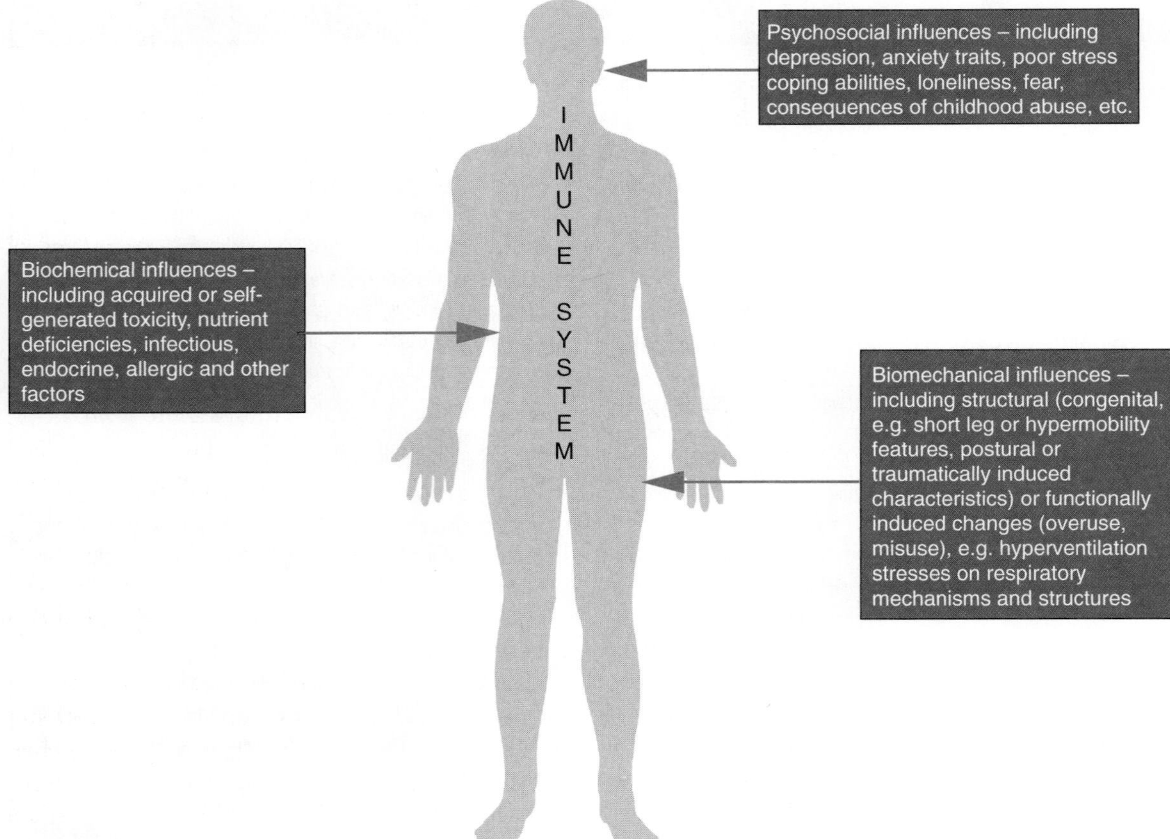
Psychosocial influences – including depression, anxiety traits, poor stress coping abilities, loneliness, fear, consequences of childhood abuse, etc.
IMMUNE SYSTEM
Biochemical influences – including acquired or self-generated toxicity, nutrient deficiencies, infectious, endocrine, allergic and other factors
Biomechanical influences – including structural (congenital, e.g. short leg or hypermobility features, postural or traumatically induced characteristics) or functionally induced changes (overuse, misuse), e.g. hyperventilation stresses on respiratory mechanisms and structures

The interacting influences of a biochemical, biomechanical and psychosocial nature do not produce single changes. For example:

- a negative emotional state (e.g. depression) produces specific biochemical changes, impairs immune function and leads to altered muscle tone.
- hyperventilation modifies blood acidity, alters neural reporting (initially hyper and then hypo), creates feelings of anxiety/apprehension and directly impacts on the structural components of the thoracic and cervical region – muscles and joints.
- altered chemistry affects mood; altered mood changes blood chemistry; altered structure (posture for example) modifies function and therefore impacts on chemistry (e.g. liver function) and potentially on mood.

Within these categories – biochemical, biomechanical and psychosocial – are to be found most major influences on health.

FIGURE 13-2 ■ Biochemical, biomechanical, and psychosocial influences on health. (From Chaitow L, Delany J: *Clinical application of neuromuscular techniques, vol 1, The upper body,* London, 2000, Churchill Livingstone.)

INJURY AND TRAUMA

Many factors can cause mechanical injuries, or **trauma.** A physical injury or wound caused by an external or internal force is known as **physical trauma. Mental/emotional trauma** causes an emotional wound (e.g., posttraumatic stress disorder). The two types of trauma often overlap, which further supports the need for multidisciplinary care for individuals who have experienced trauma. Mental trauma is best managed by mental health professionals; however, massage has a very beneficial influence on the stress response. The massage approach usually focuses on inhibiting excessive dominance of the sympathetic autonomic nervous system, although withdrawal and hopelessness can be addressed by reducing excessive parasympathetic activity. Mental/emotional trauma is discussed further in Chapter 16.

The four types of physical trauma are:

- **Direct trauma** (blunt trauma caused by contact with an object, such as occurs with car accidents and gunshot wounds)
- **Indirect trauma** (caused by sudden force overloading, such as occurs in falls and whiplash injuries)
- **Chronic or overuse trauma** (occurs as a result of repeated overload, frictional resistance, or both, such as with carpal tunnel syndrome and tendinitis)
- **Acute reinjury of a chronic condition or earlier trauma** (e.g., a sudden tear in a persistent lesion that strains muscles related to a chronic low back condition)

THE HEALING PROCESS

Trauma usually triggers the body's innate healing mechanisms. Healing mechanisms work through the development and resolution of the inflammatory response. Inflammation protects the body from infection and repairs damaged tissue by stimulating new cell growth; these cells then synthesize new fibers for repair.

Different tissues heal at different rates. Skin heals quickly, whereas ligaments heal slowly. Stress can influence healing by slowing the repair process. Sleep and proper nutrition are necessary for proper healing. Medications are commonly used for injuries, particularly analgesics and antiinflammatories, and their effects need to be considered. Pain medication reduces pain perception, allowing the patient to continue performing even though the healing process is not yet complete. This approach interferes with successful healing and can lead to chronic conditions. Antiinflammatories may slow the healing process, particularly connective tissue healing.

HOW PHYSICAL TRAUMA OCCURS

To gain an understanding of injuries and the appropriate massage applications, the massage therapist must understand tissue susceptibility to trauma and the mechanical forces involved.

Tissues have relative abilities to resist a particular load. A **load** can be one or a group of outside or internal forces acting on the body. A **force** can be defined as a push or pull. The **resistance** to a load is called a **mechanical stress,** and the **internal response** is a **deformation,** or change in dimensions (*deformation* is also defined as a mechanical strain). The stronger the tissue, the greater magnitude of load it can withstand. All human tissues have viscous and elastic properties, which allow for deformation.

Tissue such as bone is brittle and has fewer viscoelastic properties than soft tissue such as muscle. The loads (forces) applied to bone and soft tissues that can cause injury are tension, compression, bending, shearing, and torsion. Interestingly, these same forces are created by massage application. When tissue is deformed to the extent that its elasticity is almost fully exceeded, a **yield point** has been reached. When the yield point is exceeded, mechanical failure occurs, and tissue damage results.

Because these same forces are applied therapeutically during massage to encourage tissue repair, care must be taken not to superimpose extensive force that may aggravate the injury. Choosing the type of force that offers the most therapeutic value is also important. In general, for massage during the acute and subacute healing phases, do not use the same forces that caused the injury. For example, if a sprain is caused by a torsion load, then kneading, which applies a torsion force, may not be a good technique to use until healing progresses beyond the acute and subacute stages and stability has been restored in the area. With a chronic injury, the massage therapist may need to introduce the same force that caused the injury to achieve results. Therefore, if an ankle sprain caused by a torsion force has healed badly, massage reintroduces torsion force (kneading) to restore normal tissue function.

TYPES OF INJURY

The two basic types of injury are traumatic injury and repetitive injury. **Traumatic injury** occurs when the body is damaged because of a defined event. **Repetitive injury** occurs over a period of time. Traumatic injury is easier to treat than repetitive injury. Traumatic injury generally is classified as mild (grade 1), moderate (grade 2), or severe (grade 3). The most common traumatic injuries are wounds, contusions, sprains, muscle pulls and tears, strains, dislocations, fractures, and nerve impingements. The acute, subacute, and remodeling stages of healing for these injuries are well defined.

Repetitive injury results from an accumulation of minor trauma and overuse. Symptoms occur when adaptive processes are no longer effective. Bursitis and plantar fasciitis are examples. Repetitive injury is difficult to treat. The onset is gradual, and the acute, subacute, and remodeling healing stages are not clearly defined.

Both traumatic and repetitive injury can become chronic if the healing process is not completed successfully. Chronic injury symptoms may be thought of as a healing process that for some reason has been unable to resolve and is stuck in the later stages of subacute healing. Common causes of this condition are an impaired repair process, a return to activity too soon, and failure to comply with rehabilitation requirements.

Among traumatic injuries, those to the nerves, ligaments, and cartilage are the most difficult to heal. If treated properly, wounds and bone fractures heal the best. Repair and regeneration of the tissue are carried out through the process of inflammation and repair. The injury also affects the sensory nerves in the connective tissue, causing productive pain, which serves to protect the injured area.

Massage is most suitable as an active treatment process for mild and moderate injuries. Severe injury requires medical intervention and possibly surgery. Massage becomes more of a supportive method, rather than a direct care process, during healing and rehabilitation (Box 13-2).

BOX 13-2 **Appropriate Massage Approaches During the Phases of Healing**

Acute Phase
Pain management
Sleep support

Subacute Phase (Early)
Pain management
Sleep support
Management of edema
Management of compensation patterns

Subacute Phase (Later)
Pain management
Sleep support
Management of edema
Management of compensation patterns
Support for rehabilitative activity
Support for mobile scar development
Support for tissue regeneration process

Remodeling Phase
Support for healing and rehabilitation activities
Encouragement of appropriate scar tissue development
Management of adhesions
Restoration of muscle activation sequence firing patterns, gait reflexes, and neuromuscular responses
Elimination of reversible compensation patterns
Management of irreversible compensation patterns
Restoration of tissue pliability

Modified from Fritz S: *Sports and exercise massage: comprehensive care in athletics, fitness, and rehabilitation,* St Louis, 2006, Mosby.

ILLNESS

Illness involves some sort of invasion by pathogens (bacteria, viruses, or fungi) that causes infection, immune system dysfunction (hyperactivity or hypoactivity), or organ and body system failure. Examples of illnesses include colds, sinus infection, digestive upset, cardiovascular disease, Epstein-Barre syndrome, diabetes, multiple sclerosis, and fibromyalgia.

Illnesses can be acute, subacute, or chronic. Infection typically stimulates a body-wide inflammatory response, which includes a fever. A fever of up to 102°F might not be treated with medicine, but rather supported with lots of fluids and rest. Artificially reducing a productive fever (i.e., a fever that results from an unimpeded healing process, also called a *low-grade inflammatory response*) can prolong infection. However, a fever that persists longer than 2 or 3 days or a fever over 102°F should be evaluated by a doctor.

Massage is appropriate during illness if it is applied correctly and can help manage some symptoms. The typical treatment plan is a general, pleasurable, nonstraining, nonspecific, full body massage that supports sleep and restorative mechanisms, particularly parasympathetic dominance.

Energy-based modalities can be used during an infection if the individual is generally healthy. As always, additional caution is required when working with the very young and very old.

Autoimmune disease often involves an increased, sustained, and/or inappropriate inflammatory response. Antiinflammatory support includes an antiinflammatory diet (Box 13-3), possible use of antiinflammatory medications, and other antiinflammatory treatment strategies, such as cold hydrotherapy.

Massage is appropriate for autoimmune disease as long as the application does not generate inflammation and does not strain adaptive capacity. The general massage protocol described in Unit Two is appropriate, as long as care is taken not to overuse mechanical force targeting the connective tissue. Be especially cautious with shearing (friction) and compressive forces, which could cause tissue damage, such as bruising.

REALISTIC EXPECTATIONS FOR RECOVERY

The idea that a person or body part will be "good as new" after recovering from an illness or injury is misleading. Even the best healing outcome results in some sort of compensation and adaptation. Injured areas are prone to tissue changes, such as decreased connective tissue pliability; altered muscle firing patterns with a tendency toward synergistic dominance; reflexive activity to other aspects of the kinetic chain function; susceptibility to subclinical (chronic) inflammation and swelling; a tendency to develop traumatic arthritis or arthrosis; and changes in muscle size and strength patterns. Recurring illness increases the susceptibility to further episodes and other illnesses. Recovery from repeated illness or injury eventually takes its toll, and adaptive mechanisms become strained.

Massage can be an effective part of the treatment plan for all these conditions and can reduce the adaptive strain on the body of cumulative compensation. For example, if a patient has had three or four mild to moderate ankle sprains, the ongoing treatment plan would always include attention to the ankle. If a person has a chronic condition, such as fibromyalgia, massage that supports restorative sleep would be beneficial for long-term care. Massage is very effective at this level of maintenance care.

BOX 13-3 Elements of an Antiinflammatory Diet

- **Eat:** Fruits, vegetables, whole grains (organic if possible), eggs (hormone free, free range, vegetarian diet), fish (e.g., salmon and sardines, which are low in heavy metals), chicken and turkey (free range, hormone free), yogurt with live cultures (unsweetened), extra virgin olive oil, flaxseed oil.
- **Avoid:** Dairy (except yogurt), pork, beef, processed meat, refined grains and sugar, artificial food, most fats and oils (especially hydrogenated oils), and all foods containing trans fatty acids.
- **Use therapeutic foods and herbs:** Those especially valuable for controlling inflammation are ginger, turmeric, pineapple, and papaya.
- **Drink:** 64 ounces of pure water daily.

Modified from Fritz S: *Sports and exercise massage: comprehensive care in athletics, fitness, and rehabilitation*, St Louis, 2006, Mosby.

HEALING TIME

The healing of illness and injury can take some time. For injuries, after swelling has subsided, healing depends on the blood supply. A good blood supply helps move nutrients, oxygen, and infection-fighting cells to the damaged area to work on repair. People who are active and have a healthy lifestyle tend to have a better blood supply and to heal faster than smokers, individuals with chronic illness, or those with a sedentary lifestyle. Ultimately, healing time varies from person to person. Although healing mechanisms can be supported, healing cannot be forced; it just takes time. Healing of an acute infection depends on the effectiveness of the immune system.

For a person who is reasonably healthy, the following are average healing times for various injuries and illnesses:

- Fractured finger or toe: 3 to 5 weeks
- Fractured clavicle: 6 to 10 weeks
- Sprained ankle: Minor, 5 days; severe, 3 to 6 weeks
- Mild contusion: 5 days

- Strains and muscle pulls: A few days to several weeks (depends on the severity and location of the injury)
- Mild shoulder separation: 7 to 21 days
- Major shoulder separation: 6 to 12 months
- Common viral infection: Cold and flu, 7 to 14 days
- Common bacterial infection: 14 days
- Minor surgery: 14 to 21 days
- Major surgery: 6 to 12 months

JUST BETWEEN YOU AND ME

People ask all the time, "How long before I'm back to normal?" The response I give is, "Minor issue, 3 months; moderate issue, 6 months; major issue, 12 months." We do not give ourselves enough time to heal. Life is so demanding, and healing is a full-time job. Most of us can't put life on hold until the body repairs itself, so healing is compromised. I don't have an answer for this, but I feel strongly that the lack of time for healing is a major reason for chronic problems.

Any injury or illness can take longer to heal if the patient returns to normal activity too soon. During the convalescent period, the patient should sleep if he or she has severe pain or fatigue without activity. When the symptoms are at a moderate level with the patient at rest, the patient should increase activity slowly, performing simple range-of-motion exercises. If pain or fatigue increases beyond the moderate level, the patient should stop and rest. Over time, the patient can return to activity at a very low intensity and build up to the previous level. Attention must always be paid to warning signs of overdoing. Soreness, aching, tension, anxiety or depression, and/or an increase in symptoms must be acknowledged, or the patient may end up with an even more serious problem.

Knowing when to return to activity is more difficult during recovery from an illness than after an injury. Typically, the symptoms of a viral or bacterial illness above the clavicle (e.g., a head cold or sinusitis) are less serious. Activity is okay but should not cause fatigue. With a serious illness, the recovery period must be supervised by the treating physician.

At the same time, it is necessary to put mild to moderate pain, discomfort, and fatigue into perspective. The seriousness of these symptoms is often misinterpreted. People need to overcome an excessive sensitivity to pain and fatigue to best rally the healing mechanism. It is important to know when to rest and when to get on with life.

JUST BETWEEN YOU AND ME

I learned about the relative importance of pain from Dr. David Gurevich, a wonderful old medical doctor from Russia who taught at my school and who worked with me when I had a significant low back condition. One day he took my face in his hands, looked me in the eye, and said very gently, "Sandy, it is only pain. This pain will not harm you, you will not die. Your life may not be good, but you will not die. It is up to you." That was a wake-up call. My back still bothers me, and I have to keep at the maintenance exercises, ice applications, and stretches. But I am not dead, and I have decided that my life will be good.

TREATMENT OF ILLNESS AND INJURY

The massage therapist's roles in the rehabilitative process are different from those in maintenance and recovery described in Unit Two. Rehabilitative roles include supporting the general healing and restorative processes, managing soreness related to healing and rehabilitation, and managing compensation patterns related both to the condition and the treatment.

Illness and injury are treated in a variety of ways, which include medication, surgery, and physical medicine. Physical medicine consists of various therapeutic modalities that use mechanical, electrical, and thermal interventions. These modalities control or reduce swelling, reduce pain, and help maintain strength. Standard therapies, such as ultrasound, electrical stimulation (E-stim, or transdermal electrical nerve stimulation), paraffin baths, hot/cold whirlpool treatments, and massage have a proven track record for supporting recovery from an injury. Acupuncture also has been shown to produce positive effects.

Some modalities exert a beneficial effect by influencing blood and lymphatic flow and modifying the pain response. Massage is especially effective in this regard. Swelling in response to injury is particularly problematic because it contributes to a spinal cord reflex that inhibits muscle function and interferes with rehabilitative exercise. Massage supports lymphatic drainage and is especially beneficial in the management of swelling in the superficial tissues. The lymphatic drainage application is time consuming, and the massage therapist typically has more time than other professionals to apply the method. Some facilities have pneumatic compression devices that rhythmically compress and release against the tissue or use rhythmic suction. These devices are helpful in encouraging fluid movement but are less able to be specifically applied to the individual needs of the patient. Manual lymph drainage often is more effective.

At times, too much emphasis is placed on therapy when the most effective healing methods are time, rest, and proper nutrition. The patient's adaptive capacity may be limited at this time, therefore the massage therapist, along with others treating the patient, needs to respect the body and not overdo treatment.

PRICE THERAPY

The standard treatment procedure for an injury in the acute phase is **protection, rest, ice, compression, and elevation (PRICE)** (Box 13-4). The massage therapist's applications should support this treatment, even though the massage therapist is not likely to be the professional coordinating the procedure.

The first treatment for any acute injury is to reduce any swelling. Swelling causes pain and loss of motion, which in turn limits the use of muscles, which can then weaken, shorten, and resist repair. Never apply heat to an acute injury. Heat increases circulation and swelling.

Avoid the use of **nonsteroidal antiinflammatory drugs (NSAIDs)** if possible, but follow the doctor's recommendations. Ask questions about the appropriateness of using these drugs, because they interfere with the normal acute healing response and can cause nausea, stomach pain, stomach bleeding, and ulcers. In rare cases, prolonged use can disrupt normal kidney and liver function. The risk of these effects increases with age. Individuals with liver problems should consult their doctor before using products containing acetaminophen.

It is important to continue rehabilitation even when it seems as if the symptoms may have resolved. Symptoms may significantly diminish during the second stage of healing, but the area is not fully healed until the third stage (remodeling) has been completed. The old saying rings true: healing takes time (often as long as a year to be complete).

BOX 13-4 The Components of PRICE Therapy

As the acronym shows, PRICE therapy has five primary components:

- *P*rotection: Immobilize the affected area to encourage healing and to protect it from further injury. The patient may need to use elastic wraps, slings, splints, crutches, or a cane.
- *R*est: Avoid activities that increase pain or swelling in the injured area. Rest is essential to tissue healing; however, it does not mean complete bed rest. The person can do other activities and exercises that do not stress the affected area.
- *I*ce: Apply ice to the injured area to reduce pain, muscle spasms, and swelling. Ice packs, ice massage, and slush baths all can help. The recommended regimen is 20-minute applications 4 to 6 times a day.
- *C*ompression: Because swelling can result in loss of motion in an injured joint, apply compression to the area until the swelling stops. Wraps or compressive elastic bandages (e.g., Ace bandages) are best.
- *E*levation: To reduce swelling, raise the affected area above the level of the heart and above jointed areas that lie between the injury and the heart. For example, a sprained ankle should be elevated above the knee, which in turn is placed higher than the hip. Using this position at night, if possible, is especially important.

Modified from Fritz S: *Sports and exercise massage: comprehensive care in athletics, fitness, and rehabilitation,* St Louis, 2006, Mosby.

THE RECOVERY PROCESS

Recovering from a traumatic injury or an illness (e.g., a viral infection or a heart attack) presents a challenge. The way each person understands and responds to pain and limitation is a very individualized experience that is based on many factors. However, certain responses and psychological skills can help most people take an active role in their recovery.

People often initially feel overwhelmed by health issues. The ability to cope greatly improves if the patient works closely with the doctor and other healthcare providers to develop a clear plan for recovery.

Successful recovery begins with the patient becoming informed about the condition. It is important to know the implications of the health condition, a realistic expectation of recovery time, and a plan to recover safely and effectively. The patient must see himself or herself as an active participant in the treatment process. The patient may not understand every scientific detail of treatment, therefore careful, accurate explanations of the massage method are necessary, including how it affects the underlying physiology and its relationship to the healing and rehabilitation program as a whole. The information provided by the massage therapist must not conflict with explanations of other healthcare professions. Be ready to answer the patient's questions respectfully, but keep your answers within the scope of massage practice. If the question is outside that scope, suggest that the patient consult someone with specific information in that area.

How the patient responds to the health condition also is very important. An illness or injury usually is not expected, planned, or welcomed. Health concerns have very different meanings for different people. For some, an illness or injury might be life-threatening; for others, it is a nuisance. Health issues also can interfere with a job or responsibilities at home. Therefore the patient must understand the coping skills needed to help him or her through the stress of recovery, using professional help if necessary (see Unit One).

Directing or redirecting the patient's response to the recovery process may help the person maintain a positive outlook during healing. A few suggestions you can make to the patient include:

- Consider the condition as something that will heal and go away or, if the condition is chronic, something that can be managed.
- Mentally and physically befriend the pain as a guide to recovery. Pushing too hard may cause relapse, but fearing pain may lead to a too-passive approach to recovery.
- Be positive every day about one's ability to cope with and recover from the condition.
- Use the desire to recover to help integrate the sense of self with mental and physical healing power.
- Connect with emotions and let them be the guide through the healing process. If the person becomes emotionally overwhelmed, encourage activity that is enjoyable and distracting. When the person feels emotionally strong, that energy should be used to progress in recovery.

The patient should express needs and concerns about the healing and rehabilitation process directly to the healthcare team. However, some of these discussions probably will occur first with the massage therapist, who tends to spend longer uninterrupted time with patients and who experience blood chemistry changes (i.e., lower cortisol and increased serotonin, dopamine, endorphin, and oxytocin levels) that promote personal bonding during massage. While our hands are busy, we can listen to the patient as the person relaxes and becomes ready to talk. Identify any negative mental responses, chart them, and report them to the supervising medical professional, who will evaluate for appropriate intervention. Then let go and be supportive of the treatment plan developed for the patient.

It helps greatly if the patient is creative, humorous, and positive in his or her approach to the daily inconveniences caused by illness or injury. A person receiving healthcare needs to ask for and receive help and to be surrounded by emotionally and physically supportive people.

Several specific mental techniques can also aid recovery. These methods usually are presented by the psychologist and can be supported by the massage therapist.

- *Progressive relaxation:* The person is directed to start with the head and work down, first flexing the muscles in each body part (producing tension) and then relaxing them. The person then is instructed to mentally and physically memorize the feeling of relaxation. Progressive relaxation methods are easy to incorporate into a massage.

- *Breathing:* Breath control can help modify stress and the response to pain. Massage can support a functional breathing pattern.
- *Visualization:* Using imagery can enhance healing by creating a positive internal atmosphere; this is done by focusing on a scene that creates a positive, nurturing, and healing state of mind during the massage. The use of music that the patient finds peaceful reinforces this technique as it is practiced. The massage therapist usually does not guide the visualization but can support the effectiveness of the method. A relaxed patient can concentrate on total body healing by visualizing a color or sound that represents healing as it moves slowly through the entire body, cell by cell. Others prefer to focus on the illness or the injured area by creating a healing image (e.g., blood vessels sending out healing roots) or by holding the image and "seeing" the area heal. Some people combine these techniques and images. Some individuals prefer to visualize only, whereas others like to combine visualization with mental statements, such as, "I am healing," "I am calm," or "I will get better." Visualization also is helpful as a form of distraction from pain. Use imagery to pull away from the body to a scene or favorite experience. This technique also may help facilitate sleep.
- The massage therapist can also visualize and use an energetic intention for healing during the massage. Ethically it may be most appropriate not to disclose the details of the process of intention to the patient, because of the risk of upsetting the patient's belief system. The massage therapist can share the visualization with the patient, by having the person explain what he or she is doing, and then provide the massage. The massage therapist incorporates the patient's healing vision into the intention. We do not understand how all this works, but the concept of healing intention does support healing. For the patient, this process often may take the form of prayer and meditation. This thought form places intention in the spiritual realm, and the massage therapist must not superimpose his or her personal spiritual practices on the patient.

PSYCHOLOGICAL INFLUENCES ON HEALING

The prospect of prolonged recovery from an illness or injury can be daunting for anyone. Healing has both psychological and physical stages. The psychological stages are shock, realization, mourning, acknowledgment, and coping. Physically, a person must progress through the stages of initial pain, swelling, and loss of the previous level of control. The patient also faces the challenge of re-establishing strength, stamina, and confidence before trusting the body to function at an acceptable level. Psychological factors influence the patient's return to health without fear of relapse or reinjury.

THE ROLE OF MASSAGE

The role of the massage therapist during recovery is to continue to support the healing process for up to 1 year and to manage any lingering pain or compensation. Successful completion of a healing and rehabilitation program challenges both the physical and psychological capacities of the therapist to the fullest. Patience, commitment, and persistence are necessary for any professional working in a healthcare setting. Massage therapists require solid emotional stability and a bit of professional detachment and neutralization so that they do not allow the emotional storms of the patient to affect them personally. Remember, the healing and rehabilitation process is about the patient, not about you. Being neutral does not mean eliminating compassion and empathy; rather, it supports nonjudgmental care.

CHRONIC CONDITIONS

A **chronic condition** is defined as a disease, injury, or syndrome that shows either little change or slow progression. **Acute illness** and **acute injury** are short-term conditions that resolve through normal healing processes and, if necessary, with the aid of supportive medical care. Compared with chronic conditions, acute conditions are relatively easy to deal with because healing produces measurable results. Dealing with chronic illness is difficult for the person who has it, for the physician and the healthcare team, and for the massage therapist. In many situations, little can be done except to make day-to-day living with the condition more tolerable. Cure is an option in some cases, but even then, total recovery is a long process that requires work, commitment, and support.

The dynamics of family relationships, work and career demands, emotions, and coping skills play an important role in the etiology of a chronic illness. Chronic illness affects every aspect of a person's life and the lives of those around the individual. An entire family's dynamic functioning pattern may be set up around a chronically ill family member, therefore shifting health patterns may be difficult. All relationship dynamics may change if the chronically ill individual improves. Family and friends may actually demonstrate enabling behavior, perpetuating the condition. If a chronic condition improves, personal and professional responsibilities that the patient has been able to avoid because of the health issue must be addressed. As mentioned previously, a benefit gained by chronic illness is called *secondary gain.* This process may be subconscious and therefore difficult for the patient to recognize or change. The dynamics of secondary gain reach far beyond the physiology of the disease, and professional counseling may be required to resolve the situation.

A person deriving secondary gain probably has internal conflict. Most people do not want to be in pain and have limited function, but the situation provides some sort of solution to an existing problem. This is the key to understanding secondary gain; fundamentally, the process is a solution, and until the underlying problem can be solved in another way, the health condition will persist until it is no longer effective. This usually is not a conscious or planned process. Rather, it develops as a learned behavior or accidental conditioned response. For example, a child with asthma realizes that her parents do not argue when she has an asthma attack. The learned response is: asthma attack = no fighting. It does not take long for these experiences to become a habit and become subconscious and perpetuating.

Working with chronic conditions does not often produce measurable improvements. More often, a slowed deterioration is seen or, at best, a stabilization. For this reason, the treatment of individuals with chronic conditions does not easily fit into the current medical system, which is geared more toward acute and traumatic care.

Long-term debilitating diseases such as Parkinson's disease, multiple sclerosis, systemic lupus erythematosus, rheumatoid arthritis, fibromyalgia, asymptomatic human immunodeficiency virus (HIV) infection, acquired immunodeficiency syndrome (AIDS), and disk problems that cause back pain all respond well to the short-term, symptomatic relief massage provides. Massage also can reduce general stress, helping the individual to better cope with the condition.

Chronic illness follows an uneven cycle, with good and bad periods. On good days the person may overexert and deplete an already weakened energy reserve. The immune system may be compromised, leaving the individual more susceptible to infections, such as colds and influenza. Because most chronic illness patterns are marked by good days and bad days, the intensity of the massage session must be geared to the patient's condition that day. For example, when symptoms are more active, it may be better to give massages more often for shorter periods.

One approach to rehabilitation of chronically ill individuals is a hardening or toughening program. **Hardiness** is the physical and mental ability to withstand external stressors. Individuals with chronic illnesses often reduce their activity levels, isolate themselves, and become less hardy. Massage, hydrotherapy, and specially designed exercise programs can increase a person's hardiness.

People with chronic illnesses usually are under a doctor's care and may be taking medications. The massage therapist must work closely with the medical professionals to understand the effects of the various treatments and medications. The Evolve website has a comprehensive section on medications and presents some guidelines for determining the interplay of massage with various medications. Because medications often change, it is vital to have access to resources for updated information about medications.

Mind/body approaches, behavior modification, relaxation techniques, empowering practices, spiritual healing, and other types of interventions and alternative types of care are helpful to those with chronic illnesses. All these approaches tend to empower the patient, rallying the powerful internal resources human beings have. These methods are being incorporated into multidisciplinary care. The only caution about alternative interventions is that some of those who offer such services do not have the patient's greatest good as their top priority. Instead, they prey on the misery of the chronically ill. These people usually offer cures, charge high fees for treatment sessions, require frequent sessions, and try to convince the patient that their way is the only way, making the patient dependent on them. This type of behavior is unethical and is a major underlying concern of medical professionals.

A massage therapist who wants to work with the chronically ill must have realistic expectations. Instead of trying to develop a massage approach to cure the health condition (which is out of the scope of massage practice anyway), the therapist should focus on helping the patient feel better for a little while.

A clinical reasoning process is necessary in order to make appropriate decisions on the type of care most beneficial for a person with a chronic illness. Treatment plans revolve around therapeutic change, condition management, or palliative care. Because of the nature of chronic illness, the emotional factors involved, and possible secondary gain, the treatment process most often chosen is condition management, with palliative care provided during acute episodes of the illness. This does not mean that an actual plan for therapeutic plan is not possible; it simply is not as common in these cases.

The massage therapist's expectations must be realistic and professionally detached from the actual outcomes for a patient with a chronic illness. Often the patient's current situation is the best that can be achieved under the existing circumstances. If each pattern presented by a patient is seen as a solution to a problem, rather than as the problem, it is easier to understand why approaches that relieve the symptoms and support healing often are met with resistance. For example, a patient with chronic fatigue syndrome consumes 4 or 5 cups of coffee after noon and finds that she cannot sleep at night because caffeine is known to disturb sleep. Massage in this case would be ineffective at supporting sleep. The patient will not stop drinking coffee in the afternoon, because she cannot function at work if she does not drink the coffee. So what do you do? There is no easy answer, particularly when survival mechanisms reinforce short-term solutions, even if these behaviors create long-term problems.

For the massage therapist, a valuable goal in working with people with chronic conditions is to help the patient rediscover that each person is in charge of her or his own life, and the illness or injury is not. The health condition may have been allowed to take over the person's life and personal power. "Healing" may be the act of reasserting and reclaiming control of one's life, not getting rid of the condition. The benefit of massage may be that it provides enough relief to enable the patient to find the inner resources necessary for dealing constructively with the effects of a chronic health condition, thereby enhancing the patient's quality of life and the lives of those around the individual.

evolve 13-1

The following terms and expressions specific to Chapter 13 have already been used to search PubMed for the latest research literature available. The *Click Here for Massage* feature associated with this chapter on your textbook's Evolve website allows you to hyperlink to a continually updated PubMed search of research literature that corresponds to this subject.

Hyperlink Search Terms

Massage chronic condition
Massage healing
Massage illness injury
Massage recovery
Massage trauma

SUMMARY

This chapter provides an overview of the processes of illness and injury. Injury and illness are different. An injury is primarily a local condition and typically involves trauma, whereas illness is more of a system breakdown. Various risk factors increase the likelihood that a person will be injured or become ill. Healing requires time and effort. If the healing process does not resolve a condition, it can become chronic. Most chronic conditions can be managed. Massage is a beneficial aspect of healthcare that can support healing mechanisms and the management of chronic conditions.

WORKBOOK

1. Using yourself as the patient, do a risk factor assessment based on the following:

   Fatigue ______

   Inappropriate exercise or repetitive motion activities ______

   Postural deviation ______

   Muscle weakness ______

   Lifestyle ______

   Psychological and emotional factors ______

2. Develop a massage treatment protocol for each of the following types of trauma. First identify the type of trauma (e.g., direct, indirect, chronic, acute reinjury of a chronic condition). Then develop the treatment protocol, and finally, justify the application.

   Bruise on the back caused by a fall ______

   Laceration from a construction accident ______

   Tendinitis from computer work ______

   Plantar fasciitis caused by jogging ______

   Recurrence of shoulder bursitis after moving boxes ______

   Recurrence of neck pain, reason unknown, 6 months after a car accident involving whiplash ______

3. Analyze the similarities and differences of the treatment protocols in question 2. ______

4. Compare and contrast the massage applications for the following:

   Acute injury ______

   Acute illness ______

   Subacute injury ______

   Subacute illness ______

   Remodeling injury ______

   Recovery from illness ______

   Chronic injury ______

   Chronic illness ______

Chapter 14 Concept Map

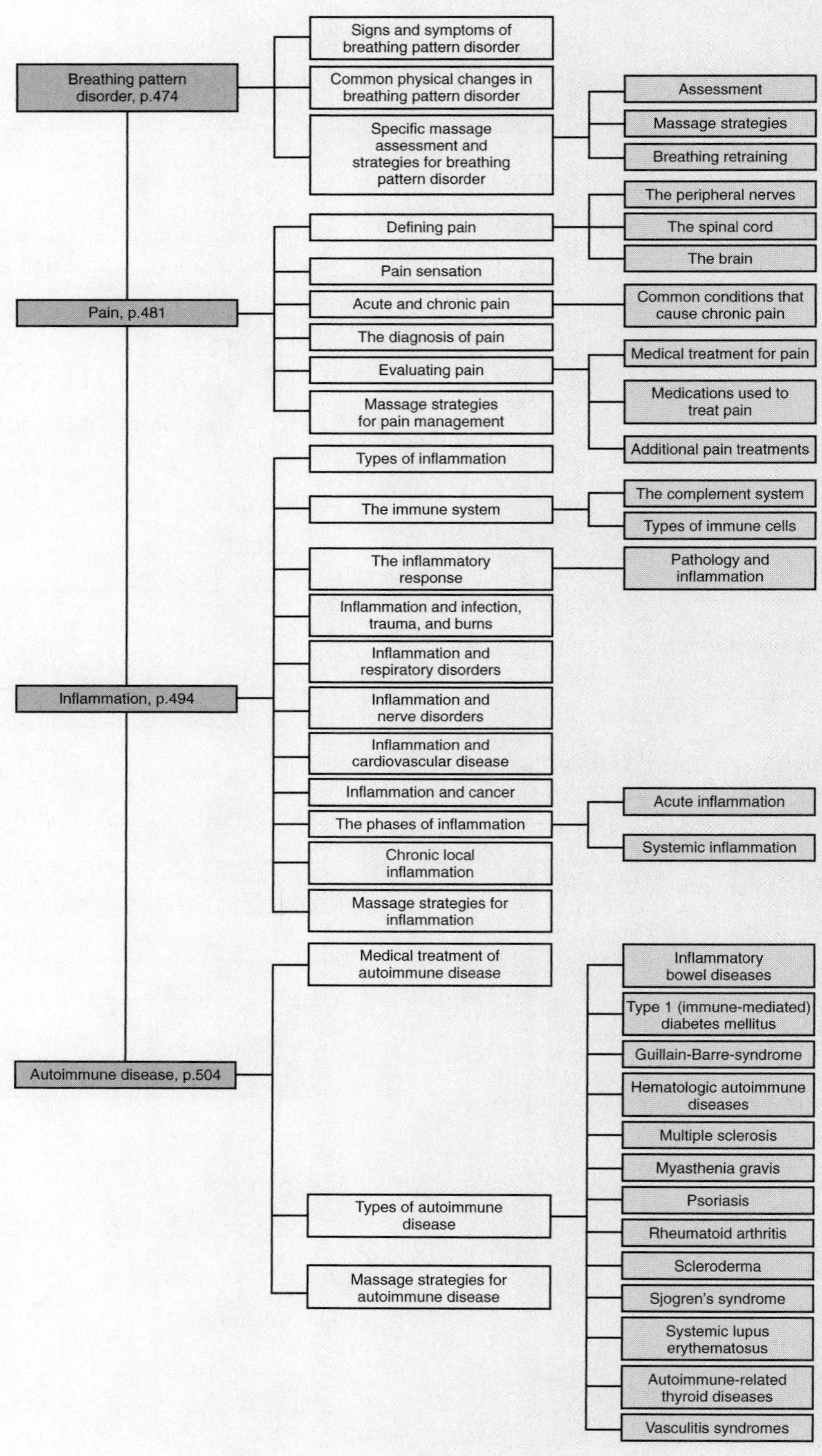

Breathing pattern disorder, p.474
Signs and symptoms of breathing pattern disorder
Common physical changes in breathing pattern disorder
Specific massage assessment and strategies for breathing pattern disorder
Assessment
Massage strategies
Breathing retraining
Pain, p.481
Defining pain
The peripheral nerves
The spinal cord
The brain
Pain sensation
Acute and chronic pain
Common conditions that cause chronic pain
The diagnosis of pain
Evaluating pain
Medical treatment for pain
Medications used to treat pain
Additional pain treatments
Massage strategies for pain management
Inflammation, p.494
Types of inflammation
The immune system
The complement system
Types of immune cells
The inflammatory response
Pathology and inflammation
Inflammation and infection, trauma, and burns
Inflammation and respiratory disorders
Inflammation and nerve disorders
Inflammation and cardiovascular disease
Inflammation and cancer
The phases of inflammation
Acute inflammation
Systemic inflammation
Chronic local inflammation
Massage strategies for inflammation
Autoimmune disease, p.504
Medical treatment of autoimmune disease
Types of autoimmune disease
Inflammatory bowel diseases
Type 1 (immune-mediated) diabetes mellitus
Guillain-Barre-syndrome
Hematologic autoimmune diseases
Multiple sclerosis
Myasthenia gravis
Psoriasis
Rheumatoid arthritis
Scleroderma
Sjogren's syndrome
Systemic lupus erythematosus
Autoimmune-related thyroid diseases
Vasculitis syndromes
Massage strategies for autoimmune disease

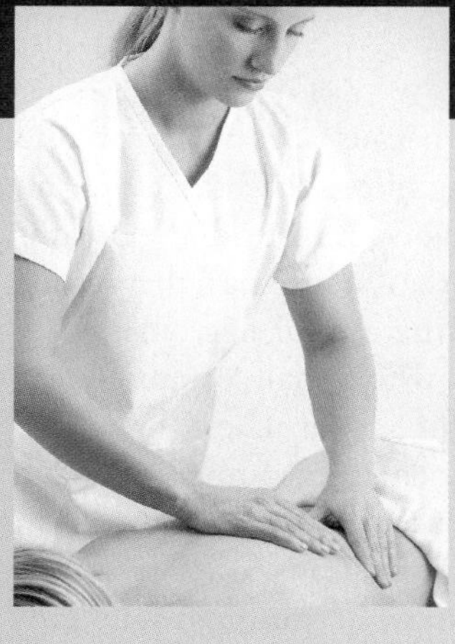

CHAPTER 14

GENERAL MASSAGE TREATMENT FOR PREDISPOSING AND PERPETUATING FACTORS AND SYMPTOM MANAGEMENT

Key Terms

Aching pain
Acquired immunity
Acupuncture
Acute inflammation
Acute pain
Adjuvant drugs
Asthma
Autoimmune diseases
Biofeedback
Bohr effect
Breathing pattern disorder
Burning pain
Chemokines
Chronic inflammation
Chronic pain
Complement system
Counterirritation
Cytokines
Deep pain
Deep second-degree burn
Distraction
Endotoxin
Fibrosis
Hypnosis
Imagery
Immune complex
Immune system
Inflammation
Inflammatory mediators
Innate immunity
Lipopolysaccharide (LPS)
Localized pain
Lymphocytes
Macrophages
Muscle pain
Neurogenic pain
Neutrophils
Nonsteroidal antiinflammatory drugs (NSAIDs)
Pain
Pain threshold
Pain tolerance
Pathogens
Perceptual dominance
Plasmapheresis
Platelets
Pricking (bright) pain
Projected pain
Psychogenic pain
Radiating pain
Referred pain
Regeneration
Remodeling
Replacement
Second-degree burn
Sensitization
Sepsis
Somatic pain
Superficial second-degree burn
Transcutaneous electrical nerve stimulation (TENS)
Visceral pain

For definitions of key terms, refer to the Evolve website.

OBJECTIVE

Upon completion of this chapter, the reader will have the information necessary to:

1. Develop appropriate treatment plans for massage application targeted to the four underlying predisposing and perpetuating factors.

Some recurring and underlying dysfunctions and predisposing factors appear over a broad spectrum of pathologic health conditions, both as causal factors and as symptoms. This chapter discusses the underlying dysfunctions that influence the success of a patient's treatment and that best respond to massage.

Four primary underlying processes predispose a person to or perpetuate health dysfunction and symptoms: breathing pattern disorder, pain, inflammation, and immune function. Complementary health methods are very effective at addressing these underlying issues, which are common among many health conditions. General normalization of the homeostatic process in the body influences these four processes, creating an environment that supports healing and sustains health. Therapeutic massage is beneficial in addressing all four conditions and therefore effective in the care of most health concerns. Management of these four primary factors also forms the foundation of preventive healthcare, and here, again, therapeutic massage plays an important part in achieving and maintaining health.

Breathing pattern changes support either sympathetic or parasympathetic dominance. A breathing pattern disorder typically creates sympathetic dominance, which can increase various symptoms. Massage effectively addresses the mechanical aspect of breathing, allowing the breathing process to be as normal as possible. This is an important aspect of the management of most stress-related conditions.

Pain management is a major element of medical treatment, and massage can be an effective method both of managing pain symptoms and supporting the patient's ability to cope with pain. Research now indicates that inflammation is a major underlying factor in most illnesses and a perpetuating factor in chronic pain. Massage can support the resourceful inflammation that is needed for healing, reduce the tendency for an excessive inflammatory response by decreasing sympathetic arousal, and manage symptoms related to the pain and swelling that accompany inflammation. Finally, massage can support normal immune function so that the body's self-regulating processes are able to function properly.

BREATHING PATTERN DISORDER

Breathing pattern disorder is a complex set of behaviors that leads to overbreathing and upper chest breathing function. It is considered a functional syndrome, because the anatomy and physiology are working effectively; therefore, no specific pathology is involved. Instead, the breathing pattern is inappropriate, a situation that results in confused signals to the central nervous system (CNS), which sets up a whole chain of subsequent events. A tendency for upper chest breathing commonly leads to biochemical imbalances as a result of exhalation of excessive amounts of carbon dioxide (CO_2). This in turn leads to relative alkalosis of the bloodstream, which automatically produces a sense of apprehension and anxiety and many physiologic changes. Women may be more at risk of this condition as a result of hormonal influences, because progesterone stimulates the respiratory rate (Figure 14-1).

A disruption of autonomic nervous system (ANS) function that results in generalized sympathetic dominance is an underlying factor in the development of nonoptimal breathing function. A person in pain is prone to breathing dysfunction. Increased upper chest breathing results in chemical changes that temporarily reduce the pain but in the long run may make it worse. Individuals with any sort of respiratory disease are also susceptible to nonoptimal breathing function. Respiratory illness, such as a cold, can shift the breathing function to an upper chest pattern, and it sometimes may not reverse after the illness has resolved. Chronic respiratory disease, such as asthma, perpetuates breathing dysfunction. People with anxiety and depression often display nonoptimal breathing function. Also, a person can get "stuck" in the breathing pattern required for physical activity (e.g., athletics), which means the individual sometimes is unable to reverse the pattern to a resting phase.

Increased ventilation is a common component of the fight-or-flight response, but when breathing increases while actions and movements are restricted or do not increase accordingly, the person is breathing in excess of metabolic need. Blood levels of CO_2 fall, and recognizable symptoms (e.g., irritability or digestive upset) may occur. Cerebrovascular constriction, a primary response to disordered breathing, can reduce the amount of oxygen available to the brain by about 50%. Along with heightened arousal and anxiety and reduced cerebral oxygenation, the oxygen in

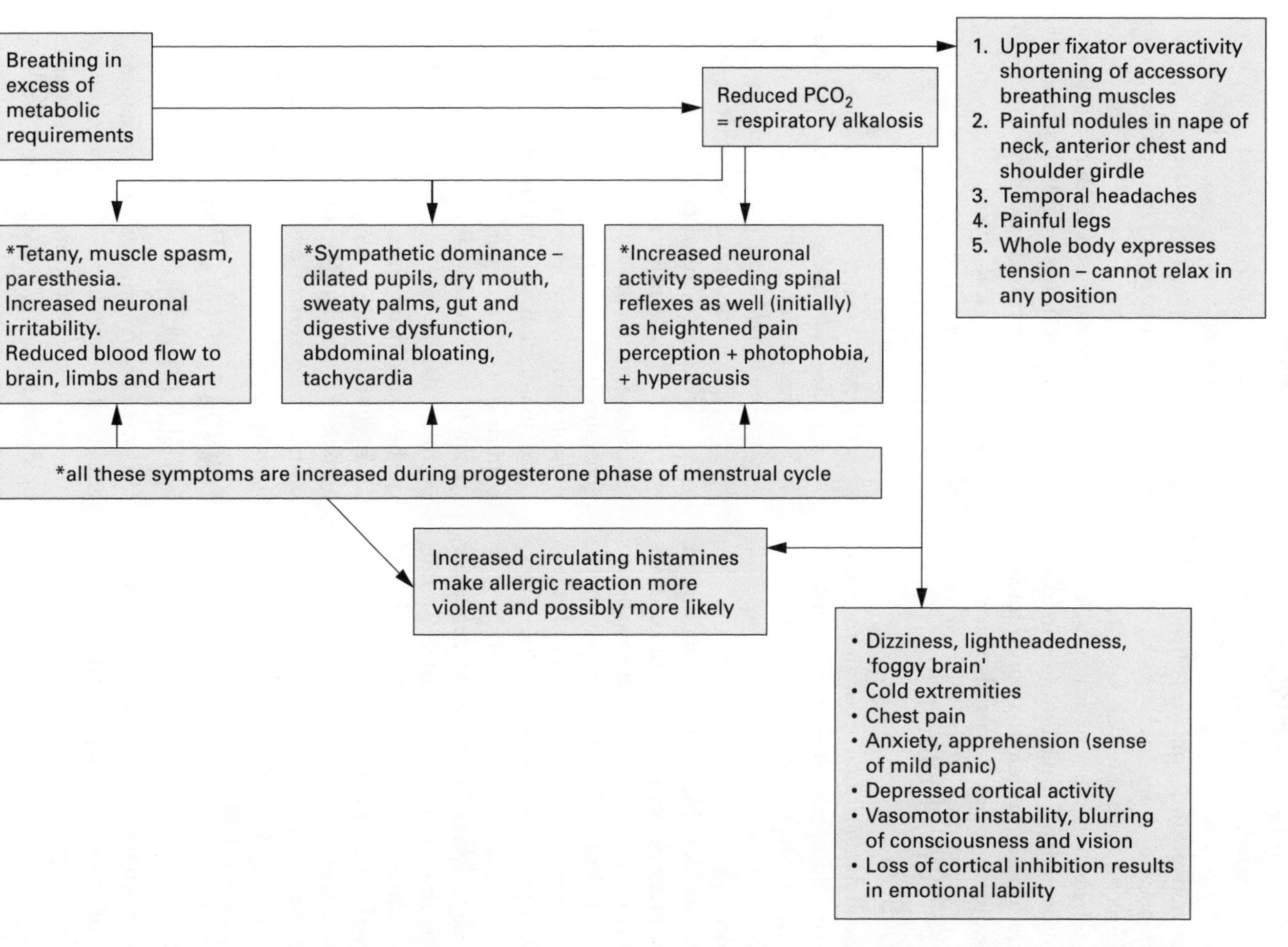

FIGURE 14-1 ■ Negative health effects of a dysfunctional breathing pattern, such as hyperventilation. (From Chaitow L, Delany JW: *Clinical application of neuromuscular techniques, vol 1, The upper body,* Edinburgh, 2000, Churchill Livingstone.)

the bloodstream tends to become more tightly bound to its hemoglobin carrier molecule, leading to decreased oxygenation of tissues **(Bohr effect).**

In addition to all these events, the threshold of peripheral nerve firing is decreased, which leads to an increased perception of pain. The fascia contains a vast network of capillaries, autonomic nerves, sensory nerve endings, and smooth muscle cells. The ANS seems to be able to regulate tension in the fascia by causing the smooth muscles to contract. An elevated pH (alkalinity) caused by disordered breathing can produce smooth muscle contraction and even spasm in fascial tissues.

SIGNS AND SYMPTOMS OF BREATHING PATTERN DISORDER

The biochemical changes that occur in response to disordered breathing can cause many signs and symptoms. The massage therapist should continually monitor the patient for them during each massage session.

- *Cardiovascular effects:* Palpitations, missed beats, tachycardia, sharp or dull atypical chest pain, angina, vasomotor instability, cold extremities, Raynaud's phenomenon, blotchy flushing of the blush area, capillary vasoconstriction (face, arms, hands)
- *Neurologic effects:* Dizziness, unsteadiness or instability, feelings of faintness (in rare cases, actual fainting); visual disturbance (blurred or tunnel vision); headache (muscle tension and vascular migraine); paraesthesia (i.e., numbness, uselessness, heaviness, pins and needles, burning, limbs that feel out of proportion or as if they "don't belong"), commonly of the hands, feet, or face but sometimes of the scalp or whole body; hypersensitivity to light or noise; dilated pupils (wearing dark glasses on a dull day); sensation of giddiness
- *Respiratory effects:* Shortness of breath, typically after exertion; irritable cough, tightness or oppression of the chest; difficulty breathing, "asthmatic," air hunger, inability to take a satisfying breath; excessive sighing, yawning, or sniffing
- *Gastrointestinal effects:* Difficulty swallowing, dry mouth and throat; acid regurgitation, heartburn, exaggeration of symptoms of hiatal hernia as a result of aerophagia (air swallowing), nausea, flatulence, belching, abdominal discomfort, bloating
- *Muscular effects:* Cramps, muscle pains (particularly occipital, neck, shoulders, and between scapulae; less commonly, lower back and limbs), tremors, twitching, weakness, stiffness or tetany (seizing up), increased fascial tone
- *Psychological effects:* Tension, anxiety, "unreal feelings," depersonalization, feeling "out of body," panic, phobias, agoraphobia (fear of being in open spaces)
- *General effects:* Feelings of weakness; exhaustion; impaired concentration, memory, and performance; disturbed sleep, including nightmares; emotional sweating (axillae, palms, sometimes whole body); "thick-headed" sensation

Massage therapists also should be alert for generalized body tension characterized by increases in motor and fascial tone and chronic inability to relax. In addition, individuals prone to breathing pattern disorder are particularly prone to spasm (tetany) in muscles involved in the "attack posture"; that is, they hunch the shoulders, thrust the head and neck forward, scowl, and clench the teeth. The massage therapist needs to be able to address the mechanism of breathing effectively, both to help correct dysfunction and to support optimal function.

COMMON PHYSICAL CHANGES IN BREATHING PATTERN DISORDER

If the accessory muscles of respiration (the scalenes, sternocleidomastoid, serratus posterior superior, pectoralis minor, levator scapulae, rhomboids, abdominals, and quadratus lumborum) are constantly activated for breathing when forced inhalation and expiration are not required, dysfunctional muscle patterns typically occur.

Therapeutic massage can help normalize these conditions and support more effective breathing (Box 14-1). Breathing well is very difficult if the

BOX 14-1 Massage Interventions for Common Soft Tissue Changes in Breathing Pattern Disorder

- With breathing pattern disorder, an imbalance develops between increasingly weak abdominal muscles and increasingly tight erector spinae muscles, coupled with a weak or overly taut pelvic floor structure.
  - *Massage addresses this condition by:* Correcting muscle firing sequences, reducing motor tone in tight and short muscles, and supporting therapeutic exercise of weak muscles.
- Increased fascial tension is also a factor in this disorder.
  - *Massage addresses this condition by:* Using connective tissue methods and techniques that reduce the activity of the sympathetic autonomic nervous system.
- The upper ribs are elevated, there is a sensitive costal cartilage tension, and the thoracic spine is disturbed because of lack of normal motion of the articulation with the ribs. Sympathetic outflow from this area may be affected.
  - *Massage addresses this condition by:* Increasing the pliability of surrounding tissues and providing gentle mobilization of the jointed areas. Chiropractic or osteopathic manipulation may be helpful, and massage can prepare the soft tissue before manipulation and soothe the tissue afterward.
- Accessory respiratory muscles increase in motor tone and shorten, especially the scalenes, upper trapezius, and levator scapulae.
  - *Massage addresses this condition by:* Providing inhibitory pressure at the attachment and in the muscle belly, coupled with muscle energy methods and lengthening of short muscles.
- Fibrosis and trigger points develop in the accessory muscles of breathing.
  - *Massage addresses this condition by:* Using mechanical force applications, which increase tissue pliability and reduce activity in the trigger points that are most medial and most proximal and that recreate active symptoms
- The cervical spine becomes progressively rigid, and a fixed lordosis is a common feature in the lower cervical spine. Reduced mobility of the second cervical segment and disturbance of vagal outflow from this region are likely.
  - *Massage addresses this condition by:* Reducing soft tissue restriction, which increases the effectiveness of any type of joint mobilization or manipulation.
- Upper crossed syndrome patterns develop, which can lead to lower crossed syndrome patterns as well.
  - *Massage addresses this condition by:* In general, lengthening the short areas, increasing tissue pliability, and supporting therapeutic exercise in the areas that are weak and long.

mechanics are not working efficiently. Many who have attempted breathing retraining have been frustrated by their inability to change the breathing pattern; this happens because the muscle patterns have not changed. Individuals with this problem may have more success after the soft tissues of the body and the mechanisms of breathing have been normalized.

Massage influences breathing in two distinct ways:

- It supports balance between the sympathetic and parasympathetic ANS functions. This generally is accomplished by using a relaxation focus for the general protocol described in Chapter 11 (and shown in the Appendix, p. 761). It normalizes and then maintains effective thoracic and respiratory muscle function.

The massage protocol that follows specifically targets these circumstances. If the assessment indicates a tendency for breathing pattern dysfunction, these applications are integrated into the general protocol to work more specifically with breathing function. It is strongly recommended that the reader study this condition further by using the textbook *Multidisciplinary Approaches to Breathing Pattern Disorders.**

SPECIFIC MASSAGE ASSESSMENT AND STRATEGIES FOR BREATHING PATTERN DISORDER

The massage therapist can assess for breathing pattern disorder and use the information to develop appropriate treatment plans. The patient should be referred to the physician for specific diagnosis. Some conditions benefit from treatment by a respiratory therapist.

Assessment

1. Observe the patient for the following:
   - Breathes through the nose or mouth
   - Frequently sighs or yawns
   - Holds the breath for short periods

*Chaitow L, Bradley D, Gilbert C: *Multidisciplinary approaches to breathing pattern disorders*, 2002, Churchill Livingstone.

- Shows chaotic combinations of the preceding factors
- Repeatedly clears the throat, gulps air, or sniffs
- Swallows frequently

2. Observe and palpate for overuse of the upper chest breathing muscles during normal relaxed breathing.

    Stand behind the patient and place the person's hands over the upper trapezius area so that the tips of the fingers rest on the top of the clavicles. As the patient breathes, determine whether the accessory muscles are used for relaxed breathing. If the shoulders move up and down as the patient breathes, the accessory muscles probably are being recruited. In normal relaxed breathing, the shoulders should not move up and down. The patient also is using the accessory muscles if the chest movement is concentrated in the upper chest rather than the lower ribs and abdomen. Any use of the accessory muscles for breathing results in increased tension and a tendency to develop trigger points. These conditions can be identified with palpation. Connective tissue changes are common, because the breathing dysfunction often is chronic. The connective tissues palpate as thick, dense, and shortened in this area.

3. Assess the inhale to exhale ratio.

    Have the patient naturally inhale and exhale and observe for a consistent exhale phase that is longer than the inhale phase. In normal relaxed breathing, the inhalation phase is shorter than the exhalation phase. The reverse of this pattern is the basis for breathing pattern disorder. The ideal pattern is 2 to 4 counts for inhalation and 6 to 12 counts for exhalation. Targeted massage and breathing retraining methods can restore normal relaxed breathing.

4. Assess the patient's ability to hold the breath.

    Have the patient hold the breath without strain to assess for tolerance to CO_2 levels. The patient should be able to hold the breath comfortably for at least 15 seconds (30 seconds is ideal).

5. Assess rib mobility.

    With the patient in each of the following positions–supine, prone, side-lying, or seated–palpate and gently mobilize the thorax to assess for rib mobility. The ribs should have a springy feel and should be a bit more mobile from the sixth to the tenth ribs.

6. Assess for shortness of the accessory muscles of breathing and for functional problems.

    Muscles that should be assessed for shortening and for an increase in both muscle and motor tone are the quadratus lumborum, psoas, pectoralis major, latissimus dorsi, upper trapezius, levator scapulae, scalenes, and sternocleidomastoid, as well as the thoracic and cervical paraspinal muscles. Functional assessments should be performed (involving muscle activating firing sequences) to establish the relative functional efficiency of the scapulohumeral rhythm, as well as hip extension and abduction.

7. Apply skin palpation methods (e.g., drag) to assess for viscerosomatic and reflexive dysfunction.

    Areas that redden or are hot, sweaty, or develop goose bumps are active. A trigger point evaluation should be done in muscles shown by previous assessments to be dysfunctional. For this purpose, use appropriate palpation methods, especially drag palpation.

Massage Strategies

Massage focused on breathing dysfunction specifically targets the following muscles, because they tend to shorten with this disorder:

- Scalenes
- Sternocleidomastoid
- Serratus anterior
- Serratus posterior superior and inferior
- Levator scapulae
- Rhomboids
- Upper trapezius
- Pectoralis major and minor
- Latissimus dorsi
- Psoas
- Quadratus lumborum
- All abdominals
- Pelvic floor muscles
- Calf muscles

The intercostals and the diaphragm, the main muscles of breathing, also are addressed. All these muscles should be assessed for shortening and increased motor tone, weakness, and agonist/antagonist interaction. Muscles that orient mostly transverse (e.g., the serratus anterior, serratus posterior superior and inferior, rhomboids, and pelvic floor muscles) are difficult to assess with movement and strength testing. Palpation is more accurate for these muscles.

Muscles assessed as short need to be lengthened. If a neuromuscular cause is the primary reason for the shortening, use muscle energy methods, inhibitory pressure, or both at the muscle belly and the attachment and lengthen either by moving the adjacent joints apart or, more likely, by introducing tension, bend, or torsion force directly on the muscle tissues. For the scalenes, sternocleidomastoid, serratus anterior, pectoralis minor, latissimus dorsi, psoas, quadratus lumborum, diaphragm, rectus abdominis, and pelvic floor muscles, follow the recommendations in the specific release section in Chapter 13. Perform these muscle releases only if the muscles are assessed as short, cause symptoms, and appear to directly restrict breathing. Only work specifically with the most dysfunctional muscles during any session if the patient's ability to adapt is compromised. Address the more superficial muscles first (e.g., the latissimus dorsi, rectus abdominis, pectoralis major, trapezius). Work each area as needed and as it becomes convenient during the general massage session. Use the least invasive technique possible to restore a more normal muscle resting length.

When the breathing pattern has been dysfunctional for some time (longer than 3 months), connective tissue changes are common. Focused connective tissue massage is effective for this.

Once the soft tissue is more normal, gentle mobilization of the joints of the thorax is appropriate. If the thoracic vertebrae and ribs are restricted, chiropractic or other joint manipulation methods may be appropriate, and referral is indicated. Massage therapists can use indirect functional techniques to help increase the mobility of the area.

Because breathing is a whole body function, the methods and sequences used to address the breathing function need to be integrated into a full body approach. A protocol that could be added to the general massage session proceeds as follows (it also is demonstrated on the DVD that accompanies this text):

- Increase your attention to the general massage of the thorax. Posterior, anterior, and lateral access to the thorax is used primarily to address the general tension or dysfunctional patterns in the respiratory muscles of this area. Address the scalenes, psoas, and quadratus lumborum if they are symptomatic. Massage the legs, especially the calves.
- Normalize the muscle activating/firing sequences if possible. If treatment is ineffective after two or three attempts, it is less likely that optimal function can be restored during the current session. Attempt it again during the next massage session.
- Use appropriate muscle energy techniques to lengthen and stretch the shortened muscles of the cervical, thoracic, and lumbar regions and the legs.
- Gently move the rib cage with broad-based compression. Incorporate indirect functional techniques to support mobility. Assess for areas that move easily (ease) and those that are restricted (bind). With the patient in the supine position, identify the amount of rigidity in the ribs by applying bilateral compression to the thorax beginning near the clavicles and moving down toward the lower ribs, maintaining compressive force near the costal cartilage. With the patient in the prone position, identify rigidity in the ribs on both sides of the spine at the facet joints, beginning near the seventh cervical vertebra and moving down toward the lower ribs, maintaining compressive force near the facet joints. With the patient in the side-lying position, use compression against the lateral aspect of the thorax to assess rib mobility in both the facet and costal joints. Begin applying the compression near the axilla and move down toward the lower ribs. Apply the compression with sufficient force that you can feel the ribs spring, but not so much as to cause discomfort.

A normal response is a feeling of equal springiness and mobility bilaterally. A feeling of stiffness or rigidity indicates immobility.

- Identify the area of the greatest mobility (ease) and the area of the greatest restriction (bind). Position the patient so that a broad-based, compressive force can be applied to the areas of ease. Apply compression gently and slowly until the area begins to bind. Hold this position and have the patient cough. Coughing acts as a muscle energy method and supports mobility through activation of the muscles. Repeat 3 or 4 times.
- If areas of rigidity remain, the following direct functional technique may be useful:
  1. Apply broad-based compression to the area of immobility (bind) using the whole hand or forearm.
  2. Have the patient exhale, then slightly increase the intensity of the compressive force while following the exhalation.
  3. Hold the ribs in this position.
  4. Have the patient push out against the compressive pressure.
  5. Instruct the patient to inhale while you continue to hold the compressive focus against the ribs.
  6. Have the patient exhale while you increase the compressive force, following the action of the ribs. You should note an increase in mobility.
- Gently mobilize the entire thorax with rhythmic compression. Reassess the area of greatest bind. If the areas treated have improved, a different area is located and the sequence is repeated. Three or four areas can be done in a session.
- Palpate for tender points in the intercostals, pectoralis minor, and anterior serratus. (Patients are not very tolerant of this, so be direct and precise.) Use positional release to release these points by moving the patient (or having the patient move) into various positions until the pain in the tender point diminishes. The procedure for positional release in this area has been adapted as follows:
  1. Locate the tender point.
  2. Gently initiate the pain response with direct pressure. (Remember, the sensation of pain is a guide only; the pain point is *not* the point of intervention.)
  3. Slowly position the body, actively or passively, until the pain subsides. This positioning can be local, achieved by moving the patient's ribs. It also can be more general, accomplished by moving the arm, the head, or the whole body and involving many different areas (including having the patient move the eyes) to find the position where pain diminishes (see the DVD).
  4. Maintain the position up to 30 seconds or until the patient feels the release while lightly monitoring the tender point.
  5. Slowly reposition the patient to neutral and then into a lengthening position for the tender point. If the release position was accomplished primarily by moving the ribs, direct tissue stretching usually is most effective.

Breathing Retraining

Once the thorax and breathing function begin to normalize (usually after four to six focused sessions), the patient can be taught simple breathing exercises. The main focus is the process of exhalation; do not even address the inhalation process. When the exhale pattern normalizes, the inhale pattern usually does as well. The respiratory therapist may need to be involved in the breathing retraining program. Make sure that you arrange the appropriate collaboration.

The four basic principles of restoring normal, energy-efficient, physiologically balanced breathing are:

1. Awareness of faulty breathing patterns
2. Relaxation of the upper chest, shoulders, and accessory muscles and improved use of the body (e.g., posture)
3. Retraining of an abdominal/low chest breathing pattern
4. Awareness of normal breathing rates and rhythms both at rest and during activity

Three common activities can normalize the inhale to exhale ratio: yelling, crying, and laughing. Blowing up balloons is a good exercise to support the exhale function, as is playing a horn, flute, or similar musical instrument. Singing, chanting, or simply toning the vowel sounds (a, e, i, o, u) are variations that support the exhale function. Each of these activities, sustained for 3 to 5 minutes, can be a valuable part of any breathing retraining program.

Many additional resources are available for retraining breathing patterns. Find one that is comfortable and use it regularly. The pursed lip exhale is helpful as a retraining exercise. The patient inhales as he or she typically would, holds the breath for a couple of seconds, and then exhales slowly and gently (as if trying to make a candle flame about a foot away flicker) by blowing the air through pursed lips.

Methods that might inhibit the muscles that contribute to upper chest breathing include the following:

- On inhalation, pushing the elbows or forearms down on the arms of a chair
- On inhalation, putting the arms behind the back, grasping the wrist with the other hand, and pulling down
- Reclining with the hands behind the head ("beach pose") to open the chest and reduce shoulder movement during inhalation
- On inhalation, interlocking the hands on the lap and applying finger pad pressure to the dorsum of the hands to inhibit shoulder movement
- Putting one hand behind the back and the other hand around the back of the head

Combining a slow breathing pattern with a stretching and flexibility program that targets the short muscle areas can be helpful for the patient. The patient also can practice holding the breath, until the breath can comfortably be held for 30 seconds.

Rescue breathing techniques for risk situations that are likely to trigger symptoms (e.g., laughing, crying, high-intensity exercise, prolonged speech, humid or hot conditions, flying) include the following (Figure 14-2):

- Raise both arms over the head, interlace the fingers, and turn the hands palm up. Breathe slowly, concentrating on the exhale. This position inhibits the accessory breathing muscles and supports diaphragm function.
- Perform short breath holds (to allow CO_2 levels to rise) followed by low chest/low volume breathing. Great care must be taken to teach patients to hold the breath only to the point of slight discomfort and to avoid deep respirations on letting go.
- Cup the hands over the nose and mouth and breathe into the hands for 1 to 2 minutes. This helps the patient identify and separate symptoms from triggers.
- Sit in front of a fan. The sensation of air moving over the trigeminal nerve outlet on each side of the face helps deepen and calm respiration.

Remind patients to forget about their breathing between practice sessions, because keeping aware of one's breathing all the time is unnatural and uncomfortable. Encourage short, effective practice sessions.

PAIN

Pain is a major issue in healthcare, and pain management is most effective when pursued as a multidisciplinary intervention. Pain is a universal experience. The degree to which a person reacts to pain depends on the individual's biologic, psychological, and cultural makeup. Past encounters with painful conditions also can influence pain sensitivity. Patients who are prone to recurring injury in the same area can experience increasing pain sensation for the same or even a less significant injury **(sensitization).** Sensitization also can occur with pain associated with illness.

Pain that persists beyond the expected duration of healing can become a chronic condition. No longer is the pain just the symptom of another disease; now, it is a separate condition unto itself. The massage therapist needs to understand pain and how to use massage methods effectively to manage pain. This information expands on the content in Units One and Two and provides specific massage strategies for pain management.

The massage professional especially needs to understand the mechanisms of pain. Pain

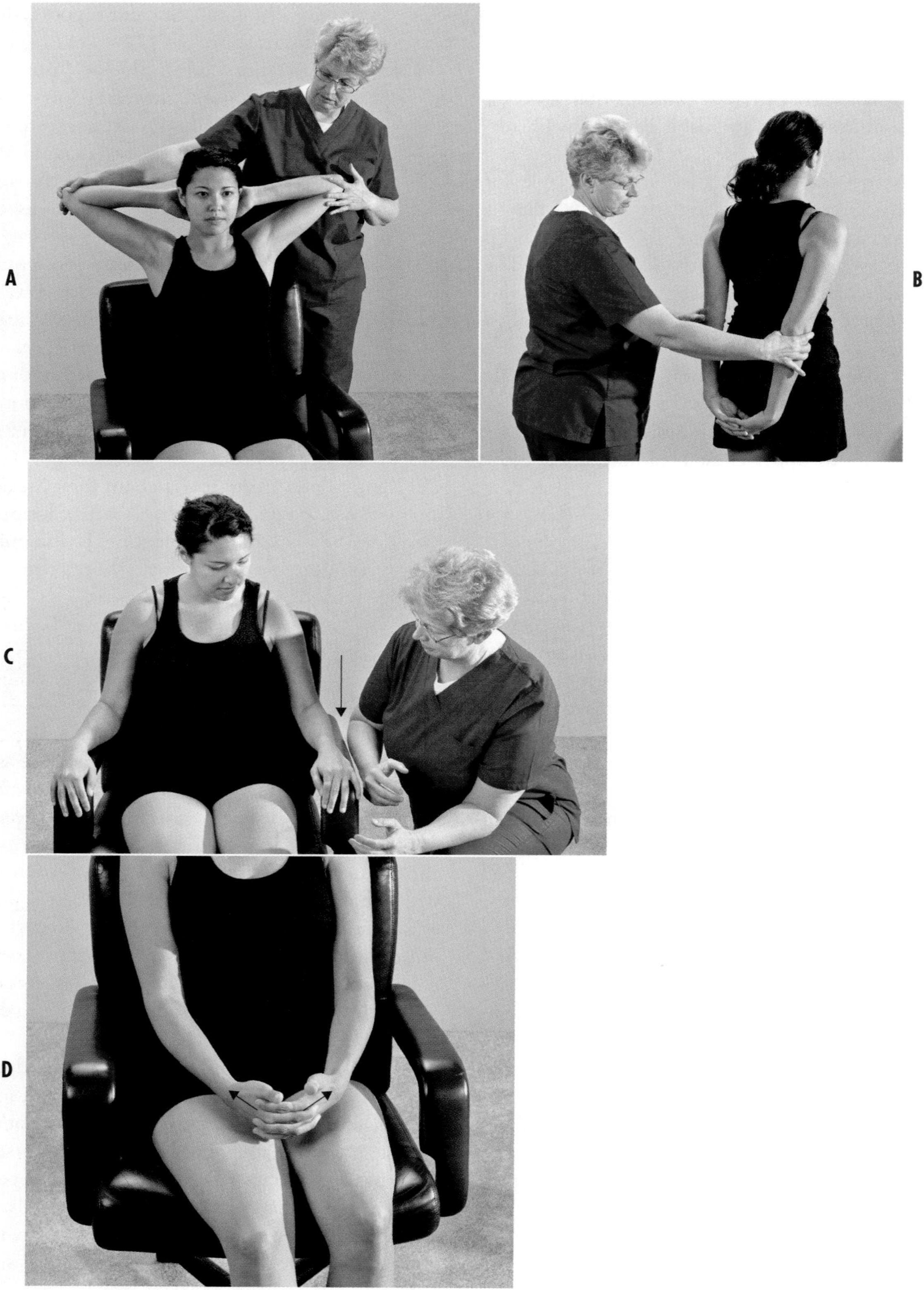

FIGURE 14-2 ■ Breathing retraining: ways to position the body and activate muscle groups to inhibit upper chest breathing and support normal breathing function. **A,** This position opens up the chest and lifts the lower ribs. **B,** This position opens the chest and inhibits the breathing muscles that produce inhalation. **C,** Pressing the forearm down on the arm of the chair inhibits the upper chest muscles. **D,** Pressing the fingers into the top of the hand inhibits the shoulder muscles, supporting belly breathing.

BOX 14-2 Health Conditions Related to Breathing Dysfunction

Allergies
Anxiety
Asthma
Cardiovascular
Chronic bronchitis
Chronic obstructive pulmonary disease (COPD)
Constipation
Depression
Emphysema
Fatigue syndromes
High blood pressure
Insomnia
Lymphatic stagnation
Pain syndromes
Panic attacks
Posture, spinal stabilization
Sinusitis
Sleep apnea
Snoring

receptors are found in almost every tissue of the body and may respond to any type of stimulus. When stimuli for other sensations, (e.g., touch, pressure, heat, and cold) reach certain intensities, they also stimulate the sensation of pain. Injured tissue may release prostaglandins, making peripheral nociceptors more sensitive to the normal pain response (hyperalgesia). Aspirin and other **nonsteroidal antiinflammatory drugs (NSAIDs)** inhibit the action of prostaglandins and reduce pain.

Pain is caused by excessive stimulation of a sensory organ. Additional stimuli for pain receptors include excessive distention or dilation of a structure, prolonged muscular contractions, muscle spasms, inadequate blood flow to tissues, and the presence of certain substances. Through their sensitivity to all stimuli, pain receptors perform a protective function by identifying changes that may endanger the body.

The point at which a stimulus is perceived as painful is called the **pain threshold.** This varies somewhat from individual to individual. One factor affecting the pain threshold is **perceptual dominance,** in which the pain felt in one area of the body diminishes or obliterates the pain felt in another area. Not until the most severe pain is diminished does the person perceive or acknowledge the other pain. This mechanism is often activated with massage applications that produce a "good hurt" as a pain management strategy.

Pain tolerance is the length of time or the intensity of pain that the person endures before acknowledging it and seeking relief. Like the pain threshold, pain tolerance is likely to vary from one individual to another. A person's tolerance for pain is influenced by a variety of factors, including personality type, psychological state at the onset of pain, previous experiences, sociocultural background, and the meaning of the pain to that person (e.g., the ways in which it affects the person's lifestyle). Factors that reduce pain tolerance include repeated exposure to pain, fatigue, fear, sleep deprivation, and stress. Warmth, cold, distraction, alcohol consumption, hypnosis, and strong spiritual beliefs or faith all serve to increase pain tolerance.

The origins of pain can be divided into two types, somatic pain and visceral pain. **Somatic pain** arises from stimulation of receptors in the skin (superficial somatic pain) or from stimulation of receptors in skeletal muscles, joints, tendons, and fascia (deep somatic pain). **Visceral pain** results from stimulation of receptors in the viscera (internal organs).

Pain usually is classified as acute, chronic, intractable, phantom, or referred pain.

DEFINING PAIN

As mention previously, pain is caused by the stimulation of nociceptors. These receptors usually are stimulated by chemicals such as substance P, bradykinin, and histamine, which excite the nerve endings. Pain is elicited by three different classes of stimuli: mechanical, chemical, and thermal stimuli. Also, the brain inhibits or enhances a reaction to pain. This explains how patients can ignore pain and fear, and anxiety can exaggerate pain. Soft tissue pain is caused by the chemicals released during tissue injury o
irritation arising from cumulativ
flammation, or extreme hot or c
psychological stress, called *auton*
can cause pain by causing hyp

muscles and shifts in fluid flow that affect oxygen and nutrient delivery and waste removal.

Visceral pain occurs when the viscera sends impulses to the limbic and hypothalamic areas of the brain; this also causes emotional reactions of anxiety, fear, anger, and depression.

Pain basically results from a series of exchanges involving three major components: the peripheral nerves, the spinal cord, and the brain.

The Peripheral Nerves

The peripheral nerves make up a network of nerve fibers that branch throughout the body. Attached to some of these fibers are special nerve endings (nociceptors) that can sense an unpleasant stimulus, such as a cut, a burn, or painful pressure.

Millions of nociceptors are found in the skin, bones, joints, and muscles and in the protective membranes around the internal organs. They are concentrated in areas more prone to injury, such as the fingers and toes. As many as 1300 nociceptors may be found in just 1 square inch of skin. Skin stimulation during massage that is intense enough to produce the "good hurt" response causes the nociceptors to fire. This is one of the mechanisms of counterirritation; it also is a major massage benefit for pain management.

The muscles, protected beneath the skin, have fewer nerve endings. The internal organs, protected by skin, muscle, and bone, have even fewer. Some nociceptors sense sharp blows, others sense heat. One type senses pressure, temperature, and chemical changes. Nociceptors can also detect inflammation caused by injury, disease, or infection.

Massage that addresses these receptors must involve enough depth of pressure and intensity to elicit a sensory response without causing unnecessary pain or a guarding response.

When nociceptors detect a harmful stimulus, they relay pain messages, in the form of electrical impulses, along a peripheral nerve to the spinal cord and brain. The speed at which the messages travel can vary. Sensations of severe pain are transmitted almost instantaneously. Dull, aching pain (e.g., an upset stomach, earache, or achy [illegible]nt) is relayed on fibers that transmit more [illegible].

The Spinal Cord

When pain messages reach the spinal cord, they connect with specialized nerve cells that act as gatekeepers. These gatekeepers filter the pain messages on their way to the interpretive areas of the brain, where the pain is felt and understood and coping strategies are developed.

For severe pain that is linked to bodily harm, the "gate" is wide open, and the messages take an express route to the brain. Nerve cells in the spinal cord also respond to these urgent warnings. They trigger other parts of the nervous system into action, especially the motor nerves, which signal muscles to move away from harm (this process is known as a *reflex arc*). Weak pain messages (e.g., a scratch) may be filtered or blocked by the gatekeepers. People often do not realize that they have these minor injuries, and the massage therapist may be the first to notice them.

The pain messages can also change in the spinal cord. Other sensations may overpower and diminish the pain signals. This is called **counterirritation** (or *hyperstimulation analgesia*). Massage is an effective intervention for creating counterirritation to suppress pain sensation.

Nerve cells in the spinal cord also release chemicals such as endorphins and substance P that amplify or diminish the strength of a pain signal that reaches the brain for interpretation. Massage can influence these chemical responses, although research has not yet identified the exact mechanism.

The Brain

When pain messages reach the brain, they are first processed by the thalamus, which is a sorting and switching station. The thalamus quickly interprets the messages as pain and forwards them simultaneously to three specialized regions of the brain: the physical sensation region (somatosensory cortex), the emotional feeling region (limbic system), and the thinking (cognitive) region (frontal cortex). Awareness of pain therefore is a complex experience of sensing, feeling, and thinking. Pain tolerance comes from the interplay of these functions. Massage can influence all these areas: somatic sensation through nerve stimulation; the limbic system by calming sympathetic dominance and providing nurturing; and the cognitive areas through education, reframing, and providing symptom relief.

The brain responds to pain by sending messages that trigger the healing process. Signals are sent to the ANS, which sends additional blood and nutrients to the area. Pain-suppressing chemicals send stop-pain messages. The use of pain-suppressing medication that mimics the body's own chemicals is controversial and may even slow healing. However, the stress of severe acute pain can slow the healing process, and intractable chronic pain suppresses the immune system. In these cases, pain medication is appropriate and supports healing.

PAIN SENSATION

Pain comes in many forms of physical sensation: sharp, jabbing, throbbing, burning, stinging, tingling, nagging, dull, and aching. These were described in the assessment section of Unit Two. Pain also varies from mild to severe. Severe sharp pain produces a greater physical and emotional response than mild pain. Severe pain can be incapacitating, making it difficult or impossible to function.

The location of pain can affect the response to it. A headache that interferes with the ability to focus or work may be more bothersome than, for example, arthritic pain in the ankle. Therefore the headache receives a stronger pain response. An individual's emotional and psychological state, memories of past pain experiences, upbringing, and attitude also affect how the person interprets pain messages and tolerates pain.

The emotional state can also improve a person's tolerance of severe pain. People can condition themselves to endure pain that would incapacitate others. Many people who have achieved a higher tolerance for pain may not realize the difference between "good hurt" and "bad hurt" during massage, and this makes them vulnerable to tissue damage from a massage application that is too intense.

ACUTE AND CHRONIC PAIN

Acute and chronic pain are different. **Acute pain** is triggered by tissue damage. This type of pain generally accompanies injury or surgery and is location specific. Acute pain can be mild and last just a moment (e.g., pain caused by an insect sting), or it can be severe and last for weeks or months (e.g., pain from a burn, pulled muscle, or broken bone). [1]

Within a fairly predictable period, and with treatment of the underlying cause, acute pain generally fades away.[1] Massage targets acute pain with symptom management and healing support. It is fairly easy to treat.

In **chronic pain,** the original illness or injury shows every indication of being healed, yet the pain remains and may be even more intense. The pain may be constant, or it may vacillate. Chronic pain also may be caused by vascular conditions that reduce blood flow to an area of the body.

The cause of chronic pain is not well understood, and no sign of disease or damage to the body tissues may be evident that is linked to the pain. This situation is extremely frustrating for the medical team and the patient. Chronic pain that is not related to physical disease or injury or any other physical cause is called **psychogenic pain.** This type of pain is also referred to as a pain disorder with psychological factors. Mental and emotional disorders may cause, increase, or prolong pain. Headache, muscle pain, back pain, and stomach pain are the most common types of psychogenic pain. Physicians and mental health specialists work together to treat patients with this disorder. Massage is one of the more effective interventions for managing chronic pain.

Touch, vibration, and joint and muscle movement stimulate mechanoreceptors, diminishing the pain information received by the brain. Massage stimulates the entire region of the body, along with localized pain areas. A large number of mechanoreceptors are stimulated, dramatically reducing the discomfort of working deep somatic tissues. This is the reason full body massage is better for pain management than localized spot work.

Common Conditions That Cause Chronic Pain

Neck pain and back pain (especially pain in the lower back) are two of the most common health problems in adults. Fortunately, most neck and back pain is temporary, caused by short-term stress on the muscles or ligaments that support the spine rather than by a serious injury or medical condition such as nerve damage or kidney disease. Massage is most effective in pain management related to musculoskeletal neck and back pain.

Long-term illnesses and injuries are the most common causes of chronic pain. Other causes include damage to the CNS or peripheral nervous system (PNS) and vascular conditions. Ongoing conditions that may cause chronic pain include ear infections, migraine headaches, and peripheral neuropathy (e.g., carpal tunnel syndrome). Initial injuries (e.g., sprain, muscle strain) and underuse and overuse injuries (e.g., back pain, Achilles tendinitis, and heel pain) also may become chronic.

Chronic pain caused by damage to the CNS (i.e., brain, brainstem, or spinal cord) or PNS is called **neurogenic pain.** Central pain syndrome, trigeminal neuralgia, and phantom pain are types of neurogenic pain.

Long-term illnesses that may result in chronic pain include the following:

- Cancer (chronic pain often is caused by tumors that infiltrate and compress organs or bones and by treatments, such as radiation and chemotherapy, that cause edema)
- Degenerative disease (e.g., osteoarthritis, osteoporosis)
- Fibromyalgia (Box 14-3)
- Complex regional pain syndrome (formerly called *sympathetic reflex dystrophy*)
- Inflammatory disease (e.g., rheumatoid arthritis)
- Central pain syndrome: A neurologic condition caused by damage to the CNS, this condition may occur in people who have suffered a spinal cord injury, brain injury, or stroke and in patients with multiple sclerosis (MS). It is characterized by steady pain (usually described as a burning, aching, or cutting sensation) and brief bursts of sharp pain. Central pain syndrome may develop years after the CNS is damaged.
- Trigeminal neuralgia: Also called *tic douloureux,* this condition is caused by damage to the fifth cranial nerve (the trigeminal nerve). It is characterized by severe, stabbing pain on one side of the jaw or cheek that typically lasts a few seconds and recurs throughout the day. Talking, brushing the teeth, touching the face, chewing, and swallowing may trigger an attack. Trigeminal neuralgia may persist for days or months, disappear, and recur months or years later.

THE DIAGNOSIS OF PAIN

The general practice physician often initially diagnoses pain conditions. Patients may be referred to a specialist such as a neurologist for diagnosis and treatment. Diagnosis is based on the patient's history, reported signs and symptoms, underlying conditions, physical and neurologic examination, and other types of diagnostic tests.

The diagnostic test may include:

- Imaging tests (i.e., computed tomography [CT], magnetic resonance imaging [MRI] scan), and bone scans
- Spinal tap (i.e., lumbar puncture), to diagnose infection, MS
- Electrophysiologic studies of the nerves and muscles
- Thermography (measures the temperature of surface tissue) used to detect altered blood flow to a painful area, which may indicate a vascular condition.
- Blood test
- Urine tests

EVALUATING PAIN

Pain is a primary indicator in many disease processes. Therefore the massage therapist must have a basic protocol for evaluating pain so that appropriate referrals can be made for diagnosis when necessary.

Pain has many characteristics. Location, for example, can be divided into four categories:

- **Localized pain** is pain confined to the site of origin.
- **Projected pain** typically is a result of proximal nerve compression; this type of

BOX 14-3 Fibromyalgia and Myofascial Pain

A number of researchers have studied the connection between myofascial trigger point activity and fibromyalgia.

- Yunus (1993) states that, "Fibromyalgia and myofascial pain syndrome (MPS) [trigger point–derived pain] share several common features, [and] it is possible that MPS represents an incomplete, regional, or early form of fibromyalgia syndrome since many fibromyalgia patients give a clear history of localized pain before developing gerneralised pain."
- Australian researchers Granges and Littlejohn (1993) studied the overlap between trigger points and tender points in fibromyalgia syndrome (FMS). They concluded that:
  - Tender points in FMS represent a diffusely diminished pain threshold to pressure, whereas trigger points are the expression of a local musculoskeletal abnormality.
  - In diffuse chronic pain states such as FMS, trigger points probably contribute only in a limited and localized way to lowering the pain threshold to pressure.
  - Taken individually, trigger points are an important clinical finding in some patients with FMS; nearly 70% of FMS patients tested have at least one active trigger point.
  - Of FMS patients with active trigger points, about 60% reported that pressure on the trigger point reproduced a localized and familiar FMS pain.
- Researchers at Oregon Health Sciences University studied the history of patients with FMS and found that more than 80% reported that before the onset of generalized symptoms, they suffered from regional pain problems (which almost always involve trigger points). Physical trauma was cited as the major cause of pre-FMS regional pain. Only 18% had FMS that started without previous regional pain (Burckhardt, 1993).
- Research at the University of California in Los Angeles has shown that injecting active trigger points with the pain-killing agent Xylocaine produced marked benefits in FMS patients in terms of pain relief and reduction of stiffness; however this relief was not significantly apparent for at least 1 week after the injections. FMS patients reported more local soreness after the injections than patients with only myofascial pain, but the FMS patients improved after this initial soreness resolved. This reinforces the opinion of many practitioners that myofascial trigger points contribute a large degree of the pain experienced in FMS (Hong, 1996).
- Travell and Simons (1993) found that, "Most of these [fibromyalgia] patients would be likely to have specific myofascial pain syndromes that would respond to myofascial therapy."

Modified from Chaitow L, Delany J: *Clinical application of neuromuscular techniques, vol 1, The upper body,* London, 2000, Churchill Livingstone.

pain is perceived in the tissue supplied by the nerve.

- **Radiating pain** is diffuse pain (i.e., not well localized) around the site of origin.
- **Referred pain** is felt in an area distant from the site of the painful stimulus.

Pain also can be divided into five types:

1. **Pricking (bright) pain:** Pricking, or bright, pain results when the skin is cut or jabbed with a sharp object. It is short-lived but intense and easily localized.
2. **Burning pain:** Burning pain is slower to develop, lasts longer, and is less accurately localized. It occurs when the skin is burned, and it often stimulates cardiac and respiratory activity.
3. **Aching pain:** Aching pain occurs when the visceral organs are stimulated. It is constant, not well localized, and often referred to areas of the body far from the point of damage. This type of pain is important, because it may be a sign of a life-threatening disorder of a vital organ.
4. **Deep pain:** The main difference between superficial and deep sensibility is the different nature of the pain evoked by noxious stimuli. Unlike superficial pain, deep pain is poorly localized, nauseating, and frequently associated with sweating and changes in blood pressure. Deep pain can be elicited experimentally from the periosteum and ligaments by injecting them with hypertonic saline. Pain produced in this fashion initiates reflex contraction of nearby skeletal muscles. This reflex contraction is similar to the muscle spasm associated with injuries to bones, tendons, and joints. The steadily contracting muscles become ischemic, and ischemia stimulates the pain receptors in the muscles. The pain, in turn, initiates more spasms, creating a vicious cycle called the *pain-spasm-pain cycle.*
5. **Muscle pain:** If a muscle has sufficient blood supply as it contracts and then relaxes, pain does not occur. Pain can occur regardless of the cause if the blood supply to a muscle is occluded (closed off) and can persist until blood flow is reestablished. Also if a muscle with an adequate blood supply contracts continuously without periods of relaxation, pain can occur because the sustained contraction compresses the blood vessels supplying the muscle, resulting in decreased blood availability.

Nonverbal behaviors such as facial grimacing, flinching, tearing, abnormal gait or posture, muscle tension, and guarding of the body are common indicators of pain. Verbal and emotional signals indicating pain may include crying, moaning, groaning, irritability, sadness, and changes in voice tone.

Pain scales, which involve rating the pain on a scale of 1 to 10 or describing it as mild, moderate, or severe (Figure 14-3), are helpful for measuring pain perception. Only the patient can determine the severity. Pain is rarely the same at all times. It is felt (perceived) differently over time and differs with various precipitating and aggravating factors. Pain can range from excruciating to mild and may be difficult for the patient to verbalize. Without a diagnosis or logical reason for the pain (e.g., a recent burn or mild ankle sprain or areas of exhaustion with delayed onset muscle soreness), the massage therapist should assume that the pain is a symptom of an underlying condition that requires evaluation by the appropriate healthcare professional.

Medical Treatment for Pain

Managing pain challenges the healthcare system because there are so many reasons for pain. A painful condition may have multiple causal factors, and a multidisciplinary approach offers the best treatment results. Treatment for pain depends on the type of pain and the underlying cause. Because pain is a subjective experience, patients and the healthcare team need to work together to find the best treatment plan. Complete pain relief is not always possible, and the patient needs to have realistic expectations and be willing to make the necessary lifestyle changes identified in the treatment plan. Since pain (especially chronic pain) can create feelings of helplessness it can be difficult to actively engage the patient in pain management strategies.

Treatment plans for pain management usually start with the least invasive measures and become increasingly intense as needed. **Transcutaneous**

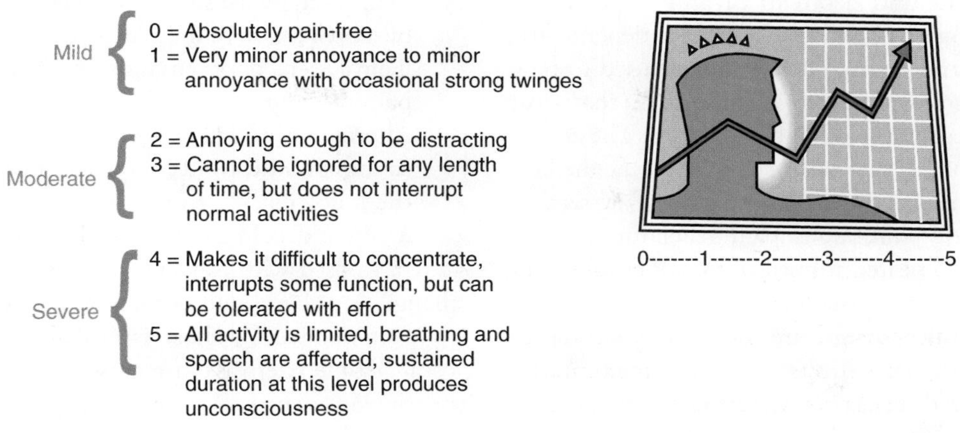

The Pain Scale
Mild
0 = Absolutely pain-free
1 = Very minor annoyance to minor annoyance with occasional strong twinges
Moderate
2 = Annoying enough to be distracting
3 = Cannot be ignored for any length of time, but does not interrupt normal activities
Severe
4 = Makes it difficult to concentrate, interrupts some function, but can be tolerated with effort
5 = All activity is limited, breathing and speech are affected, sustained duration at this level produces unconsciousness
0-------1-------2-------3-------4-------5

FIGURE 14-3 ■ Pain scale. (From Salvo S: *Massage therapy: principles and practice*, ed 2, Philadelphia, 2003, WB Saunders.)

electrical nerve stimulation (TENS), uses brief pulses of electricity applied to nerve endings to block pain transmission. and is safe and noninvasive. This procedure has proved effective for many different types of chronic pain. The mechanism of action appears to be that the small electrical impulses interfere with pain signals.

Surgery may eliminate some types of chronic pain. Joint replacement surgery for hip pain and diskectomy to relieve nerve compression are examples of surgical intervention. Cordotomy involves severing of the nerve fibers on one or both sides of the spinal cord and may be used in severe cases of lower body pain when other treatments are ineffective. This procedure eliminates the sensations of pain and temperature.

Brain or spinal cord stimulation may be used to treat widespread, severe pain. This invasive procedure involves surgical implantation of electrodes in the brain or spine, which the patient controls by means of an external transmitter. Technologic advancement in this type of device has increased its effectiveness.

Medications Used to Treat Pain

Medication for pain control is very effective for short-term acute pain and should be used to alleviate surgical pain and other forms of acute pain related to injury. However, long-term use of pain medication almost always will produce undesirable side effects. Over-the-counter (OTC) analgesics (e.g., NSAIDs) may be used to treat chronic pain. People will often self-treat with over-the-counter medication; however, individuals should not use these medications to relieve pain for longer than 10 days without consulting a physician. These medications can mask serious underlying causes of pain or result in side effects such as nausea, abdominal pain, gastrointestinal bleeding, reduced blood clotting ability, dizziness, tinnitus (ear ringing), and rash.

Prescription medications commonly used to treat chronic pain include:

1. Muscle relaxants: side effects—drowsiness, dry mouth, and constipation.
2. Prescription-strength NSAIDs: side effects—indigestion, diarrhea, stomach pain, and reduced blood coagulation.
3. Opioids: side effects—tolerance requiring increased use to achieve same result, dependence, addiction, confusion, constipation, dry mouth, excessive sleepiness, excessive sweating, high blood pressure or low blood pressure, nausea, and vomiting.
4. Opioid analgesics delivered by a patch worn on the skin—side effects—cause life-

threatening hypoventilation (reduced breathing rate and depth of breathing) tolerance, and physical and psychological dependence. This transdermal dosing can be used to treat moderate to severe chronic pain that does not respond to other medications. The advantage of this delivery system is that the medication is slowly released into the system to provide continuous pain relief for up to 3 days. Repeated administration of opioids may result.

5. **Adjuvant drugs** are used to increase or support the effects of other medications. Adjuvant drugs include antidepressants, anticonvulsants, and corticosteroids.
6. They may be used to treat chronic pain that does not respond to other pain relievers and to reduce the side effects of other medications.
7. Complementary and alternative pain treatments

Many alternative approaches are also used for pain treatment. These methods are often used in combination with a specific medical treatment. In some cases these methods can be used instead of medical treatment, which reduces the potential for side effects. One of the mechanisms of action is the placebo effect. Research shows that about 1/3 of people respond favorably to treatment with a placebo (e.g., sugar pill, saltwater injection). The precise way in which a placebo works is unknown. Pain relief may result from the power of suggestion, distraction, or optimism or from a neurochemical reaction in the brain (Box 14-4).

Some alternative methods and their effects include:

1. Appropriate exercise can strengthen muscles throughout the body, build bone mass, and enhance feelings of well-being.
2. Massage therapy can reduce pain, improve function, and prevent recurrences.
3. Spinal manipulation (adjustment) can be used to relieve chronic pain caused by musculoskeletal conditions (e.g., osteoarthritis).
4. **Acupuncture** consist of fine needles inserted at selected points in the body. Acupuncture is now a widely accepted and proven method of pain relief. It should be performed by a licensed acupuncturist.
5. Cold or heat application often is an aspect of hydrotherapy used to help manage pain. Heat often relieves sore muscles and is comforting. Cold lessens pain sensations by numbing the painful area and reducing inflammation. Alternate heat and cold for added relief. Precautions for heat and cold applications include the following:
   - Avoid cold application if you are diagnosed with Raynaud's disease.
   - Hot baths and hot saunas are not recommended for those with diabetes or multiple sclerosis, women who are pregnant, or anyone with abnormally high or low blood pressure.
   - Do not use a heating pad on bare skin.
   - Do not go to sleep with the heating pad turned on.
   - Elderly people and young children may be exhausted by too much heat and should avoid long full-body hot treatments such as baths and saunas.
   - Do not use heat over a new injury. Wait at least 24 hours.
   - Do not use heat or cold over any treatment area receiving radiation therapy and for 6 months after treatment has ended because skin in the area is too fragile.
   - Do not use heat or cold over any area where circulation or sensation is poor or altered by the action of medication.
   - Do not use the heat or cold application for longer than 15 to 20 minutes before allowing the temperature to return to normal. Then repeat.

Counterirritants also can be used for pain relief. Creams, lotions, liniments, and gels are available that contain menthol or capsicum. When rubbed into the skin, these increase blood circulation to the affected area or produce a warm (or sometimes cool), soothing feeling that lasts several hours to produce counterirritation. Precautions for the use of counterirritants include the following:

- Do not rub the product near the eyes or over broken skin, a skin rash, or mucous membranes (e.g., inside the mouth or around genitals or rectum).

BOX 14-4 The Power of Placebos

If a person believes that a form of treatment will relieve pain, it will do so far more effectively than if the person believes that the treatment cannot help. In studies involving more than 1000 people with chronic pain, dummy medications reduced the level of pain by at least 50% of that achieved with *any* form of pain-killing drug, including aspirin and morphine (Melzack and Wall, 1989). The researchers stated that, "This shows clearly that the psychological context—particularly the physician's and patient's expectations—contains powerful therapeutic value in its own right in addition to the effect of the drug itself."

Facts About Placebos

- Placebos are far more effective against severe pain than mild pain.
- Placebos are more effective in people who are severely anxious and stressed than in people who are not, which suggests that the antianxiety effect of placebos is at least part of the reason for their usefulness.
- Placebos work best against headache-type pain (over 50% effectiveness).
- In about one third of all people, most pains are relieved by placebo.
- A placebo works more effectively if injected than if taken by mouth.
- Placebos work more powerfully if accompanied by the suggestion that they are indeed powerful and that they will rapidly produce results.
- Placebos in capsule or tablet form work better if two are taken rather than one.
- The effects of placebos are related to size and color:
  - Large capsules are more effective as placebos than small ones.
  - Red placebos are the most effective at helping with pain problems.
  - Green placebos are most effective at helping with anxiety.
  - Blue placebos are the most sedating and calming.
  - Yellow placebos work best for depression.
  - Pink placebos are the most stimulating.
- Placebos have been shown to be effective in a wide variety of conditions, including anorexia, depression, skin diseases, diarrhea, and palpitation.
- Effects are not dependent on injection or oral dosing of the placebo; all forms of treatment (e.g., manipulation, acupuncture, surgery) exert some degree of placebo effect.

Recognition of the placebo effect allows us to realize the importance of the power of suggestion in all of us, and some people are more influenced than others. It is essential that health professionals avoid assuming that because a placebo works in a person, he or she is not genuinely suffering pain or the reported relief is false (Millenson, 1995).

A person's attitudes and emotions are powerful aids (or hindrances) to recovery. Feelings of hope and expectation of improvement, coupled with a relationship with caring helpers, whether professional or otherwise, assist recovery and coping.

Modified from Chaitow L, Delany J: *Clinical application of neuromuscular techniques, vol 1, The upper body,* London, 2000, Churchill Livingstone.

- Do not use menthol or capsicum in the treatment area during radiation therapy.
- If aspirin is being used, do not use these preparations unless monitored by the physician. Many menthol preparations contain an additional ingredient similar to aspirin. A small amount of this aspirin-like substance may be absorbed through the skin.

Other types of treatment that can be used to manage chronic pain include relaxation and behavior modification therapy, meditation, hypnosis, and biofeedback. **Biofeedback** is a method people can learn to control certain body functions such as the heart rate, blood pressure, and muscle tension with the help of special equipment. Biofeedback sometimes is used to help people learn to relax as the primary method of pain management. Learning the various methods requires the help of a licensed biofeedback technician.

Mental processes such as imagery, distraction, and hypnosis can be taught to patients to control pain. **Imagery** is the use of imagination to create mental pictures or situations and can be thought of as focused daydreaming or self hypnosis. **Distraction** is the process of turning the attention to something other than the pain. People use this method without realizing it when they watch television, listen to music or read to "take their minds off" their pain. This is used to manage mild pain or with medication to manage brief episodes of severe pain, such as pain related to medical procedures. Any activity that occupies the attention can be used for distraction. Distractions can be internal (e.g., counting, singing, praying, or repeating statements such as "I can cope") or external (e.g., doing crafts such as needlework, model building, or painting). Visiting with friends or family is another useful distraction technique.

Hypnosis is a set of techniques designed to enhance concentration, minimize one's usual distractions, and heighten responsiveness to suggestions to alter one's thoughts, feelings, behavior, or physiological state. The way in which these methods affect pain is not completely understood but used appropriately is safe. This state can be elicited by a person trained in hypnosis, often a psychologist or psychiatrist. Hypnotherapists can easily teach most people how to place themselves in a hypnotic state, make positive suggestions to themselves, and leave the hypnotic state.

MASSAGE STRATEGIES FOR PAIN MANAGEMENT

As part of a healthcare team, the massage professional can contribute valuable manual therapy for various pain conditions. This type of therapy involves the use of direct tissue manipulation and reflex stimulation of the nervous system and the circulation. As a therapeutic intervention, massage may help reduce the need for pain medication, thereby reducing the side effects of the drugs.

All medications, including OTC drugs, have some side effects. For patients in extreme pain, the massage therapy must be monitored by a doctor or other appropriate healthcare professional. Most people experience pain in less severe forms occasionally throughout life. Massage may provide temporary, symptomatic relief of moderate pain brought on by daily stress, replacing OTC pain medications or reducing their use (Tables 14-1 and 14-2).

It is important that the massage therapist understand the distinction between the management of acute pain and the management of chronic pain.

- Intervention for acute pain is less invasive and focuses on supporting a current healing process.
- Chronic pain is managed with either symptom relief or a more aggressive healing and rehabilitation approach that incorporates a therapeutic change process.

Various mechanisms that influence pain are affected by massage, including the neurotransmitters that perpetuate and, more important, inhibit the pain response. The neurochemicals most recognized by patients are the endorphins. Endorphins are part of a group of peptides that act as the body's internal pain modulator, somewhat like morphine. Endorphins are a component of

TABLE 14-1 Pain Assessment Factors

Factors	Questions to Ask
Location	Where is the pain located?
Quality	What does the pain feel like (e.g., dull, sharp, shooting, throbbing, searing, tingling)?
Intensity	How severe is the pain? (See pain rating scales.)
Precipitating factors	When does pain occur (e.g., when exercising, bending, after eating, with position change)? Is it sudden or gradual?
Aggravating factors	What makes the pain worse (e.g., moving, standing, sitting)?
Alleviating factors	What makes the pain better (e.g., pain medications, positioning, relaxation, rest, distraction)?
Associated manifestations	What other signs or symptoms accompany the pain (e.g., nausea, vomiting, lack of appetite, agitation, depression, drowsiness, fatigue, sleeplessness)?
Observed behaviors	What behaviors are displayed (e.g., agitation, restlessness, rubbing, guarding, moaning, grunting, crying, sighing, wincing, grimacing, clenching the teeth)?

Modified from Stillwell SB: *Mosby's nursing PDQ for critical care,* St Louis, 2005, Mosby.

TABLE 14-2 **Harmful Effects of Unrelieved Pain**

Domains Affected	Specific Responses to Pain
Endocrine	Increased ACTH, cortisol, ADH, epinephrine, norepinephrine, GH, catecholamines, renin, angiotensin II, aldosterone, glucagon, interleukin-1; decreased insulin, testosterone
Metabolic	Gluconeogenesis, hepatic glycogenolysis, hyperglycemia, glucose intolerance, insulin resistance, muscle protein catabolism; increased lipolysis
Cardiovascular	Increased HR, CO, PVR, SVR; hypertension, coronary vascular resistance, myocardial oxygen consumption, hypercoagulation, DVT
Respiratory	Decreased flows and volumes, atelectasis, shunting, hypoxemia, cough, sputum retention, infection
Genitourinary	Decreased urinary output, urinary retention, fluid overload, hypokalemia
Gastrointestinal	Decreased gastric and bowel motility
Musculoskeletal	Muscle spasm, impaired muscle function, fatigue, immobility
Cognitive	Decreased cognitive function and mental function
Immune	Depression of immune response
Developmental	Increased behavioral and physiologic responses to pain, altered temperament, higher somatization, infant distress behavior, possible altered development of the pain system; greater vulnerability to stress disorders, addictive behavior, and anxiety states
Future pain	Debilitating chronic pain syndromes (e.g., postmastectomy pain, postthoracotomy pain, phantom pain, postherpetic neuralgia)
Quality of life	Sleeplessness, anxiety, fear, hopelessness, thoughts of suicide

Modified from McCaffery M, Pasero C: *Pain: clinical manual,* ed 2, St Louis, 1999, Mosby.
ACTH, Adrenocorticotropic hormone; *ADH,* antidiuretic hormone; *GH,* growth hormone; *HR,* heart rate; *CO,* cardiac output; *PVR,* peripheral vascular resistance; *SVR,* systemic vascular resistance; *DVT,* deep vein thrombosis.

the so-called runner's high. Actually, a combination of neurotransmitters and hormones works together to alter pain perception, both inhibiting and enhancing it.

Massage seems to alter the chemical interaction. The pain-inhibiting chemicals influenced by massage are the endorphins, serotonin, gamma aminobutyric acid (GABA), and dopamine. The pain-facilitating chemicals influenced by massage are adrenaline, noradrenaline, cortisol, and substance P. The research on just how all this works is still scant, but our current knowledge is sufficient for developing strategies and justifying the use of massage for pain modulation.

Massage also influences the CNS and PNS (somatic and autonomic). As described previously, massage applications that result in counterirritation function by activating the gate control for the transmission of pain signals. Reducing mechanical pressure on peripheral somatic nerves by increasing pliability in the tissues modulates pain sensation. Massage also can reduce the stimulation of nociceptors in tissues. In addition, it can alter the firing of proprioceptors. When this occurs, joint function and the muscle tension/length relationship normalize, reducing pain. Supporting parasympathetic dominance increases pain tolerance.

Using lymphatic drainage to reduce the hydrostatic pressure caused by edema decreases interstitial fluid and eases the pressure on pain receptors. Similar results are obtained when tissue density is diminished through the use of connective tissue methods to increase ground substance pliability or to reduce adhesions from random connective tissue fiber distribution.

As mentioned, pain can also occur if circulation is not appropriate. Ischemic tissues are sensitized to pain. Massage exerts a powerful influence on blood movement. Both the arterial and venous circulations are involved, and massage can target normalization. Furthermore, massage has a compassionate and comforting quality that can increase pain tolerance.

Massage application targeted to pain management incorporates the following principles:

1. A general, full body application using a rhythmic, slow approach should be performed as often as feasible for 45 to 60 minutes per session. The palliative care protocol is followed for this.
   Goal: To achieve parasympathetic dominance and reduced cortisol production.
2. The pressure depth is moderate to deep, and a compressive, broad-based application is used. Be sure to avoid any poking, frictioning, or pain-causing methods.
   Goal: To support the production and utilization of serotonin and GABA and to reduce the production of substance P and adrenaline.
3. Drag is slight unless the connective tissue is targeted. Drag is targeted to lymphatic drainage and skin stimulation.
   Goal: To reduce swelling and create counterirritation through skin stimulation.
4. Nodal points with a high neurovascular component are massaged with a depth of pressure sufficient to create a "good hurt" but not so deep as to cause defensive guarding or withdrawal. These nodal points are the location of cutaneous nerves, trigger points, acupuncture points, and reflexology points. The feet, hands, face, and head are excellent target locations, as is the area along the spine.
   Goal: To support the gate control response and the release of endorphins and other pain-inhibiting chemicals.
5. The direction of massage varies but always deliberately targets fluid movement.
   Goal: To improve circulation.
6. Agitation-quality mechanical force (e.g., shear, bend, and torsion) is applied for some soft tissue conditions; that is, it is meant to "stir" the ground substance, not to cause inflammation.
   Goal: To increase tissue pliability and reduce tissue density.
7. Mechanical force (e.g., shear, bend, and torsion) is applied to address adhesion or fibrosis, but it must be specifically targeted and limited in duration.
   Goal: To reduce localized nerve irritation or remove restriction interfering with circulation.
8. Muscle energy methods and lengthening are applied rhythmically and gently and are targeted to shortened muscles.
   Goal: To reduce nerve and proprioceptive irritation and normalize muscle motor tone and circulation inhibition.
9. Stretching to introduce tension force is applied slowly, without pain, and targeted to shortened connective tissue.
   Goal: To reduce nerve and proprioceptor irritation.
10. The massage therapist provides focused, attentive, and compassionate care but maintains appropriate boundaries.
    Goal: To support entrainment, normalization of bioenergy, and palliative care.

Additional methods that modulate pain sensation and perception that can be incorporated into the massage include simple applications of hot and cold hydrotherapy, analgesic essential oils, calming and distracting music, and (possible) north pole magnet application. These methods were discussed in Unit Two.

INFLAMMATION

Inflammation has been recognized for thousands of years and has been described consistently by the classic signs of heat, redness, pain, and swelling. The inflammatory process is a normal and important process and is how the body protects itself from an infection and to stimulate tissues to heal. When the inflammatory process does not resolve itself in the normal way then chronic inflammation occurs, which has many health consequences. Inflammation works primarily through the immune system, which is discussed later in the chapter.

TYPES OF INFLAMMATION

In general, inflammation can be categorized as acute or chronic and local or systemic. Acute inflammation can be very painful due to nerve compression by swollen tissue and the chemical messengers that are released to activate nerve cells in the injured area to communicate tissue damage to the brain. The result is a protective response such as muscle guarding, which can feel like muscle cramping, spasm, and aching. The guarding response results from soft tissue becoming more stiff and taut to reduce movement in the injured area. Fortunately, acute inflammation usually lasts only a few days during the acute and subacute healing phases and remains localized to a specific area. This type of response is typically treated with ice and rest of the affected area.

During an acute inflammatory reaction, the movement of fluids helps carry immune cells and natural tissue remodeling substances to the area as part of the healing response. These substances stimulate blood clotting to stop bleeding and close up the injured area. For local acute inflammation, full body, palliative massage applications are used to support healing. The area of injury usually is avoided in the initial stages of healing, when acute inflammation is present; in these cases the massage application follows the strategies for wounds described in Chapter 17.

If the acute inflammatory reaction is severe it can become systemic. Examples include a large crush injury or a large burn area. In these instances a major acute whole body response occurs, resulting in a systemic inflammatory reaction.

The body deals with extreme traumatic injury by mounting a large-scale inflammatory reaction. If this process does not occur properly, major problems can develop, including multiple organ failure. Damaged tissue releases chemicals that attract white blood cells to the scene of the injury. The immune system activates various types of immune cells during this process. The severe tissue damage that occurs with a crush injury, massive bleeding, or a serious burn causes physical and chemical changes in the skin, the underlying organs, or both. Cell components and blood vessels physically break apart. Small pieces of tissue can enter the bloodstream and become lodged, preventing the delivery of oxygen to the body's vital organs.

All of the blood is routed through the lungs so that it can become enriched with oxygen. Because the lungs receive the entire blood supply, this organ system often is the first to shut down after massive trauma. Other organ systems then begin to fail, such as the brain, heart, and kidneys. (This obviously is a condition that requires intensive emergency medical care, not massage.)

Chronic inflammation is a different situation, and massage can be an effective part of the treatment plan for this disorder. **Chronic inflammation,** which lasts for weeks, months, or longer, can cause lasting damage to many body tissues, and many health problems have been linked to an overactive, uncontained inflammatory response, which can be linked to various autoimmune diseases. For example, chronic inflammation can lead to Crohn's disease, a disorder involving severe abdominal pain and intestinal problems. Like Crohn's disease, other diseases such as MS, rheumatoid arthritis, and even some forms of cancer are the consequence of unchecked, ongoing inflammation. (Massage for these conditions is discussed later in the textbook.)

To appreciate the importance of inflammation, both productive and nonproductive, the massage therapist must have a basic understanding of the human immune system.

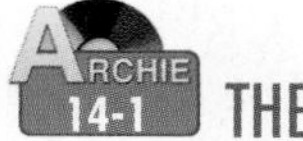

THE IMMUNE SYSTEM

The **immune system** responds to foreign substances in the body. Cells in the skin are actually considered part of the immune system, and tears and nasal mucus contain natural chemicals that digest bacterial substances. The immune system defends the body from attack by invaders recognized as foreign.[2] It can recognize and respond to substances called antigens whether they are infectious agents or part of the body (self-antigens). The immune system is an extraordinarily complex system that relies on an elaborate and dynamic communications network that links the many different kinds of immune cells that patrol the body. [2]

The immune system is based on two protective mechanisms, which function to prevent an infection from developing. The first response relies on inborn defenses, collectively known as **innate immunity.** The second response draws on **acquired immunity;** this means that the body deals with a pathogen based on previous exposure, and it mounts a specific response to fight the infection. Acquired immunity involves the production of antibodies and certain specialized immune cells that are tailored to destroy or neutralize microbes or other foreign substances.

Occasionally immune cells overreact and end up doing harm to the body's cells and tissues. Most of the time this condition resolves fairly quickly on its own. However, if it does not, various autoimmune diseases may develop.

The Complement System

An important aspect of immune function is the **complement system,** which consists of various molecules found in the blood in an inactive form. Complement molecules become active when they detect pathogens, injury, or other immune triggers. When activated, complement proteins cause a range of responses associated with starting and maintaining inflammation. This is the point where inflammation and immunity become integrated. The blood vessel walls become more permeable (leaky), various types of immune cells move to the area of inflammation, and other substances that promote inflammation are produced. A molecule called *C-reactive protein* (CRP) interacts with the complement system. The presence of CRP in the blood is a telltale sign of inflammation, because it is not present in appreciable amounts in the blood of healthy people.

Types of Immune Cells

Most immune system cells are white blood cells, of which there are many types. **Lymphocytes** are one type of white blood cell.[2] Lymphocytes are divided into two major classes, T cells and B cells. All lymphocytes start out in the bone marrow; however, B cells mature in the marrow before entering the bloodstream, whereas T cells travel to the thymus and mature there. B cells and T cells perform different roles. When activated, B cells acquire the ability to make antibodies that attack foreign substances. An antibody binds to an antigen and marks the antigen for destruction by other immune system cells. In contrast, some T cells (i.e., killer T cells) sense the presence of infected cells and do away with them directly. Other T cells (i.e., helper or suppressor T cells) assist killer T cells and also help keep the immune response under control. Once activated, helper T cells produce immune substances that tell B cells to produce antibodies. Helper T cells are divided into two types, Th1 and Th2. Most healthy people have more Th1 cells than Th2 cells; this balance is often reversed in severely injured people.

T cells are critical immune system cells that help destroy infected cells and coordinate the overall immune response. The T cell has a molecule on its surface called the T-cell receptor. This receptor interacts with the molecules that make up the *major histocompatibility complex (MHC).* MHC molecules, which are present on the surface of most other body cells, help T cells recognize antigen fragments.

Other types of white blood cells are called **macrophages** and **neutrophils.** These cells circulate in the blood and identify foreign substances (antigens) such as bacteria, then engulf and destroy them by making toxic molecules. If production of these toxic molecules continues beyond what is necessary to destroy the pathogens not only are the foreign substances destroyed, but surrounding healthy tissue is also destroyed, which results in the body attaching itself. For instance, macrophages and neutrophils that invade blood vessels produce toxic molecules that damage blood vessels. In rheumatoid arthritis, macrophages and neutrophils that invade the joints cause a non productive inflammation, which produces warmth and swelling and damages the joint.

When a virus, for example, infects a cell, a special molecule binds to the virus (antigen) and displays the presence of antigen on the cell's surface, in essence calling for the immune system to respond. Cellular response is the action of the blood cells, primarily white blood cells, that deal with pathogens. Natural killer cells are a subset of lymphocytes that can eliminate virus-infected cells. Cells such as macrophages and neutrophils begin to phagocytize, or to surround and destroy, pathogens. Basophils and mast cells (from connective tissue) release chemicals that initiate inflammation. Eosinophils release chemicals that slow or stop the inflammatory response (how the body maintains homeostasis). Chemical response includes not only the chemicals released by the previously mentioned cells but also substances found throughout the body. The skin and mucous membranes maintain a certain degree of acidity that prevents entry of foreign pathogens. Mucus is sticky and contains enzymes that destroy these microorganisms, and saliva, tears, and urine actually wash them out of the body.

The organizational structures and responses of the immune system can break down. The imbalances that occur in that circumstance are immune deficiencies, hypersensitivities, and autoimmune diseases. Immune deficiency is a condition in which the body is unable to mount the proper immune response to a pathogen. An analogy is an office that has too much work and not enough workers to get the job done. The work piles up, the workers get further and further behind, and eventually the office system breaks down. Some immune deficiencies are present at birth. These congenital problems affect the development of lymphocytes and result in severe inability to respond to disease. Other immune deficiencies arise later in life, such as acquired immunodeficiency syndrome (AIDS). Chronic stress also suppresses the immune system. Stress can be caused by physical mechanisms (e.g., chronic pain), other forms of chronic disease, or unresolved emotional or spiritual disturbances. When immunosuppressed, the body is more likely to be susceptible to a variety of bacterial, viral, and toxic pathogenic activity.

The immune system also can become overactive, a condition called hypersensitivity or allergy. Few persons die of allergies, but they can make life miserable. Allergy can be understood by equating the immune system response to creating mountains out of molehills. Anaphylactic shock is the exception, and although rare, it is life-threatening. Anaphylactic shock is a severe, usually immediate reaction to a substance that causes respiratory distress, anxiety, and weakness. In extreme cases, anaphylactic shock also can involve arrhythmia and can result in death if not treated immediately. Autoimmune diseases occur when the body cannot distinguish self from nonself; self-antigens are treated as foreign antigens. When the recognition of self breaks down, the immune cells begin to attack the self. Some of the autoimmune diseases are multiple sclerosis, Graves' disease, rheumatoid arthritis, and juvenile diabetes.

JUST BETWEEN YOU AND ME

I am just fascinated by the communication setup of the immune system. Communication of any kind is a wonderful yet complex process. Teaching (and writing textbooks) is a communication process. So many steps are required to make sure that the end result is an understood message. Miscommunication results in an inappropriate response. So many times, I have given what seemed to me to be clear descriptions and instructions to students; yet, when I observed their use of the information, I realized that the interpretation of that information was very different from what was intended. So where did the communication process break down? In the delivery? In the processing? Who knows? It's just amazing that we understand each other at all. Now, back to the immune system: it is amazing, too, but mistakes and misunderstandings do occur.

Normally during various immune responses T-cells secrete cytokines and chemokines. Cytokines are proteins that may cause surrounding immune system cells to become activated, grow, or die. They also may interfere with normally functioning tissues. For example, cytokines play a part in the condition called scleroderma by contributing to the thickening of the skin.

Chemokines are small cytokine molecules that attract cells of the immune system, targeting the immune response. However, if chemokines mistake normal tissue for pathogenic tissue the inflammation results in autoimmune diseases. In some autoimmune diseases, B cells mistakenly make antibodies against self antigens (autoantibodies) instead of foreign antigens and healthy tissue is attacked, which interferes with the normal function of the tissues or causes destruction of the tissues. For example, muscle weakness occurs in the condition called myasthenia because autoantibodies attack a part of the nerve that stimulates muscle movement.

When many antibodies attack antigens in the bloodstream, they form an immune complex. An immune complex is a bundle of these cells structures and is harmful when they accumulate, because they cause inflammation and block blood flow. Normally the body removes immune complexes before they can cause damage. Specialized molecules of the immune system (complement system) remove immune complexes. These molecules make immune complexes more soluble and prevent the formation. If they do form, then the immune system can reduce the size of immune complexes so that they do not accumulate in the organs and tissues of the body, causing damage. In rare cases, some people inherit defective genes for a complement molecule and cannot make a normal amount or type of complement molecule. As a result, their immune systems are unable to prevent the accumulation of immune complexes in tissues and organs. Immune complexes are a causal factor in systemic lupus erythematosus.

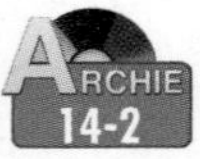

THE INFLAMMATORY RESPONSE

The inflammatory response is a part of an effective immune response as long as it does not become overactive or sustained (chronic). **Inflammatory mediators** are molecules inside and outside the body that play a role in inflammation. An exogenous inflammatory mediator is called an **endotoxin** (or a **lipopolysaccharide [LPS]**). Endotoxins, which are found in the outer covering of some types of bacteria, signal to immune cells that bacteria are present, causing an increase in inflammation. Cells have receptors on their surface, called *toll-like receptors* (TLRs), that can sense the presence of several different microbial stimuli, such as endotoxins.

During inflammation, monocytes and macrophages become activated by various immune system molecules such as cytokines and interferons (IFNs), and also by endotoxins and other microbial signals. Activated macrophages develop different properties, one of which is the capacity to stop dividing. Another feature of activated macrophages is the vigorous production of inflammatory molecules such as tumor necrosis factor (TNF) and interleukins (ILs), clotting factors, prostaglandins, free radicals, nitric oxide, and tissue remodeling enzymes. Activated macrophages also promote the growth of new blood vessels.

Neutrophils are among the most important cells in the first stage of an inflammatory response. Neutrophils and other leukocytes can devour infectious organisms. By doing so, these cells buy time for the healing phase of an inflammatory response to begin. Neutrophils can kill organisms because they carry molecular weapons called *free radicals* that are poisonous to bacteria. Typically, these poisons are hidden in specialized storage sacs kept separate from body tissues.

When a neutrophil senses an infection or injury, it undergoes a dramatic maneuver called a *respiratory burst,* gulping oxygen to make lots of free radicals, such as the molecule superoxide, along with protein-chewing enzymes that rip up the outer walls of bacterial cells. Neutrophils and other cells (e.g., macrophages) continue to produce these toxins and loosen up the tissue to help the substances spread quickly through an injured site or, in the case of systemic inflammation, throughout the body. Lymphocytes become activated, and antibodies are produced.

Platelets are essential components of the blood. They stimulate clotting to prevent blood loss. Platelets are not actually cells, but rather cell fragments that become activated (i.e., they change their shape) in response to injury signals. Platelets are an integral part of the inflammation process. Activated platelets shed certain molecules that directly activate inflammation inside blood vessels. Platelets also produce a variety of inflammatory mediators, such as growth factors, adhesion molecules, and cytokines.

JUST BETWEEN YOU AND ME

Wow; that was a lot of information about the inflammatory response. Better go back and read it again, because those aspects of the immune system and inflammatory mechanisms are what go wrong when a mess-up in the process results in a pathologic condition.

Pathology and Inflammation

Autoimmune diseases develop when the immune system mistakes its own tissues as foreign material and mounts an inappropriate attack on the body. Overblown inflammation is a common thread in these chronic conditions. In the case of autoimmune diseases, overproduction of cytokines and chemokines leads to inflammation of a body tissue. Examples of these disease are MS, type 1 diabetes, Crohn's disease, lupus, and rheumatoid arthritis. (Because autoimmune disease is so common, it is discussed in detail later on.)

MS, the most common nerve disease in young adults, is a chronic inflammatory disorder of the nervous system that is believed to be the result of a misguided autoimmune attack on myelin, a protective coating on nerve cells. The myelin is slowly eroded by the body's immune system, leading to problems with muscle coordination (because muscles require the action of nerves) and vision. For some reason, as the disease progresses, inflammation diminishes, but lasting damage has already been done to body tissues. Researchers suspect that the autoimmune trigger in MS may be infection by a virus or other microorganism, but this has not been proven beyond doubt.

INFLAMMATION AND INFECTION, TRAUMA, AND BURNS

Microorganisms that infect people and cause illness are called **pathogens.** Some pathogens cause disease by prompting a serious inflammatory response in a particular organ, such as the brain or kidneys. Two well-known examples of infections that cause inflammation in the brain are meningitis and encephalitis.

Trauma is a major cause of inflammation because of tissue damage and the resulting potential for infection. In addition to car accidents (the primary cause), physical trauma is caused by burns, gunshots and stabbings, falls, impacts from heavy objects, lightning strikes, and countless other injuries. Surgery is a kind of controlled trauma. Surgeons cut open tissues, which leaves the body prone to infection and inflammation. This means that surgery patients face many of the same recovery risks as trauma and burn victims.

To recover from trauma, the body must achieve a careful balance between stimulating inflammation to protect against infection and stopping the inflammation in time for healing to begin. If inflammation persists too long after an injury, organ systems begin to uncouple from one another, and the body becomes a disorganized system. If this happens, the body becomes ever more defenseless and is at great risk for developing a dangerous systemic inflammatory condition called **sepsis,** which can throw the body into a deadly state of shock.

Severe burns cause serious tissue damage and fluid loss. Because skin performs so many vital functions in the body, when skin is lost or damaged, these functions can become severely weakened. Burns can be caused by heat, chemicals, electricity, sunlight, or nuclear radiation. The most common kinds of burns are caused by scalds, building fires, and flammable liquids and gases. First-, second-, and third-degree burns affect varying depths of skin, which consists of three layers: the epidermis on top, the dermis just below, and the hypodermis on the bottom.

A burn that causes blisters is a **second-degree burn.** This type of burn typically is characterized as superficial or deep.

- A **superficial second-degree burn** involves only the most superficial dermis. It manifests as blistering or sloughing of overlying skin, causing a red, painful wound. The burn typically blanches but shows good capillary refill. Hairs cannot be pulled out easily. Healing occurs within 14 days, usually without surgical intervention or scarring.
- A **deep second-degree burn** involves more of the dermis. It may manifest as blisters or a wound with a white or deep red base. Sensation usually is diminished, and healing takes longer than 14 days. Hypertrophic scarring occurs if the healing phase lasts longer than 2 weeks, therefore wound débriding and skin grafting are recommended by 2 to 3 weeks.

INFLAMMATION AND RESPIRATORY DISORDERS

Asthma is the major respiratory disease linked to inflammation. It is caused by the actions of inflammatory cells such as mast cells, eosinophils, neutrophils, T lymphocytes, epithelial cells, and macrophages. Inflammation of the airways produces the classic symptoms of asthma: coughing, wheezing, chest tightening, and difficulty breathing.

As with many other inflammatory reactions, the key molecules involved in causing the symptoms of asthma are histamine, leukotrienes, and various cytokines. These molecules stimulate the production of mucus, which clogs the airways, making breathing difficult. Inflammatory molecules also cause changes in the lining of the blood vessels and the structure of the smooth muscle of the airway vessels. In general, these inflammatory molecules appear to create "jittery lungs" that are too responsive and tend to overreact to various forms of stimuli.

Because of the prominent role inflammation plays in asthma, medicines that block inflammation can be effective treatments for this disorder. Antiinflammatory drugs used to treat asthma include certain forms of steroid molecules (i.e., inhaled corticosteroids) and a relatively new class of drugs call *leukotriene inhibitors* (e.g., Accolate and Singulair). These medications block the production of inflammatory leukotrienes and help minimize the biologic effects, which include attracting eosinophils, crimping airway vessels, and stimulating the production of excess mucus. Other respiratory disorders linked to inflammation are chronic bronchitis, pneumonia, and pleurisy.

INFLAMMATION AND NERVE DISORDERS

The central nervous system consists of the brain and spinal cord. For the most part, it is protected by a blockade of cells and other components called the *blood-brain barrier.* If the brain is injured or infected, inflammatory responses can result. More than anywhere else in the body, the brain very carefully controls the extent of an inflammatory reaction in itself. The release of too many cytokines or other inflammatory molecules can lead to permanent damage to brain cells.

Neurons resemble other cells in the body in many ways; however, unlike other cells, they have long, tendril-like structures called *axons* and *dendrites.* These thin extensions are the most vulnerable to damage from inflammatory chemicals. Axons can be compared to telephone wires; when they are severed or damaged, a communication breakdown throughout the body can result. Some neurologic conditions in which excessive inflammation destroys axons are MS, various viral and bacterial infections, amyotrophic lateral sclerosis (ALS), encephalitis, head trauma, and epilepsy. In many cases the severity of these diseases can be linked to the extent of axon damage. Researchers have also linked inflammation to Alzheimer's disease.

Scientists think that reducing inflammation with medicines may be an effective way to treat some of these debilitating nerve disorders. Antinflammatory medications have proved effective at stalling early stage MS, and a recent study indicated that inflammation-blocking medication may help delay the onset of Alzheimer's disease.

INFLAMMATION AND CARDIOVASCULAR DISEASE

Inflammation may be a causative factor in heart attacks and strokes. Atherosclerosis, a common factor in heart attacks and strokes, is a condition in which fatty plaques build up on the insides of blood vessels, restricting flow. In recent years scientists have come to appreciate the role inflammation plays in this artery-clogging process. A diet high in saturated fat and cholesterol can induce changes in the structure of the blood vessel walls by increasing the manufacture of a sticky protein called *vascular cell adhesion molecule-1* (VCAM-1).

Researchers think that tiny fat droplets can stimulate inflammation in blood vessels, signaling the production of VCAM-1. Fat and other particles cause white blood cells to stick to vessel linings, disrupting blood flow. Local disruptions in blood flow can prevent oxygen from reaching vital organs; this can cause heart attacks and strokes, especially at branch points in vessels where the flow already is somewhat restricted.

Inflammation also promotes heart disease through the production of so-called foam cells. Monocytes in the blood vessels, which have the ability to ingest various substances, ingest droplets of cholesterol and turn into foam cells. These cells congregate to form a fatty plaque, or lesion.

INFLAMMATION AND CANCER

Some types of cancer arise from tissue irritation, infection, and inflammation. In fact, inflammatory cells such as neutrophils can help tumor cells multiply and spread. Some tumors have been compared to wounds that will not heal.

Cells in a tumor act territorially, producing substances that attract nutrients and support structures to advance their survival. Among these molecules are chemokines, which draw neutrophils to a tumor. In turn, cancer cells can move through the body by attaching to the adhesion molecules that help propel the movement of the neutrophils. As in wound healing, neutrophils, macrophages, lymphocytes, monocytes, and other white blood cells produce tissue remodeling ingredients. These molecules spur the continued growth of cancer cells. On-site production of growth factors stimulates the growth of blood vessels to nourish the tumor and perpetuate the cycle.

Melanoma, which is the result of excessive exposure to ultraviolet light from the sun and other sources, is thought to be caused partly by uncontrolled inflammation of the skin.

A growing body of evidence supports the theory of a link between infection, inflammation, and many types of cancers. Among the cancers known to be associated with infection are certain types of lung, colon, pancreatic, and bladder tumors. Chronic infection with the hepatitis C virus is a significant risk factor for liver cancer, and chronic infection with the ulcer-causing microorganism *Helicobacter pylori* is the leading cause of stomach cancer.

Substances that block inflammation (e.g., aspirin and other NSAIDs) have been shown to prevent certain kinds of colon, lung, mouth, and stomach cancers.

THE PHASES OF INFLAMMATION

Acute Inflammation

A local inflammatory process can be described in three phases. Systemic inflammation follows a similar pattern. A local inflammatory process occurs as follows:

- *Vascular (acute) phase:* This phase of inflammation typically lasts 24 to 48 hours but in some cases may last up to a week. The arteries, veins, and capillaries dilate, resulting in redness, heat, and escape of blood plasma, causing edema. Function typically decreases, and the number of fibroblasts and macrophages increases. The fibroblasts increase in size and synthesize ground substance and collagen; this process begins within 4 hours of injury and can last 4 to 6 days. Collagen initially forms a weak, random mesh of fibers. Pain is caused by the pressure from swelling and the chemical irritation that stimulates the pain receptors.
- *Regeneration and repair (subacute) phase:* The process of regeneration and repair usually begins 2 to 6 days after injury and lasts approximately 3 or 4 weeks. New capillaries are formed and are laid down in a random orientation unless the area is mobilized, disturbing this process. Fibroblastic activity and collagen formation increase. Scar tissue at this stage is highly cellular and fragile.

  NOTE: In the acute and subacute stages, collagen is laid down in a random, disorganized pattern, usually in a plane perpendicular to the long axis, and therefore has little strength. The collagen develops abnormal cross-links, leaving the tissue with less flexibility. Immature connective tissue is less dense and more easily disrupted, therefore care must be taken with the amount of pressure and drag applied during massage to prevent reinjury of the tissue.
- *Remodeling phase:* In the early stages of **remodeling,** the collagen matures into a lattice that is completely disorganized in a gel structure. It can be palpated as thickened or fibrous tissue. A relative decrease in cellularity and vascularity occurs as collagen density increases. After approximately 2 months, fibroblastic activity declines, as does collagen synthesis. Random orientation of collagen provides little support for tensile loads. Rehabilitation exercises are necessary to induce the collagen to reorient along the lines of imposed stress. Two months to 2 years later, collagen may develop a functional linear alignment in response to stimuli provided by movement and use patterns.

Ineffective healing often is the result of immobilization and lack of proper rehabilitation during the subacute and remodeling phases. This leads to significant adhesion formation, osteoporosis (loss of bone density), and atrophy of muscles, joint capsules, and ligaments.

JUST BETWEEN YOU AND ME

One of the biggest errors massage therapists make is being too aggressive with massage in the subacute phase of healing. Inappropriate massage can pull apart fragile tissue that has formed; this is like picking a scab. We all know not to pick scabs, because it disturbs the healing process and increases scar formation. So for massage therapists, the word to the wise during the first 2 weeks after an injury (including surgery) is *be careful*. Don't friction the area, don't stretch it aggressively, and don't dig or poke around it.

Another big error in massage application is not being aggressive enough during the remodeling phase. This is the time to stretch and deform tissue to encourage the final formation of a mobile, pliable scar.

Systemic Inflammation

The Acute Phase. An acute systemic inflammatory process typically occurs in response to invasion by a pathogen, such as the influenza virus. The first response is fever, which creates a hostile environment for the pathogen. The ground substance of the connective thickens to slow the migration of the organism through the body; this results in general stiffness and aching. Fatigue, sluggishness, and headache occur as a result of shifts in blood movement, and neurochemical changes slow the person and increase sleep requirements, which are necessary for effective healing.

The use of medication to bring down the temperature tends to lengthen the healing time, as does lack of sleep. A productive fever (100° to 102° F) should be supported. A person with an acute immune response should drink fluid, stay warm, and rest. This phase typically lasts 3 to 7 days.

The Subacute Phase. In the subacute phase, the fever diminishes but the fatigue and achiness may remain. The body continues to need rest for up to 14 days.

The Recovery Phase. During the recovery phase, the person begins to resume normal activity levels. However, if he or she overdoes things, the fatigue and aching increase. This phase can last up to 3 months.

JUST BETWEEN YOU AND ME

Chronic illness, such as chronic fatigue syndrome, can be thought of as a body stuck in the subacute healing phase. A link exists between a bad bout with a viral infection and the development of various chronic illnesses, such as fibromyalgia. Just as with local chronic injury, the common reasons the body is unable to resolve the illness are poor lifestyle choices, inadequate rest, and too much stress.

CHRONIC LOCAL INFLAMMATION

Chronic local inflammation can result from repeated episodes of microtrauma or chronic irritation of the tissue. This is an inflammatory process that is no longer productive. Repetitive strain injuries frequently result in limitations on or curtailment of an activity because of local chronic inflammation. The injuries may result because the person placed constant, repetitive stress on bones, joints, or soft tissues; forced a joint into an extreme range of motion; or engaged in prolonged, strenuous activity. Overuse and repetitive stress injuries may be relatively minor; still, they can be disabling.

Chronic local inflammation leads to stimulation of pain receptors; this causes compensatory adaptations that either facilitate muscles, causing hypertonicity, or inhibit muscles, causing weakness. With joint inflammation the flexors of the joint typically become hypertonic and the extensors become inhibited. The body's innate logic is apparent: the flexed position affords more joint capsule space for the increased fluid and prevents the greater pressure and pain that would occur if the joint were in an extended position. Extended positions frequently (but not always) are associated with increased force caused by weight bearing, therefore flexion occurs subconsciously as a form of guarding.

Chronic local inflammation can sensitize the mechanoreceptors, and normal mechanical stimuli then cause the mechanoreceptor to be a pain producer.

JUST BETWEEN YOU AND ME

As I said before, think of chronic inflammation as an injury that is stuck in the subacute phase, and the body cannot resolve it. This occurs for many reasons, such as poor rest habits, poor nutrition, returning to activity too soon, and so forth. So what is a massage therapist to do? Careful, controlled use of friction (shear and torsion forces) can generate just enough controlled acute inflammation to jump start the healing process, and if the person rests, attends a rehabilitation program, and eats right, maybe the inflammatory response will begin to resolve. Be patient; this whole process takes up to a year to complete. The skill in application is trying to figure just how much acute inflammation to create. Here's how I do it: The local area should get warm and red. It should be tender to the touch the next day but should not be sore when the area is moved. The tenderness to touch should dissipate in 48 hours. Friction is applied again on the third day; if the area is not sore to the touch, increase the intensity. If the area is sore when moved or remains sore to the touch longer than 3 days, reduce the intensity.

MASSAGE STRATEGIES FOR INFLAMMATION

Therapeutic massage seems to be beneficial for prolonged inflammation. Plausible theories for this benefit include the following:

1. The stimulation from massage activates a release of the body's own antiinflammatory agents.
2. Certain types of massage increase the inflammatory process (i.e., therapeutic inflammation) to a small degree, triggering the body to resolve the inflammation process.
3. Massage may facilitate the dilution and removal of the irritant by increasing lymphatic flow.

In general, massage often is contraindicated during acute systemic inflammation, because the patient is very ill. Once the acute crisis has resolved, massage begins as palliative and then progresses to a restorative approach. The approach is a general, nonspecific massage. If massage is used during acute systemic inflammation, it is palliative and lasts less than 30 minutes. Areas that ache as a result of bed rest are targeted. Gentle, energy-based modalities are comforting.

Massage for chronic systemic inflammatory disease is beneficial as long as the patient's adaptive mechanisms are not strained. Massage can manage pain symptoms and support fluid movement. It can also reduce sympathetic ANS dominance and thereby indirectly support the body's ability to resolve nonproductive inflammation. Massage also supports restorative sleep.

For local inflammation, massage can support the tissue repair process. The processes of inflammation trigger tissue repair, which is the replacement of dead cells with living cells. In a type of tissue repair called **regeneration,** the new cells are similar to those they replace. Another type of tissue repair is replacement. In **replacement,** the new cells are formed from connective tissue and are different from those they replace; this results in a scar. Often, fibrous connective tissue replaces the damaged tissue, resulting in a condition called **fibrosis.** Most tissue repair is a combination of regeneration and replacement. A goal in the healing process is to promote regeneration and keep replacement to a minimum. Massage has been shown to slow the formation of scar tissue; it thus supports regeneration and keeps scar tissue pliable when it does form.

As we discussed earlier, inflammation is a multiphase process (Table 14-3). General massage is used to manage pain and edema and restore mobility. Initially rest is important in treatment. Massage used to create parasympathetic dominance helps support restorative sleep. During the subacute phase, massage supports rehabilitation.

Massage also can address localized chronic inflammation and fibrosis. Careful and targeted use of methods that superimpose acute inflammation can help resolve these conditions. The key is to create just enough acute injury to jump start the resolution of the inflammatory process. Deep frictioning techniques and connective tissue stretching methods are the most common approaches used to create these areas of controlled acute inflammation.

The benefit derived from therapeutic inflammation depends on the body's ability to generate healing processes. If healing mechanisms are suppressed, methods that create therapeutic inflammation should not be used. Therapeutic inflammation is not used in situations in which sleep disturbance, compromised immune function, a high stress load, or systemic or localized inflammation is already present. This method is also contraindicated if any condition that involves

TABLE 14-3 Phases of the Inflammatory Process

Acute Phase (Inflammatory Reaction)	Subacute Phase (Repair and Healing)	Chronic Phase (Maturation and Remodeling)
Vascular changes Exudation of cells and chemicals Clot formation Phagocytosis, neutralization of irritants Early fibroblastic activity Inflammation Pain before tissue resistance	Removal of noxious stimuli Growth of capillary beds into area Collagen formation Granulation tissue formation Fragile, injured tissue Diminishing inflammation Pain synchronous with tissue resistance	Maturation of connective tissue Contracture of scar tissue Remodeling of scar Alignment of collagen to stress Absence of inflammation Pain after tissue resistance
Protection Phase	**Controlled Motion Phase**	**Return to Function Phase**
Control effects of inflammation through selective rest and immobilization Promote early healing and prevent negative effects of rest Provide passive movement, general massage with caution	Promote healing and development of mobile scar Begin cautious mobilization of scar tissue along fiber direction toward injury Progress carefully in intensity and range with nondestructive active, resistive, open and closed chain stabilization, and muscular endurance exercises	Increase strength and alignment of scar Develop functional independence Begin progressive stretching, strengthening, endurance training, functional exercises, and specificity drills Provide cross-fiber frictioning of scar tissue with directional stroking along lines of tension away from injury

impaired repair and restorative functions (e.g., fibromyalgia) is present, unless the application is carefully supervised as part of a treatment program. People may not have enough adaptive capacity to resolve inflammation, therefore caution is advised when considering the use of methods that create inflammation.

Possible patient use of antiinflammatory medications is another factor that must be considered. If a person is taking such medication, either steroidal or nonsteroidal, the effectiveness of therapeutic inflammation is negated or reduced, and restorative mechanisms are inhibited. When these medications are used, any methods that create inflammation are to be avoided (Box 14-5).

AUTOIMMUNE DISEASE

The word *auto* is the Greek word for self. If a person has an autoimmune disease, the immune system mistakenly targets the cells, tissues, and organs of the person's own body.

There are many different autoimmune diseases, and each affects the body in a different way. For example, in MS, the autoimmune reaction is directed against the nerves; in Crohn's disease, it is directed against the gut. In other autoimmune diseases, such as systemic lupus erythematosus (lupus), the tissues and organs affected vary from person to person. In one individual, the skin and joints may be involved, whereas in another, the skin, kidneys, and lungs may be affected. Ultimately, the damage to certain tissues may be permanent, such as occurs in autoimmune-related thyroid disease or in type 1 diabetes mellitus, in which the insulin-producing cells of the pancreas are destroyed.

Many of the autoimmune diseases are rare. As a group, however, autoimmune diseases affect millions of people. No autoimmune disease has ever been shown to be contagious; unlike infections, these diseases do not spread to other people. They are not related to hepatitis, tuberculosis, or the human immunodeficiency virus, nor are they a type of cancer.

Genetic tendency contributes to a person's susceptibility to autoimmune diseases. Development of a disease may be influenced both by genetics and by the way the person's immune system responds to certain triggers or environmental influences.

Some diseases, such as psoriasis, can occur in several members of the same family. This suggests

BOX 14-5 Goals for Massage in the Phases of Healing

Acute Phase
Manage pain
Support sleep

Early Subacute Phase
Manage pain
Support sleep
Manage edema
Manage compensation patterns

Later Subacute Phase
Manage pain
Support sleep
Manage edema
Manage compensation patterns
Support rehabilitative activity
Support mobile scar development
Support tissue regeneration

Remodeling Phase
Support rehabilitative activity
Encourage appropriate scar tissue development
Manage adhesions
Restore firing patterns, gait reflexes, and neuromuscular responses
Eliminate reversible compensation patterns
Manage irreversible compensation patterns
Restore tissue pliability

Modified from Fritz S: *Sports and exercise massage: comprehensive care in athletics, fitness, and rehabilitation,* St Louis, 2005, Mosby.

that a specific gene or set of genes predisposes a family member to psoriasis. Individual family members with autoimmune diseases may inherit and share a set of abnormal genes, although they may develop different autoimmune diseases. For example, one first cousin may have lupus, whereas another may have dermatomyositis, and one of their mothers may have rheumatoid arthritis.

Some autoimmune diseases are known to begin or worsen as a result of certain triggers, such as viral infections. In rheumatic fever, the person produces antibodies to antigens of streptococcal bacteria. Some experts theorize that the streptococcal antigens are structurally similar to antigens of the heart, and antistreptococcal antibodies, combining with antigenic sites on the heart, damage the muscle and heart valves. Sunlight not only acts as a trigger for lupus, it also can worsen the course of the disease. On the other hand, psoriasis improves with exposure to sunlight.

It is important to be aware of the factors that can be avoided, which helps prevent or minimize the amount of damage from the autoimmune disease. Other, less well understood influences that affect the immune system and the course of autoimmune diseases include exposure to chemicals and heavy metals, aging, chronic stress, hormones, and pregnancy.

Diagnosis of an autoimmune disease is based on the person's symptoms, the physical examination findings, and laboratory tests. Autoimmune diseases can be difficult to diagnose, particularly early in the course of the disease. Symptoms of many autoimmune diseases (e.g., fatigue) are nonspecific. Laboratory test results may help, but they often are inadequate for confirming a diagnosis.

If a person has skeletal symptoms, such as joint pain, and a positive but nonspecific laboratory test result, the diagnosis may have the confusing name of early or undifferentiated connective tissue disease. In this case, a physician may want the patient to return frequently for follow-up. The early phase of any autoimmune disease may be a very frustrating time for both the patient and the physician. In other cases, symptoms may be short lived and inconclusive laboratory test results may reveal nothing of a serious nature; however, the symptoms may recur sometime in the future.

Sometimes a specific diagnosis can be made. If the disease is diagnosed shortly after the onset of symptoms, early, aggressive medical therapy can be started. For some diseases, patients respond completely to treatment if the cause of the disease is discovered early in its course.

MEDICAL TREATMENT OF AUTOIMMUNE DISEASE

Although autoimmune diseases are chronic, the course they take is unpredictable. A doctor cannot foresee what will happen to the patient based on how the disease starts. Patients should be monitored closely by their doctors so that environmental factors or triggers that may worsen the disease can be discussed and avoided, and any new medical therapy can be started as soon as possible.

Frequent visits to a doctor are important so that the physician can manage complex treatment regimens and watch for medication side effects.

Autoimmune diseases are often chronic, requiring lifelong care and monitoring even when the person may look or feel well. Currently, few autoimmune diseases can be cured or made to disappear with treatment. However, many people with these diseases can live normal lives if they receive appropriate healthcare.

Physicians most often help patients manage the consequences of inflammation caused by the autoimmune disease. For example, for individuals with type 1 diabetes, physicians prescribe insulin to control blood sugar levels so that elevated blood sugar does not damage the kidneys, eyes, blood vessels, and nerves. In some diseases, such as lupus or rheumatoid arthritis, medication occasionally can slow or stop the immune system's destruction of the kidneys or joints.

Diseases of the immune system currently are treated with a variety of nonspecific immunosuppressive drugs and steroids. Immunosuppressive medications or therapies slow or suppress the immune system response in an attempt to stop the inflammation involved in the autoimmune attack. Immunosuppressive drugs include corticosteroids (prednisone), methotrexate, cyclophosphamide, azathioprine, and cyclosporin. Unfortunately, these medications also suppress the immune system's ability to fight infection and have other potentially serious side effects.

In some people, a limited number of immunosuppressive medications may result in disease remission. However, even if an autoimmune disease goes into remission, patients are rarely able to discontinue the medications. The possibility that the disease may re-emerge when the immunosuppressive medication is discontinued must be balanced against the long-term side effects of the drug. The current goal is to find treatments that produce remissions or reduce symptoms and have the fewest side effects.

TYPES OF AUTOIMMUNE DISEASE

As noted previously, there are many autoimmune diseases. Although the treatment strategies are similar, it is important for the massage therapist to have an understanding of the major autoimmune diseases.

Inflammatory Bowel Diseases

More than 1 in 500 people have some type of inflammatory bowel disease. The term *inflammatory bowel disease* describes two autoimmune disorders of the small intestine, Crohn's disease and ulcerative colitis. Symptoms of Crohn's disease include persistent diarrhea, abdominal pain, fever, and general fatigue. Symptoms of ulcerative colitis include bloody diarrhea, pain, urgent bowel movements, joint pain, and skin lesions. Both diseases carry a risk of significant weight loss and malnutrition.

The side effects of the medications used to treat these diseases can either decrease or increase symptoms. For example, daily use of high-dose corticosteroid (prednisone) therapy, which is needed to control severe symptoms of Crohn's disease, can predispose patients to infections, osteoporosis, and fractures. For patients with ulcerative colitis, surgical removal of the lower intestine (colon) eliminates the disease and the increased risk of colon cancer.

Treatment focuses on symptom management. Antidiarrheal pills or bulk formers are used for mild cases. Antiinflammatory medications are effective for more serious cases,. Corticosteroids are reserved for acute flare-ups of these diseases. In some cases, surgery may be required to remove obstructions or repair a perforation of the colon. With proper management, patients can continue to function normally. For patients with ulcerative colitis, the risk of colon cancer increases with time.

Massage is appropriate for generalized stress management. Typically the general, nonspecific, restorative massage is used as the basic approach. Because osteoporosis is one of the more serious side effects of the medications used to treat these diseases, the massage therapist must monitor the pressure levels used during massage.

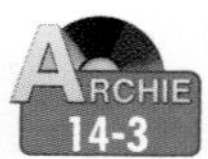

Type 1 (Immune-Mediated) Diabetes Mellitus

As mentioned earlier, type 1 diabetes mellitus results from autoimmune destruction of the insulin-producing cells of the pancreas. The body needs insulin to keep the blood sugar (glucose) level under control. High levels of glucose are responsible for the symptoms and complications of the disease. However, most of the insulin-producing cells are destroyed before the patient develops symptoms of diabetes. Symptoms include fatigue, frequent urination, increased thirst, and possible sudden confusion.

Type 1 diabetes mellitus usually is diagnosed before the age of 30 and may be diagnosed as early as the first month of life. Together with type 2 diabetes (not considered an autoimmune disease), type 1 diabetes is the leading cause of kidney damage, loss of eyesight, and leg amputation. Close control of blood sugar levels reduces the rate at which these events occur.

Type 1 diabetes, which involves a genetic predisposition, occurs in about 1 in 1000 people. Among individuals who have a close relative with this disease, those at high risk for developing it can be identified. Efforts are underway to evaluate prevention strategies for these family members at risk.

Symptoms of type 1 diabetes include increased thirst, increased urination, weight loss, fatigue, nausea, vomiting, and frequent infections. The disease is relatively easy to control with proper medical attention, including the use of insulin, and acute complications are increasingly rare. However, long-term complications, such as disorders of the eye, kidneys, circulatory system, and nerve fibers, are common. If left untreated, diabetes can be fatal.

Massage is appropriate for individuals with type 1 diabetes, and the restorative stress management approach is used as a base. Neuropathic symptoms can be reduced temporarily with massage using various pain control strategies. Cautions for massage include fragile skin, adaptive strain, and areas where insulin is injected. Do not massage around the injection site within 12 hours of injection or if any evidence of inflammation is present.

Guillain-Barré Syndrome

Guillain-Barré syndrome is an acute illness that causes severe nerve damage. Two thirds of all cases occur after a viral infection. Symptoms include tingling in the fingers and toes, general muscle weakness, difficulty breathing and, in severe cases, paralysis. Treatment involves supportive care until the condition stabilizes, then rehabilitation therapy to relieve pain and facilitate retraining of movements. A process called **plasmapheresis,** in which plasma and nerve-damaging antibodies are removed from the blood, is used during the first few weeks after a severe attack and may improve the individual's chances of a full recovery. Most patients recover after a period of months, but some permanent impairment remains in about 10% of cases. The mortality rate is 3% to 4%. Massage for these patients is palliative in nature.

Hematologic Autoimmune Diseases

Blood also can be affected by autoimmune disorders. In autoimmune hemolytic anemia, red blood cells are prematurely destroyed by antibodies. Other autoimmune diseases of the blood include autoimmune thrombocytopenia purpura (a disease of the platelets) and autoimmune neutropenia (a reduction in neutrophils).

Palliative care massage approaches may be indicated, depending on the specific condition. Massage treatment should be closely monitored by the physician.

Multiple Sclerosis

MS is a disease in which the immune system targets nerve tissues. Most often, damage to the CNS occurs intermittently, allowing a person to lead a fairly normal life. MS usually first appears between the ages of 20 and 40; it affects women twice as often as men.

MS is the leading cause of disability among young adults. Symptoms include numbness, weakness, tingling or paralysis in one or more limbs, impaired vision and eye pain, tremor, lack of coordination or unsteady gait, and rapid, involuntary eye movement At the extreme, the symptoms may become constant, resulting in a progressive disease with possible blindness, paralysis, and premature death.

A history of at least two episodes of a cluster of symptoms is necessary for a diagnosis of MS.

Because MS affects the CNS, symptoms may be misdiagnosed as mental illness and depression, and fatigue is a common symptom.

MS is a difficult disease to treat. The drug baclofen is used to suppress muscle spasticity, and corticosteroids help reduce inflammation. Some medications, such as beta interferon, are helpful to people with the intermittent form of MS. The disease is degenerative and often follows a fluctuating course. The average life expectancy is 35 years after the onset of symptoms. Most people with MS can function effectively; however, a rare form of acute MS can be fatal within weeks.

Massage is appropriate for patients with MS. However, the technique must change in duration, intensity, depth of pressure, and drag according to the patient's current situation. Methods that create inflammation must be avoided.

Myasthenia Gravis

Myasthenia gravis is a chronic autoimmune disorder characterized by gradual muscle weakness, which often appears first in the face. Symptoms include drooping eyelids, double vision, and difficulty breathing, talking, chewing, and swallowing. The drug edrophonium, along with daily rest periods, can improve muscle strength. Treatment can induce remission, and individuals with this disease can lead productive lives.

The symptoms of myasthenia gravis, especially in the early stages, may prompt the person to seek massage treatment. The massage therapist should be able to recognize vague symptoms as indicators of a potentially serious disease and refer the person for diagnosis.

Palliative massage is appropriate for these patients. The general protocol may be too intense and may strain adaptive mechanisms.

Psoriasis

Psoriasis is an immune system disorder that affects the skin and occasionally the eyes, nails, and joints. Psoriasis may affect very small areas of skin or may cover the entire body with a buildup of red scales called *plaques.* The plaques have different sizes, shapes, and severity and may be painful as well as unattractive. Bacterial infections and pressure or trauma to the skin can aggravate psoriasis. Most treatments focus on topical skin care to relieve the inflammation, itching, and scaling. Oral medications (i.e., steroids and immune suppressants) are used for severe cases. Psoriasis is common and may affect more than 1 in 50 Americans. The disease often runs in families.

With patients with psoriasis, the massage therapist should avoid areas of broken and irritated skin. However, massage over scaly patches is appropriate if the skin is not broken. As with other autoimmune diseases, the massage is restorative and stress reducing in nature. Symptomatic relief of joint pain is possible.

Rheumatoid Arthritis

In people with rheumatoid arthritis (RA), the immune system predominantly targets the lining (synovium) that covers various joints, causing pain, swelling, and joint stiffness. These features distinguish rheumatoid arthritis from osteoarthritis, which is a more common degenerative wear-and-tear arthritis. RA also can affect the heart, lungs, and eyes. Of the estimated 2.1 million Americans with RA, approximately 71% are women. Symptoms include inflamed and/or deformed joints, loss of strength, swelling, and pain.

This condition typically is treated with rest, exercise, and antiinflammatory medications when necessary. Joint replacement for severely deformed joints is an option and often is performed for the finger joints.

The massage application for patients with RA has a general, nonspecific, stress-reducing focus. It should not increase inflammation.

Scleroderma

Scleroderma results in thickening of the skin, blood vessels, and organs. The disease involves activation of immune cells, producing scar tissue in the skin, internal organs, and small blood vessels. It affects women three times as often as men overall, and the rate is 15 times higher for women during childbearing years.

Scleroderma cannot be cured, but timely intervention can improve the person's quality of life. Almost every patient with scleroderma has Raynaud's syndrome, which involves spasms of the blood vessels in the fingers and toes. Symptoms of Raynaud's syndrome include increased sensitivity of the fingers and toes to the cold, changes in skin color, pain, and occasionally ulcers of the fingertips or toes. In people with scleroderma, thickening of skin and blood vessels can result in loss of mobility. Other symptoms include joint stiffness in the hands, pain, sore throat, and diarrhea.

The drug D-penicillamine has been shown to reduce skin thickening. Symptoms involving other organs (e.g., the kidneys, lungs, esophagus, intestines, and blood vessels) are treated individually.

Massage may increase skin pliability for a short time in these patients. Methods that increase inflammation should not be used. As with most medical conditions, full body, general, palliative massage is appropriate.

Sjögren's Syndrome

Sjögren's syndrome (also called *Sjögren's disease*) is a chronic, slowly progressing inability to secrete saliva and tears. Symptoms include dryness of the eyes and mouth, swollen neck glands, difficulty swallowing or talking, unusual tastes or smells, thirst, tongue ulcers, and severe dental caries. The disease can occur alone or with RA, scleroderma, or lupus. Nine of 10 cases occur in women, most often at or around midlife. The disease has a benign course, but in rare cases malignant cancer of the lymph nodes may develop. Interventions including drinking adequate fluids to keep the mouth and eyes moist, using eye drops, and good oral hygiene and eye care.

No specific massage strategies are necessary for these patients, nor is massage contraindicated.

Systemic Lupus Erythematosus

An inflammatory disease of the connective tissues, systemic lupus erythematosus can afflict every organ system. It is up to nine times more common in women than in men. The condition is aggravated by sunlight, and symptoms include fever, weight loss, hair loss, mouth and nose sores, malaise, fatigue, seizures, and symptoms of mental illness. Ninety percent of individuals with lupus experience joint inflammation similar to that seen in RA, and 50% develop a classic butterfly-pattern rash on the nose and cheeks. Raynaud's phenomenon (extreme sensitivity to cold in the hands and feet) appears in about 20% of people with lupus. In severe cases, the immune system may attack and damage several organs such as the kidneys, brain, or lungs.

Antiinflammatory medications can help control the arthritis-like symptoms, and skin lesions may respond to topical treatment (e.g., corticosteroid creams). Oral steroids, such as prednisone, are used for the systemic symptoms. However, if a patient is not closely monitored, the side effects of the medications can be quite serious. Wearing protective clothing and sunscreen when outdoors is recommended.

Once a disease with a high mortality rate, lupus has become a chronic disease as a result of new treatment approaches. Now, about 97% of individuals live at least 5 years after diagnosis, and 90% live at least 10 years. In 1954 just 50% lived longer than 4 years.

General restorative massage that targets symptom management is appropriate for patients with lupus. Cautions include massage interactions that may increase the side effects of medications. The side effects of long-term steroid use include osteoporosis and fragile tissue.

Autoimmune-Related Thyroid Diseases

Hashimoto's thyroiditis and Graves' disease result from immune system destruction or stimulation of thyroid tissue. Symptoms of low thyroid function (hypothyroid) or overactive function (hyperthyroid) are nonspecific and can develop slowly or suddenly; they include fatigue, nervousness, cold or heat intolerance, weakness, changes in the amount or texture of the hair, and weight gain or loss. The diagnosis of thyroid disease is readily made with appropriate laboratory tests.

Hashimoto's thyroiditis is a type of autoimmune disease in which the immune system destroys the thyroid, the gland that helps set the rate of metabolism. It attacks women 50 times more often than men. Low levels of thyroid hormone cause mental and physical slowing, greater sensitivity to cold, weight gain, coarsening of the skin, and goiter. Thyroid hormone replacement therapy is an effective treatment, and most patients regain normal health with treatment.

Graves' disease is one of the most common autoimmune diseases. It affects about 13 million people, women about seven times as often as men. Patients with Graves' disease produce an excess amount of thyroid hormone. Symptoms include weight loss as a result of increased energy expenditure; an increase in the appetite, heart rate, and blood pressure; tremors, nervousness, and sweating; and frequent bowel movements. The normal course of treatment involves antithyroid drug therapy, surgical removal of the thyroid gland, or treatment with radioactive iodine, followed by administration of the appropriate dose of thyroid replacement hormone. If left untreated, Graves' disease can be fatal.

Many of the symptoms of thyroid disease can be misdiagnosed. Quite a few of these symptoms involve muscle and joint aching, fatigue, and anxiety, which may prompt a person to seek massage treatment. If massage therapists recognize the cluster of symptoms indicating thyroid disease, it is important that they refer the person for diagnosis. Thyroid disease can be treated effectively with proper medical care. Massage is effective at managing the various symptoms and, as with all autoimmune diseases, it can support the body's self-regulating mechanisms.

Vasculitis Syndromes

The vasculitides are a broad, heterogeneous group of diseases characterized by inflammation and damage to the blood vessels, thought to be brought on by an autoimmune response. Blood vessels of any type, size, and location can be involved. Vasculitis may occur alone or in combination with other diseases, and it may be confined to one organ or involve several organ systems.

In these cases general massage is indicated; however, the patient must be closely monitored for any type of blood clot formation or vessel blockage. Caution is necessary (Box 14-6).

BOX 14-6 Autoimmune Diseases

Antiphospholipid syndrome
Autoimmune disease of the adrenal gland
Autoimmune hemolytic anemia
Autoimmune hepatitis
Autoimmune neuropathies
Autoimmune thrombocytopenia
Autoimmune uveitis
Behcet's disease
Crohn's disease
Dermatitis herpetiformis
Dermatomyositis
Graves' disease
Hashimoto's thyroiditis
Multiple sclerosis
Myasthenia gravis
Pemphigus vulgaris
Pernicious anemia
Polymyositis
Primary biliary cirrhosis
Psoriasis
Rheumatoid arthritis
Scleroderma
Sjogren's syndrome
Spondyloarthropathies
Systemic lupus erythematosus
Temporal arteritis
Type 1 (immune-mediated) diabetes mellitus
Ulcerative colitis
Vasculitides
Vitiligo

MASSAGE STRATEGIES FOR AUTOIMMUNE DISEASE

Suggestions for massage for patients with specific autoimmune diseases have been provided throughout this section. In general, massage is appropriate for people with autoimmune diseases. Typically these are chronic diseases that fall into the condition management category. The medications used for treatment have significant side effects, and the use of some alternative methods, such as massage, may allow the doctor to reduce the dosage or eliminate some of these drugs (e.g., pain medications).

Autoimmune diseases generally are stress responsive and involve an inflammatory process. The various medications used to treat them can cause the blood to thin (i.e., fail to coagulate), increasing the potential for bruising. The development of fragile bones also is a possibility. The massage methods used for these patients need to be palliative and restorative, stress management, full body techniques (with possible regional contraindications, such as psoriasis) that do not strain the patient's adaptive capacity or increase inflammation.

evolve 14-1

The following terms and expressions specific to Chapter 14 have already been used to search PubMed for the latest research literature available. The *Click Here for Massage* feature associated with this chapter on your textbook's Evolve website allows you to hyperlink to a continually updated PubMed search of research literature that corresponds to this subject.

Hyperlink Search Terms

Massage autoimmune disease
Massage breathing disorder
Massage inflammation
Massage pain

SUMMARY

This chapter described the four major predisposing and perpetuating processes and symptoms that massage can target regardless of the specific disease: breathing dysfunction, pain, inflammatory processes, and autoimmune disorders.

Regardless of the diagnosis, the massage therapist can identify these areas and design treatment plans to support general restorative function. These four conditions are interrelated and can become cyclical. Pain can perpetuate breathing disorder, which increases sympathetic arousal, perpetuating inflammation, which can get out of control and cause immune dysfunction, giving rise to autoimmune disease, which strains the self-regulating mechanism, perpetuating inflammation and causing pain, which increases the tendency for breathing disorder. Life stresses increase the tendency for breathing disorder, which perpetuates chronic inflammation, which results in pain that increases stress, which strains the immune function, and so on and so forth. Fortunately, intervention that targets these four predisposing and perpetuating factors can break this vicious cycle, and massage is an effective intervention for all these conditions when combined with other types of supportive care.

REFERENCES

1. http://pain.health.ivillage.com/painbasics/painbasics3.cfm
2. http://www.thyroid-info.com/autoimmune/work.htm

WORKBOOK

1. Identify three health conditions with which you would like to work (e.g., insomnia, migraine, headache, fibromyalgia, cancer, infertility, multiple sclerosis). For each condition, identify how breathing dysfunction, pain, inflammation, or autoimmunity is involved in the condition. Then design a massage treatment recommendation that addresses the various aspects of breathing dysfunction, pain, inflammation, or autoimmunity that you have indicated are involved in this specific condition.

____
____
____
____
____
____

2. Analyze the three treatment approaches you devised in question 1. Identify areas that are similar in their treatment recommendations and create a master massage treatment approach.

____
____
____
____
____
____

3. List all the health conditions discussed in this chapter that could be addressed effectively using the master massage treatment plan you created in question 2.

____

____

____

____

____

____

Chapter 15 Concept Map

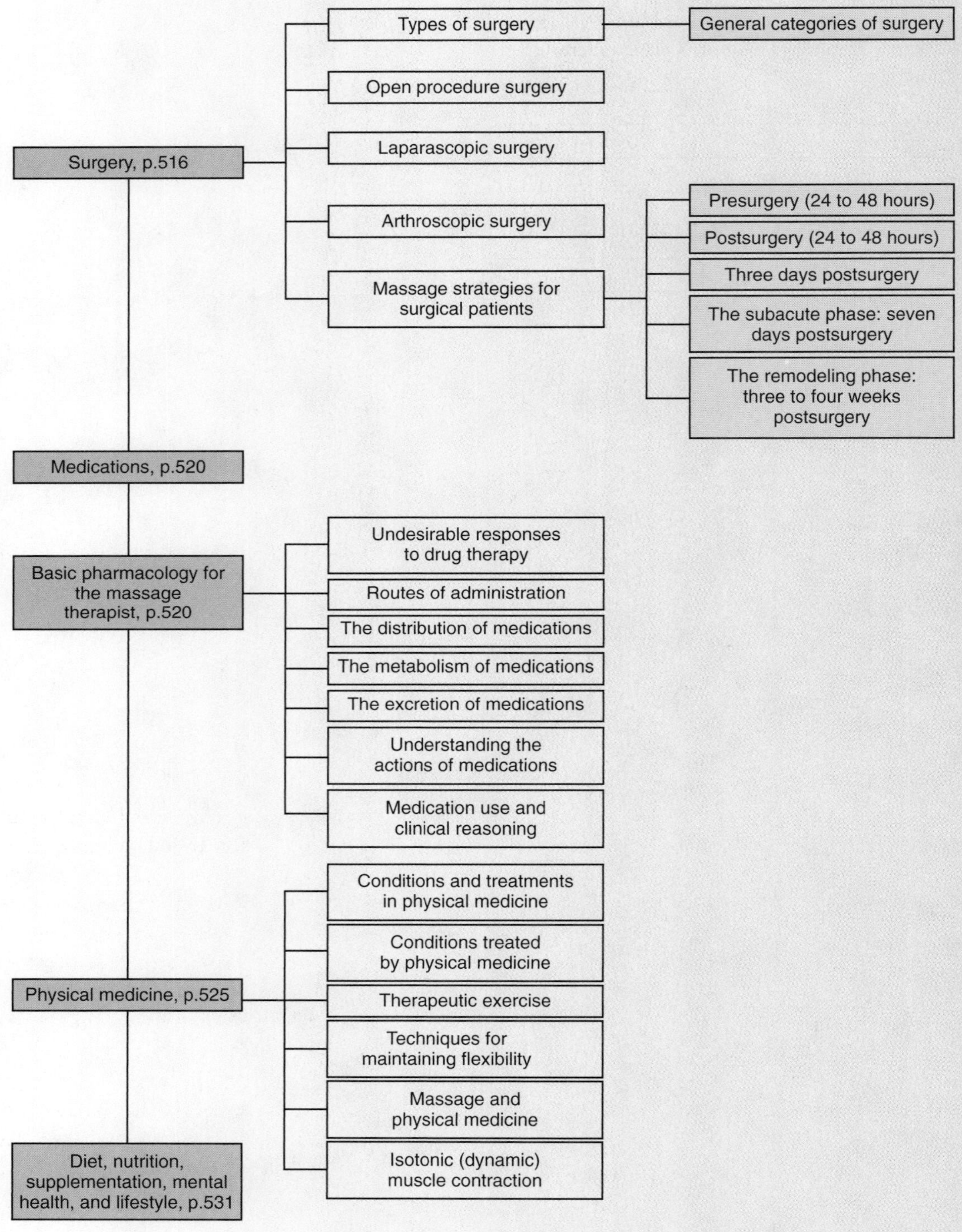

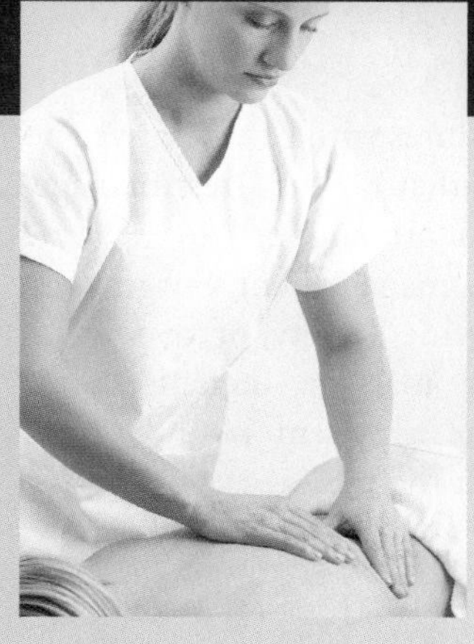

CHAPTER 15

MEDICAL TREATMENT FOR ILLNESS AND INJURY

Key Terms

Active assistive range-of-motion (AAROM) exercise
Arthroscopic surgery
Laparoscope
Laparoscopic surgery
Major surgery
Minimally invasive surgery
Passive range-of-motion (PROM) exercise
Proprioceptive neuromuscular facilitation (PNF)
Surgery
Synergistic effect

For definitions of key terms, refer to the Evolve website.

OBJECTIVES

Upon completion of this chapter, the reader will have the information necessary to:

1. Explain the importance of the appropriate use of surgery and medications to treat illness and injury.
2. List indications and contraindications for massage related to medical treatments.
3. Perform appropriate presurgical and postsurgical massage applications.
4. Alter massage to effectively complement the use of medications.
5. Apply massage as an aspect of physical medicine.

Advances in medical treatment, including surgical procedures, medications, and rehabilitative exercise, have prolonged life and improved its quality for many individuals. Massage therapists need to understand medical treatments in order to make appropriate decisions about the advisability of massage and the methods to apply to support these interventions. The variety of possible medical treatments is huge. Addressing each surgical procedure or medication individually is beyond the scope of this text. The massage therapist must research the specific procedures each patient has undergone and then develop a treatment plan based on that information. This chapter explains the basic premise of medical treatments and provides the foundation for effective research. In addition to reference texts and journals, the Internet has become a vast resource for looking up information. One caveat: when consulting websites, the massage therapist must make sure to verify that the information is from a reliable, unbiased source.

evolve 15-1

Box 15-1 on the Evolve website lists some excellent websites for looking up information on medical treatments. Most large hospitals and universities also have websites that provide information on various types of medical treatments.

SURGERY

Surgery is a medical treatment that typically involves opening the body to allow the surgeon access to areas that need repair, alteration, or removal. Historically, the most significant risk factors with surgery were anesthesia, blood loss, and infection. All of these now can usually be managed successfully, and this allows for more advanced and complicated procedures. Surgery always involves risk, and often more conservative care is attempted before surgery is considered as a final option. Significant advances in surgical procedures, such as microsurgery, laparoscopic surgery, and arthroscopic surgery, have reduced the risks and healing time and have improved the chances of a successful outcome. In addition, advances in computer technology are contributing to the development of safer, more effective surgical procedures.

TYPES OF SURGERY

Major surgery is the term used for surgical procedures that involve large incisions and a longer healing time. **Minimally invasive surgery** is a closed or local procedure rather than an open, invasive one. Minimally invasive procedures generally involve the use of laparoscopic devices, as well as remote-control manipulation of instruments with indirect observation of the surgical field through an endoscope or similar device. Because minimally invasive surgery involves less trauma to the body, the number of long hospital stays may drop, and the number of short stays and day surgeries may increase.

The massage therapist must understand the general types of surgery and must be able to support surgical procedures with preoperative and postoperative massage that targets stress management, pain management, support for wound healing, and scar tissue management. Surgery can be performed for a wide variety of conditions (Box 15-1), and the massage therapist must research any procedure a patient is undergoing before proceeding with the massage.

General Categories of Surgery

As mentioned previously, the massage professional must have a basic understanding of the general types of surgical procedures. These include open procedure surgery, laparoscopic surgery, and arthroscopic surgery.

Open Procedure Surgery. Until recently, open procedure surgery was the primary method of performing surgery. An incision is made large enough to allow the surgeon to see the target area and perform whatever procedures are required. The tissues are then sutured back together. This type of surgery is still performed when necessary, but newer, more technologically advanced surgical procedures are replacing the open procedure whenever possible.

Laparoscopic Surgery. In **laparoscopic surgery,** the abdomen first is inflated with carbon dioxide to provide more room for the procedure. Next, a small incision is made at the navel, and a **laparoscope** (an instrument similar to a small telescope on a flexible tube) is inserted into the abdomen so that the area can be viewed. Three small additional holes are made in the lower abdomen to allow the insertion of surgical instruments to obtain tissue samples or perform additional procedures. When the procedure is complete, the carbon dioxide gas is released and the incisions are stitched.

Laparoscopic surgery has been called band-aid surgery. It has a lower rate of complications, a shorter hospital stay, and a better cosmetic result than the open procedure. However, the complexity of a surgical case sometimes may require use of the open technique.

BOX 15-1 Common Surgical Procedures and Related Terms

- Ambulatory surgery: Surgery performed on an outpatient basis. The surgery may be hospital based or performed in an office or surgical center.
- Cardiovascular surgery: Surgery performed on the heart or blood vessels.
- Cryosurgery: The use of freezing as a surgical technique to destroy or excise tissue.
- Curettage: The process of scraping (usually of the interior of a cavity or tract) to remove new growth or other abnormal tissue or to obtain material for tissue diagnosis.
- Débridement: The removal of foreign material and dead or contaminated tissue from or adjacent to a traumatic or infected area until surrounding healthy tissue is exposed.
- Digestive system surgery: Surgery performed on the digestive system or its parts.
- Elective surgery: Surgery that could be postponed or omitted without danger to the patient. Elective surgery includes procedures to correct medical problems that are not life-threatening, as well as those performed to alleviate conditions that cause psychological stress or other potential risk to patients (e.g., cosmetic or contraceptive surgery).
- Electrosurgery: The process of cutting tissue using a high-frequency current applied locally with a metal instrument or needle. This type of surgery reduces blood loss.
- Endocrine surgery: Surgery performed on any endocrine gland.
- Extracorporeal circulation: The diversion of blood flow through a circuit outside the body but continuous with the bodily circulation.
- Intraoperative period: The period of time during which a surgical procedure takes place.
- Laser surgery: The use of a laser either to vaporize surface lesions or to make bloodless cuts in tissue. It does not include laser coagulation of tissue.
- Microsurgery: Surgery that is performed with the aid of a microscope.
- Minor surgery: Surgery that treats minor problems and injuries and does not in itself pose a danger to life.
- Neurosurgery: Surgery performed on the nervous system or its parts.
- Obstetric surgery: Surgery performed on a pregnant woman for conditions associated with pregnancy, labor, or the puerperium. It does not include surgery on the newborn infant.
- Ophthalmologic surgery: Surgery performed on the eye or any of its parts.
- Oral surgery: Surgery performed to treat disease, injuries, and defects of the oral and maxillofacial region.
- Ostomy: The surgical construction of an artificial opening (stoma) to allow external fistulization of a duct or vessel by insertion of a tube with or without a supportive stent.
- Otorhinolaryngologic surgery: Surgery performed on the ear and its parts, the nose and nasal cavity, or the throat, including surgery of the adenoids, tonsils, pharynx, and trachea.
- Prosthesis implantation: The surgical insertion of a prosthesis.
- Reconstructive surgery: Surgery performed to restore or improve defective, damaged, or missing structures.
- Surgical decompression: Surgery performed to relieve pressure.
- Thoracic surgery: Surgery performed on the thoracic organs, most commonly the lungs and heart.
- Transplantation: The transfer of a tissue or organ within an individual, between individuals of the same species, or between individuals of different species.
- Urogenital surgery: Surgery performed on the urinary tract or its organs and on the male or female genitalia.

Data from National Library of Medicine-Medical Subject Headings.

Arthroscopic Surgery. **Arthroscopic surgery** involves the use of fiberoptic cameras and small surgical instruments to visualize the intraarticular structures of the joint and to treat many abnormalities or injuries. Arthroscopy can be used both to examine and repair joint problems in one operation. First used primarily on the knee joint, arthroscopy now can be used for the diagnosis and treatment of problems in the shoulder, elbow, wrist, hip, and ankle. Besides reducing the invasiveness of joint surgery, arthroscopy also reduces the recovery time. Because less pain and swelling result, less disruption occurs in other structures around the joint. This allows weight-bearing, range-of-motion, and strengthening exercises to begin earlier. The healing and rehabilitation process should be easier, and the return to activity also is accelerated.

The technique of arthroscopic surgery involves the placement of small incisions (portals) around the joint (Figure 15-1). One of the standard arthroscopic incisions is a small fluid outflow (or in some cases inflow) portal. Fluid is introduced into the joint to allow better visualization and separation of structures and to remove any blood that might be present from the surgical incisions

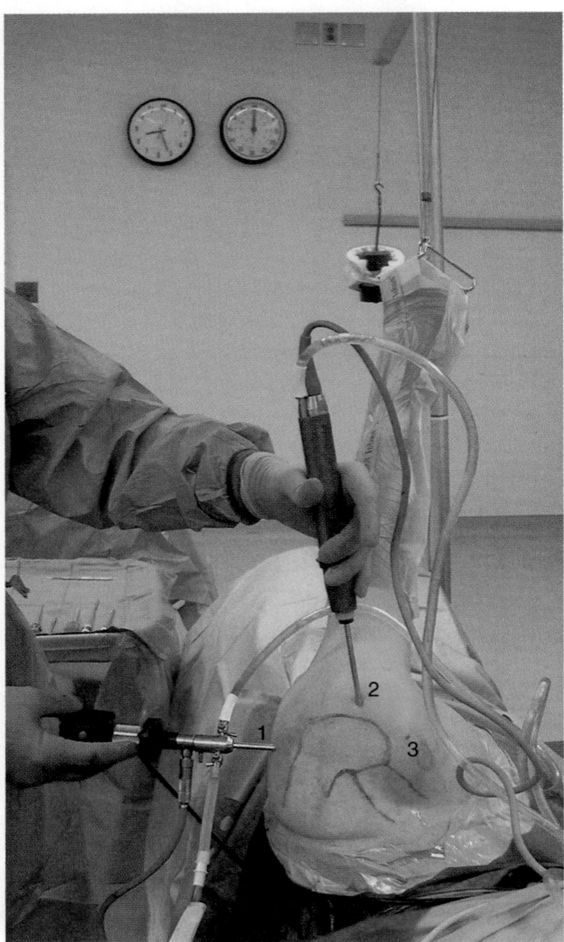

FIGURE 15-1 ■ Arthroscopic portals: *1,* Posterior; *2,* anterior; and *3,* lateral. (From Miller MD, Cole BJ: *Textbook of arthroscopy,* Philadelphia, 2004, WB Saunders.)

or injuries. Another standard portal is used to place the arthroscopic camera for most of the work inside the joint. The arthroscope is inserted through a small incision in the side of the joint. A beam of light and a small camera transmit an enlarged image of the joint's interior to a TV monitor. Repairs are made through the portal incisions, which are so small that stitches usually are not required to close them. Risks associated with arthroscopy include nerve injury, infection, bleeding, and stiffness. Some complex procedures still require traditional open surgery, but many can be enhanced by the use of an arthroscope.

Almost all arthroscopic surgeries are now performed on an outpatient basis. In most cases, special adhesive strips are placed over the arthroscopic portals to allow the skin incisions to heal and to minimize scarring. A loose, sterile dressing is then applied, which can be removed in 3 to 4 days. The patient is allowed to bear weight as tolerated with the use of crutches and may wean off the crutches when he or she can walk without a limp. Rehabilitation should begin as soon as the surgeon permits it so that the joint does not stiffen and the muscles do not atrophy. Most patients recover fully (Figure 15-1).

MASSAGE STRATEGIES FOR SURGICAL PATIENTS

Presurgery (24 to 48 Hours)

In the presurgical period, the targeted outcomes for massage are to reduce anxiety and support restorative sleep. A calm, rested patient requires less anesthesia and copes better with the stress of the surgical procedure. Do not work directly on the targeted surgical areas with deep pressure, intense drag, or any methods that may cause tissue damage. Use a palliative approach. Target breathing function, parasympathetic dominance, and neurochemical balance.

Postsurgery (24 to 48 Hours)

Massage in the postsurgical period follows a combined sequence for wounds, pain management, and lymphatic drainage. Depending on the extent of the procedure, massage can begin within 24 to 48 hours. It focuses on controlling pain, reducing anxiety, and supporting restorative sleep. The massage is kept relatively short but is given more frequently (e.g., twice a day). It targets areas that are achy other than the surgical site. Often the neck, shoulders, and low back are sore from bed rest or from positioning during surgery. Massage of the head, face, hands, and feet usually is effective for calming the person. Do not use methods that cause pain. Do not work near the surgical site. Because infection control is very important, always maintain meticulous sanitation. For uncomplicated surgeries, especially laparoscopic and arthroscopic procedures, the patient goes home the day of surgery or the next day.

Three Days Postsurgery

For most types of surgery, especially laparoscopic and arthroscopic procedures, the patient is home and ambulatory by 3 days after the procedure. Massage remains palliative, with a focus on lymphatic drainage to manage postoperative edema if the physician approves. Do not work directly on the surgical site; however, careful, gentle work around the area is appropriate. This is considered acute care, and the surgical sites are wounds (see massage for wounds in Chapter 17). Sanitation and infection control are top priorities. If the patient has been instructed to perform range-of-motion exercises, massage supports the movement pattern. Work with reflex patterns. The paired functional areas (Figure 15-2) are as follows:

- Right shoulder, left hip, and vice versa
- Right elbow, left knee, and vice versa
- Right wrist, left ankle, and vice versa
- Right hand, left foot, and vice versa

The functional muscle units are:

- Flexors with opposite side flexors and same side extensors
- Extensors with opposite side extensors and same side flexors
- Internal rotators with opposite side internal rotators and same side external rotators
- External rotators with opposite side external rotators and same side internal rotators
- Adductors with adductors and abductors with abductors

The trunk paired patterns are:

- Neck flexors with trunk flexors
- Neck extensors with trunk extensors
- Neck lateral flexors with trunk lateral flexors

Because massage is contraindicated in the surgical area, paired areas can be addressed to create beneficial reflex responses (Box 15-2).

If the patient can move the surgical area, the effect of the massage is enhanced if the person moves the area gently while the targeted reflex areas are massaged. It is important to be intentional and deliberate in the focus. For example, in the arthroscopic knee surgery case in Box 15-2, when massaging the right biceps, be thinking about the left hamstring. Using these reflexes does not mean that you are massaging the arm for the benefit of the arm; the arm is massaged to influence the leg. Continue lymphatic drainage and massage daily if possible.

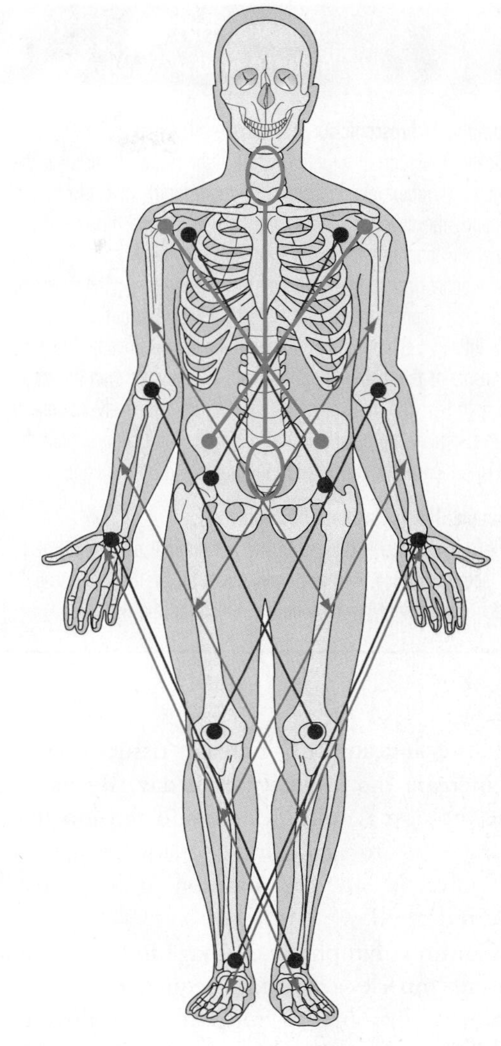

FIGURE 15-2 ■ Areas of symmetry: Arm/thigh. Forearm/leg. Hand/foot. Shoulder/hip. Elbow/knee. Wrist/ankle. Cervical spine/sacrum. Shoulder girdle/pelvic girdle. (From Fritz S: *Sports and exercise massage: comprehensive care in athletics, fitness, and rehabilitation*, St Louis, 2006, Mosby.)

The Subacute Phase: Seven Days Postsurgery

By the subacute phase, the stitches (if any) should be out and gentle scar tissue work can begin in the surgical area. Use massage strategies for wounds. Do not pull on the incision. Use gentle bending and shear force about 1 inch

BOX 15-2 Surgery on Part of a Paired Area

Example: Arthroscopic surgery on the left knee
Reflexive massage is targeted to the right elbow. It includes the biceps (to reflexively influence the hamstring), the triceps (to influence the quadriceps), and the wrist and finger flexors at the elbow (to influence the calf). Lymphatic drainage and techniques that support circulation are applied to the entire arm. The massage application then moves to the left elbow and is targeted to reflexively influence the right hamstring and the left quadriceps. The wrist extensors at the elbow target the calf. The process then moves to the right leg. The hamstrings on the left are reflexively influenced by massage of the quadriceps on the right. The quadriceps on the left is influenced by massage of the hamstring on the right.

Example: Hernia in the right groin
Reflexive massage is applied to the left anterior and lateral neck, the pectoralis major and pectoralis minor on the left, the scapula region on the right, and the neck extensor on the right.

from the incision to increase tissue pliability and increase the intensity each day. By day 14, if the incision is fully healed, add tension force. At day 18 to 20, add torsion force and work directly on the incision unless this is contraindicated.

Continue lymphatic drainage in the area and reset all muscle activation sequences and gait reflexes if appropriate. Support all healing and rehabilitation exercises. Massage should be offered three or four times a week if possible.

The Remodeling Phase: Three to Four Weeks Postsurgery

During the remodeling phase, resume use of the full body general protocol presented in Unit Two. Continue to manage edema, as well as muscle activation sequences, reflex patterns, and any other compensation. Address scar tissue during each massage. Normalize all residual muscle guarding. Continue this focus for at least 6 months. Provide massage twice a week if possible, although weekly sessions are adequate.

Each of the phases of healing may take longer if the patient is more fragile, such as an elderly person (Figure 15-3).

MEDICATIONS

Medications are chemical agents that influence the physiologic processes of the body. This topic can be overwhelming, because it encompasses prescribed medications, over-the-counter (OTC) medications, and a huge variety of nutritional supplements and herbs. Do not expect that you will be able to remember all the indications for and side effects of medications. Massage often is targeted to reducing the side effects of medications. More conservative intervention includes consideration of lifestyle changes as well.

Some medications have very harmful side effects; in some cases, the side effects may even be worse than the symptoms. Other medications can become problematic when taken for a long time. The patient may have a better outcome if less risky methods, such as massage, can replace a medication or can allow the doctor to reduce the dosage. The Evolve website expands on this section, and the student needs to become familiar with the content on basic pharmacology. Massage therapists must have a basic understanding of this information to make appropriate massage treatment decisions for patients taking medications.

JUST BETWEEN YOU AND ME

When it comes to medications, you will be constantly looking up stuff. Get the books listed and find a website that works for you. Whenever a patient is taking a medication. you have to look it up. Don't rely on memory.

BASIC PHARMACOLOGY FOR THE MASSAGE THERAPIST

Pharmacology is the science of drugs, including the development of drugs, their mechanisms of action, and the conditions for which they are used. It also deals with assessment of their efficacy (through clinical trials) and their safety (through an oversight system called *pharmacovigilance*). Pharmacists are the medical professionals who specialize in pharmacology.

The terms *medication* and *drug* often are used interchangeably. *Medication* refers specifically to

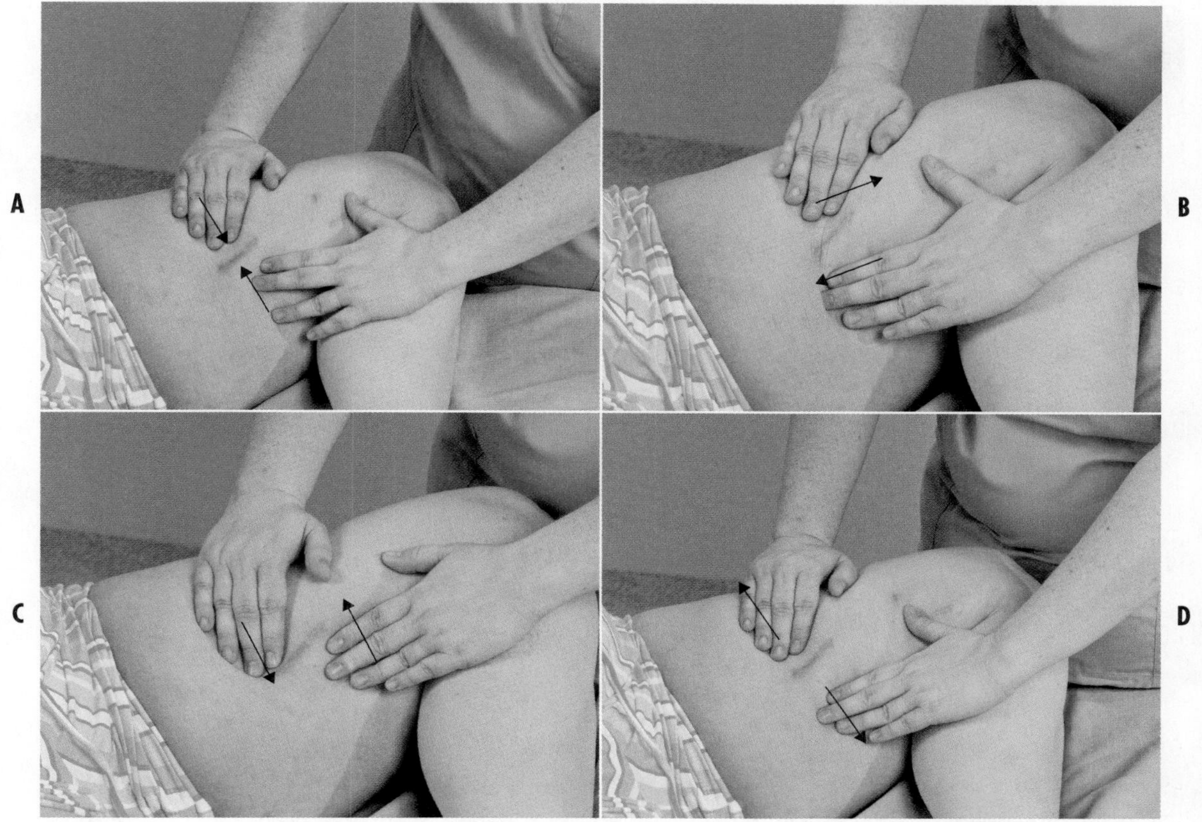

FIGURE 15-3 ■ Example sequence for scar tissue management in a postoperative area. **A,** Early postoperative period (phase I): *Gently* move skin together during acute healing (3 to 7 days). Observe precautions for sanitation, fragile tissue, stitches, staples, and dressings. **B,** Later postoperative period: Move tissues back and forth during early subacute healing (7 to 14 days). Do not move tissues beyond bind. Observe precautions for infection and fragile tissue. **C,** Add shear force at approximately 10 days after surgery. Continue to observe precautions for fragile tissue, infection, and swelling. **D,** Add tension force to stretch tissue about day 14. Continue precautions.

pharmaceutical agents used in the treatment of disease, whereas *drug* can encompass a broader scope of chemical use, including drugs of abuse (e.g., cocaine) and OTC medications. The following discussion typically uses the term *drug.* The section focuses on the possible interaction between the influences exerted by massage and the effects of drugs.

Herbs and vitamins are considered in this discussion because they work in the body through mechanisms similar to those of drugs. After all, food, herbs, and vitamins metabolize into chemicals that are used and/or discarded by the body. Vitamin products usually are standardized, and the effects of specific doses and types can be studied. Herb products made from the unaltered plant substance can vary tremendously in the concentration and strength of the active chemical. Some herbal products are *standardized,* which means that the active elements are consistent in each dose of the herb. Many believe that whole plant sources of herbs contain components that enhance and buffer the effects of the active chemicals, reducing the chances of undesirable side effects; this may or may not be the case. All chemicals taken into the body—medications, OTC drugs, drugs of abuse, environmental pollutants, food, vitamins, supplements, herbs, and manufactured food ingredients (e.g., artificial sweeteners, coloring, preservatives)—have the potential to produce beneficial or negative effects.

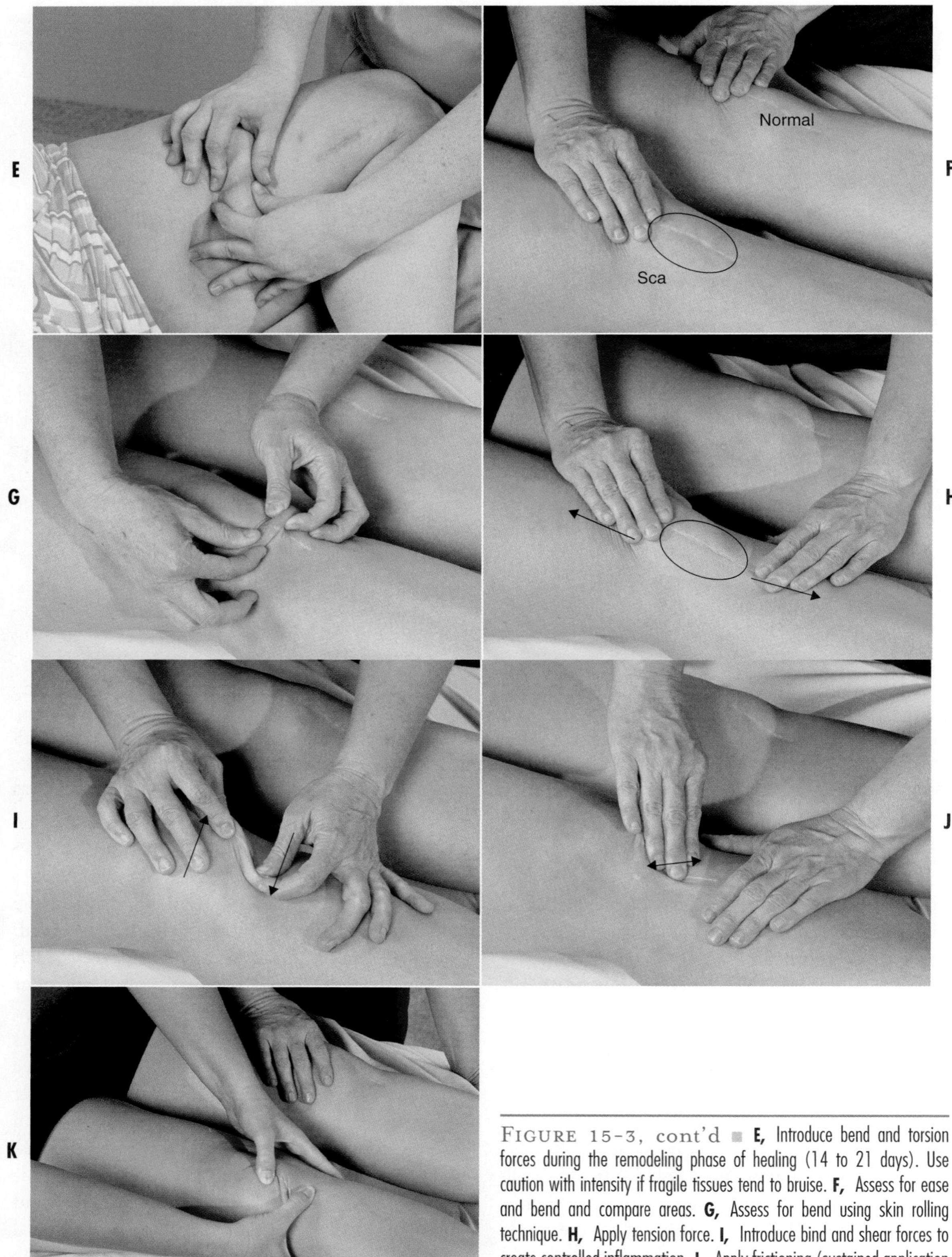

FIGURE 15-3, cont'd ■ **E,** Introduce bend and torsion forces during the remodeling phase of healing (14 to 21 days). Use caution with intensity if fragile tissues tend to bruise. **F,** Assess for ease and bend and compare areas. **G,** Assess for bend using skin rolling technique. **H,** Apply tension force. **I,** Introduce bind and shear forces to create controlled inflammation. **J,** Apply frictioning (sustained application of a shear force) to introduce therapeutic inflammation. **K,** Teach the patient self-management.

Many drugs began as herbal products, therefore pharmacology and herbology are intrinsically linked. Food contains carbohydrates, fats, proteins, fiber, enzymes, vitamins, minerals, and other bioactive elements that can be used to treat various health conditions. For example, foods such as blueberries are high in antioxidants that the body can use to control inflammation and eliminate free radicals. Nutrition can and should be an aspect of therapeutic treatment using chemicals. Certain foods, herbs, and vitamins can interact with drugs, and this interaction can be either supportive or detrimental. For example, grapefruit, a nutritionally valuable food, should not be eaten while taking certain medications. Potentially severe side effects can occur if St. John's wort, SAMe, or 5-HPT is taken along with a selective serotonin reuptake inhibitor (SSRI) medication. Vitamins typically work best when taken with food, but the absorption of certain medications is inhibited if the medication is taken with food. The entire potential interaction process can get extremely complicated. Regardless, the product (food, herb, vitamin, mineral, or drug) has to be taken into the body and used, and the waste products must be eliminated.

evolve 15-2

Refer to the Evolve website for more detailed information on pharmacology and massage.

In general, medicines work in the body by three modes of action. They:

- Replenish or replace deficient or missing substances
- Alter the activity of cells
- Destroy infectious microorganisms or abnormal cells

An understanding of these simple modes of action can help the massage therapist make informed decisions about the potential influence of massage on the action of the medication. For example, massage appears to influence the action of dopamine. Dopamine deficiency is one of the causal factors of Parkinson's disease. Individuals with this disease are given medication to replenish the deficient dopamine. Massage seems to increase blood levels of dopamine or to enhance dopamine's availability, thereby sustaining its action. In this case, massage and the medication both address deficiency.

Massage application can cause localized inflammation. Some medications, such as antiinflammatories, alter the cellular function related to inflammation. If massage is used to create a therapeutic inflammatory effect but the person is taking antiinflammatory drugs, the effects of the massage will be altered.

If a person is taking an antibiotic to treat a bacterial infection, the person's immune system is compromised and the adaptive capacity is strained. Massage can support the immune response, especially by encouraging parasympathetic dominance and restorative sleep, or it can interfere with immune function by being too aggressive and further straining adaptive capacity.

No concrete scientific studies have identified the potential interaction of massage effects with the effects of drugs. Therefore the massage therapist must use the clinical reasoning process to make safe, justifiable decisions on how to alter a massage application for a patient taking medication.

UNDESIRABLE RESPONSES TO DRUG THERAPY

Most drugs are not entirely free of unwanted effects. However, drugs that are frequently prescribed, that are highly potent, or that have a narrow therapeutic index are likely to carry a greater risk of such effects. Undesirable responses to a drug are described as follows:

- Adverse reaction: Any undesirable effect of a drug.
- Side effect: Frequently used interchangeably with *adverse reaction;* an unwanted but predictable response to a drug.
- Toxic effect: Usually occurs when an excess amount of a drug has accumulated in the patient; this may happen as a result of an acute high dose, chronic buildup over time, or increased sensitivity to the standard dose.
- Drug allergy (hypersensitivity): A condition in which the body responds to a drug as if it were an antigen and mounts

an immune response against it; this may be an immediate response or a delayed reaction.

ROUTES OF ADMINISTRATION

For a drug to work, its active ingredients must get into or absorbed by the body by some means. The means by which a drug is introduced into the body (e.g., injection, topical application, orally) is called the *route of administration.*

THE DISTRIBUTION OF MEDICATIONS

The distribution of a drug is the process by which the drug is transported to the target site. Once a drug has been absorbed from the stomach and/or intestines (gastrointestinal [GI] tract) into the bloodstream, it is circulated to some degree to all areas of the body that receive blood flow.

Organs with a high blood flow (e.g., the brain, heart, and liver) are the first to accumulate drugs; connective tissue and less vascular organs are the last. The size of the organ, binding of the drug to various components of blood and tissue, and the permeability of tissue membranes also affect absorption. The more fat-soluble a drug is, the greater is its ability to pass across the cell membrane. Levels of a drug in bone, fat, muscle, and skin may take some time to rise, and the person's level of activity and the local tissue temperature may also affect drug distribution to the skin and muscle.

The blood-brain barrier restricts the passage of drugs from the blood into the central nervous system (CNS) and cerebrospinal fluid. The capillaries of the CNS differ from those in most other parts of the body. They lack channels between endothelial cells, through which substances in the blood normally gain access to the extracellular fluid. Lipid-soluble drugs pass fairly readily into the CNS, whereas drugs that are not lipid soluble have few or no CNS effects.

Protein binding (attachment of a drug to blood proteins) is an important factor that influences drug distribution. Many drugs are bound to blood proteins (e.g., serum albumin, the main blood protein) and are not available as active drugs.

The placenta permits passage of lipid-soluble and nonionized compounds from the mother to the fetus, but it prevents the passage of substances that are not lipid soluble.

THE METABOLISM OF MEDICATIONS

Drugs in the blood and tissues must be inactivated and excreted from the body. This process occurs by means of alteration of the chemical structure of the drug to promote its excretion. The transformation of the drug molecule into a chemically related substance that is more easily excreted from the body is called metabolism, biotransformation, or detoxification. For example, the alcohol molecule is metabolized in the liver by the enzyme alcohol dehydrogenase and becomes acetaldehyde, which causes dilation of the blood vessels and, after accumulation, is responsible for a hangover. Acetaldehyde is subsequently metabolized by the enzyme aldehyde dehydrogenase and becomes acetate, a substance very similar to acetic acid or vinegar.

Most drug metabolism occurs in the liver, where hepatic enzymes cause various biochemical reactions. However, drugs can also be metabolized in the kidneys, intestinal mucosa, lungs, plasma, and placenta.

THE EXCRETION OF MEDICATIONS

Excretion is the process by which a drug is eliminated from the body A drug's *half-life* is the rate of excretion. The half-life is the amount of time required to eliminate half of the drug from the body.

UNDERSTANDING THE ACTIONS OF MEDICATIONS

A massage therapist needs to understand why a patient is taking a medication and the action of that medication to determine the drug's potential interaction with the physiologic effects of massage, as well as what adjustments to the massage may be necessary. To do this, the therapist must obtain the answers to the following questions:

- What is the name of the drug (both the generic name and the brand name)?
- Why is the patient taking it?
- What does the drug do?
- When and how is the drug taken?
- What are the possible side effects (reactions of the body to the drug)?

- Does the drug react with any other medications, foods, or drinks?
- Are there any activities that should be avoided while taking this drug?
- Are there any signs that indicate the drug is working?

Most of the answers to these questions can be found in a drug consult. The patient may be able to supply information, and supervising medical personnel also can explain drug actions.

MEDICATION USE AND CLINICAL REASONING

Massage therapists must use a clinical reasoning approach to determine the best massage treatment when a patient is taking medication. The best way to teach this is by example. Using the antidepressant sertraline (Zoloft) as an example, Box 15-3 shows how information about a medication might appear in a web-based source. The box also presents an example of how the massage therapist would analyze the information to determine whether massage would be effective for a patient taking this drug.

evolve 15-3

Aspirin, a nonsteroidal antiinflammatory drug (NSAID), is analyzed on the Evolve website.

JUST BETWEEN YOU AND ME

It is important that the massage therapist understand the reason a medication was prescribed; that is, the condition the medication is treating. Because some medications can be used for different purposes, the massage therapist would have to ask the patient clarifying questions or get more information from the doctor.

JUST BETWEEN YOU AND ME

The analytic example for aspirin is found on the Evolve website. As you read through it, it may seem that the information on aspirin would scare a person to death before the side effects ever kicked in. Obviously, I'm being sarcastic, but it goes to show how complex things can get.

The examples in Box 15-3 and on the Evolve website provide models for investigating the interaction between massage and medication. This process needs to be completed for each medication a patient is taking. Because many people take multiple medications, the interactions are a complicating factor. No standardized resource is available describing the interaction of massage and medications. Massage therapists can manage these issues only by acquiring an understanding of the physiologic effects of massage and making informed decisions.

With medical patients, complex decisions must be made about the appropriate massage applications, and these should be conservative decisions made to reduce risk. Conservative decisions are not based on fear. Applications can be altered so that the massage therapist can work safely with most people whose conditions are treated with medication; however, the massage therapist must be well informed, or the patient could be harmed. Once you have researched the potential interaction between massage and a medication, ask the supervising medical professional for approval of the massage treatment plan.

PHYSICAL MEDICINE

Physical medicine and rehabilitation are the healthcare specialties that focus on the restoration of health and functional ability after an acute illness or injury such as stroke, spinal cord injury, heart surgery, amputation, joint replacement, sports injuries, and spinal disorders.

Patients with acute and chronic pain and musculoskeletal problems such as back and neck pain, tendinitis, pinched nerves, and fibromyalgia typically are treated with physical medicine. People who have experienced catastrophic events that resulted in paraplegia, quadriplegia, or traumatic brain injury; and individuals who have had strokes, orthopedic injuries, or neurologic disorders such as multiple sclerosis, polio, or amyotrophic lateral sclerosis (ALS) depend on physical medicine for rehabilitation and for adaptation training, such as the use of wheelchairs and other supportive devices.

BOX 15-3 Assessing the Interaction of Drug Therapy and Massage

Sertraline (Zoloft) is used to treat depression, obsessive compulsive disorder (i.e., bothersome thoughts that will not go away and the need to perform certain actions over and over), panic attacks (sudden, unexpected attacks of extreme fear and worry about these attacks), posttraumatic stress disorder (disturbing psychological symptoms that develop after a frightening experience), and social anxiety disorder (extreme fear of interacting with others or performing in front of others that interferes with normal life). It is also used to relieve the symptoms of premenstrual dysphoric disorder, including mood swings, irritability, bloating, and breast tenderness. Sertraline sometimes is used to treat headaches and sexual problems. It belongs to a class of medications called *selective serotonin reuptake inhibitors (SSRIs)*. It works by increasing the amount of serotonin, a natural substance in the brain that helps maintain mental balance.

(NOTE: Interspersed with the following information are questions in boldface. The answers to these questions can help the massage therapist determine the likely effects of massage in a person taking sertraline.)

The instructions for sertraline are as follows:

Sertraline comes as a tablet and a concentrate (liquid) to take by mouth. It is usually taken once daily in the morning or evening. To treat premenstrual dysphoric disorder, sertraline is taken once a day, either every day of the month or on certain days of the month, and it should be taken around the same time every day. Do not take more or less of it or take it more often than prescribed by your doctor.

The doctor may prescribe a low dose of sertraline and gradually increase the dosage until the desired effect occurs.

It may take a few weeks or longer to feel the full benefit of sertraline. Continue to take sertraline even when feeling well. Do not stop taking sertraline without talking to the doctor.

- **What special precautions should be followed when taking this medication?** (This question addresses the issue of how sertraline interacts with other medications the patient is taking.)

  Before taking sertraline, the patient should:
  - Tell the doctor and pharmacist if allergic to sertraline or any other medications. Before taking sertraline liquid concentrate, tell the doctor if allergic to latex.
  - Do not take sertraline if taking monoamine oxidase (MAO) inhibitors, including phenelzine (Nardil) and tranylcypromine (Parnate), or have stopped taking them within the past two 2 weeks, or if taking pimozide (Orap).
  - Do not take disulfiram (Antabuse) while taking sertraline concentrate.
  - Tell the doctor and pharmacist what other prescription and nonprescription medications, vitamins, nutritional supplements, and herbal products are being used. Be sure to mention any of the following: anticoagulants ("blood thinners") such as warfarin (Coumadin); antidepressants (mood elevators) such as amitriptyline (Elavil), amoxapine (Asendin), clomipramine (Anafranil), desipramine (Norpramin), doxepin (Adapin, Sinequan), imipramine (Tofranil), nortriptyline (Aventyl, Pamelor), protriptyline (Vivactil), and trimipramine (Surmontil); aspirin and other nonsteroidal antiinflammatory drugs (NSAIDs) such as ibuprofen (Advil, Motrin) and naproxen (Aleve, Naprosyn); cimetidine (Tagamet); diazepam (Valium); digoxin (Lanoxin); lithium (Eskalith, Lithobid); medications for anxiety, mental illness, Parkinson's disease, and seizures; medications for irregular heartbeat such as flecainide (Tambocor) and propafenone (Rythmol); oral medications for diabetes such as tolbutamide (Orinase); sedatives; sleeping pills; sumatriptan (Imitrex); and tranquilizers. The doctor may need to change the dosages of medications or monitor the patient carefully for side effects.
  - Tell the doctor if there is a history of depression, bipolar disorder (mood that changes from depressed to abnormally excited), or mania (frenzied, abnormally excited mood), or thoughts about or attempts at suicide either in the patient or family. Also tell the doctor about any heart attacks, seizures, liver, or heart disease.
  - Tell the doctor if pregnant, plan to become pregnant, or are breast-feeding.
- **What changes in the massage are necessary because of this medication?**
  - Sertraline may make a person drowsy. The patient should not drive a car or operate machinery until he or she knows how this medication affects them. *[Massage can also make a person drowsy. Therefore the massage may need to be altered so that it is more stimulating toward the end of the session, or the massage therapist may need to allow extra time for the patient to become more alert.]*
  - Avoid alcoholic beverages when taking sertraline.
  - Mental health may change in unexpected ways, especially at the beginning of treatment and anytime the dosage is increased or decreased. Contact the doctor immediately if any of the following symptoms occur: new or worsening depression; suicidal thoughts; extreme worry; agitation; panic attacks; difficulty falling or staying asleep; irritability; aggressive behavior; acting without thinking; severe restlessness; and frenzied, abnormal excitement. *[It is important that the massage therapist watch for these symptoms and immediatley refer the patient to a physician if they are noted.]*
- **What side effects can this medication cause?**

  Sertraline may cause the following side effects:
  - Upset stomach
  - Diarrhea
  - Constipation
  - Vomiting

BOX 15-3 Assessing the Interaction of Drug Therapy and Massage—cont'd

- Dry mouth
- Gas or bloating
- Loss of appetite
- Weight changes
- Drowsiness
- Dizziness
- Excessive tiredness
- Headache
- Pain, burning, or tingling in the hands or feet
- Excitement
- Nervousness
- Shaking hands that you cannot control
- Difficulty falling asleep or staying asleep
- Sore throat
- Changes in sex drive or ability
- Excessive sweating

The massage therapist must evaluate the side effects and determine whether massage might increase or decrease any of them. Massage may diminish the symptoms of headache but could increase the symptoms of fatigue. Massage also may help normalize sleep.

Some side effects can be serious. The following symptoms are uncommon; if any of them occur, call the doctor immediately.

- Blurred vision
- Seizure
- Abnormal bleeding or bruising
- Hallucinations (seeing things or hearing voices that do not exist)

Medications may also thin the blood; in such cases, the pressure used during massage may need to be altered. Eliminate focused point compression and maintain a broad-based contact to reduce the potential for bruising.

- **What storage conditions are needed for this medicine?**
  - Keep this medication in the container it came in, tightly closed, and out of reach of children. Store it at room temperature and away from excess heat and moisture (not in the bathroom). Throw away any medication that is outdated or no longer needed.

  In case of emergency/overdose:
- In case of overdose, call the local poison control center at 1-800-222-1222. If the victim has collapsed or is not breathing, call local emergency services at 911.
- Symptoms of overdose may include:
  - Changes in sex drive or ability
  - Diarrhea
  - Difficulty falling asleep or staying asleep
  - Dizziness
  - Drowsiness
  - Excessive tiredness
  - Excitement
  - Fainting
  - Hair loss
  - Hearing voices or seeing things that do not exist (hallucinating)
  - Rapid pounding or irregular heartbeat
  - Seizures
  - Shaking hands that you cannot control
  - Unconsciousness
  - Upset stomach
  - Vomiting

If the massage therapist recognizes any of these side effects, the patient must be referred immediately to a physician.

- **How will massage affect the action of this medication? What changes in the massage are necessary because of this medication?**

The mode of action of sertraline focuses on the neurotransmitter serotonin, and some studies indicate that massage also increases the levels of this neurotransmitter. Therefore, if a patient taking sertraline is given a massage, the effect may be the same as if the patient had taken too much medication; this is called a **synergistic effect.** The massage therapist must be alert to this possibility and monitor the patient. If the synergistic effect occurs, the massage must be altered, probably to a shorter massage that requires more active participation by the patient.

Similarly, some of the indicated uses for sertraline are related to mood, and massage also influences mood. Again, monitoring is required, and if the patient receives a massage regularly, the medication dosage (or the massage application) may need to be changed to target mechanisms other than neurochemical response. Also, the massage therapist should be alert to the patient's mood and behavior and should refer the person to a physican if inexplicable changes become evident.

These patients also may have a greater tendency to bruise, therefore the massage therapist should avoid point compression and maintain an even, broad-based compressive force.

Note: Information found in this box has been modified from the following sources
http://www.emedicinehealth.com/sertraline_zoloft/page5_em.htm
http://www.rxlist.com/cgi/generic/sertral_pi.htm
http://www.drugs.com/zoloft.html
www.pfizer.com/pfizer/download/uspi_zoloft.pdf
Retrieved 9-16-2007

Various healthcare professionals work in physical medicine. A physician who specializes in physical medicine and rehabilitation is called a *physiatrist* (fi-zee-a′-trist). Other professions involved in this discipline include neuropsychologists, physical therapists, occupational therapists, speech-language pathologists, and rehabilitation nurses.

CONDITIONS AND TREATMENTS IN PHYSICAL MEDICINE

Many different conditions are treated with physical medicine. Physical medicine involves the use of various modalities and exercise, and massage is one of the methods included in the physical medicine treatment plan. Treatment modalities include assistive therapies to improve independence and deep heat therapies.

Assistive therapies to improve independence include:

- Injection of botulinum toxin
- Corticosteroid injections into joints and soft tissues
- Epidural steroid injections

Deep heat therapies include:

- Superficial heat and cold applications
- Massage, traction, and manipulation Therapeutic exercise
- Transcutaneous electrical nerve stimulation (TENS)

evolve 15-4

See the Evolve website for a complete list of conditions treated by physical medicine.

CONDITIONS TREATED BY PHYSICAL MEDICINE

The following are some of the conditions treated by physical medicine techniques:

- Arthritis and connective tissue disorders
- Cervical spine disorders
- Conditions requiring orthotics
- Conditions requiring prosthetics
- Conditions requiring rehabilitation protocols
- Limb musculoskeletal conditions
- Lumbar spine disorders
- Medical diseases and conditions
- Movement disorders
- Muscle pain syndromes
- Muscular dystrophy
- Myopathy
- Nerve disorders
- Peripheral neuropathy
- Plexopathy
- Spinal cord injury
- Traumatic brain injury

Because massage is considered a treatment modality in physical medicine, it makes sense that the healthcare environment is beginning to include massage in more treatment protocols. Physical medicine is a logical focus for the massage therapist's work.

THERAPEUTIC EXERCISE

Therapeutic exercise is a type of treatment that massage easily complements. Massage before and after exercise may improve the quality of the patient's performance and diminish symptoms related to exercise, such as postexercise soreness.

Therapeutic exercises aimed at achieving and maintaining physical fitness fall into three major categories, each having a specific purpose (Table 15-1):

- Endurance training that requires an isotonic (dynamic) exercise technique
- Muscle strength training that requires an isometric (static) exercise technique
- Techniques to maintain flexibility

The muscle shortens during isotonic exercise, also called *active range-of-motion (AROM) exercise.* Isotonic muscle contraction causes the heart rate to rise and increases cardiac output. Eccentric isotonic training does not produce an increase in muscle strength, but concentric isotonic training does. However, isometric exercise is the most effective exercise for increasing the muscle's contractile force. Isotonic exercise is suitable for endurance training but not for training to improve muscle strength. In endurance training, large

TABLE 15-1 Some Therapeutic Exercise Routines Practiced in Hospital

Department	Disease/Condition	Therapeutic Exercise
Cardiac	• Ischemic heart disease (CID) • Post MI • Stable angina • Stable chronic heart failure	• Active range of motion; isotonic (dynamic) muscle training (e.g., after a 5-minute warmup, exercise until the heart rate reaches that attained at 50% of VO_2 max) to train endurance • Resistive isometric (static) training, which must be carried out with great caution and adjusted to the level of the physical fitness of each individual patient
Endocrine	• Obesity • Diabetes	• Isometric exercise to increase muscle strength • Graded physical training
Pulmonary	• Chronic bronchitis • Asthma • Emphysema	• Breathing techniques • Relaxation techniques • Stretching exercises to mobilize respiratory muscles Note: The level of physical effort should be limited because exercise may provoke bronchospasm.
Surgery	• Surgical conditions	• Preoperative and postoperative exercises
Orthopedics	• Fractures • Amputations	• Mobilizing and stretching of joints • Isometric training of muscle strength and isotonic exercise to train endurance
	• Spinal deformities	• Janda exercises upper and lower crossed patterns • Treadmill exercise • Elaborate rehabilitation exercises assisted by the physical therapist • Core muscle training
Burns	• N/A	• Treatment of muscle contractures • Myofascial release • Flexibility training (stretching) to mobilize joints
Gynecology and obstetrics	• Pregnancy and postdelivery • Postmastectomy • Osteoporosis • Urinary incontinence	• Gentle fitness training • Prenatal and postnatal exercises • Relaxation techniques • Training to reduce lymphatic edema • Isometric exercises for the pelvic floor
Neurology	• Cerebrovascular accident (CVA)	• Training of muscle strength • Training of balance and coordination • Later training and maintenance of general physical fitness
	• Multiple sclerosis • Parkinson disease	PNF and physical fitness training • Increasing and maintaining flexibility Training of physical fitness
	• Myopathies	Isometric and isotonic training
• Psychiatry	• Anxiety • Depression	Relaxation techniques: • Autogenic training • Aerobic fitness training

Reprint with permission from emedicine.com

muscle groups are engaged in a continuous aerobic activity.

Therapeutic Exercise in Healthy Individuals

For healthy people, exercises such as walking, running, jogging, dancing, stair climbing, cycling, swimming, rowing, skating, and cross-country skiing should be performed at 60% to 90% of the maximum heart rate.

The American College of Sports Medicine (ACSM) recommends that healthy men and women participate in endurance training for 20 to 60 minutes 3 to 5 days a week. Endurance training should be structured to include 5 minutes of warm-up activity, 30 minutes of training, and 5 minutes for cool-down.

Therapeutic Exercise in Patients

Patients at risk, especially those with cardiac or respiratory disease, need a less intense training regimen. For these individuals, the training heart rate should not exceed that attained at 50% to 60% of the maximum oxygen uptake.

For elderly patients and patients at risk, the intensity, frequency, and duration of therapeutic exercise should be established for each patient individually.

Isometric (static) muscle training is also called *resistive strength training* (RST) or *resistive exercise* because resistance is applied to the contracting muscle, preventing it from shortening. Daily application of this technique for only 6 seconds using two thirds of the maximum contractile force results in the optimum increase in muscle strength. The effect is enhanced by progressively increasing the resistance, frequency of training, and duration of resistance.

Isometric training must be done with great caution because it causes a rise in the heart rate as a result of decreased vagal tone and increased discharge of cardiac sympathetic nerves. Within a few seconds of the start of isometric exercise, both the systolic and diastolic blood pressures rise.

Caution for massage application: Most muscle energy methods involve contraction of a muscle against a resistance force, and in a fragile patient, these methods can increase the heart rate and raise the blood pressure. Muscle energy methods should not be used unless specifically prescribed by the supervising medical professional.

Exercise Regimens

For healthy men and women, the ASCM currently recommends at least one set of 8 to 12 repetitions of 8 to 10 RST exercises that condition the major muscle groups. These should be done at least twice a week.

For patients receiving healthcare, the intensity, frequency, and duration of isometric exercise must be established for each person individually according to the results of the previous medical evaluation. Because this form of training must be done with great caution, the best course may be not to extend the duration of an isometric contraction beyond 6 seconds, especially in patients with cardiovascular disease. The pause between two isometric contractions should last 20 seconds or longer.

Alternative Muscle Training Technique

Proprioceptive neuromuscular facilitation (PNF) is an excellent technique for muscle strength training. It is based on the application of resistance to muscle contraction to facilitate enhancement of the muscle's contractile force. PNF is suitable for patients with upper motor neuron lesions accompanied by spasticity; it also may be used to initiate muscle contraction in patients with partial peripheral nerve damage and extreme muscle weakness. PNF is different from the muscle energy methods used in massage. PNF is a specific sequence of movements performed to stimulate muscle and neurologic functions; muscle energy methods, on the other hand, are used to facilitate the stretching of shortened soft tissue.

TECHNIQUES FOR MAINTAINING FLEXIBILITY

Active assistive range-of-motion (AAROM) exercise is used when the patient has very weak muscles or when joint pain limits movement. With AAROM exercises, it is important to avoid forcing the joint, the soft tissue, or both beyond the point of pain.

For patients who cannot exercise actively, **passive range-of-motion (PROM) exercise** is used. These exercises stretch immobile muscles and joint capsules to prevent joint stiffness and muscle contracture. Joint flexibility is achieved through slow, steady stretching of large muscle groups and joint capsules, either manually or with the help of mechanical devices. As a preliminary exercise before isotonic or isometric training, PROM exercises should be performed during the first warm-up. They also should be done during the last cool-down phases.

These methods are elements of therapeutic massage, and they also offer opportunities for the massage therapist to assist the physical therapist. However, the physical therapist or physiatrist must establish the safe limits of movement based on the patient's condition. The massage therapist never forces a joint movement.

Recumbent and Convalescing Patients

Maintenance in recumbent and convalescing patients is achieved through AAROM or PROM exercises. These exercises are done to preserve full joint mobility and prevent joint stiffness and muscle contractures.

Mechanical Aids for Improving and Maintaining Physical Fitness

Examples of mechanical aids used for physical fitness training include electrically braked cycle ergometers, treadmills, rowing apparatuses, bed bicycles, arm cycles, pulleys, free weights, weight-training machines, indoor stair steppers, medical exercise balls, and a pool.

MASSAGE AND PHYSICAL MEDICINE

Areas of physical medicine, especially therapeutic exercise protocols, in which massage would be beneficial are easy to identify. The massage therapist must be able to understand the outcomes set by the physiatrist and the medical supervisor and then develop massage treatment plans that support the patient in achieving those goals.

DIET, NUTRITION, SUPPLEMENTATION, MENTAL HEALTH, AND LIFESTYLE

A patient's diet and nutritional status, use of supplements, mental health, and lifestyle factors must be taken into account along with treatments such as surgery, medications, and physical therapy. A dietitian or nutritionist may develop an intervention plan based on dietary changes and may supervise the use of various supplements, including herbs. Some general practice physicians value these methods and incorporate them into their practice. Chiropractors often are highly skilled in the use of nutrition to treat conditions that fall within the chiropractic realm of care.

Physical fitness programs, support groups, and stress management programs tend to support healthy lifestyle changes. Psychologists work with people to help them learn to cope effectively with life's challenges and to make beneficial lifestyle choices. The concept of the medical spa (see Unit One) typically incorporates all of these components.

Massage complements and supports many of the therapies that treat illness, maintain wellness, and encourage prevention. Many chronic and degenerative illnesses have a gradual onset, and if intervention is launched early in the disease course, the progress of the condition may be reversed or at the very least slowed. It seems prudent to incorporate a healthy lifestyle into daily activities, not only for those sick enough to be treated in the healthcare system, but for all of us.

evolve 15-5

The following terms and expressions specific to Chapter 15 have already been used to search PubMed for the latest research literature available. The *Click Here for Massage* feature associated with this chapter on your textbook's Evolve website allows you to hyperlink to a continually updated PubMed search of research literature that corresponds to this subject.

Hyperlink Search Terms

Massage diet nutrition
Massage lifestyle
Massage medication
Massage mental health
Massage physical medicine

SUMMARY

The value of combining traditional and complementary healthcare approaches with alternative medicine techniques is becoming ever more apparent. Massage therapists need to be proficient at determining safe and best practices. We are not doctors, but to provide appropriate massage that complements medical treatment, we must understand what they do.

REFERENCES

www.eMedicine.com
http://www.webmd.com
http://www.vitamins.com
http://www.medicinenet.com
http://mayoclinic.com

1. Develop a letter to an orthopedic surgeon explaining how massage benefits patients both before and after surgery.

2. List and explain at least 10 adaptations of massage applications for patients who have had surgery or are undergoing drug therapy.

   Example: Patient is not comfortable on massage table at massage office. Will need to work with patient in a reclining chair or at the home.

WORKBOOK

3. Choose one of the conditions treated with physical medicine and develop a hypothetical case study (use the Unit Four case studies as examples). Devise a treatment plan for massage that supports other medical treatments. Make sure the person in your case study is taking at least one medication that would influence the massage. Finally, using the treatment plan, develop four session notes (use the subjective, objective, assessment, and plan [SOAP] format). Base these notes on individual massage sessions and include factors involving physical medicine and lifestyle.

___

___

___

___

___

___

___

___

___

___

___

___

___

___

___

___

CHAPTER 16 CONCEPT MAP

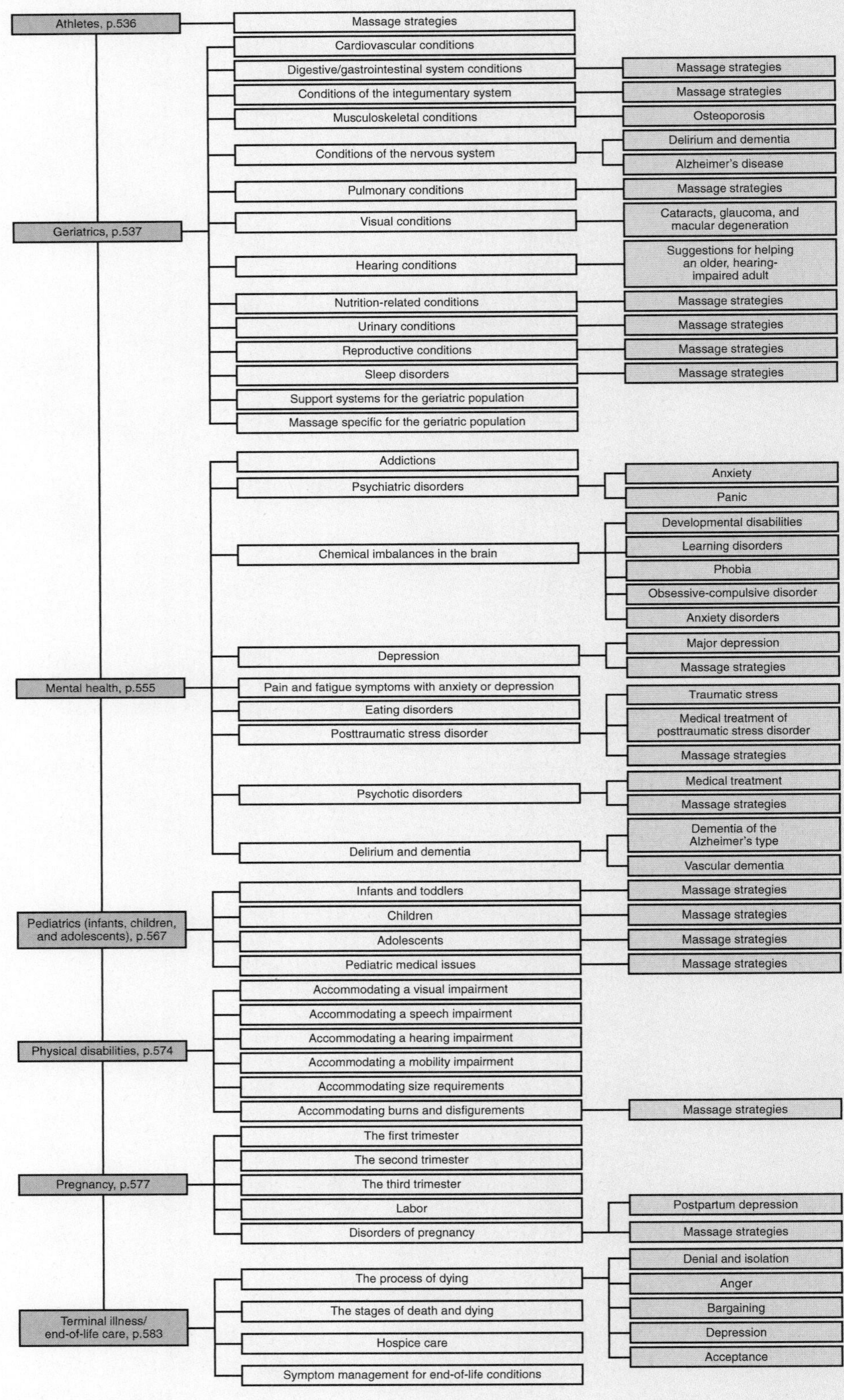

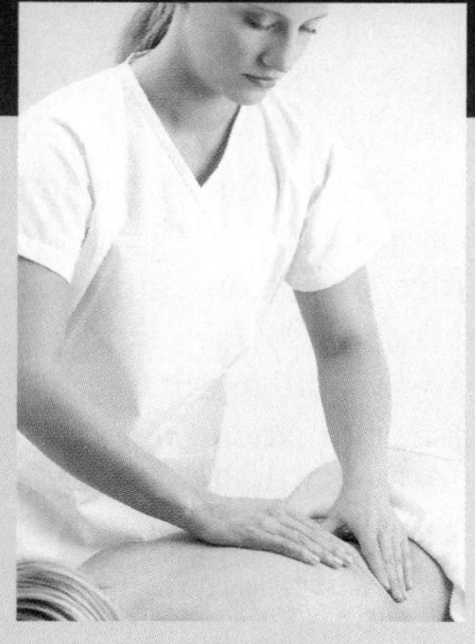

CHAPTER 16

POPULATION SIMILARITIES IN HEALTHCARE

Key Terms

Agoraphobia
Agnosia
Alzheimer's disease (AD)
Anxiety
Aphasia
Apraxia
Athlete
Autism
Bereavement
Cataracts
Cognition
Critical incident
Delirium
Dementia
Depression
Diagnostic and Statistical Manual of Mental Disorders (DSM-IV)
Glaucoma
Hospice care
Macular degeneration
Osteoporosis
Palliative care
Panic
Panic attack
Pediatric population
Phobia
Posttraumatic stress
Posttraumatic stress disorder (PTSD)
Pre-eclampsia
Presbyopia
Psychiatrist
Psychologist
Titration
Trauma
Traumatic stress
Urinary incontinence

For definitions of key terms, refer to the Evolve website.

OBJECTIVES

Upon completion of this chapter, the reader will have the information necessary to:

1. Identify common health concerns of specific populations.
2. Develop generic treatment plans based on a population and then suggest modifications to address individual situations.
3. Adjust the professional relationship based on population commonalities.

In previous chapters, we have considered healthcare in various ways and discussed how massage can support medical intervention. In this chapter, the content is organized by groups, or populations, of people. There are enough commonalities within these groups to allow the development of general strategies for massage application. As always, however, these strategies are only a place to start in the development of the massage treatment plan. The groups discussed include athletes, older people (geriatrics), people with mental health conditions, infants and children (pediatrics), people with physical disabilities, pregnant women, and people with a terminal illness (end-of-life care).

In Chapter 17, the information is categorized by general medical condition:

- Back pain
- Cardiovascular conditions
- Chronic pain and fatigue
- Headache
- Infection
- Musculoskeletal and orthopedic conditions
- Neurologic conditions
- Cancer
- Respiratory conditions
- Sleep disturbances
- Wounds and contusions

Chapters 16 and 17 work together to help you understand the complexities of medical care and how this care and massage can interact to produce benefits. For example, an athlete (this chapter) can have cancer (Chapter 17), a child can have headaches, and the elderly can have infections. Combinations also can occur within populations. For example, a person with a mental health issue can be an athlete, the elderly can have physical disabilities, and children can be terminally ill. These endlessly varying combinations of treatments, illnesses, injuries, and populations are what make working in healthcare so challenging, and they absolutely demand clinical reasoning skills. This chapter focuses on helping the massage therapist understand healthcare based on groups of people who share commonalities. People who fit into these population categories are not necessarily sick or injured, but they have a greater likelihood of illness or injury. Prevention is the ideal strategy, but sometimes effective intervention is necessary.

ATHLETES

(NOTE: The author's accumulated knowledge in the area of sports is the result of her extensive work with professional football teams and individual athletes. The textbook *Sports and Exercise Massage: Comprehensive Care in Athletics, Fitness, and Rehabilitation* covers this content in depth, therefore only a brief overview is presented here.)

An **athlete** is a person who participates in sports as either an amateur or a professional (Figure 16-1). Athletes require precise use of their bodies. The athlete trains the nervous system and muscles to perform in a specific way. Often the activity involves repetitive use of one group of muscles more than others, which may result in hypertrophy, changes in strength and movement patterns, connective tissue formation, and compensation patterns in the rest of the body. These factors contribute to the soft tissue difficulties that often develop in athletes. The physical activity of an athlete goes beyond fitness and is performance based. Fitness is necessary for everyone's wellness. The challenge for athletes is that fitness is not the goal; performance is the goal. Performance strain makes this population vulnerable to physical strain and mental strain, which increase the athlete's potential for injury and illness.

MASSAGE STRATEGIES

Massage can be very beneficial for athletes if the professional performing the massage understands the biomechanics required by the sport. If not, massage can impair optimum function in the athletic performance. The intense physical activity involved in sports can make an athlete more prone to injury. Athletes enter the medical environment when they are injured. This population is complex, and in some ways massage is more difficult to manage for these individuals than for other groups. Injuries in athletes typically are the musculoskeletal type, and illness often occurs secondary to immune suppression caused by excessive physical activity without adequate recovery. Everything discussed in this text is applicable to athletes, depending on the individual situation. The biggest mistake massage therapists make is to assume that athletes are robust and healthy; this is not always true, and in fact they are a very fragile group of people. They often are overmassaged, or inappropriate methods are used on them, leading to tissue damage. The interval of 48 hours before and after competition or heavy exercise is a particularly vulnerable period for athletes. At these times, the palliative care protocol is appropriate. The general protocol presented in Chapter 11 is a good method for athletes who want a massage for general maintenance or recovery. This approach is similar to the one

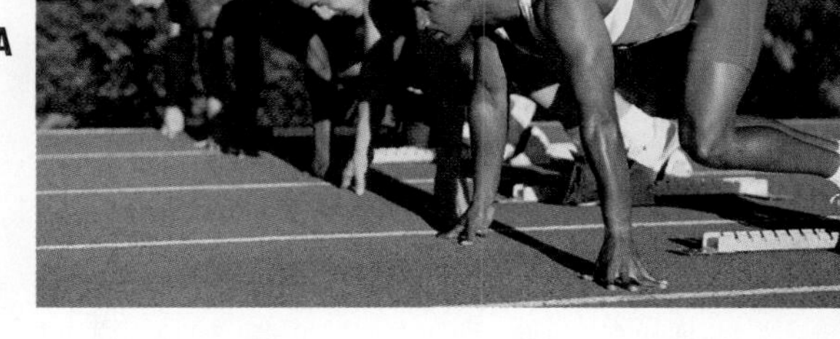

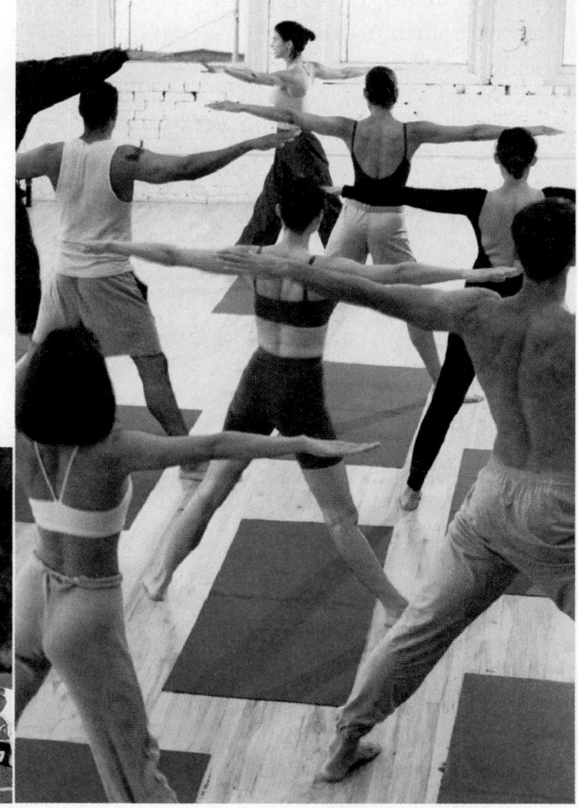

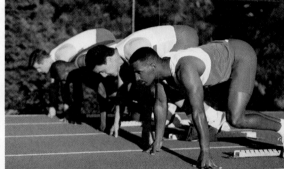

A B

FIGURE 16-1 ■ A sampling of the athletic population.

described in *Sports and Exercise Massage: Comprehensive Care in Athletics, Fitness, and Rehabilitation.*

GERIATRICS

In general, the geriatric population consists of individuals 65 years or older. Aging is not an illness but a natural process of being alive. As we age, our bodies do not function as efficiently as when we were 25 years old. Medical treatment can alleviate or reduce the symptoms of the natural aging process. In addition, as aging progresses, people have a greater tendency to develop age-related diseases, such as cardiovascular disease, some types of cancer, and dementia. The older body does not heal as quickly and is less able to fight off infection. Aging is unavoidable. However, with appropriate health habits and the benefits of advances in medical care, a person can age well and lead a long, high-quality life.

To develop appropriate massage treatment plans that can address age-related symptoms, the massage therapist must understand the natural changes that occur with aging. Lifestyle greatly influences how well people age, and lifestyle changes can slow or even reverse some age-related changes. Exercise, diet, sleep, not smoking, moderate use of alcohol, supportive relationships, and ongoing mental stimulation all support effective aging. In many parts of the world, people over 65 years of age constitute the fastest growing population group. Geriatrics is a medical specialty, and improving the quality of life for those over age 65 is a major research topic.

Getting older is a natural process that begins at conception and continues throughout the life cycle and eventually ends in death. Everyone ages differently. Someone can be considered old based on their chronologic age (i.e., 65 or 75) but may actually be much younger based on physiologic indicators, such as blood pressure, muscle mass, strength, and organ function. The specifics of why aging occurs remain a mystery. Genetics, nutrition, stress, exercise, healthcare, and lifestyle habits all influence the aging process. Although several theories have been proposed to explain the physical changes that occur during aging, none adequately explains why these changes take place. Some theories emphasize hereditary factors and others focus on the cells and their properties. The most accepted physiological factors of aging are the following:

- Loss of cellular mass
- Decreased cellular divide and reduplication
- Change in connective tissues including hardening, decreased lubrication, increased fibers adhesion all resulting in a decrease in flexibility
- Accumulation of waste material in body cells
- Cumulative effects of inflammation

It is important to remember that symptoms attributed to a disease or injury and typical age-related signs of aging are two separate things. In general, changes caused by normal aging result in slowing down in bodily functions. Physical changes that are part of the normal aging process eventually happen to everyone, usually do not cause serious disability, and can be accommodated. One example of this is age-related changes in vision that can be altered by using reading glasses. In contrast to normal aging, disease or injury leads to a temporary or permanent loss of function.

Understanding the typical aging process can be useful in targeting therapeutic massage to manage age-related issues as long as one remembers that aging is a highly individual experience. When providing massage, remember that most older adults are in relatively good health and older people are able function effectively even at an advanced age. The second half of life can bring many changes. People who cope well with age-related change know their own abilities and limits and want to make their own decisions and do as much for themselves as possible. Most people who live to an advanced age will experience various types of loss (e.g., loss of a career, a spouse, ability to drive, independence, robust health, hearing, and friends). Loss is loss regardless of the type and involves the grieving process discussed in the section on end of life care.

Aging also can result in many gains (e.g., experience, wisdom, grandchildren, time to explore interests, time to share with others). Massage can reduce some of the physical symptoms related to aging and enhance the quality of life and sooth the pain of loss.

JUST BETWEEN YOU AND ME

My grandmother lived to be 96 years old, and she lived in her own home. She gave up her driver's license at age 88. This was a difficult decision, because she then was unable to go back and forth to the store and the senior center. She had macular degeneration, which took much of her eyesight, and she developed diabetes. But all and all, she aged pretty well. The important point to share with you is this: She *hated* being treated as if she were helpless or a kid. She would ask for help if she needed it, and she insisted on paying in some fashion. I spent many a day working for my grandmother for $5 a day; I finally learned that my grandma intended to maintain her integrity. *Do not* treat the elderly like children. Interact with each person as an individual, and give these valued members of our society the respect they deserve.

Massage for the geriatric population has two goals (Figure 16-2):

- Managing the symptoms and supporting the medical treatment of age-related changes
- Supporting the medical treatment of elderly individuals who are ill or injured

Table 16-1 presents the various natural processes of aging. Massage can be beneficial as a health-promoting activity by supporting a healthy lifestyle.

CARDIOVASCULAR CONDITIONS

Changes in the cardiovascular system are age related. However, other factors contribute to these changes, including disease and lifestyle habits such as exercise, diet, and the ability to cope with

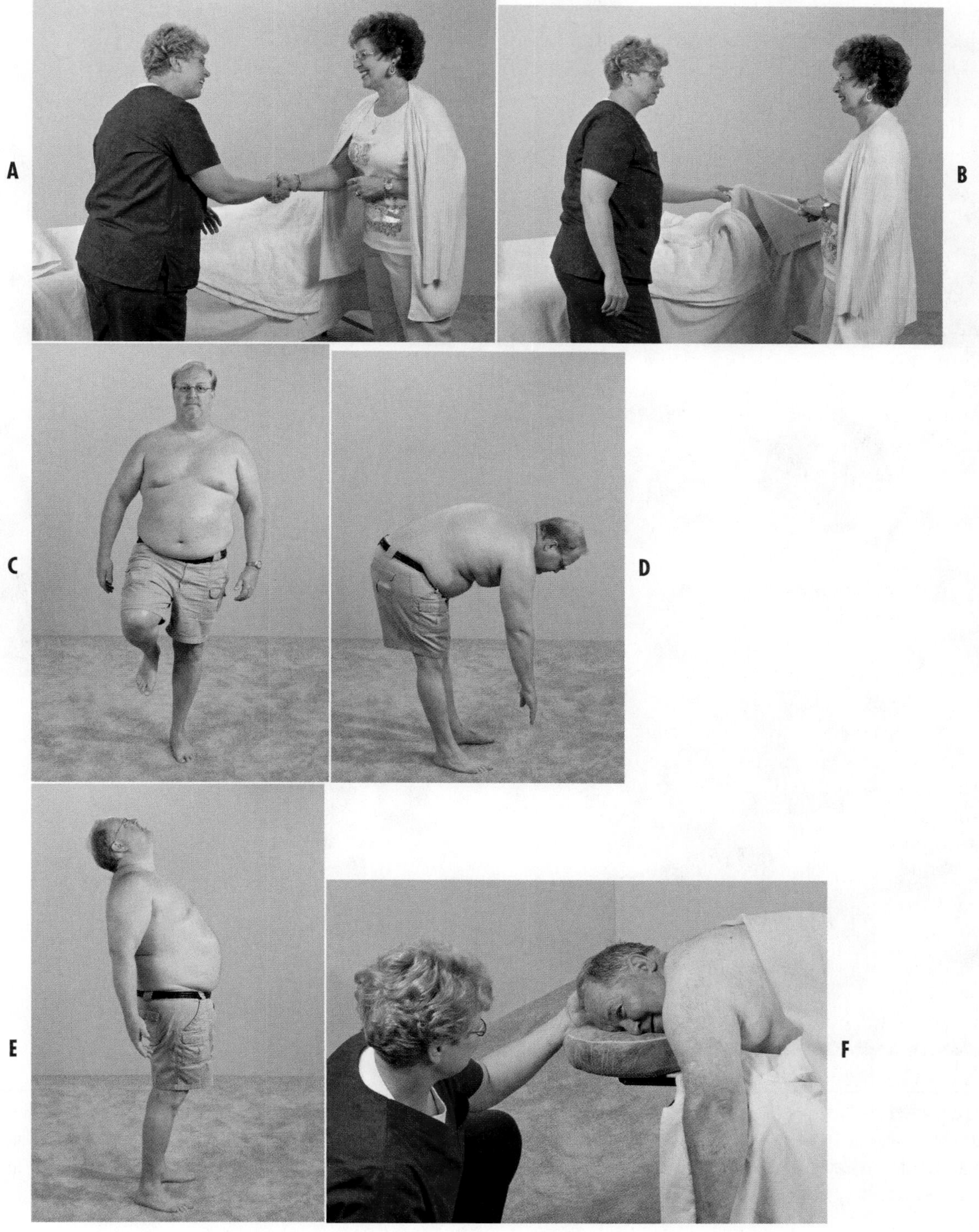

FIGURE 16-2 ■ Geriatric massage: examples of interactivity with the mature population during massage. The methods used are based on indicated outcomes. The palliative protocol (see Chapter 11) and the photo sequence in the Appendix provide a good foundation for massage. Assessment and interventions are incorporated, observing cautions for the geriatric population in these protocols. **A,** Greet. **B,** Explain. **C,** Assess balance. **D,** Assess movement changes. **E,** Assess changes in flexibility. **F,** Discuss and respect.

Continued

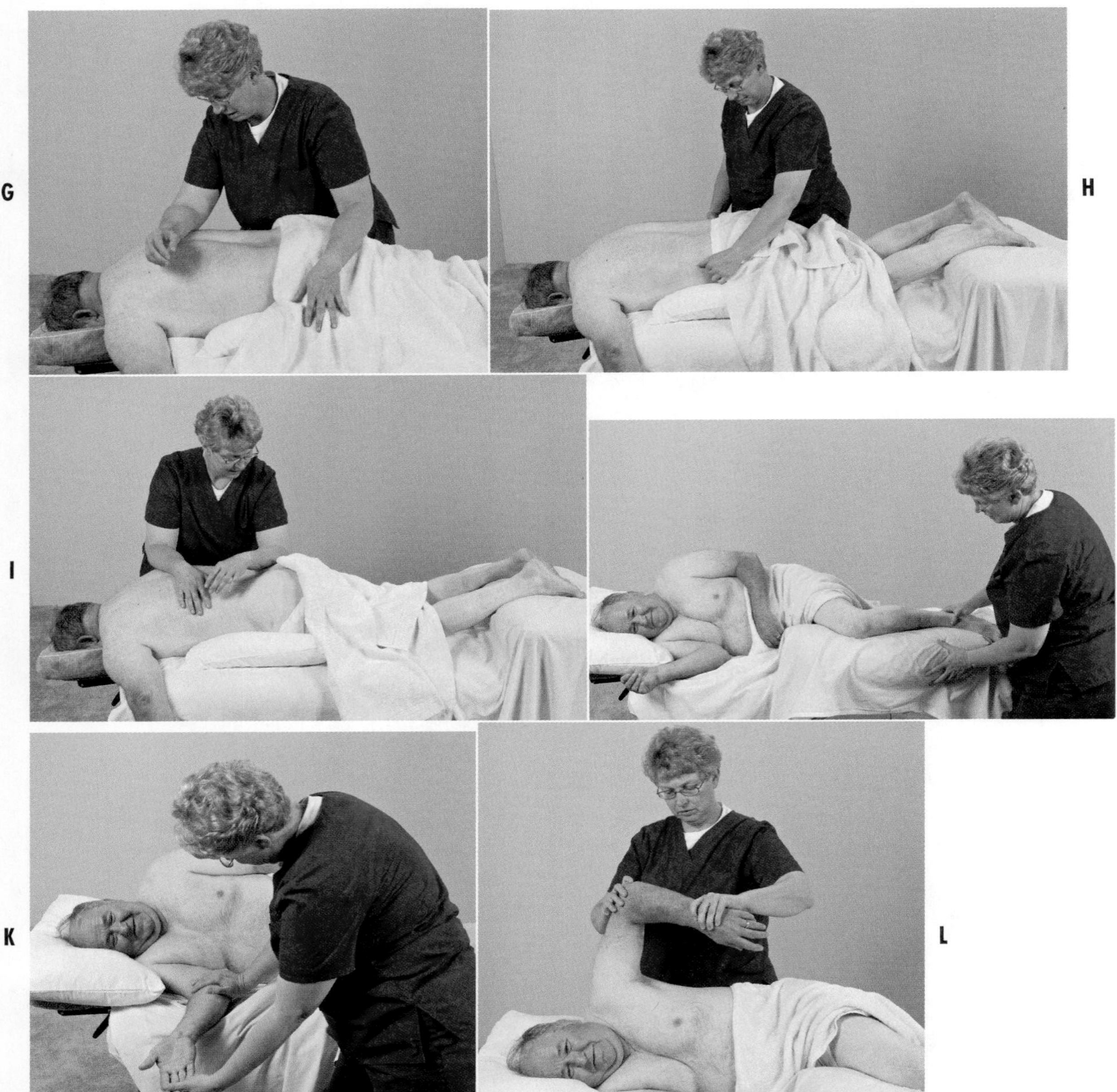

FIGURE 16-2, cont'd ■ **G,** Massage. **H,** Respectfully move undergarments on male and female clients. This population commonly feels more secure with the undergarments left on. **I,** Low back and neck aches are common, but be cautious of osteoporosis. **J,** The side-lying position is better than the prone position. Use a bolster for support. **K,** Listen to clients' stories and learn from them. **L,** Use caution with range of motion; never force movement.

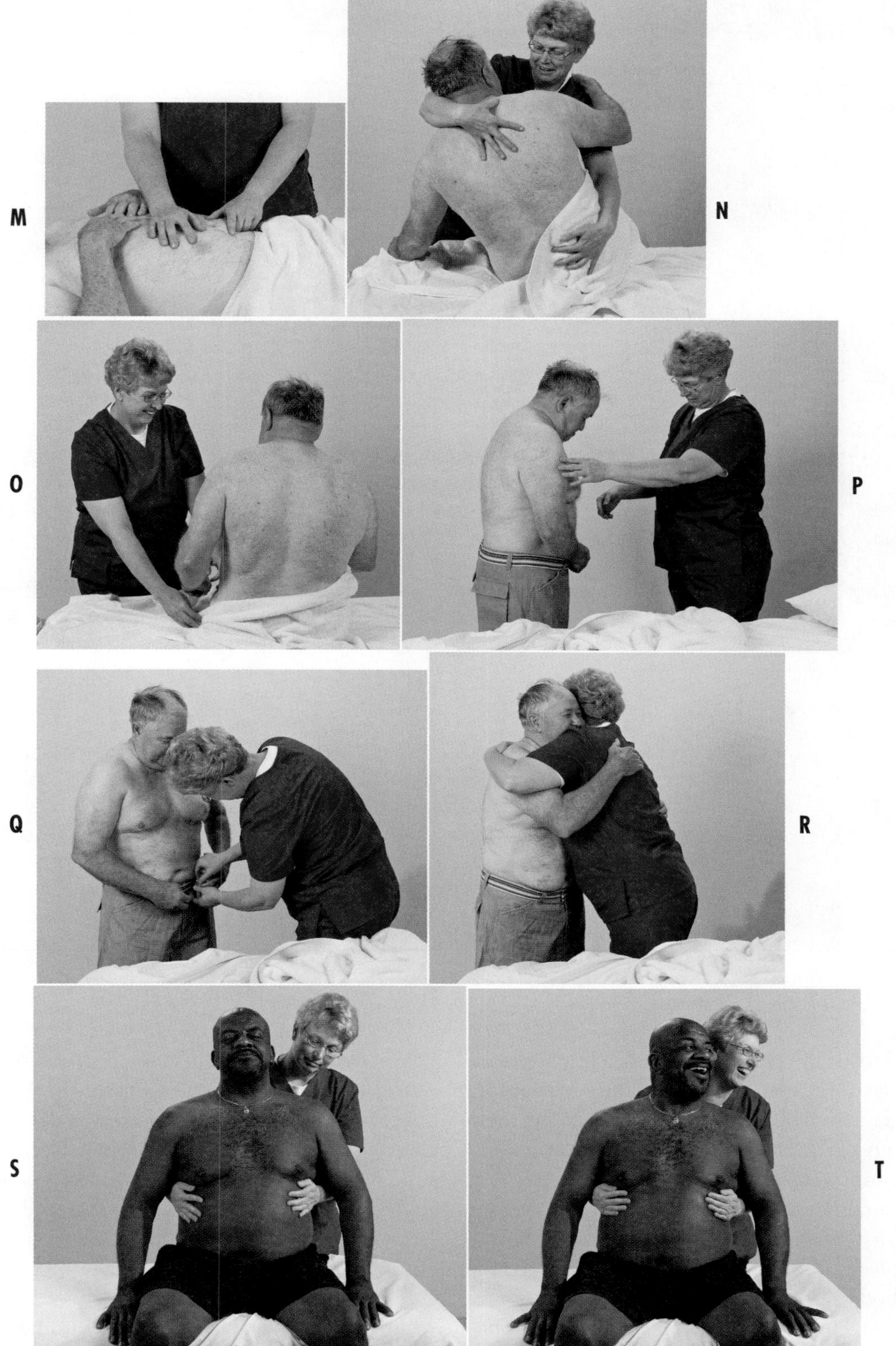

FIGURE 16-2, cont'd ■ **M,** Be aware of fragile tissue and surgical sites. **N,** Assist, if necessary, when the client rises from the table. **O,** Check for dizziness. **P,** Wait to help. **Q,** Help the client dress if necessary. **R,** Hugs initiated by clients are okay. **S,** Normal changes related to aging can be serious. **T,** But not *too* serious.

TABLE 16-1 Physical Changes that Occur with Aging

Body System	Age-Related Changes	Health-Promoting Activities
Cardiovascular	Arteriosclerosis and buildup of atherosclerotic plaque reduce blood flow to major organs; hypertension is common; cardiovascular disease is the no. 1 killer of women and men in their 60s.	Regular exercise; weight control; diet rich in fruits, vegetables, and whole grains; monitoring of cholesterol and blood glucose levels
Central nervous system (CNS)	Brain shrinks by 10% between ages 30 and 90; learning new material takes longer; attention span and language remain the same; depression, vascular disease, and drug reactions may be factors.	Aerobic exercise to increase blood flow to the CNS and maintain mental activities
Endocrine	After age 50 women experience a sharp decline in estrogen and men a more gradual decline in testosterone.	Possible hormone replacement therapy or use of natural supplements
Gastrointestinal	Gastric juices and enzymes decline by age 60; decreased peristalsis, increase in constipation; some nutrients not absorbed well.	High-fiber diet to prevent constipation; exercise and folic acid to reduce risk of colon cancer
Musculoskeletal	Muscle mass decreases; tendency to gain weight; gradual loss of bone density; deterioration of joints.	Strength training to increase muscle mass; stretching to maintain flexibility; exercise, vitamin D, and calcium supplements
Pulmonary	At about age 55 the lungs become less elastic and the chest wall gradually stiffens, making breathing more difficult.	Smoking cessation; regular aerobic exercise
Sensory organs	Potential for eye disease and vision changes increases; hearing is intact through mid-50s but declines by 25% by age 80.	Avoidance of exposure to loud noise and use of hearing aids; maintenance of good dental hygiene; avoidance of sun damage to skin; annual eye examinations; diet rich in dark green, leafy vegetables to prevent cataracts and macular degeneration
Sexuality	*Men:* Impotence is not a symptom of normal aging; men over age 50 may have some altered function. *Women:* Menopause causes vaginal narrowing and dryness, which may make intercourse painful.	*Men:* Maintenance of cardiovascular health with exercise, weight control, and no smoking *Women:* Use of vaginal lubricants or estrogen
Urinary	Kidneys become less efficient; bladder muscles weaken; one third of seniors experience incontinence; prostate enlargement is common.	Pelvic floor exercises, medication, or surgery for incontinence; annual prostate-specific antigen (PSA) monitoring for men

stress. Heart disease is ranked as the leading cause of death among men and women; therefore proper management of cardiovascular disease can help maintain the health of an aging population and reduce mortality rates.

Structural changes occur in the heart as a result of the aging process. Older people have a slower heart rate, and during physical exercise the older body is less able to maintain the maximum heart rate. Heart tissue cells enlarge, and fat deposition and connective tissue formation increase; as a result, the heart is stiffer, and the time and oxygen needed for the relaxation phase of the cardiac cycle increase. Consequently, cardiac output declines, increasing the older person's susceptibility to congestive heart failure.

Mild arteriosclerosis is considered part of the aging process. The arteries thicken and become less elastic as a result of the calcification and buildup of connective tissue. The blood vessels' ability to dilate and contract declines. To maintain an adequate blood supply throughout the body, the heart must work harder to overcome the resistance caused by the stiffened vessels. The diastolic pressure typically remains the same, but the systolic pressure may rise with age. Older adults have a higher incidence of orthostatic hypotension, which means that they can become lightheaded or dizzy when changing positions.

Older people who develop diabetes are at increased risk of developing vascular disease, including renal disorders, retinopathy, neuropathy, myocardial ischemia, angina, myocardial infarction, cerebrovascular accidents, and peripheral vascular disease. Wound healing declines, and a tendency to develop ulcers emerges.

Massage Strategies

Methods that support circulation are applied with caution and with a physician's supervision for individuals with congestive heart failure and diabetes. Extreme caution is necessary for those with congestive heart failure; do not provide massage without a physician's supervision. Abrupt positional changes must be avoided.

DIGESTIVE/GASTROINTESTINAL CONDITIONS

Digestive changes are commonly experienced by the geriatric population. The teeth and mouth areas are important areas to consider. People over age 55 tend to develop decay of the tooth near the gum line. Brushing the tongue helps remove the cause of this decay. Reduced saliva production and side effects of some medications commonly taken by older people can cause drying of the mouth. Many individuals wear dentures or have tooth loss. This can interfere with the ability to effectively chew food, which results in difficulty in digestion. The elderly need fewer calories to maintain body weight because physical energy needs usually are reduced with advanced years, and the basal metabolic rate declines.

The emotional state of the individual needs to be considered since the digestive system is sensitive to emotional states. A person who is anxious, lonely, depressed, or worried may experience gastrointestinal symptoms and unfortunately the elderly often experience these emotional states. How effectively the body handles ingested glucose and how well it maintains an appropriate blood glucose level after eating or during fasting is an important physiologic variable influenced by age.

Age-related changes in the gastrointestinal system also include a decrease in the production of hydrochloric acid, which affects the digestion of calcium and iron. Absorption of vitamin B_{12} declines, affecting the functioning of the nervous system and the formation of red blood cells and resulting in excessive fatigue. This condition is treated with vitamin B_{12} injections. Food passes through the small intestine more quickly, resulting in poorer absorption of vitamins and minerals, but peristalsis in the colon decreases, making the older person more susceptible to constipation and diverticular disease. Poor eating habits, reduced fluid intake, and some medications (e.g., antidepressants, narcotics, diuretics, antacids containing aluminum or calcium, and antiparkinsonism drugs) also contribute to constipation. Aging people have an increased incidence of several gastrointestinal diseases, such as gastroesophageal reflux disease (GERD), peptic ulcers, diverticulosis (related to lack of dietary fiber), cholelithiasis (gallbladder disease), and colorectal cancer.

The liver decreases in size and function. Although it can still perform vital functions, it takes longer to metabolize drugs and alcohol. As a result of these factors, the risk of adverse drug reactions is greater in older adults.

Massage Strategies

Massage can support parasympathetic dominance, which in turn supports digestion. If constipation occurs, abdominal massage may increase peristalsis, supporting elimination. Massage is generally calming and supportive, which can reduce the symptoms of emotionally based gastrointestinal upset.

CONDITIONS OF THE INTEGUMENTARY SYSTEM

Changes in the appearance and function of the integumentary system usually are due to a combination of ordinary age-related changes and environmental factors, especially the amount of sun exposure over time. Exposure to ultraviolet light from the sun frequently is the cause of wrinkles, age spots, blotches, and leathery, dry, loose skin, all of which are associated with aging.

The cells in the epidermis reproduce more slowly as people age. As a result, the skin is thinner and more susceptible to bruising. The skin also becomes prone to tearing and blistering, which increase the risk of infection. In addition, the wound healing process takes longer. The synthesis of vitamin D, a major function of the epidermis, significantly decreases in aged skin, and a decrease in the number of melanocytes increases photosensitivity in aging people. Seborrheic keratosis, one of the most common benign skin disorders found in the elderly, appears in the form of waxy, greasy papules that vary from a flesh color to dark brown. The papules typically are found in areas of sun exposure, such as the trunk, back, face, neck, extremities, and scalp. They are not dangerous but can be removed for cosmetic purposes.

The dermis loses mass during the aging process, resulting in the paper-thin or transparent skin seen in older adults. With the loss of mass the dermis also loses much of its vascular supply. Consequently, the older body has more difficulty regulating temperature. leading to an increased susceptibility to both hypothermia and hyperthermia. Any situation in which an older adult would be exposed to extreme cold or heat should be avoided. During massage, ask the person whether he or she is too cold or too hot, and take the necessary steps to make the individual more comfortable.

The number of collagen cells in the dermis also declines with age, causing the skin to sag and wrinkle. Atrophy of the subcutaneous layer increases the skin's susceptibility to trauma. Both sweat and sebaceous glands decrease with age; as a result, aging people have difficulty tolerating higher temperatures because they perspire less. The skin has less natural lubrication, and dry skin is one of the most common complaints of older people. Massage therapists must make sure to use adequate lubrication during the massage.

Pain receptors are distributed throughout the skin. Because of age-related changes in the receptors, older people have a higher threshold of pain; that is, the skin is not as sensitive as in youth, and awareness of surface pain declines. This has safety implications. Older people need to be alert to the fact they are not as skin sensitive to pain, heat, or cold as they once were, and the skin can be harmed before the person realizes that damage has been done. For example, the individual may not notice a cut or burn. When the padding of fat between the bones and the bottom of the foot becomes thinner, as does the skin on the toes, discomfort, bruises, or calluses commonly occur. The feet also become less sensitive to temperature changes with age.

Other changes occur in the skin appendages, the nails and the hair. Hair changes in color and growth. The nails of older people take longer to grow and are more brittle. Nails, particularly toenails, thicken as a result of trauma or nutritional causes. Splitting of the nails makes them susceptible to fungal infections.

Massage Strategies

The massage therapist must take care to use sufficient lubricant so that drag is reduced on fragile skin. This also helps moisturize dry skin. Keeping the older patient warm is important, but electric blankets or other heating devices must be used with caution to prevent injury. Pressure levels should be monitored to prevent bruising. The massage therapist should also monitor the skin and appendages for changes and notify the primary healthcare provider about changes that may seem to require medical investigation.

MUSCULOSKELETAL CONDITIONS

As the body ages, changes occur in the muscles, bones, and joints that affect the person's appearance, strength, and mobility. Joint pain is common as aging occurs. Most of the symptoms are the result of wear and tear on the joint structures and surrounding soft tissue. Lack of activity aggravates disability caused by musculoskeletal changes. Changes in the skeletal system can result in a loss of height, stooped posture, and limitation in mobility. Paradoxically, even through it may hurt to move the joints, inactivity causes further degeneration and more pain. Changes in the muscle system tend to affect agility, stability, strength, dexterity, breathing, urination, and defecation. Muscular disabilities usually are preventable with physical training and postural exercise. One of the primary ways of ensuring mobility is to practice appropriate exercises. The value of walking as a means of maintaining mobility and cardiovascular fitness cannot be overemphasized.

The amount of musculoskeletal change that occurs as a result of aging depends on diet, exercise, and heredity. Cartilage loss and degeneration cause osteoarthritis, which commonly occurs in the weight-bearing joints. Aching feet are common, and for the elderly the loss of elasticity in body tissue associated with aging alters the complex connective tissue structure that binds and supports the foot's multiple joints. When connecting ligaments lose their ability to stretch or are unable to support the arch structure, older people have pain and foot problems.

Aging brings a decrease in the strength and speed of muscle contractions in the extremities but only a slight decline in overall muscle endurance. Muscular changes in aging individuals are directly related to the person's activity level. Research shows that musculoskeletal disease is not an inevitable result of the aging process and can be somewhat reversed with appropriate exercise.

Osteoporosis

Osteoporosis, a serious condition of bone demineralization, affects 40% to 50% of women over age 50 (Figure 16-3).

Osteoporosis is the primary cause of hip fractures. The spinal vertebrae also can collapse, producing the stooped posture called "dowager's hump." Sometimes bones break because of the sheer weight of the body on them. People often say they fell and broke a bone, when in reality the bone fractured, causing the fall. Multiple factors contribute to the development of osteoporosis, but it is most common in postmenopausal women (Box 16-1).

Weight-bearing exercises, appropriate exposure to sunshine, and calcium and vitamin D supplements are recommended to prevent demineralization of the bones. Medications are available to treat individuals diagnosed with osteoporosis,

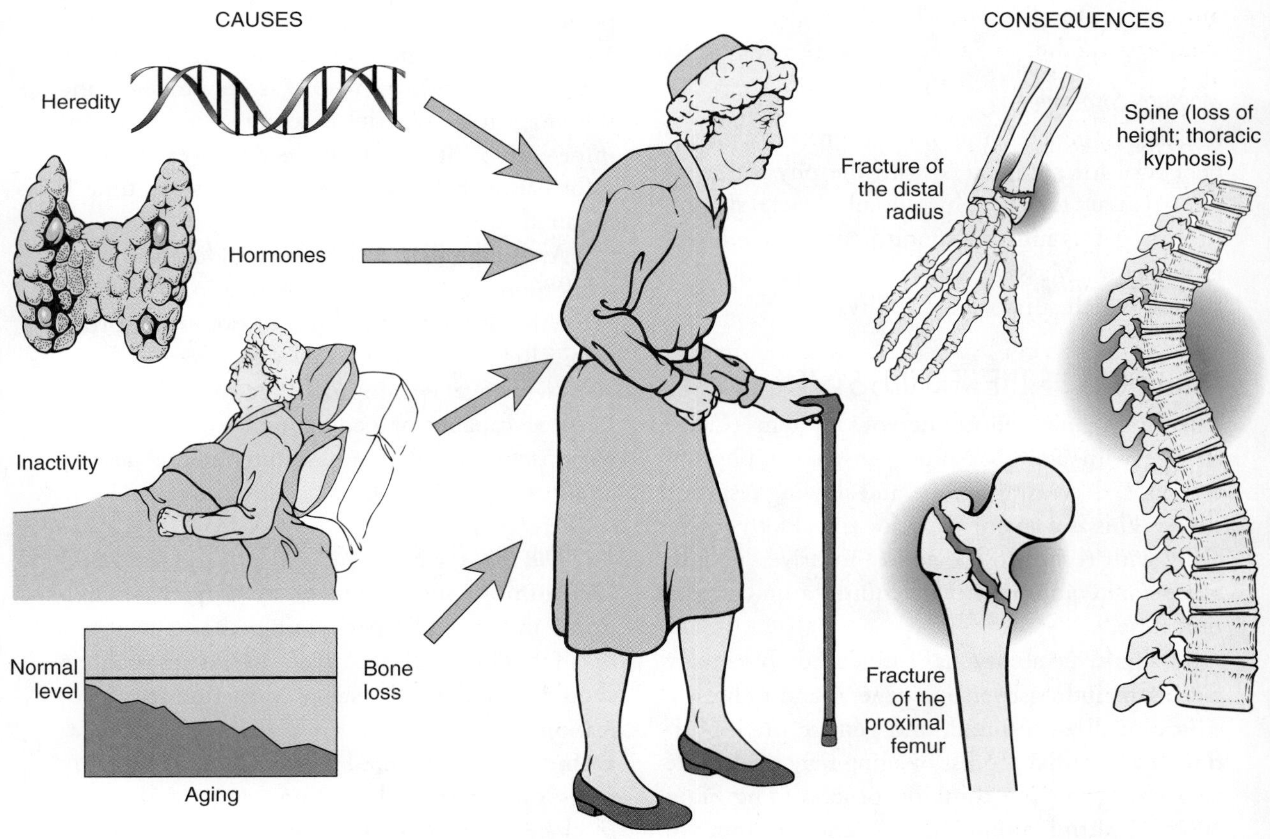

FIGURE 16-3 ■ Causes and consequences of osteoporosis. (From Damjanov I: *Pathology for the health-related professions*, ed 3, St Louis, 2006, WB Saunders.)

BOX 16-1 Risk Factors for the Development of Osteoporosis

- Female (women have a five times greater risk than men)
- Small-boned frame, thin
- Family history of osteoporosis
- Estrogen deficiency before age 45, either from early menopause or removal of the ovaries
- Estrogen deficiency resulting from an abnormal absence of the menstrual cycle (e.g., eating disorders, excessive aerobic exercise, fibrocystic ovaries)
- Race (Caucasian and Asian women are at highest risk)
- Aging
- Extended use of anticonvulsant drugs, prednisone, and excessive thyroid hormone medications
- Sedentary lifestyle, smoking, excessive alcohol intake, lack of calcium and vitamin D when growing up

including calcitonin nasal spray, Fosamax, Actonel, and Evista.

Massage Strategies

Massage in general supports movement, which is beneficial for compliance with the physical exercise necessary for a healthy musculoskeletal system. Pressure levels must be monitored if osteoporosis is a factor. Massage increases the pliability of tissues, which supports flexibility.

CONDITIONS OF THE NERVOUS SYSTEM

The brain and central nervous system (CNS) change with aging, resulting in slower physical reactions, decreasing agility, and slowing response times. This is a major issue for the elderly, especially with regard to the ability to drive safely or to operate equipment that requires a quick reaction time.

Cognitive ability is influenced by many factors, including a person's general state of health, educational background, and genetic predisposition. The normal process of aging may contribute to a change in the thinking process. The brain begins to shrink around age 50 (and continues to do so) because of a loss of fluid within the neurons and the shrinkage of dendrites. Thinning of the dendrites makes the transmission of messages from one neuron to the next more difficult. Older neurons process input more slowly, therefore retrieving old information and learning new information take longer. The reaction time also slows, and aging people are more easily distracted.

Normal aging can result in slowing of the nervous system function and can influence the learning process. New skills and information can be acquired throughout the life span, but as a person ages, learning takes more time and repetition.

Intelligence involves inherited biologic capacity and cumulative knowledge gained through experience. Decline related to inherited intelligence begins to become noticeable around 40 years of age and can become problematic as one reaches the 60s and 70s. On the other hand, the intellectual functioning that depends on experiences increases with age. Older learners can maintain and recall about as much information in primary memory as when they were younger but accessing information may be slower. How much can be new information that is remembered and the amount of repetition required to retain the information change as we age. Fewer items of information can be processed and more time is required to recall the information.

An unfamiliar task causes older people to work more slowly, and they do best in an environment that is familiar and free of excessive distractions. Recent research shows that loss of brain cells with age is minimal, and the older brain remains capable of generating new neurons in response to stimulation. Ongoing mental activity and learning new tasks is important.

Delirium and Dementia

Delirium is a sudden loss of memory, disorientation, and trouble performing the daily tasks of life. This indicates that an acute problem should be addressed, such as a reaction to a medication, an infection, or a dietary deficiency. **Dementia** is considered loss of cognitive function (cognition) due to disease or trauma and results in changes in the brain. **Cognition** is the act or process of thinking, perceiving, and learning. Cognitive functions that may be affected by dementia include memory, decision making, verbal and written communication, and changes in temperament. Dementia is not a normal aging process but is the result of a physiologic disorder. It is important that dementia be correctly diagnosed. Depression, common in the elderly, can mimic dementia symptoms as can malnutrition especially those who are isolated. Risk factors that can result in an individual developing dementia include:

- Advanced age
- Genetic predisposition (Alzheimer's disease, Huntington's disease)
- Untreated infectious disease (syphilis)
- Cardiovascular disease (e.g., hypertension, atherosclerosis)
- Metabolic disease
- Substance abuse
- Brain tumor
- Head injury
- Kidney failure, liver disease, thyroid disease
- Vitamin deficiencies (e.g., vitamin B_{12}, folic acid, vitamin B_1 [thiamine])

Most people remain mentally competent until the end of their lives. Many conditions can cause signs and symptoms of dementia, including depression; reactions to medications and over-the-counter drugs; alcoholism; malnutrition; thyroid, liver, heart, and vascular disorders; and Parkinson's disease. Increased fluid retention in the brain can be a factor, a condition that can be treated. Numerous factors can interfere with mental judgment and motor skills, giving the impression of decreased mental status. A comprehensive medical evaluation is necessary to rule out conditions that manifest symptoms similar to those of dementia.

Dementia-related changes in cognition may or may not be reversible. The degree of reversibility depends on what is causing the dysfunction and how quickly the underlying cause is treated. Individuals with irreversible dementia caused by a progressively degenerating condition such as Alzheimer's disease eventually become unable to care for themselves.

The changes in brain function may occur gradually or quickly. The gradual changes are more difficult to identify and contributing disease may go untreated. Dementia may result in behavioral and personality changes, depending on the area or areas of the brain affected.

Dementia related to advance age has increased because of greater awareness, more accurate diagnosis, and because increased longevity is creating a larger population of the elderly. Since the fastest growing population are those over 70, healthcare systems are going to be challenged as demand for treatment increases. Intensive research focus is in progress to identify various treatments to slow the decline. Long-term care facilities are adapting to the increased demand for care of this population. Physicians are specializing in geriatric care. The potential for massage to be integrated into the complex care plans for individuals with dementia is increasing. It will be important for a proactive approach to care to be organized, or this group of individuals may receive inadequate care.

Alzheimer's Disease

Alzheimer's disease (AD) is the most common irreversible condition related to dementia. AD affects the cerebral cortex and the hippocampus, which lose mass and shrink as the disease advances. AD is a condition in which cellular destruction is related to the buildup of amyloid plaques and neurofibrillary tangles (NFTs) within the brain. NFTs are twisted, abnormal remnants of a protein found inside normal brain cells. These tangles disrupt normal cell activity, and patients with AD have an excessive number in the cerebral cortex. A protein called beta amyloid occupies the center of these plaques. Surrounding the protein are fragments of deteriorating neurons, especially those that produce acetylcholine, a neurotransmitter essential for processing memory and learning. As a result, patients with AD have less acetylcholine in the cerebral cortex. Acetylcholine is necessary for cognitive function, and the reduced amounts in the brain contribute to the loss of cognitive function, especially memory, problem solving, movement coordination, and pattern recognition, which is necessary for activities such as reading. In advanced stages of the disease, all memory and mental functioning may be lost. Patients may survive 8 to 10 years with AD and some have been known to live 25 years. Death usually occurs as a result of a secondary infection, heart disease, or malnutrition. Loss of independence and changes in the environment, such as being placed in long-term care, often result in anger, confusion, and agitation in patients with AD. These individuals need well-managed orientation to a new environment and constant reassurance. Family interaction can be stressed by caring for a loved one with AD. There are support services that can help caregivers cope.

AD can be confirmed only through examination of the brain during an autopsy. As with most types of dementia the patient shows a gradual onset and progressive difficulty with memory, functional abilities, and changes in behavior and personality, and has no evidence of other causes of these disturbances, the physician makes the diagnosis of AD.

The Stages of Alzheimer's Disease. AD can be divided into three stages:

- *First stage:* Memory loss affects job performance and activities of daily living. The individual increasingly experiences confusion and disorientation and mood or personality changes. As the symptoms increase, the person has difficulty making decisions and paying bills, gets lost easily, withdraws from others, and loses things. Eventually it becomes evident that the problems need to be evaluated by a physician.
- *Second stage:* The second stage occurs 2 to 10 years after diagnosis. Memory loss and confusion increase, and the attention span shortens. The person has difficulty recognizing friends and family members. Symptoms now include restlessness; tendency to wander and get lost; and problems with reading, writing, and numbers. Mood changes, including irritability, temper, and frustration, increase. Motor problems develop, resulting in lack of dexterity, which decreases ability to produce fine motor movement required for activities such as playing a musical instrument or buttoning a shirt. Agility declines and contributes to trip and fall injury.
- *Terminal stage:* The onset of the terminal stage varies and is characterized by a contributing decline and increased severity of symptoms. The person does not recognize family, loses weight, is unable to care for himself or herself, has incontinence of the bladder and bowels, and requires complete care.

Medical Treatment of Alzheimer's Disease. Currently, AD has no cure and treatment is targeted to symptom management and slowing the progression of the disease. Research is beginning to discover causes of AD and the outlook is hopeful. Medications are available for the treatment of early stage Alzheimer's disease. These medications help increase the level of acetylcholine in the brain by inhibiting the enzyme that breaks it down. As a result, AD patients in the second stage of the disease are able to maintain function longer and the medication may even slow the progression of the disease. Unfortunately, people with liver disease, peptic ulcer disease, chronic obstructive pulmonary disease (COPD), or a slow heart rate (bradycardia) should not take these medications.

Side effects of these medications include:

- Diarrhea
- Dizziness
- Drowsiness
- Fatigue
- Nausea
- Vomiting

Memantine (Namenda) is the only medication approved by the FDA to treat moderate to severe symptoms of AD. This medication helps protect nerve cells in the brain from excess glutamate, a neurotransmitter that plays a role in neurodegenerative diseases. Clinical studies have shown that memantine can improve memory and function and prolong the ability to perform some tasks independently. Side effects include headache, constipation, confusion, and dizziness.

Depression that occurs in the early stages of AD is commonly treated with antidepressant medications, such as a selective serotonin reuptake inhibitor (SSRI) or tricyclic. Agitation and belligerence sometimes are treated with antipsychotic medications. These medications produce side effects including drowsiness, dry mouth, constipation, sedation, confusion, and increased muscle tone. Loss of independence and changes in the environment, such as being placed in a nursing home, can cause distress, anger, confusion, and agitation in patients with AD. These individuals need well-managed orientation to a new environment and constant reassurance. Family involvement and support services can help patients and their caregivers cope.

Massage Strategies

Massage is inappropriate for patients with delirium, because the condition is caused by some underlying problem that needs medical treatment. Dementia, including Alzheimer's disease, does respond to the stress-reducing effects of massage. The massage would follow the protocol for palliative care, with the outcome goals of reducing agitation, stimulating circulation, and supporting sensory processing. Massage can be targeted to manage some side effects of medication, such as constipation and increased motor tone.

PULMONARY CONDITIONS

The amount of oxygen delivered to the bloodstream and the rate of blood flow decline with age and the lung tissues seem to lose some of their ability to make the oxygen-to-blood transfer to the bloodstream. As a result, older people take in a lot of oxygen that is not used and because respiration (breathing) is slower in older people, less oxygen enters the blood per minute. The end result is that there is less oxygen in the system, which decreases the amount of cellular work that can be done.

Around age 40, the functioning of the respiratory system declines. The lungs lose their elasticity as a result of changes in elastin and collagen, and they become smaller and flabbier. The alveoli (air sacs) enlarge, their walls become thinner, and the number of capillaries declines. As a result, the effective area for gas exchange is reduced. The chest wall may stiffen from osteoporosis of the ribs and vertebrae and calcification of the costal cartilage. The respiratory muscles become weaker, which makes moving air into and out of the lungs more difficult. To compensate, older adults rely more on accessory respiratory muscles. This may contribute to breathing pattern disorder. Because of weakening of the respiratory muscles and stiffening of the chest wall, coughing deeply enough to clear mucus from the lungs becomes more difficult.

Massage Strategies

Massage application includes the strategies for breathing pattern disorder (see Chapter 14). Caution is required for methods that mobilize the ribs if osteoporosis is a concern.

VISUAL CONDITIONS

Although a decline in vision is usually associated with aging, studies indicate that this is not true. A surprisingly high percentage of older people retain adequate visual function. By age 40, **presbyopia** begins to develop, a condition that makes it difficult to focus on detailed objects close at hand. This requires the use of corrective lenses to accommodate age-related farsightedness. The ability to refocus from far to near or near to far declines quickly. Also, the ability to follow a moving object diminishes. By age 50, structural and functional changes in the eye become noticeable and particularly affect the near vision required for reading. The lens loses some of its ability to change shape to accommodate to distance. The pupils become smaller with age, which means that less light is allowed into the retina, and focusing becomes less accurate. Older people need as much as six times more light to read. However, increasing the amount of light does not completely compensate for visual decline, because the elderly also are more sensitive to glare. Glare is probably one of the most painful experiences for the aging eye. The eye is less able to respond to abrupt changes from light to dark or dark to light. Going from a well-lit waiting room into a dim hallway can be treacherous for an older person. Lateral (side) vision decreases with age, and adapting to darkness is more difficult.

The ability to see colors changes as we age. Trouble often occurs with the blue end of the light spectrum. An elderly person may have difficulty discriminating between shades of blue and between blues and greens. This situation translates into daily life activities and can become a major safety concern. For example, red and yellow pills are easier for an elderly person to see than blue or blue-green ones. If the individual takes medication incorrectly, health status is affected. Loss of the ability to differentiate closely related colors can also affect older people's depth perception, which may make them more susceptible to falls and accidents and interfere with ability to drive. Stairs become a potential hazard because they cannot see the edges clearly.

Tear production normally declines. Tear glands do not make enough tears, or the tears are of poor quality and do not keep the eyes moist enough.

Cataracts, Glaucoma, and Macular Degeneration

Eye diseases and disorders that occur frequently in older people include cataracts, glaucoma, and macular degeneration. **Cataracts** are cloudy or opaque areas in the lens that cause blurring of vision, rings or halos around lights and objects, and a blue or yellow tint in the visual field. Surgical extraction of the affected lens with implantation of an artificial lens improves vision in 95% of cases. The procedure is performed in an outpatient facility. After the procedure, the patient must avoid bending or lifting heavy objects for 3 to 4 weeks; wearing an eye shield at night and glasses during the day helps protect the eye until it heals.

In **glaucoma,** the outflow of aqueous humor is blocked; this causes the intraocular pressure to rise, which damages the optic nerve. If left untreated, glaucoma causes progressive loss of peripheral vision and ultimately can lead to blindness. The disease can be treated with medication, and the progression can be slowed or stopped, but the disease cannot be cured. Regular eye examinations are necessary to monitor the intraocular pressure, because glaucoma produces few or no symptoms.

The macula is the part of the eye responsible for sharp vision and color. In **macular degeneration,** the macula is damaged or breaks down, causing progressive loss of the central field of vision. Macular degeneration is the leading cause of blindness in the elderly. Currently the disease has no cure, but extensive research is underway, and treatments are being developed. A diet high in antioxidants is important, and the doctor may recommend antioxidant supplementation.

Massage Strategies

Massage strategies for visual difficulty are nonspecific and involve general stress management and circulation support that is not specific for visual concerns. However, the massage therapist needs to make various accommodations for those with visual impairment. Avoid blue and green color schemes. Make sure the lighting is adequate, without excessive glare, and that the area is free of tripping hazards. Offer to assist with paperwork.

HEARING CONDITIONS

Hearing loss can have a profound psychological effect on aging individuals, causing depression, social withdrawal, and feelings of isolation. A direct relationship has been demonstrated between hearing loss, isolation, and the development of depression in older adults. Hearing loss occurs gradually. Changes in auditory ability begin around age 30, and by age 65, about 25% have a hearing impairment. Of adults age 80 or older, 65% have hearing impairment.

People often try to compensate for hearing trouble by increasing the volume of sound. However, a comfortable level for people with hearing loss is very uncomfortable for individuals with normal hearing. An auditory problem common among aging people is the inability to understand conversation because of a high level of background noise. The older a person becomes, the less background noise is required to cause this inability to hear. For example, television tends to interfere with hearing when the person is trying to talk or converse. Hearing aids, which can be used to amplify speech, increase background noise, resulting in sensory overload.

Age-related hearing loss usually is the result of dysfunction or loss of cochlear hairs; this results in an inability to hear high-frequency sounds and in difficulty understanding speech. Consonants such as *g, f, s, t,* and *z* produce high-pitched sounds that are more difficult to hear and differentiate. Sounds with a low-frequency pitch, such as the vowels *(a, e, i, o,* and *u)* may be heard more easily. Inability to hear different frequencies, combined with background noise, interferes with an older person's ability to hear. Hearing impairment is compounded by ear canal impaction, long-term exposure to intense noise, and certain drugs (e.g., aspirin).

Another hearing disorder common among older people is tinnitus, which is a ringing or buzzing in the ear. It can be caused by impaction of ear wax, an ear infection, the use of antibiotics, or a nerve disorder. Tinnitus can cause the person to have difficulty understanding conversational speech and can make sleeping difficult because of the continuous sensation of ringing in the ears.

The level at which auditory loss becomes a handicap depends on many things. Some people can interpret speech sounds through listening habits and lipreading.

Suggestions for Helping an Older, Hearing-Impaired Adult

The massage therapist can take several steps to help a hearing-impaired adult:

- Stand in the person's line of vision and gently touch the individual to get attention.
- Use gestures, pictures, and large, bold print to communicate.
- Talk in short sentences into the better ear.
- Do not increase the volume of your speech; this also raises the frequency of the voice, and most older people have trouble hearing higher frequencies. Speak more slowly, lower the tone of your voice, and talk in distinct syllables.
- Eliminate or reduce background noise. Communicate in a quiet room with the door closed. If the patient has a hearing aid, make sure it is on. Do not get too close to the hearing aid, because it will make a squealing sound.

Massage Strategies

The communication suggestions in the preceding section should help the massage therapist work more effectively with the elderly. No direct application of massage is targeted particularly to reduce hearing loss, but stress management and relaxation can reduce the person's distress over not being able to hear as well. Make sure the massage environment is quiet, and do not use music or white noise in the background if it increases the person's difficulty hearing.

NUTRITION-RELATED CONDITIONS

Because of the many environmental, social, economic, and physical changes of aging, older people are at greater risk of poor nutrition, which can adversely affect their health and energy level. As we age, our senses of taste and smell decline subtly. Deterioration and atrophy of the taste buds are part of the aging process. The ability to taste salty and sweet flavors is diminished, although the ability to detect bitter and sour flavors remains relatively the same. As a result, food tastes bland and unappetizing. Patients on salt-restricted diets and patients with diabetes must be careful about using salt and sugar.

Estimates indicate that 25% of the aging population suffers from malnutrition. Nutrition screening should be part of routine primary care so that nutritional deficiencies can be detected and corrected; this can help prevent some diseases and can aid the treatment of chronic disease. Patients with chronic conditions (e.g., cardiovascular disease, hypertension, and diabetes) can benefit from nutrition assessments and interventions. Malnourished people have more infections, their injuries take longer to heal, and medical treatment is more extensive and expensive.

Massage Strategies

Massage promotes effective digestion by supporting parasympathetic function.

URINARY CONDITIONS

Urinary incontinence, the involuntary loss of urine, is a significant problem for the elderly. However, it is not a normal part of the aging process. Changes in the urinary system make older people more vulnerable to incontinence, but contributing factors (e.g., infection, confusion, difficulty with mobility, and side effects of medications) cause the problem to develop. Incontinence is an emotional as well as a physical problem.. Often people are too embarrassed to admit they have this condition, or they believe it is just part of aging.

As the body ages, structural changes in the kidneys cause the urinary system to become less efficient. The result is a more diluted, less concentrated urine. The kidneys require more water to excrete the same amount of waste. Clearing medication from the body takes longer, and this reduced filtration rate puts older adults at higher risk of toxic levels of medication building up in the bloodstream.

Fibrous connective tissue replaces the smooth muscle and elastic tissue in the bladder. This thickening of the bladder wall reduces the bladder's ability to expand and leads to increased frequency of urination and urinary retention. Urinary retention puts older adults at increased risk of urinary tract infections. Often sleep is interrupted by the need to go to the bathroom during the night. The older brain does not recognize the sensation of bladder fullness as quickly. The shorter interval between awareness of the need to void and involuntary urination can cause anxiety. Older adults often reduce their fluid intake to prevent possible embarrassment. Unfortunately, this causes dehydration and increases the risk of urinary tract infections.

Another age-related change is loss of muscle tone in the urethra. Furthermore, in aging women the pelvic floor muscles relax as a result of decreased estrogen levels or previous pregnancy and childbirth. Once the condition is diagnosed, pelvic floor muscle exercises, medication, or surgery may be recommended.

Massage Strategies

Incontinence can be aggravated by stress, and massage reduces stress. More important, the massage therapist needs to recognize the potential for incontinence and make the restroom readily available. Bowel incontinence can also be an issue. Be prepared to deal effectively with any incontinence issues and follow standard precautions during cleanup.

REPRODUCTIVE CONDITIONS

The physical capacity and desire for sex continue throughout life, even into the late 80s and beyond. Estimates indicate that about 90% of lost interest in sex is due to psychological causes, not physical impairment. Circulation to the genitals is important for both female and male sexual function. Medications have been developed for males to treat erectile dysfunction caused by circulation problems. Similar medications for females are being studied. Smoking and the use of alcohol are two of the biggest contributors to impairment of circulation to the sex organs.

With menopause, circulating levels of the female hormones estrogen and progesterone decline, whereas androgen levels increase. The vagina shrinks in width and length and becomes less elastic. The cervix, uterus, and ovaries also decrease in size. Vaginal secretions diminish, reducing lubrication, and in some cases vaginal dryness may result. Bacterial or yeast infections may occur because the vaginal secretions are less acidic. The physician may prescribe application of an estrogen cream to the vaginal tissue to treat dryness and thinning. The benefits and risks of estrogen replacement therapy are determined on a case-by-case basis.

Even though sperm production may decline after age 50, men remain virile well into old age. Changes occur in the level of the hormone testosterone, which can affect the prostate gland. The gland enlarges over time and presses down on the urethra, causing difficulty during urination. Surgery may be required to remove excess portions of the gland.

Some changes in sexual functioning do occur with age. It takes longer for the penis to become erect, longer for an orgasm to occur, and longer to recover.

Some medications and illnesses can interfere with sexual functioning. Medications used to control high blood pressure, antihistamines, antidepressants, and some stomach acid blockers, as well as diabetes, arthritis, and hardening of the arteries, can have an adverse effect on sexual functioning. Often people who have had heart surgery or a heart attack are concerned about sexual activity. It is important that people feel comfortable and unembarrassed about discussing their concerns openly with their physician. At any age, sexuality may be expressed in other forms, such as touching, holding, caressing and, of course, humor.

Massage Strategies

Massage that supports stress reduction and increased circulation may support sexual function. People frequently discuss these issues with the massage therapist once they become comfortable. A contributing factor seems to be the pleasure aspect of massage. Should the person discuss sexual topics, provide accurate, factual information and refer the individual to the appropriate professional (likely the physician). Because of the parasympathetic and circulatory effects of massage, both males and females may experience an erectile tissue response. Simply explain the physiologic nature of this response and do not confuse it with sexual attraction.

SLEEP DISORDERS

Complaints of difficulty sleeping increase with age. Older people may spend slightly more time sleeping than younger people do, but the quality of sleep declines. Older people often are light sleepers and experience periods of wakefulness in bed. Rapid eye movement (REM) sleep is the sleep stage in which people experience dreaming. Non-REM sleep is the period of deepest sleep. The amount of time spent in the deepest stages of sleep decreases with age. Sleep disturbances and sleep that leaves a person feeling tired are not part of the aging process and may indicate some underlying emotional or physical problem. Lack of sleep can result in restlessness, disorientation, thick-speech patterns, and mispronounced words. These symptoms often are mistaken for signs of dementia. Other factors that might influence sleep patterns are medications, caffeine, alcohol, depression, and environmental or physical changes.

Simple modification of behavioral patterns may resolve sleep problems. Taking fewer naps, making sure that exercising is done several hours before bedtime, changing eating times, reducing the amount of alcohol and caffeine ingested, and changing medications or the time they are taken all may resolve some of the causes of sleep disturbance.

If behavioral approaches are not effective, medications may be considered for short-term use only, because they have a high incidence of physical and psychological dependence. The elderly population is especially susceptible to the side effects of these medications, especially next-day drowsiness and temporary memory loss.

Massage Strategies

Massage is very effective for supporting restorative sleep. The modified palliative protocol is used for this purpose.

SUPPORT SYSTEMS FOR THE GERIATRIC POPULATION

At any given time, only 5% of the elderly population lives in long-term care facilities. According to the National Institute on Aging, most older people live close to their children and are in frequent contact with them. Most people prefer to live in their own home as long as possible. People are admitted to a nursing home because they no longer can perform activities of daily living, such as bathing, dressing, eating, walking, and maintaining bladder and bowel continence. They also have difficulty with grocery shopping, housekeeping, and money management.

The risk of injury from falling increases with age; falls cause the greatest number of injuries in people over age 70. Aging individuals are at greater risk of falling because of sensorimotor changes in vision and mobility, changes in the proprioceptive and vestibular mechanisms, osteoporosis, and stroke. Falls in older patients usually result in fractures because a large percentage of the elderly population has osteoporosis. Sometimes the fracture occurs first, causing the fall. Serious fractures (e.g., hip fractures) require immobilization of the patient for extended periods and can lead to a wide range of debilitating complications, such as decubitus ulcers, pneumonia, placement in a long-term care facility, and even death.

Many resources are available that enable seniors to maintain their independence. Outreach programs, such as Meals-on-Wheels, deliver nutritious meals to the homes of older adults. Senior centers serve as a focal point for many activities and a source of information. Transportation services provide rides to doctors' appointments, shopping centers, and community events. Home health agencies provide several types of services, including personal care, shopping, transportation, and meal preparation. Some home health agencies provide a range of services, such as patient education; intravenous therapy; medical-social services; physical, speech, and occupational therapies; and nutrition and dietary counseling. Advancements in technology now allow people to receive services at home that formerly could be provided only in a hospital or physician's office.

Adult day care centers provide socialization, recreation, meals and, in some centers, physical therapy, occupational therapy, and transportation. These centers provide supervision for older adults who need care during the day but whose families take care of them in the evening. The centers also serve as respite for caregivers. Assisted living facilities are intended for older adults who need help with some activities of daily living, such as bathing, dressing, and walking. Skilled nursing facilities provide 24-hour medical care and supervision. Residents also receive care that may include physical, occupational, and speech therapy. The objective of treatment is to improve or maintain the person's abilities (Box 16-2).

MASSAGE SPECIFIC FOR THE GERIATRIC POPULATION

People in their advanced years can benefit greatly from massage. Although the massage methods remain consistent, elderly people present specific concerns and require appropriate adjustments in the massage application.

The aging process is normal. Muscle tissue diminishes, as does fat and connective tissue. Connective tissue in general is affected during the aging process. It becomes less pliable, is slower to reproduce, and more easily forms fibrotic tissue. Bones are not as flexible and are prone to breaking. Joints become worn, and osteoarthritis is common. The skin is thinner, circulation is not as efficient, and fluid in the soft tissue is reduced. Medications may be prescribed to control blood pressure and other conditions, producing many side effects. The vertebral column tends to collapse a bit during aging. The spaces provided for the nerves are reduced, and bones and soft tissue structures can put pressure on the nerves, resulting in sciatica and thoracic outlet syndrome. The feet hurt because the intricate joint structure of the foot has broken down. Circulation to the extremities is diminished, often resulting in a burning type of pain. These conditions are not life-threatening, but they surely can cause a person to feel miserable.

If only temporarily, massage can help ease the discomfort of these conditions. The general protocol and the modified palliative protocol both can serve as a basis for developing an appropriate massage approach for a healthy elderly person. Cautions for thin skin, reduced tactile sensation, pain awareness, reduced muscle mass, and circulatory changes, including increased bruising and sensitivity to heat and cold, are just a few conditions that require alteration in the massage. With changes in the joints, the person may need additional bolstering to be comfortable. Many of the elderly take several medications. They also are more sensitive to the dosage level of medication and less able to self-regulate homeostatic processes. The massage professional must be attentive to the physiologic interactions between the effects of massage and the medications. Regular massage may allow the dosages of some medications to be reduced.

Elderly people often are depressed. This frequently is a chemical depression as well as a situational condition. Massage stimulates neurochemicals that can lift mild depression temporarily. Dementia conditions, such as Alzheimer's disease, have shown temporary improvement after massage. Wandering behavior has decreased, and an increased awareness of the current environment has been observed.

BOX 16-2 Support Systems for the Elderly

- Alzheimer's Association: (1-800-272-3900).
- American Council of the Blind (1-800-424-8666): Provides referrals to state and other organizations that provide services and equipment for the blind
- American Speech-Language-Hearing Association (1-800-638-8255): Offers information on hearing aids, hearing loss, and communication problems in older people and provides a list of certified audiologists and speech pathologists.
- Arthritis Foundation Information Line (l-800-283-7800): Makes referrals to local chapters and provides information.
- Eldercare Locator (1-800-677-1116): Helpline run by the National Association of Area Agencies on Aging; provides information on contacting local chapters that oversee services to older adults.
- Hospice Helpline (1-800-658-8898): Provides information about hospice and makes referrals to local hospice organizations.
- National Institute on Aging Information Center (1-800-222-2225): Provides information on geriatric health issues.
- Meals on Wheels Association of America (703-548-5558).

Dehydration, lack of appetite, and weight loss can be problems with advanced age; however, the parasympathetic stimulation produced by massage can increase appetite and improve digestion for elderly clients. Proper hydration is very important, and the massage therapist should encourage elderly patients to drink water. Sleep also can be improved by massage. Many elderly people have periods of insomnia or disrupted sleep patterns. Improved sleep supports restorative mechanisms and increases vitality.

Many elderly people are alone. Their spouses have passed away, and their families are busy with their own lives. We all need to be touched. If a person is not physically and emotionally stimulated, neurologic function begins to deteriorate. The interaction with a massage therapist can provide both physical and emotional stimulation for the elderly. If nothing else, the physical contact with another human being provides sensory stimulation, with beneficial results. Many elderly people want to talk. This social interaction may be just as important as the physical interaction of the massage.

The massage therapist also needs to appreciate changes in vision, hearing, and cognitive processing speed and to use the communication skills recommended in this chapter. Any additional health concerns are addressed as appropriate in the massage, keeping in mind that healing occurs more slowly and adaptive mechanisms are not as effective. The massage application should not tire or stress the person.

If a person does not have adequate cognitive skills (e.g., has dementia), he or she will be unable to give informed consent for the massage. The guardian, physician, or other healthcare professional must then give the necessary permission. Massage therapists working in long-term care facilities need to be aware of and to follow all required policies and procedures.

MENTAL HEALTH

Mental health is necessary for fitness of body, mind, and spirit. It is an important aspect of physical healing regardless of the cause of illness or injury. The stresses of life strain mental health mechanisms. Mental health conditions usually have biologic factors, and pharmacologic treatment is an important aspect of mental healthcare, coupled with behavioral therapy and counseling. Psychologists and psychiatrists are the primary healthcare professionals who treat mental health conditions, although nursing specialties and licensed counselors also are involved. A **psychiatrist** is a doctor of medicine trained in psychological issues; psychiatrists can prescribe medications. A **psychologist** is a person with expert training in the diagnosis of psychological problems and the treatment of those problems using behavioral therapy and other types of therapies. Psychologists do not prescribe medications.

In the United States, the major classification system for mental health disorders is published in the ***Diagnostic and Statistical Manual of Mental Disorders,*** which was developed by the American Psychiatric Association. The manual, now in its fourth edition, is commonly referred to as the ***DSM-IV.*** Healthcare therapists are expected to use this classification system when completing patient reimbursement forms for both private and public insurance providers.

Massage can be a very effective part of mental healthcare, especially for stress management. Massage affects the brain chemicals by encouraging the release and/or utilization of serotonin, dopamine, and the endorphins, which alter mood. It also affects the release of various action hormones that influence mood. Massage has a strong normalizing effect on the autonomic nervous system and can support other medical interventions for psychiatric disorders.

People with physical health issues often have mental health concerns. Excessive stress can manifest as a number of disorders, such as cardiovascular problems, including hypertension; digestive difficulties, including heartburn, ulcer, and bowel syndromes; respiratory illness; susceptibility to bacterial and viral illnesses; endocrine dysfunction, particularly adrenal or thyroid dysfunction; delayed or diminished cellular repair; sleep disorders; and anxiety and depression, to mention just a few.

It has long been recognized that depression and anxiety often have aspects of somatization. At the same time, the stigma attached to seeking help for emotional problems often delays recognition and treatment of these disorders. People often avoid mental healthcare because of this social stigma. In addition, mental health issues are seen very differently in different ethnic cultures. A problem that might be treated with psychiatric intervention in one culture may be addressed with a religious practice in another.

The treatment of emotional problems has always been a major part of medicine. Research suggests that in 40% to 70% of those who seek medical care, a primary emotional problem is either the main reason for the visit or a major component of the physical complaint. As the understanding of neuroscience has improved, effective pharmacologic agents have been developed to treat specific psychiatric syndromes. However, they do not replace interactive mental healthcare. Many psychiatric disorders are underdiagnosed or misdiagnosed. Unless the correct questions are asked, anxiety disorders and depressive disorders are often missed. These patients continue to experience myriad puzzling somatic complaints, and they often are referred for massage or some other generalized palliative care.

At times we are all challenged psychologically. It is important to understand how our minds work and the interaction of the mind/body connection. Current research has shown the link between the mind, the body, and health. A dedicated massage therapist will seriously consider taking some psychology courses at a community college or other educational center and keeping up-to-date on research findings.

The actual massage approach is no different when working with individuals receiving mental health treatment. An understanding of psychotropic pharmacology is important, because massage and these medications affect the body in similar ways. The massage interaction should be supervised closely by a psychologist or psychiatrist. Mental health issues best addressed with massage as part of the treatment plan include addictions, psychiatric disorders (e.g., anxiety, panic, depression, eating disorders), chemical imbalances in the brain, posttraumatic stress disorder, and psychotic disorders (Box 16-3).

ADDICTIONS

Individuals withdrawing from chemical and alcohol addictions may find that massage helps reduce stress levels. The type of chemical to which the person is addicted determines the type of stressful experiences they experience. The massage therapist adjusts the massage to calm an anxious patient or to give a boost to a depressed patient. Heavy connective tissue massage should be avoided during withdrawal phases. Toxins released from this type of massage may overtax a system already burdened with withdrawal detoxification.

PSYCHIATRIC DISORDERS

Psychiatric disorders, such as anxiety, panic, depression, and somatoform and eating disorders, involve the interplay of a combination of autonomic nervous system functions and hormones, neurotransmitters, neuropeptides, and other brain chemicals.

Anxiety

Anxiety is an uneasy feeling usually connected to increased sympathetic arousal responses. Anxiety disorders are very common in the general population. About one third of otherwise normal individuals have experienced a panic attack, and 1% to 2% of the population have symptoms severe enough to be diagnosed as indicative of a panic disorder. Severe fearfulness of leaving the home and severe specific phobias occur in 2% to 5% of the general population, and about 20% of people have milder phobias. About 5% of the general population has symptoms of generalized anxiety. Anxiety symptoms are often misdiagnosed and undertreated. Those with anxiety disorders often also experience depression. Although the primary care provider often treats the symptoms of anxiety adequately, the depression frequently is not identified.

A variety of medical conditions can produce symptoms that mimic anxiety disorders. These include cardiovascular disease (e.g., paroxysmal tachycardia and mitral valve prolapse); endocrine or metabolic disorders (e.g., hypoglycemia or thyroid disease); multiple sclerosis; acute organic brain syndromes; pulmonary disorders, including

BOX 16-3 Classifying Mental Disorders

Surgeon General's Report on Mental Health

The Surgeon General's Report on Mental Health describes a half-century of advances in the understanding of mental disorders and the brain and in our appreciation of the centrality of mental health to overall health and well-being. The report in its entirety provides an up-to-date review of scientific advances in the study of mental health and of mental illnesses that affect at least one in five Americans. The statements and conclusions throughout this report are documented by reference to studies published in the scientific literature. Several important conclusions may be drawn from the extensive scientific literature summarized in the report.

The past 25 years have been marked by several discrete, defining trends in the mental health field. These have included:

1. The extraordinary pace and productivity of scientific research on the brain and behavior
2. The introduction of a range of effective treatments for most mental disorders
3. A dramatic transformation of our society's approaches to the organization and financing of mental health care
4. The emergence of powerful consumer and family movements

To access the entire report, go to http://www.surgeongeneral.gov/library/mentalhealth/toc.html

Modified from http://www.gpoaccess.gov

Social Security Disability Criteria

According to the Social Security disability eligibility mental health issues are described as follows:

Organic mental disorders: Psychological or behavioral abnormalities associated with a dysfunction of the brain. History and physical examination or laboratory tests demonstrate the presence of a specific organic factor judged to be etiologically related to the abnormal mental state and loss of previously acquired functional abilities.

Schizophrenic, paranoid and other psychotic disorders: Characterized by the onset of psychotic features with deterioration from a previous level of functioning.

Affective disorders: Characterized by a disturbance of mood, accompanied by a full or partial manic or depressive syndrome. Mood refers to a prolonged emotion that colors the whole psychic life; it generally involves either depression or elation.

Mental retardation: Mental retardation refers to significantly subaverage general intellectual functioning with deficits in adaptive functioning initially manifested during the developmental period (i.e., the evidence demonstrates or supports onset of the impairment before age 22).

Anxiety-related disorders: In these disorders, anxiety is either the predominant disturbance or it is experienced if the individual attempts to master symptoms; for example, confronting the dreaded object or situation in a phobic disorder or resisting the obsessions or compulsions in obsessive compulsive disorders.

Somatoform disorders: Physical symptoms for which there are no demonstrable organic findings or known physiological mechanisms.

Personality disorders: A personality disorder exists when personality traits are inflexible and maladaptive and cause either significant impairment in social or occupational functioning or subjective distress. Characteristic features are typical of the individual's long-term functioning and are not limited to discrete episodes of illness.

Substance addiction disorders: Behavioral changes or physical changes associated with the regular use of substances that affect the central nervous system.

Autistic disorder and other pervasive developmental disorders: Characterized by qualitative deficits in the development of reciprocal social interaction, in the development of verbal and nonverbal communication skills, and in imaginative activity. Often, there is a markedly restricted repertoire of activities and interests, which frequently are stereotyped and repetitive.

From http://www.ssa.gov/disability/professionals/bluebook/12.00-MentalDisorders-Adult.htm; accessed July 21, 2007.

hypoxemia and pulmonary embolism, and infectious diseases, such as tuberculosis. Medications and nonprescription drugs that may cause anxiety symptoms include CNS stimulants such as amphetamines, cocaine, caffeine, monosodium glutamate, theophylline, and neuroleptics.

Several different conditions are included under the heading of anxiety disorders. These include generalized anxiety disorder, situation-specific anxiety, panic disorder with or without agoraphobia, obsessive compulsive disorder, social phobia and specific phobia, and posttraumatic stress disorder.

Generalized Anxiety Disorder. In generalized anxiety disorder, the person finds it difficult to control the worry and anxiety. Anxiety, worry, or physical symptoms cause significant distress or impairment in social, occupational, or other important areas of functioning. Symptoms include the following[1]:

- Restlessness
- Being easily fatigued
- Difficulty concentrating
- Irritability
- Muscle tension
- Sleep disturbance

Situation-Specific Anxiety. Certain types of anxiety arise in response to specific situations, such as the following:

- *Separation anxiety.* Anxiety occurs when the person is separated from an important person (or pet). This may express itself in fearfulness, disruptive behavior, physical complaints, or increased demands for attention.
- *Stranger anxiety.* Although normal in childhood, this is manifested by distress or increased complaints when a person is confronted by unfamiliar people.
- *Anxiety about dependency.* These individuals are threatened by any situation that makes them feel dependent. They may devalue those who offer help.
- *Anxiety about loss of control.* This type of anxiety occurs when important decisions are taken out of a person's hands, such as when he or she requires medical care. In the medical setting, the individual may try to regain a sense of control by arguing about the diagnosis, failing to comply with treatment, failing to keep appointments, and remaining oppositional. These people often express similar behavior in any situation in which they feel out of control.
- *Anticipatory anxiety.* This type of anxiety is directed toward future events. The person projects into the future and becomes overly concerned about events that may or may not occur.

Panic

Panic is an intense, sudden, overwhelming fear or feeling of anxiety that produces terror and immediate physiologic change that results in immobility or senseless, hysterical behavior. A **panic attack** is an episode of acute anxiety that occurs at unpredictable times with feelings of intense apprehension or terror. Symptoms of a panic attack include a feeling of shortness of breath that leads to hyperventilation, dizziness, sweating, trembling, and chest pain or heart palpitations. Many people think they are having a heart attack, and this needs to be ruled out with proper diagnosis. Most symptoms can be directly related to overactivation of the sympathetic autonomic nervous system. This is where massage is so effective, because applied appropriately, it can reduce sympathetic arousal and calm the patient.

Agoraphobia is diagnosed when two symptoms occur:

- The person feels anxiety about being in places or situations in which escape might be difficult or embarrassing or in which help may not be available in case of another panic attack.
- Situations are avoided or endured with marked distress.

Panic Disorder

Panic Disorder Without Agoraphobia. Although panic attacks occur and are accompanied by concern about additional attacks, the patient is not immobilized to the point of avoiding triggering situations.

Agoraphobia Without a History of Panic Disorder. In this situation, the patient has a fear of developing paniclike symptoms without having experienced the symptoms that meet the criteria for panic disorder.

Panic Disorder with Agoraphobia. In panic disorder with agoraphobia, a discrete period of intense fear or discomfort occurs in which four or more of the following symptoms develop abruptly and reach a peak within 10 minutes. At least one of the attacks must have been followed by fear of having additional attacks, worry about the consequences of the attack, or a significant change in behavior related to the attacks[2]:

- Palpitations, a pounding or accelerated heart rate
- Sweating, trembling, or shaking
- Sensation of shortness of breath or smothering

- Feeling of choking, chest pain, or discomfort
- Nausea or abdominal distress
- Feeling of dizziness or lightheadedness; fainting
- Feeling of unreality or of being detached from oneself
- Fear of losing control or of going crazy
- Fear of dying

CHEMICAL IMBALANCES IN THE BRAIN

Certain mental heath conditions arise from an imbalance of brain chemicals. Hyperactivity, attention deficit disorder (ADD), bipolar disorder (formerly called manic-depressive disorder), schizophrenia, seasonal affective disorder (SAD), obsessive compulsive disorder (OCD), and clinical depression are just a few of the disorders caused by an imbalance of brain chemicals.

Medication is an important part of the treatment of these individuals. The massage therapist should never make a person feel guilty for taking medication or suggest that medication is not necessary. Medications must be monitored carefully by a physician, with the smallest effective dosage given to avoid side effects. Massage cannot replace medication, but the person who receives massage regularly may be able to reduce the dosage and duration of medication treatment in some cases. In other situations, the side effects of certain medications can be managed with massage.

Developmental Disabilities

Massage for people with developmental disabilities has the same effect as for everyone else. Care must be taken to communicate at the patient's level of understanding but not below functioning level. Adults with developmental disabilities are not children and should not be treated as such.

Autism is believed to be a developmental disorder characterized by impaired social interaction and communication and a restricted repertoire of interests. Contrary to popular belief, most children and adults with autism do want to be touched. A very reliable, structured touch with firm, consistent pressure usually is preferred. Massage applied in a very deliberate way within the patient's comfort level has been shown to increase social interaction somewhat and reduce anxiety.

Learning Disorders

The organized, systematic, sensory stimulation of massage may help treat the difficulty in processing sensory input that occurs in some learning disorders. Having a learning disorder is stressful. (AUTHOR'S NOTE: I have dyslexia, as well as an inner ear dysfunction that makes hand-eye coordination difficult. Thank goodness for assistants, computers, spell check, and editors.) Life is more difficult when a person must deal with any special situation. Stress from dealing with the environment aggravates the learning difficulty. Self-esteem is hard to maintain when a person has been made to feel stupid in school because he or she could not write, spell, or read. People with learning disabilities are not stupid; they just need to learn differently. Massage helps reduce their stress, thereby facilitating learning and enabling them to feel more positive about themselves.

Phobia

Phobia is an excessive or unreasonable fear. Exposure to the feared object or situation almost invariably provokes anxiety or a panic attack. Affected individuals avoid such situations or endure them with intense anxiety; this avoidance interferes with their normal routine, occupational functioning, or social activities or relationships.

A *specific phobia* is an excessive or unreasonable fear in the presence of or in anticipation of a specific situation or object (e.g., a fear of water or snakes). Exposure to the phobic stimulus almost invariably provokes an immediate anxiety response. A *social phobia* is a marked and persistent fear of one or more social or performance situations in which the person is exposed to unfamiliar people or to possible scrutiny by others. The person fears that he or she will act in a way that will be humiliating or embarrassing.

Obsessive Compulsive Disorder

The person has either obsessions or compulsions. Obsessions are recurrent, intrusive, and inappropriate thoughts, impulses, or images that cause marked anxiety or distress, which the individual attempts to ignore or suppress. Compulsions are repetitive behaviors that the person feels driven to perform in response to an obsession. With both obsessions and compulsions, the individual recognizes that the obsessions or compulsions are excessive or unreasonable.

Anxiety Disorders

Research indicates that different areas of the brain and different neurochemical mechanisms are involved in the various mental health disorders. Medication is being more specifically targeted to the individual conditions. In general, however, antianxiety agents, such as buspirone and the benzodiazepines, are used for generalized anxiety disorders, whereas disorders involving panic often respond to the newer antidepressants, especially the SSRIs. Older antidepressants, such as the monoamine oxidase inhibitors (MAOIs), are very effective but tricky to use because of their dangerous interactions with certain foods and medications.

Phobias and social anxiety are treated with a combination of antianxiety medications and behavioral treatments such as relaxation training and desensitization to the feared stimulus. Certain kinds of social anxiety, such as performance anxiety, respond to beta blockers, a type of antihypertensive agent. OCD responds both to treatment with SSRIs and to behavioral training, which enable the patient to stop and interrupt obsessive thinking or compulsive rituals.

In addition to medication, a variety of other treatments often are effective for these disorders. These include reassurance, explanation and patient education about treatments, systematic exposure to feared situations, and relaxation and visualization techniques to assist in immediate reduction of anxiety. For treating phobias, systematic desensitization often used is together with medication. Other techniques include providing support, encouraging the patient to use mechanisms such as exercise that have previously been helpful in stressful situations. Family counseling sometimes is useful to help individuals maintain progress, so that the family does not inadvertently encourage dependence or regression.

Massage Strategies

Massage targets normalization of breathing dysfunction, reduction of sympathetic arousal, and general relaxation. The massage typically is a full body, painless approach in which deep, rhythmic, broad-based gliding and kneading are used. The pressure levels need to be intense enough to produce a pleasurable sensation of a "big squash," and the massage should last 45 to 60 minutes.

DEPRESSION

Depression is one of the most common conditions seen in healthcare. It affects 10% to 20% of the population at any given time; 4% to 8% of the population has full-blown clinical depression. The incidence of depression has gradually increased, and more people are becoming depressed at an earlier age.

Symptoms of depression include a decrease in functional activity, mood disturbances, exaggerated feelings of emptiness, hopelessness, and melancholy. The person also can have periods of high energy with no purpose or outcome. Although everyone feels depressed by disappointment or loss, these feelings usually go away after a short time as the situation or the grieving process resolves. Depression as a disorder is more pervasive and disabling and does not resolve itself. Research suggests that this type of depression is related to biochemical changes in the brain. Studies also have shown that a low level of the B vitamins can affect a person's tendency to develop depression. Depression is associated with a worse outcome when it occurs with physical illness, such as coronary artery disease. Depressive symptoms can exist in schizophrenia, dementia, and anxiety disorders. Depression is found in bipolar disorder, in which an elevated mood, increased energy, a decreased need for seep, and poor judgment alternate with the more classic symptoms of major depression.

A number of common illnesses and prescription and over-the-counter drugs can cause depression. Illnesses in which depression is common include cancer, viral disease, endocrine abnormalities, anemia, stroke, and liver disease. Medications that can cause depression include oral contraceptives, steroids, some beta blockers, and L-dopa. Drugs that can trigger depression include alcohol and narcotics. Withdrawal from amphetamines or cocaine also results in depression.

Major Depression

For a diagnosis of major depression, five or more of the following symptoms must be seen during the same 2-week period. One of the symptoms is a depressed mood or a loss of interest or pleasure in usual activities. These symptoms cause significant distress, are not due to substance use, and are not caused primarily by bereavement:[2]

- Depressed mood most of the day, nearly every day
- Diminished interest or pleasure in most activities
- Significant weight loss or a decrease or increase in appetite or weight gain
- Insomnia or hypersomnia nearly every day
- Motor agitation or retardation nearly every day
- Fatigue or loss of energy
- Feelings of worthlessness or excessive guilt
- Decreased ability to think or concentrate
- Recurrent thoughts of death, suicide, or a suicide attempt or specific plan

The treatment of depression includes medication, focused psychotherapy, and emotional and social support. Many medications are available and effective for treating depression. Support can come from family, friends, and the healthcare team, including the massage therapist. Emotional and social support are the mainstays of treatment for depression.

Massage Strategies

Massage is an effective support treatment for a comprehensive treatment plan for depression. Massage application would normalize breathing dysfunction, reduce sympathetic arousal, and promote general relaxation and restorative sleep. Typically the massage is a full body, painless massage using deep, rhythmic, broad-based gliding. The pressure levels need to be intense enough to produce a pleasurable sensation of a "big squash," and the massage should last 45 to 60 minutes. The massage therapist must be aware of changes in the progression of the depression. More so than anxiety, depression can truly be life-threatening, because depressed patients may commit suicide. If the patient's mood changes significantly, either for the better or the worse, the change should be reported immediately to the medical supervisor. A decision to commit suicide may result in reduction of the depressive symptoms. Do not assume the patient is getting better if symptoms significantly diminish.

PAIN AND FATIGUE SYMPTOMS WITH ANXIETY OR DEPRESSION

Anxiety and depressive disorders are commonly accompanied by fatigue and pain syndromes. These syndromes are multicausal and often chronic, nonproductive patterns that interfere with well-being, activities of daily living, and productivity. Some of these syndromes are fibromyalgia, chronic fatigue syndrome, infection with the Epstein-Barr virus, complex regional pain syndrome (formerly called sympathetic reflex dystrophy), headache, arthritis, chronic cancer pain, neuropathy, low back pain syndrome, idiopathic pain, somatization disorder, and intractable pain syndrome. Acute pain, as well as acute episodes of chronic conditions, can be factors in these syndromes. Panic behavior, phobias, and a sense of impending doom, along with a sense of being overwhelmed and/or hopeless, are common with these conditions. Mood swings; breathing pattern disorder; sleep disturbance; concentration difficulties; memory disturbances; outbursts of anger; fatigue; and changes in habits of daily living, appetite, and activity levels are symptoms of these conditions and syndromes. Massage therapists may recognize mental health concerns in their patients with pain and fatigue syndromes, and they should refer these patients to the medical team for evaluation and mental health intervention.

EATING DISORDERS

Eating disorders involve mood disorders, physiologic responses to food, and control issues. They are complicated situations that usually require professional intervention. Individuals who have anorexia nervosa (a starving disorder) lose a great deal of weight. Bulimia is more difficult to recognize; this disorder involves binge eating and purging by vomiting and use of laxatives. The regurgitated stomach acids damage the teeth and gums, and the massage professional may notice this effect when working with the patient. These individuals should be referred to the primary healthcare provider for diagnosis. The general palliative care massage protocol is effective for people with eating disorders.

POSTTRAUMATIC STRESS DISORDER

Trauma is the result of physical injury by violent or disruptive action or by a toxic substance. It also is the result of psychic injury caused by a short-term or long-term severe emotional shock. In these cases, the person has experienced, witnessed, or been confronted by traumatic events that involved the threat of death or serious injury or a threat to the physical integrity of oneself or others. The person's response involved intense fear, helplessness, or horror. **Posttraumatic stress** can be a normal survival mechanism. **Posttraumatic stress disorder (PTSD)** is a pathogenic version of that mechanism. Not everyone develops PTSD after a traumatic event. History is replete with traumatic events, both of natural and human origin, that have left physical and mental scars on the victims and survivors and have affected their psychological functioning and adaptation to everyday life thereafter.

War, natural disasters, abusive relationships, rape, and severe auto accidents are just a few of the events that can result in posttraumatic stress. The early concepts of traumatic stress disorder focused on emotional reactions to environmental stimuli, such as earthquakes, fires, and occupational burnout. Traumatic stress has had many names over the past 50 years, including shell shock, traumatic neurosis, combat fatigue, and operational exhaustion, but researchers and clinicians are still trying to define it. In the 1970s, traumatic stress disorders were viewed as the result of psychosocial stress such as that observed in Holocaust victims, Vietnam veterans, and victims of rape and abuse; they also were seen as the result of occupationally induced stress, such as that seen in police officers, nurses, paramedics, firefighters, and physicians. Because of the psychiatric morbidity associated with Vietnam veterans, the term *posttraumatic stress disorder* was finally used to describe this condition.

People with PTSD persistently re-experience the traumatic event in one or more of the following ways:

- Through recurrent and distressing recollections of the event, including images, thoughts, or perceptions.
- Through recurrent, distressing dreams of the event.
- By acting or feeling as if the event is recurring (state-dependent memory); this includes a sense of reliving the experience, illusions, hallucinations, or dissociate flashback episodes, including those that occur on awakening or when intoxicated.

Symptoms are accompanied by intense psychological distress, including persistent symptoms of increased sympathetic arousal. The person shows persistent avoidance of stimuli associated with the trauma, as well as numbing of general responsiveness by means of reactions such as avoiding thoughts or conversations associated with the trauma, avoiding activities that remind the person of the trauma, inability to recall aspects of the trauma, diminished interest in significant activities, feelings of detachment or estrangement from others, restricted ranges of mood, and a sense of a troubled future.

Traumatic Stress

Traumatic stress differs from general stress, cumulative stress, and even distress. Researchers are trying to understand the interaction between the individual and the stressor events, including such variables as the individual or group personalities, the coping processes involved, and the psychobiologic mechanisms affected by trauma.

People seem to have a natural reaction to a traumatic event, behaviorally, emotionally, physiologically, and psychologically. A traumatic stress reaction begins with the response to the event and continues as long as symptoms are present. Symptoms may be swift in onset, as in an acute reaction, which follows minutes after a critical incident. This response is a normal grief response, one that would be expected after a tragedy. If intense symptoms persist or if the symptoms appear sometime after the tragedy and continue, a cumulative or delayed stress reaction is present, and the symptoms may last months or decades. Avoidance behavior may occur, and the emotional response may impair the person's ability to function and to relate to other people.

Many factors determine how and whether a person is affected by traumatic stress. These include age, experience, expectations, interpretations, and perceptions of the traumatic event. Adaptation to a traumatic life event may be affected by personality, coping resources, and support resources. Traumatic events that overwhelm coping mechanisms set the stage for a person to react automatically with excessive emotional responses to subsequent stressors.

Little was known about the underlying physiologic mechanisms of traumatic response until the research done by Hans Selye, who described the pituitary-adrenalin-cortical response to experimental stressors. He also described the general adaptation syndrome, in which he detailed the characteristic responses to major personal threats as the alarm-resistance-exhaustion reaction. He categorized stress as *eustress*, or good stress, such as that caused by marriage, and *distress*, or bad stress, such as that caused by divorce.

The limbic system plays an important role in guiding the emotions that stimulate the behavior necessary for self-preservation and survival. It is responsible for such complex behaviors as feeding, fighting, fleeing, and reproducing. It assigns to life experiences feelings of significance, truth, and meaning. The limbic system is also the primary area of the CNS in which memories are processed, and it is the most likely location of an explanation for the memory disturbances that follow trauma.

The hippocampus, which records the spatial and temporal dimensions of experiences in memory, does not fully mature until the third or fourth year of life. This is one reason trauma experienced by young children can result in lifelong behavioral changes. The hippocampal localization system remains vulnerable to disruption, and severe or prolonged stress can suppress hippocampal functioning. The amygdala is involved in the acquisition of a conditioned fear response. Trauma can cause long-term alterations in neuronal excitability, which may lead to lasting neurobiologic and behavioral changes caused by alterations in the temporal lobe.

Diminished serotonin activity in traumatic stress is at the core of the reduced functioning of the behavioral inhibition system, which in turn is responsible for the continuation of emergency responses to minor stresses long after the actual trauma has ended. In a well-functioning person, stress produces rapid, specific hormonal responses, and the body then returns to a normal state. However, chronic, persistent stress blunts this effective stress response and causes sensitization and overreaction by the response system. When overarousal occurs, rage, panic, and agitated behavior result. Memory and ongoing functions of memory are at the core of the psychological disruptions seen with chronic traumatic stress disorders. Events of the past continue to be experienced as if in the present.

Medical Treatment of Posttraumatic Stress Disorder

A **critical incident** is defined as any event with sufficient impact to produce a significant emotional reaction in people at the time of occurrence or later. These events are considered outside the range of ordinary human experience. The event may lead to the development of PTSD if the issues caused by the event are not resolved by the person effectively and quickly. Early intervention at the time of the crisis can prevent or reduce the tendency for posttraumatic stress to evolve into PTSD. Individuals and groups in crisis need an opportunity to do the following:

- Experience and express their feelings of fear, panic, loss, and pain within a safe environment
- Become fully aware and accepting of what has happened to them
- Resume activity and begin reconstructing their lives with the social, physical, and emotional resources available
- Express their feelings to someone who will listen with concern and sympathy
- Understand the reality of what has happened, a bit at a time
- Make contact with relatives, friends, and other resources needed to begin the process of social and physical reconstruction

Massage Strategies

Massage performed as part of crisis intervention is palliative, with the intention of general reduction of the sympathetic nervous system arousal. The American Massage Therapy Association (AMTA) provides massage as part of critical incident care through a massage emergency response team (MERT): "MERT prepares volunteer massage therapists for professional response when a disaster occurs. It's an invaluable opportunity for you to grow personally and professionally as you provide critical assistance to emergency workers and volunteers through your state chapter. Enrollment in MERT is reserved for AMTA Professional Active members only."*

> **JUST BETWEEN YOU AND ME**
>
> My massage school has an educational partnership with a hospital run by the Department of Veterans Affairs (the VA). My students learn so much from working with the veterans. Posttraumatic stress disorder (PTSD) is one of the conditions treated with massage. Students often feel overwhelmed by the patient's condition and history. I tell them to keep their hands moving, their mouths shut, and to support the patient with empathy, not by trying to fix things. The relaxation and compassion provided during the massage are enough.

Chronic Posttraumatic Stress Disorder. A variety of psychopharmacologic medications (e.g., clonidine, the benzodiazepines, MAOIs, and tricyclic antidepressants) affect the physiologic arousal system and can reduce the long-term effects of trauma and shock. They also seem to have some use in the treatment of PTSD. Medications can be used to relieve depression and to improve sleep, suppress intrusive memories, and calm explosive anger. Psychotherapy through individual counseling and support groups is an important aspect of the treatment of PTSD. This type of therapy can do the following:

- Provide therapeutic support
- Help the person develop the ability to express emotions
- Promote interest in meaningful activities
- Help the person explore feelings of helplessness
- Help the person put feelings into perspective
- Evoke positive emotions
- Reduce the cycle of numbing, intrusive thoughts, distortion, and dissociation

Crisis Intervention/Preventive Care for Traumatic Stress. The basic principles of crisis intervention are (1) to intervene immediately after the event and stabilize the victim or the community; (2) to facilitate understanding of what has happened; (3) to focus on problem solving within the realm of what is possible for the victim; and (4) to encourage self-reliance to restore a sense of independent functioning.

Multidisciplinary care is necessary to treat PTSD effectively. Medication, psychotherapy, behavioral modification, and relaxation training all are helpful, but the condition is complex and difficult to treat.

Massage Strategies

Because therapeutic massage is beneficial for normalizing the effects of the physiologic manifestations of stress, it can be an effective tool in the management of or recovery from PTSD.

The massage approach targets normalization of breathing dysfunction, reduction of sympathetic arousal, and promotion of general relaxation. The massage typically is a full body, painless approach using deep, rhythmic, broad-based gliding. The pressure levels need to be intense enough to produce a pleasurable sensation of a "big squash," and the massage should last 45 to 60 minutes. Various physical conditions associated with the trauma can be addressed individually. Somatization is common and includes headache, neck and shoulder pain, and back ache. If the person was injured during the trauma, residual physical conditions may exist that massage can address.

Should the person experience a state-dependent memory, the massage therapist typically slows the massage and deliberately and gently changes its focus or location. Do nothing abruptly, and allow the patient to regain a sense of control

*www.amtamassage.org.

in the current time frame. Do not attempt to engage in a dialog or to change the patient's cognitive process, but do report the event to the medical supervisor. If the patient does not become calm within a few minutes, call for help but do not leave the person.

Rather than having an intense emotional reaction, a patient with PTSD more often dissociates and disengages from the current experience of the massage. The breathing usually changes, becoming either slower or faster, and the eyes become distant and internally focused. The body may feel wooden or empty to the massage therapist. If dissociation occurs, slow the massage and deliberately and gently change its focus or location. Do nothing abruptly, and allow the patient to regain a sense of control in the current time frame. Do not attempt to engage in a dialog or to change the patient's cognitive process, but do report the event to the psychiatrist or psychologist, as well as what you were doing when the patient experienced the disassociation. Occasionally the psychologist or psychiatrist will want to sit in on a session, and if dissociation or state-dependent memory occurs, they will engage the patient in a dialog to help the person gain a better understanding of the situation. Subsequently, in psychotherapy, they will develop coping strategies to help the person function better.

PSYCHOTIC DISORDERS

Schizophrenia usually is first identified during the late teens and early 20s. It often is preceded by a period in which a person whose previous functioning was reasonably good becomes disorganized, withdrawn, and suspicious. The person shows increasingly impaired reality awareness. A person with schizophrenia also shows a deterioration in the ability to work, to have interpersonal relationships, and to carry out self-care activities compared with previous levels of functioning. For a diagnosis of schizophrenia, two or more of the following symptoms must be present during a 1-month period:

- Delusions. The patient exhibits fixed, false ideas that are inconsistent with his or her culture or religion and cannot be corrected by rational argument. The delusions may be bizarre and sometimes are associated with a depressed or elevated mood.
- Hallucinations: These are perceptual experiences that occur in the absence of an actual stimulus. Auditory and visual hallucinations are most common.
- Disorganized speech: This symptom often reflects both the individual's difficulty concentrating and the bizarre content of the person's thoughts.
- Gross disorganization or catatonic behavior: In this situation, the patient may become severely withdrawn, mute, and unresponsive to questions or requests and may even be incontinent.
- Negative symptoms: The patient shows flattening of emotional expression, the absence of speech, and absence of interest in any activities or participation in any activity.

Psychotic thinking sometimes may be associated with other disorders besides schizophrenia. These include delirium, dementia, toxic states, and mood disorders. It also may be seen with psychosis associated with severe depressive illness or bipolar disorder, especially during the manic phase when grandiose delusions are very common.

Medical Treatment of Psychotic Disorders

Antipsychotic medications have become increasingly refined, and newer medications produce fewer adverse effects than the older drugs. With the older drugs, many people who had some remission of hallucinations and delusions were troubled by motor stiffness, involuntary motor restlessness and, at times, acute motor spasms. Also, the older drugs usually were not helpful for negative symptoms. Many patients who use the newer antipsychotic medications are able to live independently and hold jobs, and they have a much brighter affect and higher energy level. Despite these improvements, many people with residual schizophrenia still have poor judgment, engage in intermittent drug or alcohol abuse or dependence, have difficulty managing money, and receive marginal healthcare. This often happens because of poor compliance with treatment, confusion about the need for medical follow-up, poor coping and problem-solving skills, and problems trusting authority figures.

A treatment team often is necessary to help a person with schizophrenia remain stable. This team usually includes a case manager, family members, a primary care team to keep track of the medical aspects of the patient's condition and, whenever possible, a community advocate, who keeps track of resources in the community, educates health and mental health providers, and serves as a source of legal and financial advocacy if necessary.

Massage Strategies

No specific recommendations are made for massage, which typically is used less often for treatment of schizophrenia than for other mental health conditions. However, people with schizophrenia may also have health conditions that can be helped by massage, such as low back pain. In such cases the massage therapist must understand the communication challenges they face with these individuals, the effects of the medication coupled with massage, and ways to manage the erratic behavior. The massage approach should target a stress management outcome.

> **JUST BETWEEN YOU AND ME**
>
> I have worked with people who have schizophrenia. Because the massage was provided to manage headaches and back pain, the actual behavior related to the schizophrenia was an incidental factor in the massage. One person in particular was a bit paranoid, and it was really important to him that all the window blinds be closed. He would get up every few minutes to look out the window. I accommodated this need. Another person had a specific ritual about making appointments; he had a code number that I had to use every time I called him. Massage was helpful in both cases for the headaches and the back pain, but not for the schizophrenia.

DELIRIUM AND DEMENTIA

Delirium can occur secondary to medication or drug intoxication, metabolic conditions, medication or substance withdrawal, or acute physical illness that involves a disturbance in consciousness, which shows the following characteristics:

- Disturbance of consciousness, with reduced clarity of awareness of the environment and reduced ability to focus, sustain, or shift attention
- A change in cognitive abilities, such as memory deficit, disorientation, language disturbance, or the development of a perceptual disturbance
- A disturbance that develops over a short period and tends to fluctuate over the course of the day

Dementia is a chronic disturbance of memory, judgment, and intellectual functioning without prominent clouding of consciousness. The onset is often insidious. Two of the most common forms of dementia are dementia of the Alzheimer's type and vascular dementia.

Dementia of the Alzheimer's Type

The criteria for dementia of the Alzheimer's type include multiple cognitive deficits manifested by both memory impairment and one or more of the cognitive disturbances of aphasia, apraxia, and agnosia.

- **Aphasia** is the impairment of language, which affects the production or comprehension of speech and the ability to read or write. Aphasia is always caused by injury to the brain, most often from a stroke, particularly in older individuals. However, brain injuries that cause aphasia may also arise from head trauma, brain tumors, or infections. Aphasia can be very mild or so severe that it makes communication with the patient almost impossible. It may affect mainly a single aspect of language use (e.g., the ability to retrieve the names of objects), the ability to put words together into sentences, or the ability to read. More often multiple aspects of communication are impaired, while some channels remain accessible for a limited exchange of information.[3]
- **Apraxia** is a motor disorder in which volitional or voluntary movement is impaired without muscle weakness. The ability to select and sequence movements is impaired. Oral apraxia affects the ability to move the muscles of the mouth for purposes other than speech. A person with oral apraxia has trouble coughing, swallowing, wiggling the tongue, or puckering the lips when asked to respond.

Verbal apraxia, or apraxia of speech, is an impairment in the sequencing of speech sounds. Apraxia is different from dysarthria in that no muscle weakness is involved. The errors heard in dysarthric speech are usually consistent and predictable, whereas the errors in apraxic speech are unpredictable. Apraxic speakers grope for the correct word; they may make several attempts at a word before they get it right.[4]

- **Agnosia** manifests as a disorder involving the ability to identify objects and perceive where objects are located with respect to other objects. There are basically three different forms of visual agnosia; the person may have difficulty recognizing objects, or faces, or words.

In dementia of the Alzheimer's type, the disturbance in the person's ability to function is marked by (1) cognitive deficits that significantly impair social or occupational functioning and that represent a significant decline from a previous level of functioning and (2) a progression characterized by gradual onset and continuing cognitive decline.

Vascular Dementia

The criteria for vascular dementia are similar to those for the Alzheimer's type. In this condition, however, focal neurologic signs and symptoms or laboratory evidence of cerebrovascular disease is present, and the clinical course usually shows episodic rather than gradual decline.

Massage Strategies

Dementia is most common in the elderly. Because in an elderly person delirium often occurs along with a permanent memory problem, it is crucial that the primary care provider take a careful history and do a thorough mental status and physical examination to differentiate how much of the memory problem is related to an irreversible process and how much is related to an acute medical problem. (These conditions were discussed in more depth in the section on geriatrics.)

As mentioned previously, massage is not appropriate for delirium unless it is used as a method to calm the patient. Massage has been shown to be helpful for dementia. Specific strategies are discussed in the section on geriatrics.

PEDIATRICS (INFANTS, CHILDREN, AND ADOLESCENTS)

The **pediatric population** includes the age range that starts with infancy and runs through the end of adolescence (approximately 18 years) (Figures 16-4 to 16-6). This population is identified for special consideration because the very young are more prone to illness, and adolescents experience extreme physical changes. Massage is a valuable treatment option for various conditions that develop within this population. Massage therapists are likely to find themselves teaching parents and other caregivers how to use massage to benefit a child.

The first group includes infants from birth to 3 years of age, which includes the toddler phase. A baby grows rapidly and completes the developmental process of the nervous system until at least 24 months of age. Males often develop more slowly than females; therefore this text describes this grouping conservatively. The next group, childhood, includes children from age 3 to the onset of puberty. Puberty can begin anywhere from 8 or 9 years of age to 15 years. Childhood typically is a stable health period, and the child grows physically and accumulates experience. Adolescence, the final group in this section, begins at the onset of puberty and lasts until physical maturation.

All massage for infants and for minors up to 18 years of age must be done with specific parental informed consent and supervision. In the medical setting, supervision can be provided by medical personnel.

The medical concerns of this population include most of the potential injuries and illnesses discussed in the text. Identifying any trends based on age is difficult, but some patterns do exist. For example, infants are prone to infection or may be dealing with birth trauma issues. Many genetic disorders are identified at this time.

Children are more apt to suffer an injury, such as falling, but there are increasing concerns with early development of stress-related diseases

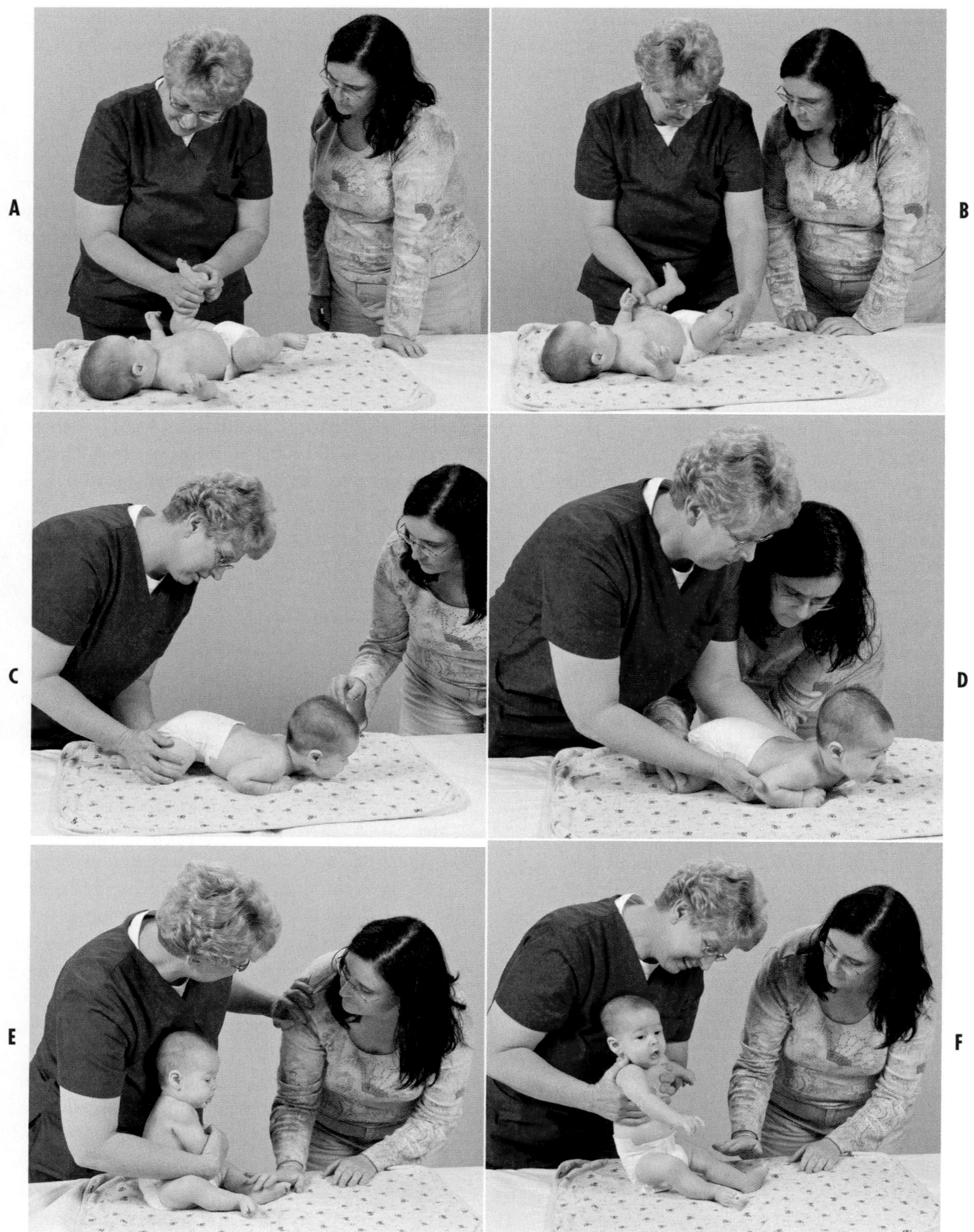

FIGURE 16-4 ■ Infant massage for an injured or ill baby. It is important to be attentive to the concerned care the parents are giving the baby and to teach simple application methods to support medical healing. **A,** Connect with the baby. **B,** Assess the baby and explain your findings and what you intend to do to the parent. **C,** Application of therapeutic massage. **D,** Teach the parent to provide massage. **E,** Connect with the parent to establish a trusting professional relationship. **F,** Return the baby to the parent's care.

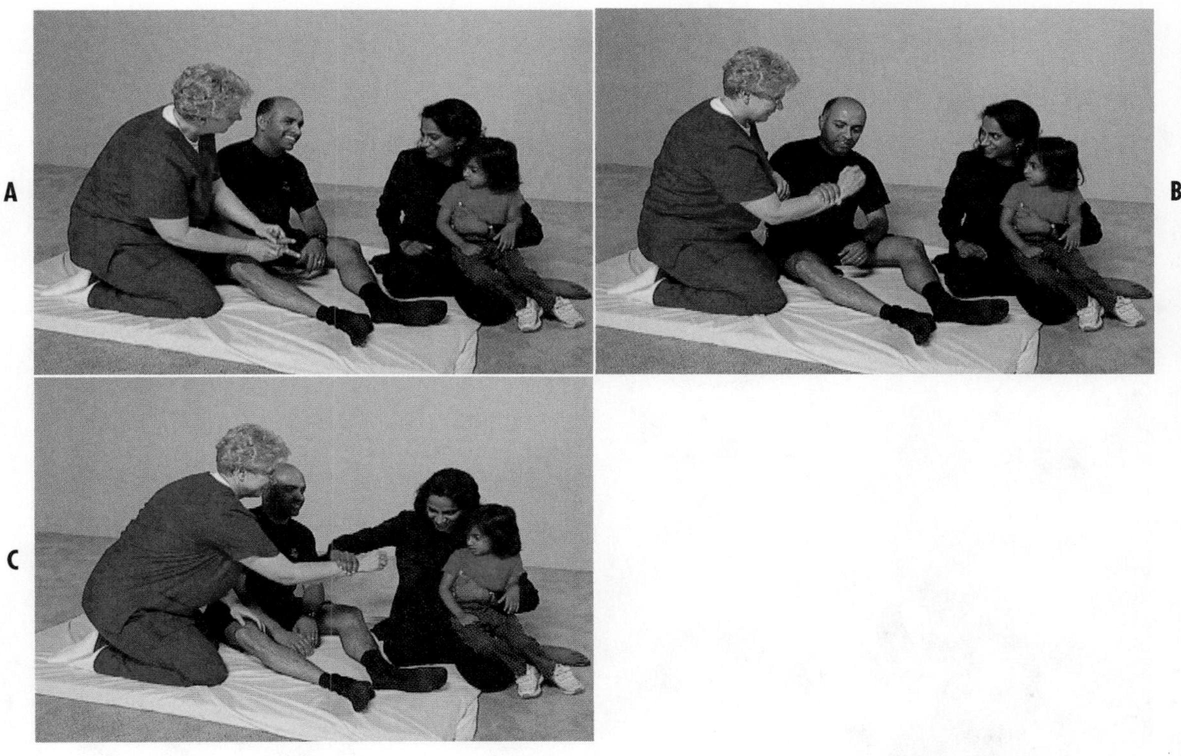

FIGURE 16-5 ■ Interaction with a toddler, who is more inclined to stay near mommy and daddy.

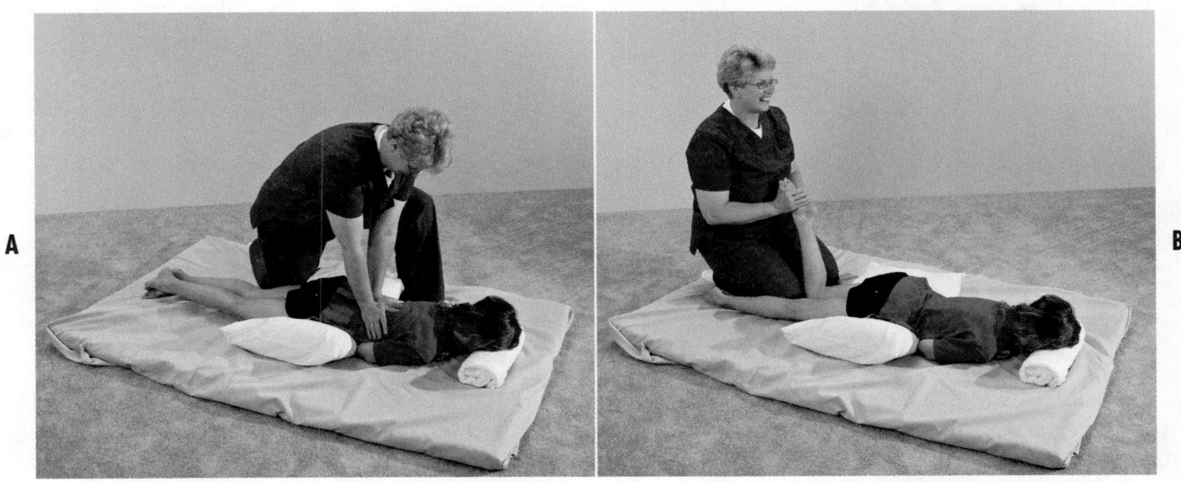

FIGURE 16-6 ■ Massage for a young adolescent. Massage can be provided traditionally on the massage table, or a mat can be used. Supervision by a parent or guardian is necessary. Children should wear loose clothing, and the massage should be provided over the clothes. **A,** Typically, begin with the adolescent in the prone position. **B,** Interact with the observing parent (not pictured).

Continued

C

D

E

F

G

H

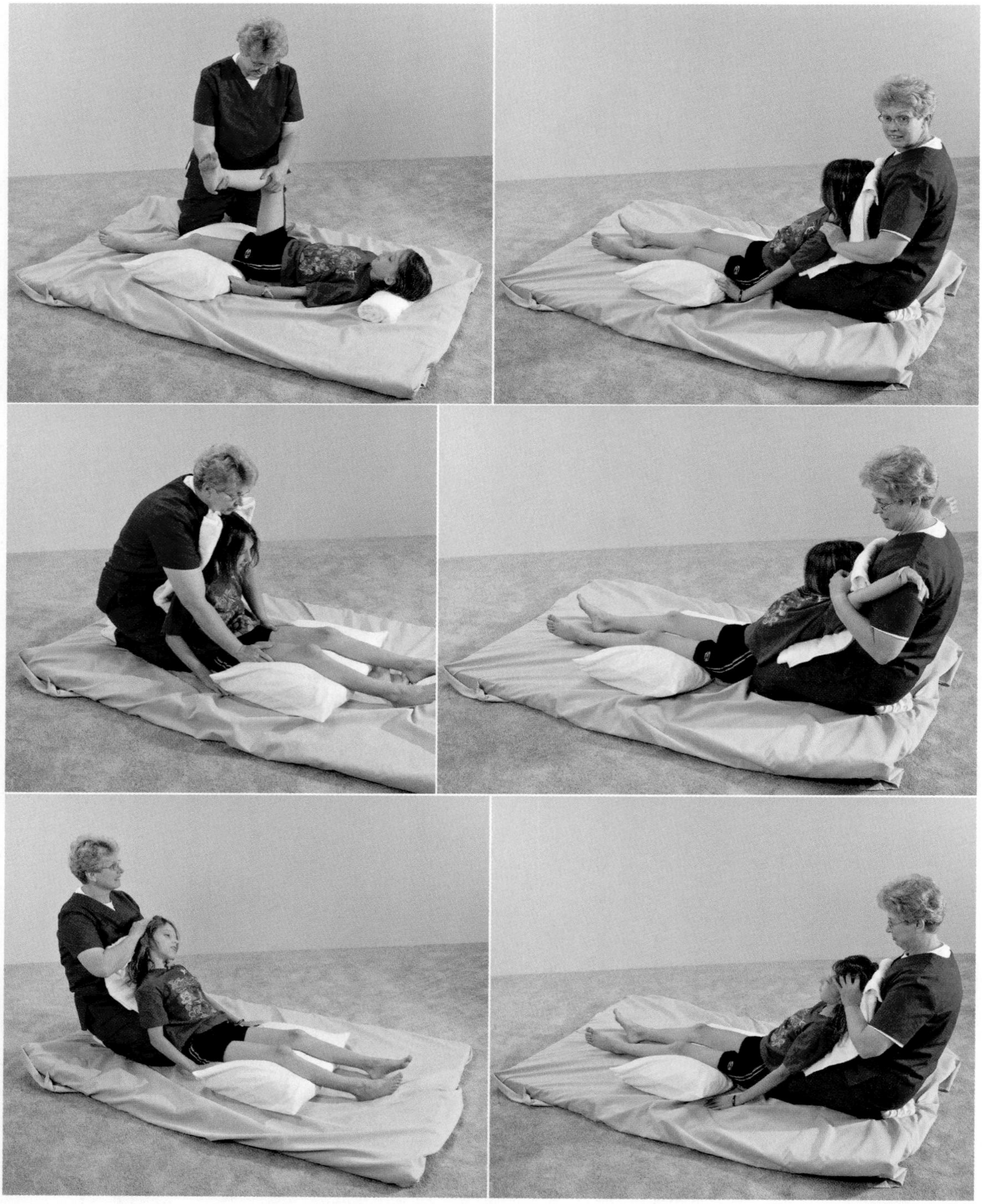

FIGURE 16-6, cont'd ■ **C,** Explain the methods to the adolescent. **D,** Demonstrate a position to the observing parent (not pictured). **E,** Listen to the adolescent as he or she explains symptoms. **F,** Therapeutic application of muscle energy method and lengthening. **G,** Interact with the observing parent (not pictured). **H,** Soothing massage.

such as headaches and stomachaches. Learning disabilities usually are identified at this age. Also, some types of cancer occur more often in children, and asthma, juvenile diabetes, or rheumatoid arthritis may develop during the childhood phase.

Adolescents are most often injured in car accidents or suffer sports-type injuries. They also can have substance abuse problems, eating disorders, and early symptoms of autoimmune disease. Because of stress and lifestyle choices, adolescents are prone to suppressed immune function, and they are susceptible to viral infection. Type 2 diabetes is appearing in adolescents at an alarming rate. Girls may have menstrual difficulties, and adolescent sexual activity increases the potential for sexually transmitted disease.

INFANTS AND TODDLERS

Most authorities designate babies from birth to 18 months of age as infants. For the purposes of this textbook, the classification is expanded to 3 years of age because infants are still developing neurologically until that time.

Compared with other mammals, human infants are born about halfway through the gestation period, while the head is still small enough to pass through the birth canal. Otherwise, babies would stay in the safe haven of the womb at least another year. The womb is a much safer place to be unless the pregnant mother uses tobacco, drugs, alcohol, or other chemicals that cross the placental barrier or if she does not provide adequate nutrition and care for herself and thus her baby. Neonatal intensive care units are filled with infants struggling because the prenatal care and lifestyle of the parents, especially the mother, did not support infant development. Many studies indicate that massage for these challenged little babies is effective at reducing stress and supporting development. (This is also discussed later.)

Protection, nutrition, connection, bonding, stimulation, and soothing acceptance are crucial for human infants. Infants are born with a need for sociability, along with the more basic needs for food, shelter, and so forth. The people of most cultures massage their infants. Although this practice has been almost lost in the westernized world, it is being revived. Research by Dr. Tiffany Field and her associates shows that premature infants who are massaged fare much better than those who are not. Massage provides an organized, logical approach to sensory stimulation, which is important for infants because part of their growth is learning to sort and organize sensory stimulation.

As mentioned, physiologically, an infant's growth pattern is not complete until 3 years of age. By 12 months of age (when, if our heads were not so big, a child would just have been born), the infant can move independently from place to place but still is utterly dependent on the protection of a parent figure or family group. Two-year-olds are still babies, even though they are considered toddlers. Three-year-olds are quite different in both function and body form. By the time a toddler can control bladder and bowel functions reliably (about age 3), cognitive functions are better able to be organized. Now is the time to work on learning the meaning of "no," picking up toys, and sharing, and the baby is ready to pass into childhood.

Understanding the limitations of these walking babies is important. Many 2-year-olds have been spanked for not sharing toys or not putting toys away, when physically and developmentally they are incapable of understanding the concept. Touch then becomes negative in connotation. Lots of hurt happens at this age. The parents' expectations often are too high, resulting in frustration on the part of both parents and child. The wonderful and challenging twos are a great time to take time out and give the baby a massage. If the child is approached appropriately, this experience can be calming for both parent and child, and touch then becomes a very positive experience (Box 16-4).

Massage Strategies

When working with any person, the massage therapist needs to "meet" the person where he or she is at that moment. This is most important when working with infants and toddlers. A fussy baby or a 2-year-old in a tantrum is caught up in the physiologic process. It takes time for both the nervous and endocrine systems to calm down. When verbal skills are not sufficient to express the problem, crying may be a way to burn off internal

BOX 16-4 Developmental Sequence for Babies

- *Birth to 2 months:* Babies focus on the caregiver's face when the person talks; arm and leg movements appear to be uncoordinated; weak neck muscles mean that babies cannot control head movements.
- *3 to 4 months:* Babies begin to develop head control and can lift the chest when placed on the stomach. Babies should have some supervised play time on the stomach but should always be placed on the back to sleep.
- *4 to 5 months:* Babies roll from side to back and/or from back to side.
- *6 to 7 months:* Babies can turn over completely (front to back and/or back to front).
- *7 months:* Babies can pull themselves up to stand but have trouble sitting down again.
- *7 to 8 months:* Babies can sit up steadily with the support of their arms.
- *8 to 10 months:* Babies can creep on their stomachs or begin to crawl on their hands and knees. (Some babies do not learn to crawl until after they learn to stand.) The crawling phase is important in neurologic development and should be encouraged. Keep the use of walkers and other standing devices to a minimum to support crawling.
- *9 to 11 months:* Babies can walk when led by the hands or holding onto furniture.
- *12 to 15 months:* Babies can stand without holding onto anything and begin walking.
- *18 months:* Toddlers walk well, both forward and backward; they can creep down stairs and get on and off a low chair; they can throw a ball without losing balance.
- *24 months:* Children are able to run and climb.
- *36 months:* Children are refining large motor skills; they can alternate feet while climbing stairs, ride a tricycle, jump, and balance on one foot. They can throw a ball overhand.

From www.missourifamilies.org

agitation that has built up through the day. A parent or massage therapist who expects the infant to settle into the massage immediately may be disappointed. Relaxing takes time. Repetitive long strokes and rhythmic movement of the limbs can initiate a calming response in an infant. Bilateral pressure (on the sides) is calming. Swaddling provides this type of consistent, even pressure that reduces neural activity. If the baby stiffens with the massage, the tactile stimulation most likely is too intense, too light, uneven, or painful. An infant's nervous system is very sensitive. Confining the massage to the feet or rhythmic rocking may be preferable to stroking for infants who seem highly sensitive to tactile stimuli. When just the right combination of methods is found, the infant will respond calmly to the touch.

It is appropriate to teach parents to massage their own babies. Massage may be especially helpful for parents who have trouble bonding with their infants. Bonding is the attachment process that occurs between parent and child. Although bonding is considered primarily an emotional response, it is theorized that some biochemical and hormonal interaction may support the process. The hormone oxytocin is present in both the mother and the father and may be a factor in the bonding process. Massage, through skin stimulation, increases the level of oxytocin.

A confident touch is important; babies can detect nervousness immediately. To them, this is not a "safe" touch, and they will not respond and may even try to withdraw. The parents may then feel rejected by the infant.

In infants born to mothers addicted to drugs and alcohol, the nervous system is especially challenged. Research is underway to determine whether the gentle, organized, tactile approaches of massage can help these special babies. The initial findings are promising. In well-baby care, a shorter massage time (15 to 30 minutes) is sufficient. The massage should follow an organized sequence, be rhythmic, and typically consists of slow gliding and gentle kneading with a lubricant. It should exert sufficient pressure to stimulate the relaxation response. A light touch should be avoided, because it is arousing and can trigger the tickle response. The massage is never painful, and it is important to monitor for pain behavior such as flinching, changes in facial expression, and changes in breathing. The massage typically lasts 15 to 30 minutes, depending on the baby's tolerance. The lubricant should be very basic and safe for baby's skin. Lubricants with scents or other additives should be avoided.

A typical logical sequence for infant massage is buttocks and back, neck, head and face, chest, abdomen, arms, legs, and feet. Another sequence might be feet, legs, abdomen, chest, arms, buttocks and back, neck and head, and face. Spend about 2 minutes in each area (a little more or less, depending on the baby and the time available), which is about a 20-minute massage. If the baby seems to respond to massage in one area more than another, then adjust the duration accordingly. Babies enjoy daily massage. This is one reason caregivers need to learn how to massage the baby.

Remember, each baby is different. Listen to their little bodies and structure the massage to best meet their needs.

CHILDREN

Providing massage services for children is not much different from providing massage for adults. For the purposes of this textbook, children are people ranging in age from 3 years to the onset of puberty. Children love physical contact. It is interesting that the horsing around and wrestling during play looks a lot like massage. Because children and adolescents may have shorter attention spans than adults, a 30-minute massage usually is sufficient. However, if the child enjoys a longer time frame, up to 60 minutes is appropriate.

From age 3 to puberty, physical growth occurs mostly in height and length of limbs. Both physical and emotional growing pains are common. Physical growing pains occur because the long bones grow more rapidly than the muscle tissue, resulting in a pull on the periosteum or connective tissue bone covering, which is a very pain-sensitive structure. Children need physical activity, but they do not get enough of it in the typical Western society. Children watch television and play video games rather than running around in general physical play. The result is a tendency to become overweight and an increase in the general stress response. Sympathetic dominance is balanced by physical activity.

Another strategy for reducing stress feelings is eating, especially carbohydrates and fat. This can become a vicious cycle that results in childhood obesity, a major health concern.

At the other extreme are children who are involved in so many activities they do not have unstructured time to simply grow and be a child. These children often display stress-related symptoms.

Massage Strategies

Massage can help growing pains by gently lengthening the muscles, stretching the connective tissue, and providing symptomatic relief of pain through the effects of counterirritation, hyperstimulation analgesia, gait control, and release of endorphins. Use the general protocol as a pattern for massage application. It may need to be shortened based on how long the child is comfortable with the massage process. The modified palliative care protocol also is appropriate. If respiratory illness or stress symptoms are present, the methods for addressing breathing pattern disorder can be beneficial.

ADOLESCENTS

Adolescents live in bodies that are changing every second. At adolescence, growth in height accelerates under the influence of increased hormonal levels, and sexual maturation occurs as well. Hormonal levels fluctuate constantly, and mood swings are common. Natural sleep-wake patterns often are disrupted. It is not uncommon for a teenager to be up all night and want to sleep all day. Daily life is emotionally and physically stressful for adolescents.

Massage Strategies

Massage may help an adolescent become more comfortable with his or her ever-changing body. It certainly helps with physical growing pains. Use special caution when working with adolescent boys. The reflexive physical sexual response is sensitive, and almost anything can trigger an erection. The massage therapist should be sensitive to this and should not use a smooth sheet over the groin area when working with male adolescents. Instead, keep the sheet bunched in this area to disguise any physical response to the massage. Use the general protocol as a starting point for massage and modify as necessary.

PEDIATRIC MEDICAL ISSUES

When infants, children, or adolescents become ill or are injured, the various medical treatments target the nature of the medical concern. Medication dosages are adjusted based on size and age. Surgeries are a bit more difficult because the body is smaller. Communication is more difficult for infants and toddlers. Ill or injured children are more logical about pain and treatment procedures than most adults. They may not totally process the abstract nature of being hurt or ill, but they often do better with the day-to-day aspects of rehabilitation and treatment than adolescents or adults.

Massage Strategies

The massage therapist working with ill or injured children must rediscover the simple, direct language of children and simply give the massage that best meets the outcomes determined by the treatment plan (e.g., pain management, stress management, scar tissue management, sleep support). Be as concrete as the child. Listen to the child and ask for direction and input. It is amazing how much children understand. For example, when determining pressure levels for a particular area, give the child three choices and demonstrate each on the body: light, medium, and deep. Then let the child choose. Another approach is to have the child press or massage the massage therapist's arm the way the child wants to be massaged. The therapist then models the application in terms of speed, depth of pressure, and so on. Kids are much better at this than adults.

Adolescents love massage as a general rule. Normal adolescent concerns about body changes may cause some embarrassment, but once that has passed, the same methods used for adults are appropriate for this group. As always, the massage application is individualized based on health issues and treatment outcomes.

Everything is more intense at this age. Adolescence often is the time of drama and overreaction. Certainly if health issues are a factor, there will be emotional concerns as well as physical ones. Massage therapists just need to do their job as presented in this text. Do not expect adolescents to be adults, but remember that they are not children anymore, either.

PHYSICAL DISABILITIES

When employed in the medical/healthcare setting, massage therapists commonly work with people who have physical disabilities. Sometimes the reason for massage is directly related to the disability. For example, a patient may have phantom limb pain with amputation, scar tissue management may be needed for people who have been burned, a person may be confined to a wheelchair or motorized scooter because of respiratory disease, or size concerns may be a factor, such as with bariatric surgery for weight loss. Other times the person receiving the massage has health concerns unrelated to the disability, but they require some sort of accommodation because of the disability. Rather than providing specific protocols, this section discusses ways to accommodate various physical challenges. Impairments are just another factor to be considered in the treatment plan for the individual. Hopefully, by now you have learned that there is no specific massage for any one condition or any population group. Massage for babies needs to accommodate the fact that the patient is a baby. The same holds true for the elderly, and now for those who have visual problems, hearing loss, or require the use of a wheelchair, and so on.

According to the guidelines of the Americans with Disabilities Act, a physical disability or impairment is any physiologic disorder, condition, cosmetic disfigurement, or anatomic loss that affects one or more of the following body systems: neurologic, musculoskeletal, special sense organ, respiratory (including speech organs), cardiovascular, reproductive, digestive, genitourinary, hemic and lymphatic, skin, and endocrine. Extremes in size and extensive burns also may be considered physical impairments.

People with physical impairments can benefit from massage for all the same reasons that any other person can. These individuals often require ongoing medical treatment for rehabilitation and support services to treat illness related to the disability. They may develop compensation patterns in response to the disability. For instance, a person in a wheelchair could have increased neck and shoulder tension from moving the chair. In addition, dealing with a physical impairment can make routine daily functions more stressful. The following are some guidelines that may help the massage therapist provide supportive services for these individuals:

- The massage therapist must never presume to know, understand, or anticipate a person's need for assistance. It is important to ask!
- A concerned massage therapist does not try to pretend that the disability does not exist, but rather responds professionally. After the individual has provided the necessary information about the disability and the accommodation required, the massage therapist should accept the impairment as part of how the person functions and structure the treatment plan to meet the outcomes determined for massage application.
- People with a physical disability often require some sort of accommodation, such as barrier-free access, restroom support, Braille labeling, noninterference with service animals, and so forth. Healthcare facilities typically are equipped with various accommodations necessary to aid patients with these types of challenges.

The following suggestions target the one-on-one interaction that occurs between the massage therapist and the patient during massage.

ACCOMMODATING A VISUAL IMPAIRMENT

Many people with a visual impairment have some type of sight. Comparatively few people have no vision at all. When assisting a patient with a visual impairment, the therapist should never push or pull on the person. Instead, if guiding is necessary, the therapist should stand just in front and a bit to the left of the client, who can then touch the massage therapist's right elbow when following.

Useful directions should also be given to a person with a visual impairment. If asked where something is, the massage therapist should not point and say "over there." Instead, directions such as left, right, about 10 steps, and so on are much easier to follow. It is not necessary to speak more loudly to individuals with a visual impairment; they usually can hear just fine.

The conversation should begin with the massage therapist addressing the person by name so that he or she is aware that the therapist is speaking to them. The therapist then should state his or her name but should not touch the patient until the person is aware of the therapist's presence in the room.

If a person with a visual impairment places anything anywhere, it should not be moved. If a door is opened, the direction of the opening (toward or away from the person) and the location of the hinges (left or right) should be explained. It is best to let the person open the door himself or herself so as to be better oriented to its position.

If a service dog is harnessed and working, be it a guide dog for someone with a visual impairment or any other support service, do not pet, feed, or in other way interact with the dog. This distracts the dog and makes its important job more difficult.

ACCOMMODATING A SPEECH IMPAIRMENT

It may be difficult to understand a person with a speech problem. The massage therapist should ask the person to repeat anything that is unclear until it is understood and then should repeat what was said so that the person can clarify if necessary. If the therapist cannot understand what is being said, the person should be informed of this. If necessary, a notepad can be used to put communication in writing. Although having an accent is not a speech impairment, it can make communication difficult. Not speaking the same language also hinders communication. An interpreter may be necessary.

ACCOMMODATING A HEARING IMPAIRMENT

To gain the attention of a person with a hearing impairment, the therapist should lightly tap the person once on the shoulder or discreetly wave a hand. If no interpreter is present, all talking should be done in a normal tone and rhythm of speech. If an individual can lip read, it is important that the massage therapist always face the person and not cover his or her own mouth when talking. A normal voice tone and speed should be used. If the therapist normally speaks quickly, the speed should be slowed a bit. If necessary, a notepad can be used to put communication in writing.

Hearing aids amplify sound; they do not make sound clearer. Reducing background noise helps the hearing impaired to hear better. With this in mind, it may be wise to ask before using any music during the massage session. Getting too close to a hearing aid can make it squeal, therefore be cautious when massaging near the ears.

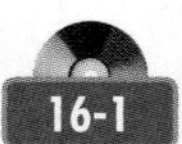

ACCOMMODATING A MOBILITY IMPAIRMENT

There are many types of mobility impairment and many reasons for it. Just because a person is paralyzed does not mean that a particular area has no feeling. Furthermore, just because a person uses a wheelchair does not mean that the person is paralyzed.

When speaking to a person in a wheelchair, it is best to do so from eye level. Looking up strains the individual's neck. The process obviously requires the massage therapist to sit down.

A wheelchair must never be pushed unless the person in the chair gives permission. The individual also will give directions for pushing the wheelchair over barriers.

When a patient is transferred from a wheelchair to the massage table (Figure 16-7), the person can give the best directions on how to proceed. A transfer to a mat on the floor may be easier to accomplish, in which case the massage should be given there. The most efficient transfer is a lateral transfer to a table that is the same height as the wheelchair. If the massage table does not have motorized height adjustment, a shift in body mechanics by the massage therapist is necessary. Many healthcare environments have equipment available that assists in transfers. If necessary, massage can be provided in the chair.

Special care must be taken in giving a massage to a person with paralysis because normal feedback mechanisms may not be functioning. A person who has undergone amputation and uses a prosthesis may or may not want the device removed during the massage. Others readily remove the prosthesis. Ask permission before massaging the amputated area. If the client is comfortable with this, massage can be especially beneficial if a prosthesis is used. Often the outcome goal for the massage is relief of phantom pain, which requires massage at the site of the amputation.

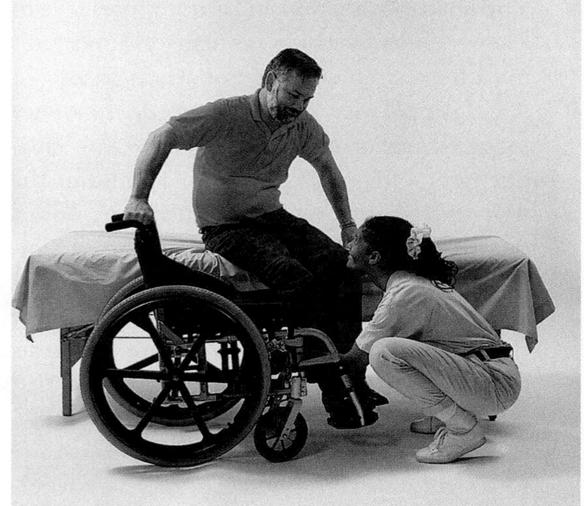
A

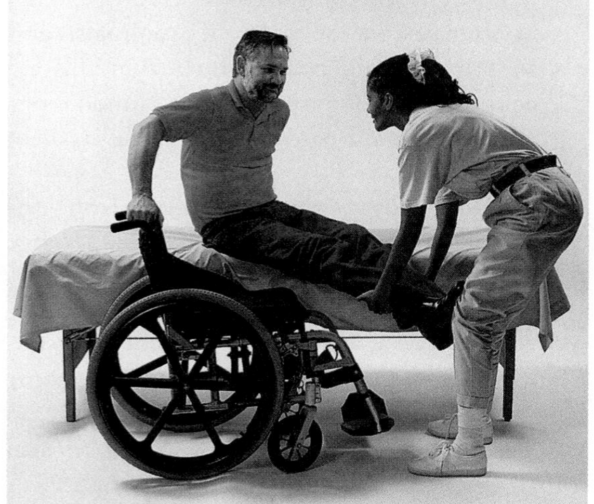
B

FIGURE 16-7 **A,** A transfer from a wheelchair to the massage table. **B,** A low table that allows a lateral transfer is best. (From Fritz S: *Mosby's fundamentals of therapeutic massage*, ed 3, St Louis, 2003, Mosby.)

ACCOMMODATING SIZE REQUIREMENTS

If the person is short, a stool may be needed to help reach the massage table, clothing hangers, or restroom fixtures. The massage professional should casually sit down to establish eye contact with the patient so that the person does not have to look up, which strains the neck.

A very large person may not trust the massage table and may be more comfortable on a floor mat. Getting up and down from the floor may be difficult. Sometimes seated massage is the better option. Ask the patient what is preferable. If the therapist is nervous about doing the massage on the massage table, the patient must be told (disclosure) because the therapist's anxiety will affect the quality of the massage.

ACCOMMODATING BURNS AND DISFIGUREMENTS

People who have been burned may face an assortment of challenges ranging from impaired mobility to disfigurement. As burns heal, scar tissue replaces functional epithelial tissue. All the functions of the skin are compromised, including excretion, sensation, and protection. Scar tissue tends to contract and pull, which can make the area of the healed burn feel shortened or tight and binding. Severe contractures sometimes develop, which are treated medically. Myofascial release and other connective tissue techniques can soften and gently stretch connective tissue. Massage of this type may reduce the effect of this shrinkage somewhat.

Many disfigurements tend to draw our attention because the mind is designed to notice differences. Although most disfigurements do not limit an individual function in any way, they can create social difficulties. Attempting not to notice a disfigurement usually fails. The disfigured person recognizes that the situation exists and has various levels of comfort with the condition. Honest communication is effective in redirecting the attention from the disfigurement to the person over time. The therapist might offer a simple statement such as, "I can't help but notice (the particular disfigurement). I'm not uncomfortable, but the difference naturally draws my attention."

Massage Strategies

It is not possible to describe specific massage strategies for people with physical disabilities. Clinical reasoning is the only method appropriate for determining the best way to provide massage to these individuals. The massage treatment plan depends on the treatment orders, the determined outcomes for the patient, any other medical treatment the patient is receiving, and accommodations that may be necessary for the disability.

JUST BETWEEN YOU AND ME

Plain and simple: We all have to get past our own "stuff." When interacting with a person with a disability, we get nervous. Somewhere in our minds we wonder, "What if this were me?" People with various disabilities and disfigurements know that they have them. They know the rest of us notice. I remember being at a resort and sitting by the pool. A young boy about 8 years old was playing next to me. He had a severe facial disfigurement. Being the enlightened person I am, I chatted with him and pretended not to notice his face. After a bit he said, "My face is different. Do you want to know why?" He then launched into a discussion of his condition. I learned that day that you can't get beyond something if you don't understand it. The unknown is scary. As professionals, it is our responsibility to understand. So, ask questions. If the patient is unable to explain the condition for one reason or another, ask your supervisor.

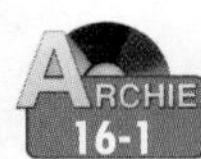

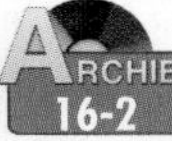

PREGNANCY

Pregnancy is not an illness; it is a natural event. However, it typically is managed in the healthcare environment (Figures 16-8 and 16-9). Early prenatal care provided by qualified healthcare professionals is very important for pregnant women. Prenatal care is needed to ensure that proper nutrition is provided for the mother, that the pregnancy is progressing normally, and to identify any potential problems early. If a woman is planning to become pregnant, she should build up and maintain her health for about 6 months beforehand. This means eliminating all alcohol, drugs, and nicotine; normalizing her weight; developing a moderate exercise program; and eating a nutritious diet. These activities help prepare the best environment for the baby's growth. Smoking, alcohol, and drug use are very dangerous to the unborn child. Excessive stress also is dangerous to the developing infant and can be the cause of miscarriage and inability to conceive. Stress management massage that supports parasympathetic dominance may support conception and is used as part of a couples' infertility treatment.

Pregnancy is divided into three distinct segments: the first, second, and third trimesters. A pregnant woman undergoes extensive physical

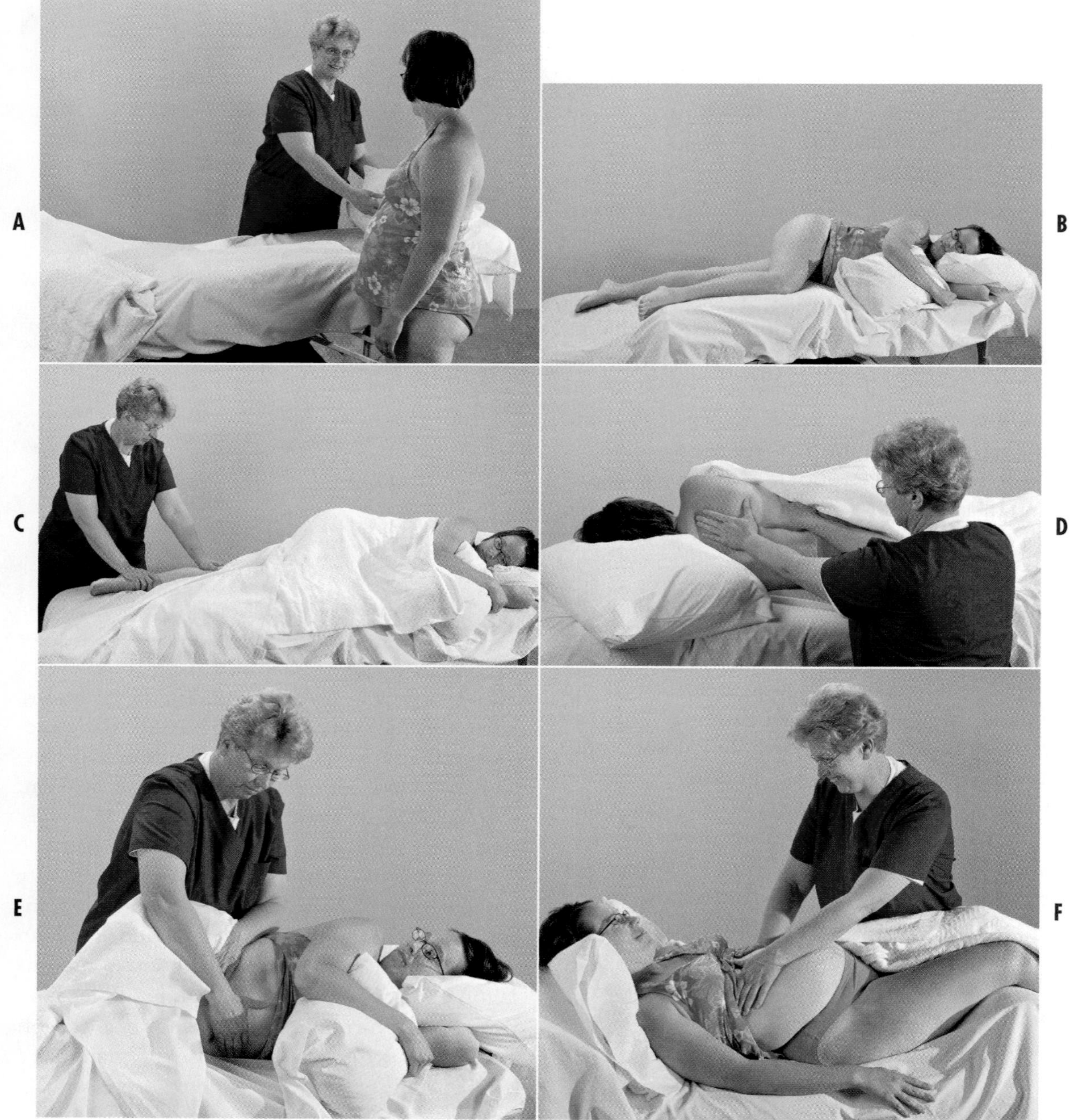

FIGURE 16-8 ■ Prenatal massage. Under most circumstances, pregnancy is a normal condition that results in chemical and postural changes that can be managed with general massage that accommodates the various stages of pregnancy. **A,** Greet the client and explain the cautions and accommodations for prenatal massage. **B,** After the first trimester, the client will be most comfortable in the side-lying position with appropriate bolstering. **C,** Use the palliative protocol (see the Appendix) as the basic approach. Include lymphatic drainage if edema is present, and use methods to relax muscles that are achy because of postural change. Always be alert for signs and symptoms indicating that the patient should be referred to a physician. **D,** Massage of the back is very beneficial. **E,** Massage of the abdomen is appropriate as long as it is gentle. **F,** Breathing can be affected during the third trimester, and gentle massage to the thorax is helpful.

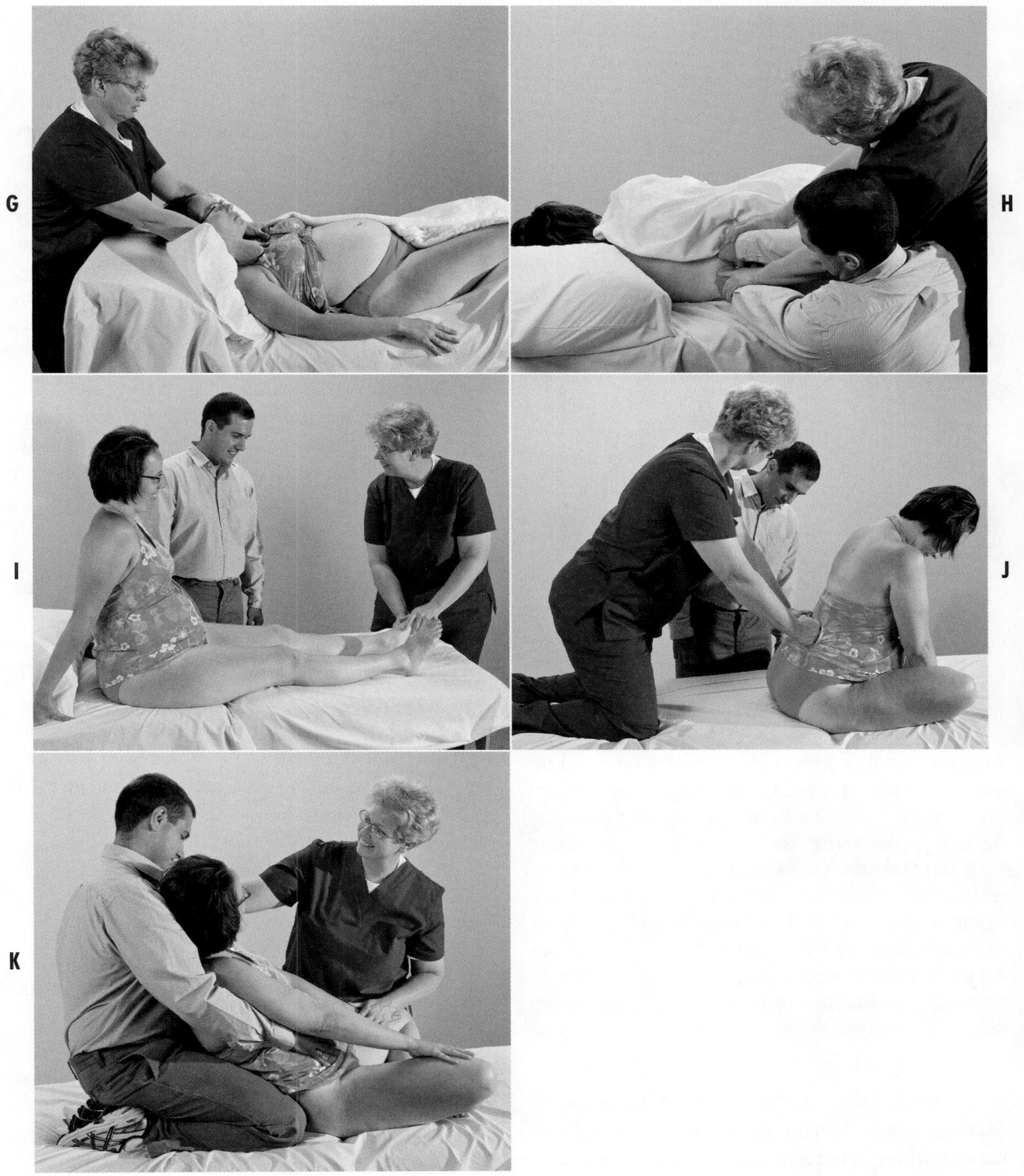

FIGURE 16-8, cont'd ■ **G,** Massage of the patient in the supine position must be limited in the third trimester; the side-lying position is preferred. **H,** Teach the partner the massage methods. **I,** Foot massage is excellent during pregnancy. **J,** Demonstrate methods for use during labor. **K,** Support the bonding process.

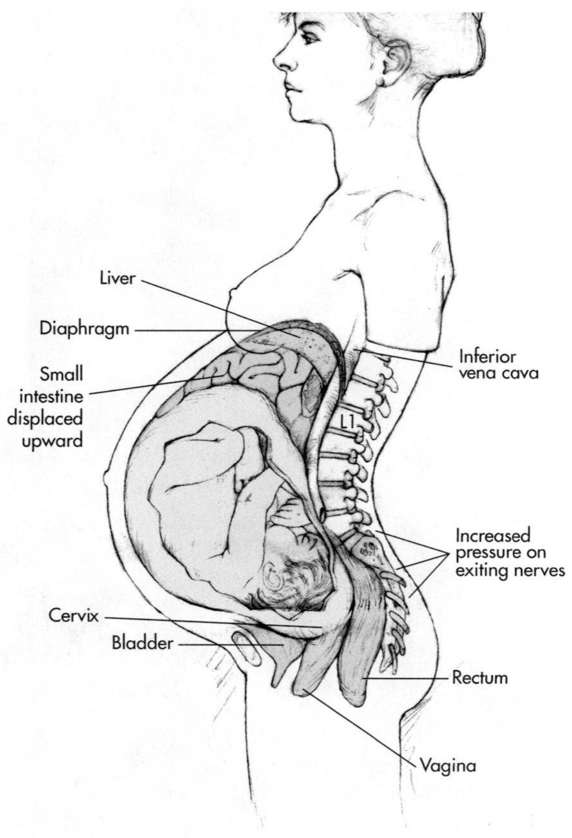

FIGURE 16-9 ■ A fetus in utero. Note the degree to which the pregnant uterus displaces other abdominopelvic structures and puts pressure on important regions such as the pelvic diaphragm and the respiratory diaphragm. Venous return from pelvic and lower limb structures is more difficult because of pressure on the inferior vena cava, and women commonly develop hemorrhoids and varicose veins in the lower limbs. Breathing may be difficult because of pressure on the diaphragm and the inability to depress it fully to permit filling of the lungs. Back and lower limb pain is common because of pressure on the nerves that exit the lumbar and sacral plexuses. (From Mathers LH et al: *Clinical anatomy principles*, St Louis, 1995, Mosby.)

and emotional changes during each of these stages. Massage is appropriate during all stages of pregnancy and is altered as necessary to accommodate the comfort of the mother to be. The assumption in this section is that the pregnancy is planned and desired, but remember, this is not always the case. Unplanned pregnancy can be very stressful.

THE FIRST TRIMESTER

Massage given during the first trimester is general wellness massage, which may help balance the mother's physiologic responses to the pregnancy. During the first 3 months (the first trimester), the woman's body must adjust to tremendous hormonal changes, which are likely to cause physical symptoms and mood swings. This is also a very vulnerable time for the developing baby. Positioning during the massage is not a concern unless the breasts are tender. Deep massage work on the abdomen is avoided so as not to disrupt the attachment of the baby to the uterine wall. Surface stroking can be pleasurable to the client. A number of symptoms are common during the first trimester.

- Nausea, or the sensation of feeling sick, and vomiting are commonly referred to as *morning sickness.* Morning sickness tends to be most severe in the early morning but can occur in the evening and may last all day and night. Symptoms usually diminish by the tenth week of pregnancy and usually are gone by the end of 14 weeks. Only rarely do they last through the entire pregnancy.
- Frequent urination is common because of the presence of the hormone progesterone, which causes relaxation of the smooth muscle of the bladder. This tendency usually declines by the second trimester.
- Constipation is common, and again the hormone progesterone is responsible. It causes relaxation of the smooth muscle of the large intestine, which slows the movement of fecal matter through the system and increases the absorption of water from the colon. Constipation may continue throughout pregnancy. Mechanical pressure from the enlarging uterus contributes to the problem.
- Blood pressure often falls in early pregnancy, specifically the diastolic pressure. This is also due to the presence of progesterone, which relaxes the muscular wall of the blood vessels. The mother to be may be fatigued and feel lightheaded or faint, especially during prolonged standing. Blood pressure usually returns to normal during the fourteenth week of pregnancy.
- Breast changes begin during this stage. There is a sense of increased fullness and some tenderness and heightened sensitivity, which may continue throughout the pregnancy.

- Musculoskeletal changes result from the influence of estrogen, progesterone, and relaxin. Relaxin is produced as early as 2 weeks into the pregnancy and is at its highest levels in the first trimester; it then falls 20% and remains at that level until labor. Relaxin affects the composition of collagen in the joint capsules, ligaments, and fascia, allowing greater elasticity. This enables more movement in the joints and creates more room in the abdomen. Although all the joints are affected, the most vulnerable ones are those of the pelvis (e.g., the symphysis pubis and the sacroiliac [SI] joint) and those that bear weight (e.g., the ankle and the joints of the foot). Massage application should avoid excessive stretching.
- Taste and smell are altered in the early stages of the pregnancy. Certain smells and food become disagreeable to the woman. Avoid using scented massage lubricants and essential oils.

THE SECOND TRIMESTER

The second trimester usually brings a leveling of the hormones, and the woman feels better. During this time she may start to "show" and feel the first movements of the baby. If the pregnancy was planned, this is a joyful time. If not, the physical evidence of the growing baby may cause additional stress for the mother. The following symptoms are common during the second trimester:

- Toward the end of the second trimester, the connective tissue, under the influence of relaxin, begins to soften to allow the pelvis to spread.
- The joints seem to become sloppy. The muscles of the legs, gluteals, and hip flexors must provide joint stabilization, and tension and pain can develop. Overstretching of tissue during massage must be avoided.
- Carpal tunnel syndrome caused by fluid retention is common among pregnant women and may be perpetuated even after the birth as a result of caring for the infant. Localized lymphatic drainage may temporarily help.
- Edema is common at any time during the pregnancy because of the retention of fluid. As the pregnancy advances, edema of the legs occurs in up to 40% of women. The mechanical obstruction created by the uterus and its contents causes an increase in venous pressure distally, which results in edema. Lymphatic drainage massage should be applied cautiously. The woman's body is having trouble maintaining fluid distribution, and mechanical methods, such as lymphatic drainage, may increase the strain on the system. Full body lymphatic drainage should be avoided. Limited use of these methods on targeted areas, such as the ankles, may reduce discomfort from fluid pressure.

  Excessive edema may indicate **pre-eclampsia**, a very serious complication that requires medical attention. The diagnosis of pre-eclampsia is made when blood pressure increases, generalized edema is present, and high concentrations of protein are found in the urine. Some common elements that may predispose a woman to pre-eclampsia are:
  - First pregnancy
  - Multiple pregnancy
  - Chronic or long-term hypertension
  - Chronic renal disease
  - Malnutrition
  - Diabetes
- Supine hypotension occurs as the fetus grows and compresses the aorta and inferior vena cava against the lumbar spine. This may cause the woman to feel faint when she is lying on her back. Massage is best provided in the side-lying position with bolstering.
- Shortness of breath is also common. This is due to the combination of mechanical change in the thorax, the position of the diaphragm, and physiologic changes.

When providing massage, support for the abdomen is important. The side-lying position is most comfortable, and lying on the left side produces the least amount of abdominal congestion from the expanding uterus. There is little need to be extensively concerned with position as long as the expectant mother is comfortable.

Be attentive for strain in the back muscles during positioning. Keep the head in alignment with the spine. Using a support so that the shoulder lies comfortably and does not fall forward or toward the ear is helpful. Support between the knees helps keep the hips in the neutral position and relieves stress in this area. A support under the top arm may also be comfortable. Allow the client to change position often. As in the first trimester, deep work on the abdomen must be avoided.

THE THIRD TRIMESTER

During the last (third) trimester, the weight of the growing baby, the postural shifts, and the movement of the internal organs may cause discomfort for the pregnant woman. Because many of the internal organs are pushed up and back, the diaphragm does not work as efficiently. The mother uses her neck and shoulder muscles to breathe, possibly causing discomfort or thoracic outlet symptoms. Breathing pattern disorder may develop. Massage offers temporary relief of these symptoms.

About 2 weeks before birth (in the first pregnancy), the baby turns head down and drops into the birth canal. This provides more space for the diaphragm to work and breathing becomes easier, but pressure on the bladder causes frequent urination. Impingement on lymph vessels may cause the legs and feet to swell. Edema or fluid accumulation may be a symptom of more serious complications, and the client should be referred to a physician immediately if these are noted. Low back ache may develop as a result of the postural shift. The breasts have enlarged in preparation for lactation. A woman may not feel very attractive at this point and most likely is not very comfortable physically. Fatigue and sleep disturbances may result.

Massage is gentle, supports comfort, and assists circulation. If a comfortable position cannot be found, allow the client to change position often and use the restroom as needed. General massage may help the woman feel better for a little while and support comfortable sleep.

LABOR

Labor occurs as the baby moves down the birth canal. Education and birthing classes are important, especially for first pregnancies. It may be appropriate to teach the woman's support person some massage techniques before the onset of labor. Massage given by the support person helps that person to feel useful and involved with the pregnancy and birthing process. Massage of the lower back and stroking of the abdomen may provide comfort and a point of focus during labor. Massaging the feet often is helpful. Massage can relax the body and divert the attention of the nervous system, thereby providing distraction during early labor. Labor proceeds easier and faster if the woman is relaxed and works with her body.

During a phase of labor called *transition*, women frequently do not want to be touched. Transition occurs just before the second stage of labor, with the actual movement of the baby down the birth canal. The contractions at this time are very hard and have not yet been replaced by the urge to push. After delivery, massage may help the woman's body return to normal, may reduce the stress of taking care of a new baby, and may give the client some time to take care of herself.

DISORDERS OF PREGNANCY

Although pregnancy and delivery are considered normal physiologic functions, problems can occur. Early recognition and referral are important. Warning signs of a pregnancy at risk require immediate referral. Some of these warning signs include the following:

- Vaginal bleeding
- Severe, continuous abdominal pain
- Breaking of water or rupture of membranes
- Pre-eclampsia, edema, dizziness, elevated blood pressure, severe headache
- Fever and frequent, painful urination, which can indicate a urinary tract infection
- Excessive vomiting of such severity and frequency that no food or fluids can be retained
- Excessive itching, which may suggest liver or kidney dysfunction

Postpartum Depression

Postpartum major depression occurs in as many as 1 in 10 childbearing women. This condition is serious, and a healthcare physician should treat the individual. This depression often goes undiagnosed. The tendency to depression occurs because of hormonal changes, stress from the pregnancy and birth, lack of sleep, caregiver's stress, lack of support, and many other factors. Solid evidence is mounting that maternal depression is not good for babies' development. Babies do not learn as well when they listen to the flatter, less melodic voices of depressed women. Adults' perky, high-pitched baby talk sets the stage for intellectual development.

When possible, the depression is best treated with both medical and mental healthcare, sleep, exercise, bright light, upbeat music, appropriate vitamin or mineral replacement, and healthy food. Massage can also be an effective aspect of treatment. Exercise is particularly difficult in the postpartum period; both time and energy often are lacking. However, exercise has been proven to help specifically with postpartum depression. One hour of aerobic exercise daily can be as powerful as even the strongest antidepressant medications. Even 10 minutes a day can make a noticeable difference.

An hour of quiet rest with no responsibilities can significantly improve the depression symptoms. If treatment of the depression without medicines does not produce satisfactory results, it is important that antidepressant medicines be used.

Massage Strategies

Unless specific circumstances or complications are involved, massage for pregnant women should be a general massage. Do not massage vigorously or extremely deeply, do not overstretch, and do not massage the abdomen other than with superficial stroking. Avoid massage on the inside of the ankle, because a reflex point in that area may stimulate uterine contractions (this area is located on the spleen meridian). Watch for fever, edema, varicose veins, and severe mood swings. Teach the partner to do massage. After birth, postpartum depression can become a serious problem for some women. Refer a client with these conditions to her physician immediately.

Massage has been shown to be effective as part of a total treatment program for postpartum depression. General relaxation massage with a focus on breathing function is the typical massage approach. If the symptoms change, refer the patient immediately. Early intervention is necessary to protect both the mother and infant.

At times pregnancy is not a joyous event, as in an unwanted pregnancy. The practitioner must not try to convince the woman that she really does want the baby or try to change her mood. She must be supported with caring, quiet touch and listening.

Interrupted pregnancies also are difficult. Whether the cause is spontaneous abortion in the first 3 months, induced abortion, or miscarriage, an interrupted pregnancy is a strain on a woman's body and emotional well-being. If a client has had an interrupted pregnancy, watch for emotional changes at what would have been the projected time of birth. Extra caring and support are helpful then.

TERMINAL ILLNESS/END-OF-LIFE CARE

One of the most challenging aspects of the massage therapist's practice is caring for dying patients and their families. Most healthcare professionals are not prepared to handle the emotional stress of dealing with a patient who is going to die. Questions about our personal views on life and death may emerge, and we must deal with our own issues about mortality before we can help someone else.

THE PROCESS OF DYING

It is well recognized that most people in Western society have been poorly socialized about death and dying. Death education is rarely incorporated into the curricula of elementary or secondary school programs and is infrequently introduced in the home environment. Unless adults have made specific efforts to discuss death and dying with young people during childhood or adolescence, children develop strong fears about death that they carry into adulthood.

Patients who are dying and their families often feel that healthcare providers "avoid' or "abandon" them during the dying process. This may be true, and it may reflect the response of healthcare professionals to fears and anxieties about their own mortality. You have an obligation to examine your attitudes and feelings about death and dying carefully before providing massage for those who are dying. If you can care for these people in an empathic way and with respect, what a gift massage can be for those who feel isolated and abandoned.

THE STAGES OF DEATH AND DYING

Elisabeth Kübler-Ross interviewed patients with terminal illnesses over $2^1/_2$ years. She described her experiences in her book, *On Death and Dying*, which was published in 1969. It was the first publication that specifically addressed the need to talk with people who were dying in order to learn more about their feelings. The book also identified specific emotional phases, or "stages," that the individuals she interviewed experienced during the dying process. The commonality of these stages does not negate the uniqueness of death for each individual. People do not necessarily experience each stage, nor do they necessarily proceed in the order presented here.

Denial and Isolation

When people discover that they have a terminal illness, they respond to the news with a statement of denial, "It can't be true." The lack of realization that this could be happening to them may be so intense that they deny treatment suggestions and, in fact, seek other healthcare providers to support their denial. This is a time of adjustment. They must acknowledge that their condition is terminal. Over time, people begin to realize that the diagnosis is accurate and may seek to retreat from the world. They are uncertain with whom they want to share the information, and sometimes they try to protect their loved ones by sheltering them from knowing about the terminal illness.

Anger

As people begin to realize that the illness is terminal and that they have a limited amount of time to live, they often express anger and resentment. A frequently asked question is, "Why me?" The anger is directed at many different targets, and people can be angry with their healthcare providers about the lack of medical treatment to cure the disease. They express feelings of frustration and even jealousy toward their friends and family, who will go on living after they have died. Individuals may also have angry feelings toward God for "allowing" them to die. Family members and healthcare providers find it difficult to be with a dying patient in this stage, because the person may be aggressive or defiant. The dying person also is frustrated by the perceived loss of control over his or her life.

Bargaining

Bargaining occurs when a person realizes that the condition is terminal and that the hope for cure is not a viable one. Therefore, they hope for more time. This state is an attempt to prolong the inevitable death and to eliminate or reduce the pain and physical suffering they may be experiencing. An aspect of bargaining most often shown during this stage is the promise of good behavior for a reward of more time for a specific reason, such as to attend a special event or to experience an important milestone. It is not always clear with whom the person is bargaining. Sometimes the person bargains with the healthcare providers and other times with God.

Depression

As the disease progresses, the person becomes more acutely aware that the condition is terminal. He or she can no longer deny that the illness is life threatening and that life, as the person has known it, will change. Physical discomfort becomes more pronounced, and fatigue and weakness limit daily activities. In addition, the person may be undergoing treatments that have debilitating adverse effects, such as nausea and vomiting. The individual also may feel uncomfortable with the physical appearance; he or she may have lost weight and hair and may have undergone skin changes. A combination of the physical and mental stresses the illness has caused leaves the person feeling tired and depressed.

People become depressed about losing or "leaving behind" people and pets they love. They and their loved ones experience anticipatory grief as they begin to acknowledge that death is approaching. Often, at this stage the person begins to detach himself or herself from significant others as part of this process. With the realization that time no longer is unlimited, the dying person is forced to reflect on what he or she wishes they had done "but never got around to." Although everyone acknowledges cognitively that death is inevitable, most people believe they have plenty of time to do what they desire. Depression stems from the realization that their time to die is approaching and they have yet to live their lives.

Acceptance

In the final stage described by Kübler-Ross, the individual comes to accept the fact of dying. Although this is not a happy time, the person often has a sense of peace and contentment and may feel a need to organize personal affairs. The person attends to financial concerns, especially those related to beneficiaries, and to funeral arrangements. Often a shift of energy occurs, from seeking curative medical treatments to making plans for the family's future security.

This is also a time to complete "unfinished business." Dying people may reflect on their lives with their loved ones as they recall events they shared. Good-byes, spoken and unspoken, occur.

The massage therapist does not need to fix any of the situations that occur as a result of the dying process. Just give the massage. It is enough.

JUST BETWEEN YOU AND ME

This is tough stuff. But you know what? We're all going to die. That said, when working with people who are dying, don't get confused: they are dying, not you. It's not about you yet; it's about them.

HOSPICE CARE

When nothing further can be done to prolong life, care focuses more on comfort measures; this is **hospice care**. The experts in terminal illness are the dedicated hospice physician, nurses, and staff members who treat death with dignity. It has been said that the staff members of hospices are midwives to the dying.

Dramatic advances in medical care over the past century have had the unintentional side effect of redefining death. Instead of being the natural culmination of life, it now is an unwanted outcome of disease and a failure of medical intervention. A century ago, most Americans died in their homes. Nowadays, of the 2 million deaths that occur in the United States each year, more than 80% occur in a healthcare institution (65% in hospitals and 15% in nursing homes). The causes of death have also changed over the past 100 years. In 1900, 5 of the 10 leading causes of death in the geriatric population were infectious diseases; in 1995, only pneumonia and influenza remained in the top 10.

Our enhanced ability to successfully manage and significantly extend life for patients with chronic disease such as diabetes, congestive heart failure, coronary artery disease, and renal failure and to successfully treat previously fatal diseases such as cancer, bacterial infections, and tuberculosis has complicated the natural process of dying. Individuals and healthcare providers regard prolonging life and curing disease as the fundamental goals of modern medicine. Somewhere in the quest for life, we have forgotten how to die.

Providing for a peaceful death is an important medical concern. Caring for those who are dying is not easy. It requires the ability to address and balance the needs of the individual, the family, and the support system; the ability to communicate about intimate and spiritual issues; expertise in pain and symptom management; and the ability to coordinate and function within an interdisciplinary team. A fundamental requirement is the willingness to come to grips with our own mortality and the mortality of those we love. Massage is an extremely valuable part of end-of-life care provided by hospice. This section addresses some of these issues.

As defined by the World Health Organization, **palliative care** is the active total care of people whose disease is not responsive to curative treatment. Comprehensive palliative care plans include control of pain and other distressful symptoms, as well as psychological, social, and spiritual support. The current disease model for palliative care traditionally has been cancer, but palliation is also appropriate for people with other chronic illnesses such as congestive heart failure, COPD, renal failure, and degenerative neurologic conditions such as Alzheimer's disease, amyotrophic lateral sclerosis, and Parkinson's disease.

Hospice is not a place but a special concept of care designed to provide comfort and support to those who are dying and their families when a life-limiting illness no longer responds to cure-oriented treatments. The word hospice derives from the same linguistic root as *hospital* and *hospitality*. The term goes back to medieval times, when it described a place of shelter and rest for weary travelers on long journeys. It was first used to describe specialized care for terminally ill patients in 1967, when the modern hospice movement began in England. Today the term *hospice* refers to a steadily growing concept of humane and compassionate care. Hospice care neither prolongs life nor hastens death. Hospice staff and volunteers offer a specialized knowledge of medical care and address all symptoms of a disease, with a special emphasis on controlling pain and discomfort. In addition, hospice care deals with the emotional, social, and spiritual impact of the disease on the person and the family and friends, and it offers a variety of bereavement and counseling services to families before and after death. Hospice services are available to people of any age, religion, race, or illness.

JUST BETWEEN YOU AND ME

One of the clinical outreach programs available to my students involves a residential hospice. A student was scheduled to provide massage for a gentleman who that day was restless and agitated. In previous sessions he had very much enjoyed having his feet massaged, so this is what the student began to do. In a few minutes the gentleman began to calm down and became very peaceful. The student finished the foot massage and, because the man was sleeping quietly, left the room and reported to the hospice nurse that the client was resting quietly. The nurse went back to the room with the student to check on the client. She then gently told the student that the man must have died quietly while she was massaging his feet. What a gift these two people, a dying elderly man and a young student, gave each other! This is one of the most touching stories I know about the gift of massage.

Hospice provides interdisciplinary team care (physicians; nurses; social workers; home health aides; clergy and spiritual advisors; speech, language, occupational, and physical therapists; massage therapists; and volunteers to help dying patients, primarily in the home). Some hospices are located in long-term care facilities and residential programs. Hospice care is covered under Medicare, Medicaid, most private insurance plans, health maintenance organizations (HMOs), and other managed care programs.

SYMPTOM MANAGEMENT FOR END-OF-LIFE CONDITIONS

Physical Pain

Severe, chronic pain seldom occurs alone; rather, it usually is accompanied by a number of other symptoms, including anxiety, depression, fearfulness, insomnia, anorexia (loss of appetite), withdrawal, and thoughts of suicide. All these symptoms are compounded by memories of pain already experienced, currently perceived pain, and anticipation of pain yet to come. Unmanaged or inadequately managed severe, chronic pain is a complex problem that needlessly aggravates the symptoms of the underlying disease.

Pain can be relieved safely without any danger of death or addiction. Hospice caregivers and most doctors are familiar with the proper use of analgesic drugs. When these drugs are given in the correct dosage at the right time, pain can be relieved without sedating the person. Good pain management does not shorten the course of life. Some types of pain require multimodality approaches to pain relief. Recent advances in pain management ensure that pain can be relieved by using commonly available medications and/or a combination of approaches that may include chemotherapy, radiation therapy, nerve block, physical therapies, including massage, and other complementary methods.

If pain is not relieved by the lesser-strength analgesics (e.g., aspirin, nonsteroidal antiinflammatory drugs [NSAIDs], codeine, and hydrocodone), it is best to change to a stronger analgesic to bring the pain under continuing (24 hour) control. Pain that is only partly or occasionally controlled tends to increase in severity. In most cases, an adequate dose of a stronger analgesic (e.g., morphine) prescribed on a regular basis brings the pain under control.

When morphine and other opioid analgesics are prescribed for the management of pain, the dosage sometimes is raised to make sure that pain is well controlled 24 hours a day, 7 days a week. Opioids given to relieve pain generally do not lead to the development of tolerance. As a disease (such as cancer) progresses, more opioid may be needed to control the pain on a continuing basis. Once pain is under control and the dose of opioid analgesic holds steady for several days, the dosage sometimes can be lowered without the pain recurring. Levels of opioid can be raised safely as needed to control increasing pain. This change in dosage to meet individual needs is known as **titration.** The fact that the dosage of opioid can be lowered once pain is controlled is one of the paradoxes of treating severe, chronic pain.

Several excellent, long-acting opioid analgesics are available. Morphine and related opioids can control pain for 24 hours when given on a regular basis twice daily. Other long-acting opioid preparations that offer transdermal (through the skin) delivery are available with a 72-hour (3-day) period of action.

When opioids are prescribed on a regular basis at a dosage sufficient to relieve pain, no empirically based evidence indicates that they lead to addiction. When they are prescribed to manage severe, chronic pain, there is no problem discontinuing the drug once pain is under control. Withdrawal from an opioid analgesic is not a life-threatening condition, unlike withdrawal from a number of other commonly prescribed medications, such as barbiturates. The symptoms of withdrawal from opioids generally are mild and fairly easy to manage with commonly available medications.

Morphine does not initiate the final phase of life or lead directly to death. Morphine provides not only relief of severe, chronic pain, it also provides a sense of comfort. It makes breathing easier. It lets the patient relax and sleep. It does not cloud consciousness or lead to death. Morphine does not kill, and it effectively reduces suffering.

Mouth Care

Dry mouth and lips are a common consequence of diminished fluid intake and medications. Lip lubricants, lemon glycerin swabs, and artificial saliva are helpful. Sips of water and ice chips also may be helpful.

Anorexia

Loss of appetite is very common in dying people and may not require intervention if the individual is near death and does not express a desire to eat. Earlier in the course of a serious illness, improved appetite and nutrition may contribute to energy levels, well-being, and functional capacity. Patients should be encouraged to eat whatever is most appealing without regard to fat, sugar, and salt restrictions if possible. If they don't want to eat, don't force them.

Elimination/Constipation

Elimination problems in the dying can be handled in a variety of ways.

- Various laxatives and stool softeners can be used to treat constipation.
- Diarrhea often is due to fecal impaction or antibiotic-associated colitis. It is a particularly distressing and exhausting symptom in the terminally ill. Once common causes have been ruled out, kaolin-pectin or psyllium may be effective at reducing diarrhea. Loperamide or tincture of opium may be used if these measures fail.
- The differential diagnosis of urinary incontinence in the terminally ill includes functional incontinence, overflow incontinence due to fecal impaction or other source of obstruction, vaginal atrophy, infection, and spinal cord or neurological disease. A urethral catheter may be necessary for patient comfort and to ease the burden of personal care tasks for the caregivers.

Psychiatric Symptoms

Some common psychiatric problems that occur with dying include the following:

- Depression: Studies have shown that most terminally ill patients with a serious desire to die have a co-existing and untreated major depression. A trial of antidepressant therapy and a psychiatric consultation are appropriate treatment measures.
- Anxiety: Anxiety secondary to pain or dyspnea can be managed by treating the underlying symptom, but persistent anxiety often is a manifestation of depression. Antidepressants and benzodiazepines with a short half-life are appropriate initial steps in management. *Dyspnea* refers to the subjective symptom of breathlessness. A cool breeze on the face from an open window or a fan may reduce dyspnea. Anxiety heightens dyspnea, and relief of anxiety is very important in its management. Oxygen may help relieve anxiety as well as relieving dyspnea directly. Sedatives, including benzodiazepines or barbiturates, may be prescribed. Opioids are effective for managing dyspnea caused by a variety of factors. Frequent reassurance and companionship are very important.

SIGNS OF APPROACHING DEATH

This section presents a general description of what is expected when death is near. What actually occurs varies greatly, depending on the cause of death, the person's general health, medications used, and any other significant factors.

- The most obvious sign of impending death is a generalized decrease in activity and diminished interest in food and water.
- Body temperature drops by a degree or more.
- The blood pressure begins to fall gradually.
- Circulation to the extremities declines, and the hands and feet begin to feel cool compared to the rest of the body.
- Breathing changes from a normal rate and rhythm to a new pattern of several rapid exchanges of air followed by a period of no respiration (Cheyne-Stokes respirations).
- Skin color changes from normal to a duller, darker, grayish hue.
- The fingernail beds acquire a blue tinge.
- The person stops responding to questions and no longer speaks spontaneously.
- The person may fall into a coma, which may last from minutes to hours before death occurs. A person in a coma may still hear what is said even if he or she no longer seems to respond to verbal or even painful stimuli. Those who are nearby should always behave as if the person is aware of what is going on and is able to hear and understand.

BEREAVEMENT

Bereavement is the process of grieving. The experience of loss and separation begins well before the actual death of the patient, and the health professional can contribute a great deal toward an effective bereavement process. The opportunity to provide direct care to the dying person is an important means of expressing love and connection; overzealous delivery of professional services can take this role away from loved ones, who may begin to worry about their own lack of expertise. Family members can be taught simple, comforting massage application. They may need to be encouraged to say good-bye, to try to think of the things they want to be sure to have said, and to make an opportunity to say them. This process should occur even if the patient is unresponsive or unable to speak, because often the loved one seems to understand the tone of the words or the meaning of a touch or embrace. Families should be given information about what the actual death may be like and what various signs and symptoms mean. The time immediately after death is a shock no matter how anticipated the event, and families need privacy and quiet time together without undue staff intrusion.

Respectful treatment of the body, with attention paid to cultural norms and rituals, and allowing family members to participate in washing and dressing the body may all contribute to initiation of a healthy grieving process.

Grieving

Loss and the grief that follows it are recognized as causal factors for distress, depression, and disease. No one is ever fully prepared to lose a loved one.

Most recognize the importance of grieving for family and friends after the death of a loved one. Healthcare providers grieve as well. The intimate nature of compassionate care creates emotional bonds, yet support for healthcare providers to help them grieve is almost nonexistent. As more massage therapists work with people at the end of their physical life, it is important for us to not only appreciate grief in others, but also learn how to grieve ourselves.

Grieving is painful, physically and emotionally. Grieving individuals experience a roller coaster of emotions; one day they feel okay, and the next day they are overwhelmed with sadness. The grieving process is different for everyone. Although it often seems endless, it gets easier with time. Grieving is a natural response to loss, and done well, it results in healing. Grief is the normal response of sorrow, emotion, and confusion that comes from losing someone or something important. It is a natural part of life. Grief is a typical reaction to death, divorce, job loss, a move away from family and friends, or loss of good health as a result of illness. Grieving is a normal process; depression is an illness. Depression is more than a feeling of grief after losing someone or something beloved. Clinical depression is a whole body disorder.

Individuals who are not dealing effectively with loss and who are suffering from grief can begin to heal when they familiarize themselves with the symptoms of grief and commit to the essential steps of the healing process. The stages of grief are denial, anger, bargaining, depression, acceptance, and hope for the future. On average, it takes 18 to 24 months to go through all these stages. However, grief lasts as long as it takes to accept and to learn to live with the loss. For some people, grief lasts a few months. For others, grieving may take years. The length of time spent grieving is different for each person. There are many reasons for the differences, including personality, health, coping style, culture, family background, and life experiences. The time spent grieving also depends on the relationship with the person lost and if there was time to prepare for the loss.

Grief does not occur just with the death of a loved one (including pets). These reactions also occur with the loss of a living situation (house to apartment or care facility) or sometimes even with retirement. Even if retirement has been something a person has been anticipating with gladness, the transition can be somewhat difficult. Grieving saps a tremendous amount of emotional and physical strength. As soon as feasible, grieving individuals should get active in something they really enjoy. They might develop a new interest or hobby.

Bereavement has been shown to pose significant health risks, ranging all the way from immune system disorders to sudden death and increased death rates from all causes. Immune system disorders associated with bereavement include a lower activity level of lymphocytes, diminished natural killer cell activity, and feeble T-cell strength, among others. Corticosteroid levels increase significantly, causing immune system sluggishness. Decreased antibody response increases the person's susceptibility to all kinds of illnesses.

The Grieving Process. Although everyone's grieving process is different, there are basic emotions that most people experience. The first emotion, shock, usually accompanies the news of a death. An individual may go numb or be unable to comprehend what is happening. A person in shock may practice everyday tasks but is unable to feel anything. Denial typically follows shock. Even though a person knows the loved one is gone, he or she may not be able to accept the truth.

As soon as people accept the death of a loved one, they often develop feelings of guilt. They either become upset over their last interaction with the loved one or they wish they could have done something to prolong the loved one's life. Sadness inevitably follows guilt and may last for a week, a month, or even years. During this stage, individuals may feel alone and experience frequent crying episodes.

Eventually grieving people begin to move forward and brace themselves for life without the loved one. Acceptance is the first clear sign of healing and is usually accompanied by a positive attitude toward life. From this point on, individuals remain in a state of growth, where they learn to turn their loss into something meaningful (Box 16-5).

BOX 16-5 Physical Symptoms of Grief

- Sleeplessness
- Dizziness
- General malaise
- Upset stomach
- Heaviness in the chest
- Loss of appetite
- Mood swings
- Assuming the loved one's mannerisms
- Inability to finish simple jobs
- Need to take care of others
- Need to repeat memories of the loved one
- Feeling the loved one's presence
- Unexpected crying spells

Each person who experiences a death or other loss needs to achieve the following:

1. Accept the loss
2. Feel the physical and emotional pain of grief
3. Adjust to living in a world that is different
4. Move on with life

The following tips can help a person protect the immune system during the grieving process:

- Get plenty of rest and maintain a normal sleep pattern at night.
- Eat a balanced diet.
- Get plenty of fluids but avoid those that contain alcohol or caffeine. Both alcohol and caffeine increase dehydration.
- Exercise regularly. Walking is one of the best exercises.
- Maintain a social support system.
- Make use of professional services, such as the doctor, psychologist, and massage therapist.

MASSAGE IN THE HOSPICE SETTING

To work successfully with people dealing with a terminal illness, massage therapists must be aware of their personal feelings about death. Every massage professional who wants to work with clients during this very important, challenging, and special time of life should become a hospice volunteer and take specialized hospice training.

No one knows when a person is going to die. However, two very powerful psychological forces influence living and dying: hope and the will to live. Attitudes about death vary. Adults usually have more fears about death than children do. They fear pain, suffering, dying alone, the invasion of privacy, loneliness, and separation from family and loved ones. They worry about who will care for and support those left behind. Elderly people usually have fewer of these fears than younger adults. They may be more accepting that death will occur and have had more experience with death and dying. Many have lost family members and friends. Some welcome death as freedom from pain, suffering, and disability.

Massage has much to offer in comfort measures for the terminally ill. Being bedridden and immobile is painful. Massage can distract the sensory perception and provide temporary comfort measures. It provides continued human contact.

Massage can become an important stress reduction method and a means of support for family members and caregivers. Caring for someone who is terminally ill can be very stressful. This support person may need to receive massage simply to have someone take care of him or her for an hour. Teaching simple massage methods to caregivers provides them with a means of meaningful and structured interaction with their loved one, as well as a means of connecting with and supporting each other.

The massage professional should be an integral part of the team that works to make this time of passage as gentle as possible. This means that once the decision to work with someone who is terminally ill has been made, it is important to stay with the process until the client dies, if possible. The massage therapist probably will grow to care for the person and will mourn and grieve when death comes.

As always, it remains the client's choice as to what is wanted, and he or she must give informed consent. The individual who is dying needs to retain as much personal empowerment as possible. It should not be discouraging if all that is done during a massage session is to stroke the person's hands.

JUST BETWEEN YOU AND ME

I was proofreading draft material for this chapter while lying in the emergency department getting checked out for cardiac issues related to some chest pain and other symptoms. How synchronistic with my own reality at the time was that information about aging and physical disability, mental health, and end-of-life care. Life is just so interesting!

While I was tucked away in a corner of the ER, hooked up to various monitors, I heard a new baby's cry and saw the anguish on the parents' faces because something was wrong. An emergency medical team brought in a victim of a car accident who had either a head or spinal cord injury, from what could be observed and heard. A gentleman with an irregular heartbeat was in the same room as me, and (likely from stress) his wife complained about everything. Some people do that when stressed. The staff forgot to feed me; they apologized and said that they were dealing with two critical cases, and I believed them.

The ER doctor was so young—at least it seemed that way to me—but he checked on me and explained what was going on, and he did a good job. I overheard one of the nurses explaining to him how to perform some test on the guy next to me, and to the doctor's credit, he thanked her.

The nurses were excellent, even if a bit rushed, and the nurse's aide laughed at my jokes. Laughing is good. I overheard the crying when the doctor had to inform a family that one of their loved ones had died. Crying is good, too. That same doctor then had to come in and check on me. How do they do that and stay sane? He asked me what I did for a living. (He assumed that I was in healthcare, because I had on my scrubs, thinking that I would be seeing clients that afternoon.) I shared with him that I was a massage therapist, and he had heard of me. We talked a bit about the benefits of massage, and he was very supportive. He looked like he needed a massage, too.

As I sat writing this, I inadvertently pulled off one of the leads for the cardiac monitor (a medical device) I was wearing. I stuck it back on, and hopefully, it won't skew the test results. A lead also came off while I was in the ER. Apparently someone was watching the monitors, because three nurses and the doctor came running. They thought I had died, I guess. But I hadn't; not yet, anyway. Someday I will, and I hope I do a good job of it.

Tests never did reveal the cause of the chest pain, but the doctors and nurses made a point of telling me that I did the right thing by coming in, because my family has a history of heart disease, and cardiac symptoms are not typical in women. In retrospect, I can appreciate the whole thing as a learning experience. What better way to understand patients—the physical, emotional, and spiritual influences—than by being one? It was scary, and the medical staff, although not perfect (and who is?), were excellent and helped me not to feel so vulnerable.

P.S. Four months later I did have cardiac bypass surgery. So it just goes to show that medicine is an imperfect science staffed by people who are doing the best they can at that point in time.

evolve 16-1

The following terms and expressions specific to Chapter 16 have already been used to search PubMed for the latest research literature available. The *Click Here for Massage* feature associated with this chapter on your textbook's Evolve website allows you to hyperlink to a continually updated PubMed search of research literature that corresponds to this subject.

Hyperlink Search Terms
Massage athletes
Massage end of life
Massage geriatrics
Massage mental health
Massage pediatrics
Massage physical disabilities
Massage pregnancy
Massage terminal illness

SUMMARY

This chapter discussed people who share common experiences related to healthcare issues. The massage therapist needs to consider the populations with which they work and make appropriate accommodations for the individuals served. Populations, conditions, and treatments overlap considerably in healthcare. A person can be elderly, have visual and hearing difficulties, and yet be an athlete. A female can be pregnant, anxious, and speak a language different from that of the caregiver.

Hopefully, this chapter provided information sufficient to help you begin to understand the complexities of the human experience, especially when it is complicated by injury, illness, or dysfunction. No specific massage protocol exists for a jogger, a person in a smoking cessation program, a girl experiencing the cramps of her first menstrual cycle, a toddler throwing a temper tantrum, an autistic adult under stress from social interaction, a baby with a tummy ache, or a depressed spouse who has lost his mate after a long life together. There is no such thing as addiction withdrawal massage, sports massage, geriatric massage, infant massage, PTSD massage, and so on. People benefit from appropriate massage based on their individual needs. The massage therapist in the healthcare environment must rely on clinical reasoning skills to develop beneficial and safe treatment protocols.

REFERENCES

1. Cognitive Behavior Therapy Center for OCD and Anxiety: http://www.cbtmarin.com/disorder_general.asp
2. American Psychological Association.
3. National Aphasia Association: www.aphasia.org/Aphasia
4. The Speech-Language Pathology Website: http://home.ica.net/~fred/index.htm

WORKBOOK

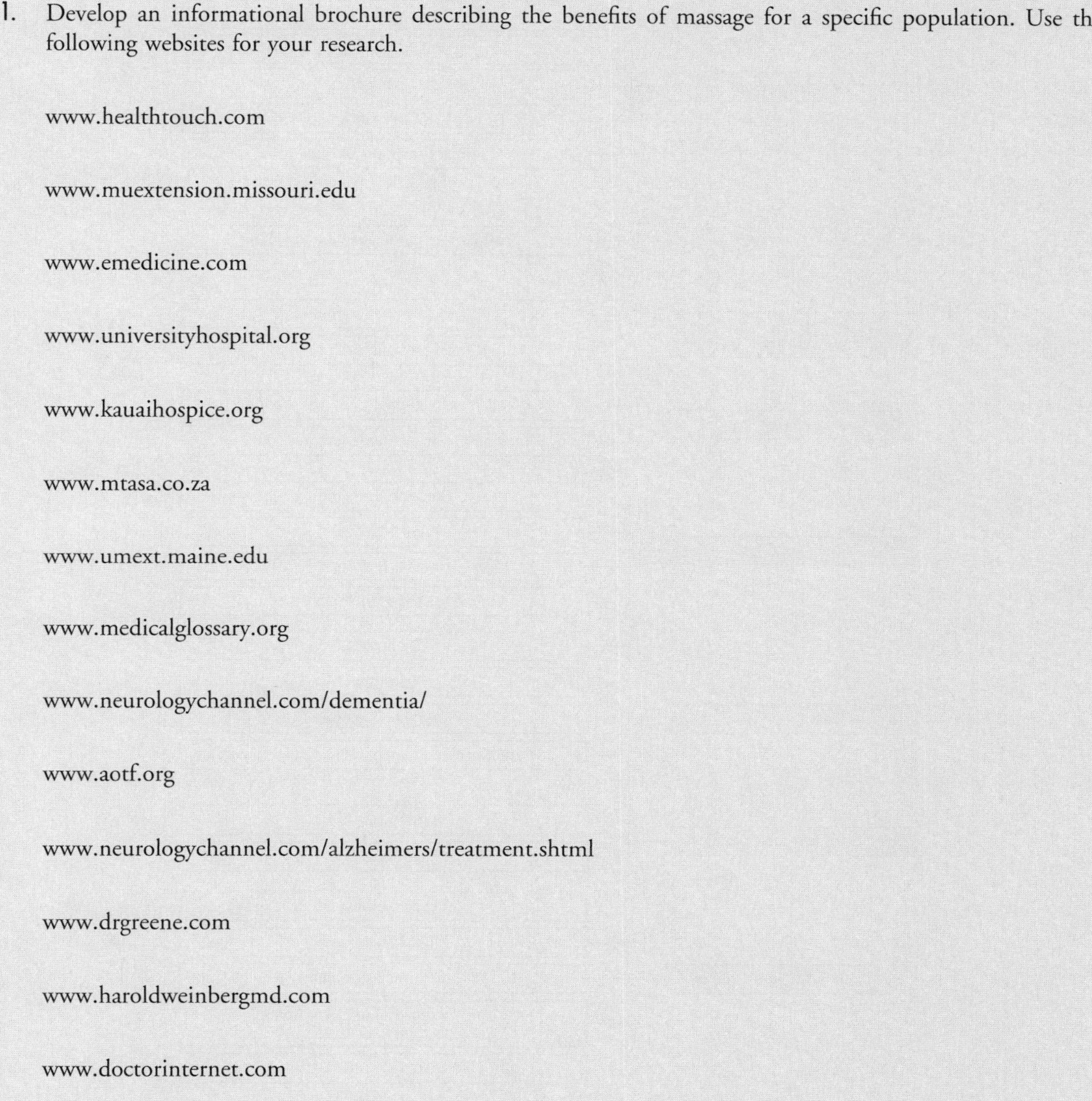

1. Develop an informational brochure describing the benefits of massage for a specific population. Use the following websites for your research.

   www.healthtouch.com

   www.muextension.missouri.edu

   www.emedicine.com

   www.universityhospital.org

   www.kauaihospice.org

   www.mtasa.co.za

   www.umext.maine.edu

   www.medicalglossary.org

   www.neurologychannel.com/dementia/

   www.aotf.org

   www.neurologychannel.com/alzheimers/treatment.shtml

   www.drgreene.com

   www.haroldweinbergmd.com

   www.doctorinternet.com

Chapter 17 Concept Map

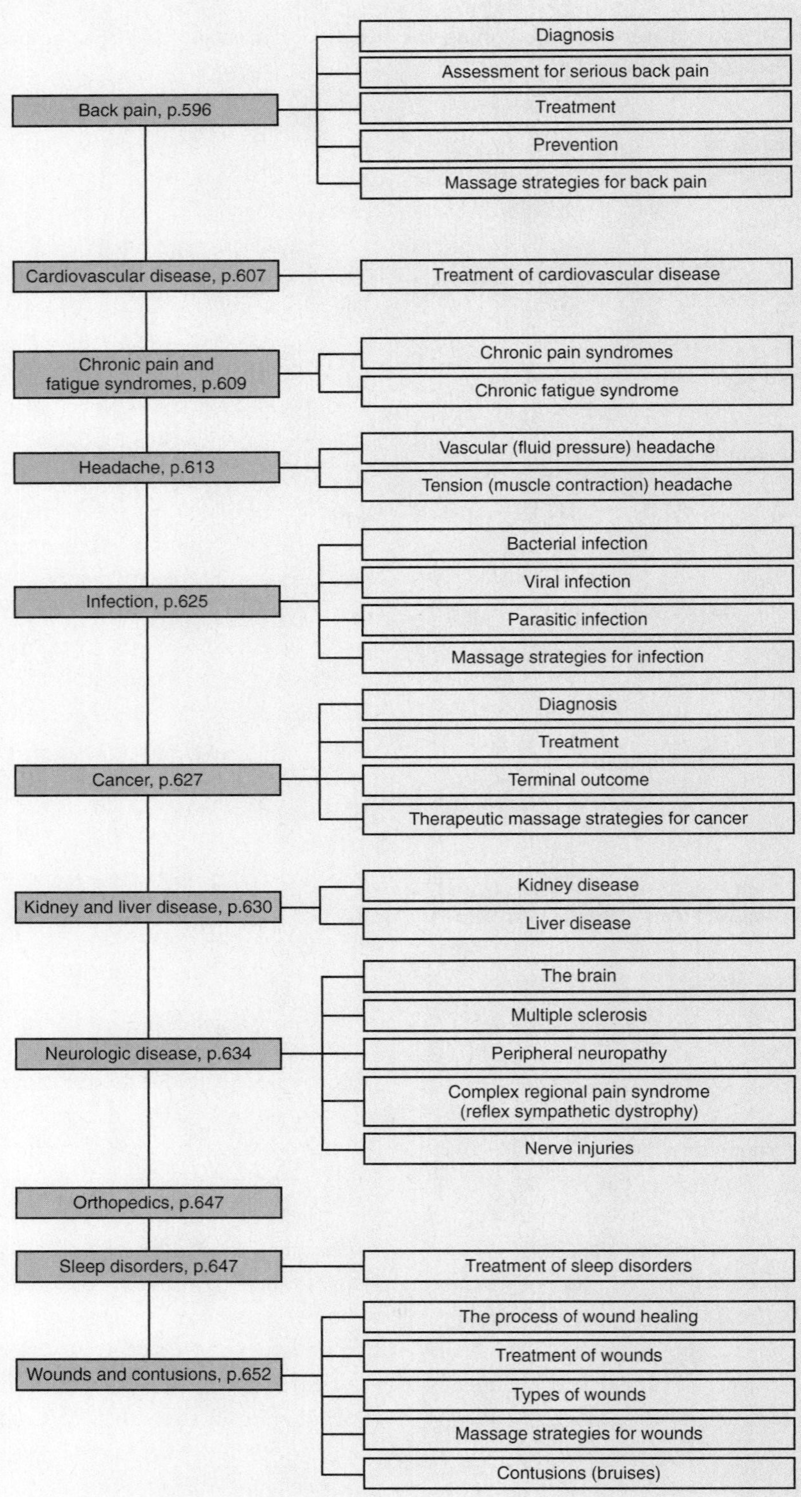

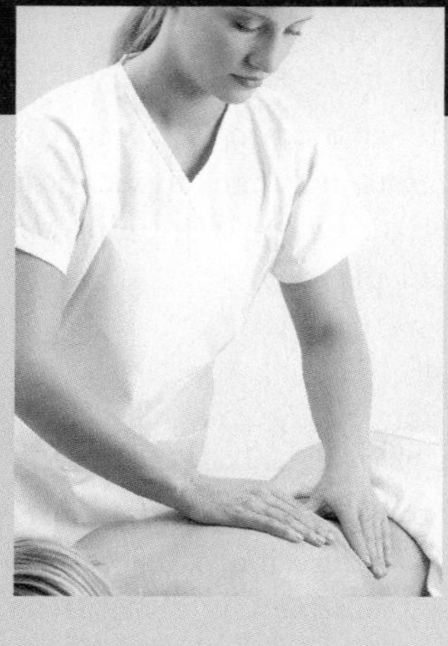

CHAPTER 17

COMMON CATEGORIES OF ILLNESS AND INJURY AND THE CLINICAL REASONING PROCESS

Key Terms

Atrophy
Contractures
Degenerative joint disease
Disk herniation
Entrapment
Nerve impingement
Nerve injuries
Nerve root compression
Stress fractures
Subluxation
Tendinitis

For definitions of key terms, refer to the Evolve website.

OBJECTIVES

Upon completion of this chapter, the reader will have the information necessary to:

1. Understand the mechanisms of various pathologic conditions for which massage may be an appropriate aspect of treatment.
2. Develop valid massage strategies targeted to individual diagnosed conditions.
3. Perform specific massage procedures that address common conditions.

This chapter discusses healthcare concerns by common conditions, especially those for which massage is most beneficial. Similar illnesses and injuries are categorized into general treatment protocols; the change is in the targeted location. For example, a sprained knee and a sprained wrist are similar injuries; only the anatomy is different. A wound, whether on the leg or the foot, is still a wound, and breast cancer, prostate cancer, liver cancer, and lung cancer are all types of cancer. For massage therapists, an understanding of the generalities of sprains, wounds, and cancers and their medical treatment initially is sufficient for developing a massage treatment plan. The clinical reasoning process individualizes the massage application according to each patient's specific situation.

It may seem to you that the same information is repeated over and over. However, the intent of this chapter is to help you build a foundation of knowledge that allows you to develop massage treatment applications targeted specifically for each patient, applications that safely and effectively support the outcomes determined during the assessment and treatment plan processes. Clinical reasoning aids in this development process. The chapter covers considerable territory, and it is supported extensively on the Evolve website.

Anyone can get an infection, a bruise, or a sprain. Some people are more prone to cardiovascular disease, such as the elderly, but anyone can develop heart or vascular disease. To understand the pathology of a condition, you have to have an understanding of normal anatomy and physiology (see Unit Two). The treatment of various medical conditions is based on the type of illness or injury and the patient's general health status. Remember, the health status of the very young and the very old typically is more fragile than that of a 25-year-old. A person undergoing chemotherapy is more fragile and susceptible to infection or fatigue than a relatively healthy child. A child who is sleep deprived from staying up too late becomes more susceptible to accidents and the resulting wounds, contusions, fractures, sprains, or strains. A person who suffers cracked ribs in a car accident may develop breathing pattern disorder, which can lead to anxiety, which supports a predisposition to a posttraumatic stress response to the car accident.

JUST BETWEEN YOU AND ME

I could write these circle patterns all day. That is why this textbook, the instructors with whom you are working, and/or the professional experience you have acquired eventually have to lead you to a problem-solving (i.e., clinical reasoning) approach to massage care. People ask me all the time, "I have a patient with [fill in a problem]. What type of massage should I do?" The answer is, I have no clue; I can only make educated guesses based on commonalties in certain population groups, the causal factors, the treatments and prognoses for various disease and injury patterns, and the person's current health status. Ugh; I am constantly making it up as I go. And you know what? So will you if you end up wanting to be really good at massage.

The potential patterns and interactions are endless. Therefore this chapter and the affiliated Evolve site material address healthcare concerns according to the illness and injury model rather than the population model used in Chapter 16. This chapter also suggests massage application strategies and can be used as a starting point for individualizing treatment plans.

BACK PAIN

Back pain is one of the most common complaints in healthcare. Because there are many contributing and causal factors, back pain is difficult to treat. The anatomic structures of the back, which include bones, ligaments, fascia, muscles, nerves, and tendons, can all cause back pain individually or in combination. Joint and bone diseases such as arthritis and osteoporosis can lead to degeneration, inflammation, and compression of the spine. Although infrequent, infections such as spinal meningitis and tuberculosis can create back pain. Referred pain is also an issue, such as with kidney infection.

Back pain is common and most people will have at least one occurrence of some sort of back problem in their lives. Many individuals will experience multiple acute episodes within the context of a long-term chronic condition. Physically demanding occupations that require repetitive bending and lifting have a high incidence of back injury leading to disability. A sedentary lifestyle and being overweight increase the stress on the lower back and contribute to poor posture.

While work-related injury, coupled with decreased physical fitness from a sedentary lifestyle, is the most common cause of back injury, other predisposing factors are: advancing age; wear and tear on the spinal structures; traumatic injury such as falls, disk degeneration, and spinal stenosis; static positions such as standing or sitting for extended periods; and activities that involve twisting the torso (e.g., gardening and raking). These can increase symptoms for existing back pain or can be the primary cause of back pain. Many back issues are related to sport and recreational activities, such as golf, baseball, and horseback riding. Using poor body mechanics when lifting and carrying heavy loads or sleeping on a soft mattress can perpetuate back pain.

DIAGNOSIS

The evaluation of back pain begins with a patient history. Diagnostic tests involve a physical examination that includes range-of-motion and flexibility testing, as well as neurologic tests for motor, sensory, or deep tendon reflex loss; testing using straight leg raises; and tests for other indicators of disk disease. Diagnostic tests include: x-ray, magnetic resonance imaging (MRI), bone scans, electromyography (EMG), myelograms, and computed tomography (CT) scans. Blood tests can identify Paget's disease, tuberculosis, cancer, and infection. A urinalysis identifies kidney or other urologic involvement.

The most common causes of back pain are spondylolysis, **stress fractures,** defects in the intervertebral disks, muscle strain in the back, and mechanical pain caused by poor posture. Back pain has different causes in younger and older patients. A younger patient generally does not have degenerative changes in the spine, and the back pain usually is due to a specific illness, injury, or event. The incidence of spondylolysis is higher in the young than in the old. In older people, back pain often is related to disk degeneration. Also, older patients generally have more degenerative disease of the spine, pathologic spinal conditions, and weight-control problems that can lead to back pain.

Most back pain is the result of a combination of mechanical factors, including improper weight-lifting techniques, overstretching, torsion, direct trauma, static positioning, repetitive loading, hard repetitive contact, sudden violent muscle contraction, and spondylolysis or spondylolisthesis. The possibility of a disk condition and related nerve irritation must be considered in any long-lasting episode of back discomfort, especially if the pain radiates into the leg.

A quick assessment for serious back injury can be made with the forward trunk flexion and the backward trunk extension (Figure 17-1). If the patient feels greater pain during flexion, disk involvement is possible. If extension increases pain, the patient may have a stress fracture of the vertebrae.

ASSESSMENT FOR SERIOUS BACK PAIN

The symptoms of back pain vary, depending on the source. Some of the most common symptoms are as follows:

- Back strain/mechanical or musculoskeletal pain: The pain could be caused by strain on the muscles or ligaments of the spine.
- Degenerative disease of the joints between the bones of the spine.
- Herniated disk: In this condition, a disk has bulged out from its proper place as the shock absorber between the vertebrae or bones of the spine. The disk thus may impinge upon nerves, causing severe pain (Figure 17-2).
- Sciatica: This is a condition of impingement upon the sciatic nerves, which causes pain in the buttocks, the back of the thigh, and sometimes farther down into the lower leg and foot.
- Spinal stenosis: In this condition, a narrowed spinal cord exerts pressure on the nerves, causing pain, numbness, and weakness, especially in the legs.
- Radiculopathy: This condition is marked by irritation of the nerve roots, which causes weakness or pain, numbness or tingling, or a combination of these.

Other symptoms of back pain may include swelling, stiffness, and limited motion. Nearly all back injuries are muscular in nature. Most back problems are due to tense muscles or to strain caused by a sudden overloading of muscles during activity. About 95% of low back pain is the result of muscular problems caused by lack of exercise, weak muscles, or being overweight (Figure 17-3). Breathing disorders cause back pain or can occur because of back dysfunction.

TREATMENT

The treatment plan for back pain varies among healthcare professionals. It is important to realize that neurosurgeons, orthopedists, osteopaths, chiropractors, and massage therapists have

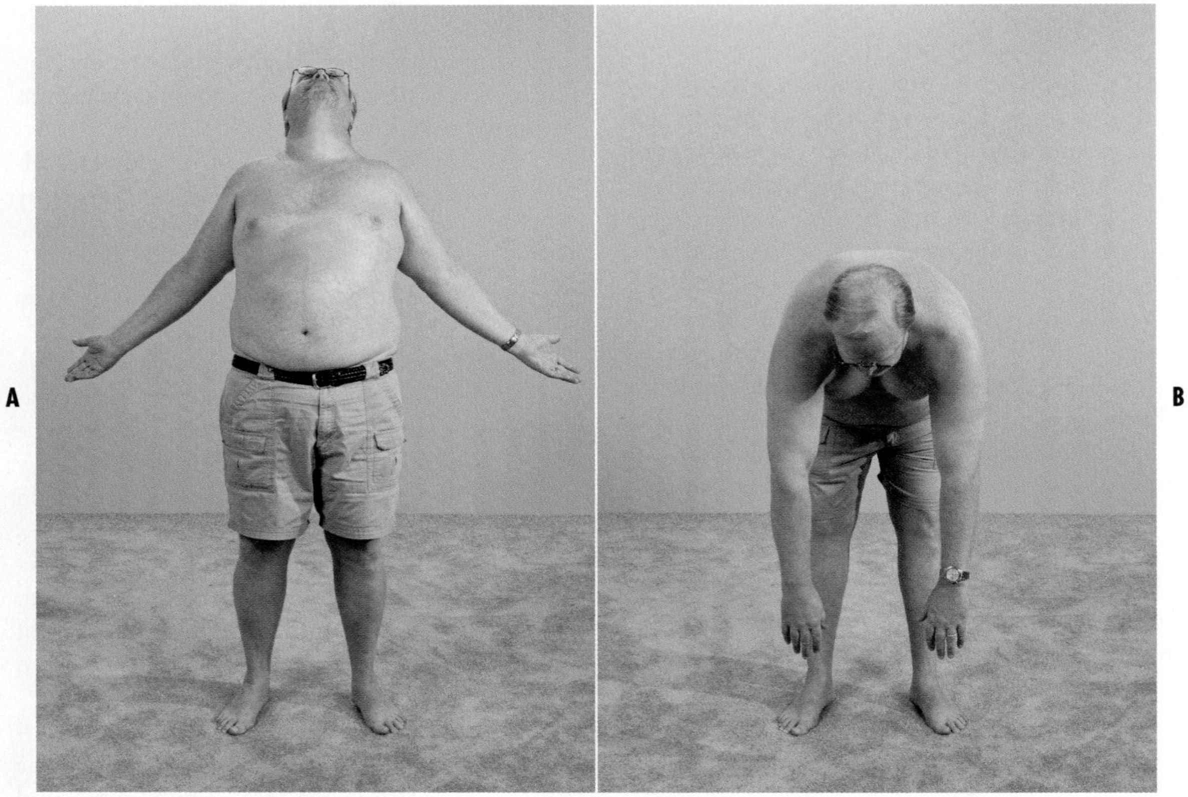

A B

FIGURE 17-1 ■ **A,** The patient may have a stress fracture of the vertebrae if this position increases pain. **B,** Disk involvement is possible if this position increases pain.

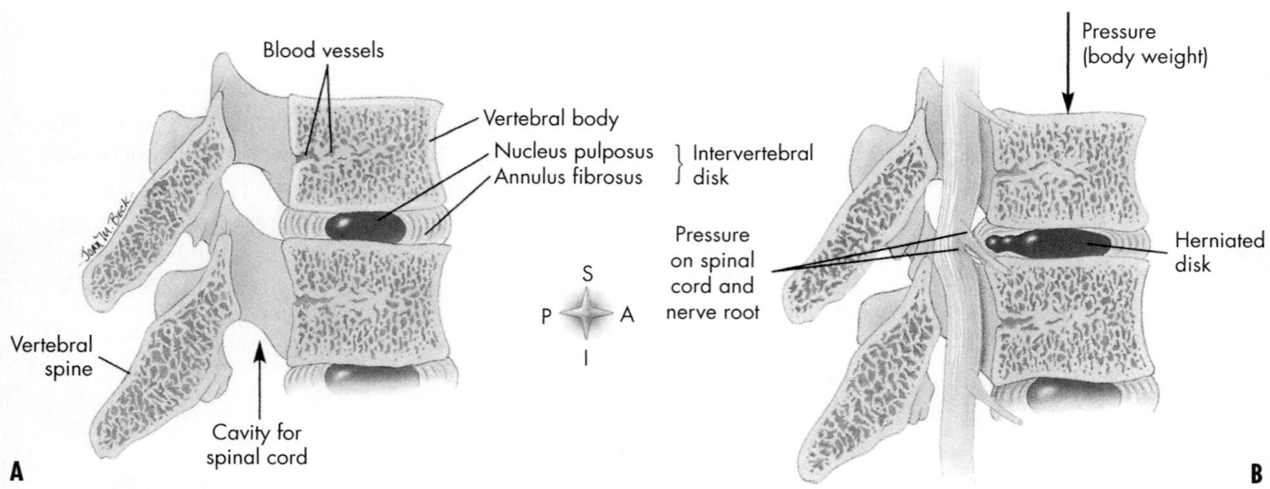

FIGURE 17-2 ■ Sagittal section of the vertebrae. **A,** Normal disks. **B,** Herniated disks. (From Thibodeau GA, Patton KT: *Anatomy and physiology,* ed 6, St Louis, 2007, Mosby.)

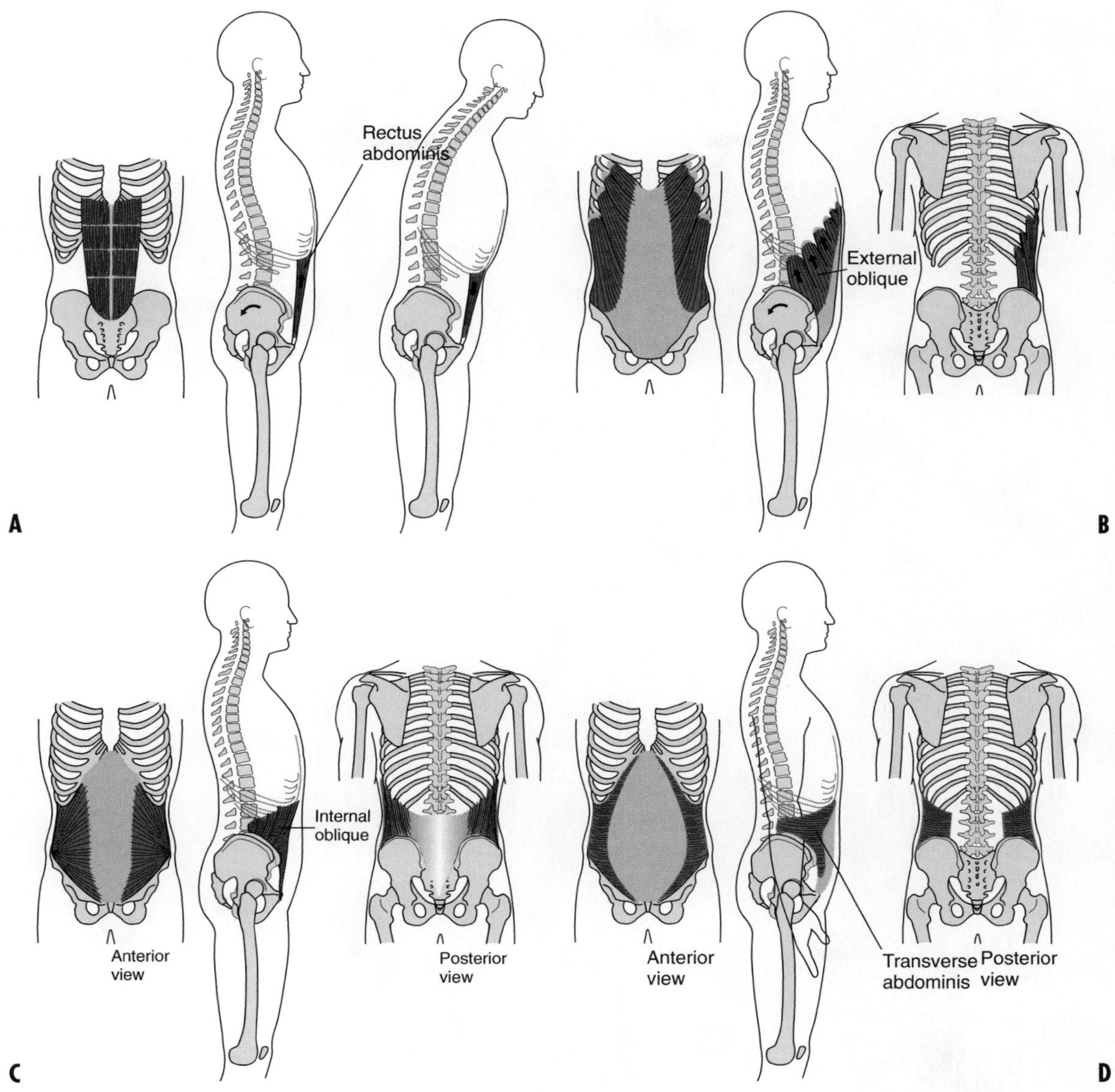

FIGURE 17-3 ■ The major muscles involved in low back pain. (From Saidoff DC, McDonough A: *Critical pathways in therapeutic intervention: extremities and spine,* St Louis, 2002, Mosby.)

Continued

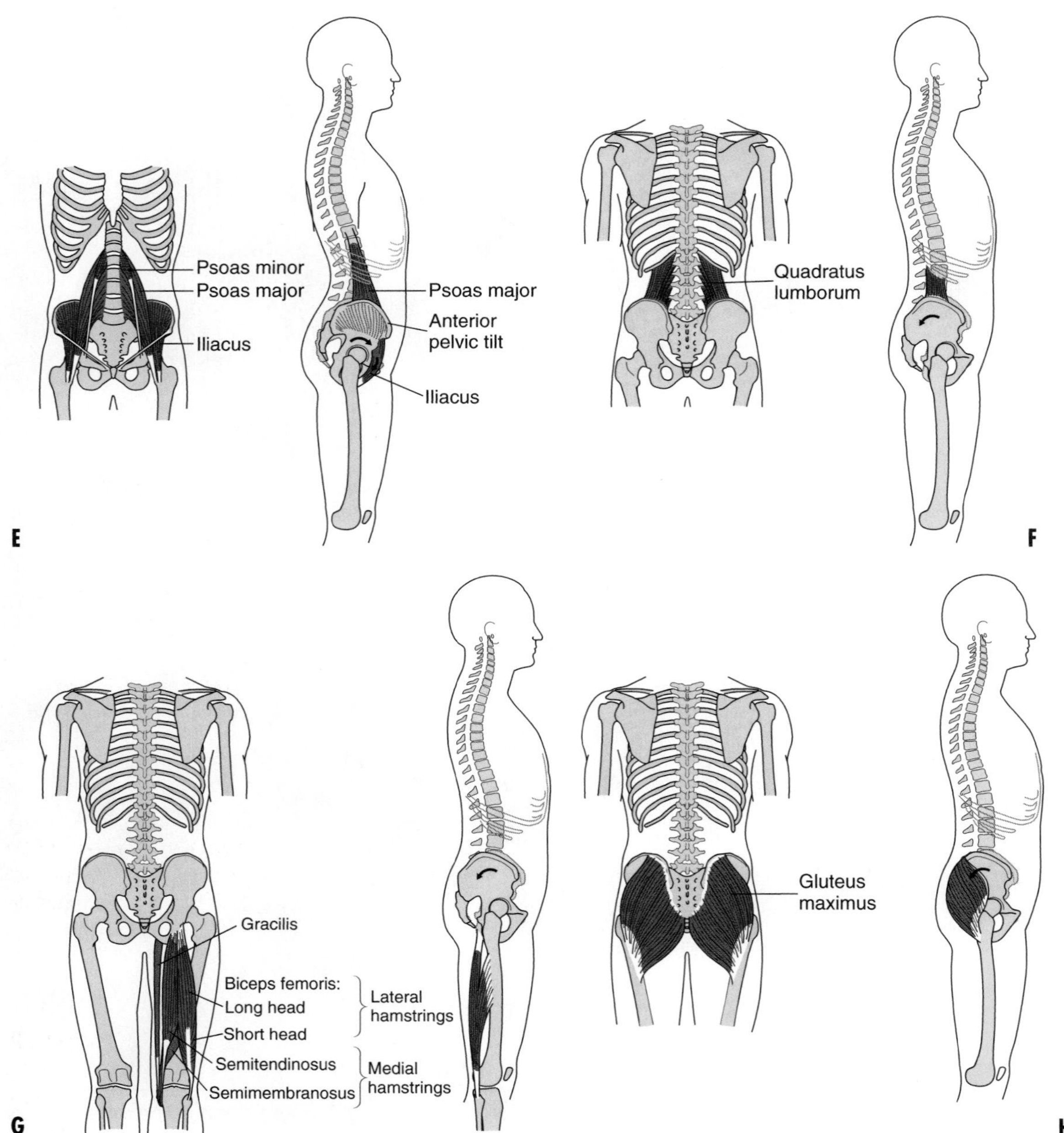

FIGURE 17-3, cont'd

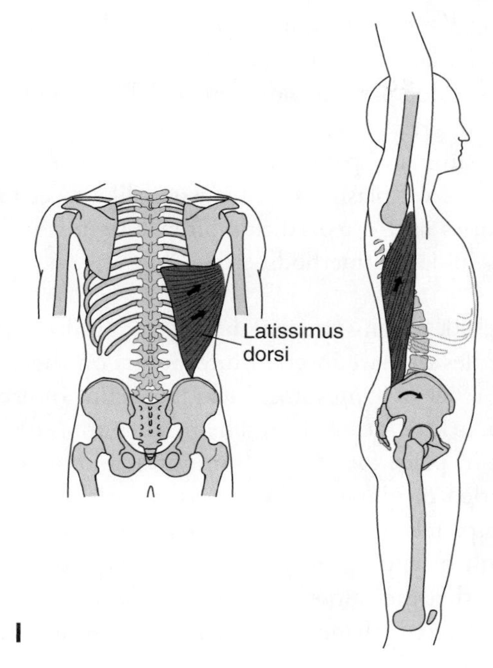

FIGURE 17-3, cont'd

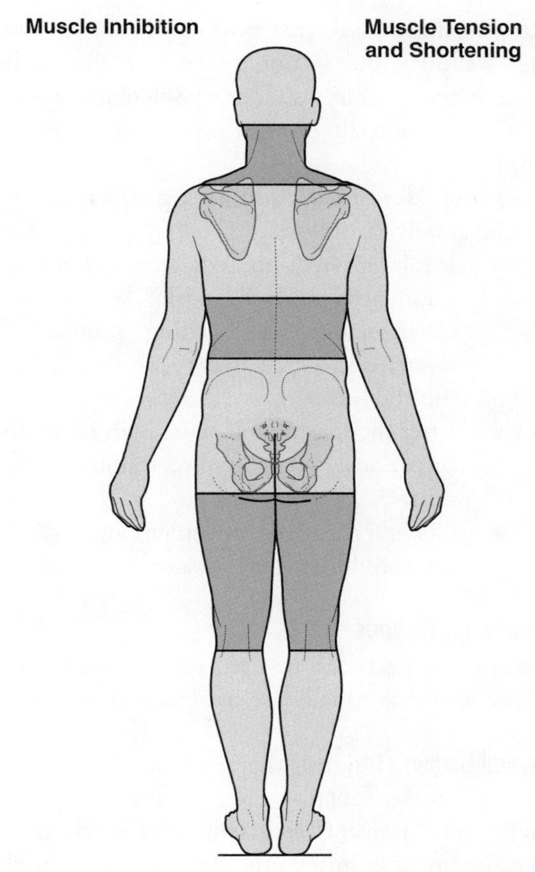

FIGURE 17-4 ■ Areas of muscle inhibition (light shading) and muscle tension and shortening (dark shading). (From Fritz S: *Sports and exercise massage: comprehensive care in athletics, fitness, and rehabilitation,* St Louis, 2005, Mosby.)

unique approaches, training, and philosophies with regard to the treatment of general back pain.

Regardless of the medical approach, a comprehensive rehabilitation program is necessary. This program must include core stability training and a flexibility program, especially for the hamstrings, the piriformis, the external rotators of the hip, and the hip flexors, including the psoas and the gluteal muscles. Patients in rehabilitation programs should progress from single-plane to multiplane exercises that emphasize dynamic stabilization.

Chiropractic or osteopathic mobilization for abnormal facet function can be helpful. Muscle activation sequences for the trunk, hip extension, and knee flexion usually are dysfunctional and need treatment.

Most people with back pain can recover without surgery. Treatment includes pain medications, antiinflammatory drugs, steroid injections, hot and cold hydrotherapy, rest, traction, support, massage, and physical therapy. Exercises to stretch and strengthen muscles can help prevent further problems. Walking and swimming are both good exercises for strengthening and protecting the spine. Losing weight and improving posture are also beneficial. Fortunately, most simple backaches go away within a few days or weeks, with or without treatment. A therapeutic exercise program that strengthens the lower back and the abdominal muscles (the core) can prevent back pain and help prevent the recurrence of pain (Figure 17-4).

Bed rest for longer than a couple of days only weakens the muscles and increases the potential for lingering dysfunction. A patient with back pain needs to get out of bed as soon as possible. The condition should be treated with ice and with alternating hot and cold applications. Orthopedists often advise those with back pain to avoid activities that put severe stress on the back. Swimming, walking, and stationary cycling all can be done without sharp, sudden movements, severe arching of the back, or twisting or rotation of the trunk.

Most cases of back and neck pain are treated conservatively, as follows:

- Ice is applied immediately and for 48 hours after straining a muscle. Ice slows inflammation and swelling, numbs soft tissue, and slows nerve impulses in the injured area.
- After the spasms and acute pain have subsided, heat can be applied to loosen tight muscles.[1]
- General pain-free movement and stretching should be done as soon as possible.

Treatment Options

Various methods can be used to treat back pain. These methods usually are used in combination.

Physical Therapy. Physical therapy is used to reduce pain, increase function, restore normal movement, and prevent recurrences of back pain. Because most injuries are the result of muscle weakness, almost every back problem will require some sort of strengthening program.

Exercise. Using therapeutic exercise to strengthen muscles that support the spine can correct certain back problems causing pain. In addition, exercise can help to strengthen other regions of the body, including the arms, abdomen, and legs, further helping to reduce back strain. Exercise also plays a part in strengthening bones for greater support and reduced risk of injury when events such as falls and collisions occur. Because most injuries are the result of muscle weakness, increased strength is the answer to almost every back problem. Strengthening of the core is essential.

Electrotherapy. Sometimes called "stim," this category of treatment includes various forms of hydrotherapy, thermotherapy, and ultrasound therapy. These treatments are used to improve circulation to the area and reduce muscle spasm.

Massage. Massage therapy increases circulation to the injured area and reduces muscle pain.

Spinal Manipulation. Chiropractors and osteopaths manipulate the structures of the spine. This is often referred to as "adjustment." The intent is to relieve pressure on nerves and, as a result, reduce or eliminate pain. Musculoskeletal conditions such as whiplash and joint issues like facet joint injuries and osteoarthritis often respond well to manipulation methods.

Acupuncture. This ancient healing art utilizes thin needles that are inserted into points on the body for relief of symptoms, including pain. Insertion causes little or no pain. The needles are generally left in place for 15 to 30 minutes, and are often twirled or vibrated after insertion. Although not completely understood, pain relief may be the result of endorphin release. There is also indication that the smooth muscle bundles in the fascia are affected, changing the degree of fascial tone in the area.

Medication. Various over-the-counter and prescription NSAIDs are recommended for pain relief. Chronic back pain caused by nerve root damage can manifest as numbness, burning, aching, throbbing, or stabbing pain. This type of pain is sometimes treated with tricyclic antidepressants. Side effects include drowsiness, dry mouth, and constipation.

Antiinflammatory drugs, nonnarcotic or narcotic pain relievers, and muscle relaxants can be used to relieve acute back pain. If necessary, short-term use of an oral steroid, such as prednisone, is prescribed to reduce inflammation during acute episodes of back pain. With this steroid, patients are started on a high dose and the dosage is gradually reduced over 5 or 6 days.

Injections. Steroids can be injected with an anesthetic for selective nerve root blocking and can significantly reduce inflammation and pain caused by a variety of conditions, including herniated disks, degenerative disk disease, and stenosis. The side effects, however, can be serious and include loss of bone mass, headaches, and compromised wound healing.

Surgery. Surgery is a treatment of last resort. Even with the many advances in surgical techniques and methods, it is common for more conservative measures to be used as treatment before surgery is indicated. Surgery can be used successfully for progressive or severe neurologic dysfunction. Symptoms of such conditions include: muscle weakness, spinal cord compression, and bowel, bladder, and sexual dysfunction. Sometimes surgery is used for pain that has not responded to other treatments. Depending on the condition during surgery, the disk may be removed or part of the spine fused, with rods, plates, or screws stabilizing the spine. A diskectomy is the removal of a herniated disk to relieve pressure on a nerve root. A laminectomy is performed when the primary problem appears to be spinal stenosis. This procedure involves removal of the lamina to make room for the nerves. The surgeon may also remove bone spurs at the same time. A spinal fusion uses bone grafts between two or more vertebrae to cause the vertebrae to grow together, or fuse. Fusing the vertebrae reduces mechanical back pain and pressure on the nerve root.

Advances in surgical treatment have increased the success rate and reduced the complications of back surgery; however, surgery still is the treatment of last resort. The success rate for low back pain surgery is questionable, and it is considered the final option, to be used only after more conservative treatments have failed. New microscopic surgical procedures are less invasive and show promising results.

Other approaches also have been used. For example, surgically implanted pumps deliver a constant dose of pain-relieving medication to the spinal area, and spinal cord stimulators modulate the pain response so that the patient experiences less pain.[1]

PREVENTION

People with back pain, and even those without it, need to take the following steps to prevent further problems:[1]

- Learn proper body mechanics, particularly if an activity they commonly perform involves repetitive bending, lifting, and twisting.
- Exercise regularly, keeping the back muscles strong and flexible.
- Maintain good posture.
- Avoid standing or sitting in one place for long periods.
- Maintain a proper weight for their body size.
- Eat a healthy diet.

evolve 17-1

See the Evolve website for specific types of back pain and treatment strategies.

MASSAGE STRATEGIES FOR BACK PAIN

Massage strategies for back pain are pictured in the Appendix.

Therapeutic massage best addresses back pain of a muscular origin, such as simple back strain and overuse without joint or disk involvement. Massage also is useful as part of a comprehensive treatment program for more complicated conditions, such as disk dysfunction. Joint dysfunction usually requires manipulation by the physician, physical therapist, or chiropractor. Massage is an adjunct treatment before and after adjustment. More complex back pain often results in muscle tension and spasm (i.e., guarding), which are the body's attempts to stabilize the structure. If these muscles are excessively tense, stiffness, pain, and possibly increased irritation of the joint structure may occur as a result of the muscles pulling structures together, causing compression. In these cases unequal forces are applied to the joint structure, because the flexors, adductors, and internal rotators exert more pull than the extensors, abductors, and external rotators.

Massage can reduce muscle tension caused by guarding, but it should not seek to eliminate it. The guarding response is appropriate. Pain control methods are appropriate as well. These two strategies combined should support more normal movement and enhance the effectiveness of other treatments. Manipulation of the joints is easier if massage is applied to the surrounding soft tissue. Massage after joint manipulation can reduce any spasm that may result. Complex back pain that is more than muscle-related pain requires multidisciplinary treatment, in which massage plays a supportive role.

Massage for simple back pain is best combined with hot and cold hydrotherapy and application of a counterirritant ointment. The patient should rest and perform gentle range-of-motion exercises and stretching activities. Rest without movement is not advisable, because this can worsen the situation.

Massage is targeted to the core complex of muscles: the abdominals, psoas, quadratus lumborum, hamstrings, and gluteal group. Firing pattern dysfunction is almost always present, and gait reflexes usually are disrupted.

Specific Massage Strategies for Back Pain

Midback Pain. Muscle-oriented pain in the midback usually is caused by short anterior serratus, pectoralis minor, and pectoralis major muscles and weak core muscles. The rhomboids and trapezius usually are long, and protective spasms and trigger point activity are seen at the attachments. The biggest mistake massage therapists make with this condition is to massage the long areas in the area of the pain; this only makes them longer. Massage targeted to the long structures consists of local pain control using only surface rubbing with a counterirritant ointment and hyperstimulation analgesia. Use all muscle energy methods and inhibitory pressure on the muscle belly and lengthen the short tissues in the anterior chest. (See anterior serratus and pectoralis minor release in Chapter 10.)

If connective tissue bind exists in the pectoralis region, address this with appropriate mechanical forces by kneading, compressing, or stretching the tissues. Therapeutic exercise needs to strengthen the inhibited muscles (e.g., the rhomboids). The scalene muscles can impinge upon part of the brachial plexus, resulting in a pain pattern to the midscapular region. Massage addresses the impinging tissue in the neck that recreates the symptoms.

If the patient feels as if he or she wants to "crack" the back, the paraspinal muscles usually are the problem. (See release of the paraspinal muscles, multifidi, and rotators in Chapter 10.)

If the patient is sniffling, coughing, sneezing, or has been laughing a lot, they may experience midback pain, and the posterior serratus inferior is often the cause since it stabilizes the lower ribs. This muscle shortens, and because of its fiber direction, it is very difficult to stretch. An aching sensation just below the scapula at the location of the muscle is one of the symptoms. Compression into the muscle belly with local tissue stretching usually relieves the symptoms.

Low Back Pain in the Lumbar Area. Various low back pain syndromes can develop. The most serious is referred pain for kidney or bladder illness or injury, infection, or a ruptured disk. These conditions require medical treatment.

Sacroiliac Joint Pain. Dysfunction of the sacroiliac (SI) joint, a major cause of pain, requires a multidisciplinary approach. Usually one side is more painful than the other. The joint can be jammed or fused and thus interfere with movement of the pelvis during gait. The restricted pelvic movement creates increased movement at L4-5, the S1 area, the hip, or both. Pain occurs in the lumbar area, hip abductors, and around the coccyx/sacrum on the affected side (Figure 17-5).

Assessment for SI joint dysfunction is fairly simple. Stand behind the patient and stabilize the person lightly near the scapula. Have the patient stand on one foot (the side that is least sore) by bringing up the opposite knee so that the hip is flexed to about 90 degrees (as if marching). Then instruct the patient to lean back against your hands and slightly arch the back. Check for pain. Then have the patient stand on the opposite foot (i.e., on the side that hurts) and repeat the sequence. If the SI joint is dysfunctional, the patient's pain will increase, because the movement compresses the joint surfaces, recreating and increasing the symptoms. This condition requires proper mobilization of the joint by the physical therapist, physician, or chiropractor.

Massage supports the mobilization process by reducing muscle guarding and increasing tissue pliability. Once the joint has been adjusted, the mobilization sequence for the SI joint (see Chapter 10) can be incorporated into the general massage. The latissimus dorsi muscle opposite the symptomatic SI joint is part of the force couple that stabilizes the SI joint. The lumbar dorsal fascia must be pliable but not so loose as to affect stability.

Usually the symphysis pubis is somewhat displaced in conjunction with SI joint dysfunction. A simple resistance method can address this condition. With the patient supine with the knees bent, the massage therapist provides resistance against the patient's attempt to pull the knees together. This activates the adductors, which then can pull the symphysis pubis into better align-

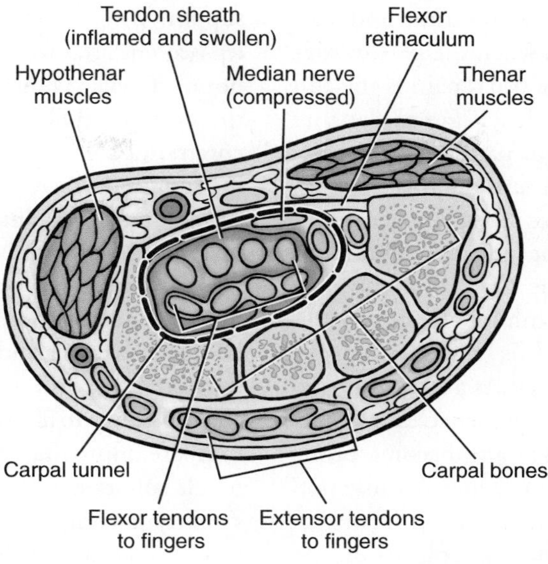

FIGURE 17-5 ■ The sacrum can move within the pelvis relative to the two pelvic bones. (From Muscolino JE: *Kinesiology: the skeletal system and muscle function,* enhanced edition, St Louis, 2007, Mosby.)

ment. Sometimes a pop is heard when the symphysis pubis resets, but this is neither necessary nor desirable for effective results.

Reflexively and functionally, the sternoclavicular (SC) joint is a factor in SI joint pain. Assess for corresponding pain in the SC joint and apply massage to inhibit muscle tension and increase tissue pliability and joint mobility.

Often the sacrotuberous and sacrospinous ligaments are short or the hamstring and gluteus maximus attachments near these ligaments are binding. These ligament structures are difficult to reach. When they are located, a compressive force is applied to the ligaments and the muscle attachment while the patient activates the hamstrings and gluteus maximus. The result should be increased pliability of the ligament, and the muscles should be lengthened and should move more freely, without bind.

If a functional long leg is present, the SI joint can become jammed on the long leg side. Typically the pelvis is rotated anteriorly on the symptomatic side and posteriorly on the nonsymptomatic side, with the quadratus lumborum short on the nonsymptomatic side. For mild cases, an effective approach consists of the indirect function techniques for pelvic rotation combined with quadratus lumborum release (see Chapter 10). The physical therapist or chiropractor can rotate the pelvis into proper alignment, and the massage therapist can deal with the soft tissue compensation. Gait patterns and firing patterns need to be assessed and normalized (see Chapter 9).

Quadratus Lumborum Pain. A primary symptom is pain in the lumbar region just above the iliac crest. Typically, the pain is felt more on one side than the other and the patient has a rotated pelvis and functionally uneven legs. Coughing and sneezing increase the pain. SI joint pain is a common element of quadratus lumborum pain. The patient often has a history of long/short leg syndrome or of stepping into a hole or coming down hard on one leg on an uneven surface (as in stepping off a curb) during running or other activity. This causes the leg to be driven up into the joint, and the muscle spasms as the SI joint jams. The paired muscle group is the scalenes, which need to be addressed in conjunction with the quadratus lumborum. Include the scalene and quadratus lumborum releases in the general massage application.

Psoas-Related Low Back Pain. The main symptoms of low back pain related to psoas dysfunction are a deep aching in the lumbar area, difficulty moving from a seated to a standing position and vice versa, and pain that occurs when the person rolls over when lying down. The psoas pain is the end result of a series of events that begin at the core muscles. The most common pattern is weakness of the transverse abdominis and oblique muscles, which renders the trunk muscle activation sequence ineffective. The rectus abdominis becomes dominant, and the psoas shortens. The gluteus maximus becomes inhibited, and the hip extension function instead is assumed by the erector spinae and hamstrings. As a result, the hip extension muscle activation sequences are abnormal. The hamstrings shorten and become prone to injury. The gastrocnemius begins to function as a knee flexor and shortens. This interferes with ankle mobility. Uneven forces are placed on the knees, and the calf muscles usually stick together and pull at the Achilles tendon. Eventually problems with the plantar fascia can develop.

The massage strategy is to normalize the firing patterns and reduce tone in the shortened muscles (i.e., the psoas, hamstrings, and calf). (See psoas and hamstring treatment in Chapter 10.) However this sequence only treats the symptom. The problem is core instability. A proper strength and conditioning sequence must deal with core strength. The muscles targeted in the strengthening program are inhibited by the short, tense erector spinae, psoas, hamstring, and calves, and a vicious cycle is created. Before corrective exercises begin, the short muscles need to be treated and normal resting length restored as much as possible. This can take up to a month of concentrated effort with massage two to three times a week and a sequential stretching program. Then core training begins. The massage is reduced to two times a week, and daily stretching continues.

The full body massage protocol is necessary for this regimen, with attention paid to reflex paired body areas (i.e., hamstrings/biceps, quadriceps/triceps, calf/forearm, quadratus lumborum/scalenes, and psoas/sternocleidomastoid. The rectus abdominis needs to be inhibited and the psoas released. Include thorough massage of the feet, and connective tissue strategies for binding structures.

Assess for breathing dysfunction and address it using the strategies in Chapter 14.

With psoas-related back pain, the muscle-stabilizing patterns of the connective tissue support mechanism in the lumbar area into the leg become strained. The latissimus dorsi, lumbar dorsal fascia, with the gluteus maximus and the iliotibial (IT) band on the opposite side is a common pattern. This is due to adaptive stabilizing function. Massage treatment inhibits the latissimus dorsi and gluteus maximus and increases pliability in the lumbar fascia and IT band.

To further complicate the back pain treatment, underlying joint instability may be present in the lumbar area and SI joint. If too much mobility is restored, joint pain may occur. Introduce change slowly to allow the body to adapt. If symptoms are improving and then suddenly return, too much soft tissue stability was released and joint stability is compromised. Back off and return to general massage until the condition improves.

Acute Treatment for Back Pain Using Massage

The side-lying position is recommended for treatment. If the prone position is used, support the patient with pillows under the abdomen and ankles. *Do not* keep the patient in the prone position for an extended period—15 minutes is the maximum. When moving the patient from the prone to the side-lying position, have the person slowly assume a hands and knees position and then slowly arch and hunch the back (cat/camel move, valley/hill). Next, have the patient stretch back toward the heels with the arms extended. Then slowly have the person move to the side-lying position and add bolsters for stability.

Pain Control Mechanisms for Acute Back Pain. *Do not* do deep work or use any method that causes guarding, flinching, or breath holding. Use rocking and gentle shaking combined with gliding and kneading of the area with the most pain and symptomatic muscle tension. This most likely will be on the back, even though the causal muscle tension and soft tissue problem usually are in the anterior torso. Massage the hamstrings and adductors, gluteals and calves. They usually are short, tight, and firing out of sequence. Do not attempt to reset the firing patterns while acute symptoms are present. Include massage of the reflex points of the feet that relate to the back. Place the patient in the supine position after working with both the left and right sides and bolster the knees. The rectus abdominis and pectoralis muscles likely are short and tense. Massage as indicated in the general protocol. The psoas muscles and adductors are likely short and spasming, but it is best to wait 24 to 48 hours before addressing these muscles. Continue rocking and shaking.

Subacute Treatment Using Massage

24 to 48 Hours after Onset. As part of the general massage protocol, repeat the acute massage application but begin to address second- and third-layer muscle shortening, connective tissue pliability, and firing patterns. Use direct inhibition pressure on the psoas, quadratus lumborum, paraspinals, and especially the multifidi, always monitoring for a guarding response. *Do not* cause guarding or changes in the breathing. The hip abductors probably will have tender areas of shortening, but lengthen the adductors first. Gently begin to correct the trunk, gluteal, hamstring, and calf firing patterns. Include massage application for breathing dysfunction, because it commonly is associated with low back problems. Do not overdo the treatment.

Three to Seven Days. Continue with subacute massage application as part of the general massage, increasing the intensity of the massage as tolerated. In addition, normalize the gait and eye reflexes and gently mobilize the pelvis (for low back pain) and the ribs (for upper back pain). (See the pelvis mobilization sequence in Chapter 10.) The patient should not feel pain during any active or passive movements. Positional release methods and specific inhibiting pressure can be applied to tender points. The inhibiting pressure should recreate but not increase the symptoms. Work with the trigger points that are most medial, proximal, and painful. Do not address latent trigger points or work with more than three to five areas. Continue to address breathing function. The patient should be doing gentle stretches and appropriate therapeutic exercises.

Postsubacute Treatment Using Massage

Continue with general massage and address the muscles that remain symptomatic. Begin to assess for body-wide instability, compensation patterns, and other conditions that may contribute to acute back pain. Usually core muscle firing is weak, and synergistic dominance of the rectus abdominis and psoas is present.

If breathing is dysfunctional, midback pain may be present as well. Continue to normalize the breathing pattern disorder. For chronic back pain, continue with postsubacute treatment and support rehabilitative exercises, including breathing retraining.

Low back pain massage is illustrated in the Appendix.

CARDIOVASCULAR DISEASE

Cardiovascular/respiratory disease is the number one cause of death in the United States. Coronary artery disease is caused by the buildup of plaque (which is composed of cholesterol, calcium, and fibrous tissue) inside a coronary vessel. This results in narrowing of the coronary arteries (stenosis), which reduces coronary blood flow, thereby decreasing the delivery of oxygen to the heart. Coronary artery disease most often is caused by arteriosclerosis, atherosclerosis, and thrombus formation in one or more of the coronary arteries.

Arteriosclerosis, which means hardening of the arteries, refers to arteries that have become brittle and have lost elasticity. The arteries gradually lose elasticity as a person ages. If they cannot enlarge, the blockage becomes more serious. Although arteriosclerosis has several causes, the most common and important is atherosclerosis, the deposit of fatty plaques in medium and large arteries. In atherosclerosis, small fat deposits from cholesterol in the blood build up at stress points in the arteries. These stress points occur where the arteries branch out or incur damage. The fat combines with connective tissue sent to repair the damage and forms plaque. As this process continues, blood flow diminishes. Symptoms do not usually appear until a major blockage occurs. The body compensates by enlarging the artery, if possible. Sometimes the artery enlarges, forms an aneurysm, and ruptures. Problems also occur when the plaque breaks off and completely blocks (occludes) the vessels. In the brain, this is called a stroke or brain attack.

Partial occlusion of a vessel in the heart causes the transient chest, arm, and neck pain of angina. Total occlusion causes the crushing or squeezing pain of infarction. Blockage of the artery diminishes the amount of oxygen and nutrients reaching the heart tissues.

evolve 17-2

See the Evolve website for specific types of cardiovascular and respiratory disorders.

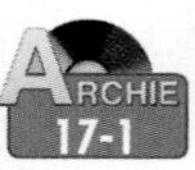

TREATMENT OF CARDIOVASCULAR DISEASE

Some of the many risk factors for coronary artery disease can be controlled through diet, weight management, and avoidance of smoking. Treatment frequently includes the use of beta blockers and calcium channel blockers to slow the heart rate and reduce the strength of the contractions. In addition to lowering blood pressure, calcium channel blockers dilate the coronary arteries. Angioplasty, a surgical procedure, unclogs the arteries.

Cardiovascular disease is treated with medication, surgery, and lifestyle changes (e.g., diet, exercise, and smoking cessation). Numerous studies show that regular exercise protects the heart. It lowers the risk of developing coronary artery disease and reduces cardiac injury during a heart attack. It also reduces several cardiovascular risk factors, including hypertension, diabetes mellitus, obesity, blood lipids, the risk of thrombosis (blood clotting), and endothelial (blood vessel) dysfunction (Figure 17-6).

An analogy can be drawn for this situation. Think of rust as representing free radicals, and the antioxidants as representing Rustoleum, which can stop the spread of rust. Antioxidants are molecules that can remove free radicals by filling their incomplete bonds and forming a new, less reactive molecule, thereby preventing free radical–mediated cellular illness and injury. Research supports the cardioprotective effects of regular exercise, as well as the benefits of nutritional antioxidant supplementation in protecting the heart during a heart attack.

Massage Strategies

In general, cardiovascular disease presents contraindications to and cautions for therapeutic massage. Cardiovascular issues that influence massage include blood disorders, deep vein thrombosis, side effects of medications, and cognitive heart failure.

Various blood disorders need to be considered, especially those in which platelet function is diminished. Massage may be contraindicated in these cases, depending on the severity of the condition.

Deep vein thrombosis is a major concern and a contraindication to massage. The term *phlebitis* refers to inflammation of a vein caused by injury, infection, or swelling. Phlebitis diminishes blood flow, which may cause thrombin clots to develop, a condition known as *thrombophlebitis.* The superficial leg veins are the most common sites, primarily the saphenous veins. Varicose veins may increase the incidence of thrombophlebitis. Clots also may form in the deep veins, especially in the legs and abdomen; this is deep vein thrombosis. These clots can break off and travel to the lung, causing a pulmonary embolism.

If a contraindication does not arise from the cardiovascular disease itself, the medication taken to control the disease may pose problems. For example, blood thinners increase the risk of bruising and hemorrhage. Nonetheless, therapeutic massage often is indicated as part of a supervised treatment program for cardiovascular disease. The key is supervision by a qualified healthcare provider, because cardiovascular diseases can be complex in the presenting pathologic condition and the treatment protocols. The general stress management and homeostatic normalization effects of therapeutic massage are desirable for most cardiovascular difficulties, as long as the treatments are supervised as part of a total therapeutic program.

The most important aspect of massage is linked to exercise. Massage supports the exercise program required for cardiofitness, healing, and rehabilitation by managing muscle soreness and joint aching. It also contributes to increased compliance with exercise programs. The massage needs to be altered to account for medications, age, and the patient's general adaptive capacity. Otherwise, the methods discussed in Unit Two are appropriate.

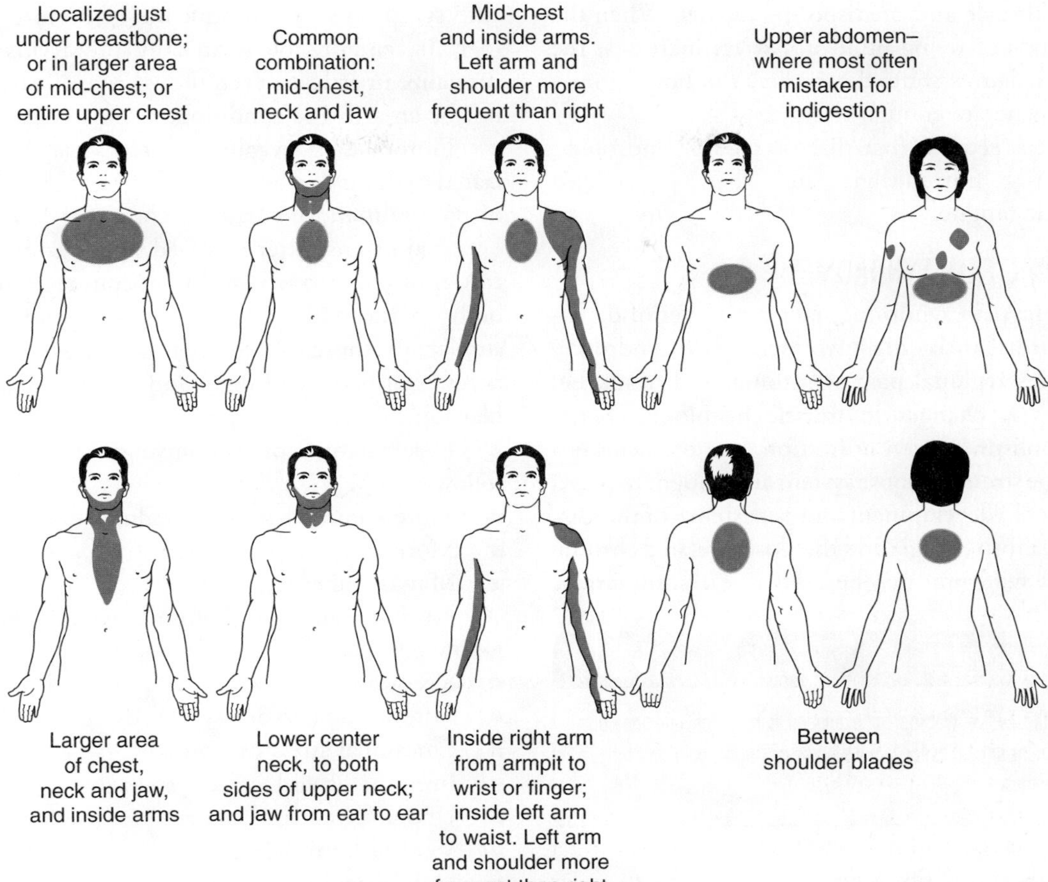
Localized just under breastbone; or in larger area of mid-chest; or entire upper chest
Common combination: mid-chest, neck and jaw
Mid-chest and inside arms. Left arm and shoulder more frequent than right
Upper abdomen– where most often mistaken for indigestion
Larger area of chest, neck and jaw, and inside arms
Lower center neck, to both sides of upper neck; and jaw from ear to ear
Inside right arm from armpit to wrist or finger; inside left arm to waist. Left arm and shoulder more frequent than right
Between shoulder blades
Most common warning signs of heart attack
• Uncomfortable pressure, fullness, squeezing or pain in the center of the chest (prolonged)
• Pain that spreads to the throat, neck, back, jaw, shoulders, or arms
• Chest discomfort with lightheadedness, dizziness, sweating, pallor, nausea, or shortness of breath
• Prolonged symptoms unrelieved by antacids, nitroglycerin, or rest
Atypical, less common warning signs (especially women)
• Unusual chest pain (quality, location, e.g., burning, heaviness; left chest), stomach or abdominal pain
• Continuous midthoracic or interscapular pain
• Continuous neck or shoulder pain
• Isolated right biceps pain
• Pain unrelieved by antacids; pain unrelieved by rest or nitroglycerin
• Nausea and vomiting; flu-like manifestation without chest pain/discomfort
• Unexplained intense anxiety, weakness, or fatigue
• Breathlessness, dizziness

FIGURE 17-6 ■ Early warning signs of a heart attack. (From Goodman C, Snyder T: *Differential diagnosis in physical therapy*, ed 3, Philadelphia, 2000, WB Saunders.)

CHRONIC PAIN AND FATIGUE SYNDROMES

Chronic pain and fatigue syndromes are common, difficult to diagnose, and complicated to treat. "Type A" perfectionists and "type B" caregivers are prone to chronic pain and fatigue syndromes. Type A individuals work, work, and work until they burn out; type B people give, give, and give, nurturing their spouses, children, family, and friends, until they break down. Anyone whose lifestyle has very little downtime is at risk. These syndromes are related not so much to mental state as to lifestyle and predisposing factors. When the demands of living build up, stress increases, the hypothalamus shuts down, and the body simply can't generate enough energy.

This section first discusses pain syndromes, primarily fibromyalgia and then generalized chronic fatigue.

CHRONIC PAIN SYNDROMES

Chronic pain syndromes take a number of different forms, including myofascial pain syndrome, complex regional pain syndrome, and headache. However, changes in muscle histology, energy metabolism, oxygen utilization, and the neuroendocrine stress-response system are thought to play a role in the development and persistence of this disorder. Fibromyalgia and the closely related chronic fatigue syndrome may be endocrine dysfunctions.

evolve 17-3

See the Evolve website for expanded information and massage treatment strategies for various types of chronic pain and fatigue syndromes.

Currently, fibromyalgia is thought to be a neurochemical dysfunction of the pain processing system. It has been considered a chronic musculoskeletal syndrome characterized by pain, aching, tenderness, and stiffness in the neck, shoulders, chest, legs, and lower back. The pain of fibromyalgia generally is accompanied by sleep disorders, fatigue, gastrointestinal disorders, and depression. The pain may be aching, burning, or throbbing and tends to move around the body (migratory pain). Many people also experience muscle tightness, soreness, and spasms. The pain often is strong in the morning, relieved throughout the day, and then worsens at night.

Fibromyalgia symptoms can be constant or occur intermittently for years or a lifetime. The latest research indicates that fibromyalgia may be the result of biochemical imbalances that cause the physical symptoms, but the specifics remain elusive. Because it is a syndrome (i.e., a collection of signs and symptoms) rather than a disease, fibromyalgia cannot be diagnosed by a set of specific symptoms or reproducible laboratory findings. It tends to be treated by physicians who specialize in arthritis even though the disease may not be an arthritic condition.

Fibromyalgia's vague symptoms may be associated with diminished blood flow to certain parts of the brain and increased amounts of substance P, a neurotransmitter involved in the communication of pain, touch, and temperature from the body to the brain. Many of the symptoms are similar to those of chronic fatigue syndrome, myofascial pain syndrome, and temporomandibular joint (TMJ) syndrome.

Risk factors for fibromyalgia include the following:

- More common in young adults
- More common in women
- May be inherited

Possible causes of fibromyalgia include the following:

- Sleep disorders
- Autonomic nervous system dysfunction
- Emotional stress or trauma
- Immune or endocrine system dysfunction
- Upper spinal cord injury
- Viral or bacterial infection
- Unhealthy lifestyle choices

Symptoms vary, depending on the person's level of stress and physical activity, the time of day, and the weather. According to the National Institute of Arthritis and Musculoskeletal and Skin Diseases, patients with fibromyalgia have combinations of many chronic and frustrating symptoms. Patients with fibromyalgia experience pain and tenderness when pressure is applied to certain areas of the body. These areas are the back of the head, elbows, hips, knees, neck, upper back, and upper chest.

Common symptoms of fibromyalgia include the following:

- Sleep apnea
- Morning stiffness
- Restless legs
- Temperature sensitivity
- Cognitive and memory problems, sometimes referred to as "fibro fog"
- Gastrointestinal symptoms, such as abdominal pain, bloating, gas, cramps, alternating

diarrhea and constipation, and irritable bowel syndrome
- Chronic headaches, including facial and jaw pain
- Heightened sensitivity to odors, loud noises, bright lights, various foods, medicines, and changes in the weather
- Dysmenorrhea and dyspareunia
- Frequent urination, a strong urge to urinate, and dysuria
- Rapid or irregular heart rate and shortness of breath
- Sensation of edema in the hands and feet, even though swelling is not present
- Numbness or tingling sensations

The pain, sensitivity, and cognitive functioning problems experienced by fibromyalgia patients are thought to be due to a decreased blood flow to specific areas of the brain. The thalamus seems to be particularly sensitive to these blood flow changes.

Other probable contributing factors for fibromyalgia include the following:

- High levels of "substance P," a central nervous system neurotransmitter involved in pain processing.
- Low levels of several neurochemicals: serotonin, norepinephrine, dopamine, and cortisol.
- Low levels of nerve growth factor.
- Low levels of somatomedin C, a hormone that promotes bone and muscle growth.
- Low levels of phosphocreatine and adenosine, muscle-cell chemicals.

Treatment of Chronic Pain Syndromes

With chronic pain syndromes, the goals of treatment are to reduce pain, improve sleep, and relieve symptoms. Management of fibromyalgia requires the integration of both pharmacologic and nonpharmacologic approaches. Medications used include tricyclic antidepressants, selective serotonin receptor antagonists, analgesics, benzodiazepines, and antiinflammatory agents. Antidepressants are first taken at the lowest possible dosage and then gradually increased, if necessary. Their overall benefit for relieving pain, fatigue, and sleeplessness appears to be limited. Many people are unable to tolerate the side effects of these medications (i.e., nausea, loss of appetite, and insomnia), even at low doses, and they therefore stop taking them.[1]

Small doses of aspirin or acetaminophen may provide some pain relief and may relieve muscle stiffness. Restoration of a normal hormone balance, including thyroid, adrenal, and reproductive hormones, may help. Appropriate treatment may be necessary for bacterial, viral, fungal, or parasitic infections, which may be present as a consequence of the body's diminished immune functions. Nutritional support, particularly with B complex vitamins, magnesium, zinc, and malic acid, may be helpful.

Most treatment regimens include a combination of medication, lifestyle changes, exercise, physical therapy, and behavior modification.[1] Therapeutic massage also is beneficial.

Tender trigger points can be injected with a local anesthetic (e.g., lidocaine) and/or a corticosteroid, and the involved muscle is then stretched. The local anesthetic increases blood flow to the muscle, and the corticosteroids reduce inflammation. However, this treatment is not well tolerated, because the injections can be painful, and improvement may take 2 to 4 days.[1]

Medical and Physical Therapy. Depending on the symptoms, heat, ice, massage, whirlpool treatments, ultrasound therapy, and electrical stimulation may be used to reduce pain.[1] Physical therapists also can design an exercise program to improve flexibility, fitness, and posture.

Behavioral/Cognitive Therapy. Counseling or another type of talk therapy may help people with chronic pain learn better methods of coping with their illness; it also can help enhance their self-esteem and reduce stress and attempts at perfection. Behavioral/cognitive therapy effectively streng-thens a person's belief in his or her own abilities. It enables the person to develop tools for dealing with stress and helps change the belief that the person is helpless against the pain.[1] Behavior modification involves learning coping skills, relaxation exercises, and self-hypnosis.

Lifestyle changes that can help alleviate symptoms include taking steps to support restorative sleep, avoiding caffeine (which can aggravate sleep disorders), and following an exercise program. The restoration provided by sleep is essential, and a minimum of eight to nine hours of sleep every night is important. Appropriate medications or nutritional supplements should be used for this purpose, if necessary. This is the aspect of the disorder in which massage may be most beneficial.

Massage Strategies for Chronic Pain Syndromes

Therapeutic massage for chronic pain syndromes follows the general protocol. This includes methods for pain management, breathing pattern disorder, and local treatment of active tender points, typically using trigger point methods. Be careful not to overdo the massage application, because the adaptive mechanisms are strained when a person has chronic pain. Avoid any methods that might cause inflammation.

CHRONIC FATIGUE SYNDROME

According to the CDC, those with chronic fatigue syndrome (CFS) experience debilitating fatigue that is present for at least 6 months and that substantially curtails the person's activity level. CFS affects millions of people globally and it is likely that many more people with similar fatiguing illnesses who do not fully meet the strict research definition of CFS suffer.

The condition is not related to any known clinical condition or medication for which fatigue is a symptom or side effect. At least four of the following symptoms should be present concurrently with the persistent or relapsing fatigue: substantial impairment in short-term memory or concentration; sore throat; tender lymph nodes; muscle pain; multijoint pain without swelling or redness; headaches of a new type, pattern, or severity; nonrestorative sleep; and postexercise fatigue lasting more than 24 hours.

In addition to the eight primary defining symptoms of CFS, a number of other symptoms have been reported by some CFS patients including abdominal pain, bloating, chronic cough, diarrhea, dizziness, dry eyes or mouth, earaches, irregular heartbeat, chest pain, jaw pain, morning stiffness, nausea, night sweats, depression, irritability, anxiety, panic attack, shortness of breath, skin sensations, tingling sensations, and weight loss. It is interesting that this same symptom pattern occurs with disordered breathing, and normalizing the breathing process would be a logical massage intervention strategy.

Stress of all types and particularly physiologic stress impact immune reactivity via complex interactions involving the hypothalamus, the pituitary gland, and the adrenal glands, as well as the autonomic nervous.

Researchers might have found evidence that CFS is a real neurologic condition. A pilot study found that patients with CFS had a set of proteins in their spinal cord fluid that were not detected in healthy individuals. These proteins might give insight into the causes of CFS and could be used as markers to diagnose patients with CFS (http://www.eurekalert.org/pub_releases/2005-12/bc-pss112905.php).

Treatment of Chronic Fatigue Syndrome

Currently, no curative treatment is available for CFS. Treatment targets the symptoms and possible underlying causes. The first step is to manage sleep with sleep medications and fatigue with a combination of antidepressants and stimulant drugs. Antidepressants are used because most patients with chronic illness and pain have low levels of serotonin and dopamine; this makes for sleep disruption, a low pain threshold, and irritability. Antidepressant therapy makes the patient feel more motivated and alert. A combination of methods is used to address pain and autonomic dysfunction. Most patients with CFS can be treated with reasonable success.

Pharmacologic Therapy. People with CFS appear particularly sensitive to the effects of medications, especially those that target the central nervous system (CNS). The usual treatment strategy is to begin with a very low dose and to increase the dosage gradually as necessary.[2] The following medications frequently are used:

- Low-dose tricyclic agents: Tricyclic agents sometimes are prescribed for CFS to improve sleep and to relieve mild, generalized pain.[2]

These drugs include doxepin (Adapin, Sinequan), amitriptyline (Elavil, Etrafon, Limbitrol, Triavil), desipramine (Norpramin), and nortriptyline (Pamelor). Side effects include dry mouth, drowsiness, weight gain, and an elevated heart rate.

- Antidepressants: Antidepressants often are used to treat depression in patients with CFS. However, some physicians have found that patients with CFS who are not depressed benefit as much or more than depressed patients from treatment with selective serotonin reuptake inhibitors (SSRIs).[2] Examples of antidepressants used to treat CFS include fluoxetine (Prozac), sertraline (Zoloft), paroxetine (Paxil), venlafaxine (Effexor), trazodone (Desyrel), and bupropion (Wellbutrin). A number of side effects may occur, and these vary depending on the specific drug used.
- Nonsteroidal antiinflammatory drugs (NSAIDs): These drugs may be used in prescription or over-the-counter (OTC) strength to relieve pain and fever.[2] Some OTC NSAIDs include naproxen (Aleve, Anaprox, Naproxen), ibuprofen (Advil, Bayer Select, Motrin, Nuprin), and piroxicam (Feldene). These medications generally are safe when used as directed, but they can cause a variety of side effects, including kidney damage, gastrointestinal bleeding, abdominal pain, nausea, and vomiting.
- Antiallergenic drugs: Some patients with CFS have a history of allergy, and these symptoms may flare periodically. Nonsedating antihistamines may be helpful for these individuals. Examples include astemizole (Hismanal) and loratadine (Claritin). Some of the more common side effects associated with their use include drowsiness, fatigue, and headache. Sedating antihistamines also can be beneficial in helping patients fall asleep.
- Antihypotensive drugs: Fludrocortisone (Florinef) sometimes has been prescribed for patients with CFS who tested positive for excessively low blood pressure. An increased salt and water intake also is recommended for these patients. High blood pressure may be an adverse reaction to this treatment.

Many people report symptom relief with massage, acupuncture, and chiropractic care. Physical activity and exercise can help relieve symptoms for some individuals, but for others, physical activity and exercise can worsen symptoms. An expert in therapeutic exercise, such as a physical therapist or exercise physiologist, should design and monitor the exercise program.

Massage Strategies for Chronic Fatigue Syndrome

The massage application for CFS should follow the general protocol but should not be fatiguing or strain the patient's adaptive function. The modified palliative massage may be more appropriate than the general protocol. Include applications for pain management, breathing function, and restorative sleep.

HEADACHE

Figures 17-7 to 17-9 illustrate the sequence for massage treatment for headache.

One of the most common health complaints is headache, a symptom with a multitude of causes. Headaches can be caused by stress, muscle tension, chemical imbalance, medications, circulatory and sinus disorders, and tumors. Because the brain has no sensory innervations, headaches do not originate in the brain. The pain of a headache is caused by pressure on the sensory nerves, vessels, meninges, or muscle-tendon-bone unit. This pressure is caused primarily in two ways: it may be fluid pressure, which has a variety of causes, including dilation of blood vessels, or it may be caused by soft tissue shortening, which can be caused by connective tissue changes and muscle contraction. All headaches should be evaluated by a physician so that serious underlying conditions can be ruled out.

Headaches can be classified simply as the vascular type or the tension (muscle contraction) type. The most common type of vascular headache is the migraine headache.

VASCULAR (FLUID PRESSURE) HEADACHE

In general, vascular (or fluid pressure) headaches include sinus headache, migraine headache, cluster

Text continued on p. 620.

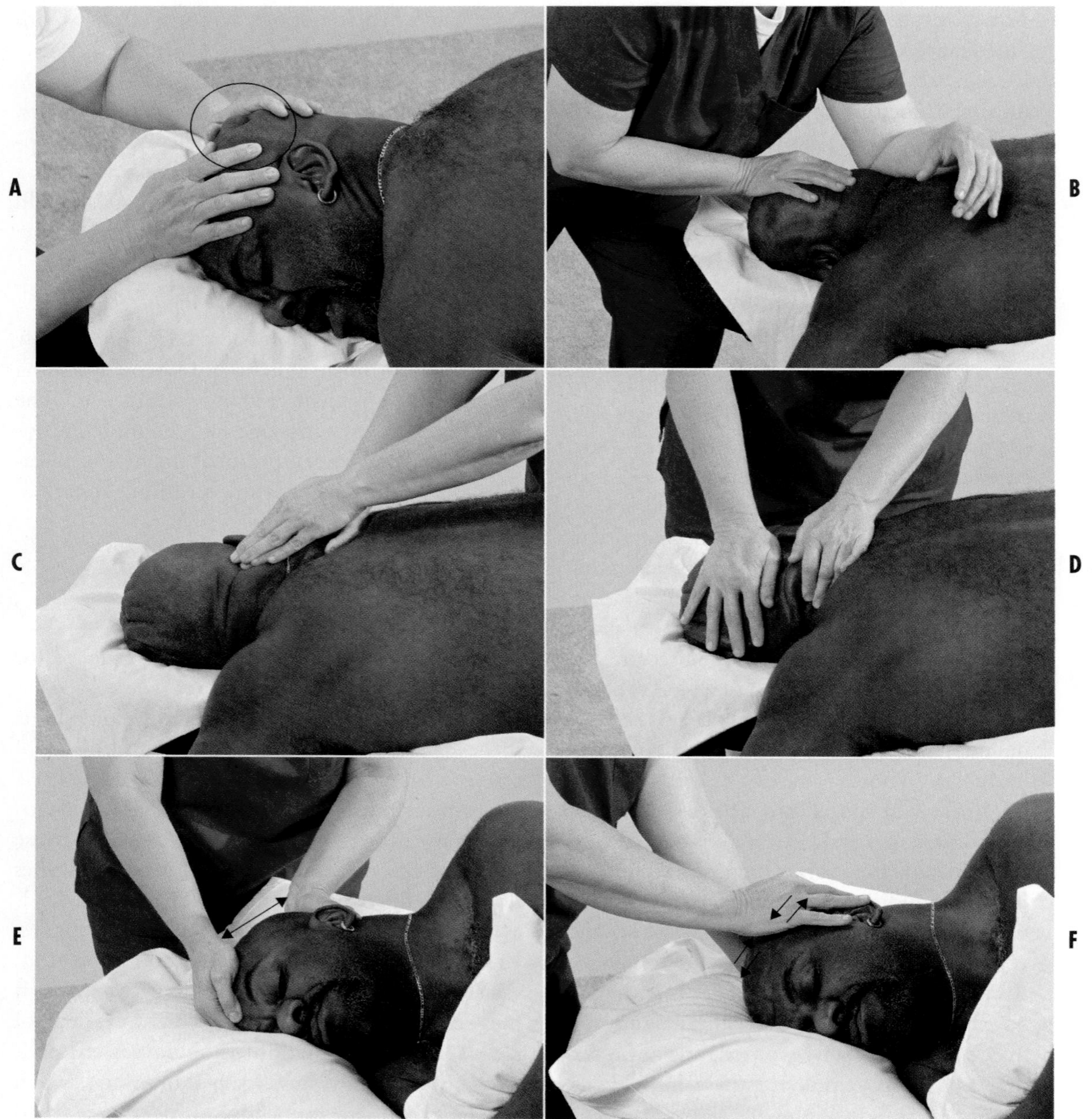

FIGURE 17-7 ■ Massage strategy for tension headache. This headache is the type most successfully treated with massage. The soft tissues are short and binding and have increased motor and fascial tone. Trigger points can occur, and areas of reduced blood flow are common. Massage successfully addresses these issues. **A,** Assess the area and identify potential contraindications and cautions that would alter treatment. This patient has a compression fracture from a 20-year-old bullet wound. Although the area has healed completely, it is prudent to alter the pressure in the immediate area. **B,** Massage the areas that could contribute to headache symptoms. During massage, assess for trigger points that refer pain into the symptom pattern and address with various methods (e.g., positional release and inhibitory pressure). **C,** Using inhibitory pressure to address trigger points. **D,** Continue to massage the area to increase tissue pliability and circulation. Make sure to address all soft tissue that could be contributing to the headache while the patient is in the prone position (as pictured), as well as in the side-lying and supine positions. **E,** Incorporate pulsed muscle energy methods to address motor tone in the neck muscles. **F,** Use various directions of movement during pulsed muscle energy methods.

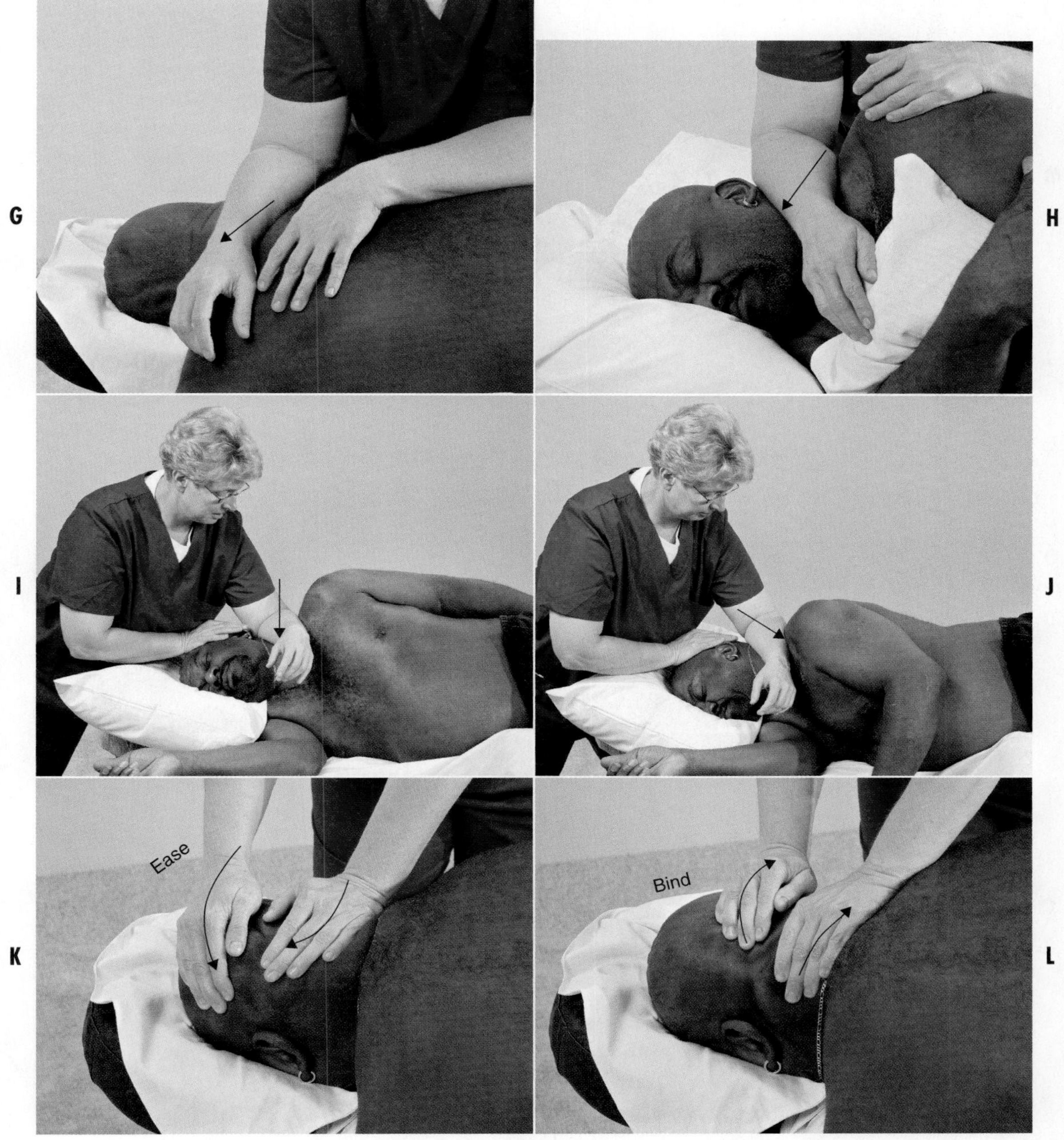

FIGURE 17-7, cont'd ■ **G,** After the area has been massaged, generally begin specific releases using inhibitory pressure (these attachment are at the occipital base). Keep contact broad based for best results. **H,** Release the suboccipitals and attachments of sternocleidomastoid if appropriate. **I,** Scalenes: Move the head to focus on specific points. **J,** Lower attachments of scalenes and upper trapezius. **K,** Assess for ease and bind of tissue. Treat bind areas by moving tissue to ease and holding for 15 to 30 seconds. **L,** Next, move tissue into bind and hold for 15 to 30 seconds. Repeat this procedure in different areas that relate to headache pain pattern.

Continued

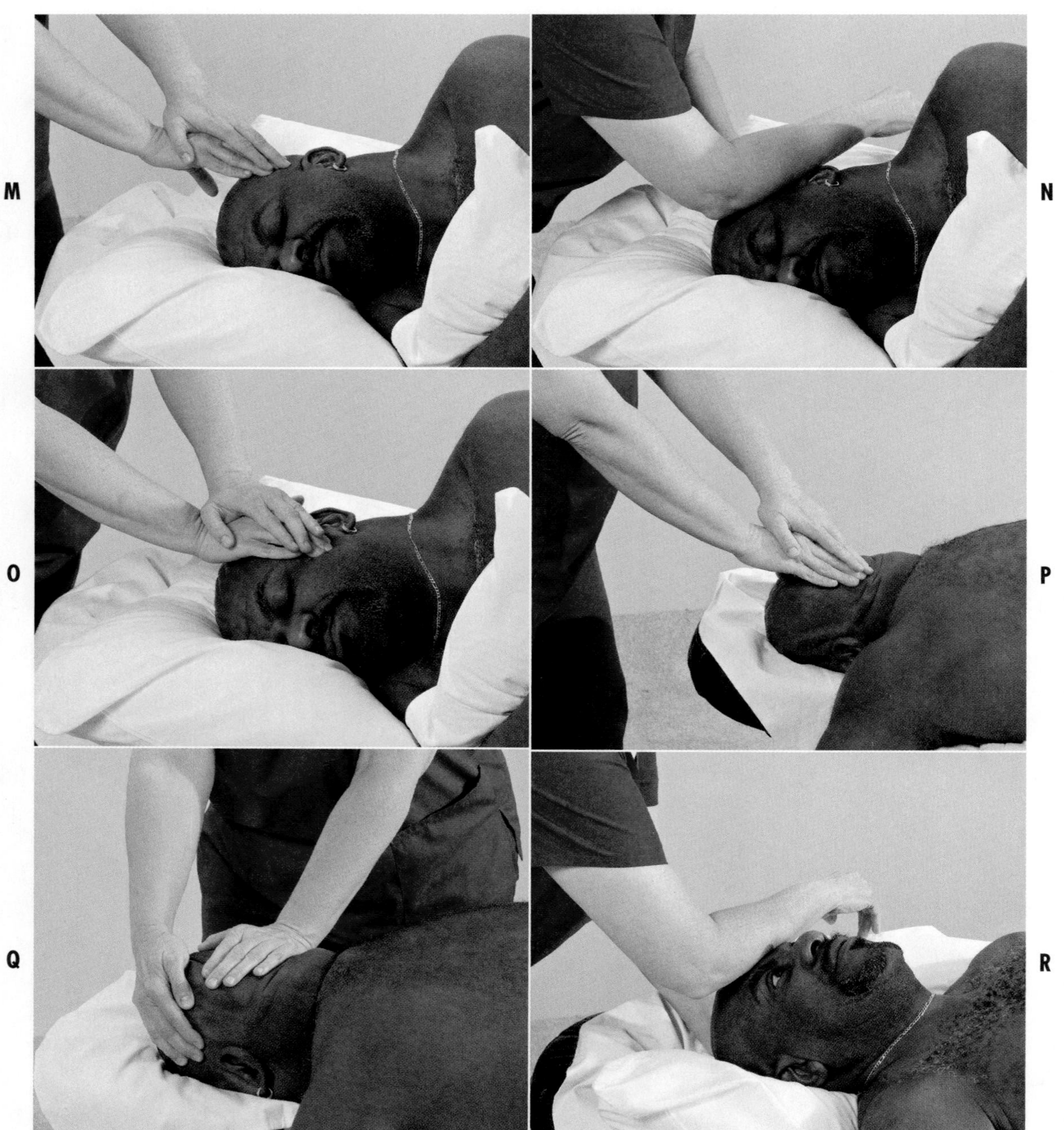

FIGURE 17-7, cont'd ■ **M,** Inhibitory pressure on the small muscles around the ears. **N,** Inhibitory pressure on the temporalis. **O,** Inhibitory pressure on the masseter. **P,** Inhibitory pressure or friction on the occiput attachment. **Q,** Massage after inhibitory pressure to increase circulation and stretch tissues. **R,** Inhibitory pressure on the frontalis with eye movement.

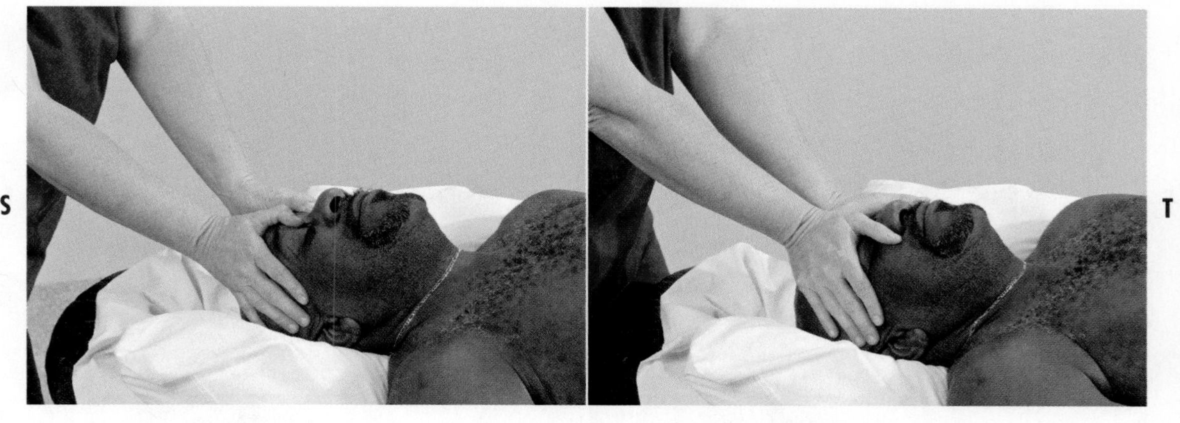

FIGURE 17-7, cont'd ■ **S,** Massage the face and address tender points. **T,** Finish with focused, soothing, intentional work and continue with the massage.

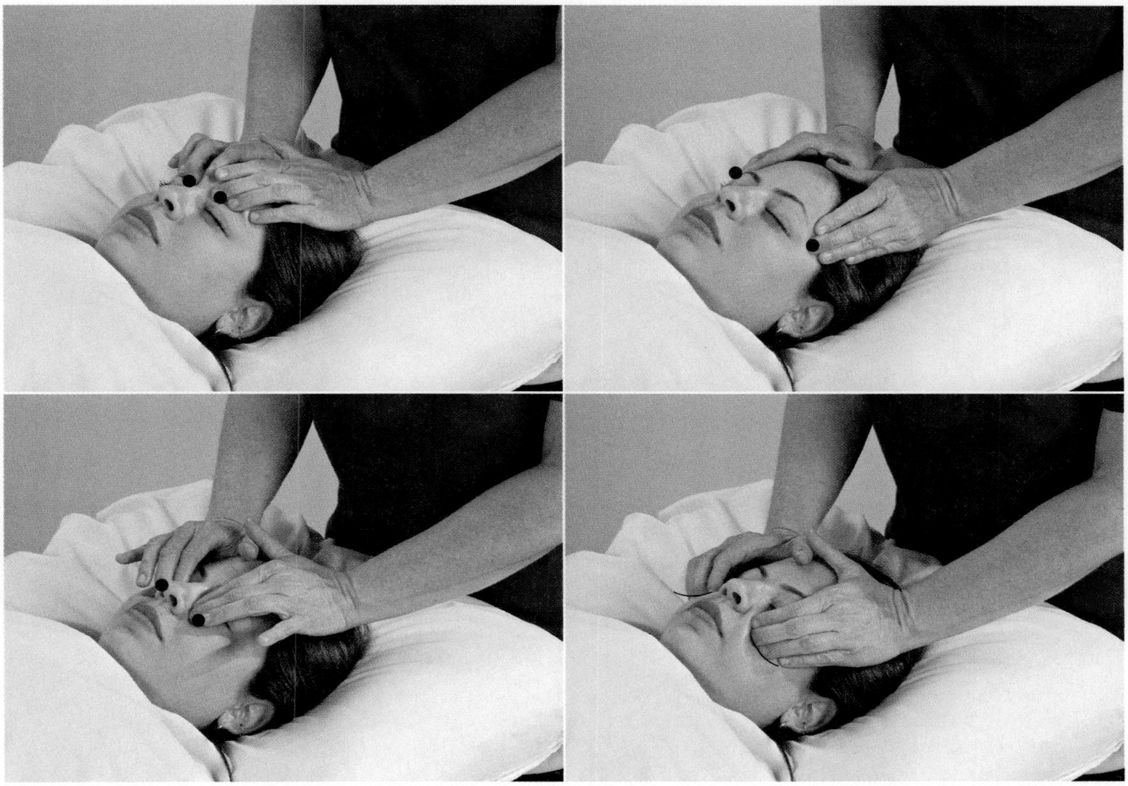

FIGURE 17-8 ■ Massage strategy for sinus headache. **A-C,** Apply rhythmic compression to points. **D,** Apply rhythmic compression up and under the cheek.

Continued

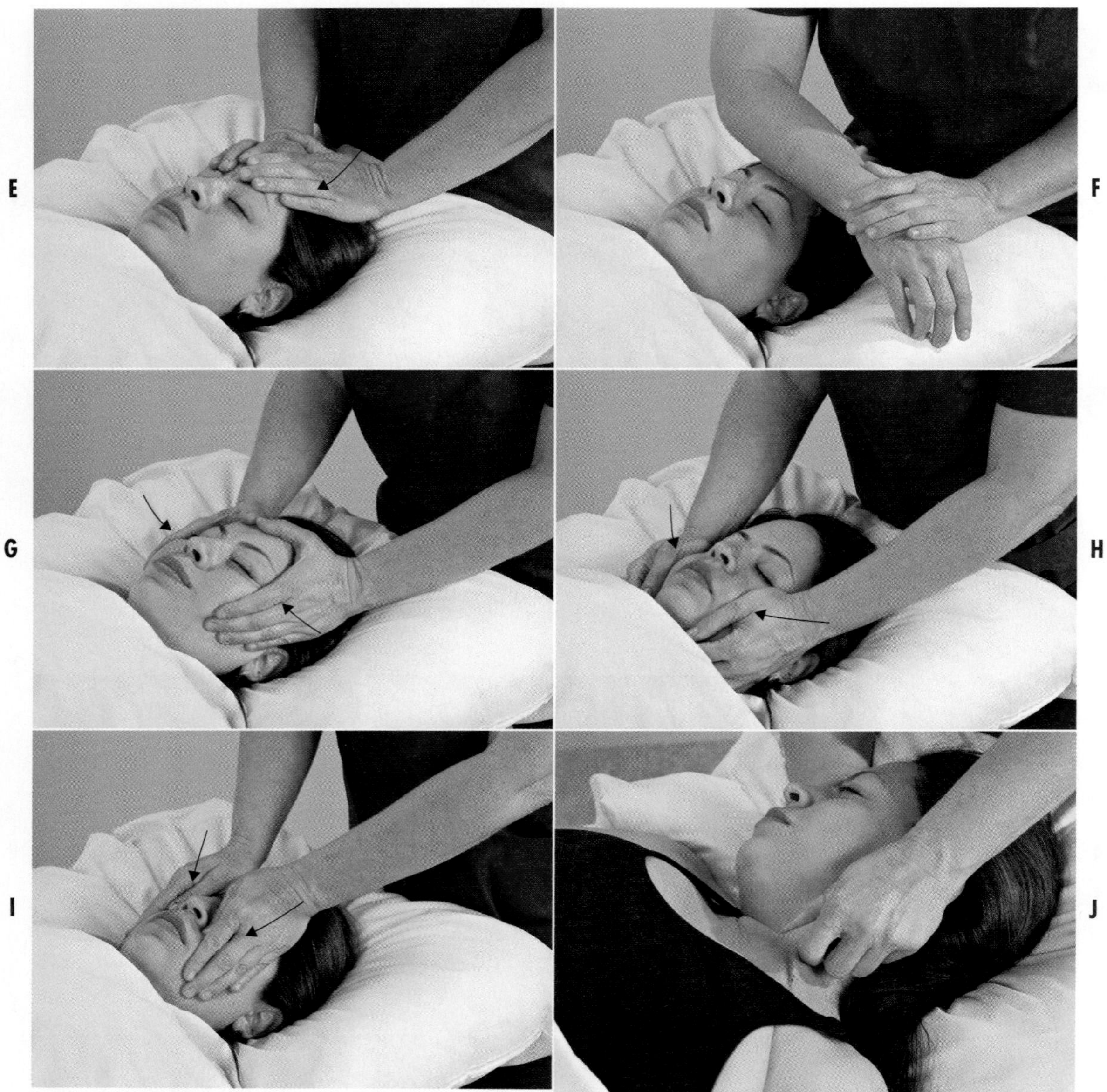

FIGURE 17-8, cont'd ■ **E,** Apply broad-based, rhythmic compression to the top of the head. **F,** Apply rhythmic compression to the forehead. **G,** Apply rhythmic compression to the sides of the face. **H,** Apply rhythmic compression to the cheek and jaw. **I,** Apply rhythmic compression to the face, hands cupped over the eyes. **J,** Incorporate sternocleidomastoid release if pressure occurs in the eyes and the base of the skull.

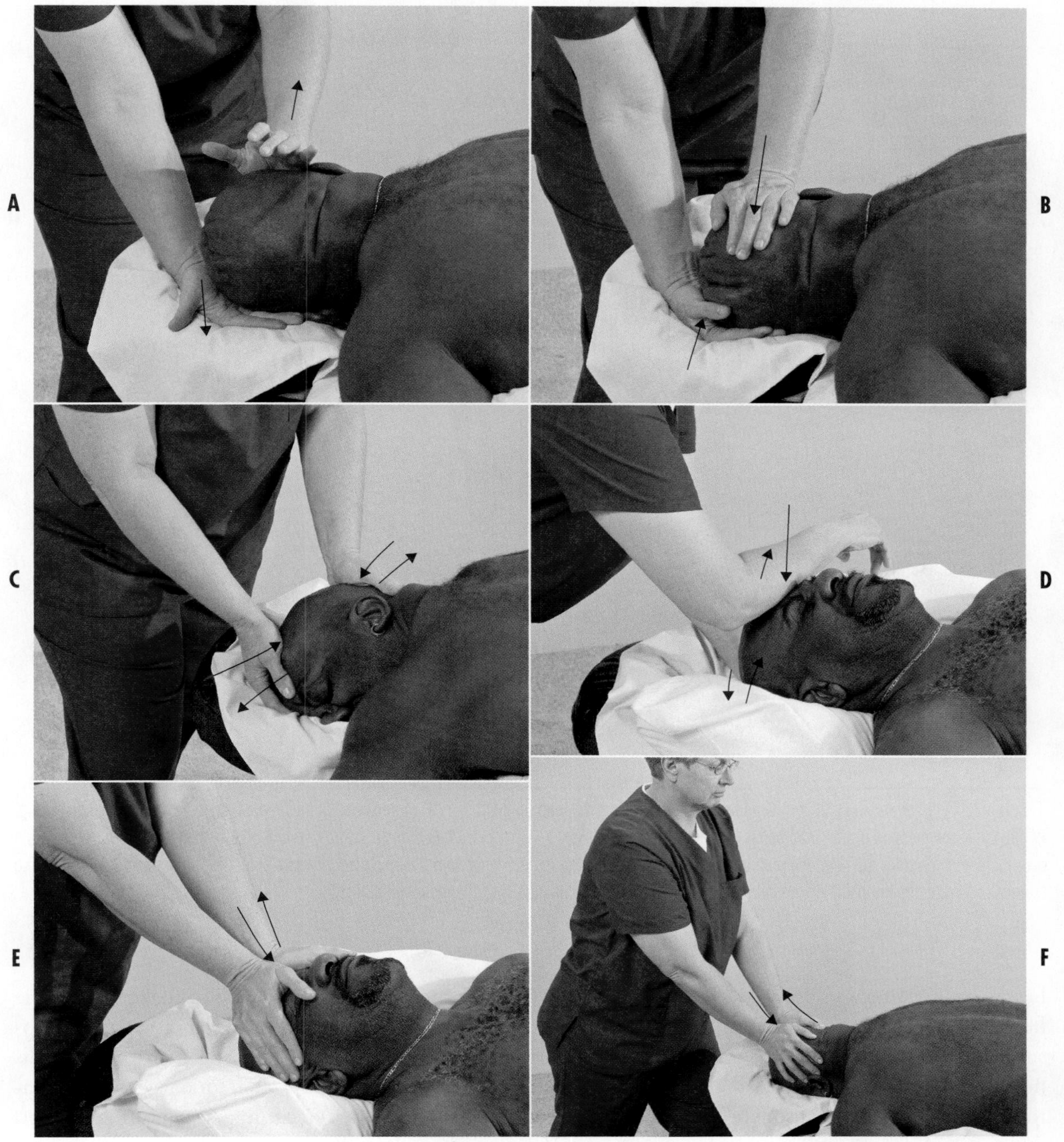

FIGURE 17-9 ■ Massage strategy for vascular headache. Vascular headache is difficult to manage with massage. It often is beneficial to address tension headache and then incorporate the following pumping methods if they feel beneficial to patient. If a person has a full-blown vascular headache, tension headache methods may be too intense. If that is the case, use only pumping methods. **A,** Applying rhythmic pumping compression to the lateral sides of the head. **B,** Use broad-based contact to prevent painful poking. Repeat 5 or 6 times. **C,** Rhythmic compression and release in various positions, posterior and anterior. **D,** Compressive pumping, posterior and anterior. **E,** Compressive pumping, anterior. **F,** Compressive pumping, posterior.

Continued

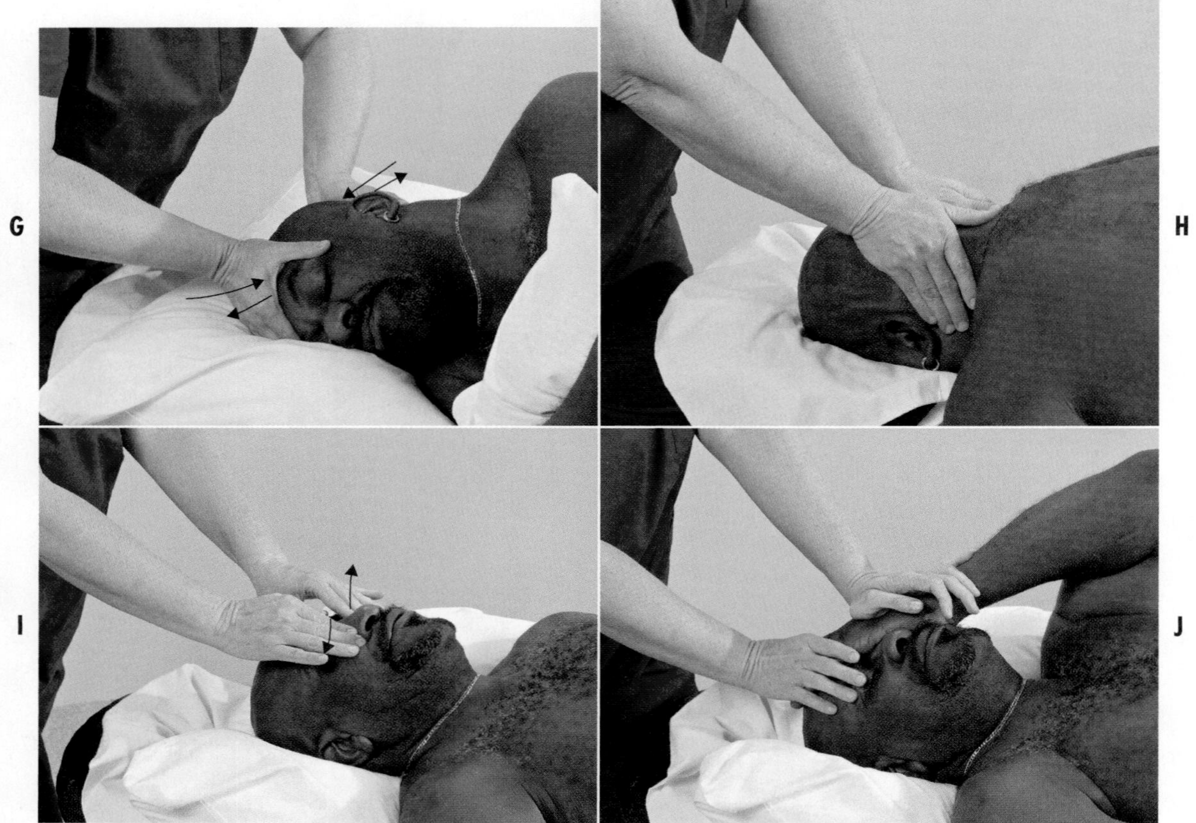

FIGURE 17-9, cont'd ■ **G,** Compressive pumping, posterior and anterior. **H,** Intersperse pumping applications with compressive gliding. **I,** Rhythmic compression of the facial bones also addresses the sinuses. **J,** If a person has a cluster headache or headache pain in the eye, compression over the eye can soothe the pain. Pressure and pain in the eyes can be referred pain from the sternocleidomastoid muscle. If assessment (i.e., pinching the muscle) recreates the pain, include muscle release methods and continue with the rest of the massage.

headache, caffeine withdrawal headache, and toxic headache. Pain is experienced as an ache or pressure that pushes outward from the inside of the head. The person may feel as if the head is going to explode. Vascular headaches are difficult to manage with massage.

Cluster headaches occur on one side of the head, possibly with intervals of remission and recurrence for long periods. These headaches usually occur at night and are associated with symptoms such as red eyes and sinus drainage.

Although the cause of migraine headaches is unknown, they are believed to be caused by excessive dilation of the cerebral blood vessels. Any visual distortion (e.g., flashing lights) is thought to be caused by vasoconstriction that precedes the vasodilation and pain. A migraine headache produces a throbbing or pulsating pain that often is one sided (unilateral).[1] It frequently is accompanied by nausea; vomiting; sensitivity to light, sound, and smells; sleep disruption; and depression. Attacks often recur, and they tend to become less severe as the person ages. Migraine headaches afflict millions of people. They may occur at any age, but usually begin between the ages of 10 and 40 and diminish after age 50. Some people experience several migraines a month, while others have only a few migraines throughout their lifetime and women are more susceptible than men.[1]

As mentioned, the cause of migraine headaches has not yet been determined, but considerable research is underway in this area. The condition may result from a series of reactions in the CNS caused by changes in the body or in the environment. A family history of the disorder often is a factor, which suggests that migraine sufferers may inherit sensitivity to triggers that produce inflammation in the blood vessels and nerves around the brain, causing pain.[1]

Some illnesses that must be ruled out as a cause of the headache include bowel problems, mold allergies, vitamin deficiencies, hypertension, TMJ misalignment, food allergies or intolerances, dehydration, spinal subluxation, coffee or caffeine intoxication, and aspartame (NutraSweet, Equal) toxicity. All of these can cause migraine symptoms and usually can be treated very easily. Common triggers for migraine headaches include the following[1]:

- Alcohol (e.g., red wine)
- Weather, altitude, time zone changes
- Caffeine
- Monosodium glutamate (MSG)
- Nitrates
- Glare and bright light
- Hormonal changes in women
- Hunger
- Lack of sleep
- Medications (OTC and prescription)
- Perfume and other scents
- Stress

Migraines are categorized according to their symptoms. The two most common types are migraine with aura and migraine without aura. Less common types include basilar artery migraine, carotidynia, headache-free migraine, ophthalmoplegic migraine, and status migraine.[1]

These types of headaches can become debilitating. Some people experience the primary headache pain along with nausea and vomiting and sensitivity to light and sound. The hands and feet may feel cold and sweaty, and odors may be intolerable. Once the headache has passed, migraine sufferers often feel tired and weak.

Various types of migraine headache have been described. Following are brief descriptions of migraine headache variations:

- *Migraine with aura:* An aura is a neurologic phenomenon that occurs 10 to 30 minutes before the headache. Most auras are visual, but nonvisual auras include motor weakness, speech or language abnormalities, dizziness, vertigo, and tingling or numbness, especially of the face and head. Visual aura is typically experienced as bright and shimmering lights around objects or at the edges of the field of vision, zigzag lines, wavy images, or temporary loss of vision.
- *Migraine without aura:* Migraine without aura is more common than migraine with aura and may occur on one or both sides of the head. The person can become tired or moody the day before the headache occurs. Nausea, vomiting, and photophobia (bothered by bright lights) often accompany migraine without aura.
- *Headache-free migraine:* This variation of the migraine is characterized by an aura experience without a headache. This migraine occurs in patients with a history of migraine with aura.
- *Basilar artery migraine:* This migraine involves a disturbance of the basilar artery in the brainstem. Symptoms include severe headache, vertigo, double vision, slurred speech, and poor muscle coordination.
- *Carotidynia migraine:* This headache, also called lower-half headache or facial migraine, produces a deep, dull aching. Tenderness and swelling over the carotid artery in the neck are typical. Piercing pain in the jaw or neck can occur.
- *Ophthalmoplegic migraine:* This migraine begins with pain in the eye and is accompanied by vomiting. As the headache progresses, the eyelid droops and the nerves responsible for eye movement become paralyzed.
- *Status migraine:* This migraine is rare and produces intense pain that usually lasts longer than 72 hours; the person may require hospitalization.

Treatment of Vascular Headache

There are two variations of drug treatment that are used to help alleviate the pain of a migraine:

abortive and preventive. In abortive treatment, medication is administered at the onset of a headache or while the headache is actually occurring. Patients using preventive therapy take daily medication. Preventive therapy is reserved for patients who experience severe migraines on a frequent basis. Before resorting to drug treatment, doctors suggest that women adhere to the following advice.

- Avoid alcohol and nicotine
- Avoid skipping meals
- Exercise 3 to 5 days a week
- Get plenty of rest
- Practice relaxation techniques

Prophylactic measures include preventive medication that may be prescribed for patients who have three or more headaches a month that do not respond to abortive treatment. Many of these medications have adverse side effects. If the migraines are brought under control, the dosage can be reduced or the drug may be discontinued.

Preventive medications include the following:

- Beta blockers: These drugs affect the heart rate, thus they should not be taken by patients with asthma and should be used with caution by those with diabetes. Side effects include gastrointestinal upset, insomnia, low blood pressure (hypotension), a slowed heart rate, and sexual dysfunction. Some beta blockers pass into breast milk and may cause problems in nursing infants.
- Antiseizure drugs: The side effects of these drugs include nausea, gastrointestinal upset, sedation, liver damage, and tremors.
- Calcium channel blockers: These medications inhibit artery dilation and block the release of serotonin. They should not be taken by patients with a heart condition. Side effects include constipation, flushing, low blood pressure, rash, and nausea.
- Antidepressants: Tricyclic and SSRI antidepressants most often are used, although side effects of the tricyclic antidepressants include constipation, dry mouth, low blood pressure, an increased heart rate, urinary retention, sexual dysfunction, and weight gain. The SSRIs usually are better tolerated than the tricyclic antidepressants, but they may not be as effective. Side effects include nausea, insomnia, sexual dysfunction, and loss of appetite.
- Methysergide maleate: This drug (e.g., Desyrel, Sansert) is prescribed for patients with frequent, severe migraines. Side effects include insomnia, drowsiness, lightheadedness, and hair loss. This medication should not be used by patients with coronary artery disease and must be discontinued for 3 to 4 weeks after 4 to 6 months of use because it can cause retroperitoneal fibrosis, a condition in which the blood vessels in the abdomen thicken, reducing blood flow to organs.

Strategies for abortive treatment depend on the intensity and frequency of the headache events. Mild, infrequent migraines may be relieved by OTC medications. Analgesics (e.g., aspirin, ibuprofen, acetaminophen) provide symptomatic relief of headache pain and should be taken at the first sign of a migraine. However, frequent use of analgesics (i.e., more than four times a week) can cause rebound headaches.

Severe headaches require a prescription medication. Ergots may be administered orally or as a suppository and often are taken with antinausea drugs, such as prochlorperazine (Compazine). The ergots should be taken at the first sign of a migraine because they may not be effective if the headache has moved into the throbbing stage. Side effects include gastrointestinal upset, dizziness, stroke, and high blood pressure (hypertension). Ergots should not be taken by patients with heart, vascular, liver, or kidney disease. Chiropractic adjustments and maintaining correct spinal alignment can be very beneficial for preventing headaches triggered by muscle stress and spasm. Acupressure also can be helpful, as can alternating applications of hot and cold hydrotherapy. A transcutaneous electrical nerve stimulation (TENS) unit can help reduce muscle spasm pain.

Massage strategies for vascular headaches are presented on p. 621.

TENSION (MUSCLE CONTRACTION) HEADACHE

Tension (muscle contraction) headache is caused by referred pain from trigger point activity or nerve impingement, muscle tension, and muscle guarding. The pain is experienced as pressure from the outside of the head pushing in, and the person may feel as if a tight band is encircling the head. This type of headache is effectively managed with massage.

Tension headaches are the most common type of headache. They are believed to be caused by a muscle-tendon strain at the origin of the trapezius and deep neck muscles at the occipital bone or at the origin of the frontalis muscle on the frontal bone (occipital or frontal headaches). Tension headache also can originate in the TMJ muscle complex. Connective tissue structures that support the head may be implicated in headache if they are shortened and pull the head or scalp into nerves, creating pain. Conversely, if connective tissue support structures are lax and fail to support the neck and head, nerve structures may be compressed as well.

Headaches are a common condition, and predisposing factors include the following:

- Headgear and hats that put pressure on pain-sensitive structures
- Squinting under bright lights or in the sun
- Dehydration
- Changes in blood flow
- Tendency for overbreathing
- Blood sugar changes
- Impact trauma that increases neck muscle tension
- Changes in activity that strain upper body muscles and joints

Treatment of Tension (Muscle Contraction) Headache. Most tension headaches are treated with NSAIDs, such as aspirin or ibuprofen. However, frequent use of headache medication can cause a rebound headache pattern, therefore these drugs should be used only if other methods fail.

Massage Treatment Strategies for Headache

Massage and other forms of soft tissue therapy are effective in treating tension headache but much less effective for vascular (e.g., migraine or cluster) headaches. However, soft tissue therapy can relieve secondary tension headache caused by the pain of the primarily vascular headache. Headache is often stress induced. Stress management in all forms usually is indicated in chronic headache conditions. Massage and other forms of soft tissue therapy are effective in treating tension headaches.

Strategies for Vascular Headache. As mentioned, vascular headache is a feeling of pain and pressure pushing outward from inside the head. Sometimes the headache is caused by constipation; in these cases, abdominal massage is an option. A toxic headache caused by chemicals (e.g., MSG, excessive alcohol consumption) often responds to hydration and the vascular headache strategy (see Figure 17-9). However until the liver detoxifies the substance and it is cleared from the body, the headache will linger.

Approach the massage as if excessive fluid were present in the skull and the goal of the massage is to help eliminate the fluid. Rhythmic compression on the head and face serves as a pump to move the fluid. The compressive force exerted on the head is substantial and should be broad based. The person should feel a pleasant relief from the pressure inside the head.

To perform this technique, place your flat hands or forearms on the occipital bone and frontal bone and press together firmly. Then release. Repeat this sequence rhythmically and slowly, up to 50 repetitions. Next, repeat the entire process, applying the pressure at the temporal bones.

If the pain is more in the face (e.g., a sinus headache), apply the rhythmic compression at the temples, cheeks, side of the nose, and over the eyes using either the palm of the hand or the pads of the fingers. When you apply pressure over the eyes, do not actually press on the eyeballs. Instead, cup the palm and apply pressure around the eye socket. Often a tension headache accompanies a vascular headache.

Strategies for Tension Headache. Tension headache is pain on the outside of the head and at the base of the neck. This type of headache may be a muscle or connective tissue bind headache. Inhibitory pressure is used on the muscles of the scalp (i.e., the occipital/frontalis, temporalis, and auricular [ear] muscles). Muscle energy and positional release methods can be used for these headaches by instructing the patient to move the eyebrows, clench the teeth, and move the ears. Massage the entire muscle area, paying attention to both the belly and the attachments of the muscle; the pressure should be intense enough to recreate but not to increase the headache symptoms. Tension in the suboccipital muscles, scalenes, sternocleidomastoid, and trapezius can cause referred pain by causing nerve impingement. Inhibiting pressure, along with muscle energy and lengthening procedures, is used on the muscles that create the headache symptoms.

Headaches that are more in the face can arise from the muscles of mastication or those that control eyebrow movement. They are addressed as previously described. The pressure level is intense enough to recreate the headache symptoms; this is significantly more pressure than is typically used during general relaxation massage. However, the pressure should not cause guarding, and although it is painful, it should be a "good" hurt.

The scalp has a significant number of connective tissue structures. The tendons and fascial anchoring bands of the scalp can shorten. The forces applied to these structures during massage usually are shear and bend forces with localized tension force. As with any connective tissue application, apply the forces slowly and rhythmically, into and out of bind. Again, the intensity is more than that typically used during general massage, and both the pressure and the location should feel right to the patient.

If possible, the muscles and connective tissue can be stretched by pulling the hair. Grab a large bundle of hair near the scalp and exert an even, firm pull. At the point of resistance, shift the direction back and forth, into and out of bind. Repeat the process sequentially all over the head; this should feel intense but good to the patient. If the patient has no hair or very short hair, the scalp can be rolled and twisted about the skull, into and out of bind. Next, firmly massage along all cranial sutures with a circular-type friction.

Eye muscles can be a factor in headache pain. Have the patient place the finger pads over the eyes and apply a gentle compression to the eyeballs. Maintaining the compression, the patient moves the eyes in alternating circles and a figure-eight pattern.

Thoroughly massage the neck and shoulder muscles, addressing any areas that recreate the headache symptoms.

The connective tissue structures from the skull to the sacrum, if short, can cause headache. These structures need to be addressed to increase tissue pliability and reduce bind. Effective methods include connective tissue techniques that generate mechanical forces and skin rolling approaches that exert sufficient drag from the scalp down the midline of the back to the sacrum. Begin at the head and end at the sacrum, then reverse direction and begin at the sacrum and end at the head.

Additional approaches for headache of both general types include reflexology, especially at the big toe, and acupressure.

USE OF COUNTERIRRITANTS AND ESSENTIAL OILS FOR HEADACHE

A cooling counterirritant ointment with a menthol or peppermint base, applied to the base of the neck, the temples, and the forehead, is effective for all headache types. Many products that have menthol as an ingredient are available over the counter. Essential oils can be placed on cotton balls and put in plastic bags for the patient to sniff. Sinus headaches tend to respond to eucalyptus, tension headaches respond to peppermint and lavender, and toxic headaches respond to citrus (e.g., lemon, orange, and lime). However, if the headache is a migraine type, using the various aromas can make the headache either better or worse. Therefore, the patient would need to guide the use. Various medications can relieve headache, therefore the massage therapist should ask patients whether they have taken any medications and adjust the massage accordingly.

SELF-HELP FOR HEADACHE

Because vascular headache responds to external compression, self-help techniques for these headaches may include wrapping a towel or elastic bandage tightly around the head, wearing a tight hat, or putting a weight (e.g., a rice bag) on top of the head.

Tension headache responds to compression of the muscles. As silly as this may sound and look, the person can pull a plastic clothes hanger over the head to press on the muscles causing the symptoms; this should relieve the pain somewhat. Areas of the hanger that poke should be padded. Putting a bag of sand or a rice bag on top of the head also works for these headaches.

JUST BETWEEN YOU AND ME

I have a tendency to get both migraine and tension headaches, and I have some unusual methods of coping with them. One day my youngest son came home with a couple of friends, and he brought them back to my office to meet me. I was at the computer (which tends to result in a headache). There I sat, not one but two clothes hangers on my head. One was poking my forehead, so I had a sock under it for a cushion, and I had a bag of navy beans on top of my head. I had peppermint and lavender lavished all over my neck and forehead. I chatted a moment with my son's friends without ever mentioning the contraptions on my head. As they were leaving, I heard my son say, "Mom is cool even if she acts weird." One of the kids replied, "She smells good."

INFECTION

Infection should always be diagnosed and treated by a physician.

BACTERIAL INFECTION

A bacterial infection can occur anywhere in the body. It can be a local condition, such as an infected wound, or a more general one, such as a gastrointestinal infection. If bacterial infection is present, digestive upset, including diarrhea, is common, because this is an immune response to rid the body of the pathogen. A fever under 102° F (often called a *low-grade inflammatory response*) usually is productive during infection and should not be reduced unless complicating factors exist (e.g., another immune response to infection). Usually but not always during a bacterial infection, the person may get really sick within a relatively short period. The fever and other immune responses are more extreme. If bacterial infection is detected, antibiotics may be prescribed. The rest of the treatment for bacterial infection is supportive (i.e., rest, fluids, drainage of abscesses, and support of the immune system).

Massage is not indicated in the acute phase of a bacterial infection (the first 3 to 5 days). During the subacute phase, general palliative massage is appropriate to support sleep and to soothe aching resulting from reduced activity (Figure 17-10).

VIRAL INFECTION

Viruses cause many different illnesses, which can persist or become chronic. Common viral diseases

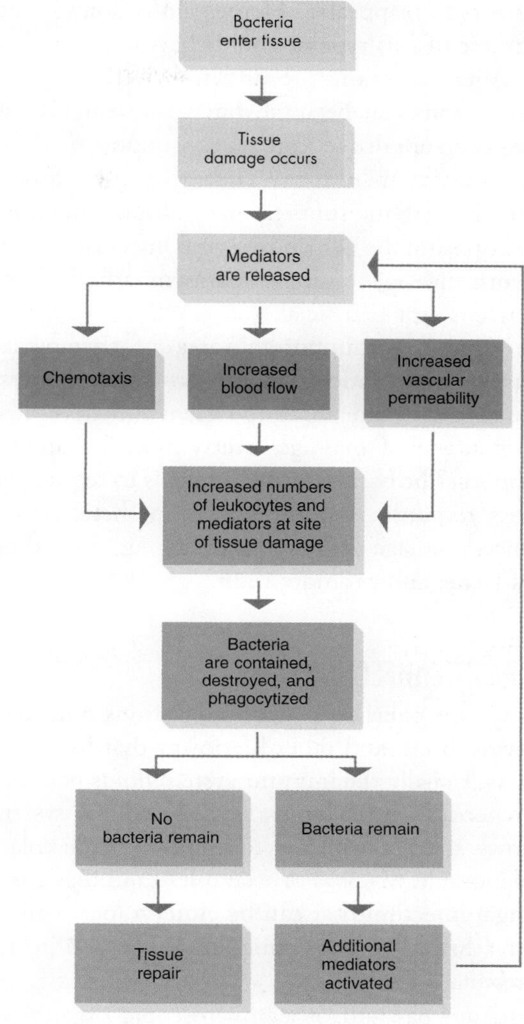

FIGURE 17-10 ■ The inflammatory response. (From Thibodeau GA, Patton KT: *Anatomy and physiology,* ed 6, St Louis, 2007, Mosby.)

are mononucleosis, viral respiratory disease, influenza, hepatitis, human immunodeficiency virus (HIV) infection, and herpes. Severe viral infection (e.g., flu, mononucleosis) has been linked with the later development of various autoimmune diseases. Viral infections tend to produce a more subtle immune response. The fever is not as high as in a bacterial infection. The onset of the illness after exposure is longer than with bacterial infections, and the symptoms begin as mild and progress to the severe stage. Recovery from a viral infection seems to take longer. Many viruses are never actually eliminated; they hide in the body, and when the immune system is suppressed, the symptom reappears. Herpes infection is an example of this type of viral behavior.

Viral infections are difficult to treat. A few medications can be used, but treatment usually involves supportive care (i.e., support for the immune system, rest, and a nutritious diet). Stress, pain, and fatigue suppress the immune function, predisposing the person to a viral infection. Therapeutic massage to support parasympathetic dominance is very beneficial.

This is an important area of therapeutic massage intervention, which works well for stress management and immune system function. The main target of massage intervention is immune support. The basic treatment plan is to reduce the stress response; support parasympathetic dominance; manage stiffness and aching, including headache; and promote sleep.

PARASITIC INFECTION

Fungi are parasitic plants and various amoebas, worms, bugs, and other life forms that live in or on us. Usually the immune system holds parasites in check, but weakening of the immune system allows these organisms to multiply and create diagnosable illness. For example, candidiasis is a fungal infection that can be either a local condition (thrush) or a systemic one if it grows in the intestinal tract.

Amoebas and other microscopic organisms, as well as round worms, tapeworms, and liver flukes (which are pretty big), are much more common than any of us would like to think. Most kids get lice, and anyone who has pets is exposed to fleas to some degree.

When people are healthy, these plants and creatures can feed on us without causing health problems. However, if an overgrowth of fungus occurs or if the number of parasitic animals increases, treatment is required. Effective medications are available, but because they basically poison the parasite and are toxic, medication-related side effects occur. Parasites are contagious (perhaps a better term is *transferable*), therefore sanitation is crucial.

Massage does not directly support treatment for parasites other than by helping to support the immune system (Figure 17-11).

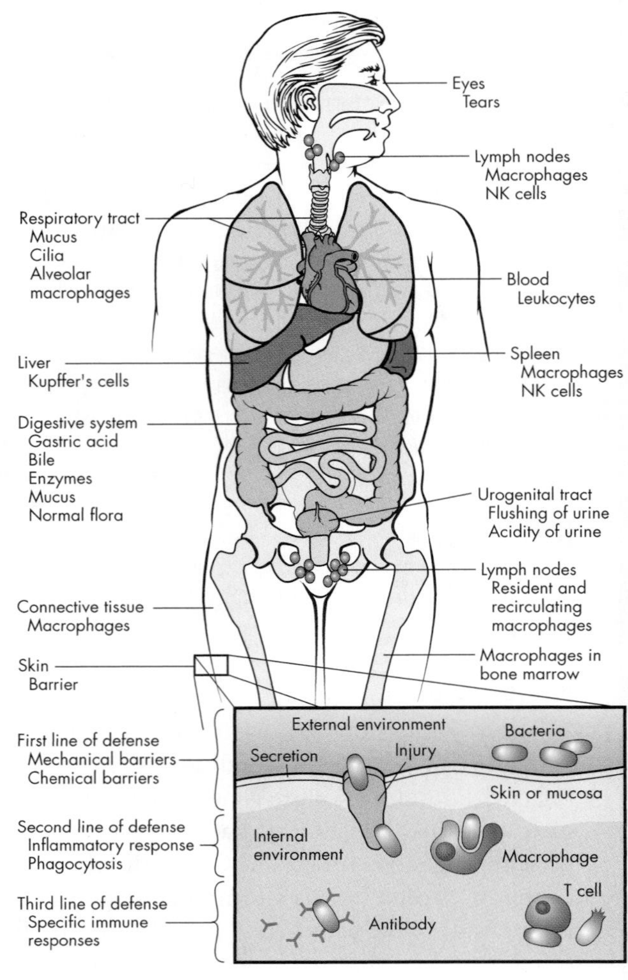

FIGURE 17-11 ■ Natural protective mechanisms of the human body. *NK*, natural killer (cells). (From Damjanov I: *Pathology for the health-related professions*, ed 3, Philadelphia, 2006, WB Saunders.)

MASSAGE STRATEGIES FOR INFECTION

Massage is contraindicated in the acute phase of an infection. In the subacute phase, *do not* overdo the massage and strain the person's adaptive mechanism. Regardless of any treatment plan, back off and apply general, nonspecific massage for no longer than 45 to 60 minutes. Use a method with a relaxation/palliative outcome and encourage rest, sleep, proper fluid intake, and nutritional support. Also, take care of yourself so that your immune system remains strong and can protect you from infection.

CANCER

Cancer is any one of a large number of diseases characterized by the unchecked development and proliferation of abnormal cells, which are able to metastasize and destroy normal body tissue. The treatment of cancer combines disease-specific scientific knowledge, public health awareness, and psychosocial support. The challenge for oncology (the study and treatment of cancer) is to successfully combine compassion and medical expertise at this critical time in a person's life.

Tumors are cell masses that are either benign or malignant and cancerous. Not all tumors are cancerous, and not all cancers form tumors. For example, leukemia is a cancer that involves the blood, bone marrow, lymphatic system, and spleen, but it does not form a single mass or tumor.

Not only do cancerous cells invade and destroy normal tissue, they also can produce chemicals that interfere with body functions.

Cancer occurs with increasing frequency throughout the middle years of life and later (Box 17-1). The three most commonly diagnosed cancers in women are expected to be cancers of the breast, lung, and bronchus; colon and rectal cancer are expected to be the most commonly diagnosed cancers in men. The most common cause of cancer death among men and women is cancer of the lung and bronchus.

BOX 17-1 Location and Types of Cancer

Anal	Mesothelioma
Bladder	Multiple myeloma
Bone	Myelodysplastic syndrome
Brain and central nervous system	Non-Hodgkin's lymphoma
Breast	Ovarian
Cervical	Pancreatic
Colon	Prostatic
Esophageal	Rectal
Gastric	Renal
Head and neck	Sarcoma
Hodgkin's lymphoma	Skin
Leukemia	Testicular
Liver	Thyroid
Lung	Uterine
Melanoma	Skin

The American Cancer Society (ACS) estimates that two thirds of patients with cancer survive for 5 years or longer after diagnosis. Many people have undergone treatment and returned to a normal life. Others live with permanent disabilities and pain. Anyone can develop cancer, and receiving the diagnosis can be devastating. The ACS estimates that half the men and one third of the women in the United States will develop cancer during their lifetime.

Cancer is caused by damage (mutations) to deoxyribonucleic acid (DNA), which causes cells to grow and divide in chaotic fashion. Lifestyle choices are known to cause cancer. Smoking, drinking more than one drink (for women) or two drinks (for men) a day, being overweight, sun damage to skin, and unsafe sexual behaviors can lead to the mutations that cause cancer. Also, the environment may contain harmful chemicals that can cause mutations in genes. Secondhand smoke and chemicals such as asbestos and benzene can cause cancer. Some DNA mutations can be inherited, although having an inherited genetic mutation does not automatically mean that a person will develop cancer. Chronic inflammation can be a factor in the development of cancer.

Medical oncology specializes in the use of systemic forms of treatment for cancer, such as chemotherapy, biologic modulators, and immunotherapy. Traditionally, the medical oncologist serves as the internist in the multidisciplinary management of cancer. For the most part, the surgical oncologist and the radiation oncologist provide specialized, short-term care. The medical oncology team is responsible for the continued and long-term follow-up of the cancer patient, including end-of-life care for patients with an incurable disease.

Cancer can take years to develop. By the time a cancerous mass is detected, 100 million to 1 billion cancer cells probably are present, and the original cancer cell may have been dividing for 5 years or longer.[3]

DIAGNOSIS

Cancer can be diagnosed only through the examination of cells under a microscope. A surgical process called a *biopsy* is performed to obtain a sample of tissue. Microscopically, normal cells look uniform, having similar sizes and an orderly organization, whereas cancer cells vary in size and have no apparent organization.[3]

Some warning signs of cancer include the following[3]:

- Sores that do not heal
- Unusual bleeding
- A change in the appearance or size of a wart or mole
- A lump or thickening in any tissue
- Persistent hoarseness or cough
- Chronic indigestion
- A change in bowel or bladder function

Cancer is no longer an automatic death sentence. More than two thirds of those diagnosed with cancer survive 5 years or longer after diagnosis. One key to survival is early detection of the cancer. Cancer screening tests include the following:

- Breast self-examination
- Mammogram
- Colon and rectal cancer screening
- Pap test for cervical cancer
- Prostate cancer screening

Some of the most common, nonspecific symptoms of cancer are fatigue, pain, anorexia, insomnia, and nausea. Occasionally a palpable mass is present. After the cancer has been diagnosed, the care of the oncology patient begins with a detailed history and physical examination. Most patients with cancer receive some type of therapy once a histologic diagnosis has been made and the extent of disease has been determined by appropriate staging (stage 1, least advanced; stage 2, moderately advanced; stage 3, critically advanced). Stage 1 cancer is the most treatable. Accurate staging provides a basis for both the medical team and the patient to weigh individual benefits and risks associated with each treatment option.

Whether treatment has a curative or palliative intent, success depends on the disease stage and the patient's acceptance of the treatment plan. If the intent of therapy is curative, both the oncology team and the patient are more apt to accept the harshness and toxicities of treatment. However, if the goals of treatment are to enhance quality of life and, when possible, to extend life for awhile, palliative treatment is more appropriate.

Over the past few years, the value of a multidisciplinary, integrated approach to the care and treatment of individuals with cancer has been increasingly recognized. In many healthcare environments, multidisciplinary cancer clinics offer people the opportunity to be evaluated by the medical oncologist, surgical oncologist, radiation oncologist, nutritionist, physical therapist, and social worker at the time of the first or second clinic visit. Therapeutic massage is fast becoming an important aspect of multidisciplinary care in these settings. Other complementary therapies (e.g., meditation, yoga, aromatherapy) also are incorporated into the care in multidisciplinary centers. The spiritual needs of individuals are considered and supported as well. In the multidisciplinary approach to patient management, each discipline performs a complementary function. In this regard, cancer care, like hospice care, is becoming a model for effective, integrated medical care in which many professionals work together to achieve the best possible outcome.

Increasingly, several types of treatments are used together (concurrently) or in sequence with the goal of preventing recurrence; this is known as *multimodality treatment* of the cancer.

TREATMENT

Surgery

The primary care physician most often refers the patient to a surgeon for biopsy and pathologic diagnosis. The surgical oncology team, therefore, often is the first to see an individual with a newly diagnosed or suspected cancer.

Surgery is used to diagnose cancer, determine its stage, and treat cancer. A common type of surgery that may be used to help with the diagnosis of cancer is a biopsy. As mentioned, a biopsy involves taking a tissue sample from the suspected cancer for examination by a specialist in a laboratory. A biopsy often is performed in the physician's office or in an outpatient surgery center. A positive biopsy result indicates the presence of cancer; a negative result may indicate only that no cancer is present in the sample.

When surgery is used for treatment, the cancerous mass and some adjacent tissue typically are removed. In addition to allowing local treatment of the cancer, surgery provides information that is useful for predicting whether the cancer is likely to recur and whether other treatment methods will be necessary.

Radiation Therapy

Radiation therapy, or radiotherapy, uses radiation to damage or kill cancer cells by preventing them from growing and dividing. Like surgery, radiation therapy is a local treatment used to get rid of visible tumors. It is not typically useful for shrinking or eliminating cancer cells that have spread to other parts of the body.

Radiation therapy can be delivered externally or internally. External radiation therapy delivers high-energy rays directly to the tumor site from a machine outside the body. Internal radiation therapy involves the implantation of a small amount of radioactive material in or near the cancer.

Radiotherapy has both curative and palliative indications in the treatment of cancer. Radiation often is given in conjunction with surgery, as well as chemotherapy. Radiotherapy is an integral and indispensable modality for pain relief and palliation of other conditions, such as metastatic disease to bone or obstructing bronchial lesions. Individuals undergoing radiation therapy have a variety of symptoms that most often are related to the organs within the direct radiation field. Radiation dermatitis and skin breakdown can occur, and patients often have associated fatigue and nausea. Patients undergoing brain irradiation, whether for a primary CNS tumor or a metastatic lesion, can experience myriad symptoms, including severe fatigue, disequilibrium, nausea, vomiting, confusion or short-term memory loss, and hair loss.

Chemotherapy

Chemotherapy is any treatment that uses drugs to kill cancer cells. More than half of all people diagnosed with cancer receive chemotherapy. For millions of people who have cancers that respond well to chemotherapy, this approach helps treat their cancer effectively, enabling them to enjoy full, productive lives. Unlike surgery and radiation therapy, which destroy or damage cancer cells in a specific area, chemotherapy works throughout the body. Chemotherapy can destroy cancer cells that have metastasized or spread to parts of the body far from the primary tumor.

More than 100 chemotherapy drugs are used in various combinations. Cancer chemotherapy may consist of single drugs or combinations of drugs. Although a single chemotherapeutic drug can be used to treat cancer, the effect generally is more potent if the drugs are used in combination.

Chemotherapy can be administered through a vein (usually through a line that remains in place), injected into a body cavity, or delivered orally in the form of a pill. Chemotherapy is different from surgery and radiation therapy in that it is a systemic treatment; that is, the cancer-fighting drugs circulate in the blood to parts of the body where the cancer may have spread, killing or eliminating cancer cells at sites far from the original cancer.

Many side effects once associated with chemotherapy now can be easily prevented or controlled, allowing many people to work, travel, and participate in many of their other normal activities while receiving chemotherapy. Unfortunately, most chemotherapeutic medications affect the body's normal tissues and organs as well as the cancer cells, resulting in treatment complications and side effects.

The way a person experiences side effects, which ones, and their severity depend on a variety of factors, including the type of cancer, the type of chemotherapeutic drug or regimen, the person's physical condition and age, and other such factors. For purposes of developing massage treatment plans, the following side effects typically are associated with chemotherapy:

- Anemia
- Fatigue
- Infection
- Nausea/vomiting
- Mouth sores
- Hair loss
- Constipation
- Diarrhea
- Constipation
- Pain
- Reproductive and sexuality problems
- Low platelet count (thrombocytopenia)

Fortunately, in the past 20 years a great deal of progress has been made in the development of treatments to help prevent and control the side effects of cancer therapy. For example, modern antivomiting drugs, called *antiemetics,* have reduced the severity of nausea and vomiting caused by chemotherapy. Blood cell growth factors are now available to protect patients from infection and to reduce the fatigue associated with anemia.

Fatigue is one of the most common complaints of people with cancer, and the incidence of chronic fatigue is higher in some cancer survivors. Fatigue is difficult to describe, and patients express it in a variety of ways, using terms such as tired, weak, exhausted, weary, worn out, heavy, or slow.

For many people diagnosed with cancer, fatigue may become a critical issue in their lives. It may influence one's sense of well-being, the performance of activities of daily living, relationships with family and friends, and compliance with treatment. Therapeutic massage is beneficial in managing some side effects of chemotherapy, such as fatigue and pain.

Biologic Therapy

Biologic therapy is a type of treatment that uses the body's immune system to facilitate the killing of cancer cells. Biologic therapeutic agents include interferon, interleukin, monoclonal antibodies, colony-stimulating factors (cytokines), and vaccines.

Hormonal Therapy

When cancer occurs in breast or prostate tissue, the body's own hormones may cause it to grow and spread. In these cases, treatment involves drugs that block hormone production or change the way hormones work and/or removal of organs that secrete hormones, such as the ovaries or testicles.

TERMINAL OUTCOME

The most common cause of death in patients with cancer is infection, followed by respiratory failure, hepatic failure, and renal failure. Usually, many months pass between the diagnosis of metastatic cancer and the development of these complications. Hospice provides an extraordinary service for cancer patients and their families and usually results in a positive and satisfying experience for the medical team as well.

THERAPEUTIC MASSAGE STRATEGIES FOR CANCER

As previously mentioned, massage is an accepted part of a multidisciplinary approach to cancer treatment. The benefits of massage are obvious: stress management; pain management, both preoperative and postoperative; management of treatment side effects; and more.

There are no specific protocols for massage and cancer care. The person undergoing cancer treatment must be evaluated each session, and the massage treatment is determined by the patient's status at that time.

The concern that massage increases the spread of cancer is unfounded. However, the prudent course is to avoid massaging over any type of tissue mass. Specific, extensive, full body lymphatic drainage may task an already compromised immune function and should not be used. Local lymphatic drainage methods may be appropriate. Avoid areas of radiation treatment, because the treatment damages the skin. Because bones under areas that receive radiation treatment can be brittle, carefully monitor levels of massage pressure. Do not use any massage methods that might cause tissue damage, because chemotherapy reduces the body's ability to repair tissues.

The general protocol may be too intense during cancer treatment, but the modified palliative protocol is appropriate. (See Chapter 11 and the Appendix for examples and text for the general and palliative protocols.)

KIDNEY AND LIVER DISEASE

The kidneys and the liver are the main detoxifying organs of the body. When the functional ability of these organs is reduced, poisoning of the body results. Diabetes harms the kidneys, and various types of hepatitis can damage the liver. These conditions are best treated by the medical team and have many contraindications for massage.

KIDNEY DISEASE

Healthy kidneys remove extra water and wastes, control blood pressure, maintain chemical balance, retain bone strength, produce red blood cells, and help children grow normally. Chronic kidney disease occurs when the kidneys are no longer able to clean toxins and waste products from the blood or to perform their functions to full capacity. Kidney failure, also called *end-stage renal disease* (ESRD), can occur suddenly or over time. Many people with kidney failure undergo dialysis or have a functioning kidney transplant.

Diabetes is the primary cause of kidney disease, and high blood pressure is the second highest cause. Another form of kidney disease is glomerulonephritis, a general term for many types of kidney inflammation. Genetic diseases, autoimmune diseases, birth defects, and other problems can also cause kidney disease.

Diagnosis

A *nephrologist,* a specialist in the treatment of kidney disease, evaluates the patient and suggests medications or lifestyle changes to help slow the progression of kidney disease. Kidney disease can be diagnosed through laboratory tests and by the symptoms. A urinalysis is an examination of a sample of urine to check for protein, blood, and white blood cells, which should not be present. Blood tests assess for creatinine and blood urea nitrogen (BUN), waste products that healthy kidneys remove from the bloodstream. High levels of creatinine and BUN in the blood or high levels of protein in the urine suggest kidney disease. People with diabetes should have a yearly urine test for microalbumin, small amounts of protein that do not show up on standard urine protein tests.

Symptoms of kidney disease can include the following[4]:

- Changes in urination: Making more or less urine than usual, feeling pressure when urinating, changes in the color of the urine, foamy or bubbly urine, or having to get up excessively at night to urinate.
- Blood in the urine (typically only seen through a microscope).
- Swelling of the feet, ankles, hands, or face: Fluid the kidneys cannot remove that may stay in the tissues.
- Fatigue or weakness: A buildup of wastes or a shortage of red blood cells (anemia) can cause these problems when the kidneys begin to fail.
- Shortness of breath: Kidney failure is sometimes confused with asthma or heart failure because fluid can build up in the lungs.
- Ammonia breath or an ammoniac or metallic taste in the mouth: Waste buildup in the body can cause bad breath, changes in taste, or an aversion to protein foods such as meat.
- Back or flank pain: The kidneys are located on either side of the spine in the back.
- Itching: Waste buildup in the body can cause severe itching, especially of the legs.
- Loss of appetite
- Nausea and vomiting
- More hypoglycemic episodes (if the person is diabetic)
- Feeling cold all the time
- Mental confusion
- Desire to chew ice or eat clay or laundry starch (pica)

Acute Renal Failure

In acute renal failure, the kidneys fail suddenly, often as a result of a toxin (e.g., drug allergy or poison), severe blood loss, or trauma. Dialysis is performed to clean the blood and give the kidneys a rest. If the cause is treated, the kidneys may be able to recover some or all of their function.

Acute kidney failure may occur for a variety of reasons. A crush-type injury may damage internal organs, including the kidneys. Overexposure to metals, solvents, and certain antibiotics and medications also can lead to this condition. An infection in the kidneys may cause them to shut down.

Obstructions in the urinary tract or renal artery can start acute kidney failure. Tumors, kidney stones, or an enlarged prostate can block the flow of urine in the urinary tract. A kidney stone develops when substances in the urine form crystals. Kidney stones can be large or small. Large ones can damage the kidneys; small ones may be able to pass in the urine. Because crystals have sharp edges, passing even small stones can be very painful. Treatment depends on the composition of the stones. A blockage in the renal artery can cut off the supply of oxygen to the kidneys.

The most obvious symptom of acute kidney failure is a decrease in urine. When urine output is low, fluid retention occurs. Excess fluid causes swelling in the legs, feet, and ankles. Because wastes are not being removed from the body, the person feels sick.

Doctors first treat any reversible illness that caused the kidney failure. Infections can be treated with medication. Blockages such as tumors or kidney stones may require surgery. Because treating the causes of acute kidney failure takes time, the body is unable to remove waste from the bloodstream, and the patient undergoes dialysis until the kidney has healed.

Sometimes patients accumulate high levels of potassium in the blood as a result of acute kidney failure; this condition is called *hyperkalemia.* Doctors can prescribe medication to bring an elevated potassium level under control. In order to help keep the wastes and electrolytes at acceptable levels, patients may be placed on a special diet that is low in protein, salt, and potassium. Fluid intake may also be restricted, and the person may undergo kidney dialysis until the kidneys can resume function.

Chronic Renal Failure

Chronic renal failure (CRF) may result from any major cause of renal dysfunction. The most common cause of ESRD is diabetic nephropathy; other causes are hypertensive nephroangiosclerosis and various primary and secondary glomerulopathies.

Symptoms include muscular twitches, peripheral neuropathies with sensory and motor phenomena and muscle cramps. The skin may appear yellow-brown; occasionally, urea from sweat may crystallize on the skin (uremic frost). Pruritus (itching) is especially uncomfortable for some patients.

Unless closely monitored, most people with ESRD develop renal bone disease (renal osteodystrophy). Renal bone disease is a complex condition that involves many more factors than can be listed in this limited space. If it goes untreated, the patient's bones are depleted of calcium, become brittle, and are likely to fracture. This condition limits the use of massage methods that involve pressure; however, energy-based modalities using very light touch (or no touch) would be appropriate.

Treatment of Kidney Disease

Controlling hyperglycemia in diabetic nephropathy and hypertension substantially reduces the deterioration of kidney function. Diet is a major factor in treatment. Because dietary restrictions may reduce necessary vitamin intake, patients should take a multivitamin preparation containing water-soluble vitamins. Additional vitamin A or vitamin E also is unnecessary.

Maintaining appropriate fluid and electrolyte levels is an important aspect of management.

Congestive heart failure, most commonly caused by sodium and fluid retention by the kidney, responds to sodium restriction and diuretics. Pruritus may respond to ultraviolet phototherapy.

Cramps, especially leg cramps, are common in people with kidney disease. Cramps are thought to be caused by imbalances in fluid and electrolytes, but they also may be caused by nerve damage or blood flow problems.

When conventional therapy is no longer effective, long-term dialysis or transplantation should be considered.

Massage Strategies for Kidney Disease

Kidney disease is complex and has many cautions for massage, as well as some indications. Developing specific strategies for patients with this disease can be difficult because so many factors are involved. When massage is appropriate, the modified palliative protocol is the basis for treatment. Massage has limited benefit for muscle cramping caused by electrolyte imbalance, but it can be soothing. Do not address edema with lymphatic drainage unless it is specifically ordered by the physician. Monitor pressure levels carefully because of the potential for brittle bones. People with kidney disease often feel sick and do not want a full body massage. In these cases, sometimes a more local massage is soothing, such as a foot massage or a massage of the head and face.

LIVER DISEASE

Liver disease has many causes. Inflammation (i.e., hepatitis) may be caused by infection (especially viral infection), exposure to toxins (including alcohol and drugs), autoimmune reactions, and heart failure. Portal hypertension and metabolic diseases, such as Wilson's disease and hemochromatosis (an excessive buildup of iron), also can cause significant liver problems. In addition, the liver can develop benign primary tumors and cancer.

The liver is responsible for many essential functions. Impairment of these vital functions by hepatic disease leads to symptoms that are often similar, regardless of the specific cause. Initially the symptoms may be mild, because the liver is a resilient organ that can compensate for a certain amount of damage. However, function eventually breaks down, resulting in some combination of the following:

- Blood clotting abnormalities (associated with a poor prognosis)
- Poisoning of the brain, with symptoms that include confusion and coma
- Ascites (fluid accumulation in the abdomen)
- Portal hypertension

Types of Liver Disease

Hepatitis can be caused by a number of factors, including infection (viral, bacterial, fungal, or protozoal), exposure to toxins (alcohol, drugs, or chemical poisons), and autoimmune disorders. The most common cause of hepatitis is viral infection. The three major viruses that cause hepatitis are hepatitis viruses A, B, and C. Hepatitis A is the most common type of hepatitis. Hepatitis A and hepatitis E are mainly transmitted by the fecal-oral route, whereas hepatitis B, hepatitis C, and hepatitis D are spread through blood or other body fluids.

Clinically, people with hepatitis may be completely asymptomatic and free of jaundice. More commonly, they complain of symptoms such as anorexia (loss of appetite), nausea, weakness, headache, muscle aches, altered smell or taste, aversion to food or tobacco, fever, abdominal pain, and jaundice. Hepatitis generally is considered acute if it resolves without permanent liver damage within 6 months.

Chronic hepatitis is liver inflammation that has persisted for longer than 6 months. Chronic hepatitis is most likely to be caused by hepatitis B or C. Symptoms vary greatly and may include fatigue, abdominal pain, and jaundice. A person may go undiagnosed until a routine checkup reveals abnormal liver function or an enlarged liver. Chronic hepatitis often leads to progressive liver scarring and cirrhosis.

Alcohol, drugs, and poisons cause hepatitis by damaging liver tissue or, indirectly, by reducing the body's defenses or stimulating an autoimmune response. Alcohol is primarily metabolized by the liver, and excess consumption can result in liver damage. Numerous medications can damage the liver; this can range from a mild, asymptomatic alteration in liver chemistries to hepatic failure and death. Acetaminophen is very toxic to the liver. Both environmental and industrial toxins can cause a wide variety of changes in the liver.

Autoimmune disease can develop in the liver. This occurs in autoimmune hepatitis, in which the immune system attacks and destroys parts of the liver. If left unchecked, persistent inflammation can eventually lead to cirrhosis. Systemic infections, such as tuberculosis, candidiasis, and toxoplasmosis, may spread to the liver. In addition, heart failure can lead to liver congestion, scarring, and ascites, because blood cannot drain from the liver properly when the heart is not pumping effectively.

Vascular disorders of the liver also can occur. Obstruction of the portal blood flow that drains the intestines, stomach, and spleen results in portal hypertension (elevated portal blood pressure). Think of the liver as a sieve that filters portal blood.

Metabolic disorders cause liver disease. Problems with metabolic processes in the liver can be either congenital (present at birth) or acquired. Some of these disorders, such as Wilson's disease and hemochromatosis, manifest as hepatitis or cirrhosis. These conditions need to be treated specifically, and proper diagnosis is essential.

Benign tumors usually are asymptomatic. The most common tumors are hemangiomas (blood-filled vascular channels). However, the liver is the most frequent site of blood-borne metastases of malignant tumors. Primary malignant liver cancer, or hepatocellular carcinoma (HCC), most often occurs in patients with cirrhosis caused by viral infection, alcoholism, and hemochromatosis.

Cirrhosis is the common endpoint of many chronic liver diseases, because inflammation and cell death eventually yield to fibrosis, or scar formation, and the liver cannot regenerate (Figure 17-12).

Patients with cirrhosis have significantly shortened life spans. Cirrhosis may not be detected for many years or may not produce recognizable symptoms except for progressive weight loss, fatigue, and chronic jaundice. Eventually, liver failure and portal hypertension develop, with deepening jaundice and bleeding. Without a liver transplant, more than 50% of patients with cirrhosis die, usually from a combination of the conditions described previously.

Massage Strategies for Liver Disease

Liver disease presents many contraindications to massage. There are few indications, other than

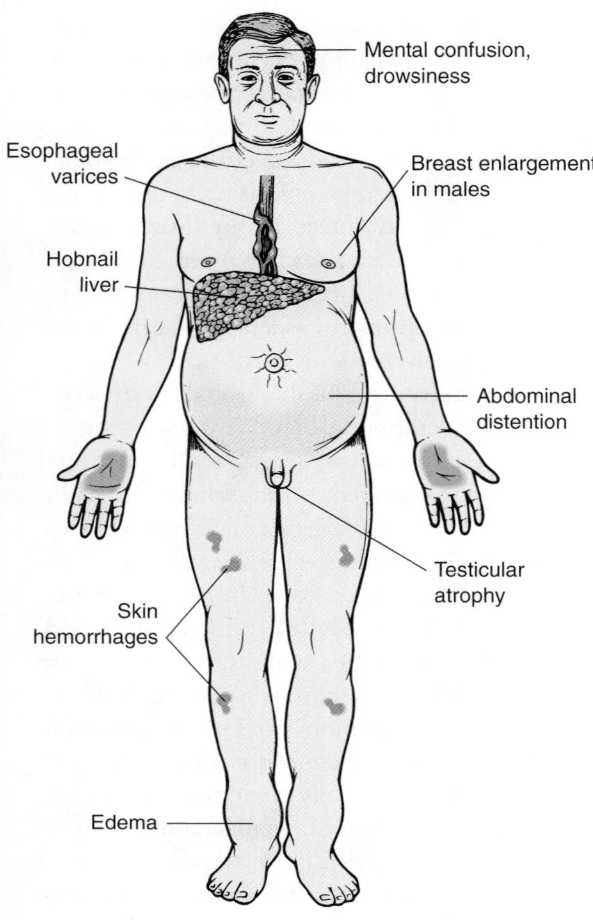

FIGURE 17-12 ■ Signs and symptoms of cirrhosis of the liver. (Modified from Frazier MS, Drzymkowski JW: *Essentials of human diseases and conditions,* ed 2, Philadelphia, 2000, WB Saunders.)

palliative care and stress management. Massage should be provided only with medical supervision. A diseased liver cannot handle increased fluid movement. Even if edema is present, lymphatic drainage massage should not be attempted unless specifically requested by the physician.

NEUROLOGIC DISEASE

This section discusses illness and injury of the nervous system. It covers brain injury, nerve deterioration, neuropathy, and nerve injury, including spinal cord injury and impingement (**entrapment** and **compression**), because massage is an effective aspect of the treatment process for these conditions.

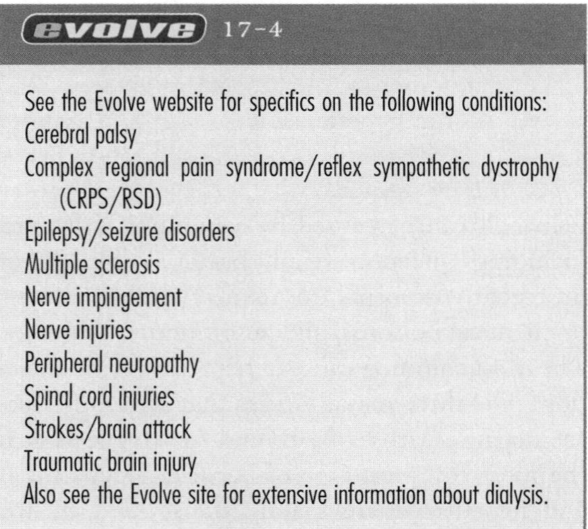

evolve 17-4

See the Evolve website for specifics on the following conditions:
Cerebral palsy
Complex regional pain syndrome/reflex sympathetic dystrophy (CRPS/RSD)
Epilepsy/seizure disorders
Multiple sclerosis
Nerve impingement
Nerve injuries
Peripheral neuropathy
Spinal cord injuries
Strokes/brain attack
Traumatic brain injury
Also see the Evolve site for extensive information about dialysis.

THE BRAIN

The central nervous system (CNS) is made up of the brain and spinal cord. The CNS ultimately controls bodily functions. The two types of cells found in the CNS are the neurons, or nerve cells, which conduct impulses, and the neuroglia, which are specialized connective-tissue cells. The function of the neurons is to receive and transmit electrical signals from and to other neurons, muscles, or glands. The neuroglia (*glia* means glue) supports and protects neurons as it holds them together. In addition, neuroglia supports the tiny blood vessels (capillaries) in the brain.

Nerve cells consist of a cell body and its nerve fibers, the axons and dendrites. The cell body contains a nucleus and its organelles. The dendrites, which look like small hairs, are extensions of the cytoplasm of the cell, and they carry signals to the cell body. The axon is an elongated projection that carries signals away from the cell body and may have branches known as *collaterals* that allow communication among neurons.

In the peripheral nervous system, the neuroglia forms a protective sheath around the axons. The neuroglia contains a fatty insulator called myelin, which is produced by Schwann cells. The outer membrane is called the neurilemma and also is formed by Schwann cells. Small gaps between segments of the myelin sheath are called nodes of Ranvier; they help to speed the nerve impulses.

Neurons are identified by their functions. A sensory neuron conducts sensory signals to the CNS, whereas motor neurons conduct motor signals away from the CNS. Association neurons, or interneurons, act as bridges in the CNS to conduct signals from one neuron to another.

The gelatin-like brain is held together by layers of membranes. The membranes are the dura, the pia, and the arachnoid. Between the pia and arachnoid membranes is the subarachnoid space, where a network of arteries is located. Damage to these blood vessels can lead to blood clots, causing damaging pressure against the brain. The brain is encircled by a cushioning layer of cerebrospinal fluid (CSF).

The brain is the largest and most complex unit of the nervous system. The brain is responsible for our intellect, emotions, and actions, and the brain interprets, regulates, and coordinates physiologic activities. The brain is divided into the cerebrum, cerebellum, and brainstem, which includes the diencephalon.

The cerebral cortex, the largest part of the brain, is divided into two hemispheres. The right hemisphere controls the left side of the body, and the left hemisphere controls the right side. In most people, the left hemisphere regulates language and speech, and the right hemisphere controls nonverbal spatial skills, such as the ability to draw or play music. If the right side of the brain is damaged, movement in the left arm and leg, vision in the left eye, or hearing in the left ear may be affected. An injury to the left side of the brain affects speech and movement on the right side of the body.

The cerebral cortex is also divided into several lobes. The left and right frontal lobes, located behind the forehead, control intellectual activity. The temporal lobes, located behind and below the frontal lobes and just behind the ears, control memory, speech, and comprehension. The parietal lobes, located at the back of the head and above the ears, control the ability to read, write, and understand spatial relationships. The areas between the frontal and parietal lobes regulate movement and sensation. The occipital lobes, located at the back of the head, control sight. The diencephalon is the location of the hypothalamus and the limbic system. The limbic system regulates appetite, thirst, temperature, and some aspects of memory, and controls sexual arousal, emotion, and mood.

The brainstem controls body functions such as consciousness, fatigue, heart rate, and blood pressure. Damage to the brainstem can cause loss of consciousness or concussion of the brain. Behind the brainstem is the cerebellum, which controls balance and coordinates fine motor skills.

Damage to the various areas of the brain can result in impairment of the functions they regulate.

Cerebrovascular Accidents/Strokes

The term *cerebrovascular accident* (CVA), or stroke, is an umbrella term that covers disorders, such as aneurysms and hemorrhages, that damage brain tissue. Thrombosis is a common cause of blood vessel damage. Stroke, or brain attack, is a major cause of death and permanent disability. A stroke occurs when blood flow to a region of the brain is obstructed, and it may result in the death of brain tissue. The medical term for a stroke is *brain infarction.* The two main types of strokes are ischemic strokes and hemorrhagic strokes.

Ischemic stroke is caused by blockage of an artery that supplies blood to the brain, resulting in a deficiency in blood flow. During an ischemic stroke, the diminished blood flow initiates a series of events, called the ischemic cascade, that may result in additional, delayed damage to brain cells. Early medical intervention can halt this process and reduce the risk of irreversible complications from the stroke.

Ulcerated plaque from arteriosclerosis or a portion of a blood clot may break away from a different part of the body and form an embolus that travels to the brain. These conditions deprive the brain of oxygen. Because brain cells consume large quantities of oxygen, any deficit can cause damage quickly.

Hemorrhagic stroke is caused by bleeding from ruptured blood vessels in the brain.

A transient ischemic attack (TIA) is a prestroke condition that mimics a stroke. A TIA resolves in less than 24 hours. In some cases, when the deficit lasts longer than 24 hours and then clears completely, the condition is called a reversible neurologic deficit or a residual ischemic neurologic deficit. The signs of a TIA are transient blindness in one eye, aphasia, numbness or weakness of the hand or foot, slurred speech, dizziness, ataxia, syncope, and numbness around the lips. The signs may last only a few minutes and then disappear. They are commonly ignored. Knowing the basic signs of TIA and referring the client immediately is important because a TIA is frequently a warning of a major stroke.

When a stroke occurs, an artery in the brain is occluded, or closed off, by a blood clot called a thrombus. A stroke lasts longer than 24 hours. The location at which the blood flow has been cut off and the length of time the cutoff has lasted determine the damage caused by the stroke. The following deficits may occur:

- Hemiparesis: Partial motor deficit on one side of the body.
- Quadriplegia: Total motor deficit in both arms and legs (usually seen in trauma).
- Sensory losses: Inability to feel pain, temperature, vibration, and so forth.

The limbs are initially flaccid (relaxed). Later, they become spastic (contracted). The forearm in flexion and the leg in extension are common sites because of the unequal innervation of extensors and flexors. The cause of the spasticity is thought to be loss of control of lower motor neurons.

Behavioral changes caused by damage in the association areas of the cortex often are present. If the left hemisphere is involved, language difficulties (such as aphasia) occur. A stroke in the right hemisphere produces inattention and lack of concern. Confusion may be present if either hemisphere is affected.

Strokes are emergencies that require immediate medical attention. Warning signs of a stroke include the following:

- Sudden numbness or weakness, especially on one side of the body
- Sudden confusion
- Sudden vision problems in one or both eyes
- Sudden difficulty walking, dizziness, or loss of balance or coordination
- Sudden, severe headache with no known cause
- Sudden difficulty speaking or understanding speech

According to the CDC, some conditions, as well as some lifestyle factors, can put people at a higher risk for stroke. The most important risk factors for stroke are high blood pressure, heart disease, diabetes, and cigarette smoking. Persons who have already had a stroke need to control the risk factors in order to lower their risk of having another stroke. All persons can take steps to lower their risk for stroke.

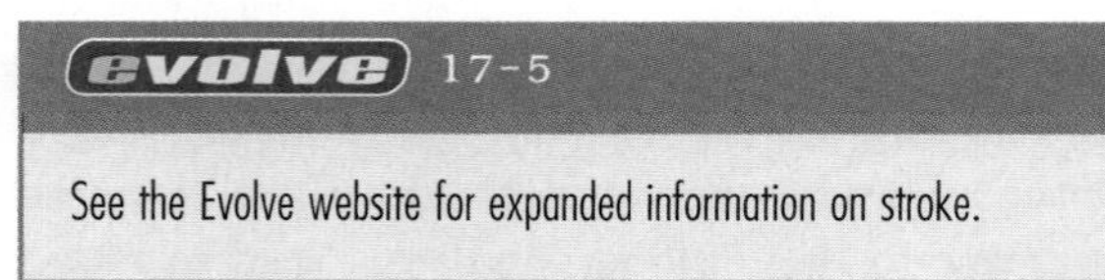

See the Evolve website for expanded information on stroke.

Rehabilitation for Stroke. Recovery and rehabilitation are important aspects of stroke treatment. In some cases, undamaged areas of the brain may be able to perform functions that were lost when the stroke occurred. Rehabilitation includes physical therapy, speech therapy, and occupational therapy. Physical therapy uses exercise and other physical means, such as massage and hydrotherapy, to help people regain the use of their arms and legs and prevent muscle stiffness for those with permanent paralysis. Speech therapy helps patients regain the ability to speak, if needed. Occupational therapy helps patients regain independent function and relearn basic skills necessary for activities of daily living.

Massage Strategies for Stroke. Massage is not used during the initial strategies of stroke treatment, but it can become an important aspect of symptom management and rehabilitation. Some of the effects of brain attack diminish as the body heals and adapts. Other effects are permanent. General restorative massage to support healing and manage stress is appropriate. Targeted massage application for muscle function depends on the damage caused by the stroke and the physical therapy methods used.

Traumatic Brain Injury

Traumatic brain injury (TBI) is damage to the brain caused by a blow to the head, resulting in bleeding, swelling, and nerve and vessel changes. The severity of the injury can range from minor, with few or no lasting consequences, to major, resulting in disability or death.

Coping with the life-changing consequences of TBI presents a great challenge for patients, families, physicians, and therapists. TBI causes shearing of large nerve fibers in the brain, microscopic nerve and vessel damage, and stretching of blood vessels in many areas. A common result is impaired cognitive function, resulting in disorganization, impaired memory, and varying degrees of inattentiveness. Visual changes or weakness on one side of the body may also occur.

Contusions (concussion) are focal injuries that cause bruises, resulting in swelling, bleeding, and destruction of brain tissue. Symptoms of a brain contusion include the following:

- Abnormal sensations
- Behavior impairment
- Loss of some or all vision
- Loss of coordination, weakness (less common)
- Memory impairment

Contusions shrink as swelling diminishes, but they can leave scars in the brain tissue that cause permanent neurologic impairment. Multiple contusions can result in cumulative brain injury, leading to more severe disability with each additional brain injury.

Treatment of Traumatic Brain Injury. The three stages of treatment for TBI are as follows:

- Acute stage: The aim is to stabilize the patient immediately after the injury. Massage is not applicable.
- Subacute stage: The aim is to rehabilitate the patient and return the person to daily living activities and work if possible. Massage is appropriate if supervised by the rehabilitation medical team.
- Chronic stage: The aim is to continue rehabilitation and treat long-term impairments. Massage is an appropriate part of long-term care.

Seizures may occur seconds, weeks, or years after a traumatic brain injury. A seizure can be a minor twitching of one finger or limb or a complete loss of consciousness accompanied by involuntary movements of the entire body. Seizures can be particularly dangerous during the initial healing stages, therefore most patients with a moderate to severe head injury receive antiseizure medication for at least the first few weeks.

evolve 17-6

See the Evolve website for more information on traumatic brain injury.

Massage Strategies for Traumatic Brain Injury. If massage is used, it is palliative in nature. Do not attempt to reduce muscle guarding in the upper body, because this is a protective mechanism to reduce movement of the head. Massage in the acute stage is most likely to be used for a minor brain contusion (concussion). However, there really is no such thing as a minor brain injury. If you are working with an individual who has had a concussion, do not aggressively move the head or neck. The massage is palliative only; do not attempt to reduce muscle guarding in the upper body.

Monitor for signs that the injury is more severe than indicated (e.g., headache, clumsiness, increased fatigue, digestive upset, and confusion). Refer the patient to the physician immediately if such signs are noted. Concussion is serious, no matter how mild.

Subacute Stage Treatment. The massage therapist must work closely with the various medical professionals involved in rehabilitation. Massage may calm the patient, which is important; however, it can just as easily agitate a patient with a brain injury.

Many patients with TBI have poor balance, lack of coordination, weakness, or cognitive impairments that put them at risk for injury. They may be impulsive and unaware of their physical limitations and may try to climb out of bed or walk by themselves when it is unsafe to do so. Agitation and restlessness may also lead to injury. A well-designed rehabilitation unit and a well-trained staff can keep these patients safe, using little or no medication.

evolve 17-7

See the Evolve website for specific information about disabilities and handicaps caused by traumatic brain injury.

Epilepsy/Seizure Disorders

According to the CDC, epilepsy is a general term that includes various types of seizures. People with diagnosed epilepsy have had more than one seizure, and they may have had more than one kind of seizure. A seizure happens when abnormal electrical activity in the brain causes an involuntary change in body movement or function, sensation, awareness, or behavior. http://www.cdc.gov/Epilepsy/

Epilepsy is primarily classified as idiopathic or symptomatic in nature. Idiopathic epilepsy has no known cause, and the person has no other signs of neurologic disease or mental deficiency. Symptomatic epilepsy results from a known condition, such as a stroke, a head injury, or cerebral palsy.

A seizure occurs when impulses from nerves are disrupted. Normally, nerve transmission in the brain occurs in an orderly way, allowing a smooth flow of electrical activity. Certain areas of the brain are more likely than others to be involved in seizure activity. The motor cortex, which is responsible for body movement, and the temporal lobes, including the hippocampus, which is involved in memory, are particularly sensitive to biochemical changes, including decreased oxygen levels, metabolic imbalances, and infections that cause abnormal brain cell activity.

Seizures may be partial or generalized in nature. What happens to a person during the seizure depends on where in the brain the disruption of neural activity occurs. After a seizure, the person may be drowsy and confused as the brain recovers from the seizure activity.

Simple partial seizures produce symptoms associated with the area of abnormal neural activity in the brain; motor signs, sensory symptoms, involuntary activity controlled by the autonomic nervous system, and altered states of consciousness can occur. Consciousness is not impaired in simple partial seizures.

During generalized seizures, seizure activity occurs simultaneously in large areas of the brain, often in both hemispheres. The three types of generalized seizures are tonic-clonic, absence, and myoclonic seizures.

- Tonic-clonic (grand mal) seizure: This type of seizure involves loss of consciousness. The tonic phase, marked by increased muscle tone, is followed by the clonic phase, which involves convulsive jerking of the body.
- Absence (petit mal) seizure: This type of seizure typically begins between the ages of 5 and 12 years and then stops unexpectedly in the teens. The loss of consciousness is so brief that the child usually does not even change position. Most absence seizures last 10 seconds or less. The person usually is unaware of what occurs during the seizure.
- Myoclonic seizure: This type of seizure is so brief it may go unnoticed. It involves sudden muscle contractions that occur very rapidly and often are confused with tics. Myoclonic seizures occur at all ages.

Treatment of Seizures

Medication. Most seizures disorders are successfully controlled with medication. Antiepileptic medication can prevent seizure activity by altering neurotransmitter activity in nerve cells, but it cannot correct the underlying condition. To control seizures, a constant level of medication must be maintained in the body. Antiepileptic drugs should not be discontinued abruptly, because life-threatening complications can occur. The medication regimen must be carefully designed to maximize the drug's effectiveness and to avoid serious complications and side effects.

Vagus Nerve Stimulator. A vagus nerve stimulator is a device that is implanted near the collarbone and attached to the vagus nerve. The device delivers small bursts of electrical energy to the brain at regular, preprogrammed intervals. For some individuals, the frequency of seizures is reduced. Most patients who are helped by a vagus nerve stimulator continue to take antiepileptic medication, but a reduced dosage may be possible.

Electrocorticography. Electrocorticography (ECoG) can be used to monitor and control seizures in patients with epilepsy. It involves placing a series of electrodes on the surface of the brain. It provides much better signals than electroencephalography, in which the electrodes are placed on the scalp, and is much less traumatic than procedures in which the electrodes actually penetrate the brain. http://physicsweb.org/articles/news/9/1/9/1

Ketogenic Diet. The ketogenic diet is used in children who do not respond to standard therapy or who cannot tolerate the side effects of antiepileptic drugs. The diet is a high-fat, low-carbohydrate diet that fundamentally alters the body's metabolism, causing it to change from using glucose as a primary energy source to using fats. The diet is most effective in children 10 years of age or younger.

Surgery. Surgery is an option for a small number of patients whose epilepsy cannot be controlled with medication. Hemispherectomy is the most drastic surgical intervention for epilepsy. It involves the removal of the entire affected side of the brain. The remaining hemisphere develops language and motor areas for both sides of the body. With intense rehabilitation, most individuals who undergo this procedure lead functional lives.

> **evolve** 17-8
>
> For specific information about cerebral palsy, including types, causes, diagnosis, and medical treatment, see the Evolve website.

Massage Strategies for Epilepsy. Yoga, acupuncture, therapeutic massage, aromatherapy, biofeedback, behavior psychotherapy, and meditation may improve the quality of life for patients with epilepsy. Some of these therapies reduce stress, which diminishes seizure activity in some patients. The general protocol is the basis for massage, and outcomes are targeted to stress management, restorative sleep, and normalization of residual muscle tension from seizure activity. Any massage therapist working with a person who has seizures should know how to respond if a seizure occurs. The most important point is to protect the person from harm caused by falls or by hitting the furniture or walls. Ask the person and the supervising medical staff what measures are necessary if the person has a seizure. Make sure you understand the instructions and how to follow them.

Cerebral Palsy

Cerebral palsy (CP) is a motor impairment that results from brain damage in a young child, regardless of the cause of the damage or its effect on the child. In cerebral palsy, faulty development or damage to motor areas in the brain impairs the body's ability to control movement and posture. This results in a number of chronic neurologic disorders. CP usually is associated with events that occur before or during birth, but it may be acquired during the first few months or years of life as the result of head trauma or infection.[1]

CP is neither contagious nor inherited, nor is it progressive. The symptoms of CP differ from person to person and change as children and their nervous systems mature into adulthood. Some people with severe CP are completely disabled and require lifelong care, whereas others show only a slight awkwardness and need no special assistance. Complications associated with CP include learning disabilities, gastrointestinal dysfunction, sensory deficits, and seizures.[1]

CP can be categorized into the following types[1]:

- Spastic CP: Stiff, permanently contracted muscles
- Athetoid CP (also called *dyskinetic cerebral palsy*): Slow, uncontrolled, writhing movements
- Ataxic CP: Poor coordination, balance, and depth perception
- Mixed CP: Presence of two or more types

Massage Strategies for Cerebral Palsy. Massage does not affect the primary cause and result of the brain injury in CP. Therapeutic massage targets the body's adaptations to the neurologic damage. People with CP benefit from the stress management, muscle normalization, and fluid movement effects of massage.

Contractures are common with CP, and massage can help maintain pliable tissue. Never force soft tissue or joint stretching, even though this type of aggressive treatment may be done by those trained to do it, such as the physical therapist. Various surgeries may also be used to manage contracture, and the scar tissue can be addressed with massage to maintain tissue pliability. Gait disturbances and the use of canes, crutches, wheelchairs, and other assistive equipment can cause disruption of muscle activation firing sequences. For example, constantly looking up at people from a wheelchair increases tension in the neck and shoulder muscles. Breathing function may be labored, and massage to support breathing patterns may be beneficial. Patients who are not independently mobile may have muscle **atrophy,** therefore pressure levels need to be monitored. Methods such as muscle energy techniques that require coordinated resistance may be difficult to perform but should not be eliminated from the massage for this reason. Also, circulation may be impaired, requiring the appropriate massage approaches.

These alterations in the massage application have more to do with the patient's lack of mobility and the equipment the person uses to support mobility than they do with the CP. If the patient has difficulty speaking, learn to listen carefully and, if necessary, ask for assistance from someone who has learned to understand the person. Also, because each person experiences unique circumstances with a brain injury, that person, when possible, is the best source of information about the goals for massage and the assistance that is needed.

MULTIPLE SCLEROSIS

Note: This material is also discussed with the autoimmune diseases.

Multiple sclerosis (MS) is an autoimmune disease of the central nervous system. MS is characterized by intermittent damage to myelin caused by the destruction of specialized cells (oligodendrocytes) that form the substance. The damage results in scarring and hardening (sclerosis) of nerve fibers. Researchers have identified how the body's own immune system contributes to the nerve fiber damage caused by multiple sclerosis. Studies have revealed how immune system B-cells damage axons during MS attacks by inhibiting energy production in these nerve fiber cells, ultimately causing them to degenerate and die, resulting in symptoms. Because different nerves are affected at different times, the symptoms of MS are erratic; they can worsen and then improve and/or develop in different areas of the body. MS can progress steadily or can manifest as acute attacks (exacerbations) that are followed by a partial or complete resolution of symptoms (remissions). http://www.eurekalert.org/pub_releases/2006-10/uoc–con101606.php

According to neurologychannel.com, MS is more common in women and Caucasians. The average age of onset is 18 to 35 years. The children of parents with MS have a higher incidence, indicating a possible genetic predisposition. Most people with MS can live a relatively normal life. After 25 years, approximately two thirds of those with MS remain mobile. The disorder eventually results in physical limitations in about 70% of patients.

evolve 17-9

For more specifics about multiple sclerosis, see the Evolve website.

Massage Strategies for Multiple Sclerosis

Massage therapy is very beneficial as part of a comprehensive, multidisciplinary treatment program for multiple sclerosis. The general protocol is the basis for massage application, which is adjusted on a session-by-session basis, depending on the person's current state. Follow the recommendations in Chapter 14 for autoimmune diseases in general, as well as those for pain management, breathing pattern disorder, and depression.

PERIPHERAL NEUROPATHY

Peripheral neuropathy is a general term that refers to disorders of the peripheral nerves. Peripheral neuropathy can be caused by poor nutrition; disease; nerve compression, entrapment, or laceration; exposure to toxins; or inflammation. In many cases, especially in people over age 60, no cause can be determined. Most people with diabetes have peripheral neuropathy.

evolve 17-10

For more information on peripheral neuropathy, see the Evolve website.

Treatment of Peripheral Neuropathy

Neuropathy is very difficult to treat. Prompt treatment of the underlying cause can reduce the risk for permanent nerve damage. For example, controlling diabetes may reduce diabetic neuropathy, and renal dialysis often improves neuropathy that develops as a result of chronic renal failure. In neuropathy caused by medication or exposure to a toxin, discontinuing the medication or eliminating exposure to the toxin may resolve the neuropathy. Vitamin supplements may be used to treat nutritional neuropathy.

Treatment options for reducing pain include medication, injection therapy, and physical therapy (which may include massage as part of the treatment). Surgery may be needed to treat some causes of neuropathy, such as carpal tunnel syndrome.

- Because analgesic medication usually is ineffective against pain caused by neuropathy, treatment often involves medications that target nerve cells. Common side effects of these medications include constipation, diarrhea, dry mouth, nausea, dizziness, and hot flashes. Occasionally anticonvulsants and antidepressants are prescribed to treat the neuropathic condition; side effects of these medications include drowsiness, dizziness, low blood pressure, and fatigue. Anticonvulsants may cause low white blood cell counts, nausea, vomiting, dizziness, nervousness, lightheadedness, drowsiness, and double vision.
- Topical treatment with capsaicin cream may be prescribed for patients with focal neuropathy, such as herpes zoster (shingles). Capsaicin stings when it is applied, and it often is combined with a local anesthetic to reduce this side effect.
- Injection therapy involves injection of a nerve block (e.g., lidocaine) into the area surrounding the affected nerves, preventing the nerve from carrying impulses to the brain and temporarily reducing symptoms. Injection therapy is often used in combination with other treatments.
- Physical therapy, including exercise, massage, and heat, may be used to treat symptoms, and acupuncture has been shown to be beneficial.

Massage Strategies for Peripheral Neuropathy

As mentioned, neuropathy is difficult to treat. General massage may be helpful for temporary symptom relief, and the general protocol should be followed. The underlying condition in neuropathy needs to be considered. For example, diabetes presents cautions for massage. Do not irritate the area of the nerve damage. Because sensory feedback is altered, be cautious about pressure levels and the intensity of connective tissue methods. Massage may reduce common side effects of medication, but more often, the medication creates cautions. Do not massage around areas of injection therapy. Dizziness is a common side effect, and massage can also make people feel unsteady, increasing the potential for balance problems. Capsicum-based ointment increases the histamine response in the skin, and massage in those areas can increase the histamine symptoms (redness, burning, and itching) (Box 17-2).

COMPLEX REGIONAL PAIN SYNDROME (REFLEX SYMPATHETIC DYSTROPHY)

Complex regional pain syndrome (CRPS), also known as reflex sympathetic dystrophy (RSD), is a chronic, painful, and progressive neurologic condition that affects the skin, muscles, joints, and bones. It usually affects people between the ages of 40 and 60, although it can occur at any age.

The syndrome usually develops in an injured limb, such as a broken leg, or after surgery. The condition can occur after minor injury, such as a sprain, and in some causes no prior causal event can be identified. Symptoms of CRPS may go away for a time and then reappear with a new injury. Two types of CRPS have been defined. Type 1 does not involve nerve injury, and type 2 (formerly called *causalgia*) involves nerve injury. The signs and symptoms are the same for both.

CRPS symptoms include the following:

- Burning pain
- Sweating
- Swelling
- Sensitivity to touch

evolve 17-11

See the Evolve website for more information on CRPS/RSD.

Massage Strategies for CRPS/RSD

Use the general protocol as a guide and alter as necessary based on what is effective and what may increase symptoms. Stress management and increased coping ability are the main outcome goals. Remember to consider all cautions presented by medication and other treatments. This is a difficult condition to treat, and the presenting symptoms, as well as responses to massage, vary tremendously from person to person.

BOX 17-2 Pain Behavior

Patients' expectations, motivations, and fears influence their behavior. Patients who equate hurt with harm develop fear-avoidance behavior, which promotes deconditioning. Pain behavior can also include maneuvers in which the patient repeatedly checks to see if the pain is still present; this can lead to habituation (a habit), sensitization, or both. Personality characteristics associated with increased muscle tension habituate and sensitize pain patterns. Pain expectancies are not only important in chronic patients but also in acute patients. Fear-avoidance beliefs, such as pain expectancies, begin with acute pain and precede other psychosocial problems that develop as acute pain becomes chronic behavior and affects both general and specific functional abilities.

The Impact of Fear-Avoidance Behavior

Problems

- Pain catastrophizing (fearing the worst) is a precursor of pain-related fear.
- Fearful patients tend to be more hypervigilant (acutely aware of possible signals of threat).
- Psychophysical reactivity is present in individuals with fear-avoidance behavior if activities are perceived as harmful even if they are not actually harmful.
- Guarded movements (e.g., an altered flexion-relaxation ratio) correlate with fear-avoidance beliefs, not actual pain.
- Anxious patients predict pain earlier in the performance of physical tasks such as range-of-motion or straight leg raise tests.
- Fear and anxiety lead to the tendency to avoid the perceived threat.
- Pain-related fear leads not only to poor physical performance but also to restrictions in activities of daily living.
- Avoidance behavior is highly resistant to treatment because the individual rarely comes into contact with the actual (nonharmful) consequences of the feared situation.

Solutions

- A cognitive-behavioral approach addresses the individual's inaccurate predictions about the relationship between specific activities and pain.
- Education of patients with pain-related fear should emphasize that the fear can be self-managed after repeated desensitization from graded exposure to the feared stimuli. (NOTE: Therapeutic massage can be a form of exposure to the pain stimuli. For sensitized individuals, compression, stretching, and other forms of stimuli applied during massage can begin to differentiate somatic sensation to help the person catalog sensations instead of interpreting every sensation as painful. Massage can also teach the difference between *hurt* and *harm*.)
- Pain expectancies are corrected with repeated performance of the movements or exercises on subsequent days.
- After multiple exposures, overpredictions of pain intensity change to match actual pain experience.

Modified from Vlaeyen JWS, Linton S: Fear-avoidance and its consequences in chronic musculoskeletal pain: a state of the art, *Pain* 85:317-332, 2000.

NERVE INJURIES

Major **nerve injuries** are caused by two main forces: compression and tension. As with injuries to other tissues in the body, a nerve injury may be acute or chronic.

Any number of traumas that directly affect the nerves can produce a variety of sensory responses, including pain. For example, a sudden nerve stretch or pinch can produce muscle weakness as well as a sharp, burning pain that radiates down a limb. Neuritis, a chronic nerve problem, can be caused by a variety of forces that usually have been repeated or continued for a long period. Symptoms of neuritis can range from minor nerve problems to paralysis.

Pain felt at a point in the body other than its actual origin is known as *referred pain.* Another potential cause of referred pain is a trigger point, which occurs in the muscular system. The most common nerve injuries include spinal cord injuries and nerve impingement. Massage applications for nerve injuries are typically palliative to reduce pain. If the nerve is impinged upon by short muscles and fascia, massage can be used to restore the normal length of these tissues and reduce pressure on the nerve.

Spinal Cord Injury

The most serious spinal cord injury damages the cervical vertebrae in the neck (commonly called a broken neck). A head-on blow may cause a compression fracture of the neck, in which the force to the top of the head compresses and shatters some of the cervical vertebrae. An equally severe injury can occur from a blow when the neck is bent down.

Injuries to the spinal cord can result in a number of neurologic problems. Studies of blood flow and metabolism indicate that spinal cord injury involves not only direct neuronal trauma but also direct and delayed vascular trauma. The most frequently injured sites are at the most mobile segments of the spine, such as the cervicothoracic junction (C7 to T1) and the thoracolumbar junction (T12 to L1-L4). About 40% of spinal cord injuries result in complete interruption of function. Other spinal cord injuries result in impairment or destruction of certain sensory and motor functions.

Injury or severing of the spinal cord is followed by a 2- to 3-week period of spinal shock in which all spinal reflex responses are depressed. The spinal reflexes below a severed cord become exaggerated and hyperactive. The neurons become hypersensitive to the excitatory neurotransmitters, and the spinal neurons may grow collaterals that synapse with excitatory input. The stretch reflexes are exaggerated, and the tone of the muscle increases.

Loss of movement of all four limbs is known as *quadriplegia.* If the lesion is lower, only the lower limbs are affected, and the condition is called *paraplegia.* Should the nerves to only one limb be affected, the condition is called *monoplegia.*

If spinal cord injury occurs above the third cervical spinal nerve, voluntary movement of all the limbs is lost. If the injury affects the phrenic nerve arising from the third, fourth, or fifth cervical nerve to supply the diaphragm, respiratory movements are affected and the person becomes dependent on a respirator (Figure 17-13).

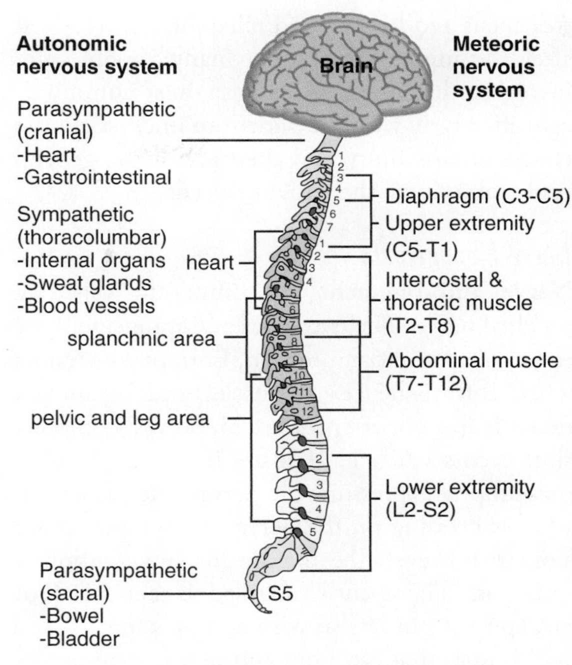

FIGURE 17-13 ■ Levels of possible injury to the spinal cord. (From Fritz S: *Sports and exercise massage: comprehensive care in athletics, fitness, and rehabilitation,* St Louis, 2005, Mosby.)

evolve 17-12

See the Evolve website for more specifics on spinal cord injury.

Massage Strategies for Spinal Cord Injury. During the acute and subacute phases, spinal cord injury is managed by the medical team. If massage is used, the bone break sequence is appropriate around the area of the injury, combined with palliative massage. Various types of paralysis require caution with pressure levels and intensity. Because the ability to regulate temperature may be impaired, do not use electric heating devices and be extremely cautious with hydrotherapy methods combined with massage.

Massage is an effective part of a comprehensive, supervised healing and rehabilitation and long-term care program. Massage can help manage secondary muscle tension caused by alterations in posture resulting from the use of equipment such as wheelchairs, braces, and crutches. Massage may temporarily influence increased motor tone below the lesion. Affected limbs can move spastically if the skin and muscles are stimulated. Discuss this issue with the patient to learn how to manage the situation if it occurs. Massage may reduce the intensity of the movement. Specifically focused massage can help manage difficulties with bowel paralysis. The circulation enhancement effect of massage can assist in the management of a decubitus ulcer.

In compensating for areas that have reduced function, the functioning areas of the body can become stressed. Massage can be an aspect of the management of this compensation. *Do not* assume that the paralysis equals no feeling in the area; this depends on the area of the break, the type of break, the damage to the spinal cord, and the body's adaptive capacity, as well as the type of medical treatment and healing and rehabilitation received after the injury. Because so many variables are involved, the massage therapist must communicate effectively with the patient to understand the effects of the injury and then adjust the general protocol to meet the patient's needs.

Nerve Impingement

Nerve impingement is commonly called a pinched nerve. The two types of impingement are entrapment and compression. Entrapment results when soft tissue (e.g., muscles and ligaments) exerts inappropriate pressure on nerves; compression occurs when hard tissue (e.g., bone) exerts inappropriate pressure on nerves. Regardless of what is pressing on the nerve, the symptoms are similar; however, the therapeutic intervention is different. Therapeutic massage is beneficial in entrapment but less so with compression.

Tissues that can bind and impinge on nerves are the skin, fascia, muscles, ligaments, and bones. Shortened muscles and connective tissue (fascia) often impinge on major and minor nerves, causing discomfort. Because of the structural arrangement of the body, these impingements often occur at major nerve plexuses. The specific nerve root, trunk, or division affected determines the condition, producing disorders such as thoracic outlet syndrome, sciatica, and carpal tunnel syndrome (Figure 17-14).

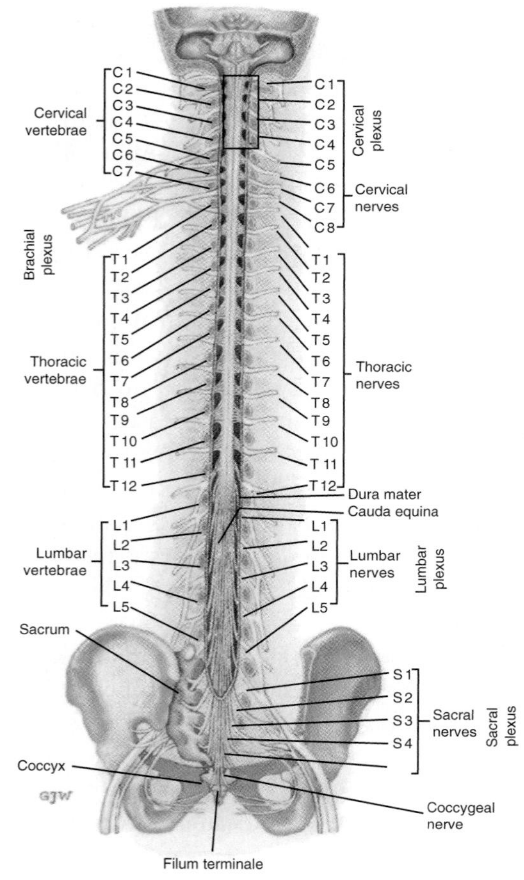

FIGURE 17-14 ■ Spinal nerves. Each of the 31 pairs of spinal nerves exits the spinal cavity from the intervertebral foramina. Note that after leaving the spinal cavity, many of the spinal nerves interconnect to form networks, which are called *plexuses.* (From Chipps EM, Clanin JJ, Campbell VG: *Neurologic disorders,* St Louis, 1992, Mosby.)

If impingement affects the cervical plexus, the person most likely has headaches, neck pain, and breathing difficulties. The muscles most responsible for pressure on the cervical plexus are the suboccipital and sternocleidomastoid muscles. Shortened connective tissue at the cranial base also presses on these nerves. Many cutaneous (skin) branches of the cervical plexus transmit sensory impulses from the skin of the neck, ear area, and shoulder. The motor branches innervate muscles of the anterior neck. Impingement causes pain in these areas.

The brachial plexus is situated partly in the neck and partly in the axilla and consists of virtually all the nerves that innervate the upper limb. Any imbalance that increases pressure on this complex of nerves can result in pain in the shoulder, chest, arm, wrist, and hand. The muscles most often responsible for impingement on the brachial plexus are the scalenes, pectoralis minor, and subclavius muscles. The muscles of the arm also occasionally impinge on branches of the brachial plexus. Brachial plexus impingement is responsible for thoracic outlet symptoms, which often are misdiagnosed as carpal tunnel syndrome. Whiplash injuries often cause impingement on the brachial plexus.

Carpal tunnel syndrome is caused by compression of the median nerve as it passes under the transverse carpal ligament on the palmar aspect of the wrist. It can occur when fluid retention causes swelling of the hand and wrist. The syndrome is common in people who use their hands in repetitive movements, usually because of inflammation that results in compression on the nerve. The symptoms are palmar pain and numbness in the first three digits. In some cases surgically opening the transverse carpal ligament can help relieve the pain (Figure 17-15).

Impingement on the lumbar plexus gives rise to low back discomfort, which is marked by a beltlike distribution of pain and pain in the lower abdomen, genitals, thigh, and medial lower leg. The main muscles that impinge on the lumbar plexus are the quadratus lumborum, multifidi, and psoas. Shortening of the lumbodorsal fascia exaggerates a lordosis and can cause vertebral impingement on the lumbar plexus.

The sacral plexus has about a dozen branches that innervate the buttocks, lower limbs, and pelvic structures. The main branch is the sciatic nerve. Impingement on this nerve by the piriformis muscle is a cause of sciatica. Shortened ligaments that stabilize the sacroiliac joint can affect the sacral plexus. Pressure on the sacral plexus can cause pain in the gluteal muscles, leg, genitals, and foot.

Various forms of massage reduce muscle spasm, lengthen shortened muscles, and soften and stretch connective tissue, restoring a more normal space around the nerve and alleviating impingement. When massage is combined with other appropriate methods, surgery is seldom necessary. If surgery is performed, the massage practitioner's role is to manage adhesions to prevent re-entrapment of the nerve in the future, maintaining soft tissue suppleness around the healing surgical area. As healing progresses, extend the focus of the massage to deal with the forming scar more directly. Always obtain the physician's approval before doing any work near the site of a recent incision. In general, work close to the surgical area can begin after the stitches have been removed and all inflammation has dissipated. Follow the massage strategies for wounds.

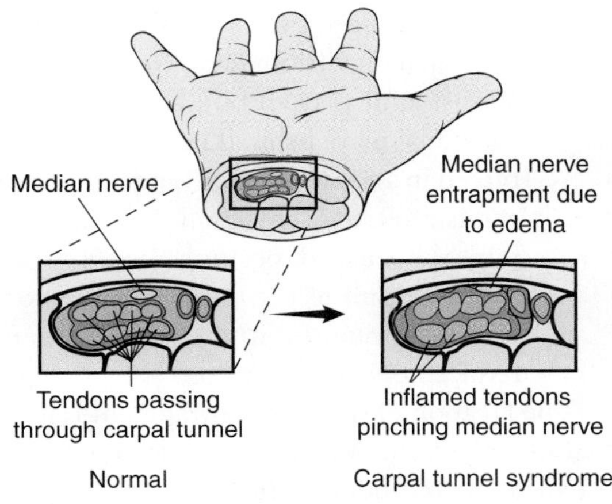

FIGURE 17-15 The physiology of carpal tunnel syndrome. (From Frazier MS, Drzymkowski JW: *Essentials of human diseases and conditions,* ed 2, Philadelphia, 2000, WB Saunders.)

Nerve Root Compression

Many different conditions can result in **nerve root compression,** including tumors, **subluxation** of vertebrae, muscle spasms (entrapment), and muscle shortening. Disk degeneration is a common cause. As the degeneration progresses and the fluid content of the disk diminishes, the disk becomes narrower. As a result, the amount of space between vertebrae is reduced. Because spinal nerves exit and enter in the spaces between the vertebrae, this situation increases the likelihood of nerve root compression. The condition most commonly occurs in the areas where the spine moves the most: the cervical area (C6 to C7), the thoracic area (T12 to L1), the lumbar area (L3 to L4), and the sacral area (L5 to S1). The result is radiating nerve pain often associated with protective and stabilizing muscle spasm, weakness, or both.

Disk Herniation

Disk herniation occurs when the fibrocartilage surrounding the intervertebral disk ruptures, releasing the nucleus pulposus (Figure 17-16). The resultant pressure on spinal nerve roots may cause pain and damage the surrounding nerves. This condition most often occurs in the lumbar region and involves the L4 or L5 disk and the L5 or S1 nerve roots. This particular back pain radiates from the gluteal area down the lateral side or back of the thigh to the leg or foot. Back strain, illness, or injury often causes disk herniation, but occasionally coughing and sneezing may precipitate the condition. Improper form during weight lifting is a common source of injury.

The symptoms of herniation are similar to those produced by a compressed disk but often

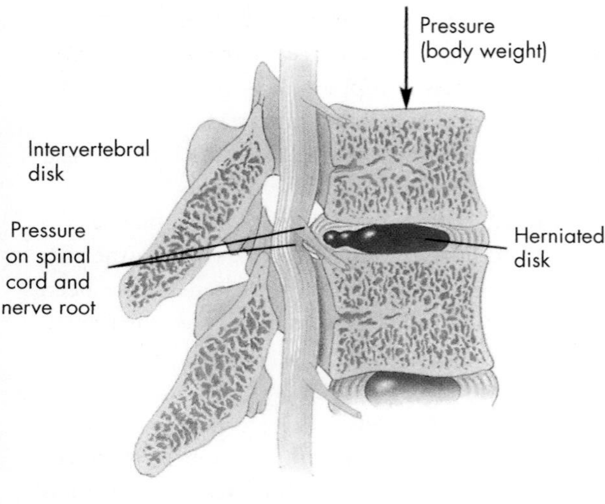

FIGURE 17-16 ■ A herniated disk. (From Thibodeau GA, Patton KT: *Anatomy and physiology*, ed 6, St Louis, 2007, Mosby.)

are more severe. In extreme cases, surgical intervention may be necessary; otherwise, conservative care is used. Conservative treatment consists of rest, exercise, and other methods, including massage to reduce spasm. Traction can be beneficial.

Massage Strategies for Nerve Impingement

Various forms of massage are important for managing the muscle spasm and pain associated with the nerve irritation caused by the ruptured disk. The muscle spasms (i.e., guarding response) serve a stabilizing and protective function. Without some protective muscle guarding, the nerve could be damaged further, but too much muscle contraction increases the discomfort. The aim of therapeutic intervention is to reduce pain and excessive tension and restore moderate mobility while supporting resourceful compensation produced by the muscle tension pattern.

Nerve impingement is a common condition, and physical healing and rehabilitation exercises are used to treat it in the general population. Repetitive strain, posture changes, and compensation for traumatic illness or injury are common causes of nerve impingement. The elderly are prone to cervical and lumbar nerve impingement as a result of age-related tissue and bone changes. Nerve pain usually radiates in a line following the pathway of the nerve. Massage applied to reduce soft tissue binding on the nerve must effectively address the soft tissue but must *not* irritate the underlying nerve. If the impingement is both entrapment and compression, the muscle tension may actually be protective, attempting to stabilize the bony structures and prevent further compression on the nerve. For effective treatment, massage application must address the soft tissue, in combination with repositioning of the underlying structure, manipulation, and therapeutic exercise.

The massage methods used to treat entrapment vary, depending on the source of the impingement.

- Muscle shortening: Use muscle energy methods, including positional release and lengthening. Direct inhibiting pressure at the spindle cell and/or Golgi tendons, combined with application of tension and bend forces, can lengthen the muscle.
- Connective tissue bind: Mechanical force (i.e., bend, torsion, and compression forces) increases ground substance pliability. Adhesion and fibrosis can be addressed with bend, shear, torsion, and tension forces to encourage more appropriate fiber alignment.
- Fluid buildup: Lymphatic drainage should be used, combined with passive and active joint movement.
- Bone misalignment: Compression usually is best managed by the physical therapist, physician, or chiropractor. In simple situations, joint play and indirect functional methods may help. The body area is placed in an ease position, and the patient exerts muscle force to pull the body back into the neutral position (see Chapter 10). The pull of the muscle on the bone can help reposition the structure and reduce nerve compression.

The location of the nerve entrapment is identified by palpation. When the area is located, the symptoms are reproduced. If the nerve is irritated in this location, sustained compression or intense stretching only increases the irritation. After the area has been located, the nature of the impingement must be identified (i.e., muscle tension, connective tissue bind, fluid buildup, structural misalignment) and then treated accordingly. When in doubt, apply all methods, but do not overwork the area. Begin with general massage around the area before targeting the actual impingement site.

If a patient has bulky muscles and dense tissues, reaching the area of impingement often is very difficult. In these cases, use muscle energy methods, especially positional release. Firing patterns and gait reflexes usually need to be normalized. If the impingement is caused by muscle spasm, short-term use of muscle-relaxing medication is effective.

ORTHOPEDICS

Orthopedic medical care targets the bones, joints, and associated muscles.

JUST BETWEEN YOU AND ME

The term *medical massage* currently is a source of confusion among therapeutic massage professionals. It has not yet been defined in a way that is generally accepted by the entire massage profession. Usually, "medical" type massage is actually orthopedic in nature. However, medical massage logically could be considered as massage appropriate for those with medical conditions; orthopedic medical conditions are only one aspect of healthcare. Make sure you don't get confused by various training courses in massage that mix up the concepts of medical massage and orthopedic massage.

Muscles comprise a large percentage of the soft tissues of the body. Muscle tissue contracts to provide movement and stability. Muscle is largely connective tissue, and it is highly vascular, therefore fluid dynamics and connective tissue mechanisms are important to an understanding of muscle dysfunction (muscle tone).

All the massage methods in this text are appropriate for use in orthopedics. Figure 17-17 shows several different types of orthopedic injuries. These types of injuries are also discussed on the Evolve website. The Evolve site presents information about myopathies, including muscular dystrophy, amyotrophic lateral sclerosis (ALS), various types of muscle soreness and stiffness, strains, sprains, **degenerative joint disease,** fractures, **tendinitis,** and more. (This material is covered in depth in *Sports and Exercise Massage: Comprehensive Care in Athletics, Fitness, and Rehabilitation* [Mosby, 2005].)

evolve 17-13

See the Evolve website for extensive information on orthopedic conditions.

SLEEP DISORDERS

Sleep is absolutely essential for normal, healthy function. Inadequate sleep can have a significant effect on health. Studies have shown that sleep is crucial to normal immune system function and to maintaining the body's ability to fight disease and sickness. Sleep is also essential for normal nervous system function, for learning, and for normal cell growth and regeneration. The amount of sleep a person needs to function normally depends on several factors, including the person's age, health status, and daily activity. Infants sleep about 16 hours, and toddlers about 13 hours a day; teenagers usually need about 9 hours a day, and adults need an average of 7 to 8 hours a day.

Restorative sleep is extremely important. Fitful, restless sleep is not restorative. Lack of restorative sleep can affect the individual's energy level. Restorative, deep, restful sleep helps bolster the immune system so that it can fight off viruses and bacteria. Many people are functioning on less than normal sleep. It is well known that sleep-deprived individuals have a shorter attention span, impaired memory, and a longer reaction time. Experiments in rats have now found that sleep deprivation interferes with learning by reducing the survival of new cells in the hippocampus.

The mechanism of feeling tired and wanting to sleep appears to be due to prolonged neural activity. Remaining awake for long periods or overworking mentally triggers the release of adenosine, which in turn slows down neural activity in the arousal center areas. Because the arousal centers control activity throughout the entire brain, the process expands outward and causes neural activity to slow down everywhere in the brain, leading to drowsiness and encouraging sleep. Caffeine in coffee or tea prevents drowsiness by blocking the link between the prolonged neural

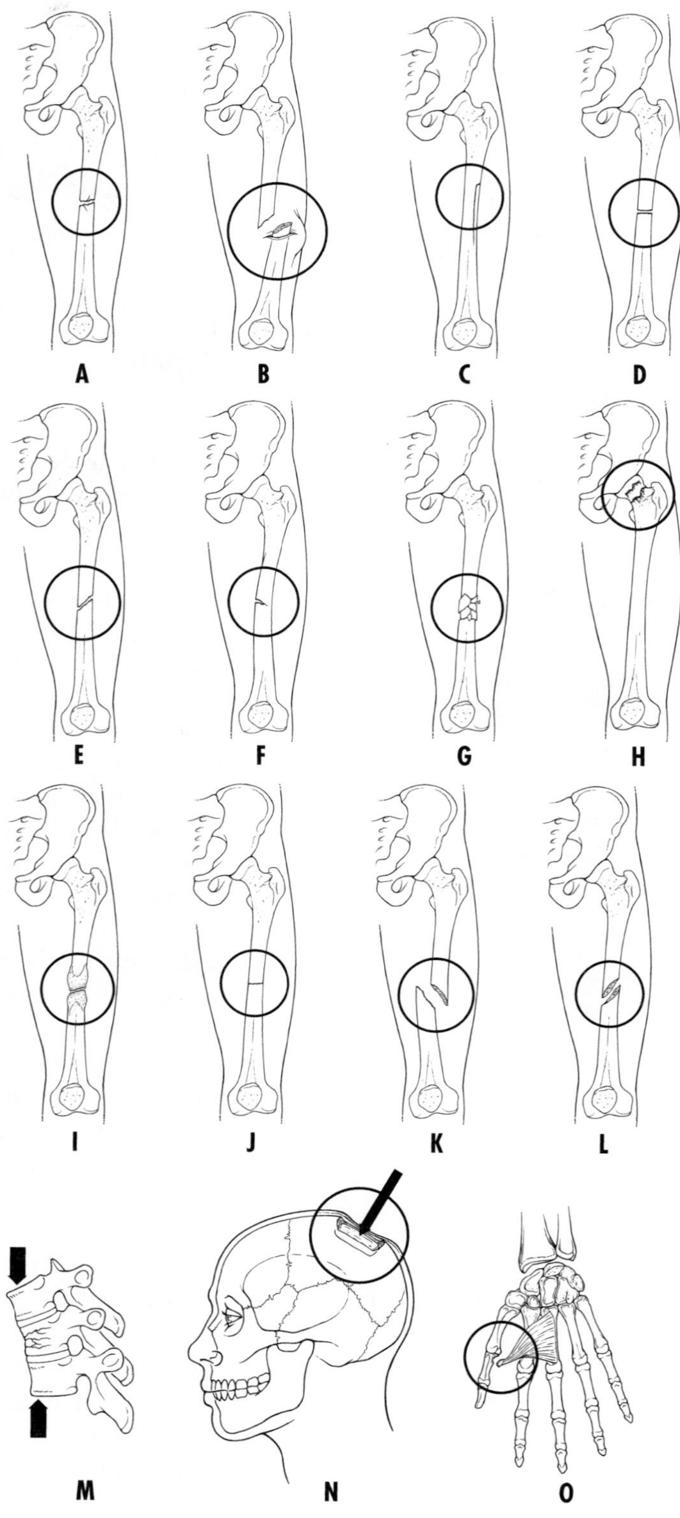

FIGURE 17-17 ■ Types of fractures (A to O). **A,** Closed (or simple). **B,** Open (or compound). **C,** Longitudinal. **D,** Transverse. **E,** Oblique. **F,** Greenstick. **G,** Comminuted. **H,** Impacted. **I,** Pathologic. **J,** Nondisplaced. **K,** Displaced. **L,** Spiral. **M,** Indirect compression. **N,** Direct compression. **O,** Avulsion.

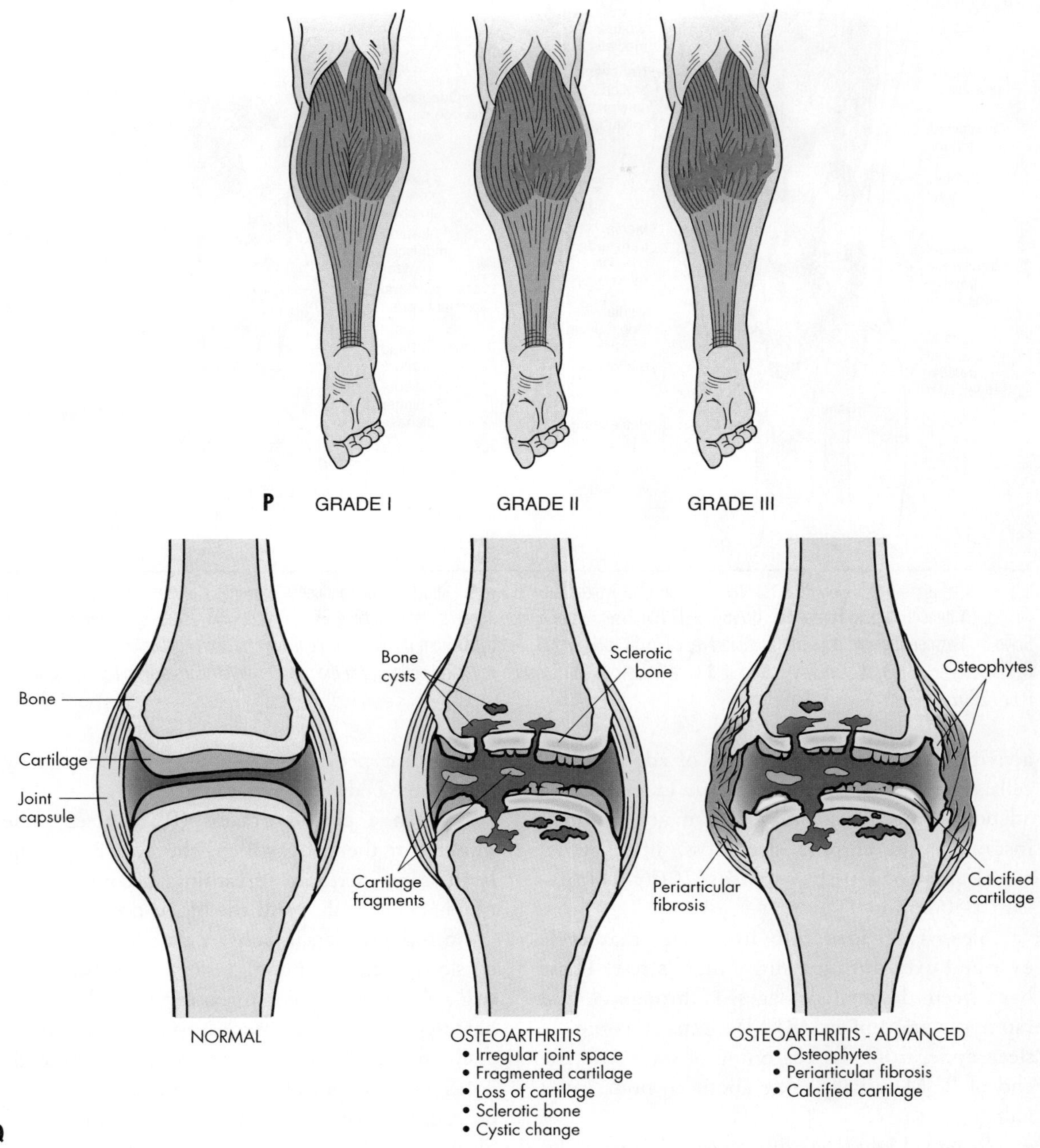

FIGURE 17-17, cont'd ■ **P,** Calf pull with degrees of severity. **Q,** Schematic presentation of the pathologic changes that occur with osteoarthritis.

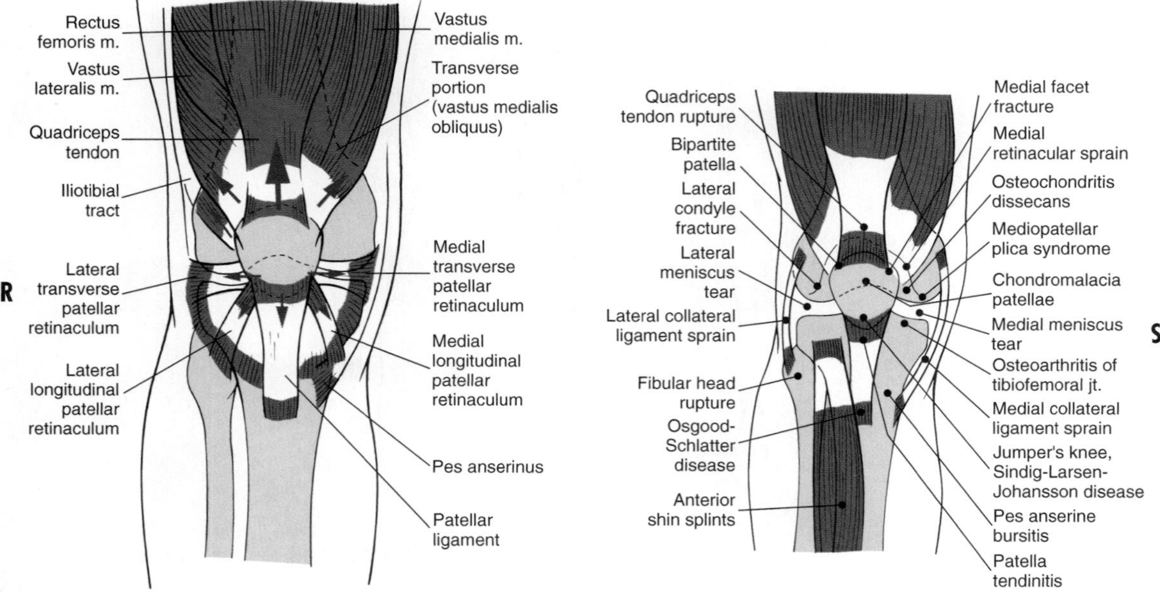

FIGURE 17-17, cont'd ■ **R,** Location of a typical knee injury. **S,** Structures that influence movement of the knee, specifically the patella. (**A** through **O** from Frazier MS, Drzymkowski JW: *Essentials of human diseases and conditions,* ed 2, Philadelphia, 2000, WB Saunders; **P** from Salvo S: *Massage therapy: principles and practice,* ed 2, St Louis, 2003, Mosby; **Q** from Damjanov I: *Pathology for the health-related professions,* ed 3, Philadelphia, 2006, WB Saunders; **R** and **S** from Saidoff DC, McDonough A: *Critical pathways in therapeutic intervention: extremities and spine,* St Louis, 2002, Mosby.)

activity and the increased levels of adenosine in cells. The researchers believe that failure of the adenosine mechanism may be a major factor in insomnia and chronic sleep loss. http://www.eurekalert.org/pub_releases/2006-01/aps-lsu010506.php

Sleep is divided into five stages that cycle over and over during a single night's rest. These have been designated stages 1 through 4 and rapid eye movement (REM) sleep. A complete sleep cycle, from the beginning of stage 1 to the end of REM, usually takes about an hour and a half.

- Stage 1: Light sleep, during which the muscles begin to relax and a person can be easily awakened.
- Stage 2: Brain activity slows and eye movement stops.
- Stage 3: Characterized by very slow brain waves (delta waves) interspersed with small, quick waves.
- Stage 4: Brain waves are all delta waves.

Stages 3 and 4 comprise deep sleep, during which all eye and muscle movement ceases. It is difficult to wake a person during deep sleep. During deep sleep, some people sleepwalk, and children may experience bedwetting or night terrors.

When a person dreams (REM sleep), the muscles of the body stiffen, the eyes move, the heart rate increases, breathing becomes more rapid and irregular, and the blood pressure rises.

Sleep disorders usually are classified as (1) lack of sleep (i.e., insomnia) or (2) disturbed sleep (e.g., obstructive sleep apnea, excessive sleep, and narcolepsy). In most cases, sleep disorders can be easily managed once they are properly diagnosed.

The treatment of a sleep disorder depends on its cause. Insomnia is the most common sleep disorder. It includes difficulty going to sleep, staying asleep, or going back to sleep when awakened early. It may be temporary or chronic. About one in three people have insomnia at some point in their lives. With insomnia, simple changes in the person's daily routine, lifestyle, and habits usually result in better sleep (Box 17-3).

TREATMENT OF SLEEP DISORDERS

Insomnia

If sleep studies have ruled out a disease-related cause, the best treatment for insomnia is improv-

BOX 17-3 Common Causes of Insomnia

- Anxiety: Anxiety may keep the mind too alert, preventing the person from falling asleep or awakening the individual in the middle of the night.
- Stress: Stress can keep the mind too active and prevents relaxation for sleep. A busy brain and excessive boredom can cause stress that interferes with sleep.
- Depression: Depression causes a person either to sleep too much or to have trouble sleeping. This may be due to chemical imbalances in the brain, or worries that accompany depression may prevent relaxation that allows sleep.
- Stimulants: Prescription drugs, including some antidepressants, high blood pressure medications, and steroids, can interfere with sleep. Many over-the-counter medications, including some brands of aspirin, decongestants, and weight loss products, contain caffeine and other stimulants. Antihistamines initially may make a person groggy, but they can worsen urinary problems, causing people to get up more during the night.
- Change in the environment or work schedule: Traveling or working a late or early shift can disrupt the body's circadian rhythms, making it difficult to get to sleep when necessary. Circadian rhythms act as internal clocks, guiding such factors as the wake-sleep cycle, metabolism, and body temperature.
- Long-term use of sleep medications: Doctors generally recommend using sleeping pills only for up to 4 weeks until the person notices benefits from self-help measures. If the sleep medication is needed for a longer period, the drug should be used no more than two to four times a week so that it does not become habit forming. Sleeping pills often become less effective over time.
- Pain: Arthritis, fibromyalgia, and neuropathies can interfere with sleep.
- Behavioral insomnia: Behavioral insomnia may occur when people worry excessively about not being able to sleep well and try too hard to fall asleep. Most people with this condition sleep better when they are away from their usual sleep environment or when they do not try to sleep, such as when they are watching TV.
- Eating too much too late in the evening: Having a light snack before bedtime is okay, but eating too much may cause a person to feel physically uncomfortable while lying down, making it difficult to get to sleep. Many people also experience acid reflux (a backflow from the stomach to the esophagus after eating). This uncomfortable feeling may keep the person awake.

BOX 17-4 Sleep Hygiene: How to Get a Good Night's Sleep

- Stay on a sleep-wake schedule: go to bed and wake up at the same time each day.
- Exercise daily but not at night before sleep.
- Avoid caffeine, cigarettes, sugar, herbal stimulants, and alcohol.
- Develop a relaxing bedtime ritual every night before going to bed, such as taking a hot bath or reading a book.
- Exposure to early sunshine helps trigger and reset the biologic clock in the brain that controls the sleep-wake cycle.
- Make sure the bedroom is neither too hot nor too cold.
- Avoid "trying" to sleep.
- If you take medications regularly (prescribed and over-the-counter), check with your doctor or pharmacist to see whether the medications may be contributing to sleep disturbances.
- Manage pain if painful conditions are bothersome.
- Limit naps; naps can make it harder to fall asleep at night.
- Minimize sleep interruptions. Close the bedroom door or establish a subtle background noise (e.g., turn on a fan).

ing "sleep hygiene" (Box 17-4). In most cases, sedatives should be used only on a short-term basis; however, some people require long-term drug therapy. Antidepressants may be effective.

Sleep Apnea

Devices also are available that a person can wear during sleep. A continuous positive airway pressure (CPAP) machine provides a constant airflow (and pressure) to the upper airway, preventing obstruction and keeping the airway open.

Those with enlarged tonsils or a large deviated septum causing obstruction may benefit from surgery. If overweight, a weight loss program can be helpful in treating obstructive sleep apnea. Avoiding sleeping on the back also can help relieve the condition. People with sleep apnea should not take sleeping pills, because the pills can prevent them from waking up enough to start breathing again.

Restless Leg Syndrome and Periodic Limb Movement Disorder

Medication, warm baths, stretching, and massage may be used to treat restless leg syndrome and periodic limb movement disorder. Nutritional changes, such as supplementation of magnesium or other deficient vitamins, may also help.

Narcolepsy

Narcolepsy has no cure, but symptoms can be managed with stimulant type medication.

Massage Strategies for Sleep Disorders

Massage is an excellent method for supporting sleep. Use the palliative protocol in Unit Two for this purpose. If supporting restorative sleep is the main outcome for the massage, addressing any specific issue will interfere with the overall relaxation response. Pain management is an important aspect of effective sleep. Massage is very effective in pain management; however, if specific methods are used (e.g., psoas release, concentrated connective tissue methods, or muscle energy methods and stretching), the outcome may be an arousing effect. Relaxation and arousal are two different massage applications that are best provided at different times. The pressure levels used during massage that targets sleep support should be moderately deep (e.g., the "big squash"). The person should be kept warm, especially the feet; a hot water bottle or warm rice or seed bag placed near the feet is soothing.

WOUNDS AND CONTUSIONS

A wound is an interruption in the continuity of body tissues (Figure 17-18). It can be external, internal, or both. Generally speaking, the deeper the wound, the more serious the consequences can be. With minor wounds, the outer layer of skin, the epidermis, is either scraped away or opened up to permit bacteria and materials to enter. In a more severe wound, the next layer down, the dermis, is injured. This layer contains connective tissue, sweat glands, hair follicles, nerves, lymph, and blood vessels, and the potential for the spread of infection increases.

A wound can be intentional (e.g., a surgical incision) or accidental, and it may be open or closed. An open wound has an outward opening where the skin is broken, exposing the underlying tissues. A closed (nonpenetrating) wound does not have an outward opening, but the underlying tissues are damaged, as in a hematoma or contusion (bruise). Closed wounds usually are the result of some type of blunt trauma to the body. An aseptic (clean) wound is not infected with pathogens; septic wounds are infected with pathogens.

Open wounds may be classified according to the appearance of their openings. An incised wound has a clean edge and is made with a cutting instrument. An incised wound may be the result of surgery, an accident, or a knife injury. A lacerated wound has torn or mangled tissues and is made by a dull or blunt instrument. A penetrating or puncture wound is caused by a sharp, slender object (e.g., a needle or an ice pick) that passes through the skin into the underlying tissues. A perforated wound is a penetrating wound that passes through to a body organ or cavity, such as a gunshot wound.

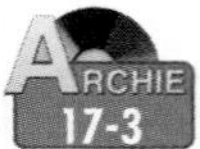

THE PROCESS OF WOUND HEALING

All wounds go through a healing or repair process that has three phases. In the first, or acute, phase, the blood vessels contract to control hemorrhage, and blood platelets form a network in the wound that acts like glue to plug the wound. After the inflammatory-mediated chemical reaction, fibrin is released into the wound, and clotting begins. The fibrin continues to collect red blood cells and the clot dries into a scab. About 12 hours later, special white blood cells arrive to clear away bacteria and dead tissue. Within 1 to 4 days, the fibrin threads contract and pull the edges of the wound together under the scab (think of this as how the body makes stitches to sew a wound closed).

The second, or subacute, phase (also called the proliferation phase) is the wound healing and new growth period, which lasts 5 to 20 days. During this phase the tissues repair themselves. New cells form, and the wound continues to contract and seal. If the wound is a clean surgical incision, complete contraction usually takes place during this phase, and little scarring or permanent fibrous tissue formation results.

The third, or remodeling, phase extends from day 21 onward. Clean, shallow wounds may contract in the first two stages; large or mangled wounds require the time and cellular activity of this third phase to build a bridge of new tissue to close the gap of the wound. The cells produce a fibrous protein substance called *collagen* (connec-

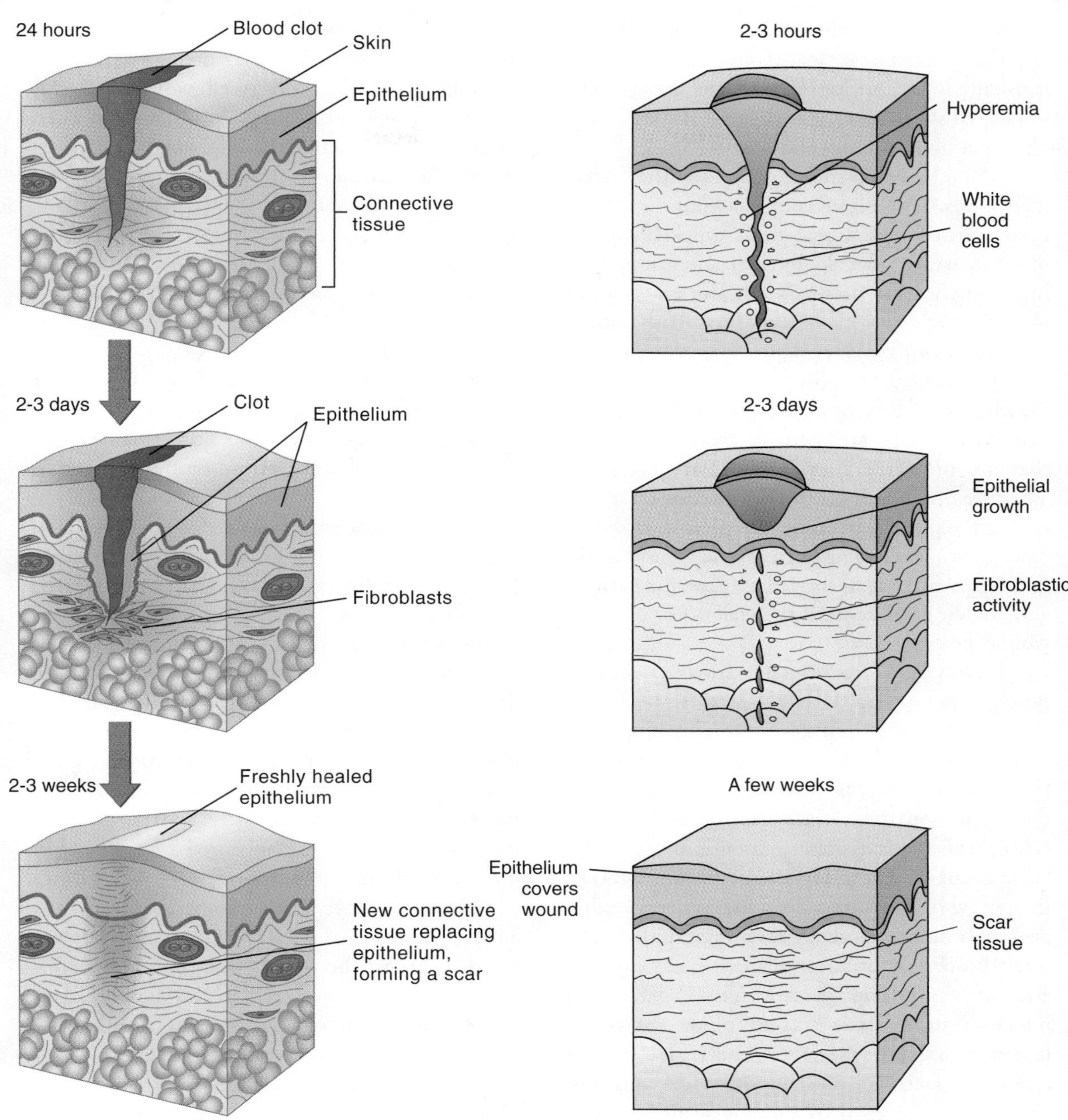

FIGURE 17-18 ■ Wound healing. Healing of skin wounds reflects mechanisms of healing in general. Wound healing is accelerated by bringing the edges of the wound together, through the use of bandaging and sutures. (Modified from Thibodeau GA, Patton KT: *Anatomy & physiology*, ed. 5, St Louis, 2003, Mosby.)

tive tissue) that gives the wounded tissues strength and forms scar tissue. Scar tissue is not true skin; it usually is very strong, but it lacks the elasticity of normal skin tissue. Scar tissue is also devoid of a normal blood supply and nerves.

Wounds are classified by the way they repair themselves. The clean surgical wound that has been sutured closed and heals quickly without much scarring does so by first intention. First intention healing occurs when the ends of the wound touch and reconnect. Frequently, small, clean lacerations may be closed with special adhesive strips called Steri-Strips. These strips reduce the chance of infection and do not leave suture scars. Steri-Strips are used on areas of the body that are protected from movement and stress. They are often used on the face. Because they are a suture replacement, only the physician should place them. They are placed on the wound in the same sequence and at the same intervals as sutures and are left in place until they fall off or until the wound heals.

Tissues that are severely damaged or purposely kept open or that fail to close heal from the bottom of the wound outward, forming granulation tissue, which then becomes scar tissue. Granulation tissue is vascular connective tissue that forms on the surface of a wound. This is called healing by secondary intention.

Several factors influence the healing process. People who are young, in good general health, and eat a nutritious diet heal more rapidly. Adequate protection and rest of the injured area also enhance the healing process. Tissue damage or infection during the second phase can delay healing and increase scarring. This is an especially important factor in determining when and how massage will be used to support wound healing and is described in depth later in the chapter.

Wounds are susceptible to infection because the normal skin barrier is broken. If there is debris in a wound as the result of the breakdown of the various cellular components, the dead (necrotic) tissue supports bacterial growth. Suppuration (pus) is dead tissue, bacteria, dead white blood cells, and other products of tissue breakdown. Necrotic tissue debris must be removed. Removal of debris is called débridement, which may occur naturally or may be performed surgically.

TREATMENT OF WOUNDS

Sometimes the physician may prefer not to use a dressing or bandage on small wounds; this is called open wound healing. Advantages of open wound healing include the following:

- It allows air to circulate freely around the wound.
- The wound is not irritated or rubbed by a dressing.
- The wound stays dry, which inhibits bacterial growth, reducing the chance of infection.
- Sutures stay dry and hold together better.
- Any pre-existing infection remains localized and is not spread by the dressing or bandage.

Wounds that are *dressed* are covered. A dressing is a sterile covering placed over a wound. Dressings usually consist of a strip of lubricated mesh gauze, a nonstick Telfa pad, or a clear dressing placed over a sutured wound. Body cavities or wounds that need to remain open for a time are dressed with long, thin packing material that often is impregnated with an antiseptic or lubricant. This is sometimes called *packing.* A good dressing must be effective and comfortable and must remain in place. If the dressing covers a hairless area, it may be anchored with tape, but no tape may touch the wound.

Sterile dressings have a number of advantages. They:

- Protect the wound from injury and contamination
- Maintain constant pressure to minimize bleeding and swelling
- Hold the wound edges together
- Absorb drainage and secretions
- Hide temporary disfigurement

A bandage should always be applied over a dressing. Bandages hold dressings in place and also help maintain even pressure, support the affected part, and help protect the wound from injury and contamination. Bandages can be gauze, cloth, or elastic cloth rolls and are bound by clips, tape, or ties. Plain elastic cloth roller bandage (e.g., Ace bandage) or elastic roller cloth with adhesive backing makes a flexible, secure cover. When an elastic roller bandage is applied as a pressure bandage, especially to the lower limbs, it is essential to keep the bandage consistent in spacing and tension to ensure even pressure. Even, gentle pressure stimulates circulation and healing. Uneven pressure causes constriction points that can create pressure sores, ulcers, or edema.

Dressings and bandages frequently appear simple to apply; however, special skill is required to apply a functional dressing. For obvious reasons, massage should never disturb or contaminate dressings and bandages.

TYPES OF WOUNDS

Wounds can be categorized into several different types (Figure 17-19).

- Abrasions: With this type of wound, the outer surface of the skin has been scraped away, and usually some minor oozing of blood and serum is seen. The wound must be cleaned to remove dirt that can cause an infection. Once cleaned, the wound should be blotted dry with sterile gauze, and pressure should be applied over the injured site for a few minutes to control bleeding. Applying a first aid or antibiotic cream to the abrasion can help prevent infection and keep the dressing from sticking. For the best protection, a bandage should cover 1 inch beyond the wound. An ice pack over the bandage can reduce swelling and ease some of the discomfort.

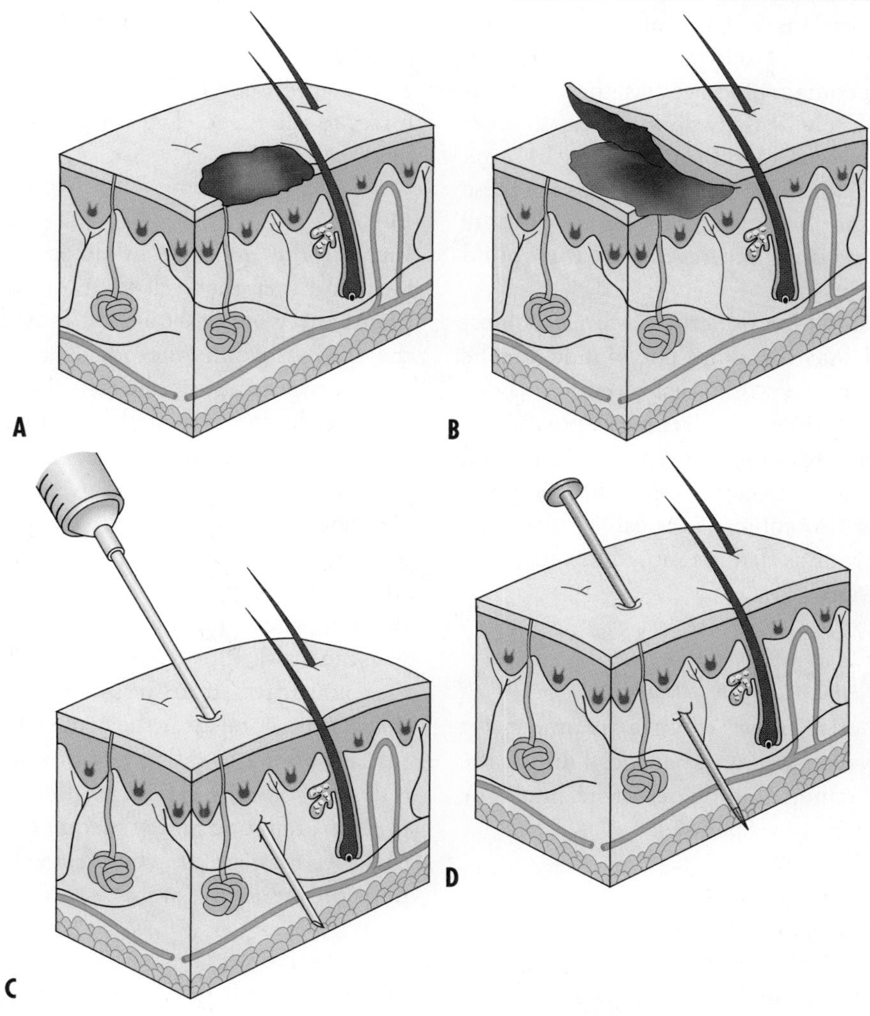

FIGURE 17-19 ■ **A,** Cross section of an abrasion. **B,** Cross section of an avulsion. **C,** Cross section of a puncture wound. **D,** Cross section of a laceration. (From Frazier MS, Drzymkowski JW: *Essentials of human diseases and conditions,* ed 2, Philadelphia, 2000, WB Saunders.)

- Avulsions: With avulsions, skin is pulled or torn off. The severed tissue should be saved and taken to the hospital to be reattached. A pressure dressing is applied over the wound until the person can receive medical care. Once a dressing has been applied, it should be left undisturbed and should not be removed to check the wound.
- Incisions: As mentioned previously, an incision is a cut with smooth edges. Incisions often are made during surgical procedures and are closed with sutures, with Steri-Strips, or by some other procedure, such as stapling.
- Lacerations: A laceration is similar to an incision, but it has jagged edges caused by tearing. Because incisions and lacerations go beyond the outer layer of skin and into the deeper layers that contain blood vessels, these wounds bleed profusely. If the wound is deep enough to cut an artery, blood squirts out with each heartbeat because of the high pressure in these vessels. Care involves applying a pressure dressing and using sutures to close the wound if necessary.
- Punctures: With a puncture, a foreign object is pushed into the skin. The wound can be superficial or deep. External bleeding may be minimal, but internal bleeding is possible. A deep puncture wound needs medical care, and a tetanus injection may be required. Some arthroscopic surgical procedures produce wounds that are more like punctures than incisions.

MASSAGE STRATEGIES FOR WOUNDS

Massage is not a direct or first treatment for wounds. However, it is most beneficial during the subacute and remodeling phases of healing. The following strategies can be used:

Days 1 to 3

- Sanitation and infection prevention are essential.
- Avoid the area during massage to protect the wound from contamination.
- Lymphatic drainage can be done above and below the wound. Do not use lymphatic drainage if any signs of infection are present, such as heat, swelling, redness (especially any type of red streaking), pus, or a sour smell.

Day 4

Use bend, shear, and tension forces around the wound, far enough away to prevent any chance of contamination. The goal is to drag the skin gently in multiple directions to prevent adhesions from forming. Connective tissue formation is random at this time. The wound edges should not be disturbed.

Days 5 and 6

Increase the intensity and depth of the forces in the area that has been treated and move closer to the wound. Decrease the intensity and gently apply bend, shear, and stretch (tension) forces to the tissue. The wound edges should not be disturbed.

Day 7

Increase the intensity in the previously treated areas and then move closer to the wound. At this point, the wound should be moving a bit from the forces loading the adjacent tissue, but the wound edges must not be disturbed. Progressively increase the intensity daily by moving closer and closer to the wound.

As soon as the wound is completely healed (14 days is typical, but it can take longer), begin to bend and shear the scar tissue and stretch it with tension.

The wound must be completely healed before you can work directly on it. Before working on the scar, address the tissue surrounding the wound; this can be done after the acute phase has passed (usually after 2 to 3 days). Work with the scar for at least 6 months. These methods can be taught to the patient or a family member (Figure 17-20). (Also see massage strategies for orthopedic conditions on the Evolve website.)

Old Scars

Old scars that have adhered to underlying tissue can be softened and stretched. All mechanical forces are used in multiple directions on the scar each session until the scar tissue and tissue at least 1 inch away from the scar become warm and

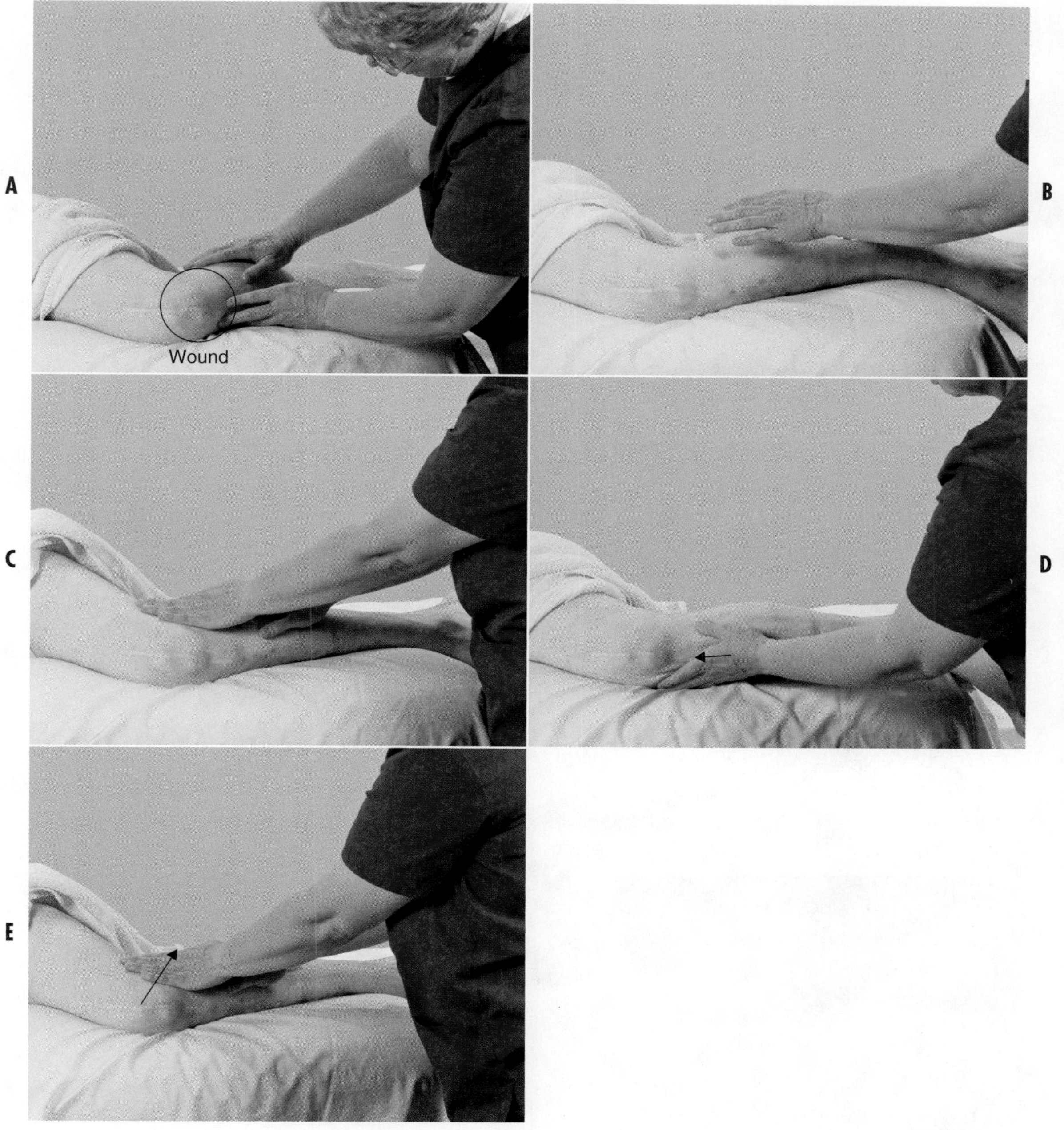

FIGURE 17-20 ■ Wounds. **A,** Assess the area. **B,** Near touch intentional method during the acute stage. **C,** Perform lymphatic drainage if the area is swollen. **D,** Push the healing edges of the tissue together. **E,** In the subacute phase of healing, begin to separate the tissue edges to support the formation of pliable scar tissue.

slightly red. The intensity should be such that the patient experiences a burning, stretching sensation. A small degree of inflammation is desirable; the area may be a bit tender to the touch after the massage, but it should not be painful to movement. Ideally, treatments should be given every other day, allowing the tissue to recover on the alternate days. These methods also can be taught to the patient or a family member (Figure 17-21).

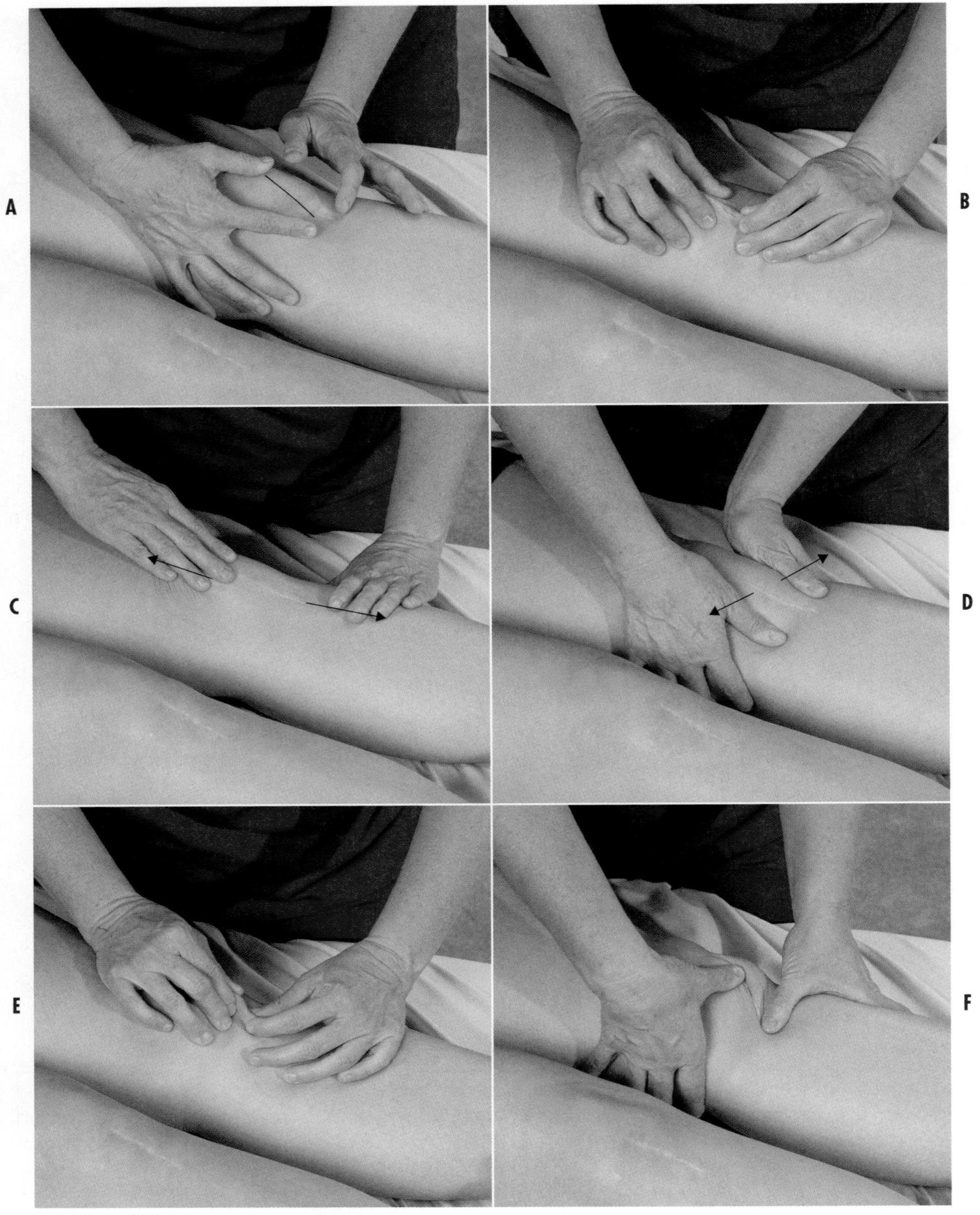

FIGURE 17-21 ■ Scars. **A,** Identify the scar; this example involves a repair of a torn anterior cruciate ligament. **B,** Assess the tissue for ease and bind. **C, D,** Apply tension force. **E,** Apply shear force. **F,** Apply torsion force.

CONTUSIONS (BRUISES)

The terms *contusion* and *bruise* can be used interchangeably to describe an injury that damages tissue and results in bleeding but does not break the skin. To clarify, the contusion is the trauma and the breaking of the blood vessels results in the bruise.

A contusion/bruise occurs because of a sudden traumatic blow to the body or some sort of sustained pressure, or in response to other types of injury (e.g., a sprain or surgery). Contusions can range from superficial and minor to extremely serious with deep tissue compression and hemorrhage.

The extent to which a person may be hampered by this condition depends on the location of the injury and the force of the blow. An impact to the muscles can cause more damage than might be expected and should be treated appropriately. If the muscle is crushed against the bone and is not treated correctly, or if it is treated too aggressively, myositis ossificans may result. The speed of healing for a contusion, as with all soft tissue injuries, depends on the extent of tissue damage and internal bleeding (Figure 17-22).

The three types of contusions are intramuscular contusions, intermuscular contusions, and bone bruises.

With an intramuscular contusion, the muscle is torn within the sheath that surrounds it. This means that the initial bleeding may stop early (within hours) because of increased pressure within the muscle; however, the muscle sheath prevents the fluid from escaping. The result is a considerable loss of function and pain, which can take days or weeks to resolve. Bruising may not appear with this type of contusion, especially in the early stages. Because no bruising is evident, the severity of the injury may not be recognized. The bruise may finally appear in the subacute phase, which indicates progressive healing.

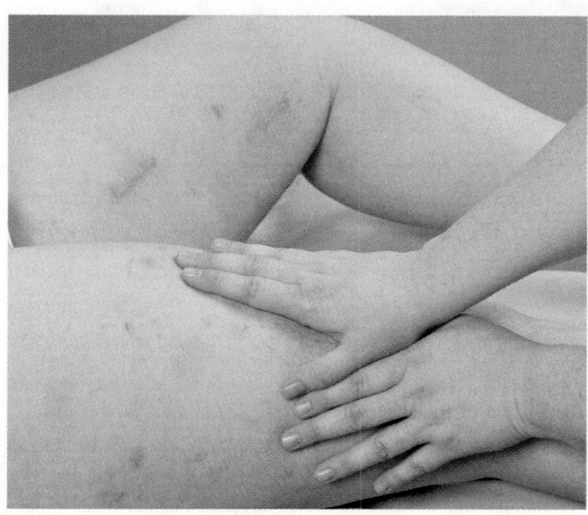

FIGURE 17-22 ■ Bruising.

Intermuscular contusions are characterized by tearing of the muscle and part of the sheath surrounding it. The initial bleeding takes longer to stop than with an intramuscular contusion. However, recovery progresses more quickly because the blood and fluids can flow away from the site of injury through tears in the muscle sheath. Bruising occurs with this type of contusion.

A bone contusion can penetrate to the skeletal structures, causing a bone bruise. Bone bruises are painful and require a fairly prolonged period of healing.

Symptoms of contusions include pain, swelling or bruising, and restricted movement. If the swelling has not resolved after 2 or 3 days, the injury likely is an intramuscular contusion. If the bleeding has spread and caused bruising away from the site of the injury, the injury is likely to be an intermuscular contusion.

Contusions are categorized as grade 1, 2 or 3, depending on their severity.

Signs of a grade 1 contusion include tightness and minor swelling, although the person still has nearly a full range of motion. Treatment includes protection, rest, ice, compression, and elevation (PRICE) and lymphatic drainage massage using skin drag methods only.

Grade 2 contusions involve painful movement, swelling, and limited range of motion. Compression causes pain. Treatment consists of ultrasound therapy and electrical stimulation, lymphatic drainage massage using skin drag methods only, and a rehabilitation program consisting of stretching, strengthening, and a gradual return to full function.

With grade 3 contusions, severe pain and immediate swelling are seen. Isometric contractions are painful and may produce a bulge in the muscle. Medical treatment is necessary.

Treatment of Contusions

Contusions are treated as follows:

- Immediate medical attention upon injury; the PRICE regimen may be used.
- Ultrasound and electrical stimulation (for 1 to 3 days).
- Lymphatic drainage massage using skin drag methods only. Wait at least 48 hours after the injury before applying massage.
- Surgery if needed to relieve pressure.

Massage Strategies for Contusions

Caution is necessary when massaging over contusions. The compressive force and depth of pressure need to be modified to avoid further injury. Lymphatic drainage–type applications usually are appropriate. Once the bruising dissipates in all three grades of contusion, kneading is used to prevent fibrosis. Over the next 3 to 6 months, continue to apply the bending and torsion forces of kneading to support the remodeling phase of healing.

CLINICAL REASONING FOR TREATMENT PLAN DEVELOPMENT

No one book can describe every medical condition that may be encountered in the healthcare setting and then provide massage treatment plans for each complication that may arise. Not enough studies of massage in relation to the treatment of various diseases have been done to allow concrete statements to be made about the appropriateness of massage and the application of massage. Also, massage application has not been completely standardized. No one knows for sure how to give the right massage for any condition.

Experts in massage do agree on a few things. For example, massage should not be given over open wounds, nor should it be given during acute kidney failure. Also, inflammation should not be increased in areas of acute inflammation, and so on. Most of this information is not based on research but on common sense and realistic caution grounded in the "do no harm" philosophy. None of the experts in the massage community, including the authors of this text, have the answers, precise protocols, and absolute indications and contraindications.

You may want protocol recipes for massage application on a condition by condition basis, but they are not available, and the ones out there (including those in this text) are opinion based, grounded in experience. Ethically it is inappropriate to create the expectation that specific protocols exist. Therefore the authors of this text and the educators in the classroom have to teach you to reason clinically; that is, to gather facts and to use those facts to make educated treatment decisions, and also to be able to justify the efficacy (benefit) and safety of those massage treatment plans.

The massage therapist absolutely must be able to use a clinical reasoning process to develop appropriate treatment plans. This process begins with fact gathering. As mentioned, the massage therapist needs certain reference texts, such as a comprehensive pathology text, a medical dictionary, a drug consult, and so forth. However, these days the Internet can be used very efficiently to gather facts. The websites listed under the Suggested Readings at the end of this chapter provide reliable information. This is important, because some information on the Web is not valid. The sites listed have all kinds of resources, such as medical dictionaries, medication descriptions, and disease signs, symptoms, and treatments.

evolve 17-14

The Evolve website makes this process so easy with links and access to extended information.

It is important to make sure that the information you collect is valid. You should research at least three different sites for the same information and compare your findings. In general, the information that is consistent on all three sites likely is valid.

The massage therapist's responsibility is to understand the signs, symptoms, prognosis, and treatments and then develop appropriate massage applications to benefit the patient without doing harm. As discussed, the massage outcome typically involves stress management, mood management, pain management, and inflammation management and supports restorative sleep. If the symptoms are musculoskeletal (e.g., low back pain of muscular origin), more specific massage applications may be used, such as the specific releases. However, in the healthcare setting other than physical therapy, physical medicine, orthopedic medicine, and chiropractic, most massage application is more general, consisting of the nonspecific, continual approaches for palliative care and condition management.

In the early stages of a massage therapist's career, it seems as if each new person (patient or client) presents a different condition. This is when the real learning takes place. Each new condition needs to be researched and the information applied to the unique circumstances of that patient. It will seem as if you spend more time looking up information than actually doing massage. This is real learning by doing, and much more applicable than lists and lists of diseases with recommendations for massage.

evolve 17-15

The Evolve website has lists of common conditions and general recommendations for massage, but that is only a place to start.

The best way to teach the clinical reasoning process is to provide a comprehensive example. This is done in two ways in this text. In this section we look at two conditions (one is found here in the text, and the other is found on the Evolve website). We describe the clinical reasoning process in a step-by-step fashion. If readers then use these examples as models and research a few more conditions, they should be able to continue the process in professional practice. In addition, Unit Four presents case studies that involve the clinical reasoning process. The conditions described in the examples and case studies are common, and massage typically is justifiable as part of a treatment process.

So let's begin. The following is an example of how to develop a justifiable treatment plan for a patient with chronic renal failure. The Evolve website presents a treatment plan for inflammatory bowel disease. The Web information example has been compiled from multiple sources but is presented as a typical information site on the Internet. Assume that the information has been compared to multiple resources and is valid. The information that follows and the web case are presented as they typically would appear on a website, with pertinent comments pertaining to massage.

evolve 17-16

The Evolve website presents comprehensive information about the conditions discussed in this chapter. First, read through all the information, then go back and identify content that would influence the massage application. As we go through the process, comments are made if the information directly affects the massage approach. Here's a hot tip: Look for information on the websites that have been designed as educational sites for patients with each condition. The content of these websites is particularly effective for the development of massage treatment plans.

JUST BETWEEN YOU AND ME

Many of you reading this text (and many of my students) want a book with all the disease and injury conditions listed and described, accompanied by a detailed, precise treatment plan. Realistically, this can't be done, because the book would be too big to carry, and the information would be only my own best-educated guess (they're pretty good guesses, based on years of experience, but still just opinion). Maybe someday such a compilation will show up on the Web, if enough of the so-called experts can agree. For now, the Evolve website and the data it presents are a great start. Use the examples as models and practice, practice, practice.

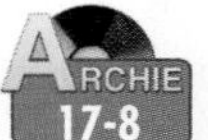

CHRONIC RENAL FAILURE

Kidney disease is a contraindication to massage, especially acute kidney failure. This example deals with chronic kidney disease and how a massage therapist would determine the appropriateness of the massage application.

Definition: Chronic renal failure is progressive and gradual loss of the kidneys' ability to excrete wastes, concentrate urine, and conserve electrolytes.

Additional names: Kidney failure–chronic; renal failure–chronic; chronic renal insufficiency; CRF; chronic kidney failure

Causes and risk factors: Chronic renal failure results from any disease that causes gradual loss of kidney function. It can range from mild dysfunction to severe kidney failure. In the early stages, there may be no symptoms and progression may be so gradual that symptoms do not occur until kidney function is significantly impaired. Progression may continue to end-stage renal disease (ESRD).

If this is the case, many people with undiagnosed kidney disease are getting massages. This is a concern.

Chronic renal failure and ESRD affect more than 2 of every 1000 people. Major causes include the following:

- Glomerulonephritis
- Diabetes
- Polycystic kidney disease
- Hypertension
- Reflux nephropathy
- Obstructive uropathy
- Kidney stones and infection
- Analgesic nephropathy

A complete history, including screening for these conditions, would be important. The two most common conditions in which massage is often indicated as part of a treatment plan are diabetes and hypertension. When working with patients who have these conditions, it would be prudent to monitor the intensity of fluid movement during the massage. Remember, increasing fluid movement during massage cannot really be avoided. The duration of the massage may need to be reduced to maybe 30 minutes and massage given more frequently, possibly three times a week.

Chronic renal failure results in the accumulation of fluid and waste products in the body, causing azotemia (the buildup of nitrogen waste products in the blood) and uremia. Uremia is the state of ill health resulting from renal failure. Most body systems are affected by chronic renal failure. Fluid retention and uremia can cause many complications.

This accumulation of fluid would seem to indicate lymphatic drainage methods; however, that is not the case. Lymphatic drainage needs to be avoided.

Symptoms

Initial symptoms of chronic renal failure may include the following:

- Nausea
- Vomiting
- Weight loss
- Feeling sick
- Fatigue
- Headache
- Hiccups
- Generalized itching

Pay attention to the itching as an indication of kidney disease. This may be a symptom that the patient would disclose to the massage therapist. If not, ask.

Later symptoms may include the following:

- Need to urinate at night
- Changes in urine output (increase/decrease)
- Bruising
- Blood in vomit or stools
- Decreased alertness
- Drowsiness
- Lethargy
- Confusion, delirium
- Coma
- Muscle twitching or cramps
- Seizures
- Uremic frost (deposits of white crystals in and on the skin)
- Decreased sensation in the hands, feet, or other areas

Additional symptoms that may be associated with this disease include the following:

- Excessive nighttime urination
- Excessive thirst
- Abnormally dark or light skin
- Paleness
- Nail abnormalities
- Breath odor
- High blood pressure
- Loss of appetite
- Agitation

If working with a patient who would have a risk factor for kidney failure, such as diabetes, the massage therapist should continually monitor for these symptoms and refer the patient to a physician if they are present.

Blood pressure may be high, with mild to severe hypertension. A neurologic examination may show neuropathy. Abnormal heart or lung sounds may be detected. A urinalysis and blood test may identify abnormalities such as:

- Creatinine levels progressively increase.
- BUN progressively increases.
- Creatinine clearance progressively decreases.
- Potassium test may show elevated levels.
- Arterial blood gas and blood chemistry analysis may show metabolic acidosis.

This disease may also alter the results of the following tests:

- Urinary casts
- Renal scan
- PTH [CO3]
- Serum magnesium
- Erythropoietin

These tests would be done, based on the symptoms, to confirm the kidney disease and/or kidney failure.

Treatment

Treatment focuses on controlling the symptoms, minimizing complications, and slowing the progression of the disease.

- Associated diseases that cause or result from chronic renal failure need to be addressed.
- Hypertension, congestive heart failure, urinary tract infections, kidney stones, obstructions of the urinary tract, glomerulonephritis, and other disorders should be treated as appropriate.
- Blood transfusions or medications such as iron and erythropoietin supplements may be needed to control anemia.
- Fluid intake may be restricted, often to an amount equal to the volume of urine produced.
- Dietary protein restriction may slow the build up of wastes in the bloodstream and control associated symptoms, such as nausea and vomiting.
- Salt, potassium, phosphorus, and other electrolytes may be restricted.
- Dialysis or kidney transplant eventually may be required.

Based on these treatments, it would be difficult to justify massage as part of the treatment process. If massage is used, it would be palliative and stress reducing.

Support Groups. The stress of illness often can be helped by joining a support group, in which members share common experiences and problems.

Prognosis

Chronic renal failure has no cure. Left untreated, it usually progresses to end-stage renal disease. Lifelong treatment may control the symptoms of chronic renal failure.

Complications of Kidney Disease

- End-stage renal disease
- Pericarditis
- Congestive heart failure
- Hypertension
- Platelet dysfunction
- Gastrointestinal tract bleeding
- Ulcers
- Hemorrhage
- Anemia
- Hepatitis B, hepatitis C, liver failure
- Decreased functioning of white blood cells
- Decreased immune response
- Increased risk of infection
- Peripheral neuropathy
- Seizures
- Encephalopathy, nerve damage, dementia
- Weakening of the bones
- Fractures
- Joint disorders
- Changes in glucose metabolism
- Electrolyte abnormalities, including hyperkalemia
- Decreased libido, impotence
- Miscarriage, menstrual irregularities, infertility
- Skin dryness, itching

Prevention

Treatment of the underlying disorders may help prevent or delay the development of chronic renal failure. Diabetics should control blood sugar and blood pressure closely and should refrain from smoking.

Massage Application and Treatment Plan

Chronic renal failure is a difficult condition for which to justify massage treatment. As the condition progresses, massage is contraindicated because moving fluid puts a strain on the failing kidneys. In the early stages of kidney disease, the big concern is that the symptoms are ignored or mistaken for something else. For example, the massage therapist may be the first to notice the slight changes in fluid retention. As explained, vague symptoms can indicate serious conditions. Early diagnosis means early treatment.

If a patient with chronic kidney failure requests massage treatment and the physician asks for an appropriate treatment plan, it would be prudent to rely on more reflexive methods, including energy-based modalities using entrainment and possibly subtle energy and magnetic field interactions between the practitioner and the patient. Although these subtle methods elude scientific validation, they are grounded in historical application. Even more, they are safe to use in these types of situations.

A massage method that uses repeated application of static touch (e.g., laying on of hands, polarity) with minimal mechanical force rhythmically applied can be soothing at the very least and might stimulate innate body healing processes. When the massage therapist does this type of work, intention is important. Focus on nurturing and comfort for the patient and on supporting the innate body wisdom.

Be cautious of appearing mystical or supernatural; this attitude can be unsettling. Although the human experience involves body, mind, and spirit, the patient's spiritual needs are best supported by the person's spiritual support system or the hospital chaplain. The potential of subtle energy fields is a physiologic phenomenon and should be presented as such.

Mechanical forces (i.e., bend, shear, tension, compression, and torsion) move fluid, therefore massage applications that create these forces must be avoided.

Patients with chronic renal failure have dry, itchy skin, and gently applying lotion to the skin can be part of the massage.

The duration of the massage should be limited to 30 minutes, and massage should be given daily.

evolve 17-17

The following terms and expressions specific to Chapter 17 have already been used to search PubMed for the latest research literature available. The *Click Here for Message* feature associated with this chapter on your textbook's Evolve website allows you to hyperlink to a continually updated PubMed search of research literature that corresponds to this subject.

Hyperlink Search Terms

Massage back pain
Massage cancer oncology
Massage cardiovascular respiratory disease
Massage chronic fatigue syndrome
Massage headache
Massage infection
And dozens more key terms and related research are located on the Evolve website.

SUMMARY

This chapter is extensively supported by the Evolve website. The massage strategies suggested are only starting points; you must use sound clinical reasoning to develop appropriate treatment plans.

You have two examples to model. Can you begin to do this? The information in all the preceding chapters has increased your knowledge of the effects of massage. After you study the text, come back and review these examples again. It is our understanding of how massage affects the body (or at least how we think it does) that determines how we use massage to help people with various healthcare conditions.

WORKBOOK

1. Identify five conditions that interest you. Research them both in written material and on the Internet. Using the model in this chapter and the one on the Evolve website, complete an analysis of the information and develop a justifiable massage application.

____

____

____

____

____

REFERENCES

www.neurologychannel.com
www.fmscommunity.org/immune.htm
www.mayoclinic.com
www.lifeoptions.org/kidneyinfo

Additional Sources

Jemal A: Cancer statistics, 2005. (Health Care Costs), *Medical Benefits,* February 28, 2005 issue.

Libenson C: Clinical challenges in functional reactivation, *Dynamic Chiropractic* 21(15): 22-24, 2003.

Sheerin F: Spinal cord injury: anatomy and physiology of the spinal cord: in the first of three articles, *Emergency Nurse,* December, 2004 issue.

http://www.migrainesolutions.com/migraine_resources/migraine_glossary.html#Migraine
http://www.headache.net/focus_index.asp?f=headache&b=headachenet
http://www.neurologychannel.com/headache/index.shtml
http://search.fasthealth.com
http://www.gssiweb.com
www.bragmanhealth.com
www.cdc.gov
www.davita.com
www.drguide.mohp.gov.eg
www.grmh.org
www.gssiweb.com
www.healthcentral.com
www.healthinfobase.com
www.ucsfhealth.org
www.wellnessctr.org
www.womenshealthchannel.com
www.allhealth.edu
www.arthritis-symtom.com
www.cancercenter.org
www.cancercenters.com
www.cancerhelp4u.com
www.chronicfatiguesyndromechat.com
www.council22.org
www.davita.com
www.drguide.mohp.gov.eg
www.ehc.healthgate.com
www.ehc.healthgate.com
www.etmc.org
www.grmh.org
www.gssiweb.com
www.health.hengryford.com
www.healthcentral.com
www.healthinfobase.com
www.hepnet.com
www.kenthospital.org
www.kenthospital.org
www.letstalkcounseling.com
www.merck.com
www.methodisthealthcare.org
www.painfoundation.org
www.sportsinjuryadvisor.com
www.sportsmedicine.about.com
www.sportsmedicine.miningco.com
www.sychowski.com
www.texaschildneurology.com
www.walgreens.com
www.wellnessctr.org
www.wfubmc.edu
www.womenshealthchannel.com

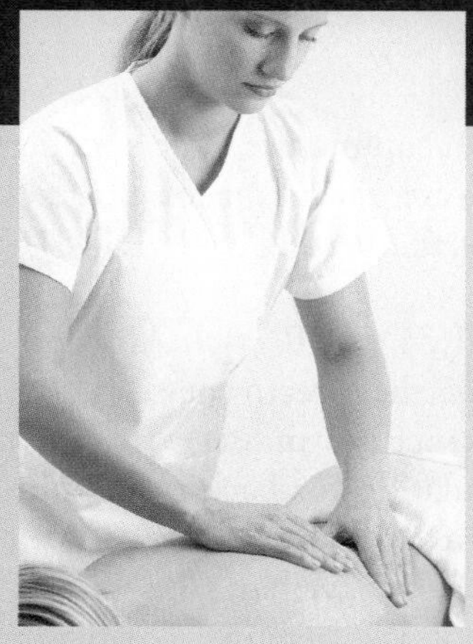

UNIT THREE REFERENCES

American Pain Society: *Principles of analgesic use in the treatment of acute pain and cancer pain,* ed 5, Glenview, Ill, 1999, The Society.

Andrews RA, Harrelson GL: *Physical rehabilitation of the injured athlete,* ed 3, Philadelphia, 2004, WB Saunders.

Astin JA, Ernst E: The effectiveness of spinal manipulation for the treatment of headache disorders: a systematic review of randomized clinical trials, *Cephalalgia* 22:617-623, 2002.

Atkinson C, Kiecolt-Glaser JK, Marucha PT et al: Hypnosis as a modulator of cellular immune dysregulation during acute stress, *J Consult Clin Psychol* 69:674-682, 2001.

Aust G, Fischer K: Changes in body equilibrium response caused by breathing: a posturographic study with visual feedback, *Laryngorhinootologie* 76:577-582, 1997.

Baechle TR, Roger WE: *Essentials of strength and conditioning,* Champaign, Ill, 2000, Kinetics.

Ballantyne F, Fryer G, McLaughlin P: The effect of muscle energy technique on hamstring extensibility: the mechanism of altered flexibility, *J Osteopath Med* 6:59-63, 2003.

Barnes P, Powell-Griner E, McFann K, Nahin R: Complementary and alternative medicine use among adults: United States, 2002, *CDC Advance Data Report No 343,* 2004.

Bennet M, Lengacher C. (1999). Use of complementary therapies in a rural cancer popula tion. http://www.indstate.edu/mary/ONF/index.htm

Berman JD, Straus SE: Implementing a research agenda for complementary and alternative medicine, *Ann Rev Med* 55:239-254, 2004.

Bernasconi P, Kohl J: Analysis of co-ordination between breathing and exercise rhythms in man, *J Physiol* 471:693-706, 1993.

Biondi DM: Physical treatments for headache: a structured review, *Headache* 45:738-746, 2005.

Born B: *The essential massage companion: everything you need to know to navigate safely through today's drugs and diseases,* Berkley, Mich, 2005, Concepts Born.

Bradley D, 1999, in Gilbert C (ed) Breathing retraining: advice from three therapists. Journal of Bodywork and Movement Therapies, 3(3): 159-167

Brandes JL: Treatment approaches to maximizing therapeutic response in migraine, *Neurology* 61(8 suppl 4): S21-26, 2003.

Brandes JL, Saper JR, Diamond M: Topiramate for migraine prevention: a randomized controlled trial, *JAMA* 25:291:965-973, 2004.

Bronfort G, Nilsson N, Haas M et al: Non-invasive physical treatments for chronic/recurrent headache. Wolfe-Harris Center for Clinical Studies, Northwestern Health Sciences University. gbronfort@nwhealth.edu

A, Duro JC, Porta M et al: Anxiety disorders in the joint hypermobility syndrome, *Psych Res* 46:59-68, 1993.

Cappo B, Holmes D: Utility of prolonged respiratory exhalation for reducing physiological and psychological arousal in nonthreatening and threatening situations, *J Psychosom Res* 28:265-273, 1984.

Cassileth B, Chapman C: Alternative and complementary cancer therapies, *Cancer* 77:1026-1033, 1996.

Cassileth BR, Vickers AJ: Massage therapy for symptom control: outcome study at a major cancer center, *J Pain Symptom Manage* 28:244-249, 2004.

Cella D, Lai JS, Chang CH et al: Fatigue in cancer patients compared with fatigue in the general United States population, *Cancer* 94:528-538, 2002.

Chair of Hygiene, DPMSC School of Medicine, University of Udine, Udine, Italy. r.quattrin @med.uniud.it *J Nurs Manage* 14:96-105, 2006.

Chaitow L: *Positional release techniques,* ed 2, Edinburgh, 2003, Churchill Livingstone.

Chaitow L: Breathing pattern disorders, motor control, and low back pain, *J Osteopath Med* 7:34-41, 2004.

Chaitow L, Bradley D, Gilbert C: *Multidisciplinary approaches to breathing pattern disorders,* Edinburgh, 2002, Churchill Livingstone.

Chen KW, Turner FD: A case study of simultaneous recovery from multiple physical symptoms with medical qigong therapy, *J Altern Complement Med* 10:159-162, 2004.

Cherkin DC, Deyo RA, Sherman KJ et al: Characteristics of visits to licensed acupuncturists, chiropractors, massage therapists, and naturopathic physicians, *J Am Board Fam Pract* 15:463-472, 2002.

Cherkin DC, Eisenberg DM, Sherman KJ et al: Randomized trial comparing traditional Chinese medical acupuncture, therapeutic massage, and self-care education for chronic low back pain, *Arch Intern Med* 161:1081-1088, 2001.

Cherkin D, Sherman K, Deyo R et al: A review of the evidence for the effectiveness, safety, and cost of acupuncture, massage therapy, and spinal manipulation for back pain, *Ann Intern Med* 138:898-906, 2003.

Chiradejnant A, Latimer J, Maher CG: Forces applied during manual therapy to patients with low back pain, *J Manipulative Physiol Ther* 25:362-369, 2002.

Cohen J, Gibbons R: Raymond Nimmo and the evolution of trigger point therapy, *J Manipulative Physiol Ther* 21:167-172, 1998.

Cohen S, Doyle WJ, Turner RB et al: Emotional style and susceptibility to the common cold, *Psychosom Med* 65:652-657, 2003.

Corey G et al: *Issues and ethics in the helping professions,* ed 6, Belmont, Calif, 2002, Brooks/Cole.

Dainese R, Galliani EA, De Lazzari F et al: Discrepancies between reported food intolerance and sensitization test findings in irritable bowel syndrome patients, *Am J Gastroenterol* 94:1892-1897, 1999.

Damas-Mora J et al: Menstrual respiratory changes and symptoms, *Br J Psych* 136:492-497, 1980.

Davidson RJ, Kabat-Zinn J, Schumacher J et al: Alterations in brain and immune function produced by mindfulness meditation, *Psychosom Med* 65:564-570, 2003.

De Domenico G, Wood EC: *Beard's massage,* ed 4, Philadelphia, 1997, WB Saunders.

Deig D: *Positional release technique,* Boston, 2001, Butterworth-Heinemann.

Edmeads J: Defining response in migraine: which endpoints are important? *Eur Neurol* 53(suppl 1):22-28, 2005.

Edvinsson L, Uddman R: Neurobiology in primary headaches, *Brain Res Brain Res Rev* 48:438-456, 2005.

Eisenberg DM, Davis RB, Ettner SL et al: Trends in alternative medicine use in the United States, 1990-1997: results of a follow-up national survey, *JAMA* 280:1569-1575.

Ernst E: Massage therapy for low back pain: a systematic review, *J Pain Symptom Manage* 17:65-69, 1999.

Ernst E: Distant healing: an "update" of a systematic review, *Wien Klin Wochenschr* 115:241-245, 2003a.

Ernst E: The safety of massage therapy, *Rheumatology (Oxford)* 42:1101-1106, 2003b.

Ernst E, Pittler MH: Experts' opinions on complementary/alternative therapies for low back pain, *J Manipulative Physiol Ther* 22:87-90, 1999.

Faling L: Controlled breathing techniques and chest physical therapy in chronic obstructive pulmonary disease. In Casabur R, editor: *Principles and practices of pulmonary therapy,* Philadelphia, 1995, WB Saunders.

Fellowes D, Barnes K, Wilkinson S: Aromatherapy and massage for symptom relief in patients with cancer, *Cochrane Database Syst Rev* 2:CD002287, 2004.

Ferel-Torey A: Use of therapeutic massage as a nursing intervention to modify anxiety and perceptions of cancer pain, *Cancer Nurs* 16:93-101, 1993.

Field T: *Touch therapy,* New York, 2000, Churchill Livingstone.

Field T: Massage therapy for skin conditions in young children, *Dermatol Clin* 23:717-721, 2005.

Field TM: Massage therapy effects, *Am Psychol* 53:1270-1281, 1998.

Ford MJ, Camilleri MJ, Hanson RB: Hyperventilation, central autonomic control and colonic tone in humans, *Gut* 37:499-504, 1995.

Fosså SD, Dahl AA, Loge JH: Fatigue, anxiety, and depression in long-term survivors of testicular cancer, *J Clin Oncol* 21:1249-1254, 2003.

Franke A, Gebauer S, Franke K, Brockow T: Acupuncture massage versus Swedish massage and individual exercise versus group exercise in low back pain sufferers: a randomized controlled clinical trial in a 2×2 factorial design, *Forsch Komplementarmed Klass Naturheilkd* 7:286-293, 2000.

Freeman LW: *Mosby's complementary and alternative medicine: a research-based approach,* ed 2, St Louis, 2004, Mosby.

Fuente-Fernandez R, Phillips AG, Zamburlini M et al: Dopamine release in human ventral striatum and expectation of reward, *Behav Brain Res* 136:359-363, 2002.

Furlan AD, Brosseau L, Imamura M, Irvin E: Massage for low back pain, *Cochrane Database Syst Rev* 2:CD001929, 2002.

Furlan L, Brosseau V, Welch et al: Massage for low back pain, *Cochrane Database Syst Rev* CD001929, 2000.

Gallob R: Reiki: a supportive therapy in nursing practice and self-care for nurses, *J NY State Nurse Assoc* 34:9-13, 2003.

Gardner WN: The pathophysiology of hyperventilation disorders, *Chest* 109:516-534, 1996.

Gerhardt H, Seifert F, Buvari P, Vogelsang H, et al: Therapy of active Crohn disease with *Boswellia serrata* extract H 15. *Z Gastroenterol* 39:11-17, 2001.

Gibbons P, Tehan P. *Spinal manipulation: indications, risks and benefits.* Edinburgh, 2001, Churchill Livingstone.

Gladstone JP, Dodick DW: From hemicrania lunaris to hemicrania continua: an overview of the revised International Classification of Headache Disorders, *Headache* 44:692-705, 2004.

Gordon C, Emiliozzi C, Zartarian M: Use of a mechanical massage technique in the treatment of fibromyalgia: a preliminary study, *Arch Phys Med Rehabil* 87:145-147, 2006.

Gorrol A, Mulley A: *Primary care medicine,* ed 5, Philadelphia, 2005, Lippincott Williams & Wilkins.

Greenman P: *Principles of manual medicine,* ed 3, Philadelphia, 2003, Lippincott Williams & Wilkins.

Griffith H, Moore SW: *Complete guide to prescription and non-prescription drugs,* Los Angeles, 2002, Price Stern Sloan.

Gross AR, Hoving JL, Haines TA et al: Cervical Overview Group: a Cochrane review of manipulation and mobilization for mechanical neck disorders, *Spine* 30:166, 2005.

Gurevich D: *Russian medical massage with Dr. David Gurevich,* Lapeer, Mich, 1992, Health Enrichment Center.

Hagen K, Hilde G, Jamtvedt G: The Cochrane review of bed rest for acute low back pain and sciatica, *Spine* 25:2932-2939, 2000.

Han J, Stegen K, De Valck C et al: Influence of breathing therapy on complaints, anxiety and breathing pattern in patients with HVS and anxiety disorders, *J Psychosom Res* 41:481-493, 1996.

Hastreite D et al: Regional variations in cellular characteristic in human lumbar intervertebral discs, including the presence of smooth muscle actin, *J Orthopaed Res* 19:597-604, 2001.

Headache Classification Committee of the International Headache Society: Classification and diagnostic criteria for headache disorders, cranial neuralgias and facial pain, *Headache* 44:2-7, 2004.

Hernandez-Reif M, Field T, Krasnegor J: Lower back pain is reduced and range of motion increased after massage therapy, *Int J Neurosci* 106:131-145, 2001.

Hides J, Jull G, Richardson C: Long-term effects of specific stabilizing exercises for first episode low back pain, *Spine* 26:243-248, 2001.

Hintz KJ, Yount GL, Kadar I et al: Bioenergy definitions and research guidelines, *Altern Ther Health Med* 9(suppl 3):A13-A30, 2003.

Hodges P, Heinjnen I, Gandevia S: Postural activity of the diaphragm is reduced in humans when respiratory demand increases, *J Physiol* 537:999-1008, 2001.

Horacek HJ Jr, Edwards D: *Brainstorms: understanding and treating the emotional storms of ADHD from childhood through adulthood,* Northvale, NJ, 2002, Aronson.

Hsieh LL, Kuo CH, Yen MF, Chen TH: A randomized controlled clinical trial for low back pain treated by acupressure and physical therapy, *Prev Med* 39:168-176, 2004.

Huan Z, Rose K. (1995). *Who can ride the dragon?*: Paradigm.

Huan Z, Rose K. (1996). *Who can ride the dragon?:* Paradigm.

Huan Z, Rose K. (1997). *Who can ride the dragon?:* Paradigm.

Huan Z, Rose K. (1998). *Who can ride the dragon?:* Paradigm.

Huan Z, Rose K. (1999). *Who can ride the dragon?:* Paradigm.

Hurwitz EL, Aker PD, Adams AH et al: Manipulation and mobilization of the cervical spine: a systematic review of the literature, *Spine* 21:1746-1759, 1996.

Irwin MR, Pike JL, Cole JC et al: Effects of a behavioral intervention, tai chi chih, on varicella zoster virus–specific immunity and health functioning in older adults, *Psychosom Med* 65:824-830, 2003.

Jonas WB, Kaptchuk TJ, Linde K: A critical overview of homeopathy, *Ann Intern Med* 138:393-399, 2003.

Keen J et al: *Mosby's critical care and emergency medication reference,* ed 2, St Louis, 1996, Mosby.

Kelman L: Women's issues of migraine in tertiary care.

Kemper KJ, Kelly EA: Treating children with therapeutic and healing touch, *Pediatr Ann* 33:248-252, 2004.

Kessler RC, Soukup J, Davis RB et al: The use of complementary and alternative therapies to treat anxiety and depression in the United States, *Am J Psychiatry* 158:289-294, 2001.

Knost B, Flor H, Birbaumer N et al: Learned maintenance of pain: Muscle tension reduces central nervous system processing of painful stimulation in chronic and subchronic pain patients, *Psychophysiology* 36:755-764, 1999.

Kraemer WJ, Adams K, Cafarelli E et al: American College of Sports Medicine position stand: progression models in resistance training for healthy adults, *Med Sci Sports Exerc* 34:364-380, 2002.

Kshettry VR, Carole LF, Henly S et al: Complementary alternative medical therapies for heart surgery patients: feasibility, safety, and impact, *Ann Thorac Surg* 81:201-205, 2006.

Landmark Health Care: *The Landmark report on public perceptions of alternative care,* Sacramento, 1998, Landmark Health Care.

Lang EV, Benotsch EG, Fick LJ et al: Adjunctive nonpharmacological analgesia for invasive medical procedures: a randomised trial, *Lancet* 355:1486-1490, 2000.

Lazar SW, Bush G, Gollub RL et al: Functional brain mapping of the relaxation response and meditation, *Neuroreport* 11:1581-1585, 2000.

Lederman E: *Fundamentals of manual therapy: physiology, neurology and psychology,* New York, 1997, Churchill Livingstone.

Lee J, Hoshino Y, Nakamura K et al: Trunk muscle imbalance as a risk factor of the incidence of low back pain: a 5-year prospective study, *Journal of the Neuromuscular System* 7:97-101, 1999.

Lewit K: Chain reactions in the locomotor system, *J Orthopaed Med* 21:52-58, 1999a.

Lewit K: *Manipulation in rehabilitation of the locomotor system,* ed 3, London, 1999b, Butterworth.

Lewit K: *Manipulative therapy in rehabilitation of the locomotor system,* ed 3, London, 1999c, Butterworth.

Liebenson C: The quadratus lumborum and spinal stability, *J Bodywork Move Ther* 4:49-54, 2000a.

Liebenson C: The trunk extensors and spinal stability, *J Bodywork Move Ther* 4:246-249, 2000b.

Linde K, Hondras M, Vickers A et al: Systematic reviews of complementary therapies: an annotated bibliography. Part 3. Homeopathy, *BMC Complement Altern Med* 1:4, 2001.

Lipton RB, Scher AI, Kolodner K: Migraine in the United States: epidemiology and patterns of health care use, *Neurology* 58:885-894, 2002.

Lum C: Hyperventilation and asthma: the grey area, *Biol Psychol* 43:262, 1996.

Lum L: Hyperventilation: an anxiety state, *J R Soc Med* 74:1-4, 1981.

Lum L: Hyperventilation and anxiety state, *J R Soc Med* 74(1):1-4, 1984 (editorial).

Lum L: Hyperventilation syndromes. In Timmons B, Ley R, editors: *Behavioral and psychological approaches to breathing disorders,* New York, 1994, Plenum Press.

Macefield G, Burke D: Paresthesia and tetany induced by voluntary hyperventilation, *Brain* 114:527-540, 1991.

Maitland G: *Maitland's vertebral manipulation,* ed 6, Oxford, 2001, Butterworth-Heinemann.

Mathew NT: Advances in cluster headache, *Neurol Clin* 8:867-890, 1990.

McCaffery M, Pasero C: *Pain: clinical manual,* ed 2, St Louis, 1999, Mosby.

McNair PJ, Stanley SN: Effect of passive stretching and jogging on the series elastic muscle stiffness and range of motion of the ankle joint, *Br J Sports Med* 30:313-318, 1996.

Melillo N, Corrado A, Quarta L et al: Fibromyalgic syndrome: new perspectives in rehabilitation and management: a review, *Minerva Med* 96:417-423, 2005.

Milgrom LR: Vitalism, complexity and the concept of spin, *Homeopathy* 91:26-31, 2002.

Morris CE, Skalak TC: Effects of static magnetic fields on microvascular tone in vivo. Paper presented at the Experimental Biology Meeting, April, 2003, San Diego, California.

Mosby's Drug Consult, St Louis, 2004, Mosby.

Mundy EA, DuHamel KN, Montgomery GH: The efficacy of behavioral interventions for cancer treatment–related side effects, *Semin Clin Neuropsychiatry* 8:253-275, 2003.

Muscolino JE: *The muscular system manual: the skeletal muscles of the human body,* ed 2, St Louis, 2005, Mosby.

Myers TW: *Anatomy trains: myofascial meridians for manual and movement therapists,* Philadelphia, 2001, Churchill Livingstone.

Neumann DA: *Kinesiology of the musculoskeletal system: foundations for physical rehabilitation,* St Louis, 2002, Mosby

Ni H, Simile C, Hardy AM: Utilization of complementary and alternative medicine by United States adults: results from the 1999 National Health Interview Survey, *Med Care* 40:353-358, 2002.

Okuyama T, Akechi T, Kugaya A et al: Development and validation of the cancer fatigue scale: a brief, three-dimensional, self-rating scale for assessment of fatigue in cancer patients, *J Pain Symptom Manage* 19:5-14, 2000.

Olsen PD, Hopkins WG: The effect of attempted ballistic training on the force and speed of movements, *J Strength Cond Res* 17:291-298, 2003.

Oncol Nurs Forum 26:1287-1294, 1999.

Oschman J: *Energy medicine in therapeutics and human performance,* St. Louis, 2003, Elsevier Science.

Oschman JL: *Energy medicine: the scientific basics,* Philadelphia, 2000, Churchill Livingstone.

Paine T: *The complete guide to sports massage,* London, 2000, A&C Black.

Paterson C, Allen JA, Browning M et al: A pilot study of therapeutic massage for people with Parkinson's disease: the added value of user involvement. MRC Health Services Research Collaboration, Department of Social Medicine, University of Bristol, Canynge Hall, Whiteladies Road, Bristol BS8 2PR, UK. c.paterson@bristol.ac.uk

Peroutka SJ: Dopamine and migraine, *Neurology* 49:650-656, 1997.

Perri M, Halford E: Pain and faulty breathing: a pilot study, *J Bodywork Move Ther* 8:237-312, 2004.

Pert CB: *Why you feel the way you feel: molecules of emotion,* New York, 1997, Scribner.

Pickar JG: Neurophysiological effects of spinal manipulation, *Spine J* 2:357-371, 2002.

Pope RP, Herbert RD, Kirwan JD et al: A randomized trial of preexercise stretching for prevention of lower-limb injury, *Med Sci Sports Exerc* 32:271-277, 2000.

Preece J: Introducing abdominal massage in palliative care for the relief of constipation, *Complement Ther Nurs Midwifery* 8:101-105, 2002.

Proctor ML, Hing W, Johnson TC et al: Spinal manipulation for primary and secondary dysmenorrhoea, *Cochrane Database Syst Rev* 2: CD002119. Accessed April 30, 2004, at www.cochrane.org

Pryor J, Prasad S: *Physiotherapy for respiratory and cardiac problems,* ed 3, Edinburgh, 2002, Churchill Livingstone.

Quattrin R, Zanini A, Buchini S et al: Use of reflexology foot massage to reduce anxiety in hospitalized cancer patients in chemotherapy treatment: methodology and outcomes, *J Nurs Manage* 14:96-105, 2006.

Reddy GK: Photobiological basis and clinical role of low-intensity lasers in biology and medicine, *J Clin Laser Med Surg* 22:141-150, 2004.

Rich GJ: *Massage therapy: the evidence for practice,* St Louis, 2002, Mosby.

Richards T, Vallbona C: Evolution of magnetic therapy from alternative to traditional medicine, *Phys Med Rehabil Clin N Am* 10:729-754, 1999.

Richardson MA, Sanders T, Palmer JL et al: Complementary/alternative medicine use in a comprehensive cancer center and the implications for oncology, *J Clin Oncol* 18:2505-2514, 2000.

Richardson MA, Straus SE: Complementary and alternative medicine: opportunities and challenges for cancer management and research, *Semin Oncol* 29:531-545, 2002.

Rowlands AV, Marginson VF, Lee J: Chronic flexibility gains: effect of isometric contraction duration during proprioceptive neuromuscular facilitation stretching techniques, *Res Q Exerc Sport* 74:47-51, 2003.

Rubik B, Pavek R, Ward R et al: Manual healing methods. In Alternative medicine: expanding medical horizons—a report to the National Institutes of Health on alternative medical systems and practices in the United States, NIH Pub No 94-066, 14-16 September 2002; Chantilly, Va, 113-157.

Rutledge JC, Hyson DA, Garduno D et al: Lifestyle modification program in management of patients with coronary artery disease: the clinical experience in a tertiary care hospital, *J Cardiopulm Rehabil* 19:226-234, 1999.

Sachse J: The thoracic region's pathogenetic relations and increased muscle tension, *Manuelle Medizin* 33:163-172, 1995.

Saidoff DC, McDonough AL: *Critical pathways in therapeutic intervention: extremities and spine,* St Louis, 2002, Mosby.

Sancier KM, Holman D: Commentary: multifaceted health benefits of medical qigong, *J Altern Complement Med* 10:163-165, 2004.

Sarrell EM, Cohen HA, Kahan E: Naturopathic treatment for ear pain in children, *Pediatrics* 111:e574-e579, 2003.

Sarrell EM, Mandelberg A, Cohen HA: Efficacy of naturopathic extracts in the management of ear pain associated with acute otitis media, *Arch Pediatr Adolesc Med* 155:796-799, 2001.

Sawyer M, Zbieranek CK: The treatment of soft tissue after spinal injury, *Clin Sports Med* 5:387-405, 1986.

Selye H: *The stress of life,* New York, 1956, McGraw-Hill.

Shephard RJ, Balady G: Exercise as cardiovascular therapy, *Circulation* 99:963-972, 1999.

Sherman KJ, Cherkin DC, Deyo RA et al: The diagnosis and treatment of chronic back pain by acupuncturists, chiropractors, and massage therapists, *Clin J Pain* 22:227-234, 2006.

Shrier I: Stretching before exercise does not reduce the risk of local muscle injury: a critical review of the clinical and basic science literature, *Clin J Sport Med* 9:221-227, 1999.

Silberstein S, Mathew N, Saper J: Botulinum toxin type A as a migraine preventive treatment, *Headache* 40:445-450, 2000.

Silberstein SD, Freitag FG: Preventative treatment of migraine, *Neurology* 60:S38-S44, 2003.

Simons D, Travell J, Simons L: *Myofascial pain and dysfunction: the trigger point manual—upper half of body,* ed 2, Baltimore, 1999, Williams & Wilkins.

Smith A, Nicholson K: Psychosocial factors, respiratory viruses and exacerbation of asthma, *Psychoneuroendocrinology* 26:411-420, 2001.

Stamenkovic I: Extracellular matrix remodeling: the role of matrix metalloproteinases, *J Pathol* 200:448-464, 2003.

Stark SD: Stretching techniques. In *The Stark reality of stretching,* Richmond, BC, 1997, Stark Reality Publishing.

Stothers L: A randomized trial to evaluate effectiveness and cost effectiveness of naturopathic cranberry products as prophylaxis against urinary tract infection in women, *Can J Urol* 9:1558-1562, 2002.

Swenson R, Haldeman S: Spinal manipulative therapy for low back pain, *J Am Acad Orthop Surg* 11:228-237, 2003.

Timmons BH, Ley R: *Behavioural and psychological approaches to breathing disorders,* New York, 2004, Plenum Press.

Trotter JF: Hepatic hematoma after deep tissue massage, *N Engl J Med* 341:2019-2020, 1999.

Tusek DL, Church JM, Strong SA et al: Guided imagery: a significant advance in the care of patients undergoing elective colorectal surgery, *Dis Colon Rectum* 40:172-178, 1997.

Van Den Bogaerde J, Cahill J, Emmanuel AV et al: Gut mucosal response to food antigens in Crohn's disease, *Aliment Pharmacol Ther* 16:1903-1915, 2002.

Waddell G: *The back pain revolution,* Edinburgh, 1998, Churchill Livingstone.

Wall P, Melzack R: *Textbook of pain,* ed 5, London, 2005, Churchill Livingstone.

Weber MD, Servedio FJ, Woodall WR: The effects of three modalities on delayed onset muscle soreness, *J Orthop Sports Phys Ther* 20:236-242, 1994.

Welch KMA: Contemporary concepts of migraine pathogenesis, *Neurology* 61:S2-S8, 2003.

West JB: *Respiratory physiology: the essentials,* Philadelphia, 2000, Lippincott Williams & Wilkins.

Whittington MA, Faulkner HJ, Doheny HC, Traub RD: Neuronal fast oscillations as a target for psychoactive drugs, *Pharmacol Ther* 86:171-190, 2000.

Whittington, MA, Traub RD, Jeffreys JGR: Metabotropic receptor activation drive synchronized 40 Hz oscillations in networks of inhibitory neurons, *Nature* 373:612-615, 1995.

Whittington MA, Traub RD, Jeffreys JGR: Synchronized oscillations in interneuron networks driven by metabotropic glutamatergic receptor activation, *Nature* 373:612-615, 1995.

Whittington MA, Traub RD, Faulkner HJ et al: Recurrent excitatory postsynaptic potentials induced by synchronized fast cortical oscillations, *Proc Natl Acad Sci USA* 94:12198-12203, 1997.

Wieting, Andary MT, Holmes TG et al: Manipulation, massage, and traction. In DeLisa JA, Gans BM, editors: *Physical medicine and rehabilitation: principles and practice,* ed 4, Philadelphia, 2005, Lippincott-Raven.

Wiktorsson-Möller M, Öberg BA, Ekstrand J et al: Effects of warming up, massage, and stretching on range of motion and muscle strength in the lower extremity, *Am J Sports Med* 11:249-252, 1983.

Winstead-Fry P, Kijek J: An integrative review and meta-analysis of therapeutic touch research, *Altern Ther Health Med* 5:58-67, 1999.

Winters J, Crago P, editors: *Biomechanics of neural control of posture and movement,* New York, 2000, Springer.

Wittink H, Michel T: *Chronic pain management for physical therapists,* ed 2, Boston, 2002, Butterworth-Heinemann.

Yahia L, Pigeon P et al: Viscoelastic properties of the human lumbodorsal fascia, *J Biomed Eng* 15:425-429, 1993.

Yang EV, Bane CM, MacCallum RC et al: Stress-related modulation of matrix metalloproteinase expression, *J Neuroimmunol* 133:144-150, 2002.

Yates A: *Compulsive exercise and eating disorders: toward an integrated theory of activity,* New York, 1991, Brunner-Routledge.

Ylinen A, Sik A, Bragin A et al: Sharp wave–associated high-frequency oscillation (200 Hz) in the intact hippocampus: network and intracellular mechanisms, *J Neurosci* 15: 30-46, 1995.

Ylinen A, Soltesz I, Bragin et al: Intracellular correlates of theta rhythm in hippocampal pyramidal cells, granule cells and basket cells, *Hippocampus* 5:78-90, 1995.

Additional Resources

http://www.biomedcentral.com/1472-6882/5/13/prepub
http://www.cancer.gov
http://www.genesishealth.com/services/physical.aspx
http://www.spineuniverse.org/
http://www.ampainsoc.org/
http://www.arthritis.org/
http://www.iasp-pain.org/
http://www.partnersagainstpain.com/
http://www.asipp.org/
http://www.painfoundation.org/
http://www.headaches.org/
http://www.aspmn.org/
http://www.mayoclinic.org

Cancer Information Service
www.cancer.gov
Toll-free: 1-800-4-CANCER (1-800-422-6237)
TTY: 1-800-332-8615

National Institute of Arthritis and Musculoskeletal and Skin Diseases
www.niams.nih.gov

Pro Health
The Effect of Cranial Manipulation on the Traube-Hering-Mayer Oscillation as Measured by Laser-Doppler Flowmetry

ChronicFatigueSyndromeSupport.com

Source
http://www.alternative-therapies.com/

Authors

Nicette Sergueff lectures throughout Europe on manual principles, diagnosis, and treatment and maintains a private practice in Corbas, France. She is an assistant professor.

Kenneth E. Nelson is a professor, and Thomas Glonek is a research professor in the Department of Osteopathic Manipulative Medicine, Chicago College of Osteopathic Medicine, Midwestern University, Downers Grove, Illinois.

American Academy of Orthopaedic Surgeons
P.O. Box 2058
Des Plaines, Illinois 60017
www.aaos.org
Telephone: 847-823-7186; 800-346-2267
Fax: 847-823-8026
e-mail: julitz@mac.aaos.org

American Academy of Physical Medicine and Rehabilitation
www.aapmr.org

American Gastroenterological Society

American Physical Therapy Association
1111 North Fairfax Street
Alexandria, Virginia 22314-1488
www.apta.org
Telephone: 703-684-2782; 800-999-2782 ext. 3395

Arthritis Foundation
1330 West Peachtree Street
Atlanta, Georgia 30309
www.arthritis.org
www.rheumatology.org
Telephone: 404-872-7100; 800-283-7800; or call your local chapter (listed in the telephone directory)

Crohn's and Colitis Foundation of America

Gatorade Sports Science Institute
www.gssiweb.com

National Anorexic Aid Society
Telephone: 614-436-1112

National Association of Anorexia Nervosa and Associated Disorders
Telephone: 847-831-3438

National Digestive Diseases Information Clearinghouse
Memorial Hospital of Union County
Marysville, Ohio 43043

www.neurologychannel.com/migraine/naturalmedicine.shtml

www.apsfa.org/migraines.htm

Mayo Clinic
www.mayoclinic.org/healthinfo www2.rpa.net/~lrandall/index.html

Detroit Medical Center
www.dmc.org/health_info

www.health-care-information.org

www.health-care-clinic.com

www.health-cares.net

www.healthfinder.gov

Spine. 2005 Jan 1;30(1):166.

PMID: 12779300 [PubMed—indexed for MEDLINE]
Spine. 2004 Jul 15;29(14):1541-8.

www.ncbi.nlm.nih.gov

www.meta.wkhealth.com

www.ncbi.nlm.nih.gov

Fernández-de-Las-Peñas C, Alonso-Blanco C, Cuadrado ML et al: Are manual therapies effective in reducing pain from tension-type headache?: a systematic review, *Clin J Pain* 22:278-285, 2006.

Conn's current therapy, ed 53, Philadelphia, 2001, WB Saunders.

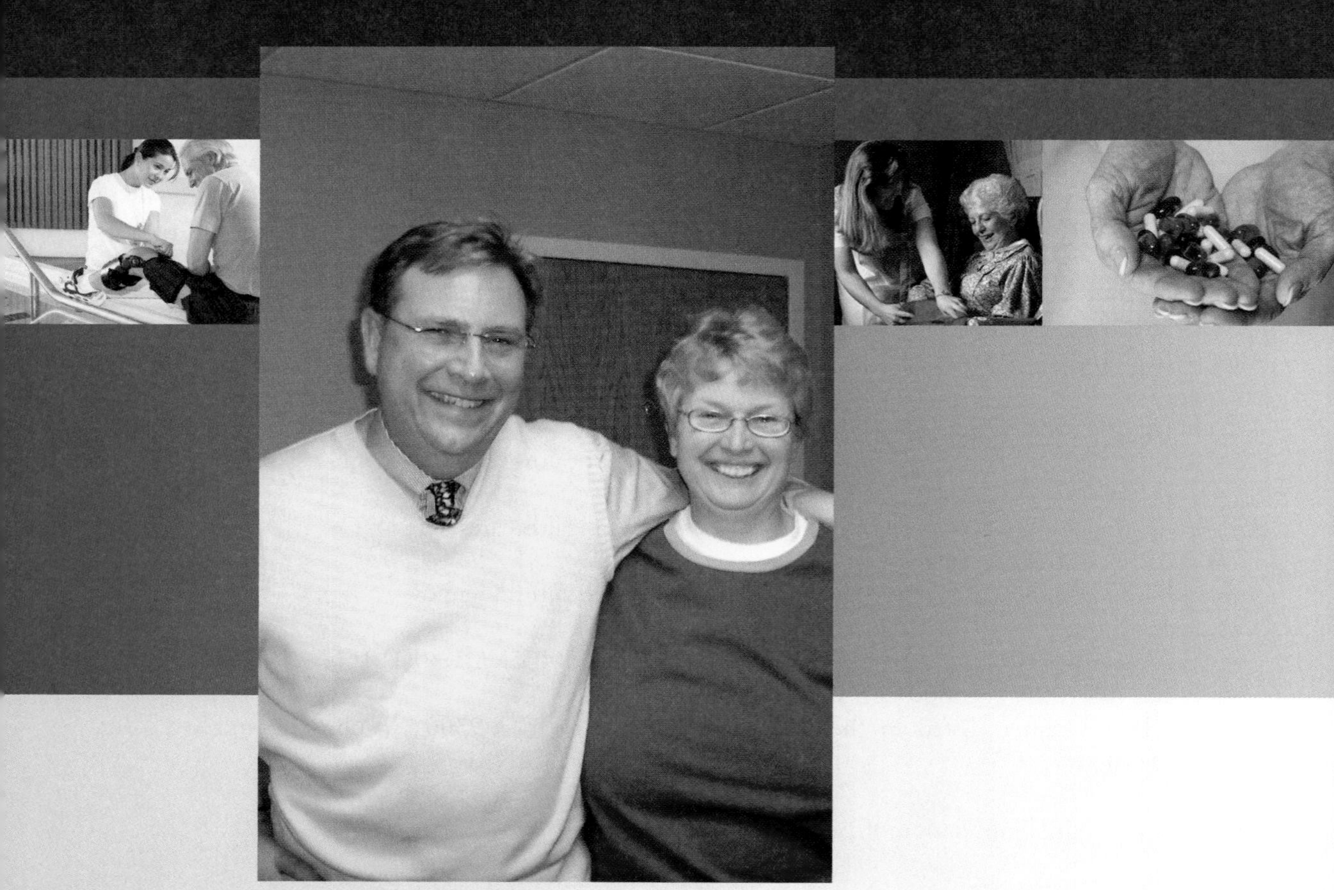

18 *Case Studies, 678*

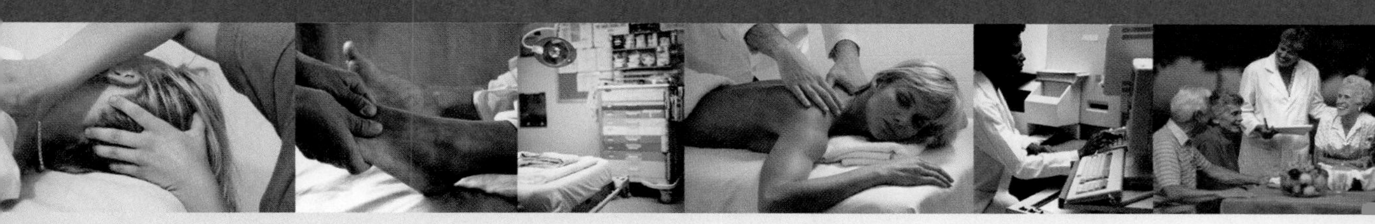

UNIT FOUR
CASE STUDIES

Most people learn best by example. This unit provides examples in case study format for the reader. Story-telling is an ancient teaching tradition. This unit combines the examples into the story-telling. The case studies presented in this unit are fictional, but they are based on Sandy Fritz's professional experiences. Each has been constructed to present a real-world scenario that demonstrates how the content in Units One, Two, and Three blends together to address massage application in the healthcare setting. Each case involves multiple health concerns that need to be considered for appropriate massage application. Although it is necessary to understand individual diseases, medication, and other treatments, massage in a recipe (i.e., this is how massage is delivered for multiple sclerosis) is just not possible. These cases present a platform for understanding how to use clinical reasoning skills to solve the various problems presented in each case.

It is possible to write hundreds of these cases with no two being the same. It is also impossible to do that in a book that has a limited number of pages. Careful study of how the cases presented are analyses using a clinical reasoning approach and a standard SOAP documentation format should help the reader grasp the process. Those who are preparing to offer massage at this advanced level will be required to move beyond recipes for massage and modality application. It is time to practice and master the concept of massage-based outcomes based on each and every unique situation.

Chapter 18 Concept Map

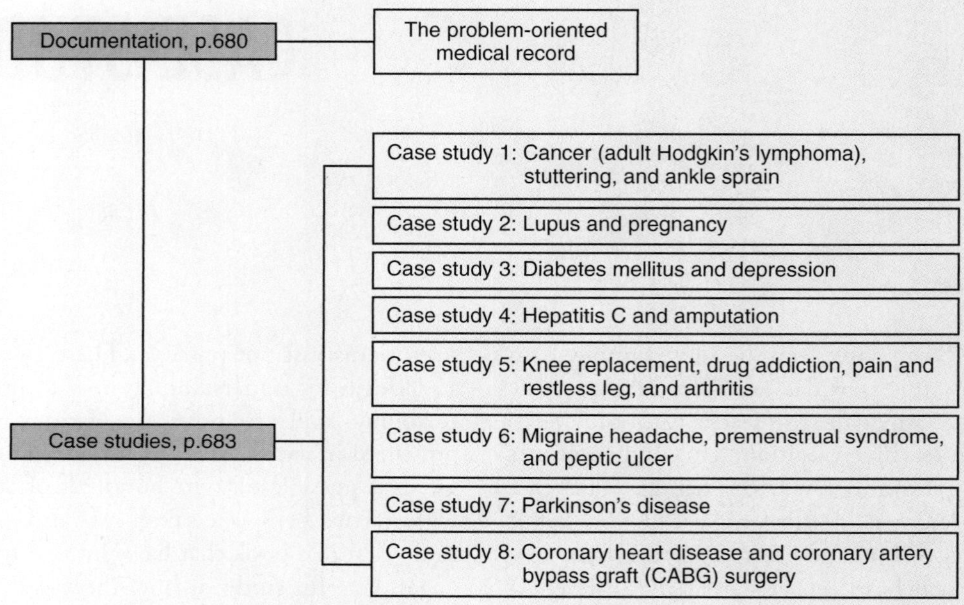

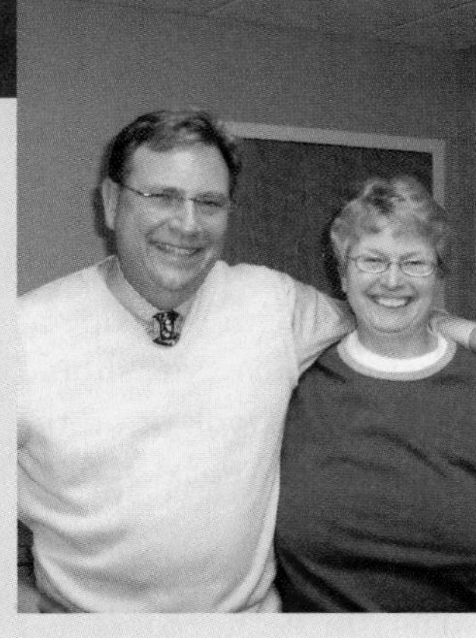

CHAPTER 18

CASE STUDIES

OBJECTIVES

Upon completion of this chapter, the reader will have the information necessary to:

1. Identify documentation styles.
2. Interpret general information on healthcare conditions relevant to massage benefits and contraindications.
3. Apply textbook content to case studies.
4. Generalize case study examples to similar healthcare conditions.
5. Write case studies.

This textbook, DVD, and the Evolve website have covered a tremendous amount of information and have taught you how to research and clinically reason to expand upon this content base. Years of teaching have shown that students struggle with the practical application of material, no matter how well it is presented. The design of the text helps the reader integrate and apply the content so as to be able to use massage effectively in each individual interaction between the patient or patient and the massage therapist.

However, as a teacher, I know this is not enough. Students routinely ask, "What do I do with a patient I'm working with who has . . ." Fill in the blank with just about any collection of conditions from a pathology text. After years of telling students to figure it out and come back to me with a plan, I realized that they needed a model or sample to follow. This unit consists of 12 such samples, or case studies. Each has been carefully designed to target common conditions presented to the massage therapist in the healthcare setting. In addition, each case describes related concerns, conditions, and complicating factors, so that the reader will come to understand that each situation is unique and requires an individualized treatment plan. The cases also reflect a category of care effectively addressed with massage, such as pain management, stress management, breathing normalization, increased mobility, and enhanced physical function. By studying each case, the student can use the model presented to help develop care plans for many different healthcare conditions.

To make this easier to understand, a standard format is provided for each case, as follows:

Title: The primary conditions to be addressed.

Similar conditions: A list of additional common conditions in which a similar massage approach is possible.

The case: A comprehensive narrative about the patient.

Research: A brief factual description of the conditions involved in the case.

Medical assessment, diagnosis, and treatment orders: A summary of the assessment, diagnosis, and treatment orders from the medical team.

Massage-specific assessment: The relevant history and physical assessment pertinent to medical treatment orders.

Clinical reasoning process: A recap of factual data; the development of treatment possibilities; analysis of treatment options; and decisions and justifications for the treatment plan.

Treatment plan development: The actual treatment plan.

SOAP charting: Five sessions are charted based on the treatment plan implemented. The charting process uses the problem-oriented medical record (POMR) approach, as exemplified in a standard charting format: subjective, objective, assessment, plan (SOAP).

If some change in a condition occurs or if some other complicating issue arises that would influence the course of the massage, it is described as a Note. These notes would not be included in the actual chart.

Evaluation of progress: A summary of the results of the massage that covers the massage-specific assessment and the five massage therapy sessions.

Recommendations for future massage care: Recommendations for a revised treatment plan based on the response to the massage.

Perspective of the massage therapist: A hypothetical discussion about what it might be like for the massage therapist to be involved in the care of this patient.

The reader will soon realize that much of the material is repeated throughout the various case studies. This happens because massage application is very similar from session to session, and the treatment plans for many different healthcare conditions are also similar, based on the general protocol and the modified palliative protocol presented in this textbook. The nuances and subtle adjustments made on a session-by-session basis reflect the skill and expertise of the massage therapist.

Any of the information in the case study that is based on material described in the text or on the Evolve Web site is cross-referenced to that specific content. For example, if the massage therapist in the case study is dealing with a preoperative and postoperative situation, the reader should review that information in the textbook or on the Evolve site. The actual procedure is not described or charted in the case.

The ability to develop justifiable treatment plans and to maintain quality medical records that document the massage intervention is necessary for continuity of healthcare, communication among healthcare professionals, and healthcare insurance authorization and reimbursement. These case studies demonstrate how treatment plans and charting might be completed and the developmental process behind the actual written documents.

The intent of this structure is that the reader will follow a case from the beginning through the re-evaluation process.

DOCUMENTATION

A number of different approaches can be used for charting and documentation.

THE PROBLEM-ORIENTED MEDICAL RECORD

The problem-oriented medical record (POMR) focuses on specific patient problems. It originally was developed by doctors and later adapted by nurses. The POMR is most effective in acute care or long-term care and home care settings.

The SOAP Format

To use the SOAP format in POMR charting, document the following information for each problem:

Subjective data: Information the patient, family members, or healthcare professionals tell you, such as the chief complaint and other impressions.

Objective data: Factual, measurable data gathered during assessment, such as observed signs and symptoms, vital signs, laboratory test values, and interventions used.

Assessment (analysis) data: Conclusions based on the collected subjective and objective data and formulated as patient problems or nursing diagnoses. This dynamic, ongoing process changes as more or different subjective and objective information becomes known. This area includes analysis of the effectiveness of the interventions used.

Plan: Your strategy for addressing the patient's problem. This plan should include both immediate or short-term actions and long-term measures.

The SOAPIE Method

A modification of the SOAP format, the SOAPIE method adds two elements: intervention and evaluation. This content was moved out of the objective area into its own sections.

Intervention: Measures taken to achieve an expected outcome. As the patient's health status changes, it may be necessary to modify the intervention plan. Be sure to document the patient's understanding and acceptance of the initial plan in this section of the notes.

Evaluation: An analysis of the effectiveness of your interventions. This content was moved out of the assessment section.

The SOAPIER Method

The SOAPIER format adds a revision section to allow documentation of alternative interventions. If the patient's outcomes fall short of expectations, use the evaluation process from SOAPIE as a basis for developing revised interventions, then document these changes.

Revision: Document any changes from the original plan of care in this section. Interventions, outcomes, or target dates may need to be adjusted to attain a previous goal.

The problem-oriented medical record style with SOAP note charting was chosen as the documentation process for this text for a variety of reasons:

- It is the style most massage textbooks present, therefore the reader is familiar with this method.
- This approach is used in many different medical settings, as well as in multidisciplinary settings.
- The method is easy to adapt to other record-keeping methods.
- It supports the clinical reasoning model.
- It organizes the information in a method that is easy to follow through multiple sessions.
- which supports the goals of this segment of the textbook.
- It provides the structure to organize data for easy conversion to electronic record keeping.

> **evolve 18-1**
>
> Four additional case studies are located on the Evolve site.

CASE STUDIES

CASE STUDY 1: CANCER (ADULT HODGKIN'S LYMPHOMA), STUTTERING, AND ANKLE SPRAIN

Similar Conditions

All types of cancer. If surgery is an aspect of treatment, preoperative and postoperative massage protocols are appropriate.

Additional Conditions

Stuttering, ankle sprain
Look for the S (SOAP) for this case.

The Case

Tara, a 26-year-old female, has been diagnosed with Hodgkin's disease. Cancer cells were found in lymph node groups on both sides of the diaphragm. She is midway though treatment that involves a combination of chemotherapy and radiation therapy.

Tara is an active preschool teacher. She is single and in a committed relationship. She enjoys outdoor activities such as hiking and biking but is not an avid exerciser. Since childhood, Tara has been interested in natural healing. This interest was fostered during summers on her great grandmother's farm (GG for great grandmother). She enjoyed working in the garden with GG and learning about natural healing with herbs. Her GG died at home in her sleep at age 95.

During a routine physical, the doctor noticed some swelling in the lymph nodes, and during the medical history, Tara indicated that she had been increasingly tired and was sweating at night. She was also itchy. Because the symptoms were vague and could be attributed to logical causes, she never considered that she was ill. The diagnosis of Hodgkin's disease was a shock, but after a few days, she pulled herself together after she had a dream about walking with GG at the farm and feeling comforted.

It was a big decision for her to use conventional treatment when she was diagnosed with Hodgkin's disease. Tara is a self-teacher, and she researched various treatment protocols before deciding that focused treatment with chemotherapy and radiation gave her the best chance for a cure. Tara also used some alternative methods, such as acupuncture, which was supported by the oncologist. She wants to include massage in her self-care program.

Tara has a strong support system of family and friends and strong spiritual beliefs. Her prognosis is very good. She is strong willed, determined to live a long and productive life, and views the development of cancer as a life experience that will provide a deep understanding of issues of life and death and the importance of determining priorities.

Although she is from a stable family, not everything has been easy for Tara. She has a tendency to stutter when stressed and was the object of teasing during grade school. She became very withdrawn during adolescence and did not have many close friends. Tara received speech therapy, which helped, but she still stutters if excited or stressed. Her GG introduced her to an old gentleman who stuttered severely, but he could sing beautifully, so he sang all the time. Between this mentor and her GG, she became determined to rise above this difficulty. Tara noticed that small children were accepting of her and that she had a talent for working with them. She volunteered often to care for children, and after high school graduation she furthered her education in early childhood education. Her dream is to have her own preschool.

ADULT HODGKIN'S LYMPHOMA

Adult Hodgkin's lymphoma is a type of cancer that develops in the lymph system, part of the body's immune system. Age, gender, and Epstein-Barr infection can affect the risk of developing adult Hodgkin's lymphoma.

Risk Factors. Risk factors for Hodgkin's lymphoma include the following:

- Being a young adult
- Being male
- Being infected with the Epstein-Barr virus
- Having a close relative (parent, brother, or sister) with Hodgkin's lymphoma

Symptoms. Possible signs of adult Hodgkin's lymphoma include the following:

- Swollen lymph nodes
- Fever
- Night sweats
- Itchy skin
- Fatigue
- Weight loss

Diagnosis. Diagnostic tests and procedures include the following:

- Complete medical history
- Physical examination (an examination of the body to check general signs of health, including signs of disease, such as lumps)

- ***Massage implications:*** Any swollen lymph nodes or any other tissue changes or growths need to be identified and avoided during the massage; treat as a regional contraindication.

- Complete blood workup
- Lymph node biopsy
  - Excisional biopsy (removal of an entire lymph node)
  - Incisional biopsy or core biopsy (removal of part of a lymph node)
  - Needle biopsy, or fine-needle aspiration (removal of a sample of tissue from a lymph node with a needle)

- ***Massage implications:*** Use preoperative and postoperative massage methods around the site of the biopsy.

- Immunophenotyping (a test in which the cells in a sample of blood or bone marrow are examined under a microscope to determine whether malignant lymphocytes (cancer) began from the B lymphocytes or the T lymphocytes)

Treatment and Prognosis. The treatment options and the prognosis for adult Hodgkin's lymphoma depend on the following:

- The patient's symptoms
- The stage of the cancer
- The type of Hodgkin's lymphoma
- Blood test results
- The patient's age, gender, and general health
- Whether the cancer is recurrent or progressive

Adult Hodgkin's lymphoma usually can be cured if detected and treated early. Three types of standard treatment are used: chemotherapy, radiation therapy, and surgery.

Laparotomy is a procedure often used for diagnosis. In this situation, an incision is made in the wall of the abdomen to check the inside of the abdomen for signs of disease. The size of the incision depends on the reason for the laparotomy. Sometimes organs are removed or tissue samples are taken for biopsy. If cancer is found, the tissue or organ is removed during the laparotomy.

Radiation Therapy. A treatment undergoing testing in clinical trials involves high-dose chemotherapy and radiation therapy with stem cell transplantation, a method of giving high doses of chemotherapy and radiation therapy and replacing blood-forming cells destroyed by the cancer treatment. Stem cells (immature blood cells) are removed from the blood or bone marrow of the patient or a donor and are frozen and stored. After therapy is completed, the stored stem cells are thawed and given back to the patient through an infusion. These reinfused stem cells grow into (and restore) the body's blood cells.

- ***Massage implications:*** Massage is used to manage the side effects of treatment and support the natural healing mechanism. Any surgical treatment for cancer would respond to the general approaches for preoperative and postoperative massage application.

Side Effects. Radiation to the chest area causes some swelling in the esophagus. The radiation irritates this area, and a patient may experience it as heartburn or a lump in the throat or chest. This can be controlled by avoiding extremes in temperature of food and liquids and by ingesting only lukewarm beverages and food. It is helpful to chew food extremely well to ease discomfort during swallowing. Patients generally are told to avoid alcohol and spicy foods, both of which can irritate the esophagus. Liquid antacids may be recommended.

Increased coughing and mucus production in the chest and throat are caused by irritation of the trachea and bronchi. Medication is available to alleviate these symptoms.

- ***Massage implications:*** The patient's position during massage may increase or decrease discomfort. Experiment with the supine, prone, side-lying, and seated positions to identify the one most comfortable for the patient.

The most common side effect of radiation treatment is an overall feeling of fatigue, likely caused by passage from the body of cellular debris from tissue breakdown. This response is not related to worsening of the cancer; it is a side effect of the radiation that resolves within 2 to 3 weeks after completion of radiation therapy.

- ***Massage implications:*** Massage is effective in supporting restorative sleep and helping the body eliminate toxins. Careful use of lymphatic drainage methods, incorporated into the palliative care massage protocol, is appropriate. Do not overmassage. Shorter, more frequent massage sessions are best; every other day is ideal.

Another side effect that must be carefully monitored are changes in the bone marrow cells. These cells reproduce very rapidly and are extremely sensitive to radiation. The treatment may depress the marrow's ability to function normally. As a result, the white and red blood cells and platelets, which are formed in the marrow, may not be released into the bloodstream in adequate amounts. Except for increased susceptibility to infection, no specific symptoms usually accompany a low white cell count. Typically, a lowered red blood cell count causes dizziness and fatigue. Very low platelet counts cause areas of hemorrhage, usually first noted on the skin, appearing as blotchy, bruised spots. In some cases it may be necessary to discontinue radiation treatment temporarily to allow the blood count to return to a normal range. This is particularly true when radiation treatment is combined with chemotherapy, because chemotherapeutic agents may significantly lower the white blood cell count. Patients who have undergone chemotherapy may already have a lowered white blood count before they begin radiation treatments. Radiation oncologists are aware of this situation when they plan treatment.

- ***Massage implication:*** Monitor pressure levels and use only broad-based, compressive force to prevent bruising. Do not use pinpoint compression. Maintain infection control and do not work with an immune-suppressed individual if the patient has a contagious condition such as an upper respiratory disorder or intestinal infection. Also, be aware of any parasitic or fungal infection (e.g., scabies or ringworm) that could be transmitted to the patient. Stay with the patient as the individual gets up from the massage table, in case the patient is dizzy.

Common physical side effects of chemotherapy include the following:

- Nausea
- Hair loss
- Loss of appetite
- Fatigue or anemia
- Infection
- Blood clotting problems
- Mouth, gum, and throat problems
- Diarrhea
- Constipation
- Nerve and muscle effects
- Skin and nail changes
- Kidney and bladder effects
- Fluid retention
- Tooth decay
- Sexual/reproductive changes

Nausea/vomiting: People who experience the side effects of nausea or vomiting can feel a bit nauseous most of the time or very nauseous only part of the time. Nausea frequently begins a few hours after a chemotherapy treatment, and some people may feel nauseated for a day or two. In addition, some people experience anticipatory nausea, in which they begin to vomit before the treatment actually begins. Many people fear they will experience uncontrolled vomiting after receiving chemotherapy, but this side effect can almost always be controlled. A number of medications (antiemetics) can control or diminish nausea. These drugs usually are administered before chemotherapy begins so that the medication has time to take effect.

The patient should avoid eating large meals and try sipping small amounts of soup, juice, or carbonated drinks that are neither too hot nor too cold. Not eating before chemotherapy does not prevent vomiting; fasting is not recommended, because it interferes with good nutrition. Prevent dehydration during bouts of nausea by drinking small amounts of clear, cool beverages about every 15 minutes. After eating, the patient should sit up in a chair rather than lie down and should avoid sudden changes in position that can cause something akin to motion sickness. Be prepared with buckets, towels, and washable linens in case of unexpected vomiting. The patient should get plenty of rest. Relaxation techniques, such as deep breathing exercises, distraction, fresh air, and exercise, can help many people stave off nausea.

- ***Massage implications:*** Be prepared for unexpected vomiting and have receptacles and moist towels or wipes available. Do not move the patient abruptly or rock or shake the upper body, which can cause inner ear disturbances. The person may be more comfortable in a seated or side-lying position. Massage should support relaxation.

Hair loss: *Alopecia,* or sudden hair loss, happens to many people undergoing chemotherapy. Hair loss affects both men and women. It is the most visible side effect of chemotherapy, and although it is not physically painful, it can be emotionally traumatic. With some anticancer drugs, hair loss is almost a certainty; with others, it may or may not occur. The extent of hair loss depends on the person and the anticancer drug or drugs taken. Facial hair, underarm hair, and pubic hair may be lost. Hair loss typically begins within three or four chemotherapy treatments. Fortunately, hair almost always grows back after the treatments are completed. Wigs are available for both men and women. Local offices of the American Cancer Society sometimes have "loan closet" programs that loan wigs to cancer patients who cannot afford to buy them.

- ***Massage implications:*** Ask the patient if he or she is wearing a wig. If so, be careful not to disturb it during the massage if the person decides not to remove it. Be sensitive about hair loss when massaging the head, and do not aggressively pull the hair. If the person has lost all hair, treat this in a matter of fact way and gently massage the scalp if it is comforting.

Loss of appetite: *Anorexia,* or loss of appetite, is fairly common for people fighting cancer because of physical as well as emotional stresses. Beware of protein or carbohydrate malnutrition. Taste alterations in many foods can also occur as a result of the effects of chemotherapy. The taste alterations are different in each individual but can affect the appetite. Some anticancer agents dry the lining of the mouth, making eating or swallowing difficult. Antinausea drugs also can cause dry mouth, which usually disappears once the medication is discontinued. Some cancer treatments cause zinc deficiency, but this may be remedied by supplementation with zinc. Nutritional supplements such as Ensure pack a lot of calories into an easy-to-digest liquid form. A number of brands and flavors of these supplements are available.

- ***Massage implications:*** Appetite may increase as a secondary response to the relaxation effects of massage.

Fatigue or anemia: Bone marrow suppression is a common side effect of some chemotherapeutic drugs. It affects the body's ability to manufacture new red blood cells, and it can make the person feel tired and fatigued almost all the time. A shortage of red blood cells means the body gets less oxygen than normal. Other symptoms may include dizziness, shortness of breath, or feeling chilled. Pale skin and muscle weakness can be aspects of anemia. Dehydration, lack of sleep, and poor quality sleep are other factors that may contribute to fatigue. The doctor may order a blood transfusion if red blood cell levels drop too low. Stress, worry, and anxiety are among the psychosocial factors that can be a significant cause of fatigue.

- ***Massage implications:*** Massage is very effective in reducing the physical manifestations of emotional stress and supporting restorative sleep. Include aspects of massage to maintain normal breathing and support sleep in the palliative care protocol. Keep the patient warm.

Infection: Bone marrow suppression also affects the production of white blood cells, which are an important component of the body's immune system. Chills, fever, sweating, diarrhea, and redness or swelling may be signs of infection. Another sign is an increased tendency to bruise. Fourteen days after treatment, the white blood cell levels usually fall to their lowest point; this is when the possibility of infection is highest. Bladder infections and other urinary tract problems can occur with chemotherapy, particularly if the individual has nausea and vomiting or other symptoms that reduce urine output. The symptoms of urinary tract infections include frequent or urgent urination, a burning sensation when urinating, off-color or bloody urine, fever, chills and fatigue, and low back or flank pain.

- ***Massage implications:*** Maintain infection control and do not work with an immune-suppressed individual if you have a contagious condition such as an upper respiratory condition or intestinal infection. Also, be aware of any parasitic or fungal infection (e.g., scabies or ringworm) that could be transmitted to the patient. Massage during an infection should be the palliative type or should be avoided completely if the person is feverish and lethargic.

Blood clotting problems: Bone marrow suppression affects the body's ability to manufacture the platelets that help blood clot; as a result, the person may bleed or bruise more easily than normal.

- ***Massage implications:*** Monitor pressure levels and maintain a broad-based, compressive force. Do not use methods that may cause tissue damage, such as direct pressure, friction, and some forms of connective tissue applications.

Mouth, gum, and throat problems: Sores in the mouth, or *stomatitis,* increase the possibility of infection from germs that live in the mouth. The tissues of the mouth and throat may become irritated, may bleed, or may become unusually dry.

The patient may have trouble swallowing or may have problems with cold sores (i.e., herpes simplex). Some people also develop a yeast infection called *thrush,* which appears as small white patches on the gums or inside of the cheeks. Inflammation or mouth pain can greatly inhibit normal eating or drinking. Mouth sores typically last 3 to 8 days, although they may affect the appetite longer. Antifungal medication controls thrush. Many yeast infections respond to lozenges or throat drops that contain clotrimazole or to mouth rinses containing Mycostatin. Acyclovir can be prescribed to prevent the recurrence of herpes simplex. Kaopectate, milk of magnesia, or other liquid drugs sometimes are recommended to reduce pain because they coat the sores and protect them from the saliva. A combination of medications may be necessary to achieve control in the most severe cases. A diet with adequate vitamins, minerals, and protein can speed the healing of mucous membranes.

- ***Massage implications:*** It may be painful for the person to speak or to be in the prone position.

Diarrhea: Chemotherapy can cause loose bowels, because the cells in the intestinal tract are vulnerable to the effects of anticancer drugs, and the body's natural response is to try to rid itself quickly of damaged cells. Diarrhea dehydrates the body; this may interfere with the elimination of waste products through the urine if the diarrhea continues for long periods, because of the body's natural tendency to conserve limited water. Diarrhea sometimes is accompanied by vomiting, and electrolyte imbalances can occur. Diarrhea can be caused by emotional stress, lactose intolerance, chemotherapy and radiation treatments directed to the abdominal region, fecal impactions, and other factors, including the use of antibiotics and sensitivities to certain foods. Diarrhea may occur a week or so after a chemotherapy treatment.

Fluid intake is important, and the patient should continually drink small amounts of water, fruit juice, soup, or even drinks such as Gatorade, a product formulated for athletes to replace lost electrolytes. The so-called BRAT diet (bananas, rice, applesauce, and weak herb tea) can be easily digested and is used by many hospitals to control diarrhea. Foods that may aggravate the bowels should be avoided, such as milk products; raw fruits and vegetables; spicy, greasy foods; and coffee and tea. Foods that are high in potassium and do not cause diarrhea include bananas, peach and apricot nectar, and boiled or mashed potatoes.

- ***Massage implications:*** Do not aggressively massage the abdomen and remember to offer the restroom. Use Standard Precautions for clean up if an accident occurs.

Constipation: Some anticancer drugs and painkilling medications can cause constipation, as can inactivity or poor diet. For example, some drugs used in chemotherapy (e.g., vincristine and vinblastine) and other symptom management drugs (e.g., narcotics and tranquilizers) can slow the normal movement of the bowels. Emotional stress can be a factor, as can lack of normal eating or drinking because of nausea or fatigue. The doctor may prescribe laxatives and stool softeners, some of which are as natural as olive oil. Regular, moderate exercise helps many people relieve this problem.

- ***Massage implications:*** Direct massage of the colon may increase peristalsis and soften the fecal matter a bit, making elimination easier.

Nerve and muscle effects: In some people, some chemotherapeutic drugs (e.g., platinum-based drugs or paclitaxel) produce side effects that affect the nervous system or the muscles. The hands or feet tingle, feel numb or weak, or even burn; this is neuropathic pain, or neuropathy. Sometimes even a very light touch can trigger nerve pain. The patient may experience a loss of balance and have trouble with motor coordination. Sometimes the muscles can feel tired or weak or sore. Pain in the jaw or stomach and hearing loss also can be symptoms. Some forms of exercise can help neuropathy, perhaps because they increase the flow of blood to the site. Simply squeezing little rubber balls or stimulating the skin on the feet by rolling golf balls under the balls of the feet might be helpful.

- ***Massage implications:*** Carefully monitor the person's response to the massage. Avoid light skin stroking during the massage. Monitor for balance issues and stay with the person as he or she gets on and off the massage table if the person is prone to problems with motor coordination. General massage with moderate, pleasurable pressure typically helps reduce symptoms for a short time.

Skin and nail changes: Chemotherapy may cause minor skin problems such as rashes, redness, acne, itching, peeling, or even a "dry look" or dry-feeling skin. *Pruritus,* an intense itching of the skin, can be caused by dehydration or by some drugs used in chemotherapy. Some chemotherapeutic drugs and radiation therapy treatments may actually cause changes in the appearance of the skin and occasionally may cause the skin to darken. Most chemotherapy makes the skin unusually sensitive to the effects of the sun. Because fingernails are just hardened skin cells, the fingernails may become more brittle than usual or change color or appearance.

- ***Massage implications:*** Use only the recommended lubricants for massage and make sure to use enough lubricant to reduce drag on the skin. Massage may increase or reduce the itching, therefore this needs to be monitored on a case-by-case basis.

Kidney and bladder effects: Some drugs used in chemotherapy can cause temporary or permanent damage to the kidneys or can irritate the bladder. A few anticancer drugs can turn the urine orange, red, or yellow or give it a medicinal smell. In men, the appearance or color of the semen may also change.

- ***Massage implications:*** Make sure the patient has easy access to the restroom and offer the restroom periodically during the massage.

Fluid retention: Some drugs used in chemotherapy, particularly the hormones (e.g., prednisone), may cause the body to retain fluid.

- ***Massage implications:*** Careful, judicious use of lymphatic drainage methods as part of the general massage may help with fluid retention. Do not overtreat. More frequent massages of shorter duration are indicated.

Tooth decay: Some chemotherapeutic drugs leave the patient vulnerable to tooth decay and to gum or periodontal infections.

- ***Massage implications:*** No direct concerns.

Sexual and reproductive problems: A person's sexual urges and desires and even the sexual organs themselves may be affected by chemotherapy. Age, general health, and the type and length of chemotherapy are factors that affect the severity of side effects. Men may experience infertility, lowered sperm counts, and other reactions. Women may find their ability to produce some hormones diminished, or the ovaries may be damaged, resulting in irregular or halted menstrual periods. Women can experience a "false menopause," with symptoms such as hot flashes, itching, and discomfort or dryness of the vagina that can make intercourse painful and leave them vulnerable to vaginal infections. Painkilling narcotics can inhibit sexual desire. Emotional stress and powerful emotions (e.g., anger, anxiety, and depression) also greatly affect sexual desire in most people, and powerful emotions may be felt not only by the person receiving chemotherapy but by the partner as well.

Many people may find sexual issues difficult to discuss, and some changes in perception and attitude may be necessary to maintain a healthy sexual relationship. Professional counseling often can be quite helpful. Most people can live without sex more easily than they can live without love. Some individuals may wish to be touched and held more frequently.

- ***Massage implications:*** Provide compassionate, nurturing massage and monitor for boundary issues, especially if the person's support system is compromised. When this is the case, the massage therapist may be the only one providing pleasurable touch. Because palliation is an important aspect of massage, it is necessary to appreciate the dynamics of transference and countertransference in the therapeutic relationship when the patient is especially vulnerable.

STUTTERING

Stuttering is commonly thought to be a speech disorder. However, it actually is an extremely complex condition that involves much more than repetitions of sounds, prolongations of syllables, and other "dysfluencies." Because stuttering affects the person as a whole, it can more adequately be described as a combination of speech, communication, and behavioral disorders. About 1% of the adult population stutters. Men account for 80% of all adults who stutter. People who stutter tend to tighten the muscles of the vocal cords when reacting to stress; this is the reason stuttering becomes worse when the person is under pressure.

People who stutter often resort to word replacement to avoid stuttering. If a person feels that he will stutter on a particular word, he often tries to find an alternative word with a similar meaning. Some people who stutter are so successful at this technique that no one realizes the difficulty. People who stutter usually do not stutter when they sing, speak in unison, whisper, talk to a pet, or speak to a small child. People who stutter tend to avoid eye contact with their listeners. They often have irregular breathing patterns and try to speak with little or no air in the lungs.

In addition to these unusual communication patterns and behaviors, many people who stutter have negative feelings and perceptions about their stuttering and about themselves, such as:

- Shame: People who stutter often are ashamed of their stuttering and go to great lengths to try to hide it.
- Guilt: People who stutter often feel guilty about not being able to achieve what they think they would be able to achieve if only they could speak fluently.
- Frustration: People who stutter often feel frustrated by their inability to communicate effectively with other people.
- Low self-esteem: Stuttering often induces a feeling of worthlessness.

All these hidden elements of the stuttering phenomenon tend to reinforce the speech disorders, and speech therapy that focuses only on the speech mechanism is bound to fail. Holistic and comprehensive stuttering therapy is necessary to address all aspects of the phenomenon.

Talking to People Who Stutter

Use the following guidelines in talking to patients who stutter:

- Do not try to finish sentences, fill in words, or interrupt.
- Avoid suggestions such as, "Slow down," "Relax," or "Take a breath." If these suggestions worked, the person would not stutter.
- Do not criticize or correct the person's speech.
- Wait patiently until the person finishes speaking. Maintain eye contact and try not to look embarrassed or alarmed.
- Talk about stuttering openly. It should not be a taboo subject. The person's friend or family member will appreciate your interest in the subject.
- Do not be afraid to say, "I'm sorry, I didn't understand what you said."
- Talk to the person who stutters in a relaxed, normal manner.

Medical Assessment, Diagnosis, and Treatment Orders

Diagnosis: Hodgkin's disease, stage IIIB

Treatment for six cycles of COPP and ABV chemotherapy, followed by radiation therapy.

Placement of a port.

Support care as needed for treatment side effects.

Patient approved for acupuncture for nausea and fatigue and massage for stress management, pain management, sleep support to combat fatigue, nausea, constipation, and fluid retention management at the cancer treatment center. Referral to clinic-based support group.

NOTE: The alternative and complementary therapies department at the cancer treatment center is supervised by a nurse practitioner who is also a massage therapist. A variety of schedules and techniques are used to deliver chemotherapy. Cancer chemotherapy may consist of a single drug or combinations of drugs that are delivered in cycles. A cycle consists of treatment with one or more drugs, followed by a period of rest.

Chemotherapeutic drugs can be administered orally (as a pill) or injected intravenously (into a vein), intramuscularly (into a muscle), intrathecally (into the spinal fluid), or into a body cavity (e.g., the bladder). Currently most chemotherapy is administered intravenously (IV); however, oral chemotherapeutic drugs are gaining wider use. In some cases it may be beneficial to administer IV chemotherapy through a venous access device (VAD), a device that is surgically implanted in a major vein to provide long-term access. Not every chemotherapy patient requires a VAD. However, for those undergoing frequent treatment, blood tests, and nutritional support, use of a VAD reduces the number of needle sticks and associated discomfort.

Several different types of VADs are available, but the two most commonly used for cancer treatment and for taking blood samples are the tunneled external catheter (Hickman catheter) and the subcutaneous implanted port (Port-A-Cath). With the Hickman catheter, the plastic tube, or catheter, exits the body, allowing external access. The Port-A-Cath is implanted completely beneath the skin in a major vein under the collarbone. The port is accessed by insertion of a special needle through the skin to deliver chemotherapy, hydration, and transfusions and to take blood samples.

For most types of cancer, radiation therapy usually is given 5 days a week for 6 or 7 weeks. (When radiation is used for palliative care, the course of treatment is shorter, usually 2 to 3 weeks.) The total dose of radiation and the number of treatments needed depend on the size, location, and kind of cancer; the person's general health; and other medical treatments being given. Administering many small doses of daily radiation rather than a few large doses helps protect normal body tissues in the treatment area. Weekend rest breaks allow normal cells to recover.

NOTE: Tara will receive chemotherapy in six 4-week cycles. Intravenous chemotherapy will be administered on Tuesdays. The first week of every cycle she will receive COPP; this is a combination of two IV chemotherapeutic drugs, one oral drug, and prednisone. The oral drug (procarbazine) is taken once a day for a week. Procarbazine has food precautions that may cause internal bleeding or dizziness. Administration of the drugs given intravenously through the Port-A-Cath is quick and painless, except for mild side effects of tingling and constipation.

The second week of the 4-week cycle, Tara will receive ABV (i.e., Adriamycin, bleomycin, and vinblastine) and will continue the prednisone. ABV is administered intravenously through the Port-A-Cath. Unfortunately, these injections cause many unpleasant side effects, such as nausea, cramps, and tiredness.

During the third week, Tara's blood cell counts will be monitored. When they drop too low, Neupogen will be used to increase the cell count. Tara will receive precautionary antibiotics on weekends, and blood will be drawn weekly to check the blood cell counts.

Massage-Specific Assessment

History: The patient is 26 years old, single, and female. She is 5′5″ tall and weighs 132 lb. Before diagnosis, her health was generally good.

Past illnesses and injuries: Typical childhood illnesses; mononucleosis at 13 with a recurrence at 15 (NOTE: A possible contributing factor for the development of Hodgkin's disease); severe lateral left ankle sprain at 17; anxiety in response to stuttering.

Symptoms related to cancer: Fatigue, night sweats, itchy skin. The patient occasionally receives a massage at the local day spa, and she indicates that she enjoys firm pressure. She likes to be quiet during the massage and appreciates it if the massage therapist does not engage in casual conversation.

Response to treatment: (NOTE: The patient is beginning her sixth chemotherapy cycle, after which she will start radiation therapy.)

- Intermittent nausea with occasional vomiting
- Intermittent constipation
- Hair loss
- Fatigue
- Mouth sores
- Fluid retention
- General aching

The skin is dry, and prednisone-related fluid retention is noted. The patient shows an upper chest breathing pattern. The shoulders are rolled slightly forward, and upper anterior thorax connective tissue shortening and binding are seen. Upper trapezius–dominant firing of shoulder abduction is present, as are trigger points in the belly of the upper trapezius. Hypermobility of the left ankle is noted, along with synergistically dominant muscle activation firing of knee flexion and hip abduction on the left.

Clinical Reasoning Process

The massage treatment orders from the physician are for stress, pain, nausea, constipation, and fluid retention management. The stress management aspect would include addressing the upper chest breathing pattern and stimulation of the parasympathetic response. Pain management for aching would involve hyperstimulation analgesia, counterirritation, and stimulation of pain-modulating neurochemicals. The constipation can be addressed mechanically with colon massage, and the fluid retention with lymphatic drainage. None of the physician's outcomes conflict with reasonable expectations for massage benefit. Dealing with the upper chest breathing, including the trigger points, requires the most adaptive ability. Lymphatic drainage can temporarily address some of the fluid retention, which is a side effect of the prednisone, but it can strain the already compromised lymphatics and other detoxification systems of the body. Physical assessment also identified adaptation to the ankle hypermobility. This area typically would not be included directly in the goals of the massage; however, increased motor tone in the gastrocnemius and quadratus lumborum, as indicated in the muscle activation sequence assessment, can influence breathing function. It would be prudent to attempt to normalize these firing patterns if the patient has sufficient adaptive capacity to respond to the treatment. Also, the tendency to stutter involves the breathing function, and increased motor tone in the muscles of the neck relates to the breathing pattern, resulting in a tendency for sympathetic dominance and subsequent anxiety, which would increase the tendency to stutter, creating a nonproductive cycle.

Conversation with the supervising nurse practitioner indicates that the patient is responding well to treatment but tends to try to maintain normal daily and work activities. She therefore is more fatigued and strained than is indicated by conversation with her. The nurse practitioner says that massage should be primarily palliative, which would ultimately address the major goals. Inclusion of methods to normalize breathing would be prudent but should be limited to no more than 10 minutes of the massage. A similar concern exists with lymphatic drainage. The nurse practitioner recommends a generalized, full body approach to lymphatic drainage as part of the general massage, but the patient should be monitored for any adverse effects the next day, such as headache, increased fatigue, or nausea.

Although the area of the port is developing some connective tissue bind, it is best to leave it alone, because it will be removed after the last chemotherapy cycle, and the surgical area can then be treated with appropriate massage support to develop a mobile scar. The patient's blood counts have been somewhat low, but she has not had any worrisome infections. Maintaining infection control is essential, because the patient is immunosuppressed.

Based on the patient's response to treatment thus far, the nurse practitioner anticipates no significant concerns with the radiation treatment. When radiation begins, she will provide a special cream to use as a lubricant over the irradiated areas during the massage.

The patient has lost her hair but uses scarves and hats instead of a wig and is not embarrassed about the baldness. Her mouth is very sore, and using the face cradle during massage is painful.

The patient has resisted attending the support group meetings, and the nurse practitioner feels that this is an aspect of the social anxiety caused by the stuttering.

Treatment Plan Development

Long-term goals: Manage side effects of cancer treatment, normalize breathing function.

Short-term goals: Reduce general body aching and support restorative sleep.

Massage therapist's objectives: Support parasympathetic dominance and normalize breathing function.

Methods to be used: Palliative approach, lymphatic drainage, and breathing pattern support.

Frequency and duration: Two times a week for 45 to 60 minutes.

Measurement of progress: Self-reporting and evaluation by nurse practitioner for symptom management.

Date of reassessment: 4 weeks

SOAP Charting

Session 1

S: No noticeable changes since assessment and treatment plan development visit.

O: Patient appears pale and lethargic but in good spirits. Shoulders move during breathing, and she sighs often. Fluid retention is mild. Massage follows treatment plan protocol. No specific massage targeting breathing to monitor how much general massage may influence upper chest breathing pattern.

A: Breathing rhythm slowed and became more even, but upper trapezius remains active during inspiration. No measurable changes in fluid retention, which is expected with generalized fluid retention caused by medication use. Tara reports less aching, and she feels sleepy. She had no episodes of increased nausea or vomiting, and she was most comfortable in the side-lying position.

P: Evaluate the 24-hour response to massage, and compare reaction to chemotherapy with massage intervention to previous reaction without massage intervention. Assess breathing pattern and ask about quality of sleep.

Session 2

S: Tara reports that she is a bit nauseous and achy. Fatigue remains the same. She feels she slept better on Monday night and was less anxious when anticipating the chemotherapy treatment. She enjoyed the massage and did not notice any adverse reactions that she could attribute to massage. She did notice that the lotion used during the massage helped relieve the sensation of dry, itchy skin. She asks if more work could be done on her shoulders, especially on the left.

O: Patient appears pale, sluggish, and labored in her movements. She often takes a series of slow, deep breaths, and when questioned about this, she indicates that it is a method to control the nausea. Palpation and observation indicate that she is retaining more fluid than last session. Palpation of the left upper trapezius indicates that the trigger points in that area are more sensitive to moderate pressure. Massage follows treatment plan recommendations combined with positional release methods and kneading for direct tissue stretching of trigger point areas. Focus on lymphatic drainage was limited, with the bulk of the massage targeting neurochemical response and parasympathetic dominance.

A: Tara responded well to the trigger point treatment and reports that she feels less "knotted up." She prefers the deeper pressure. She is less sluggish and pale after the massage and reports that the nausea has diminished. Shoulder movement during breathing decreased by 50%.

P: Maintain treatment plan protocol. Assess response to trigger point treatment and maintain ongoing monitoring of breathing function.

Session 3

S: Tara reports that she feels good today, has been sleeping better, and is taking shorter naps during the day and still feels refreshed. She tripped this morning on a rug and thinks she sprained her left ankle. This was reported to the nurse practitioner, who authorized acute sprain massage treatment. She also noticed significant improvement in the shoulder tension.

O: Tara appears less pale and more alert. She is breathing deeper, and her shoulders do not move as much during inhalation. The sighing has decreased significantly. Palpation indicates that edema has diminished from moderate to slight. The left ankle is warm to the touch and moderately swollen and has been evaluated as a grade 1 lateral sprain. Muscle guarding in the area is evident. General massage protocol, palliative focus, moderately firm pressure, lymphatic drainage on the torso only, repetitive gliding toward the injured tissue in the area of the sprain. Maintained appropriate guarding response.

A: Tara fell asleep during the massage and was allowed to wake up on her own after the massage ended. She slept an additional 30 minutes. She reports she feels relaxed and can take a deep breath. Her ankle hurts, and the nurse said she should report to physical therapy after the massage for ice and wrapping. Tara's tissues palpate as more pliable and less taut.

P: Continue with treatment plan, assess ankle and, if appropriate, request permission to massage using subacute plan.

Session 4

S: Tara reports that her left ankle is very sore and bruised. She is not feeling well today—fatigued, nauseated, and aching. She would like a basic massage with good pressure.

O: Large bruise on left ankle with moderate swelling (likely due to reduced platelet count). Lymphatic drainage for local area requested by nurse. Tara appears ill, sluggish, and despondent. General palliative massage with no specific focus and lymphatic drainage for left ankle.

A: Patient dozed on and off during the massage. Wanted to go home and nap. Was not communicative. Swelling reduced in ankle by approximately 25%. Tara reported that it was less stiff.

P: Speak to supervising nurse about Tara's emotional status and potential for depression. Continue to implement treatment plan and monitor ankle.

Session 5

S: Tara reports that ankle is slowly getting better. Her low back aches. She is looking forward to finishing the chemotherapy and starting radiation. Her shoulder is tight, and she requests the positional release approach as part of the massage. She also indicates that she is getting tired of the whole "rollercoaster" and says that for every good day, she has a bunch of bad days.

O: Tara sighs excessively and rubs her shoulders. Upper chest breathing pattern is observed. Palpation indicates short muscles in the upper trapezius, lower lumbar area, and calves. General massage with local lymphatic drainage on the injured ankle, general lymphatic drainage, positional release, kneading to stretch trigger points in upper trapezius, and broad-based compression into the quadratus lumborum region.

A: Tara reports she feels better. She is moving with less hesitancy and is not rubbing her shoulders. Breathing is more rhythmic and slower.

P: Continue with treatment plan until chemotherapy cycle is completed, then re-evaluate based on response to radiation treatment.

Evaluation of Progress

Tara has responded well to the massage. The mood swings experienced are typical but should be monitored, because a tendency for depression is common with cancer treatment. Tara attended all scheduled massage sessions and enjoyed the experience. The ankle sprain seemed to be a setback, but it is hard to tell, because she is also at the end of the chemotherapy treatment cycle, which also strains the adaptive capacity. The supervising nurse practitioner reports that the fatigue and nausea are slightly diminished from the last chemotherapy cycle. The fluid retention was only slightly affected by massage. Tara is more physically active, is sleeping better, and is experiencing less general body aching, which is the most prominent benefit of massage.

Recommendations for Future Massage Care

The treatment plan should not change significantly as chemotherapy ends and radiation begins. The fluid retention should diminish as the medications change. Caution needs to be maintained for immunosuppression and skin irritation. The fatigue probably will increase, which might increase the aching, because the patient will be less active. Massage seems to effectively address the body aching caused by reduced activity. Pressure levels directly over radiation sites should be reduced.

Perspective of the Massage Therapist

Massage therapists often find it frustrating to hold themselves in check and provide only palliative massage when other conditions might respond to treatment. Tara responded best to general massage with firm, broad-based pressure. She did not like the lymphatic drainage methods, so it was difficult to follow doctor's orders when she did not want the methods done. Because she was best able to tolerate the skin drag on the torso, interspersed with compressive gliding, the massage therapist was able to successfully incorporate this aspect of treatment, even though it was disappointing that the results were only minor. Tara did not engage in general conversation, and it was easy to respect the need to be quiet. The stuttering at times made understanding Tara difficult, which was embarrassing for both. Tara's prognosis is good, so the massage therapist does not have to deal with a patient facing ongoing deterioration and eventually death.

CASE STUDY 2: LUPUS AND PREGNANCY

Similar Conditions

Most autoimmune diseases.

Additional Conditions

Pregnancy development of pre-eclampsia.

The Case

Angelina is a 32-year-old female who was diagnosed with systemic lupus erythematosus (SLE) at age 28. She had experienced multiple vague symptoms for years, and investigation of the reason for two miscarriages finally resulted in the lupus diagnosis. She experiences a cluster of symptoms that include fatigue, headache, joint pain, lower extremity edema, and a tendency to develop infections. Her condition is considered to be in the mild to moderate range. She is of multiracial heritage, and she knows of several family members who have lupus symptoms.

Angelina is married, and she and her husband very much want children. The miscarriages were devastating for them. Angelina experienced depression after both miscarriages, and it was unclear how much of the depression was related to the lupus, the hormonal changes, and the loss. She is now pregnant again.

Angelina has been undergoing treatment for SLE since the condition was diagnosed. She has been treated with corticosteroids, immunosuppressants, and nonsteroidal antiinflammatory drugs (NSAIDs). She also is interested in complementary care. She carefully watches her diet and maintains a healthy lifestyle, focusing on managing inflammation. This careful attention to her health is motivated by her desire to have a baby. She has been doing very well for about 12 months. Steroid treatment and immunosuppression therapy were reduced and then eliminated about 6 months ago in anticipation of her getting pregnant. She currently is 12 weeks pregnant, and the pregnancy is considered a high-risk one. Fortunately, Angelina has not had any kidney involvement with the lupus.

She is anxious as well as thrilled about being pregnant. Recently the anxiety has become more pronounced, resulting in sleep disturbance and moodiness. Her obstetrician, who specializes in high-risk pregnancies, has recommended that Angelina and her husband become involved in a support group composed of other couples dealing with a high-risk pregnancy. Because the doctor does not want to use antianxiety medication unless absolutely necessary, she has prescribed a program of meditation and massage for relaxation.

Angelina has left her job as a news producer at a local TV station so that she can put all her energy into a successful outcome for her pregnancy. Her husband, Mateo, works in a family construction business that offers a comprehensive medical insurance plan. He has his own multiple stressors, but he is committed to doing what is necessary to support his wife and baby.

Research

Lupus is a complex disease, and its cause is unknown. Genetic, environmental, and possibly hormonal factors all may be involved in causing lupus. Because lupus can run in families, it likely has a genetic basis. Recent research suggests that genetics plays an important role in this disease, but as yet no specific "lupus gene" has been identified. Studies suggest that several different genes may be involved in determining a person's likelihood of developing lupus, which tissues and organs are affected, and the severity of the disease. However, scientists believe that genes are not the single determinant and that other factors also play a role. Some of these other factors that are under study are sunlight, stress, certain drugs, and infectious agents (e.g., viruses). Most likely, a number of factors work together to cause the disease.

Lupus is one of the many immune system disorders known as *autoimmune diseases.* In autoimmune diseases, the immune system turns against parts of the body it is designed to protect. This leads to inflammation and damage to various body tissues. Lupus can affect many parts of the body, including the joints, skin, kidneys, heart, lungs, blood vessels, and brain. Although people with the disease may have many different symptoms, some of the most common ones are extreme fatigue, painful or swollen joints (arthritis), unexplained fever, skin rashes, and kidney problems.

With lupus, the body's immune system does not work as it should. A healthy immune system produces proteins (antibodies) and specific cells (lymphocytes) that help destroy viruses, bacteria, and other foreign substances that invade the body. In lupus, the immune system produces antibodies against the body's healthy cells and tissues. These antibodies, called *autoantibodies,* contribute to the inflammation of various parts of the body and can cause damage to organs and tissues. The most common type of autoantibody that develops in people with lupus is the antinuclear antibody (ANA), because it reacts with parts of the cell's nucleus (command center). Researchers do not yet understand all the factors that cause inflammation and tissue damage with lupus, but many studies are underway.

- ***Massage implications:*** Stress is considered a causal factor for lupus, and stress management is a major benefit of massage.

Currently lupus has no cure. However, it can be treated effectively with medications, and most people with the disease can lead active, healthy lives. Lupus is characterized by periods of illness, called *flares,* and periods of wellness, or remission. Understanding how to prevent flares and how to treat them when they do occur helps people with lupus maintain better health. Intense research is underway, and scientists funded by the National Institutes of Health (NIH) continue to make great strides in understanding the disease, which ultimately may lead to a cure. Lupus is a primary focus of the National Institute of Arthritis and Musculoskeletal and Skin Diseases (NIAMS), a subsidiary of the NIH.

Identifying the genes that play a role in the development of lupus is an active area of research. For example, researchers suspect that people with lupus have a genetic defect in the cellular process called *apoptosis,* or programmed cell death. Apoptosis is similar to the process that causes leaves to turn color and fall from trees in the autumn; it allows the body to eliminate cells that have fulfilled their function and typically need to be replaced. If the process of apoptosis is defective, harmful cells may stay around and damage the body's own tissues. For example, in a mutant mouse strain that develops a lupuslike illness, one of the genes that control apoptosis is defective. When it is replaced by a normal gene, the mice no longer develop signs of the disease. Scientists are attempting to determine what role the genes involved in apoptosis may play in the development of human disease.

Another active area of lupus research involves the study of the complement system, a series of proteins in the blood that play an important part in the immune system. Complement system proteins act as a backup for antibodies, helping them destroy foreign substances that invade the body. If the complement proteins decline in number, the body is less able to fight or destroy foreign substances. If these substances are not removed from the body, the immune system may become overactive and begin to make autoantibodies.

Recent large studies of families with lupus have identified a number of genetic regions that appear to be associated with the risk of lupus. Although the specific genes and their function remain unknown, intensive work in mapping the entire human genome offers promise that these genes will be identified in the near future. This should provide knowledge of the complex factors that contribute to lupus susceptibility.

NIAMS-funded researchers are delineating the impact of genetic, socioeconomic, and cultural factors on the course and outcome of lupus in Hispanics, African Americans, and Caucasians. Preliminary data show that African American and Hispanic patients with lupus typically have more kidney damage than Caucasians. Researchers also have found that African American patients with lupus have more skin damage than Hispanics and Caucasians and that the death rate from lupus is higher in African Americans and Hispanics than in Caucasians.

Autoimmune diseases, such as lupus, are thought to occur when a genetically susceptible individual encounters an unknown environmental agent or trigger. In this circumstance, an abnormal immune response can be initiated that leads to the signs and symptoms of lupus. Research has focused on both the genetic susceptibility and the environmental trigger. Although the environmental trigger remains unknown, microbial agents, such as the Epstein-Barr virus and others, have been considered.

In addition, researchers are studying other factors that may affect a person's susceptibility to lupus. For example, because lupus is more common in women than in men, some researchers are investigating the role of hormones and other male-female differences in the development and course of the disease. A current study funded by the NIH focuses on the safety and effectiveness of oral contraceptives (birth control pills) and hormone replacement therapy in women with lupus. Doctors have worried about the wisdom of prescribing oral contraceptives or estrogen replacement therapy for women with lupus because of a widely held view that estrogens can aggravate the disease. However, hormone-based contraceptives and estrogen replacement therapy do not, as once feared, appear to intensify lupus symptoms.

Patients with lupus are at risk of developing atherosclerotic vascular disease (hardening of the blood vessels), which can lead to heart attack, angina, or stroke. The increased risk is due partly to lupus itself and partly to the steroid therapy used to treat it. The prevention of atherosclerotic vascular disease in individuals with lupus is a new area of study. Researchers are studying the most effective ways to manage cardiovascular risk factors and to prevent cardiovascular disease in adult patients with lupus. In childhood lupus, researchers are evaluating the safety and effectiveness of drugs called *statins,* which lower the levels of low-density lipoprotein (LDL, or bad) cholesterol as a means of preventing fat buildup in the blood vessels.

One of five patients with lupus experiences symptoms such as headaches, dizziness, memory disturbances, stroke, or changes in behavior that result from changes in the brain or other parts of the central nervous system (CNS). These individuals have *neuropsychiatric lupus.* By uncovering the mechanisms responsible for CNS damage in patients with lupus, researchers hope to move closer to improved diagnosis and treatment for patients with this form of lupus.

Promising areas of research on lupus include:

- Identifying lupus susceptibility genes
- Searching for environmental agents that cause lupus
- Developing drugs or biologic agents to treat lupus

Many researchers are focusing on finding better treatments for lupus. A primary goal of this research is to develop treatments that can effectively minimize the use of corticosteroids. Scientists are trying to identify combination therapies that may be more effective than a single treatment approach. Another goal is to improve the treatment and management of lupus in the kidneys and CNS. For example, a 20-year study supported by NIAMS and the NIH found that combining cyclophosphamide with prednisone helped delay or prevent kidney failure, a serious complication of lupus.

On the basis of new information about the disease process, scientists are using novel biologic agents to selectively block parts of the immune system. The development and testing of these new drugs, which are based on compounds that occur naturally in the body, constitute an exciting and promising new area of lupus research. The hope is that these treatments not only will be effective, but that they also will have fewer side effects. Preliminary research suggests that white blood cells known as B cells may play a key role in the development of lupus. Biologics that interfere with B-cell function or that block the interactions of immune cells are an active area of research. These targeted treatments hold promise, because they have the advantage of reduced side effects and adverse reactions compared with conventional therapies. Clinical trials are underway to test the safety and effectiveness of rituximab (also called anti-CD20) in treating people with lupus. Rituximab is a genetically engineered antibody that blocks the production of B cells. Another treatment option currently being explored is reconstruction of the immune system through bone marrow transplantation. In the future, gene therapy also may play an important role in the treatment of lupus.

Lupus can take many forms:

- Systemic lupus erythematosus (SLE) is what most people mean when they say they have lupus. The word *systemic* means the disease can affect many parts of the body. The symptoms of SLE may be mild or serious. Although SLE usually first affects people between the ages of 15 and 45 years, it also can occur in childhood or later in life.
- Discoid lupus erythematosus (DLE) is a chronic skin disorder in which a red, raised rash appears on the face, scalp, or elsewhere. The raised areas may become thick and scaly and may cause scarring. The rash may last for days or years and may recur. A small percentage of people with discoid lupus have or later develop SLE.
- Subacute cutaneous lupus erythematosus (SCLE) is a form of the disease in which skin lesions appear on parts of the body exposed to sun. The lesions do not cause scarring.
- Drug-induced lupus (DIL) is caused by medications. The symptoms are similar to those of SLE (arthritis, rash, fever, and chest pain), and they typically resolve completely when the drug is discontinued. The kidneys and brain are rarely involved.
- Neonatal lupus is a rare disease that can occur in the newborn babies of women who have SLE, Sjögren's syndrome, or no disease at all. Scientists suspect that neonatal lupus is caused by autoantibodies in the mother's blood. At birth, these babies have a skin rash, liver problems, and low blood counts. The symptoms gradually resolve over several months. In rare instances, a newborn with neonatal lupus may have a serious heart problem that slows the natural rhythm of the heart. As mentioned, neonatal lupus is rare, and most infants of mothers with SLE are entirely healthy.

It is important for women with SLE or other related autoimmune disorders to be under a doctor's care during pregnancy. Physicians can now identify mothers at highest risk for complications, which allows prompt treatment of the infant at or before birth. Also, SLE can flare during pregnancy, and prompt treatment can keep the mother healthier longer.

Symptoms. Each person with lupus has slightly different symptoms, which can range from mild to severe and may come and go over time. Some of the most common symptoms of lupus include painful or swollen joints (arthritis), unexplained fever, and extreme fatigue. A characteristic red skin rash, the so-called butterfly (or malar) rash, may appear across the nose and cheeks. Rashes may also occur on the face and ears, upper arms, shoulders, chest, and hands. Because many people with lupus are sensitive to sunlight (photosensitivity), skin rashes often first develop or worsen after sun exposure.

Common symptoms of lupus include the following:

- Painful or swollen joints and muscle pain
- Unexplained fever
- Red rashes, most commonly on the face
- Chest pain upon deep breathing
- Unusual loss of hair
- Pale or purple fingers or toes from cold or stress (Raynaud's phenomenon)
- Sensitivity to the sun
- Swelling (edema) in legs or around the eyes
- Mouth ulcers
- Swollen glands
- Extreme fatigue
- Anemia (a decrease in red blood cells)

Some people also experience headaches, dizziness, depression, confusion, or seizures. New symptoms may continue to appear years after the initial diagnosis, and different symptoms can occur at different times. In some people with lupus, only one body system is affected, such as the skin or joints. Other people have symptoms in many parts of the body. How seriously a body system is affected varies from person to person. The following body systems can be affected by lupus:

- Kidneys: Inflammation of the kidneys (nephritis) can impair these organs' ability to eliminate waste products and other toxins from the body effectively. Kidney involvement usually does not cause pain, although some patients may notice swelling in the ankles. Most often, the only indication of kidney disease is an abnormal urine or blood test. Because the kidneys are so important to overall health, lupus that affects the kidneys generally requires intensive drug treatment to prevent permanent damage.

- Lungs: Some people with lupus develop pleuritis, an inflammation of the lining of the chest cavity. This causes chest pain, particularly with breathing. Patients with lupus also may get pneumonia.
- Central nervous system: As mentioned, in some patients lupus affects the brain or CNS. This can cause headaches, dizziness, memory disturbances, vision problems, seizures, stroke, or changes in behavior.
- Blood vessels: Blood vessels may become inflamed (vasculitis), affecting the way blood circulates through the body. The inflammation may be mild and may not require treatment or may be severe and require immediate attention.
- Blood: People with lupus may develop anemia, leukopenia (decreased number of white blood cells), or thrombocytopenia (decreased number of blood platelets, which assist clotting). Some people with lupus may have an increased risk of blood clots.
- Heart: In some people with lupus, inflammation can develop in the heart itself (myocarditis and endocarditis) or the membrane that surrounds it (pericarditis), causing chest pain or other symptoms. Lupus also can increase the risk of atherosclerosis (hardening of the arteries).
- ***Massage implications:*** Lupus has an insidious onset; symptoms occur and then improve over time. Patients receiving massage for other reasons may also have lupus symptoms. The massage therapist needs to monitor the symptom pattern and refer the person to a physician when clusters of symptoms occur. Many autoimmune diseases share the vague symptoms of muscle and joint aching, lower extremity edema, fatigue, and so on. People with these symptoms commonly seek massage, and massage probably will help. However, this poses a problem: because the symptoms are managed, the person does not seek medical care, and consequently treatment is delayed. The massage therapist needs to be able to identify the clusters of symptoms common to autoimmune disease and refer the patient to a physician so that an appropriate diagnosis can be made.

Diagnosis. Diagnosing lupus can be difficult. It may take months or even years for doctors to piece together the symptoms to diagnose this complex disease accurately. Making a correct diagnosis of lupus requires knowledge and awareness on the part of the doctor and good communication on the part of the patient. A complete, accurate medical history is critical to the process of diagnosis. This information, along with a physical examination and the results of laboratory tests, helps the doctor consider other diseases that may mimic lupus or determine whether the patient truly has the disease. Reaching a diagnosis may take time as new symptoms appear.

No single test can determine whether a person has lupus, but several laboratory tests may help the doctor make a diagnosis. The most useful tests identify certain autoantibodies that are often present in the blood of people with lupus. For example, an ANA test is commonly done to check for autoantibodies that react against components of the nucleus, or "command center," of the body's cells. Most people with lupus test positive for ANA; however, a positive ANA test result can have a number of causes besides lupus, including infection or some other autoimmune disease, and occasionally this is a finding in healthy people. The ANA test simply provides another clue for the doctor to consider in making a diagnosis. In addition, blood tests can be done for individual types of autoantibodies that are more specific to people with lupus, although not all people with lupus test positive for these, and not all people with these antibodies have lupus.

Other laboratory tests are used to monitor the progress of the disease once it has been diagnosed. A complete blood count (CBC), urinalysis (UA), blood chemistries, and the erythrocyte sedimentation rate (ESR) can provide valuable information. Another common test measures the blood level of complement. People with lupus often have an elevated ESR and low complement levels, especially during flares of the disease. X-ray studies and other imaging tests can help doctors examine the organs affected by SLE.

Diagnostic tools for lupus include the following:

- Medical history
- Complete physical examination
- Laboratory tests
  - CBC
  - ESR
  - UA
  - Blood chemistries
  - Complement levels
  - ANA
  - Other autoantibody tests (anti-DNA, anti-Sm, anti-RNP, anti-Ro [SSA], anti-La [SSB])
  - Anticardiolipin antibody test
- Skin biopsy
- Kidney biopsy

Treatment. Treating lupus is often a team effort involving the patient and several types of health-care professionals. Treatment plans are tailored to the individual's needs and may change over time. A person with lupus may see a family doctor or internist or a rheumatologist. A rheumatologist is a doctor who specializes in rheumatic diseases (arthritis and other inflammatory disorders that often involve the immune system). Clinical immunologists (doctors specializing in immune system disorders) may also treat people with lupus. As treatment progresses, other professionals often help. These may include nurses, psychologists, social workers, nephrologists (doctors who treat kidney disease), hematologists (doctors specializing in blood disorders), dermatologists (doctors who treat skin disease), and neurologists (doctors specializing in disorders of the nervous system).

The range and effectiveness of treatments for lupus have increased dramatically, giving doctors more choices in how to manage the disease. It is important that the patient work closely with the doctor and take an active role in managing the disease. Once lupus has been diagnosed, the doctor will develop a treatment plan based on the patient's age, gender, health, symptoms, and lifestyle. In developing a treatment plan, the doctor has several goals: to prevent flares, to treat them when they occur, and to minimize organ damage and complications. The doctor and the patient should re-evaluate the plan regularly to ensure that it is as effective as possible.

Medications. A number of medications can be used to treat lupus.

NSAIDs: Nonsteroidal antiinflammatory drugs, which reduce inflammation, are often used for people with joint or chest pain or fever. Although some NSAIDs, such as ibuprofen and naproxen, are available over the counter, a doctor's prescription is required for others. NSAIDs may be used alone or with other types of drugs to control pain, swelling, and fever. Even though some NSAIDs can be purchased without a prescription, it is important that they be taken under a doctor's direction. Common side effects of NSAIDs can include stomach upset, heartburn, diarrhea, and fluid retention. Some people with lupus also develop liver, kidney, or even neurologic complications, which makes it especially important that the patient stay in close contact with the doctor while taking these medications.

- ***Massage implications:*** The main concern for massage application in patients taking NSAIDs is pressure levels, because these medications increase the potential for bruising. Pain perception can be altered with massage; therefore, massage may help with pain management.

Antimalarials: As the name implies, antimalarial drugs were developed to treat malaria. However, doctors have found that they also are useful for lupus. A common antimalarial used to treat lupus is hydroxychloroquine (Plaquenil). It may be given alone or with other drugs, and it generally is used to treat fatigue, joint pain, skin rashes, and inflammation of the lungs. Clinical studies have found that continuous treatment with antimalarials may prevent the recurrence of flares. Side effects of antimalarials can include stomach upset and, in very rare cases, retinal damage.

Corticosteroids: Corticosteroid hormones are the mainstay of lupus treatment. These drugs include prednisone (Deltasone), hydrocortisone, methylprednisolone (Medrol), and dexamethasone (Decadron, Hexadrol). Corticosteroids are related to cortisol, a natural antiinflammatory hormone. They work by rapidly suppressing inflammation. Corticosteroids can be given by mouth, in creams applied to the skin, or by injection. Because they are potent drugs, the goal is to use the lowest dose that provides the greatest benefit. Short-term side effects of corticosteroids include swelling, increased appetite, and weight gain. These side effects generally resolve when the drug is discontinued. It is dangerous to stop taking corticosteroids suddenly, therefore it is very important that the doctor and patient work together in changing the dosage of corticosteroids. Doctors sometimes administer very large amounts of a corticosteroid into a vein over a brief period (days); this is known as *bolus,* or *pulse,* therapy. With this treatment, the typical side effects are less likely and slow withdrawal is unnecessary.

Long-term side effects of corticosteroids can include stretch marks on the skin, weakened or damaged bones (osteoporosis and osteonecrosis), high blood pressure, damage to the arteries, high blood sugar (diabetes), infections, and cataracts. Typically, the higher the dose and the longer the drug is taken, the greater the risk and severity of side effects. Researchers are working to develop ways to limit or offset the use of corticosteroids. For example, corticosteroids may be used in combination with other, less potent drugs, or the doctor may try to slowly reduce the dosage once the disease is under control. People with lupus who are taking corticosteroids should talk to their doctor about taking supplemental calcium and vitamin D or other drugs to reduce the risk of osteoporosis (weakened, fragile bones).

- ***Massage implications:*** Corticosteroids have many side effects that present cautions for massage. A major concern is osteoporosis. The massage pressure level must be monitored closely. The edema associated with corticosteroid use may be influenced by lymphatic drainage massage, but caution is indicated if kidney involvement is a factor. More frequent massage of shorter duration (i.e., massage three times a week for 30 minutes) may be more appropriate.

Immunosuppressants: For some patients in whom the kidneys or CNS is affected, an immunosuppressive drug may be used. Immunosuppressives (e.g., cyclophosphamide [Cytoxan] and mycophenolate mofetil [CellCept]) restrain the overactive immune system by blocking the production of immune cells. These drugs may be given by mouth or by infusion (dripping the drug into the vein through a small tube). Side effects may include nausea, vomiting, hair loss, bladder problems, diminished fertility, and an increased risk of cancer and infection. The risk of side effects increases with the length of treatment. As with other treatments for lupus, there is a risk of relapse after discontinuation of the immunosuppressive drugs.

Methotrexate: In some patients, methotrexate (Folex, Mexate, Rheumatrex), a disease-modifying antirheumatic drug, may be used to help control the disease.

- ***Massage implications:*** Massage therapists must pay very close attention to infection control. They should not work with an immunosuppressed patient if they have a contagious disease. Do not support the patient in changing the treatment regimen without the doctor's supervision. Patients often disclose their intent to stop or change a treatment to the massage therapist; reinforce the importance of close supervision by the health-care team. Working closely with the doctor helps ensure that treatments for lupus are as successful as possible. Because some treatments may cause harmful side effects, it is important to report any new symptoms to the doctor promptly.

Alternative and complementary therapies: Because of the nature and cost of the medications used to treat lupus and the potential for serious side effects, many patients seek other ways to treat the disease. Some alternative approaches that people have tried include special diets, nutritional supplements, fish oils, ointments and creams, chiropractic treatment, massage, and homeopathy. These methods may not be harmful in themselves, and they may be associated with symptomatic or psychosocial benefit; however, no research to date has shown that they affect the disease process or prevent organ damage. Some alternative or complementary approaches may help the patient cope or reduce some of the stress associated with living with a chronic illness. If the doctor feels that an approach has value and will not be harmful, it can be incorporated into the patient's treatment plan. However, it is important not to neglect regular healthcare or the treatment of serious symptoms. An open dialog between the patient and the physician about the relative merits of complementary and alternative therapies allows the patient to make an informed choice about treatment options.

- ***Massage implications:*** Massage cannot replace medical treatment of lupus. Supporting stress management, reducing some side effects of treatment, and managing some symptoms of the disease are justifiable benefits of massage.

Treatment of Flares. It is important that people with lupus receive regular healthcare rather than seeking help only when symptoms worsen. The findings of regular medical examinations and laboratory tests allow the doctor to note any changes and to identify and treat flares early. The treatment plan, which is tailored to the individual's specific needs and circumstances, can be adjusted accordingly. If new symptoms are identified early, treatments may be more effective. Other concerns also can be addressed at regular checkups. The doctor can provide guidance on such issues as the use of sunscreens, stress reduction, and the importance of structured exercise and rest, as well as birth control and family planning. Because people with lupus can be more susceptible to infection, the doctor may recommend yearly influenza vaccination or pneumococcal vaccination for some patients.

Women with lupus should receive regular preventive healthcare, such as gynecologic and breast examinations. Men with lupus should have the prostate-specific antigen (PSA) test. Both men and women should have their blood pressure and cholesterol levels checked regularly. If a person is taking corticosteroids or antimalarials, an eye examination should be done at least annually to screen for and treat eye problems.

Extra effort and care are required for people with lupus to stay healthy; therefore it is especially important that they develop strategies for maintaining wellness. Wellness requires a person to pay close attention to the body, mind, and spirit. One of the primary goals of wellness for people with lupus is coping with the stress of a chronic disorder. Effective stress management varies from person to person. Approaches that may help include exercise, relaxation techniques (e.g., meditation, therapeutic massage), and setting priorities for spending time and energy.

Developing and maintaining a good support system are also important. A support system may include family, friends, medical professionals, community organizations, and support groups. Participating in a support group can provide emotional help, boost self-esteem and morale, and help develop or improve coping skills.

Warning signs of a flare include the following:

- Increased fatigue
- Pain
- Rash
- Fever
- Abdominal discomfort
- Headache
- Dizziness

Learning to recognize warning signals and maintaining good communication with the doctor can help the patient prevent flares.

- ***Massage implications:*** Monitor for the symptoms of a flare. The massage therapist may recognize the symptom cluster when updating session notes for each massage, especially as target areas of the massage are identified. Bring the situation to the patient's attention and encourage him or her to talk with the physician, or report your findings directly to the supervising healthcare professional.

Pregnancy in Women with Lupus. Although a lupus pregnancy is considered high risk, most women with lupus carry their babies safely to term. Women with lupus have a higher rate of miscarriage and premature births than the general population. Women who have antiphospholipid antibodies are at greater risk of miscarriage in the second trimester, because they have an increased risk of blood clotting in the placenta. Patients with lupus who have a history of kidney disease have a higher risk of pre-eclampsia (hypertension with a buildup of excess watery fluid in the cells or body tissues). Pregnancy counseling and prepregnancy planning are important. Ideally, a woman should have no signs or symptoms of lupus and should have taken no medications for at least 6 months before she becomes pregnant.

Some women may experience a mild to moderate flare during or after their pregnancy; others do not. Pregnant women with lupus, especially those taking corticosteroids, also are more likely to develop high blood pressure, diabetes, hyperglycemia (high blood sugar), and kidney complications, therefore regular care and good nutrition during pregnancy are essential. It also is advisable to have access to a neonatal (newborn) intensive care unit at the time of delivery in case the baby requires special medical attention.

- ***Massage implications:*** If a woman has lupus, her pregnancy is a high-risk one. A massage therapist working with a pregnant woman with lupus should know the symptoms of miscarriage and pre-eclampsia. Corticosteroid therapy increases risks during pregnancy, therefore it also is necessary to monitor for symptoms of high blood pressure, diabetes, and kidney disease. Because the patient needs comprehensive medical care during a high-risk pregnancy, the massage therapist, along with the medical team, must support regular monitoring, staying alert to any change in the patient's condition and referring the patient to the doctor immediately if changes occur.

Medical Assessment, Diagnosis, and Treatment Orders

The patient, a 32-year-old female, is 5′8″ tall and weighs 180 lb. She has systemic lupus erythematosus (SLE), which is currently in remission. Previous treatment included prednisone and mycophenolate mofetil (CellCept). She also takes an over-the-counter NSAID (Aleve) for short periods if she experiences joint pain. The patient has experienced two miscarriages within an 8-month period. The first was at 10 weeks, and the second was at 20 weeks. The patient was referred to a specialist to determine the reason for the miscarriages, and blood work indicated increased abnormalities in blood levels of antibodies. Based on additional tests and a comprehensive history, SLE was diagnosed when the patient was 28 years old. She presented moderate symptoms and depression without kidney involvement. A short-term course of antidepressants was used in conjunction with cognitive behavior therapy and grief counseling. Treatment resulted in remission of the lupus with occasional flares. The depression resolved, and the medication was gradually removed. After the patient had been in remission for 12 months with no flares, treatment was altered to allow her to conceive. She currently is taking no medications, she is 12 weeks pregnant, and all indications are that the lupus is stable and the pregnancy is progressing normally. The major immediate concern is the anxiety the patient is experiencing. The pregnancy is being closely monitored. The patient and her husband are attending a support group for couples with high-risk pregnancies, and the patient is participating in meditation classes. She is to receive a massage for stress management (60 minutes weekly) provided by the staff massage therapist. The massage application should not use any methods that would increase inflammation. Any increase in edema is to be reported immediately and evaluated before lymphatic drainage methods are approved. Prenatal massage approaches for the first and second trimester are to be used. Pressure levels should be comfortable for the patient. There is no indication of skin sensitivity or osteoporosis. Pain control methods can be incorporated for joint aching, and muscle tension headache approaches are approved. If the headache symptoms indicate a vascular headache, the patient must be referred immediately so that her blood pressure can be evaluated.

Massage-Specific Assessment

Angelina's muscle motor tone is good. She walks regularly for exercise and uses a modified yoga style of stretching. She is very aware of the inflammatory nature of her condition and follows an antiinflammatory diet.

She was in a car accident at age 22, which resulted in a whiplash injury and a bruised anterior thorax. Both appear to have resolved, although rib movement is restricted at the sternum but normal at the facet joints. Soft tissue changes have occurred in the cervical area, and the areas palpated as dense with decreased stability. The assessment for upper chest breathing pattern is positive, and this is a logical contributing factor to anxiety and sleep disturbance, which are the main targets for massage.

Angelina complains of joint aching in the area of the sacroiliac (SI) joints, hips, and feet and would like these areas targeted during massage. She indicates that her pain varies from 5 to 8 on a pain scale of 1 to 10. She also indicates that her calves are tight. She gets frequent headaches, primarily the tension headache type, which she rates as 6 to 9 on the 1-10 pain scale. Findings include connective tissue bind at the occipital base and point tenderness in the suboccipital muscles, temporalis bilateral, and frontalis, which exacerbates the headache pain. The scalenes are short bilaterally, with a short pectoralis minor on the right. The sternocleidomastoid muscles bilaterally house trigger points that refer pain into her typical headache pattern. The trunk and hip muscle activation sequences are synergistically dominant. The psoas is short bilaterally, with anterior pelvic rotation bilaterally, moderate lordosis, and a short lumbar dorsal fascia. The erector spinae fire first for hip extension, and the hamstrings are long and weak. The gluteus maximus is inhibited. Calf motor tone is increased, as is muscle tone, because of mild edema.

The patient is experiencing some morning sickness, although it is not severe. She is tired and needs a nap at midday to feel as if she can function. The doctor indicates that her symptoms seem to be more related to the pregnancy than the lupus. She is comfortable lying in all positions.

She enjoys massage and sometimes has had a massage while on vacation or as an occasional special treat at a local spa. She is enthusiastic about including massage in her care plan for the lupus and her pregnancy.

Clinical Reasoning Process

The main focus of the massage is to reduce anxiety, manage stress and pain, and support restorative sleep. The patient has experienced spa-based massage with no specific focus, therefore education about outcome-based massage that targets specific goals is necessary. The assessment indicates some postural distortion and alterations in muscle firing sequences and motor and muscle tone. The history reveals past trauma that resulted in soft tissue changes; this can perpetuate an upper chest breathing pattern, which predisposes the patient to anxiety and to some other specific symptoms (i.e., pain, moodiness, and fatigue). It would be prudent to use an approach that addresses breathing function and supports parasympathetic dominance. Because of the pregnancy, the psoas muscle cannot be addressed with direct inhibitory pressure at the muscle belly, and the aching in the SI joints indicates caution for stretching of the psoas. Reflexively paired to the psoas is the sternocleidomastoid, which has trigger points that are related to the headache patterns. Potentially, addressing the sternocleidomastoid may influence the function of the psoas. It also may be possible to inhibit the psoas near the distal attachments as it crosses the pubic bones.

Smooth muscle function in the lumbar dorsal fascia appears to be related to joint instability, breathing pattern dysfunction, and pain. The smooth muscle in the fascia typically responds to broad-based compression and tension force, and because this is a superficial structure, surface tissue compression should be safe to perform.

Local lymphatic drainage to the lower limbs should reduce the muscle tone in the calves, and motor tone should normalize with general massage application. Approval is needed to use lymphatic drainage, and the amount of edema needs to be closely monitored.

At this point, although the pregnancy is a high-risk one, it is progressing normally and would be treated as such during the massage. Ongoing monitoring for symptoms of pre-eclampsia and miscarriage is necessary throughout the pregnancy. Miscarriage is most likely in the second trimester, whereas pre-eclampsia is the concern in the third trimester.

Because the lupus has not affected the kidneys, there is no indication of osteoporosis from steroid use, and the patient is not taking any pain medications, the pressure levels can be at the patient's comfort level without risk of bruising.

Because of the patient's history of lupus and the potential for a flare during pregnancy, along with the high-risk pregnancy, the massage needs to be nonstressful and provided with ongoing caution, because her condition can change quickly.

Warning signs of a pregnancy at risk that requires immediate referral include the following:

- Vaginal bleeding
- Severe, continuous abdominal pain
- Breaking of water (rupture of membranes)
- Pre-eclampsia, edema, dizziness, elevated blood pressure, severe headache
- Fever, frequent and painful urination (possible urinary tract infection)
- Excessive vomiting of such severity and frequency that no food or fluids can be retained
- Excessive itching, which may indicate liver or kidney dysfunction (cholestasis)

Treatment Plan Development

Long-term goals: Stress management, management of pain (2 to 4 on pain scale) and lupus symptoms, and support of pregnancy through postpartum phase.

Short-term goals: Reduce physical manifestations of anxiety and joint aching and support sleep.

Massage therapist's objectives: Support parasympathetic dominance and normalize breathing function, manage mild edema in legs and feet (physician approved immediately but therapist must report any increase in fluid retention). Manage physical symptoms related to normal pregnancy.

Methods to be used: General massage, palliative care protocol, with strategies for sleep and pain. Moderate pressure and intensity. Intervention for breathing pattern disorder, prenatal massage methods.

Frequency and duration: Weekly 60-minute sessions.

Measurement of progress: Pain scales, self-reporting of sleep quality, and anxiety scale administered during support group activities.

Date of reassessment: 6 weeks.

Additional notes: Modify intensity and duration of all methods based on daily status of patient. Do not strain adaptive capacity. Work slowly to restore more efficient breathing. Alter position to support comfort as pregnancy progresses. Support attendance at group meetings and meditation. Monitor for lupus flare and complications of pregnancy.

SOAP Charting

Session 1

S: Patient reports that her condition is a bit more intense than the initial assessment visit. She feels as if she can't always get a deep breath, and she is restless when sleeping. Her calves and feet are bothering her most, and she has a tension-type headache that she assess as a 7 on the 1-10 pain scale.

O: Shoulders are moving in an upper chest breathing pattern, and patient is yawning and sighing. Calves palpate as taut with increased muscle tone but no evidence of pitting edema. Headache pain replicated with compression to frontalis, occipital, temporalis, and sternocleidomastoid. General massage to target upper chest breathing and headache. Patient found moderate to heavy compressive force most relaxing as long as she just felt "squashed," so moderate pressure was used in the thorax, calves, and arms, and heavy pressure was used on the gluteals, thighs, and upper shoulders. The scalenes, sternocleidomastoids, and suboccipital were inhibited with compression and positional release using a combination of eye and head movement and inhale and exhale movement. The muscles of the head were addressed with broad-based compression and, if tender points were identified that increased headache symptoms, direct pressure on the point combined with local tissue stretching. Short-duration lymphatic drainage to the lower limbs, combined with kneading of the calves, was provided in addition to general massage.

A: Patient reports that headache is a 2 on the pain scale, and she feels less stiff in general. Upper chest movement during breathing remains evident, and she indicates that she feels relaxed but not sleepy. She is not yawning.

P: Patient is to call next day and report the 24-hour response to massage.

NOTE: Patient called and said that she slept better, even though her headache came back, although it was not as severe. She was sore when she rubbed her upper trapezius area but not when she moved her shoulders. She was not sore anywhere else and did not experience any adverse reaction to massage.

Session 2

S: Patient reports that she feels good but still has episodes of anxiety. She particularly enjoyed having her head massaged and loved the pressure. Her calves feel stiff, and her feet ache. Sleep is about the same, with frequent waking mostly because of being uncomfortable and an increased need to use the bathroom. Pregnancy is progressing normally.

O: Assessment indicates that upper chest breathing remains evident, and rib mobility remains reduced. Calf muscle tone is similar to last massage because of edema. No logical explanation for aching feet, other than that her feet have always ached. Repeat massage as last session with less compression on upper trapezius.

A: Patient reports that she feels good. Slight increase in rib mobility at the sternum. Patient appears relaxed and dozed during the last 30 minutes of massage.

P: Call and report if any unusual response to massage. Report to obstetrician about response to massage during next visit.

Session 3

S: Patient reports she is 14 weeks pregnant, and all is progressing normally. She mentions that she feels a bit relieved, because one of her miscarriages happened when she was about 10 weeks. She still wants to take a nap in the afternoon, and urination frequency has increased, but the obstetrician feels that this is normal for pregnancy. Morning sickness is almost gone. She indicates that the area of the SI joints is especially achy today, but her calves feel less stiff. She requests massage for her feet and head. The obstetrician requests that massage be maintained according to the treatment plan, because the initial results are positive. Patient remains comfortable in the prone position.

O: No changes in status of patient's breathing. Increased trigger point sensitivity and referred pain in multifidi and gluteus medius referring to SI joint. Provide general massage with additional attention to head and feet. Address trigger points with direct inhibition and tissue stretching.

A: Patient reports that addressing the trigger points "hurts good." She feels relaxed and sleepy.

P: Reassess trigger point activity in SI joint area. Maintain general massage approach and address specific target area mentioned by patient.

Session 4

S: Patient reports that she does not feel well today. She went to the doctor because of dizziness, had a headache, and was very tired. Her blood pressure was elevated, and she is being monitored for a flare. Physician requests a general palliative massage with no specific focus, then the patient is to have her blood pressure taken again.

O: Patient appears fatigued and anxious. General palliative massage per physician request.

A: Patient reports that she feels sleepy and did fall asleep during the massage. Postmassage blood pressure check showed a normal reading. Patient was sent home to rest.

P: Evaluate patient for flare symptoms and contact physician for update.

Session 5

S: Physician reports that patient is being monitored for a flare, but her condition seems to have normalized. Continue with massage according to treatment plan. Patient indicates that she feels better and thinks she may be feeling the baby move. Her legs are stiff, and her feet hurt. She remains fatigued. She reports that she is less achy in general and sleeping better but wakes up more often to use the bathroom.

O: Upper chest breathing evident, with sighing and yawning. Mild edema in legs and feet. Evident edema in feet is a new symptom. Called obstetrician to report. Nurse indicates that edema seems to be pregnancy-related and to provide lymphatic drainage to reduce pressure and aching. General massage with lymphatic drainage to legs, and rhythmic mobilization of ribs. No direct inhibitory pressure on auxiliary breathing muscles, because patient found the pressure unpleasant. Patient used restroom halfway through massage.

A: Edema improved, feet and legs palpate less taut, and patient reports reduced stiffness. Patient also reports that she feels better and wants to go home and sleep.

P: Monitor edema and fatigue. Continue with breathing function focus. Complete assessment report and send to physician.

Evaluation of Progress

Massage appears to have reduced patient's anxiety and managed the edema. Patient is sleeping better, primarily because of decrease in pain and aching. Rib mobility and pliability of upper chest soft tissue have increased slightly. Trigger point activity in sternocleidomastoid has diminished. Headache frequency has not diminished, but pain has decreased (4 to 5 on pain scale) and does not last as long. Patient is 16 weeks pregnant, and symptoms of fatigue, increased urination, and lower extremity edema seem to be primarily related to pregnancy. Her anxiety declined markedly when she passed the first trimester mark. Because she had a miscarriage at 20 weeks in a previous pregnancy, it would be prudent to monitor anxiety levels as she approaches the 20- to 22-week mark in her pregnancy. She is just beginning to find lying on her stomach uncomfortable, therefore the side-lying position needs to be used for the rest of the pregnancy.

Recommendations for Future Massage Care

Continue with current treatment plan.

Perspective of the Massage Therapist

Care must be taken not to overwork this patient. She responds best to significant compressive force with no discomfort as an aspect of the general massage, and it is best to target only one additional area so as not to strain her adaptive capacity. When she is not tired, she responds well to direct inhibitory pressure that mimics symptoms she usually has with headache or SI joint aching, and she classified the sensation as a "good hurt." When she is fatigued, she is not tolerant of any sort of pain sensation. She responds well to massage of the head and feet, and the massage was extended to allow extra time for these areas. It seems as if some of her anxiety involves anticipation of a miscarriage. This is reasonable. She does not communicate much during the massage but did indicate that she felt better once she entered the second trimester. It has been difficult to determine which symptoms are related to the pregnancy and which to the lupus.

CASE STUDY 3: DIABETES MELLITUS AND DEPRESSION

Similar Conditions

Any depression-related conditions and various endocrine conditions.

The Case

Beth, who is 62, has difficulty controlling her type 2 diabetes. She was first diagnosed with the disease at age 42. Obesity has been a concern since the birth of her last child at age 33. She does not follow an exercise program and has difficulty managing her diet. Hypertension is a major concern, as are other risk factors for cardiovascular disease, including high cholesterol. She has mild neuropathy in her lower legs and feet. Vascular surgery was done to open clogged arteries in Beth's lower extremities, and her coronary arteries may need to be treated. She also has moderately severe osteoporosis.

Beth's children (two girls and three boys) are very concerned about the recent decline in her health. Her doctors are frustrated with her lack of compliance with lifestyle changes. Oral medications no longer control her glucose levels, and she is taking insulin. She recently moved from the family home to an assisted living facility adjacent to a long-term care facility, where her husband is receiving care for Alzheimer's disease. Beth is depressed and angry with her children, and it is suspected that she is drinking regularly.

Beth noticed that a massage therapist works at the facility where she lives, and she is interested in receiving massage. Her children and physician are supportive. Before beginning the massage sessions, the massage therapist discussed the case with Beth's physician. The doctor indicated that he was very concerned about Beth's mood and possible alcohol use and that he hopes that massage can soothe her and possibly support an exercise program. He said that he would speak to the supervising nurse at the assisted living facility about Beth's case, and he instructed the massage therapist to report any concerns to the nurse. Progress notes on the massage are to be maintained in Beth's medical files. It is hoped that her condition may improve once she has adjusted to her new living arrangements and becomes involved in the group activities. The facility has a support group for residents with diabetes. It also has a pool and an exercise room, and a variety of exercise programs are available.

Research

Diabetes is a chronic condition characterized by high levels of glucose (sugar) in the blood. It can be caused by inadequate production of insulin (a hormone produced by the pancreas to regulate blood sugar), cellular resistance to insulin, or both.

Causes and Risk Factors. As mentioned, people with diabetes have high blood glucose levels because the pancreas does not make enough insulin, or because the person's muscle, fat, and liver cells do not respond to insulin normally, or both. Diabetes affects millions of people worldwide. Risk factors for diabetes include the following:

- Family history of the disease
- Obesity
- Age 45 or older
- Gestational diabetes (during pregnancy)
- High blood pressure
- High blood levels of triglycerides
- High blood cholesterol level

The American Diabetes Association recommends that all adults be screened for diabetes at least every 3 years. A person at high risk should be screened more often. The three major types of diabetes are type 1 diabetes, type 2 diabetes, and gestational diabetes.

- Type 1 diabetes typically develops in childhood. The body makes little or no insulin, and daily injections of insulin are required. Without proper daily management, life-threatening medical emergencies can arise.
- Type 2 diabetes accounts for 90% or more of all cases of diabetes. It usually develops in adulthood, although more and more adolescents are being diagnosed with this condition. Type 2 diabetes is becoming more common because of the growing number of elderly, the increase in obesity, and widespread failure to exercise. With type 2 diabetes, the pancreas does not make enough insulin to keep blood glucose levels normal, and the body's cells are resistant to the insulin that is provided.
- Gestational diabetes is a condition of high blood glucose levels that develops during pregnancy.

Symptoms. Symptoms of type 1 diabetes include the following:

- Increased thirst
- Increased urination
- Fatigue
- Nausea
- Vomiting
- Weight loss despite an increased appetite

Symptoms of type 2 diabetes are:

- Increased thirst
- Increased urination
- Increased appetite
- Slow healing of infections
- Fatigue
- Blurred vision
- Impotence in men

- ***Massage implications:*** Monitor for these symptoms, especially those of type 2 diabetes, and refer the patient for diagnosis if diabetes is suspected. Monitor the healing rate of any injury or infection and report any concerns to supervising medical personnel. Maintain meticulous infection control procedures.

Long-term complications of diabetes include the following:

- Diabetic retinopathy (a major cause of blindness)
- Diabetic nephropathy (a major cause of kidney disease)
- Diabetic neuropathy
- Peripheral vascular disease
- Hyperlipidemia, hypertension, atherosclerosis, and coronary artery disease

- ***Massage implications:*** Neuropathy is a painful condition that is difficult to treat. Massage often provides symptomatic relief. When working with patients who have diabetes, be aware of strain on the kidney and cardiovascular system.

Ketoacidosis is a type of metabolic acidosis caused by high concentrations of keto acids, formed by the deamination of amino acids. Signs of ketoacidosis indicate a medical emergency. Obtain medical assistance immediately if any of the following are noted:

- Increased thirst and urination
- Nausea
- Deep, rapid breathing
- Abdominal pain
- Sweet-smelling breath
- Loss of consciousness

Symptoms of extremely low blood sugar (hypoglycemic coma or severe insulin reaction) include the following:

- Weakness
- Drowsiness
- Headache
- Confusion
- Dizziness
- Double vision
- Lack of coordination
- Convulsions or unconsciousness

Diabetes has no cure; the condition can only be managed. The goal of treatment is to stabilize the blood sugar. The long-term goals of treatment are to prolong life, ease symptoms, and prevent long-term complications, such as heart disease and kidney failure.

The risks of long-term complications from diabetes can be reduced. Research has shown dramatically lower rates of kidney, eye, and nervous system complications in patients who tightly control their blood glucose levels. A significant drop in all diabetes-related deaths, as well as a lower risk of heart attack and stroke, also was noted. (Tight control of blood pressure also was found to lower the risks of heart disease and stroke.)

Maintaining an ideal body weight and pursuing an active lifestyle may prevent the onset of type 2 diabetes. Currently there is no way to prevent type 1 diabetes.

Diagnosis. Medical tests for diabetes mellitus include the following:

- Urinalysis: This test may be done to check for glucose and ketones. Ketones, which are produced by the breakdown of fat and muscle, are toxic at high levels. Ketones in the blood cause a condition called *acidosis* (a low blood pH). Blood glucose levels are also high.
- Fasting blood glucose level: Diabetes is diagnosed if the value for this test is higher than 126 mg/dl on two occasions. Levels between 100 and 126 mg/dl reflect impaired fasting glucose, or prediabetes. These levels are considered to be risk factors for type 2 diabetes and its complications.
- Random (nonfasting) blood glucose level: Diabetes is suspected if this value is higher than 200 mg/dl and is accompanied by the classic symptoms of increased thirst, urination, and fatigue. (This test must be confirmed with a fasting blood glucose test.)
- Oral glucose tolerance test: A dose of glucose is administered, and diabetes is diagnosed if the glucose level is higher than 200 mg/dl after 2 hours.(This test is used more often for type 2 diabetes.)

Patients with type 1 diabetes usually develop symptoms over a short time, and the condition often is diagnosed in an emergency situation. In addition to high glucose levels, individuals with type 1 diabetes who are acutely ill have high ketone levels.

Treatment. People with diabetes need to develop basic skills for managing their condition. These skills include the following:

- How to recognize and treat low blood sugar (hypoglycemia) and high blood sugar (hyperglycemia)
- What to eat and when
- How to administer insulin or take oral medication
- How to test and record the blood glucose level
- How to test the urine for ketones (applicable only in type 1 diabetes)

- How to adjust the insulin dosage and/or food intake when changing exercise and eating habits

Diet. A person with diabetes should work closely with the healthcare provider to learn the correct amounts of fat, protein, and carbohydrates to include in the diet. People with type 1 diabetes should eat at about the same times each day and should try to be consistent with the types of food they choose. This helps prevent blood sugar levels from fluctuating between extremely high and extremely low. Patients with type 2 diabetes should follow a well-balanced, low-fat diet. A registered dietitian can be very helpful in planning dietary needs.

Weight management and exercise are important for managing diabetes. In some cases, people with type 2 diabetes who lose excess weight can stop taking their diabetes medications.

- ***Massage implications:*** Massage can support a weight loss program by substituting for the pleasure sensation and mood alteration otherwise obtained by food. Massage also supports an exercise program. Massage sessions need to be scheduled between meals, especially for type 1 patients, to prevent the patient with diabetes from having a hypoglycemic reaction after the massage.

Medication. Medications used to treat diabetes include insulin and glucose-lowering drugs called *oral hypoglycemic agents.* Because the bodies of people with type 1 diabetes cannot make insulin, these individuals require daily insulin injections. The bodies of people with type 2 diabetes make insulin but cannot use it effectively.

Insulin is usually delivered by injection, and injections generally are required one to four times a day. Some people use an insulin pump, which is worn at all times and delivers a steady flow of insulin throughout the day.

ARCHIE 18-1

- ***Massage implications:*** Do not massage over injection sites. Do not disturb the insulin pump.

Type 2 diabetes may respond to treatment with exercise, diet, and/or oral medications. Several oral hypoglycemic agents can lower blood glucose levels in people with type 2 diabetes. These drugs fall into one of three groups:

- Medications that increase insulin production by the pancreas (e.g., Glucotrol, Micronase, Glynase, Starlix)
- Medications that increase the cells' sensitivity to insulin (e.g., Glucophage, Avandia)
- Medications that delay the absorption of glucose from the gut (e.g., Precose, Glyset)

Most people with type 2 diabetes require more than one medication for good blood sugar control. Women who have type 2 diabetes and become pregnant are switched to insulin during the pregnancy and while breast-feeding.

Gestational diabetes is treated with diet and insulin.

- ***Massage implications:*** Massage may have a tendency to lower blood glucose levels. It is important to monitor for hypoglycemic symptoms, especially if the patient is taking hypoglycemic-type medications. Symptoms of hypoglycemia include dizziness, confusion, chills, sweating, hunger, headache, and pallor. A person with diabetes should always carry a syringe of glucose in case hypoglycemia develops. Advise patients with diabetes to eat before the massage. Glucose tablets are available over the counter and should be kept handy in case of an unexpected drop in glucose levels.

Exercise. Regular exercise is especially important for people with diabetes. It helps control blood sugar, reduce weight, and lower high blood pressure. People with diabetes who exercise are less likely to have a heart attack or stroke than people with the disease who do not exercise regularly. Changes in the intensity or duration of exercise may require changes in the diet or in the medication dosage to prevent blood sugar levels from going too high or low.

- ***Massage implications:*** Massage supports the exercise program by managing musculoskeletal discomfort and serving as a pleasure-based reward.

Foot Care. People with diabetes are prone to foot problems as a result of damage to blood vessels and nerves and a diminished ability to fight infection. In severe cases, the affected foot may have to be amputated. Diabetes is the most common condition leading to amputation.

- ***Massage implications:*** Foot massage encourages circulation. While massaging the feet, inspect them for changes. Report any suspect areas immediately. Do not massage over areas of tissue damage. Maintain meticulous infection control.

Osteoporosis. Osteoporosis is a disorder of the bone in which calcium and other minerals are lacking and bone protein is diminished, leaving the bones soft, fragile, and more likely to break. Osteoporosis primarily affects the spine and pelvis. The condition occurs most often in postmenopausal women as a result of the decrease in hormone levels. Causes include deficiencies in nutritional intake, absorption, or assimilation of protein and minerals; cigarette smoking; normal changes; and inactivity. Treatments include hormone therapy (primarily estrogen, progesterone, and calcitonin), increasing exercise, and including more sources of calcium, magnesium, boron, and vitamin D in the diet, along with appropriate sun exposure.

Medical Assessment, Diagnosis, and Treatment Orders

The patient, a 62-year-old female, is 5′5″ tall and weighs 195 lb. She has type 2 diabetes. She is being treated with Glucophage, Glyset, and insulin. The patient also is taking trimetazidine (Vastarel) for her blood pressure. Avoid injection sites during the massage.

The potential exists for low blood sugar symptoms. Make sure the patient is not dizzy after the massage. It is prudent to stay in the massage room with the patient after the massage and assist her off the table, making sure she is steady when standing.

The patient's fat distribution is in the abdomen and breasts. The hips and knees show arthritic changes, and she has mild neuropathy in her legs and feet. She is being monitored for kidney and eye involvement.

Currently the patient is not taking any medication for pain. However, she takes a low dose of aspirin (81 mg) daily, therefore watch for bruising.

Wound healing tends to be slow. She has a wound on her left heel from a blister that is being treated with antibiotics. Maintain meticulous infection control.

Massage will target stress management and circulation to the lower extremities and support diabetes management, including exercise.

Massage-Specific Assessment

(NOTE: Areas of the knowledge base important for working with this patient include geriatrics, weight management, cardiovascular disease, diabetes, depression, alcohol abuse, and neuropathy.)

The gait is shuffling and labored. The breathing pattern appears to be upper chest dominant, and the dysfunction probably is the result of fat distribution. Upper and lower crossed syndrome is evident. No specific muscle testing or gait assessment is to be performed, per the supervising nurse's directions, because of the patient's deconditioned status. Mild edema is present in the lower limbs, probably because of inactivity. The supervising nurse has approved lymphatic drainage for the area. The feet are cold to the touch.

Clinical Reasoning Process

Beth is a relatively fragile patient with multiple physical and emotional problems. She also is likely to have a substance abuse problem. She is deconditioned and overweight and resists exercising. Evidence indicates circulation issues and breathing disorders. The combined upper and lower crossed syndrome contributes to the breathing issues and the labored gait. However, Beth is not motivated to participate in physical rehabilitation. Massage and lengthening/stretching techniques can address the short muscles and connective tissue, but without therapeutic exercise, the results will be limited.

Beth likely will respond well to a massage that incorporates comfort measures and supports neurochemcial balance and stress reduction. It should include both circulation (venous and arterial) and lymphatic drainage techniques. Depending on tolerance, the patient may respond to some inhibiting pressure to reduce motor tone. She also may benefit from gentle lengthening and stretching to restore length-tension relationships in the muscles and to increase the pliability of the connective tissue. Breathing function may respond to the more general massage methods. Specific releases are not likely to be effective at this time.

The patient should respond to the nurturance and pleasure component on an emotional level. Combined with the neurochemical influences, mood shifts should be influenced to support less anger and depression. Both transference and countertransference are concerns. Beth's situation is difficult and likely to put a strain on the massage therapist. Most of the massage focus will be palliative, with aspects of condition management. She may be uncomfortable in the supine position; extra bolstering and the side-lying position will be necessary.

Significant changes are not likely, but some positive changes are possible. Beth requested massage, which is an indication of motivation and potential compliance. Boundaries may be a concern if Beth interprets the massage as a personal connection. Having multiple massage therapists (two or three) alternate on a regular basis would help maintain a professional therapeutic relationship, because Beth's emotional focus would be distributed among the therapists.

Treatment Plan Development

Long-term goals: Managing stress, supporting an exercise program, and encouraging circulation.

Short-term goals: Acclimate the patient to massage. Use a palliative focus with lymphatic drainage and circulation enhancement methods, especially on the lower limbs.

Massage therapist's objectives: Actively engage patient in self-care and support cooperation with care. Increase circulation to extremities.

Methods to be used: General massage protocol modified with palliative focus. Lymphatic drainage on lower limbs and circulation-enhancing techniques on legs and feet.

Frequency and duration: Two times a week for 60 minutes. (This frequency is necessary because the patient is not participating in an exercise or a stretching regimen.)

Measurement of progress: Improved lower limb circulation (diminished coldness of feet, increased potential for wound healing) and measurement of circumference of lower limbs. General mood leveling, as observed by supervising nurse. Self-reporting of comfort levels and exercise compliance.

Date of reassessment: every 6 weeks.

SOAP Charting

Session 1

S: Beth is eager for the massage. She indicates that she wants to relax and be pampered. She asks about essential oils. With the supervising nurse's permission, a lavender/orange essential oil combination is used in the massage lotion (lavender for relaxation and orange for mood regulation). Beth indicates that both her feet are swollen.

O: No change in the patient's physical condition since the intake assessment, when her ankle measurement was 10 inches. Her mood appears less sullen. General massage was provided, primarily palliative with lymphatic drainage on the legs. The thorax was decongested before the lymphatic drainage, which also supported breathing function. General massage was sufficient to increase circulation. Arterial circulation procedures were not used.

A: Beth is very happy with massage. She especially enjoyed the foot massage and having her head massaged. She was most comfortable on her side with extra bolstering at the abdomen and chest and between the knees. The supine position is also comfortable. As expected, the prone position was uncomfortable but possible for a short time if extra bolstering was used under the chest. She does not like the face cradle. The ankle measurement after massage was $9^1/_2$ inches.

P: Check with nurse supervisor for recommendations for massage. Repeat massage session with modifications necessary based on response.

Session 2

S: No specific massage recommendations from the nurse supervisor. The nurse supervisor noted that the patient's mood was less sullen for the rest of the day after the massage. Beth is very satisfied with massage and loves the essential oils.

O: No changes in ankle measurement since last session (10 inches). Beth remains excited about the massage and inquires about the essential oils. She was taught about the properties of the oils. (Orange oil has antiinflammatory, circulation enhancing, and calming effects. Lavender is an analgesic for muscle aches; it also has antibacterial, antifungal, antiviral, antiinflammatory, antidepressant, and calming properties, and it supports wound healing.) When the patient was asked whether she had a favorite flower or scent, she responded that it was rose. The nurse supervisor gave permission to include rose oil in the blend to support antiinfectious qualities and wound healing and to address depression. General massage was provided with a palliative focus, in addition to lymphatic drainage of the lower limbs with extra attention to the feet.

A: Beth enjoyed the massage and asked to take some of the lubricant with the essential oil blend. This was approved by the nurse supervisor. Beth was instructed in how to apply the lotion, especially to her feet. The ankle measurement after massage was 9 inches.

P: Check with nurse supervisor for recommendations. Repeat session with modifications as necessary. Spend more time on upper chest in areas of short muscles if tolerated.

Session 3

S: Beth reports that she feels better, but she can't really describe in what way. She says that she has more energy. The doctor's notes indicate improved wound healing on the foot. The nurse supervisor reports a reduction in late night eating.

O: Beth displays a reduction in labored movement (she walks faster with less shuffling). She is communicative, joking, and laughing. She got her hair done and had a manicure and a pedicure at the facility's salon. She is wearing some makeup. Need to put a cap on her head to protect her hair. No alteration in massage, but avoid the face because of the makeup. Good tolerance for massage focus on the pectoralis major, pectoralis minor, and anterior serratus; broad-based compression with passive movement and gentle lengthening were used. Ankle measurement before massage was $9^1/_2$ inches. Continued to use same essential oil blend. Extra attention was paid to the feet and lymphatic drainage of the legs.

A: Patient remains happy with massage and likes the pampering, indicating that it makes her feel special. Her mood remains elevated, and she has an improved, relaxed demeanor. No noticeable postural shift, but she indicates that her chest feels looser. She missed having her head and face massaged and says that she will schedule her beauty treatments after the massage. Ankle measurement after massage was 8 inches.

P: Continue with treatment plan.

Session 4

S: Beth reports that she is a bit tired and has a headache. She asks whether massage can help. The nurse supervisor indicates that Beth has a tension headache and approves the massage. Beth says that her chest was tender the day after the last massage.

O: Assessment indicates tender points in the upper trapezius, occipital, and frontalis muscles. Edema in the legs has improved but remains evident in the ankle measurement (9 inches). The feet are cold. General massage with a palliative focus was provided, with extra attention to the headache. Focal points were positional release in the upper trapezius and broad-based compression and local tissue stretching on the occipital and frontal muscles. No specific attention was paid to the thorax to allow the tenderness to dissipate. Continued to use the essential oil blend.

A: Ankle measurement was 8 inches post massage. The patient dozed through most of the massage and was a bit dizzy when she got up from the massage table. She was urged to double-check her glucose levels and report to the nurse supervisor for blood pressure monitoring and evaluation for possible hypoglycemia. She was walked to the nurse's station.

P: Check with the nurse supervisor before the next session.

Session 5

S: The nurse supervisor reports that the patient's medications have been adjusted, and that the patient had experienced mild hypoglycemic symptoms after the last massage. The doctor believes that the patient is responding well. He states that the need to reduce the medication dosage is a positive sign. Beth indicates that she feels better and her chest no longer hurts. Massage helped her headache at the last session. She also reports she has lost 3 to 5 lb. One of her new acquaintances also has diabetes and has had a partial foot amputation. However, she participates in the pool exercises and the support group.

O: Beth appeared well groomed and engaged in the massage. She asked questions about why it made her feel better. She was taught about the physiologic benefits of massage. She talked about exercise and described how tired it made her. She said the doctor and the nurse supervisor want her to join the pool exercise group and the diabetic support group, and she asked my opinion. I explained to her the importance of exercise and social support for well-being and healing. The ankle measurement was $8^1/_2$ inches before massage. The massage followed the treatment plan recommendations and the pattern of the previous session. The focus was again on the upper chest, and short soft tissue was addressed with compression. Passive movement and active assisted movement were used to stretch the tissue.

A: Beth participated in the process of lengthening short structures in the anterior thorax and reported that it felt good. She continued to explore the benefits of massage. Ankle measurement after massage was 8 inches.

P: Report the conversation about exercise and the patient's interest in the support groups to the nurse supervisor. Continue with general massage.

Evaluation of Progress

Beth showed a generalized positive response to massage. She was a bit more engaged in activities and more attentive to her appearance. She expressed more interest in essential oils, and this could become a focal point to engage her in a productive learning process. Her adaptive capacity is minimal, and any specific focus on increased motor tone or short tissue produced tenderness after the massage. There are some indications that massage is supporting the diabetes treatment (i.e., the medication adjustment and improved wound healing, as well as the interest in exploring exercise). The patient appears to enjoy the facility's amenities, such as the salon, social interaction, and massage, and she has referred some of her new friends for massage. The edema in the lower leg has diminished (the ankle measurement dropped from 10 inches to 8 inches). Some of the weight loss probably was water; regardless, the weight loss is positive.

Beth enjoys the rotation of massage therapists, and communication among the staff has been good. The nurse supervisor is supportive of adjunct methods (e.g., the use of essential oils) and appreciates that the massage therapist recognizes potential hypoglycemic symptoms and takes appropriate action. It was noted that the patient's late night eating was reduced on the day she received massage.

Recommendations for Future Massage Care

Continue with sessions two times per week for 6 weeks to support an exercise program. Maintain general focus and do not strain the patient's adaptive capacity. If the patient participates in an exercise program, reward her by continuing massage two times per week but indicate that the sessions would be reduced to once a week if she does not comply with the exercise regimen. Because Beth really enjoys the massage, the reward system may act as a positive reinforcement.

Perspective of the Massage Therapist

Multiple therapists (two women and one man) worked with Beth. She most enjoyed working with the male therapist and occasionally flirted a bit but not to the extent of concern. She was more comfortable with the older female therapist (age 36) than the younger one (age 22), but not in a way that would prevent continuing the rotation. Expectations must be realistic when working with Beth. Improvement can be achieved if she can become more engaged in her care, especially exercise, and if she can control her eating. The flirting with the male therapist appears playful, and the nurse supervisor indicates that Beth acts similarly with other male staff members. Beth's massage sessions are not physically taxing, and the massage sessions are basic. It is important not to become bored with the repetitive nature of the sessions. The general approach to massage will remain palliative and aimed at condition management. Aggressive therapeutic change methods are not indicated in this case; the patient really likes to be pampered.

Some frustration developed among the therapists when the charting was not sufficiently comprehensive to support continuing care. At times Beth had to explain the nature of the previous session. This situation needs to be addressed.

CASE STUDY 4: HEPATITIS C AND AMPUTATION

Similar Conditions

Other forms of hepatitis and liver disease, physical trauma, amputation, and use of a prosthesis.

The Case

Steven, age 34, was involved in a serious motorcycle accident 10 months ago. He suffered a concussion and was in a coma for 10 days, and his left wrist was broken. He has large avulsion wounds on his back and left thigh, and his right leg was crushed, requiring an above-the-knee amputation. In the course of treatment for the accident, Steven was found to have hepatitis C, which could have been acquired from a variety of sources. He currently is undergoing physical therapy to acclimate him to the amputation and to use of a prosthesis, as well as to resolve a residual balance problem from the concussion. There is some indication of an additional closed head injury that has resulted in a diminished ability to control mood, particularly anger. He is improving at a slow but steady rate.

Steven has generalized muscle aching as a result of his work in physical therapy and the scar tissue pulling in the healing wounds. The area of amputation is tender to deep palpation. Phantom limb pain occurs occasionally but is diminishing. The medical team is trying to reduce Steven's use of pain medication, and massage is indicated as a pain management method. Massage is also indicated for increasing scar tissue pliability.

Steven has the support of a wife, one daughter who is 8 years old, and a network of friends. Although he has lived life hard and has not been consistent with a healthy lifestyle in the past, the accident has had the effect of motivating him to approach life in a more productive way. He is in school as part of an occupational retraining program and is committed to rehabilitation and returning to an active lifestyle. He is aware of the implications of having hepatitis C; he has completed a substance abuse program and is active in a support group. His liver shows signs of involvement, but he seems to be responding to treatment and lifestyle changes.

HEPATITIS C

Research

Hepatitis C is an inflammation of the liver caused by infection with the hepatitis C virus. Hepatitis C infection occurs in approximately 1 in 70 to 100 people worldwide. Hepatitis infections can also be caused by the hepatitis A and hepatitis B viruses. Hepatitis is contagious and is transmitted in body fluids.

Hepatitis C is one of the most common causes of chronic liver disease, such as chronic liver infection, cirrhosis, and liver cancer. Hepatitis C is a major cause of liver transplantation.

- ***Massage implications:*** Hepatitis C is a contagious disease, and Standard Precautions are necessary. Gloves may need to be worn during the massage.

Risk Factors. Risk factors for hepatitis C include the following:

- Received a blood transfusion before July, 1992
- Has received blood, blood products, or solid organs from a donor with hepatitis C
- Has tattoos or body piercings (if Standard Precautions were not implemented)
- Has injected street drugs or shared a needle with someone with hepatitis C
- Has been on long-term kidney dialysis

- Has had frequent workplace contact with blood (e.g., a healthcare worker)
- Has had sex with multiple partners
- Has had sex with a person with hepatitis C
- Has shared personal items (e.g., toothbrushes, razors) with someone who has hepatitis C
- Was born to a mother who had hepatitis C

Symptoms. Many people who are infected with hepatitis C do not have symptoms. The disease often is detected during blood tests for a routine physical or other medical procedure. If the infection has been present for many years, the liver may be damaged. Most symptoms of hepatitis C are related to liver damage and include the following:

- Jaundice
- Pain in the upper right abdomen
- Loss of appetite
- Nausea and vomiting
- Low-grade fever
- Pale or clay-colored stools
- Fatigue
- Dark urine
- Itching
- Ascites (swelling of the abdomen)

- ***Massage implications:*** Comfort care and symptom management are possible with palliative massage. Use extreme caution for intensity and duration to avoid straining adaptive capacity. A slight potential exists that massage may help manage systemic inflammation; how this would affect the liver is questionable. Massage applied correctly, without straining adaptive capacity, will not harm the patient and might help somewhat.

Diagnosis. Medical tests done to diagnose hepatitis C include the following:

- Hepatitis virus serology
- Elevated liver enzymes
- Liver biopsy (shows chronic inflammation)

Treatment. Hepatitis C cannot be cured. Some patients with hepatitis C benefit from treatment with interferon (IFN) alpha or a combination of IFN alpha and ribavirin.

IFN alpha is given by injection just under the skin and has a number of side effects including flulike symptoms, headache, fever, fatigue, loss of appetite, nausea, vomiting, depression, and thinning of the hair. Treatment with IFN alpha may also interfere with the production of white blood cells and platelets.

Ribavirin is a capsule taken twice daily, and the major side effect is severe anemia (low red blood cells). Ribavirin also causes birth defects, and women should avoid pregnancy during and for 6 months after treatment.

Rest may be recommended during the acute phase of the disease, when the symptoms are most severe. All patients with hepatitis C should be immunized against hepatitis A and hepatitis B.

People with hepatitis C should avoid any substances toxic to the liver, including alcohol. Even moderate amounts of alcohol speed up the progression of hepatitis C, and alcohol reduces the effectiveness of treatment. People with hepatitis C should also be careful not to take vitamins, nutritional supplements, or over-the-counter medications without first discussing them with a doctor, because metabolizing these substances strains the liver.

AMPUTATION

Nearly every amputee feels quite depressed immediately after the surgery, except possibly those who have suffered intense pain for a period just before the amputation. This depression usually is replaced early by a will to resume an active life. Amputation results in a disabling condition. However, with modern prostheses and treatment methods, people who have had an amputation can do many of the things they could before the amputation.

- ***Massage implications:*** Massage can help maintain circulation and manage scar tissue development. It also can help regulate mood.

Note: Over the past few years, the International Standards Organization (ISO) has developed a standard method of describing amputations and prostheses that is being adapted worldwide. The term *transfemoral* now is used instead of "above the knee" to designate an amputation between the knee and the hip joint. This term has been adopted to avoid confusion with disarticulation at the hip and amputations through the pelvis. Also, use of the term *stump* for the part of the limb that is left after amputation came into question. However, because the English language has no synonym for the word *stump,* the ISO has continued to use that term.

- ***Massage implications:*** It is important to use the acceptable terminology and to be comfortable when discussing the amputation.

Amputations are caused by accidents, disease, and congenital disorders.

A congenital disorder or defect of a limb that is present at birth is not an amputation, but rather a lack of development of part or all of a limb. Sometimes amputation of part of a deformed limb or other surgery may be desirable before an artificial limb is applied.

The first surgical step in amputation is isolating the supplying artery and vein to prevent hemorrhage. The muscles are transected, and finally the bone is sawed through with an oscillating saw. Skin and muscle flaps are then transposed over the stump. Occasionally appliances used to attach a prosthesis are attached to the stump.

Surgeons preserve as much length as possible in thigh amputations because a longer stump provides better control over the prosthesis. Experienced surgeons avoid leaving unnecessary skin and muscle.

The dressing applied by the surgeon is either rigid (usually made of plaster-of-Paris) or soft (ordinary cotton bandaging). When a rigid dressing is used, it is left on for 10 to 14 days, during which time most of the healing has taken place. When the soft dressing is used, elastic bandages are used soon after surgery to aid circulation. The bandages are removed and reapplied throughout the day. Regardless of the type of dressing used, exercises are extremely important to prevent tightening of the muscles (primarily the hip flexors in transfemoral amputations) and contractures, which can affect the use of a prosthesis. Positioning that would shorten tissue at the hip needs to be avoided, such as propping the stump up on a pillow when lying down or propping it on the crutch handle when standing.

- ***Massage implications:*** Massage can manage tissue shortening and contracture. Bolstering can be used as necessary during massage, because the amount of time the limb is in the shortened position is insignificant. Bolstering the stump to facilitate lymphatic drainage is appropriate.

In general, the earlier a prosthesis is fitted, the better it is for the individual. One of the most difficult problems facing a person with an amputation and the treatment team is edema, or swelling of the stump. Edema is present to some extent in all cases, which makes fitting and wearing the prosthesis difficult. Elastic bandages or special sleeves are used to prevent or control edema when the prosthesis is not being worn. The person is taught the proper technique for bandaging during rehabilitation. Edema develops rapidly when the stump is left unbandaged, therefore replacing the bandage without delay is very important.

At least three times a day, the elastic bandage should be removed and the stump massaged vigorously for 10 to 15 minutes. The bandage then is immediately reapplied.

- ***Massage implications:*** The stump typically remains in the compression bandage during a massage session. If the massage is timed so that it occurs while a stump is unbandaged for circulation, the massage therapist can provide massage and lymphatic drainage to the stump. The stump then should be immediately rewrapped.

Some people with amputations experience the phenomenon of phantom limb; that is, they feel the body part that is no longer there. These individuals can sense an itch or an ache or can feel as if they are moving the missing part. This phenomenon seems to arise from a neural map the brain has of the body, which sends information to the rest of the brain about limbs regardless of their existence. In many cases the phantom limb phenomenon aids adaptation to a prosthesis, because it permits the person to experience proprioception of the prosthetic limb. In other cases, pain is quite severe and becomes problematic.

- ***Massage implications:*** Occasionally the source of the phantom limb pain can be traced to trigger point activity in the stump.

Massage can identify the referred pain pattern, and trigger point methods can be used to treat the condition.

People with amputations can develop ulcerating skin, infections, or local pain. Stumps can lack a durable surface that can withstand the shear forces created by walking with a prosthesis. The situation may be improved by adjusting the fit of the prosthesis; however, local soft tissue enhancement and skin resurfacing frequently are required.

- ***Massage implications:*** Massage can support various procedures to make the stump as functional as possible. General massage of the area can help increase circulation, control edema, and manage associated muscle pain and compensation patterns.

Fitting a prosthesis as soon after surgery as possible helps control edema. Fitting and alignments are difficult procedures that require a great deal of skill on the part of the prosthetist, as well as patience and cooperation from the patient. During fitting and alignment of the first prosthesis, the prosthetist must train the person in the basic principles of walking. Fitting affects alignment, alignment affects fitting, and both affect comfort and function. Extensive training is provided later by the physical therapist.

- ***Massage implications:*** Massage can be used to manage gait reflexes and muscle activation sequences to make rehabilitation as efficient as possible.

A transfemoral prosthesis has four major parts: the socket, the knee system, the shank, and the foot-ankle system. The socket fits onto the stump; it must not restrict circulation, yet it cannot be loose. Most sockets for transfemoral prostheses cover the entire stump.

A patient who is overweight will have significantly more difficulty with fitting and learning to use a prosthesis, especially a transfemoral prosthesis. Weight management and an appropriate exercise program are especially important for a person using a prosthesis.

- ***Massage implications:*** The professionals who fit and train patients to use prostheses are highly skilled. Massage therapists must take care to avoid interfering with the process and must make sure they are clear on the appropriate compensation patterns required for use of a prosthesis. The massage therapist should learn as much as possible about the individual rehabilitation program for a patient with an amputation. Any massage lubricant used needs to be cleaned off completely after massage is applied to the stump and before it is rewrapped.

Medical Assessment, Diagnosis, and Treatment Orders

Steven is 34 years old, 6′2″ tall, and weighs 205 lb. He has a muscular build that has atrophied somewhat since the accident. He is recovering his strength and stamina in rehabilitation. He has a history of substance abuse, including alcohol and various recreational drugs, and is tattooed over a large part of his body. He is receiving pegylated IFN alpha and ribavirin to treat hepatitis C, and he has experienced flulike symptoms and hair loss. He is being monitored for anemia. Medication therapy is scheduled to stop to see whether Steven has a sustained response to treatment. He is also taking an antidepressant (Celexa, a selective serotonin reuptake inhibitor [SSRI]) to regulate mood, and it seems to be helping him manage his anger and frustration.

The patient suffered multiple severe injuries in a motorcycle crash. The avulsion wounds were slow to heal, and scar tissue is extensive. The broken wrist healed well. Currently rehabilitation is focusing on helping the patient acclimate to a prosthesis for a transfemoral amputation, as well as a vestibular problem that is causing balance issues.

Massage is indicated for management of general pain and stiffness. The massage therapists should wear gloves if their hands have any broken skin. Avoid any areas of broken skin on the patient. Always observe all skin before massaging the area. Gradually increase pressure over the course of the sessions to identify the optimum pressures to reduce muscular aching. Do not specifically target fluid movement except to areas of amputation, to reduce strain on the liver. Provide massage once a week for 60 minutes (the frequency can be increased if positive results are noted). Do not specifically target gait reflexes or muscle activation sequences; these aspects are being addressed in physical therapy. Report the results of massage to the physical therapist.

Massage-Specific Assessment

Massage is limited to physical therapy treatment orders (i.e., general full body massage). Use scar tissue techniques on the thigh and back. Include the area of amputation for circulation enhancement and lymphatic drainage. No specific postural or muscle testing assessment was performed. Observation indicated elevated shoulders and forward head, likely from use of a wheelchair and crutches. The soft tissue palpates as dense and stiff with atrophy in the thighs and calves. Moderate bogginess and signs of inflammation are present in the amputation area. Specific tender points are identified in the vastus medialis and rectus femoris that refer phantom knee pain. Tenderness is identified in the left forearm and elbow, which may be related to the broken wrist and the reflex relationship between the right leg and left arm. Scar tissue on the left thigh and the back is adhered and stiff and is pulling on adjacent tissue.

Hangnails are noted on both hands, and one is bleeding. A blister is present on the left palm. Do not massage the hands until these conditions heal. Steven is loud and abrupt when talking. He was observed kicking an exercise ball when he became frustrated with a balancing exercise, but he then calmed himself down. He indicates that he wants deep pressure during the massage. He is informed that pressure levels will be applied as deeply as is safe, but that his medication can cause tissue changes, which may influence the level of pressure used.

Clinical Reasoning Process

Steven is a large man who is experiencing many challenges, including trauma; withdrawal from substance abuse; and chronic, contagious liver disease. He is having to adjust to a disability, change occupation, and manage what appear to be the residual effects of a closed head injury, including a balance problem and difficulty with mood regulation. He is taking multiple medications. It is hoped that soon the drugs for the hepatitis C will no longer be needed. The SSRI he is taking can be synergistically influenced during massage, and his response needs to be monitored. The postural and walking muscles are altered in tone and function because of the amputation and learning to use the prosthesis, as well as a wheelchair and crutches.

The treatment orders for general full body massage with approaches to increase the pliability of scar tissue initially are appropriate to see how the patient responds. As rehabilitation continues, various aspects of the kinetic chain can be introduced.

The immune system is challenged, therefore caution is necessary to protect Steven from undue exposure to infection. As always, the massage therapist must maintain Standard Precautions and should not work with the patient if the therapist has a contagious condition that could spread through casual contact, such as an upper respiratory infection.

Treatment Plan Development

Long-term goals: Support rehabilitation and immune function. Increase pliability of connective tissue in scar formation.

Short-term goals: Reduce aching and pain and support reduction in dosage of pain medication.

Massage therapist's objectives: Increase parasympathetic dominance and support pain management treatment. Support and maintain pliable scar formation.

Methods to be used: General massage protocol, modified to not specifically influence blood and lymph circulation except at amputation. Scar tissue management protocol.

Frequency and duration: Once a week for 60 minutes.

Measurement of progress: Pain scale of 1 to 10. Skinfold measurement in scars.

Date of reassessment: 8 weeks.

SOAP Charting

Session 1

S: The patient reports that he is sore in the shoulders, back, calf, and foot. The scar on his back is pulling and itching. His hands still have open wounds and need to be avoided.

O: No significant changes since the assessment session. Pain rating of 8. Stump appears red and palpates warm. Scar tissue does not lift from underlying tissue. Full body massage was provided, but the hands and inflamed areas of the stump were avoided. Sustained tension force was applied to the scars. Inhibiting pressure was applied to trigger points referring phantom pain in the right leg. Moderate compressive force was used during massage. No stretching was done other than local application to scar tissue.

A: The patient asked for more pressure. He was informed that it will be increased slowly to determine tissue tolerance. Steven indicated that it felt great to have the scars worked on. His shoulders and back feel better. The pain rating was reduced to 4 except in the stump area and the left wrist. Pliability increased slightly in the scar tissue.

P: Assess for tissue damage. If none is present, increase compressive force to the next level for depth of pressure during general massage. Assess scar tissue for pliability; if possible, add bend force to tension forces.

Session 2

S: The physical therapist reports no adverse affects from massage. Pain reduction lasted overnight. Sleep improved. The physical therapist approved an increase in the depth of pressure. Continue to follow treatment plan; avoid stump and hands. Steven indicates that he liked the massage and wants more massage on the scars. His back hurts.

O: Anterior thorax tissues are short with taut structures in the posterior thorax, especially between the scapulae. Evidence of inflammation on the stump. Scar tissue barely lifts, and burns when it does. Pain rating of 8. Repeat previous session with increased pressure to consistently address second muscle layer. Broad-based compression and gliding with no friction. No shaking or rocking. Sustain tension force into scars using direct and indirect application (into and out of bind).

A: Histamine response in scar tissue. Trigger points remain and refer phantom pain but responded to inhibiting pressure. Patient liked deeper pressure and asked that method be repeated or sustained in painful areas. Steven reports that his back feels looser. Pain rating of 4.

P: Repeat session, increasing intensity of scar tissue management.

Session 3

S: No adverse response to massage. Continue treatment plan. Physical therapist reports hearing from patient that the scars are itching and he has low back aches. He has asked for more pressure.

O: Pain rating of 8. Assessment indicates psoas shortening. Ask permission to do psoas release at the hip and not through abdomen (approved) and increase general pressure levels. Inhibiting pressure used just above the psoas' distal attachment, where it crosses the pubic bone with the iliacus. Bind remains in scar tissue. Attempted bending force but relied mostly on sustained tension force in various directions. General body massage.

A: Patient reports that his low back still hurts, but the rest feels better. Scars are itchy (histamine response). Pain rating of 4.

P: Discuss low back pain with the physical therapist. Continue with treatment plan.

Session 4

S: The physical therapist is aware of the patient's low back pain and indicates that the cause appears to be degenerative joint function at L3 to L5, with the potential for disk involvement. This condition likely existed before the accident but is aggravated by the rehabilitation and balance issues. The psoas and quadratus lumborum are providing necessary stabilization for the lumbar spine, therefore the shortening is functional and must be addressed sequentially. Inhibition near the attachment reduces tone enough for slight symptom relief. More direct access through the abdomen could reduce motor tone enough that stability would be compromised. As core stability is restored during rehabilitation, the back pain should resolve. The massage should continue to focus on general comfort measures, pain management, and scar tissue pliability. Use a counterirritant ointment on the low back during massage and teach the patient how to use the ointment.

O: Patient reports pain rating of 7 except for low back, which is an 8. Explained to patient why massage would not specifically address low back pain at this time (see explanation in S) but would address pain management in general, and that an ointment would be used to stimulate other nerve receptors and reduce the perception of pain. General massage was provided, and the patient's hands had healed, so they were included. A small wound caused by the prosthesis was noted on the stump, and the area was avoided. Scar tissue on the back is responding to treatment. Added skin rolling (bind force) to tension force. Scar on the leg remains adhered and binding. Tension force with shear force was used when possible. Additional bolster was used under abdomen when patient was in the prone position. Energy-based modalities were used on the low back.

A: Steven reports that he feels better. Pain rating of 4. His low back is stiff, but the pain is less intense. A 1/4-inch skinfold can be lifted in most sections of scar on the back. Cannot lift skin on thigh scar. Patient likes counterirritant ointment.

P: Continue with treatment plan.

Session 5

S: Steven reports that his low back is sore and stiff. Blister on the stump is worse; do not massage. The fit of the prosthesis is being adjusted. Scar on the leg is itchy. Pressure levels are good. Steven's wife indicates that he is less moody.

O: General pain rating of 6; low-back-specific rating of 8. Scar tissue pliability is improving on the back (can lift 1/4-inch skinfold in most areas). Thigh scar remains adhered and stiff. Low back pain is rated as 8. General massage included counterirritation ointment on low back. Continue force introduction (tension bind with shear) on back scar. Tension with shear force was used on thigh scar. Added massage to reflexology points on feet that correspond to low back.

A: Histamine response in scars. Scar on back continues to improve. Thigh scar really burned when worked and was itchy after massage. General pain rating of 3, specific low back pain rating of 6. Patient says he thinks his back will hurt again in the morning. Reinforce the importance of core exercises and of following the physical therapist's instructions.

P: Monitor wound on stump. Continue with treatment plan.

Evaluation of Progress

Over the five sessions, the pain rating after massage improved from a 4 to a 3, and the rating before massage improved from an 8 to a 6. The low back involvement has complicated issues and at this point is the main source of pain. The scar on the back has responded best; a skinfold of 1/4 to 1/2 inch can be lifted over the area. The thigh scar is more persistent but is beginning to soften. Steven has not missed a massage session and responds well to moderate pressure. No adverse responses to massage have been reported with regard to hepatitis. The patient's mood appears to have evened out, with fewer outbursts of anger (as reported by the physical therapist) and less moodiness at home (as reported by the wife). The extent to which the mood improvement can be directly attributed to massage is unclear. Steven likes the massage and cooperates well.

Recommendations for Future Massage Care

Massage should continue on a weekly basis indefinitely. The general stress management and pain reduction qualities of massage support Steven as he manages both chronic hepatitis C and the lingering effects of the accident. Massage can continue to normalize scar tissue and manage the soft tissue discomfort even after physical therapy is complete. Massage can also support prosthesis use by managing compensation changes in gait.

Perspective of the Massage Therapist

The massage therapist wants to do more to address the low back pain than was indicated in the original treatment plan. The low back pain developed after the treatment plan was implemented. In addition, the physical therapist had a better understanding of the entire process than the massage therapist and by regulating the massage interaction prevented a more serious development. This appeared to frustrate the massage therapist until she understood the condition better. To compensate for not being able to address the cause of the pain directly, the massage therapist used indirect methods such as reflexology and energy-based approaches.

Steven was easy to work with and would inform the massage therapist about any areas to avoid that could transmit hepatitis. The scar tissue change will continue to be slow but progressive, and care needs to be taken not to overtreat, rush the response, or cause any tissue damage. The main points for the massage therapist are to implement change very slowly and maintain the focus on stress and pain management.

CASE STUDY 5: KNEE REPLACEMENT, DRUG ADDICTION, PAIN AND RESTLESS LEG, AND ARTHRITIS

Replacement of the knee joint is a surgical procedure in which a painful, damaged, or diseased knee joint is replaced with an artificial joint (prosthesis).

Similar Conditions

Hip replacement, various locations for degenerative joint disease (DJD), pain management, and addiction.

The Case

Mrs. Freeman, a 56-year-old woman, was in an auto accident at age 32. He left leg was severely damaged, especially her knee. Osteoarthritis and degenerative joint disease have developed. Over the years, the degeneration has reached the point that the pain is debilitating and treatment options have been exhausted. The final option was a total knee joint replacement. The patient is 5′6″ tall and weighs 160 lb, with fat distribution in the hips and thighs. Although she typically is moderately active, she has become deconditioned because walking is so painful. For 3 months before surgery, she has participated in a conditioning program in a swimming pool to build up her strength to support rehabilitation after surgery. She also has been involved in a weight training program using resistance bands. She takes a high-quality multivitamin and mineral supplement. At night she takes an antiinflammatory analgesic/muscle relaxant to help her sleep (she also takes the drug during the day if she needs it). She is motivated and in good health for her age, with no indication of any disease of the cardiovascular or immune system or any other body system. She does have restless leg syndrome. She has received massage for many years to manage the knee and leg pain and the irritating sensations in her legs.

KNEE REPLACEMENT

The patient has traumatic and degenerative osteoarthritis with restless leg syndrome. These conditions have been treated with conservative measures (physical therapy and massage) and two medications, a skeletal muscle relaxant (Soma Compound with codeine) and carbamazepine (Tegretol). Because this treatment approach was unsuccessful, the patient is to have knee replacement surgery.

- ***Massage implications:*** Use caution with pressure to prevent bruising. Stay with the patient after the massage to make sure the person is not dizzy. Monitor for side effects and refer the patient to the medical staff if any occur. Massage can help constipation.

RESTLESS LEG SYNDROME

Research

Restless leg syndrome (RLS, or Ekbom syndrome) is characterized by painless, spontaneous, continuous leg movements associated with unpleasant sensations. These sensations, which have been described as tingling, pins and needles, crawling, itching, or pain, occur at rest and are relieved by movement. Sleep disturbance is common. More than one third of patients first experience these symptoms before the age of 10. Unfortunately, misdiagnosis (e.g., "growing pains" or attention deficit disorder) is common. Often the patient does not seek medical attention for the condition until after age 40, when the symptoms begin to progress.

RLS may occur in conjunction with a number of disorders:

- Abnormal iron metabolism (RLS may be associated with iron deficiency.)

- Uremia (RLS is a common complication of the neuropathy seen in kidney failure. Individuals who undergo dialysis are susceptible.)
- Diabetes mellitus (RLS may be an aspect of diabetic neuropathy.)
- Rheumatic disease (RLS is a common aspect of rheumatoid arthritis [RA]. It was found in 25% of patients with RA [compared to 4% percent of controls with osteoarthritis or seronegative arthropathy] and was associated with greater disease activity and severity.)
- Venous insufficiency (Varicose veins may cause RLS as a result of pressure on a nerve from a varicosity.)
- Genetic predisposition

Other possible causes of RLS include pregnancy, spinal stenosis, excess caffeine intake, hypoglycemia, and hypothyroidism.

Treatment. The discomfort of RLS may be relieved temporarily by massage, stretching, walking, or doing knee bends. Application of hot and cold hydrotherapy (e.g., a hot bath, a heating pad, a cold compress) also can relieve symptoms.

Medications. Drugs used in the treatment of RLS include the benzodiazepines, dopaminergic drugs, and opioids. Other drugs that may be useful include carbamazepine, clonidine, and propranolol.

Carbamazepine (Tegretol, Tegretol XR, Epitol) is an antiseizure medication. Because it interacts with a number of drugs, caution should be used in combining it with other medications. Carbamazepine also increases the metabolism (destruction) of the hormones in birth control pills and can reduce the effectiveness of birth control pills. Unexpected pregnancies have occurred in patients taking both carbamazepine and birth control pills. Carbamazepine should not be taken during pregnancy or while breast-feeding.

Side Effects. Side effects of carbamazepine include the following:

- Dangerously low red and white blood cell counts
- Severe skin reactions
- Serious liver abnormalities (e.g., hepatitis), resulting in jaundice
- Low sodium levels and thyroid abnormalities
- Minor, more common, side effects such as dizziness, unsteadiness, nausea, and vomiting

Soma Compound with codeine, a combination of carisoprodol, aspirin, and codeine, is used to treat muscle pain and stiffness. Some cautions exist for individuals who take this drug:

- The patient must not drink alcohol.
- The medication must be used cautiously if the patient also takes a blood thinner (e.g., Coumadin) or is being treated with methotrexate for arthritis or psoriasis.
- The medication may cause drowsiness. The patient should avoid taking other drugs that increase drowsiness (e.g., tranquilizers, sleeping pills, and cold or allergy medications).
- The medication may be habit forming and dangerous if taken in high doses.

Side effects that require referral of the patient to the medical staff include the following:

- Severe drowsiness
- Skin rash, hives
- Blood in the stool
- Itching
- Edema
- Ringing in the ears
- Slow heartbeat
- Seizures
- Trouble breathing
- Dizziness, especially when standing up, or fainting
- Constipation
- Nausea or vomiting
- Hiccups

- ***Massage implications:*** Remain with the patient after the massage and assist the person off the table if dizziness occurs. Monitor for side effects and refer the patient to the medical team if any are noticed.

NOTE: The patient became concerned that she was becoming dependent on the medication. She did experience withdrawal symptoms from Soma when the medication was discontinued in preparation for surgery. Aspirin has anticoagulant properties and also was stopped before surgery.

DRUG ADDICTION AND WITHDRAWAL

Mild withdrawal symptoms that can occur with discontinuation of Soma Compound with codeine include the following:

- Headache
- Nausea
- Stomach cramps
- Stomach disorder
- Flushing at times
- Feeling of dizziness when standing or sitting for a long time

The patient was given morphine for pain after surgery, and a narcotic-type pain medication (Ultram) was prescribed when she was released from the hospital.

Ultram is an opioid used to relieve moderate to moderately severe pain. Seizures have been reported as a rare side effect of treatment with Ultram. The risk of seizures may be increased in patients who have any of the following conditions:

- History of seizures or epilepsy
- Head injury
- Metabolic disorder
- Central nervous system infection
- Alcohol or drug withdrawal

Patients who take any of the following medications may also have a higher risk of seizures:

- Tricyclic antidepressants
- Monoamine oxidase inhibitors (MAOIs)
- Psychiatric medications
- Narcotic pain relievers

Ultram is in the Food and Drug Administration (FDA) pregnancy category C; this means that it is not known whether the drug is harmful to an unborn baby or whether it passes into breast milk. Patients over age 75 may be more likely to experience side effects from Ultram.

Symptoms of an Ultram overdose include difficulty breathing; shallow, weak breathing; and seizures.

Ultram may increase the effects of other drugs that cause drowsiness, including antidepressants, alcohol, antihistamines, pain relievers, anxiety medicines, seizure medicines, and muscle relaxants. Dangerous sedation, dizziness, drowsiness, or decreased breathing may occur if Ultram is taken with any of these medications. During treatment with Ultram, the patient should not take any over-the-counter medicines, including herbal products, without first talking to the doctor.

Possible serious side effects of Ultram include the following:

- An allergic reaction (difficulty breathing, closing of the throat, hives, and swelling of the lips, tongue, or face)
- Seizures

Other, less serious side effects may be more likely to occur, including:

- Dizziness, drowsiness, or headache
- Nervousness, tremor, or anxiety
- Nausea, vomiting, constipation, or diarrhea
- Itching, dry mouth, or sweating

Ultram is habit forming. Physical or psychological dependence (or both) can occur, and withdrawal effects are possible if the medication is stopped suddenly after prolonged or high-dose treatment.

- ***Massage implications:*** Monitor for side effects and refer the patient to the medical team if any are noted. Remain with the patient after the massage to assess for dizziness. Have the patient sit on the table until the person feels steady. Feedback mechanisms can be altered; adjust for pressure and stretching intensity. Ultram can be addictive.

As mentioned, Ultram is an opioid. Opioids commonly are prescribed because of their effective analgesic (pain relieving) properties. Many studies have shown that properly managed medical use of pain-killing drugs is safe and rarely causes addiction. When taken exactly as prescribed, opioids can be used to manage pain effectively. Side effects of opioids include mild dizziness, drowsiness, unclear thinking, constipation, and lowered blood pressure.

The use of opioids can cause three processes in the patient. The first is tolerance, in which higher and higher doses of the medication are required to produce the same effect. The second process is physical dependence, in which the body has become used to the drug and will produce withdrawal symptoms if the drug is discontinued. Withdrawal from opioids is extremely uncomfortable. It causes symptoms that resemble severe flu:

muscle and bone aches, chills, insomnia, involuntary leg movements, diarrhea, nausea, and vomiting. Although not fatal, opioid withdrawal usually requires treatment in a detoxification facility or careful tapering of the medication under a physician's supervision. The third process, after physical dependence, is addiction. Addiction is marked by cravings for the drug and compulsive use of the drug despite repeated, harmful consequences.

Opioids also can cause rebound pain. Rebound pain is pain that returns as the short-acting opioids wear off. Ironically, opioids also can cause changes in the nervous system that may actually heighten the perception of pain and make the patient feel more uncomfortable.

In some cases, opioids are essential drugs. Cancer patients, terminally ill patients, people recovering from surgery, and many others require these medications to function. Most people who take opioids do not become addicted, even if they become physically dependent

KNEE REPLACEMENT

Mrs. Freeman is no longer taking Tegretol, and Ultram seems to be controlling the RLS symptoms. She was released from the hospital 2 weeks ago, and massage has been approved for pain management, postoperative edema and residual swelling, scar tissue management, and support for rehabilitation, with cautions for range-of-motion activities and blood clots. Warning signs of possible blood clots in the legs include:

- Increasing pain in the calf
- Tenderness or redness above or below the knee
- Increasing swelling in the calf, ankle, and foot

Warning signs that a blood clot has traveled to the lungs include:

- Sudden increased shortness of breath
- Sudden onset of chest pain
- Localized chest pain with coughing

- ***Massage implications:*** Blood clots are medical emergencies. Refer the patient to the medical staff immediately.

Infection Control. Infection can occur after any type of surgery. To minimize the potential for infection at the time of surgery, antibiotics are given before the procedure and for 1 to 2 days afterward. Infection that develops after total knee replacement is of special concern because the prosthetic components can collect pathogens These components have no blood supply, and this makes them susceptible to infection.

Infection after total knee replacement surgery most often is caused by bacteria that entered the bloodstream during dental procedures, urinary tract infections, or skin infections. These bacteria can lodge around the knee replacement and cause an infection. *After joint replacement surgery, antibiotics should be taken before any dental work or surgical procedure that could allow bacteria to enter the bloodstream.*

The risk of infection persists for as long as the knee replacement device is in place. Once the protective outer "skin" of the bone of the femur and tibia has been cut off to mount the artificial bearing surfaces, the inside of those bones is vulnerable to infectious agents in the bloodstream. Warning signs of a possible infection include:

- Persistent fever (over 100° F orally)
- Shaking chills.
- Increasing redness, tenderness, or swelling of the knee wound
- Drainage from the knee wound
- Increasing knee pain with both activity and rest

- ***Massage implications:*** Refer the patient to the medical staff immediately if any of these signs develop.

Wound Care. Stitches or staples are used along the wound or sutures are placed beneath the skin on the front of the knee. The stitches or staples are removed several weeks after surgery. Any sutures beneath the skin do not require removal. The patient should avoid soaking the wound in water until it has thoroughly sealed and dried. A bandage may be placed over the wound to prevent irritation from clothing or support stockings. No lotions, vitamin E, essential oils, or other ointments should be used on the wound.

Diet. Some loss of appetite is common for several weeks after surgery. A balanced diet, often including an iron supplement, is important to promote proper tissue healing and restore muscle strength.

Activity. Exercise is a critical component of recovery from total knee replacement, particularly during the first few weeks after surgery. The patient should be able to resume most normal activities of daily living within 3 to 6 weeks after surgery. Some pain with activity and at night is common for several weeks. An activity program should include the following:

- A graduated walking program to increase mobility slowly (initially done inside the home and later outside)
- Resumption of normal household activities (e.g., sitting, standing, and walking up and down stairs)
- Specific exercises to restore movement and strengthen the knee, performed several times a day. The patient should be able to perform the exercises without help after a physical therapist provides instruction or after the patient completes a rehabilitation program.

Driving usually begins when the knee can bend enough to allow the patient to get into and sit comfortably in a vehicle and when muscle control allows an adequate reaction time for braking and acceleration. Most patients resume driving about 4 to 6 weeks after surgery.

Avoiding Problems after Surgery. A fall during the first few weeks after surgery can damage the replacement knee and may result in a need for further surgery. Stairs are a particular hazard until the knee is strong and mobile. A cane, crutches, a walker, handrails, or someone to assist the patient are needed until the patient's balance, flexibility, and strength have improved. The surgeon and the physical therapist will determine the assistive aids that will be needed after surgery and when the use of those aids can be safely discontinued.

More than 90% of those who have knee replacement surgery have a major reduction in knee pain and improved mobility. Rehabilitation exercises speed up the process. Long-term rehabilitation goals include a range of motion of 100 to 120 degrees of knee flexion, mild or no pain with walking or other functional activities, and independence in all activities of daily living.

Rehabilitation is a progressive program developed by the physical therapist. It is important that each exercise be done in sequence, because the specific exercise prepares the knee and related soft tissue structures for the one that follows. Warming up for postoperative knee exercises is important, because it makes the exercise easier, more productive, and less painful. It is all the more beneficial in patients with less flexible muscles. Warming up is essential to good results, and warm-up movements can be supplemented with massage.

The following sequence of rehabilitative exercises is commonly used on the surgical knee.

Week 1

Exercise 1: Seated upright, with the feet out in front, flat on the floor, contract the thigh muscles. The heels should be raised approximately 15 cm above the floor, with the toes pulled toward the knees. Hold this contraction for 5 seconds, then lower the heels slowly to the floor. Remember to keep the knee locked at all times.

Repeat ×10

Add 5 repetitions each day.

Exercise 2: Seated upright, with the feet out in front, flat on the floor, hold a soft ball or rolled towel between the knees. Squeeze the ball with both knees and hold for 5 seconds.

Repeat ×10

Week 2

Repeat the exercises from week 1, but add a light weight to exercise 1 and increase the duration of exercise 2 to 10 seconds.

Exercise 1: Seated upright, with the feet out in front, hold a rolled towel beneath the knee, with the heel resting on the floor. Tighten the thigh muscles and push the back of the knee into the towel. Hold for 3 seconds.

Repeat ×20

Exercise 2: In a seated position, hang the legs off a table. Using the thigh muscles, straighten the knee. Hold for 3 seconds.

Repeat ×20

Sets ×3

Exercise 3: Balance on one leg, with the knee bent, and hold for 30 seconds.

Repeat ×6

Week 3

Repeat the exercises from week 2, but add an ankle weight in exercise 2. For exercise 3, close the eyes or throw a ball against the wall and catch it.

Exercise 1: Wall slide. With the back against a wall and the feet shoulder width apart and approximately 18 inches out in front, slowly lower the body by bending the knees. Keep the back against the wall at all times. Then, using the thigh muscles, straighten the knees.

Repeat ×15

Sets ×5

Exercise 2: Stand on one leg, bend the knee to approximately 25 degrees, then slowly straighten the knee.

Repeat ×10

Sets ×10

Week 4

Unassisted walking for short distances

Daily life skills

Progress measurements include:

- Can go up and down stairs with no pain or stiffness (going down is more difficult than going up)
- Can bends the knee enough to pull on socks and shoes
- Can sit for an hour or so and then get up without a sense of stiffness in the knees (This may take a year or more to achieve!)
- Can get into and out of a car without having to grab the foot to force it to bend enough to clear the door
- Can stand up from a low chair or the toilet without muscle difficulty
- Can lock the knee joint straight so that standing for long periods is possible
- Can sit comfortably with the legs crossed

- ***Massage implications:*** Patients may feel some numbness in the skin around the incision. Some stiffness may be felt, particularly with excessive bending activities. Improvement of knee motion is a goal of total knee replacement, but restoration of full motion is uncommon. Never force range of motion. The motion of the knee replacement device after surgery is predicted by the motion of the knee before surgery. Most patients can expect to straighten the replaced knee nearly fully and to bend the knee sufficiently to go up and down stairs and get into and out of a car. Kneeling usually is uncomfortable but is not harmful. Occasionally, the person may feel some soft clicking of the metal and plastic when bending the knee or walking. These differences often diminish with time, and most patients find them minor annoyances compared to the pain and limited function they had before the surgery. Massage can reduce stiffness and aching and support rehabilitation. It typically takes a year before sustainable results are observed.

Indications for knee replacement include the following:

- Knee pain that has failed to respond to conservative therapy, medication, injections, and physical therapy for 6 months or longer
- Knee pain that limits or prevents activities of importance to the patient
- Decreased knee function caused by arthritis or degenerative joint disease
- Sleep disturbances caused by knee pain
- Some tumors involving the knee

Knee joint replacement usually is not recommended for individuals who have a terminal disease, are morbidly obese, have paralysis of the quadriceps muscles, or have severe peripheral vascular disease or neuropathy that affects the knee.

Risk Factors. Risk factors involved in knee replacement surgery include the following:

- Blood clots in the legs (deep vein thrombosis [DVT])
- Blood clot in the leg that breaks loose and goes to the lungs (embolus)
- Pneumonia
- Infection that results in removal of the joint
- Loosening or dislocation of the prosthesis

People who have a prosthetic device, such as an artificial joint, need to take special precautions against infection and receive prophylactic antibiotics before dental work or any invasive procedure.

Surgery. General anesthesia is used for knee replacement surgery. The orthopedic surgeon makes an incision over the affected knee, and the patella (knee cap) is moved out of the way. The ends of the two bones of the knee (the femur and the tibia) are cut to fit the prosthesis and to provide better adhesion of the prosthesis. The undersurface of the patella is cut to allow for placement of an artificial component.

The two parts of the prosthesis are implanted onto the ends of the femur, the tibia, and the patella using a special bone cement. A small drainage tube is placed during surgery to help drain excess fluids from the joint area. After surgery, the leg typically is placed in a continuous passive motion (CPM) device. This is a mechanical device that flexes (bends) and extends (straightens) the knee to prevent it from getting stiff. The CPM helps speed recovery and reduces postoperative pain, bleeding, and infection. Patients are encouraged to start moving and walking as early as the first day after surgery.

Moderate pain after surgery is expected and typically is treated with injections of narcotic medications for the first 3 days. The surgical pain gradually diminishes, and by the third day after surgery, oral medications are prescribed to control pain. Antibiotics are given to reduce the risk of infection.

To prevent diminished circulation in the legs, the patient wears antiembolism stockings or inflatable pneumatic compression stockings. When in bed, it is important for the patient to bend and straighten the ankles frequently to prevent the formation of blood clots. The patient should cough and breathe deeply to prevent lung collapse and pneumonia. A Foley catheter may be inserted during the surgery to allow monitoring of kidney function and the patient's hydration level. The catheter usually is removed on the second or third day after surgery.

Knee replacement surgery relieves pain in more than 90% of patients, and most need no assistance walking after recovery. Most prostheses last 10 to 20 years, after which they may loosen and require corrective surgery.

Rehabilitation. The hospital stay after knee replacement surgery generally is 4 to 5 days. However, the total recovery period varies from 2 to 3 months to a year. Walking and range-of-motion exercises are started immediately after surgery. The physical therapy initiated in the hospital continues after discharge until the patient's strength and motion return. Contact sports generally should be avoided, but low-impact activities (e.g., swimming and golf) usually are possible after full recovery from surgery. Some patients may need to use crutches or a walker for a few weeks or even for a few months after surgery.

- ***Massage implications:*** Massage can help manage some symptoms of postexercise soreness, as well as compensation patterns caused by gait changes that affect the rest of the body.

Medical Assessment, Diagnosis, and Treatment Disorders

Mrs. Freeman is a 56-year-old 5′6″ tall, 160-lb female. An auto accident at age 32 resulted in the left leg and knee injury. The patient has traumatic and degenerative osteoarthritis with restless leg syndrome. These conditions have been treated with conservative measures (physical therapy and massage) and two medications, a skeletal muscle relaxant (Soma Compound with codeine) and carbamazepine (Tegretol). Because this treatment approach was unsuccessful, the patient is to have knee replacement surgery.

In the short term massage is indicated for pre and post surgical outcome and then will be used to support rehabilitation.

Massage-Specific Assessment

The patient had surgery 2 weeks ago. Previously, she had been a patient for 8 years for management of the aftereffects of a car accident, degenerative changes in the left leg, and restless leg syndrome. Previous massage methods targeted normalization of motor tone in the muscles and techniques to reduce guarding that limited range of motion. The left knee would develop swelling, which would be reduced but not eliminated by localized lymphatic drainage. Gait reflexes and muscle activation sequences were addressed in most sessions to support as much normal movement as possible. General massage methods included pain control measures.

Currently the skin around the incision is numb. The incision site is healing well and shows no signs of infection. Two areas have not yet fully closed; one is midincision, and the other is distal to the patella at the end of the incision. The scar tissue is fragile. Moderate postoperative edema remains around the left knee. Mobility is improving, but stiffness develops in the leg when the patient is inactive, especially at night. Postoperative exercise stiffness is present, particularly with bending activities. Left knee flexion is 90 degrees, and right knee flexion is 130 degrees. The vastus medialis (oblique portion) is not firing during knee extension on the left, and the vastus lateralis is dominant.

Pain in the replaced knee is significantly reduced and is mostly postoperative pain. The patient reports that her shoulder and forearms are stiff and aching from using the walker, and her low back aches. RLS symptoms range from mild to moderate.

Clinical Reasoning Process

This patient has been receiving massage for a period of time. The situation will alter during the post surgical period. It seems that general massage with cautions at the surgical site is prudent. It is important to support infection control.

Treatment Plan Development

Long-term goals: Support long-term exercise and flexibility program with chronic pain management.

Short-term goals: Support stress management and edema post surgery.

Massage therapist's objectives: Create measurable changes in range of motion and tissue pliability. Address breathing function and reduce sympathetic arousal. Manage compensation.

Methods to be used: General massage protocol with lymphatic drain. Do not work near incision until approved by physician (likely 7 to 10 days). Reduce pressure level on left leg and do not do range-of-motion or resistance activities with left knee until approved by physical therapist. Monitor for bruising related to medication and alter pressure levels as necessary. Lymphatic drainage for postoperative edema. Address shoulders and forearms and low back compensation patterns.

Frequency and duration: Massage two times per week for 45 minutes; increase frequency if indicated. Begin scar tissue management at session 5.

Measurement of progress: Pain scales and functions of daily living.

Date of reassessment: 6 weeks

Additional notes: Treatment plan is to be approved by the physical therapist. Check each session before implementing a specific release to confirm that it is appropriate in conjunction with progress in the physical rehabilitation program.

SOAP Charting

Session 1

S: Patient reports that she is generally restless and bored. Rehabilitation is going well. Physical therapist indicates that massage should target compensation and postoperative edema. Incision site is itchy. Arms, shoulders, and low back are stiff and aching. Psoas assesses short, and quadratus lumborum is tender to moderate pressure.

O: Patient indicated that on a pain scale of 1 to 10, the general aching and stiffness were a 7. Palpation suggested increased motor tone in the forearms, likely related to use of the walker. Localized edema at the surgical site and fascial binding in the lumbar area were noted. Observation and palpation indicated an upper chest breathing pattern with trigger point activity in the upper trapezius and pectoralis minor. A full body, general massage was provided with the following alterations: lymphatic drainage of the left leg, muscle energy methods and lengthening of the forearms and upper trapezius, and massage protocols to support effective breathing and active release of the forearms. Tension forces were applied to the lumbar fascia (myofascial release), psoas release was done at the distal attachment, and inhibitory pressure was applied to the quadratus lumborum (quadratus lumborum release).

A: Breathing function normalized, and the patient felt as if she could take a deep breath. General aching and stiffness were reduced to a pain rating of 4. No change was seen in the edema around the left knee.

P: Consult physical therapist for massage recommendations.

Session 2

S: Patient reports minor bruising on the forearms but says that the aching and stiffness are much improved. Intensity of physical therapy is resulting in some postexercise soreness. Incision site is itchy and pulling. Patient is not as generally restless, but RLS symptoms have increased, interrupting her sleep. No specific recommendations from physical therapist. Note from physical therapist indicates that scar tissue pulling can be addressed with gentle work about 3 inches from the incision. No indication of infection or blood clots.

O: Slight upper chest breathing. Minor bruising near the elbows bilaterally. Reduce pressure in area and maintain broad-based contact. Localized edema at the surgical site. Fascial binding in the lumbar area. Binding on lateral and medial sides of the left knee. Full body general massage was provided with the following alterations: lymphatic drainage of the left leg combined with scar tissue management using tension force on the skin on the lateral and medial aspects of the knee. Muscle energy methods and lengthening of the forearms and upper trapezius. Tension forces applied to the lumbar fascia (myofascial release).

A: Patient reports that pulling and itching at the incision site are much improved. Edema has been reduced by 25% (based on knee circumference measurements before and after massage).

P: Continue with treatment plan.

Session 3

S: Patient reports increased aching in the left leg. She has a tension headache and is irritable and tired.

O: Left calf palpates as taut, swollen, and possibly warm. (NOTE: These may be indications of a blood clot.) Patient was referred immediately to the physician for evaluation. She was hospitalized and given blood thinners as a precaution.

A: Patient's condition improved within 2 days, and she was discharged from the hospital. The condition probably developed because the patient had not been wearing compression stockings diligently.

P: Continue with treatment plan. Remain cautious for blood clot symptoms.

Session 4

NOTE: This session took place 7 days after the previous massage.

S: Patient is back on her rehabilitation schedule, with no adverse effects from the possible blood clot and preventive treatment. Patient has a tension headache (pain rating of 6) and a back ache. Incision is pulling and itchy, and her feet ache.

O: Slight upper chest breathing. Localized edema at the surgical site. Fascial binding in the lumbar area and psoas shortening. Full body general massage was provided with the following alterations: lymphatic drainage on the left leg combined with scar tissue management using tension force and bending force on the skin surrounding the knee (maintaining a distance of 1 inch from the incision). Inhibitory pressure applied to the distal attachments of the psoas, with lengthening and stretching (caution for deep pressure to the abdomen due to medication patient is taking). Inhibitory pressure applied to the quadratus lumborum, and increased focus on feet. Tension headache protocol.

A: Patient fell asleep during massage, after reporting that her headache was gone. Scar tissue is more mobile, and edema has been reduced by 50% (based on knee circumference measurement before and after massage). Her back still aches but is slightly better.

P: Discuss back pain with physical therapist and recommend evaluation for core strength.

Session 5

S: Physical therapist has added core exercises and indicates that massage should include muscle activation sequence assessment and intervention for hip extension and trunk flexion. Physical therapist also requests psoas release and indicates that access from the abdomen is appropriate. Massage therapist is to continue to address scar tissue development in the left knee; physical therapist indicates that the incision area is fully closed and stable and can be worked.

Patient indicates that she is beginning to notice sustained improvement and has progressed from using a walker to using a cane. RLS symptoms are minor, and pain is insignificant. Left knee feels stiff and fat. Patient has low back aches.

O: Patient appears more confident on the knee replacement, and gait is more symmetric. Slight edema in the left knee. Left knee has 100 degrees of flexion (good) but will not move final 10 degrees of extension. Left gastrocnemius is short, with trigger point activity in the midlateral aspect and bilaterally at attachments behind the knee. Likely residual guarding activity. Knee extension firing is limited. Will attempt to reduce guarding with sustained shaking and generalized kneading. Hip extension is lumbar (erector spinae) dominant bilaterally, with short hamstrings. Trunk flexion is poor, with straining and inability to perform. General massage will be provided, along with psoas release, broad-based, inhibitory compression on the hamstrings, and inhibitory pressure on the lumbar muscles during activation of gluteus maximus. Also scar tissue management and localized lymphatic drainage in the surgical area.

A: Low back pain has improved by 75% (based on the 1-10 pain scale) but likely was symptomatic, because trunk flexion firing did not improve. Hip extension is slightly better, with less activity in the lumbar muscles, but hamstrings would not reduce in motor tone. Gluteus maximus remains inhibited. Slight increase in vastus medialis oblique (VMO) firing with 5-degree increase in knee extension.

P: Discuss with physical therapist a change in the treatment plan from postoperative care to support of rehabilitation, specifically the addition of muscle activation sequence, gait reflexes, and kinetic chain function. Patient is showing signs of developing lower crossed syndrome.

Evaluation of Progress

One setback occurred with the incident of a possible blood clot, but progress related to massage did not seem to be affected. The patient is used to massage and has realistic expectations of benefits. Scar tissue management was appropriate, and the patient progressed from postoperative care to a therapeutic focus based on the rehabilitation program.

Recommendations for Future Massage Care

Massage that focuses on physical rehabilitation after surgery should continue during the active rehabilitation period at the same frequency and duration. The frequency then should be reduced to a maintenance schedule of once a week for 60 minutes (this was the preoperative schedule).

Perspective of the Massage Therapist

The patient and the massage therapist had a long-term professional relationship before the surgery. For the massage therapist, altering the professional interaction to be accountable to the physical therapist and physician during the active intervention and rehabilitation period was a challenge and required the massage therapist to relinquish some independent decision making. There could have been some concern that the blood clot somehow was caused by massage, but given the appropriateness of the massage application, this is unlikely. More likely, the massage therapist's quick action in recognizing the changes in the calf and immediately referring the patient prevented a more serious condition.

CASE STUDY 6: MIGRAINE HEADACHE, PREMENSTRUAL SYNDROME, AND PEPTIC ULCER

Similar Conditions

Cluster headaches, mood disorders related to hormone and neurotransmitter fluctuations, gastrointestinal problems.

The Case

Cherie, a 19-year-old female who is a college freshman, is interested in becoming a physician. She lives on campus in the dorm. She began experiencing migraine headaches at age 12 at the onset of menstruation. She typically has two serious headaches a month, one at midcycle, which seems to be triggered by hormonal changes during ovulation, and again just before menstruation. She also experiences premenstrual syndrome (PMS) symptoms, including edema, bloating, irritability, and fatigue. She does not participate in regular physical exercise, but she rides her bike often around campus and rides horses when she can.

Cherie's headaches are also triggered by monosodium glutamate (MSG). When she has a headache, she is particularly sensitive to bright light and most strong smells, especially the perfumed scents found in air fresheners, candles, and so on. She often has a tension headache before the onset of the migraine. The tension headache starts at the occipital base, with trigger point referred pain patterns in the muscles of mastication (chewing) and the sternocleidomastoid.

Over the past 3 months, the frequency and severity of her headaches have increased. The doctor suspects that the lack of control over her environment (smells, fumes, sound, light), changes in her sleep cycle, and increased stress levels are the cause. Cherie also was recently diagnosed and successfully treated for a peptic ulcer, probably caused by her use of over-the-counter pain medication.

PEPTIC ULCER

Research

A peptic ulcer is an erosion in the lining of the stomach or duodenum. A peptic ulcer in the stomach is called a *gastric ulcer.* Small ulcers may not cause any symptoms. Large ulcers can cause serious bleeding. Most ulcers occur in the first layer of the inner lining. A hole that goes all the way through is called a perforation of the intestinal lining; this is a medical emergency.

Causes and Risk Factors. Normally, the lining of the stomach and the small intestines is protected from the irritating acids produced in the stomach. For a variety of reasons, the protective mechanisms may become faulty, leading to a breakdown of the lining. This results in inflammation (gastritis) or an ulcer. The most common cause of stomach inflammation is infection with the bacterium *Helicobacter pylori* (*H. pylori*). This organism lives in the gastrointestinal (GI) tract of most people with peptic ulcers. Other factors that increase the risk of ulcer development include the following:

- Long-term use of aspirin, ibuprofen, or naproxen
- Excessive use of alcohol
- Smoking cigarettes and using tobacco
- Family history of ulcers
- Blood type O

It is not clear whether stress causes ulcers.

Symptoms. The symptoms of a peptic ulcer include the following:

- Abdominal pain (not always present)
- Nausea, vomiting
- Weight loss
- Fatigue
- Heartburn, indigestion, belching, hiccups
- Chest pain
- Vomiting of blood
- Bloody or dark, tarry stools

Diagnosis. Medical tests done to diagnose a peptic ulcer include the following:

- An upper GI examination: A series of x-rays taken after the patient drinks a contrast substance (barium) that delineates the intestinal structures.
- Esophagogastroduodenoscopy (EGD): A special test performed by a gastroenterologist in which a thin tube is inserted through the mouth into the GI tract to allow examination of the stomach and small intestines. During an EGD, the doctor may take a biopsy sample from the intestinal wall to test for *H. pylori.*
- Stool guaiac cards: Used to test for blood in the stool (i.e., a fecal occult blood test)
- Hemoglobin test: Used to check for anemia

Treatment. Treatment often involves a combination of medications with different functions:

- Antibiotics (to kill *H. pylori*)
- Acid blockers (to reduce acid levels in the stomach)

- Proton pump inhibitors-reduce stomach acid
- Medications that protect the intestinal lining-coats stomach lining
- Bismuth-relieves nausea and cramping

Surgery may be required if a peptic ulcer has caused a perforation, or if the ulcer bleeds excessively and the bleeding cannot be stopped with an EGD procedure.

Prognosis. Peptic ulcers tend to recur if the cause goes untreated. This is less likely to happen if the patient follows the doctor's treatment instructions, because the *H. pylori* infection will be eliminated. If the ulcer goes untreated, peritonitis or bowel obstruction can occur. These are medical emergencies. The patient should be referred to the medical staff immediately if any of the following occur:

- Sudden, sharp abdominal pain
- Symptoms of shock (e.g., fainting, excessive sweating, or confusion)
- Vomiting of blood or blood in the stool (especially if the blood is maroon or black and tarry)
- Hard, rigid abdomen that is tender to the touch

- ***Massage implications:*** Monitor for symptoms that indicate a medical emergency. Support the medical treatment regimen to ensure the effectiveness of the medications; they need to be taken exactly as prescribed.

MIGRAINE

Research

A migraine is caused by abnormal brain activity, triggered by stress, food, or some other factor, that seems to involve various nerve pathways and chemicals in the brain. The changes affect blood flow in the brain and surrounding membranes. Migraines are different from other headaches because they are characterized by symptoms such as nausea, vomiting, or sensitivity to light.

Causes and Risk Factors. About 1 in 10 people are prone to migraines. The headaches tend to start between the ages of 10 and 46. They may run in families, and they occur in women more often than men. Migraines are classified as either with aura or without aura. An aura is a warning symptom consisting of visual disturbances. Most patients with migraines do not have auras.

The following factors can trigger a migraine:

- Allergic reactions
- Bright lights
- Loud noises
- Certain odors or perfumes
- Physical or emotional stress
- Changes in sleep patterns
- Smoking or exposure to smoke
- Skipping meals
- Alcohol
- Caffeine
- Menstrual cycle fluctuations
- Birth control pills
- Tension headaches
- Foods containing tyramine (red wine, aged cheese, smoked fish, chicken livers, figs, and some beans), MSG, and nitrates, which are most commonly found in bacon, sausage, cold cuts, hot dogs, chocolate, nuts, peanut butter, avocado, banana, citrus, onions, dairy products, and fermented or pickled foods

- ***Massage implication:*** Be cautious of the massage environment. Avoid scents, including essential oils, until it is clear how the patient may respond. Also limit live plants and monitor light and noise levels.

Symptoms. Migraine headaches range from dull to severe and usually have a throbbing, pounding, or pulsating feel. The headache is usually worse on one side of the head and lasts 6 to 48 hours. Symptoms include nausea and vomiting, sensitivity to light or sound, loss of appetite, fatigue, numbness, tingling, and weakness. Some symptoms may linger even after the migraine has dissipated, such as a feeling of mental dullness, an increased need for sleep, and neck pain.

- ***Massage implications:*** Massage is most effective before or after the actual headache event. During the active phase of the headache, the person may not want to be touched or disturbed.

Diagnosis. Migraine headache is diagnosed based on the symptoms, a history of migraines in the family, and the response to treatment. The doctor takes a detailed history to make sure the headaches are not caused by muscle tension, sinus inflammation, or a more serious underlying brain disorder. In some cases an electroencephalogram (EEG), a magnetic resonance imaging (MRI) study, or a computed tomography (CT) scan is done to rule out other causes of headache, such as a tumor or seizure condition.

Treatment. There is no cure for migraine headaches. The goal is to prevent symptoms by avoiding or altering triggers and to treat the symptoms when a headache occurs. When a migraine develops, the individual can take the following steps to try to minimize the symptoms:

- Rest in a quiet, darkened room
- Drink fluids to prevent dehydration, especially if vomiting
- Place a cool cloth on the head

Medications. Over-the-counter pain medications, such as acetaminophen, ibuprofen, and aspirin, may be helpful for a migraine. Prescription medications used to treat these headaches include ergots, triptans, isometheptene, and narcotics. If the person gets at least three headaches per month, the doctor may prescribe medication to prevent recurrent migraines. These drugs include the following:

- Beta blockers (e.g., Inderal)
- Antidepressants, including tricyclics and selective serotonin reuptake inhibitors (SSRIs)
- Anticonvulsants
- Calcium channel blockers

Many of the prescription medications used for migraines narrow blood vessels, therefore if heart disease is present, these medications may be contraindicated. The herb feverfew is known to help migraines.

Complications. Migraine headaches are not life-threatening. Stroke is an extremely rare complication of severe migraines; it occurs as a result of prolonged narrowing of the blood vessels that limits blood flow to parts of the brain for an extended period. Nevertheless, migraines can be chronic, recurrent, and frustrating and can interfere with day-to-day life.

The patient should be referred to the medical staff if the person has any unusual symptoms that he or she had not had before with a migraine; these may include speech or vision problems, loss of balance, difficulty moving a limb, or pain that rates as the most painful on a pain scale. These are signs of a potential stroke.

Massage implication: Immediately refer the patient to a physician if the headache pattern or intensity is different and the headache worsens when the person lies down. Medication side effects often occur, including an irregular heartbeat, pale or blue skin, extreme sleepiness, a persistent cough, depression, fatigue, nausea, vomiting, diarrhea, constipation, stomach pain, cramps, dry mouth, and extreme thirst. Monitor for side effects and refer the patient to the medical staff if necessary. Massage may help relieve depression, fatigue, and constipation.

Prevention. People who are prone to migraines can take a number of steps to prevent them:

- Avoid smoking, caffeine, and alcohol
- Exercise regularly
- Be sure to get restorative sleep
- Make use of relaxation and stress reduction methods (e.g., progressive muscle relaxation, biofeedback, massage)
- Join support groups

PREMENSTRUAL SYNDROME

Research

Among women of childbearing age, 70% to 90% are affected by premenstrual syndrome. For many, PMS is severe enough to interfere with daily tasks, and it can be disabling. Those who seem to be most affected include women in their late 20s to early 40s, those with at least one child, and/or those who have a family history or personal history of depression or an affective seasonal mood disorder.

PMS should not be confused with premenstrual dysphoric disorder (PMDD), a major mood disturbance that occurs in 3% to 8% of women.

The effects of PMS generally are felt during the *second half* of the menstrual cycle, that is, about 14 days after the first day of the last period. They usually do not occur for about a week after a menstrual period ends (the first half of the cycle). Symptoms of PMS include the following:

- Breast tenderness and swelling
- Bloating and weight gain
- Headache (menstrual migraine)
- Backaches
- Menstrual cramps
- Irritability
- Depression
- Unpredictable mood swings
- Decreased sex drive
- Fatigue
- Acne
- Food craving (chocolate or fat)
- Inability to concentrate
- Difficulty making decisions
- Feelings of guilt or alienation

Causes. Current theories hold that fluctuations in the hormones estrogen and progesterone cause the symptoms of PMS. Estrogen is known to cause water retention, which probably is the underlying cause of weight gain, bloating, general aching, and breast tenderness. In addition, women with PMS seem to metabolize progesterone differently from women who do not have PMS. This leads to decreased production of an antianxiety neurosteroid called *allopregnenolone.* An abnormal level of allopregnenolone can be a sign of PMDD.

Treatment and Prevention. Women who suffer from PMS can take the following steps to help prevent it:

- Reduce consumption of sugar and simple carbohydrates. Eating more fresh fruit and increasing the intake of certain minerals and vitamins sometimes can control unhealthy cravings for sugar or salt.
- Exercise regularly. Exercise can reduce the bloating and fluid retention seen with PMS by improving blood circulation. It also reduces stress and tension and increases natural production of beta endorphins, which can help prevent or combat mild depression.

PMS, the Migraine Diet, and Exercise. Women who suffer from premenstrual migraines may find that they feel better if they eat five or six small meals at regular 3-hour intervals. The diet should be high in fruits, vegetables, and whole grains and moderate in protein and healthy fats. Regular exercise is important.

Nutritionists and many medical doctors recommend that women who have PMS drink at least six glasses of water a day and reduce their intake of fat, caffeine, sugar, and salt, and that they avoid alcohol. In a healthy adult, drinking more water does not increase fluid retention; it actually helps flush fluids from the body.

Over-the-counter antiinflammatory drugs can help with mild pain and cramping, and mood-altering medications also can be used. Natural remedies include using natural progesterone suppositories or creams and eating more soy products.

Various types of hormone therapy are used for PMS and other women's health problems. Some women have unusually high levels of estrogen compared to progesterone, a condition known as estrogen dominance. In these cases, progesterone-based hormone therapy is used, which may include birth control pills. Birth control pills also regulate menstrual flow, reduce excessive bleeding, and treat acne or other PMS symptoms.

Some doctors and nutritionists believe that a diet high in minerals and complex carbohydrates (e.g., whole grains and green, leafy vegetables) can help the body rid itself of excess estrogen. Calcium, magnesium, and vitamin E supplements may be beneficial.

The National Institutes of Health has confirmed that acupuncture relieves physical pain resulting from many conditions and may be an option for both PMS and migraine pain.

Medical Assessment, Diagnosis, and Treatment Orders

The patient is experiencing migraines without aura. The family history indicates a grandmother and a maternal aunt who experienced headaches. The patient's mother has seasonal affective disorder. The frequency of the headaches has increased from two a month, which correlated with hormonal fluctuations, to three to five a month. The severity and duration of the headaches have also increased. Environmental changes, increased exposure to triggers, alterations in the sleep cycle, and stress levels are all causal factors. In addition, a mental health evaluation indicates a slight tendency to perfectionism with obsessive compulsive characteristics. A low-dose SSRI (sertraline [Zoloft]) has been prescribed. The patient is attending weekly counseling sessions (cognitive behavioral type), learning to use biofeedback to control headaches, participating in a meditation/breathing retraining class, and taking yoga. Massage has been prescribed to reduce sympathetic dominance, support restorative sleep, and address soft tissue factors involved in the tension headache component of the pain pattern. The patient also has been advised to move out of the dorm and obtain more suitable living arrangements where she can control environmental migraine triggers.

Massage Treatment Orders. Massage is to be given once a week and as needed if tension headaches occur. Each session should be a 60-minute, full body massage that addresses soft tissue factors related to the headache pattern. The massage should support restorative sleep and generalized relaxation. It also should treat tension headaches if they are present. The protocol for a circulation-based headache should be used if the symptoms are mild to moderate. Send for medication if symptoms are severe.

Massage-Specific Assessment

The patient is a 19-year-old female. She is 5′6″ tall and overweight for her height and frame (180 lb). The medical history pertinent to massage includes the following:

- Car accident at age 14 (whiplash injury)
- Nearsightedness (wears contact lenses)
- Rides horses (multiple minor falls and injuries; two major falls while jumping, which resulted in a broken clavicle at age 12 and a sprained ankle at age 16)
- Was prescribed Zoloft; takes Imitrex for migraine headache pain and ibuprofen for tension headaches
- Tendency to anxiety, worrying, and perfectionism
- Childhood experiences include death of an infant sibling when 7 years old. Mother experienced significant depression. Mother became pregnant again within a year, with normal pregnancy and birth. Cherie (almost 9 years old) undertook much of the care of her younger sister. She really does not like being separated from her.

Patient has normal gait and strength function but has a tendency to hold her head, neck, and back stiffly. She assesses positive for upper chest breathing, including thoracic rigidity and involvement of auxiliary breathing muscles during normal relaxed breathing. Especially short and active are the scalenes, upper trapezius, and anterior serratus. The pectoralis minor is extremely tender to moderately deep palpation. Patient chews gum almost constantly (except during sleep). (NOTE: This could be a behavior pattern reflecting serotonin factors and anxiety.) Sternocleidomastoid muscles are short bilaterally with a trigger point referred pain pattern to the face and eye, which mimics migraine headache. The SC joint on the right is rigid and surrounded with fibrotic tissue (broken side). Suboccipitals are tender to palpation, with a sensation of tension headache. Fascial binding is present over the cervical area; the scalp does not move easily and binds. Upper trapezius is fibrotic, with trigger point referred pain that resembles a tension headache. Lumbar dorsal fascial binding is present. Bilateral anterior rotation of the pelvis is more severe on the left, with a moderate increase in the lumbar curve (lordosis). Trunk flexion pattern is synergistically dominant with inhibited gluteus maximus. Hamstrings and lumbar muscles are dominant. Psoas is tender to palpation, and sensation from compression of psoas mimics menstrual cramps. Calves are dominant during knee flexion, with limited dorsiflexion (10 degrees out of 20 degrees possible). Core strength is adequate, but patient appears to be holding her belly in instead of allowing natural repose.

Periodic moments of breath holding are followed by sighing or yawning. Breathing generally is shallow, with an even inhale to exhale reaction (4.4 seconds).

Clinical Reasoning Process

The headaches appear to be triggered by stress, hormones, and environmental issues.

Massage best addresses the stress aspect, especially targeting breathing dysfunctions. The muscle imbalances indicate a tendency to upper and lower crossed syndrome and/or layer syndrome. Serotonin appears to be involved in the pattern, and massage can influence serotonin function.

The tension headache begins in muscles related to the head position and mastication. The constant gum chewing may influence motor tone patterns in the chewing muscle, which in turn can predispose these muscles to tension and trigger point development.

The patient also has fluid retention in the tissues related to PMS.

Massage is an aspect of a total treatment program that includes meditation, yoga, cognitive behavioral therapy, and breathing retraining. Massage can support each of these interventions through physical relaxation and normalization of identified dysfunctional areas. The interaction of the effects of the SSRI and those of massage needs to be monitored, because these two act synergistically. Logically, the breathing protocol could be integrated into the general massage; however, putting too much specific emphasis on breathing should be avoided, because overbreathers can easily become hyperfocused on breathing function and can experience rebound anxiety if they try too hard to break the habit and breathe correctly. Cherie is in a breathing retraining program, and biofeedback has a breathing component. The massage therapist should observe changes in breathing and include the breathing pattern protocol but should not attempt to focus on breathing during the massage to avoid drawing undue attention to this area.

Treatment Plan Development

Short-term goals: Reduce sympathetic dominance and trigger point referred pain related to tension headaches.

Long-term goals: Re-establish more appropriate breathing function. Normalize inhale to exhale ratio (4 counts inhale, 8 counts exhale). Reverse muscle activation sequence dysfunction for trunk and hip. Increase pliability of connective tissue that is binding and fibrotic.

Massage therapist's objectives: Address fluid retention, circulation, connective tissue bind, motor tone disruption, and muscle activation sequence problems. Support stress, breathing function, and chemical balance.

Methods to be used: General massage, following general protocol with inclusion of breathing dysfunction protocol and tension headache protocol for prevention and treatment of headache. Initially, trigger point treatment for active trigger points. Lymphatic drainage would be increased if necessary during premenstrual time frame. Sternocleidomastoid, suboccipital, and psoas releases included in session. Also, address areas with binding and fibrotic tissues using connective tissue methods. Address pelvic alignment with indirect function methods, and support normal firing patterns for trunk flexion and hip extension. Also address tension/length relationship of adductors in relation to trunk firing. Abdominal massage if bloat is present. As trigger point activity reduces, begin to address latent trigger points.

Frequency and duration: One time per week for 60 minutes, more often if tension headache occurs; provide for 12 sessions (3 months) and then re-evaluate.

Measurement of progress: Headache frequency and duration, pain scale, breathing assessment, and inhale to exhale ratio. Range of motion, muscle activation sequence assessment. Self-reporting on sleep and stress.

Date of reassessment: 12 weeks

SOAP Charting

Session 1

S: Patient reports that her neck feels tight and stiff. She is out of sorts and feeling premenstrual. She is sore from yoga. No headaches today, but she feels as if one is coming.

O: Findings from intake assessment unchanged. Evidence of slight body-wide tissue tautness related to fluid retention. General massage protocol with lymphatic drainage and abdominal massage provided. Suboccipital and scalene release with paired quadratus lumborum release. Bind and torsion forces applied to connective tissues in posterior cervical region. Slow, sustained pulling of the hair to address scalp binding.

A: Cherie really enjoyed having her scalp worked on. Also, although it was intense, she commented that the work in her neck felt good. She used the restroom midmassage after abdominal work, and gas sounds occurred during rolling of the abdomen. She commented that her head did not feel as heavy and that she was tired and wanted a nap. She felt less sore in general. Other than gas movement, no objectively measurable signs of change were noted after the massage.

P: Evaluate response to massage and adjust pressure and intensity as necessary.

Session 2

S: Patient reports that her neck was tender to the touch for 2 days but that it also was looser. She is having her period. She had one migraine, but it lasted only a day. She feels good today and continues to be sore from yoga. She went horseback riding over the weekend, and her low back is achy. She was crampy yesterday but not today. She requests that her head be massaged as before.

O: Observation indicates no improvement in posture, but Cherie is more relaxed in her speech and demeanor. She continues to hold herself stiffly, and upper chest breathing is observable. Palpation indicated reduced general edema compared to last session. Rigid thorax and fascial bind from scalp to sacral area. Firing patterns remain synergistically dominant. General massage protocol was provided with concentration on binding tissue in posterior thorax. Used combination of indirect functional methods (ease/bind)—active release/pin and stretch and tension force (myofascial release). Released psoas at distal attachment (did not want to do deep abdominal pressure during menstrual cycle if cramping is not present). Used muscle energy methods stretch for adductors and calves (contract relax/antagonist contract). Repeated neck massage from previous session and added sternocleidomastoid release.

A: Patient reported that sternocleidomastoid release was really painful and pain radiated over the side of her face and behind her eye. Pain sensation is lingering, although diminished. Her head feels lighter, and she feels less stiff. Skinfold assessment indicated a slight increase in connective tissue pliability after massage, and range of motion on ankles increased appropriate 5 degrees. Ribs remain rigid.

P: Integrate methods to increase rib mobility and address firing patterns. Do psoas release from abdomen.

Session 3

S: Cherie reports that she thought she was going to get a migraine after the massage, but it did not develop until 2 days later. Her neck was sore to the touch but seems less stiff. She has a mild tension headache today (pain rating of 6 on a pain scale of 1 to 10) and feels anxious and indicates she is really busy. She requests that her head be massaged as before.

O: Upper chest breathing is apparent with both observation and palpation. Ribs remain rigid. Palpation of the upper trapezius, suboccipitals, and scalenes replicates headache symptoms. General massage protocol was provided, along with breathing pattern protocol and tension headache protocol. Addressed connective tissue as in previous session. Added psoas release with head movement and repeated sternocleidomastoid release. Also, performed suboccipital muscle release. Used inhibiting pressure in areas that replicated headache pain, especially upper trapezius.

A: Patient responded well to positional release methods used on tender points in thorax. She indicates that headache is almost gone (pain rating of 3). Cherie was observed taking some slow, deep breaths, and she indicated that she felt more relaxed. She also remarked that the psoas release felt like her menstrual cramps, and her back feels great. Taught patient about the relationship between menstrual cramping and psoas shortening.

P: Repeat session.

Session 4

S: Patient says she thinks she is getting a migraine.

O: Cherie is holding herself stiffly, and her face is pale. She avoids eye contact, and she came in wearing sunglasses and kept them on. General massage was provided, including palliative protocol with circulatory headache protocols. Patient was urged to see the nurse after the massage.

A: Patient felt nauseous during massage and used the restroom to vomit. She reported that she felt a little better after throwing up and after the massage, but she said she would check in with the nurse before leaving.

P: Evaluate and continue with treatment plan.

Session 5

S: Patient reports that she checked with nurse after the last session and was told to go home and sleep. If her headache got worse, she was to come back in for a treatment. Cherie reports that she was able to sleep off the headache. Today she feels good.

O: Assessed firing patterns, which remain synergistically dominant. Breathing is typical for this patient. Provided general massage with focus on trunk flexion and hip extension firing. Used psoas release and added rectus abdominis release using inhibiting pressure at attachments. Sternocleidomastoid release and connective tissue methods were used to address binding tissue. Muscle energy methods were used for stretching of hamstrings and calves.

A: Hip extension normalized temporarily after psoas releases and hamstring lengthening and stretching. Trunk firing remains rectus abdominis dominant but is slightly better. Sternocleidomastoid is less tender during release procedure.

P: Patient should be entering premenstrual phase. Assess for symptoms and treat as necessary.

Evaluation of Progress

The patient is just beginning to respond to the massage intervention. This is a complex case, and progress typically is slow. The muscle releases are less painful. The firing patterns are beginning to be addressed, and the breathing function remains a long-term goal. The tension headache responded well to the massage intervention.

Recommendations for Future Massage Care

Sustained results are not likely to be noticed until the full 3-month series of 12 sessions is complete. It is important to progress slowly and to observe the monthly effects of hormonal changes. Cherie probably will need lifelong condition management–type massage.

Perspective of the Massage Therapist

Cherie is an easy patient with whom to work. Her condition is complex but straightforward. She is young, which supports adaptive capacity, and massage is being provided as part of a multidisciplinary approach, therefore boundary issues are less of a concern than if massage were the only intervention. It is important not to rush progress and to address each concern methodically—fluid retention, circulation, connective tissue bind, motor tone disruption, and muscle activation sequence problems. All of these issues interplay with the stress, breathing function, and chemical balance.

CASE STUDY 7: PARKINSON'S DISEASE

Parkinson's disease is a disorder of the brain characterized by shaking (tremor) and difficulty with walking, movement, and coordination. The disease is associated with damage to the part of the brain involved in movement.

Similar Conditions

Muscle atrophy conditions, myalgia, complications from stroke.

The Case

Mr. Anderson, a 67-year-old male, has Parkinson's disease. He was first diagnosed at age 62, and his history shows that symptoms of the disease began to appear at about age 55. His main hobby is dancing. Within the past 6 months, he has become unable to perform various dance moves, and his stiffness and movement problems have increased. He is taking levodopa and carbidopa.

Mr. Anderson is experiencing symptoms related both to the Parkinson's disease and the medications. These include mild difficulty performing daily activities, a moderate reduction in mobility and balance, and moderate changes in mood and affect (i.e., depression, fatigue, and slowness in responding to conversation). He and his wife recently returned from a cruise, and while on the ship, he received a massage. Both he and his wife noticed an improvement in his mobility, agility, and balance for a 24-hour period. He scheduled four more sessions (every other day), and he noted that after each massage, he was more mobile and his balance was better. He and his wife went dancing toward the end of the cruise, and although his performance was still impaired, he was able to perform the slower, less complex moves.

Upon their return, Mr. Anderson and his wife both related the experience with massage to Mr. Anderson's doctor, who is supportive and referred them to the physical therapist for an altered treatment plan that includes massage. The physical therapy center recently expanded its services to include therapeutic massage. Whether Mr. Anderson's healthcare insurance will cover any or all of the massage fees is unclear, but if benefit continues to be realized, the Andersons are willing to pay out of pocket. The massage therapist on the cruise ship did not adjust the massage to target Parkinson's symptoms specifically. She had given Mr. Anderson a general 45-minute massage for stress reduction. Mr. Anderson indicated that the massage was not painful and the pressure was good.

The massage therapist used oils, and Mr. Anderson was able to choose from four essential oil combinations: relaxation, sensual, energizing, and muscle aches. He had chosen the muscle aches formula but had no idea what it contained. He liked the smell and said that it was minty, like mint gum.

Research

Parkinson's disease is caused by a progressive deterioration of nerve cells in the part of the brain that controls muscle movement. Deterioration in this area of the brain reduces the amount of dopamine available to the body. Dopamine is one of the substances used by cells to transmit nerve impulses.

Insufficient dopamine disturbs the balance between dopamine and other neurotransmitters, such as acetylcholine. Without dopamine, the nerve cells cannot properly transmit messages, and this results in a loss of muscle function. The disorder may affect one or both sides of the body, with varying degrees of loss of function.

Causes and Risk Factors. The reason for the deterioration of the brain cells is unknown. The disease most often develops after age 50. It affects both men and women and is one of the most common neurologic disorders of the elderly. Parkinson's disease sometimes occurs in younger adults, but it is rarely seen in children.

The term *parkinsonism* refers to any condition that involves a combination of the types of changes in movement seen in Parkinson's disease. Parkinsonism may be caused by other disorders (secondary parkinsonism) or by external factors, such as certain medications used to treat schizophrenia.

Some people with Parkinson's disease become severely depressed as a result of the loss of dopamine in certain brain areas involved with pleasure and mood. Lack of dopamine can also affect motivation and the ability to initiate voluntary movements.

In the early stages of the disease, loss of mental capacities is uncommon; however, with severe Parkinson's disease, the person may exhibit overall mental deterioration, including dementia and hallucinations. Dementia can also be a side effect of some of the medications used to treat the disorder.

Symptoms. Early symptoms of Parkinson's disease tend to be mild and nonspecific. A slight tremor may develop, or the legs may be stiff and heavy. As the disease progresses, the following can occur:

- Shaking and tremors (tremors characteristically occur at rest, although they may occur at any time, and may become severe enough to interfere with activities; they may be worse when the person is tired, excited, or stressed)
- Finger-thumb rubbing (called *pill rolling*)
- Muscle rigidity with stiffness and difficulty bending the arms or legs
- Muscle aches and pains (myalgia) and muscle atrophy

  - Frequent falls
  - Unstable, stooped, or slumped-over posture with loss of balance
  - Gait changes, including shuffling and small steps followed by the need to run to maintain balance
  - Slow movements
  - Difficulty initiating any voluntary movement, such as when beginning to walk or getting up from a chair
  - Freezing of movement when the movement is stopped and inability to resume movement
  - Reduced ability to show facial expressions and reduced rate of blinking, resulting in staring and a masklike appearance to the face
  - Inability to close mouth, drooling
  - Slow speech with low volume and monotone
  - Loss of fine motor skills, difficulty performing small movements
  - Gastrointestinal symptoms, mainly constipation
  - Seborrhea (oily skin)
  - Depression
  - Anxiety, stress, and tension
- ***Massage implications:*** Massage can specifically address muscle aches, constipation, stress management, and anxiety.

Diagnosis. Medical tests are not usually specific for Parkinson's disease, but they may be required to rule out other disorders that cause similar symptoms. The diagnosis of Parkinson's disease may be based on the symptoms and physical examination. Symptoms can be difficult to assess, especially early in the disease and in the elderly. The physical examination may show jerky, stiff movements, tremors of the Parkinson's type, and difficulty initiating or completing voluntary movements. The reflexes usually are normal.

Treatment. There is no known cure for Parkinson's disease. Treatment is aimed at controlling the symptoms and must be tailored to the individual.

- ***Massage implications:*** Research seems to indicate that massage can influence dopamine levels and therefore can be beneficial in conditions in which dopamine is a factor.

Medications control symptoms primarily by increasing the levels of dopamine in the brain. The dosage of the medication needs to be adjusted as the symptoms change. Many of the drugs used to treat Parkinson's disease can cause severe side effects. A number of medications may be used:

  - Deprenyl may produce some improvement in mildly affected patients.
  - Amantadine or anticholinergic medications may be used to reduce early or mild tremors.
  - Levodopa is converted to dopamine by the body. It may be used to increase the body's supply of dopamine, which may improve movement and balance. Carbidopa reduces the side effects of levodopa and enhances its effectiveness.
  - Atamet and Sinemet are used to treat symptoms of Parkinson's disease. It may take a few weeks before the full benefits of this medication are observed. Stomach upset may occur and is reduced when medication is taken with food or milk.
  - Other medications that are used to help reduce symptoms or to control the side effects of primary treatment medications include antihistamines, antidepressants, dopamine agonists, and monoamine oxidase inhibitors (MAOIs).

Side effects from these medications are: drowsiness, dizziness, headache, loss of appetite, stomach upset, nausea, vision changes, or trembling of the hands. Side effects tend to subside as the body adjusts to the medication but may persist.

Refer immediately if the patient develops vomiting, difficulty swallowing, difficulty urinating, uncontrollable movements (especially twitching of the eyelid), chest pain, an irregular heartbeat, skin rash, mood or mental changes.

- ***Massage implications:*** Research all medications to determine their interaction with the effects of massage.

Surgery. Surgery to destroy tissues responsible for tremors may reduce symptoms in some people.

Lifestyle Changes. Maintaining nutrition and health is important. Exercise should continue, with the level of activity adjusted to the person's changing energy levels. Stress management is necessary, because fatigue or stress can worsen symptoms. Physical therapy, speech therapy, and occupational therapy may help promote function and independence.

Simple aids, such as railings or banisters, and special eating utensils can be helpful for a person experiencing difficulties with daily living activities. Social workers or other counseling services and support groups may help the patient cope with the disorder.

- ***Massage implications:*** Massage can support exercise and can be a valuable aspect of stress management.

Prognosis. Parkinson's disease impairs people in varying ways. Most respond to medications to some extent, but the degree of symptom relief and how long the control of symptoms lasts vary. The side effects of medications can be severe. Complications, including possible drug side effects, include the following:

- Difficulty swallowing or eating
- Difficulty performing daily activities
- Involuntary movements
- Nausea and vomiting
- Dizziness
- Changes in alertness, behavior, or mood
- Severe confusion or disorientation
- Delusional behavior
- Hallucinations
- Loss of mental functions

Medical Assessment, Diagnosis, and Treatment Orders

The patient has Parkinson's disease, which has shown a slow progression that is being managed with medication, physical therapy, and occupational therapy that especially target activities of daily living.

Massage is to be added to the treatment program and will be monitored by the physical therapist. Massage should not be fatiguing or painful to the patient. The frequency is to be determined, beginning with two 1-hour sessions per week over 6 weeks; sessions can be added, if necessary, to sustain benefit. Because the extent of insurance coverage is unclear and the Andersons are willing to pay for the massage sessions, the physical therapist indicates that Mr. Anderson would benefit from participating in the wellness center intern program in cooperation with a massage school. The treatment plan would lend itself to the development of a protocol that could be implemented by students. The lead massage therapist would monitor each session and modify the treatment plan as necessary, reporting to the physical therapist when changes are made. The massage is to be provided before regularly scheduled physical therapy sessions to support mobility. Mr. Anderson, who had been a high school science teacher, is very willing to participate in the intern program. He said that he was excited to be participating in a learning environment.

Massage-Specific Assessment

Assessment was performed by the lead massage therapist while the student massage interns observed.

History: Patient is a 67-year-old male who is 5′11″ tall and weighs 190 lb. He was a science teacher for 27 years and also coached track and field. His passion is dancing, especially ballroom dancing, and he also was an amateur performer in various musicals. He performed tap and jazz dance routines. He is no longer able to tap dance because his movements are too slow and labored, but if he could extend his ability to do ballroom dancing with his wife, he would be most pleased. He is taking medication to support dopamine function.

Currently, exercise consists of a supervised mobility program, walking, and supervised pool activities.

Mr. Anderson has the characteristic masklike appearance of Parkinson's disease. He speaks slowly but clearly. It is unclear whether his tendency to be depressed and fatigued is related to medication, Parkinson's symptoms, or his diminished ability to function. His wife thinks that if he could obtain the type of results he experienced on the cruise, with massage as part of the treatment, the depression and fatigue would improve. Mr. Anderson does not complain of pain but indicates that he feels stiff and achy (pain rating of 6 on a pain scale of 1 to 10).

Physical assessment: Mr. Anderson is moderately stooped forward and has a tendency to upper crossed syndrome posture. Gait is slightly shuffled, and movements are slow and deliberate. Palpation indicates that some muscle atrophy has occurred as his ability to move has declined. Tissues are pliable, with no evidence of fluid retention or circulation impairment. Muscle testing was not performed. Active range of motion is difficult to perform. Passive range-of-motion assessment indicated that joint function is normal for his age. Shoulder abduction, external rotation, and extension are slightly limited because of the stooped posture. Breathing is slow and shows some upper chest involvement. Counterbalancing arm swing during walking is reduced significantly.

Clinical Reasoning Process

This is a difficult situation since the disease is progressive, and eventually the patient's condition will decline. Care will need to be taken to realize that the condition will not be cured and that benefits will be short-term. This does not discount the value of massage, especially if the current quality of life is improved. The massage application is very basic and he should not have adaptive capacity strained from massage. Sessions will need to increase as symptoms increase.

Treatment Plan Development

Long-term goals: Support mobility.

Short-term goals: Support mobility.

Massage therapist's objectives: Support treatment of Parkinson symptoms. Increase ability to perform activities of daily living and pleasurable activities.

Methods to be used: Palliative massage with pressure sufficient to support dopamine utilization and using the palliative care protocol with the addition of passive movement of the joints. Pressure levels will maintain a moderate compressive force with a broad-based contact. Drag will be limited by the use of a lubricant. Reflexology will be incorporated into the massage. Essential oils to address muscle aches (e.g., birch and orange) can be added to the massage oil. Frequency will begin with two sessions per week and will be increased to three sessions if benefits are justified. Massage initially will be scheduled before physical and occupational therapy sessions, and the schedule will be adjusted if necessary.

Frequency and duration: Two times a week for 50 minutes. With increase in sessions to 3 times per week if necessary.

Measurement of progress: Range-of-motion measurements, done by the physical therapist. Reduction in upper chest breathing function, increase in soft tissue pliability. Self-reporting of improvements in mood and sleep.

Date of reassessment: Every 12 weeks.

NOTE: Mr. Anderson will be participating in the student intern program, for which massage fees are $20 per session.

SOAP Charting

Session 1

S: Patient reports that he is stiff and achy (pain rating of 7 on a pain scale of 1 to 10). He is eager for massage. He asks the massage student to remain in the massage room and assist him with disrobing and getting on the table.

O: No change since assessment. Treatment plan was implemented.

A: Mr. Anderson was able to get off the table and dress himself with noticeable improvement. He reports that he feels much better. Gait remains shuffled, but arm movement is improved.

P: Continue to implement treatment plan.

Session 2

S: Mr. Anderson reports that he felt much better the day of the massage and that his pool exercises were easier. He woke up stiff but less achy the day after the massage and was much less mobile today.

O: Mobility appears to have reverted to initial assessment parameter, as indicated by the physical therapist. Treatment plan was implemented, and massage therapist remained in the room to assist the patient with disrobing and getting on the table.

A: After the massage, Mr. Anderson said that he felt good, as in the last session, and that he was surprised he could button his shirt. Movement is less jerky, and he is more stable when standing on one foot (observed as he put on his trousers).

P: Continue to implement treatment plan.

Session 3

S: Occupational therapist reports that Mr. Anderson performs better on the days he receives a massage. Physical therapist requested an increase in sessions, and physician approved an increase to three sessions per week. Mrs. Anderson reports that her husband has an improved mood and less fatigue. Mr. Anderson indicates that he wishes he could get a massage every day.

O: Mobility again reverted to the initial assessment, but the face appears slightly less masklike. Treatment plan was implemented. Mr. Anderson requested a bit more pressure, which was approved by the instructor.

A: Mr. Anderson was more talkative during the massage than in the previous sessions. Mobility again increased, as did balance.

P: Increase frequency to three times per week.

Session 4

S: Mr. Anderson says he thinks the effects of massage lasted longer after the last session. He said it was difficult to explain, but that he just feels better.

O: Gait is more fluid than after previous session, with increased arm swing and less shuffling. Patient needs less assistance getting ready for massage. Massage treatment protocol performed.

A: Mr. Anderson dozed off intermittently during the massage. He also joked a bit and told some stories about his dancing days. He required less assistance getting off the table and getting dressed.

P: Continue with treatment plan.

Session 5

S: Patient reports that if he could get a massage every other day, he would do better. Currently he is on a Monday–Wednesday–Friday schedule, and he is much less mobile on Monday. He reports that he and his wife went dancing Friday night.

O: Patient's mobility is at initial assessment levels (this is a Monday session; the previous massage was on Friday). Performed treatment plan.

A: Mr. Anderson reports that he feels much better. He demonstrated how much more easily he can button his shirt. He required less assistance after the massage than before it.

P: Continue with treatment plan.

Evaluation of Progress

The massage intervention is a condition management process. Although immediate benefits in mobility are realized, the benefits do not last longer than 2 days.

Recommendations for Future Massage Care

The massage should continue at a minimum of three times per week indefinitely. The treatment plan likely will remain consistent, with small alterations based on the patient's current condition. Financial burden is a concern with massage of this frequency.

Perspective of the Massage Therapist

Although it was rewarding to watch Mr. Anderson's mobility improve, even though the effects of massage lasted only a couple of days, occasionally it also was frustrating to maintain a general approach to massage and avoid the temptation to work with the patient more intensely.

CASE STUDY 8: CORONARY HEART DISEASE AND CORONARY ARTERY BYPASS GRAFT (CABG) SURGERY

Similar Conditions

Any major surgery.

The Case

Sandy is a 52-year-old female with a strong family history of heart disease. For the past year, she has not been feeling "right" but has not been ill or had any significant symptoms. A physical with blood tests indicated that her thyroid levels were low. She has experienced hypothyroid problems for years. Over the past 6 months she has gained 20 pounds, mostly around her midsection. Her thyroid medication (Synthroid) was adjusted, and she was cautioned to manage her stress levels. Her family doctor "did not like the way she looked" and strongly suggested a cardiac workup, including a stress test and more extensive blood tests. Sandy had been experiencing chest discomfort, but not significantly, and it could be explained by other causes.

Sandy is a massage therapist who works with professional athletes, and she thought she had either costal arthritis or strained muscles. However, for the past 6 months, she also has been having vague symptoms of heart problems. These have included mainly sweating and intolerance to heat (which could be caused by menopausal changes), shortness of breath (which could be related to the weight gain), and increased fatigue and lack of stamina (which could be related to a heavy work schedule and low thyroid function). The blood test results showed that her cholesterol ratios were excellent, and everything else was normal. Her blood pressure was low to normal. She had never smoked, and she did not have diabetes or any other apparent risk factors for coronary artery disease. However, a suspicious result on the stress test prompted her family doctor to refer her to a cardiologist.

Based on the test results and the electrocardiogram, the cardiologist did not think that Sandy had coronary heart problems, and he wondered whether the symptoms might be related to gastroesophageal reflux disease (GERD). The only consistent symptom was chest pain that seemed like referred pain from heartburn. A 3-month trial of a long-acting nitroglycerin and a calcium channel blocker was instituted. Sandy was also instructed to lose weight and increase her cardiovascular exercise. She maintained her normal work schedule, which included working with two professional football teams, one of which won the Super Bowl. The symptoms persisted, although they neither worsened nor improved.

After the Super Bowl, Sandy went again to the cardiologist, and it was determined that the trial medications did not seem to be making a difference. A medication for GERD was tried for 3 weeks, and a heart catheterization procedure was scheduled to rule out coronary artery disease. The GERD medication did not make any difference. The cardiologist was stumped because the symptoms were so vague, and Sandy's cholesterol levels, blood pressure, and other factors did not indicate heart disease. However, because of the family history and her problems with hypothyroidism, it was deemed necessary to rule out the possibility of a buildup of arterial plaque.

During the heart catheterization procedure, a greater than 50% blockage of the left main coronary artery was found. Everyone was surprised by this finding. Sandy had suffered no heart attack and no heart damage. However, this was a serious blockage, because the main coronary artery feeds most of the heart. Because a blockage in this area cannot be treated with angioplasty, coronary bypass surgery was immediately scheduled.

Triple bypass open heart surgery was performed successfully. During surgery, it was discovered that the arteries on the left side of Sandy's heart were smaller than normal. This condition, the strong genetic tendency for heart problems, and the patient's chronic low thyroid function appeared to be the causal factors. Sandy was extremely fortunate that the condition had been identified before she had a heart attack, because infarction from blockages in the left main coronary artery typically result in very extensive heart damage or death.

The surgery was performed on a Monday, and Sandy was released from the hospital the following Friday. She described the days in the hospital as follows.

Monday: I can remember people coming in and out, and I remember begging for the pain shot. I remember my sister peering at me on and off all night. She understands the surgery. She has kept her husband from the brink of death for over 7 years; he has a cardiac condition for which surgery cannot be done. I remember my brother-in-law, too. He can be a real character, but I remember him holding my hand. He got me this stuffed animal, a turtle, that is all fuzzy, and it stayed with me the whole time. I remember my kids looking nervous. I was so thirsty, and I wanted water so badly. The nurse assigned to me for the first 24 hours was great, even though I was miserable. I don't think I could do her job.

Tuesday: The surgeon comes in and tells me I did great. I ask if he means it or if he is just working on his bedside manner. He laughs, and I can tell he cares. At this moment, I am very important to him; next month I won't be, but right now I am, and that is all that matters. His two physician assistants (PAs) and a nurse have to pull out the drainage tubes. This hurts really bad, but I am experiencing the difference between hurt and harm; the hurt is terrible, but it did not harm me. I kind of challenge the PAs, asking them tons of questions. I don't think they're used to that.

Wednesday: The surgeon comes in again. He is comforting. I ask him what my heart looked like. He explained some technical things about the smaller than normal arteries and so forth, but then he told me that I had a big, beautiful, giving heart and that my heart would be able to serve me for many more years. I think about this. This man has been inside me; he has held my heart in his hands. That's pretty intimate and intense. I have only met with him four times, and 6 weeks from now, after the final postsurgical appointment, I will probably never see him again. Yet he has touched my life forever. His skills made it possible for me to live productively for many more years.

It hurts to breathe and move—surgery hurt, not harm. Pain medication helps. It is important to do deep breathing exercises and coughing; again, it hurts bad but does not harm. I spent most of the day either sitting up or walking. I want to sleep in the afternoon. My appetite is poor, but popsicles taste great.

My son also is a massage therapist, and he was able to begin massage 2 days after surgery. My neck and back were extremely achy from the surgery and lying around. I was restless, partly from the inactivity and also from the pain. The surgeon encouraged me to have massage to help with the aching in my neck, shoulders, and back. The incision sites on my chest and leg had to be avoided, and the pressure level needed to be altered because of the anticoagulant medication I was taking.

I am using the postoperative massage application of self-massage on the incision sites on my leg and chest.

Thursday: The surgeon is pleased with my progress. I hurt, but I am also alive. My neck, shoulders, and back are so sore. Any movement feels like my chest is tearing open. Wow; never had pain like this before! Besides that, the whole thing is pulling and itching.

Took a shower today, and it felt wonderful. The dietitian came in, and we discussed dietary changes. My big task is to have a bowel movement. I massaged my own abdomen and walked. I had to force myself to eat, and finally success was achieved. This means I can go home. I used the TV remote to press a spot out of my neck that was throbbing and sore. I am grumpy today.

My son did compression and kneading on my shoulders, back, and neck; lymphatic drainage on my legs; and a foot massage. I am surprised by how much the foot massage eases the pain and calms me down. Wow! My healing essential oils are jasmine and rose. The nurses comment on how wonderful the room smells.

Friday: When the surgeon visits, we talk about the recovery and rehabilitation process and discuss the benefits of massage. He is supportive. When asked what he would expect from a massage therapist working with him, he discussed the importance of touch and compassion. He would not tolerate indifference or lack of nurturance. Obviously, sanitation is essential. Professional behavior is paramount, but it also is important to be personable. He would expect treatment orders to be followed and the massage therapist to function as a team player. The massage therapist also would need to understand the necessity of palliative care and how to alter the massage to accommodate a patient's reduced adaptive capacity, as well as have an understanding of the workings of various medical devices and medications, most especially anticoagulants. The massage therapist would need to be able to recognize signs of potential complications (e.g., temperature changes, bleeding, cognitive disruption, infection) and bring them to the attention of the nurse. Massage before and after surgery would need to be soothing and would target pain management and stress.

Massage during rehabilitation might be more comprehensive, he said, but during the critical days after surgery, it would need to be supportive, nonspecific, and gentle. He also commented on how much the staff could benefit from massage and explained a bit about the physical and emotional stress of performing surgery and being attentive not only to the patient, but also to the family and friends during the critical hours before and after surgery.

I thought he did a great job of explaining his expectations.

The nursing staff and other support staff were all excellent during my hospital stay. I have no complaints. I was cared for very well.

My mother and sister took me home and will help with the cooking, laundry, and cleaning. It is the task of my younger son, the massage therapist, to take care of me during my recuperation. My daughter has handled all the emergency stuff, made all the necessary calls, and kept everyone informed. My older son is responsible for all my spring garden work. My school office staff and instructors managed everything, and now I have 12 weeks of recovery. That's my job—to heal.

Research

Angina (also called angina pectoris) is chest pain that is caused either by a reduction in the blood flow to the heart or by certain other abnormalities of heart function. Hardening of the coronary arteries that feed the heart (atherosclerosis) usually is the underlying problem. Spasms of the coronary arteries may also cause angina.

The three main types of angina are stable angina, variant angina, and unstable angina. Stable angina is chest pain that comes on during exercise and is both common and predictable. Stable angina is most often associated with atherosclerosis. Variant angina can occur at rest or during exercise and is caused by a sudden spasming of the coronary artery, although atherosclerosis may also be present. Unstable angina is the most severe type. It occurs with no predictable pattern and can quickly lead to a heart attack. A person with significant new chest pain or worsening of previously mild angina must seek medical care immediately.

Symptoms. Common symptoms of angina include a squeezing pressure, heaviness, ache, or burning pain (resembling indigestion) in the chest that lasts for 5 to 30 minutes at a time. These sensations usually are felt behind the breastbone but may also be felt in the jaw, neck, arms, back, or upper abdomen. Some people may also have difficulty breathing or may become pale and sweaty.

The symptoms of angina usually appear during physical exertion, after heavy meals, and with heightened emotional states (e.g., anger, frustration, shock, and excitement). The symptoms can be different for men and women, and in women the symptoms often are more vague.

- ***Massage implications:*** Monitor for symptoms and refer the patient to the medical staff for proper diagnosis and treatment. People have a tendency to explain away heart-based symptoms because the whole concept of heart trouble is frightening.

Treatment. Many classes of prescription drugs are use to treat angina. Calcium channel blockers and nitrates reduce the risk of death and nonfatal heart attack in patients with a previous history of heart attack or unstable angina. Anticoagulants reduce the risk of clotting, and statins lower cholesterol levels.

- ***Massage implications:*** Aspirin is an anticoagulant, and patients who take it may have an increased tendency to bruise; monitor pressure levels. Nitrates, calcium channel blockers, and beta adrenergic blockers can cause dizziness. Monitor the patient as the person gets off the massage table.

In advanced stages of heart disease, surgical repair of the blood vessels in the heart may be recommended. Treatment may be directed toward underlying medical conditions, such as high cholesterol levels, high blood pressure, anemia, hypothyroidism, obesity, or lung disease.

Lifestyle Changes. It is critical that people with angina who smoke stop smoking, because nicotine prevents proper blood flow. Cigarette smoking damages the coronary arteries, contributing to angina. Smoking also has been shown to reduce the effectiveness of treatments for angina. Secondhand smoke should be avoided as well. Coffee probably should be avoided. Drinking five or more cups of coffee a day has been shown to increase the risk of angina, although the effects of different forms of coffee on angina are unclear.

- ***Massage implications:*** Massage can support a smoking cessation program.

Increasing physical exercise has been clearly demonstrated to reduce the symptoms of angina and to relieve its underlying causes. Exercising as little as 10 minutes a day may be as effective as beta blocker drugs for treating the symptoms of angina. A person with angina or any other heart condition, as well as anyone over age 40, should consult a doctor before beginning an exercise program.

- ***Massage implications:*** Massage can support an exercise program.

CABG SURGERY

Research

In coronary artery bypass graft (CABG) surgery, the blood is routed around clogged arteries to improve blood flow and the delivery of oxygen to the heart. The coronary arteries that bring blood to the heart muscle can become clogged by plaque, a buildup of fat, cholesterol, and other substances. This condition is called *atherosclerosis.* The plaque buildup can slow or stop the flow of blood through the heart's vessels, leading to chest pain or a heart attack. When one or more of the coronary arteries becomes partly or totally blocked, the heart does not receive an adequate supply of blood. This is called *ischemic heart disease* or *coronary artery disease (CAD),* which can cause angina.

Atherosclerosis

As mentioned, atherosclerosis is a disease of the arteries in which fatty material is deposited in the vessel wall, resulting in narrowing of the vessel and eventual impairment of blood flow. Severe restriction of arterial blood flow to the heart muscle leads to symptoms such as chest pain. Atherosclerosis has no symptoms until a complication occurs.

CAD sometimes does not cause pain until the blood supply to the heart becomes critically low and the muscle begins to die. The first symptom of CAD in this case may be a potentially deadly heart attack. Symptomless CAD is especially common in people with diabetes and in women.

The earliest symptoms of ischemic heart disease include angina (chest pain) and shortness of breath. Some people have no symptoms; mild, intermittent chest pain; or more pronounced, steady pain. In others, the CAD is severe enough to make everyday activities difficult.

Symptoms that usually prompt a person to see a doctor are a feeling of heaviness, tightness, pain, burning, pressure, or squeezing. This usually occurs behind the breastbone but sometimes is also felt in the arms, neck, or jaw. Some people have a heart attack without ever having any of these symptoms.

In cases in which no symptoms are seen but CAD may be suspected, the doctor may perform a stress test to determine whether CAD is present. CAD sometimes is suspected if a person has a family history of heart disease and a combination of other factors, including high blood cholesterol levels, diabetes, high blood pressure, cigarette smoking, hypothyroidism, and male gender. The doctor typically performs an angiogram (cardiac catheterization) to see whether any coronary arteries are blocked by plaque. A blockage can reduce the supply of blood and oxygen to the heart and over time can lead to debilitating chest pain or a heart attack.

If the blockage is too difficult to access by angioplasty or if severe blockages are seen in multiple major vessels, the doctor may recommend CABG surgery. Coronary artery bypass surgery also is a treatment option for ischemic heart disease. Coronary surgery is recommended for disease of the left main coronary artery, disease of three or more vessels (triple vessel disease), and when nonsurgical management has been unsuccessful.

Risk Factors. Coronary bypass surgery has been performed for more than 30 years, and cardiovascular surgeons have received extensive training in bypass techniques. This procedure is the most frequently performed major surgery in the United States; more than 500,000 are done each year. As with any surgery, the patient's health before surgery is a major consideration in determining the risks. Health conditions that should be considered before surgery include the following

- Age (patients over age 70 have a slightly higher risk of complications)
- Gender (women have a slightly higher risk)
- Previous heart surgery (higher risk)
- Having another serious medical condition (e.g., diabetes, peripheral vascular disease, kidney disease, lung disease)

The Procedure. Increasing blood flow to the heart muscle can relieve chest pain and reduce the risk of heart attack. To do this, surgeons take a segment of a healthy blood vessel from another part of the body and make a detour around the blocked part of the coronary artery. An incision is made in the middle of the chest, and the breastbone is separated. This allows the surgeon access to the heart and the aorta, the main blood vessel leading from the heart to the rest of the body. After the procedure, the breastbone is rejoined with wire and the incision is sewn or glued closed.

If a vein from the leg (i.e., the saphenous vein) is to be used for the bypass, an incision is made in the leg and the vein is removed. The saphenous vein, which is located on the inside of the leg, runs from the ankle to the groin. Because it normally does only about 10% of the work of circulating blood from the leg back to the heart, it can be removed without harming the patient or the leg. The affected leg commonly swells slightly during the recovery from the surgery, but this is a temporary condition that is treated by elevating the leg.

The internal mammary artery (IMA) may also be used as a graft. Arterial grafts have an important advantage; they stay open for many more years than vein grafts. The left IMA (or LIMA) runs next to the sternum on the inside of the chest wall. It can be disconnected from the chest wall without affecting the blood supply to the chest. This artery commonly is connected to the left anterior descending artery (LAD), the artery on the heart that supplies most of the muscle.

Other arteries also are now being used in bypass surgery. The most common of these is the radial artery, one of the two arteries that supply the hand with blood. The radial artery usually can be removed from the arm without impairing the blood supply to the hand.

In the surgical procedure, one end of the donor vessel is sewn onto the aorta, and the other end of the donor vessel is attached, or grafted, to the coronary artery below the blocked area. A patient may have one, two, three, or more bypass grafts, depending on how many coronary arteries are blocked.

Cardiopulmonary bypass with a pump oxygenator (heart-lung machine) is used for most CABG operations. In addition to the surgeon, cardiac anesthesiologist, and surgical nurse, a perfusionist (blood flow specialist) must be present for the surgery. During the past several years, more surgeons have started performing off-pump coronary artery bypass surgery (OPCAB). In this procedure, the heart continues beating while the bypass graft is sewn in place. In some patients, OPCAB may reduce intraoperative bleeding (and the need for blood transfusion), renal complications, and problems with postoperative neurologic deficits. The surgery can take 4 to 6 hours.

Postoperative Care and Recuperation. After the surgery, the patient is moved to a hospital bed in the cardiac surgical intensive care unit. Heart rate and blood pressure monitoring devices monitor the patient continuously for 12 to 24 hours. Medications that regulate circulation and blood pressure may be given intravenously. A breathing tube (endotracheal tube) remains in place until the physicians are confident the patient is awake and ready to breathe on his or her own. The patient may feel groggy and disoriented, and the incision sites (in the chest and also in the leg if a segment of blood vessel was taken from the leg) may be painful. Painkillers are given as needed.

The patient spends 5 to 7 days in the hospital Two or three tubes in the chest drain fluid from around the heart, and these tubes usually are removed 1 to 3 days after surgery. A urinary catheter in the bladder drains urine until the patient is able to void on his or her own. Intravenous (IV) lines provide fluids and medications. Nurses constantly watch the monitors and check the patient's vital signs (pulse, temperature, blood pressure, and respiration [breathing]).

When constant monitoring is no longer needed (usually within 12 to 24 hours), the patient is moved to a regular or a transitional care unit. Activity is gradually resumed, and the patient may begin a cardiac rehabilitation program within a few days. The chest incision makes some movements painful, such as coughing, moving from a standing to a lying position, and so on.

After surgery, it takes 4 to 6 weeks for the patient to begin feeling normal again. During recovery, the following are common:

- Poor appetite
- Swelling in the affected leg if the graft was taken from the leg
- Difficulty sleeping at night
- Constipation
- Mood swings and feeling depressed
- Difficulty with short-term memory or feeling confused (this also improves)
- Muscle pain or tightness in the shoulders and upper back

- ***Massage implications:*** Massage can be beneficial for pain management, edema, supporting sleep, mood disturbance, constipation, and muscle pain.

Many of these side effects usually disappear in 4 to 6 weeks, but full recovery may take a few months or longer. The patient usually is enrolled in a physician-supervised program of cardiac rehabilitation. This program teaches stress management techniques and diet and exercise regimens; it also helps people rebuild their strength and confidence.

- ***Massage implications:*** Massage can support a cardiac rehabilitation program and provide a method of stress management.

The full benefits of the operation may not be determined until 3 to 6 months after surgery. Sexual activity may resume 4 weeks after surgery. All activities that do not cause fatigue are permitted, and the schedule for resuming normal activities is determined with the physician.

Patients often are advised to eat less fat and cholesterol-containing foods and to walk or do other physical activity to help regain their strength. Doctors also often recommend following a home routine of increasing activity, such as doing light housework, going out, visiting friends, and climbing stairs. The goal is to return to a normal, active lifestyle.

Most people with sedentary office jobs can return to work in 4 to 6 weeks. Those with physically demanding jobs must wait longer, and in some cases, they may have to find other employment.

Possible risks in having CABG surgery include the following:

- Heart attack (5% of cases)
- Stroke (5% of cases; the risk is greatest in those over age 70)
- Blood clots
- Death (1% to 2% of cases)
- Sternal wound infection (1% to 4% of cases; most often associated with obesity, diabetes, or previous CABG surgery)

In about 30% of patients, postpericardiotomy syndrome can occur anywhere from a few days to 6 months after surgery. The symptoms of this syndrome are fever and chest pain, and the condition can be treated with medication.

The incision in the chest or at the graft site (if the graft was taken from the leg or arm) may be itchy, sore, numb, or bruised.

Some people report memory loss and loss of mental clarity, or "fuzzy thinking" after CABG. This condition is often called *cognitive disruption,* and it occurs for a variety of reasons, including blood flow changes and the use of anesthesia during surgery.

As with all surgeries, the risk of heavy bleeding exists. Also, the use of anesthesia in itself poses general risks, such as reactions to medications and problems breathing.

In most cases of CABG surgery, the grafts remain open and functioning for 10 to 15 years. CABG improves blood flow to the heart, but it does *not* prevent the eventual recurrence of coronary blockage. This requires lifestyle changes: not smoking, improving one's diet, regular exercise, and treating high blood pressure and high cholesterol levels.

ATHEROSCLEROSIS

Healing of the Sternum. Much of the healing in open heart surgery involves healing of the sternum, which is cut longitudinally during the surgery and then wired back together. It heals the same way as any fractured bone.

Fractures heal in three overlapping phases: inflammation, repair, and remodeling. Healing begins immediately with the inflammatory phase. In this phase, damaged soft tissue, bone fragments, and lost blood caused by the injury are removed by the cells of the immune system. The region around the fracture becomes swollen and tender as cell activity and blood flow increase. The inflammatory phase reaches peak activity in a couple of days but takes weeks to subside. This process accounts for most of the early pain people experience with fractures.

The repair phase begins within days of the injury and lasts for weeks to months. New repaired bone, called the *external callus,* is formed during this phase. When first produced, the callus has no calcium; it is soft and rubbery and cannot be seen on an x-ray film. Because this new bone is neither strong nor stable, the fractured bone can easily collapse and become displaced (i.e., slip out of its proper place) during this phase. At 3 to 6 weeks, the callus calcifies, becoming much stiffer and stronger, and it also becomes visible on x-ray films.

The remodeling phase (in which the bone is built back to its normal state) lasts many months. The bulky external callus is slowly reabsorbed and replaced by stronger bone; in this phase, the normal contours and architecture of the bone are restored. The bone is not likely to fracture again during this phase; however, the person may feel mild pain upon exertion.

Bones in good position, particularly in young people, may heal without a trace of a scar. If much displacement or deformity is involved or if the patient is older, an obvious bump or line at the break may always be visible on x-ray films. Bone is one of the few tissues in the body that can heal without leaving a scar. The time required for healing depends completely on the blood supply and the stability of the fracture or break. If there is no movement at the fracture site, if the bone is casted or splinted, or if a plate is affixed to the bone in the operating room, the fracture will heal without delay. If the fracture is close to the end of the bone (the metaphysis), the blood supply is strong, and the bone will heal within a few weeks. If the break is in the middle of a long bone, such as the femur (thigh) or tibia (leg), the blood supply is not quite as good, and complete healing may require several months. As mentioned, age is an important factor. Young people heal more quickly than older people.

- ***Massage implications:*** Bone healing in the sternum is compromised slightly because some movement occurs in the area during breathing and other movements that affect the ribs. Massage must not disturb the bone healing process by causing movement in the sternum or ribs. This includes movement of the ribs at the posterior vertebral attachments.

Medical Assessment, Diagnosis, and Treatment Orders

Sandy's case is a postoperative situation. Massage can be provided daily for comfort care. Short-duration lymphatic drainage on the lower legs is indicated. Avoid all surgical sites. Do not perform massage on the anterior or posterior thorax to prevent any rib or sternal movement. Use caution with pressure levels because the patient is receiving anticoagulants. Massage on the posterior neck, shoulders, arms, hands, hips, nonsurgical thigh, lower legs, and feet is appropriate. Use caution around IV sites. Avoid the prone position. The patient most often takes Plavix, Lipitor, and aspirin. She is also taking Percocet for pain.

Massage-Specific Assessment

The patient had open heart surgery 2 days ago. She no longer has a Foley catheter or drainage tubes. She has IV lines in her neck on the right and left sides. The donor site for the saphenous vein in the medial left thigh has two 3-inch incisions with one drainage site. The left groin area has significant bruising from the catheterization procedure. The incision in the thorax begins at the sternal notch and extends through the xyphoid process. Three drainage site incisions just under the rib cage have sutures. The entire area is bruised. The lower abdomen is bruised from heparin injections. The patient's breathing is shallow and painful (pain rating of 7 on a pain scale of 1 to 10). Movement is painful (pain rating of 8). The patient reports that her neck, posterior thoracic region between the scapulae, upper shoulders, and arms are sore, spasming, and aching (pain rating of 8). She is restless and cannot get comfortable.

Clinical Reasoning Process

Because the patient had surgery only 2 days ago, comfort care is indicated. General massage can be used on the areas of complaint except for the posterior thoracic region; accessing that area would require positioning that would cause movement of the posterior and anterior ribs and the sternum. Foot massage, along with lymphatic drainage on the lower legs and feet, is acceptable. Massage of the head can also be done for comfort care. Use the lotion provided by the hospital for massage. Avoid all surgical sites. An energy-based application that does not touch the surgical areas can be used. Percocet is a narcotic and can be constipating; it also can cause dizziness, nausea, and mood changes.

Treatment Plan Development

Long-term goals: Support healing and rehabilitation.

Short-term goals: Management of pain and stress.

Massage therapist's objectives: Comfort and care.

Methods to be used: Palliative care.

Frequency and duration: 30 minutes daily—up to 45 minutes if requested.

Measurement of progress: Pain scales.

Date of reassessment: 4 weeks.

SOAP Charting

Session 1

S: Patient reports that her neck, posterior thoracic region between the scapulae, upper shoulders, and arms are sore, spasming, and aching (pain rating of 8 on a pain scale of 1 to 10). She is restless and cannot get comfortable.

O: Patient had open heart surgery 2 days ago. Massage was provided in the chair to her head, neck, and shoulders using compression and kneading. Massage was provided to the lower back and hips with the patient side-lying in the hospital bed. Massage was provided to the arms, legs, and feet with the patient supine in the hospital bed. Reflexology points for the neck, shoulders, heart, chest, liver, and intestines were targeted during foot massage. Near touch energy methods were used around surgical areas.

A: Patient became calmer and said she wanted to take a nap.

P: Massage tomorrow.

Session 2

S: Patient reports that her neck, posterior thoracic region between the scapulae, upper shoulders, and arms are still sore, spasming, and aching (pain rating of 8). She is restless, cannot get comfortable, and has a headache. She asks that essential oils (jasmine and rose) be used on her feet.

O: Patient had open heart surgery 3 days ago. An IV line is still in the left hand. The entire surgical area is bruised. The lower abdomen is bruised from heparin injections. Breathing is shallow and painful (pain rating of 7). Movement is also painful (pain rating of 8). Massage was provided in the chair to her head, neck, and shoulders using compression and kneading. Massage was provided to the lower back and hips with the patient side-lying in the hospital bed. Massage was provided to the arms, legs, and feet with the patient supine in the hospital bed. Reflexology points for the neck, shoulders, heart, chest, liver, and intestines were targeted during foot massage. Used essential oil on feet (rose and jasmine). Near touch energy methods were used around surgical areas.

A: Patient became calmer and was better able to take a nap.

P: Massage tomorrow.

Session 3

S: Patient reports that her neck, posterior thoracic region between the scapulae, upper shoulders, and arms are still sore, spasming, and aching but that they are improving as she moves around more. The incision sites are pulling and itching, and she has been using self-massage in those areas.

O: Patient had open heart surgery 4 days ago. An IV line remains in the left hand. The entire surgical area remains bruised. The lower abdomen is bruised from heparin injections. Breathing is improved. Movement is painful when the patient changes from a lying down position to a seated or standing position (pain rating of 8); however, it is significantly reduced when the patient is sitting or walking. Massage was provided in the chair to the head, neck, and shoulders using compression and kneading. Massage was provided to the lower back and hips with the patient side-lying in the hospital bed. Massage was provided to the arms, legs, and feet with the patient supine in the hospital bed. Reflexology points for the neck, shoulders, heart, chest, liver, and intestines were targeted during foot massage. Rose and jasmine essential oils were used on the feet. Near touch energy methods were used around surgical areas.

A: Patient became calmer and was better able to interact with visitors.

P: Patient will be released from the hospital today. Massage will continue as part of home care.

Session 4

S: Patient reports that her neck hurts around the sternocleidomastoid. She is restless, cannot get comfortable, and has a headache from referred pain from the sternocleidomastoid.

O: Patient had open heart surgery 5 days ago. The entire surgical area is bruised. The lower abdomen is bruised from heparin injections. Breathing is improving but painful (pain rating of 7) for deep breathing and coughing. Movement is painful when turning in bed and when moving from a lying down position to a standing position (pain rating of 8). Incision sites are itchy and pulling. Massage was provided in the chair to the head, neck, and shoulders using compression and kneading. Reflexology points for the neck, shoulders, heart, chest, liver, and intestines were targeted during foot massage. Rose and jasmine essential oils in jojoba oil were used on the feet. Near touch energy methods were used around surgical areas.

A: Patient became calmer and was able to sleep.

P: Massage tomorrow.

Session 5

S: Patient reports that her neck hurts around the sternocleidomastoid. She is restless, cannot get comfortable, and has a headache from referred pain from the sternocleidomastoid. She continues to do self-massage near the incision sites, following the protocol for post-operative wound care.

O: Patient had open heart surgery 6 days ago. The entire surgical area remains bruised. The lower abdomen is bruised from heparin injections. Breathing is improving but painful (pain rating of 6) for deep breathing, more so when coughing. Movement is painful when turning in bed and moving from a lying down to a standing position (pain rating of 6). Incision sites are itchy and pulling but healing well. Massage was provided in the chair for the head, neck, and shoulders using compression and kneading. Reflexology points for the neck, shoulders, heart, chest, liver, and intestines were targeted during foot massage. Essential oils (rose and jasmine) were used on the feet. Lymphatic drainage was performed on the legs, avoiding the incision sites. Near touch energy methods were used around surgical areas.

A: Patient became calmer and was able to sleep.

P: Massage tomorrow.

Evaluation of Progress

Massage was helpful for easing the pain from the surgery in general and for reducing muscle aches that occurred as a result of the surgery and inactivity. Self-treatment of the incision sites has supported the development of pliable scar tissue. Foot massage, in particular, was calming and reduced agitation, supporting sleep.

Recommendations for Future Massage Care

Scar tissue development needs to be supported. The chest is slightly concave, and any soft tissue changes need to be addressed once the guarding is no longer productive. The ribs were displaced at the facet joint and the costal and sternal cartilage; this needs to be addressed. Breathing function needs to be normalized. Cardiovascular exercise needs to be supported. The leg from which the vein graft was harvested may swell on occasion and require lymphatic drainage. The social, economic, emotional, and spiritual ramifications of such a life-changing event, coupled with necessary lifestyle changes, may be stressful. Depression is common after heart surgery, and massage can be an aspect of managing this issue.

Perspective of the Massage Therapist

The massage therapist was not employed by the hospital but was the patient's son. He certainly had concerns about his mother's well-being. He was afraid to hurt her, and seeing his mother in such pain was difficult. He was impressed with the calming effects of foot massage and energy work.

Final Observations

This last case is for real. It happened to me, Sandy Fritz, in February, 2006, as I was finishing the manuscript for this book. I find it very interesting that circumstances played out such that I actually experienced various aspects of healthcare and the benefits and limitations of massage in the postoperative recovery period. I have a much deeper understanding of acute pain; hurt versus harm; the job of the medical staff; the emotional stress on family and friends; and the body, mind, and spirit challenges of major health events.

Four weeks after surgery, I was up and around but limited in what I could do. I was instructed to make sure I lifted nothing heavier than 10 pounds, and I was not allowed to lift anything over my head. My chest incisions and sternum were sore but improved every day. Deep breathing was uncomfortable but necessary. I had some headaches and nausea from the anesthesia and pain medication. Because of their side effects, I took pain medications only for about 4 days after coming home. I tired easily and needed more sleep.

I have felt compelled to throw out all my clothes. I have no reason why I feel this way, but I am honoring it. Goodwill is pleased.

It is now August 2006, almost 6 months.

I have found it difficult to allow my mother, sister, and kids to care for me, and I have come to truly realize how important family and friends are. This is an interesting experience, because I typically am very independent and quite a loner. My mother was most traumatized by the whole event and still comes and helps with housework and tasks. This is good for both of us.

So many people sent me well wishes and prayers of many different types, and I know that helped. One of the last things I remember before the surgery is praying for my surgeon, Dr. Rogers, and all his staff. I also sent special thoughts to the anesthesiologists who were responsible for the heart-lung machine, literally keeping me alive but unaware. I remember mentioning that I would love to have an "out of body" experience so that I could watch the surgery. The doctors told me they preferred that I stay in my body and work with them. That made sense; and, in fact, I didn't have an out of body experience. Remember, we are body, mind, and spirit.

My kids have been great, but the whole thing scared them because they wondered if they were going to lose their mom. Waiting out the duration of the surgery was really hard on them. (I wonder if some chair massage in the waiting room would have helped?)

Nowadays, the most frustrating situation is the continuing brain fog (cognitive disruption). This is common after major surgery, especially with heart surgery. Initially I felt very dull, and processing any type of information was difficult. I watched a lot of TV, which is uncommon for me. My short-term memory is still poor but improving. I have moments of being teary and overwhelmed. I did the photograph and DVD shoot in June, 2006, and as we reviewed the manuscript for this book, I realized that I don't remember writing parts of it. For some reason, I cannot untangle stuff like cords and garden hoses. My chest aches on and off and is stiff, but these sensations will not harm me. I have learned to tell the difference between somatic pain and heart pain. If I can make the pain increase with movement, then it is from the surgery—not my heart. A sense of humor is necessary. It is humbling to be in this position. This situation will improve, but it will take months, and I have to be patient. My sternum will heal before my brain does!

I doubt that I have come to grips with the seriousness of the condition, and I get nervous when I think about what might have happened. If the artery had been completely blocked, I would have had a major, probably deadly, heart attack. I expect that I will heal through this and realize the implications of a second 50 years that I probably would not have had were it not for medical miracles.

I have completed cardiac rehabilitation and am getting back to normal, at least my new normal.

It is appropriate that I have experienced this event, because I have undertaken the responsibility of writing and teaching about massage in the healthcare world. I now have had a chance to live it, which is the best learning. The experience has helped me become a better massage therapist and teacher.

My sincerest desire is to share my personal case study with the readers of this text, to support them in their quest to provide massage for people who face the challenges of dealing with a life changed by healthcare events. I hope you continue to learn and expand your skills, and that you work with each individual patient or client with compassion, empathy, tolerance, a sense of humor, and respect.

UNIT FOUR RESOURCES LIST

The sites listed below contain sources that are applicable to researching various conditions and treatments.

National Institutes of Health, National Center for Complementary and Alternative Medicine	http://altmed.od.nih.gov/nccam/
University of Texas Center for Alternative Medicine Research	http://www.sph.uth.tmc.edu:8052/utcam/
University of Washington Medicinal Herb Garden	http://www.nnlm.nlm.nih.gov/pnr/uwmhg/
Columbia University Fact Sheets on Alternative Medicine	http://cpmcnet.columbia.edu/dept/rosenthal/factsheets.html
ASPET Herbal and Medicinal Plant Interest Group	http://www.faseb.org/aspet/H&MIG3.htm#top
Herb Research Foundation	http://www.herbs.org
The Phytochemical Database	http://www.orst.edu/dept/lpi/
American Botanical Council	http://www.herbalgram.org/
National Center for Health Statistics	http://www.cdc.gov/nchs/
American Heart Association Biostatistical Fact Sheets: Cardiovascular Disease Statistics	http://americanheart.org/Heart_and_Stroke_A_Z_Guide/
United States Department of Health and Human Services Agency for Health Care Research and Quality	http://www.ahcpr.gov
The Heart: Online Exploration	http://sln.fi.edu/biosci/heart.html
You've had a heart attack—what now?	http://weber.u.washington.edu/~bmperra/heart_help.html
Children's Health Information Network	http://www.tchin.org/
Life and Health Insurance Foundation for Education	http://www.health-line.org
CPR: You can do it!	http://weber.u.washington.edu/~gingy/cpr.html#choice
Open the Door to a Healthy Heart	http://www.healthyfridge.org

Heart Failure Online	http://www.heartfailure.org
Pediatric Cardiology Almanac	http://www.neosoft.com/~r/pierce/pc.htm
Mended Hearts, Inc.	http://www.mendedhearts.org/
Minimally Invasive Heart Surgery: American Heart Association	http://www.americanheart.org/presenter.jhtml?identifier=4702
Coronary Artery Disease Treatment–Surgery: Cleveland Clinic Heart Center	www.clevelandclinic.org/heartcenter
Minimally Invasive Direct Coronary Artery Bypass (MIDCAB): Brown University Division of Biology and Medicine	www.biomed.brown.edu
HealthAnswers (Orbis-AHCN): Ask the Doctor, Infinity Heart Institute	http://www.heartinfo.org/ms/guides/16/main.html
Mayo Clinic Health Letter, May 1994	www.mayoclinic.com

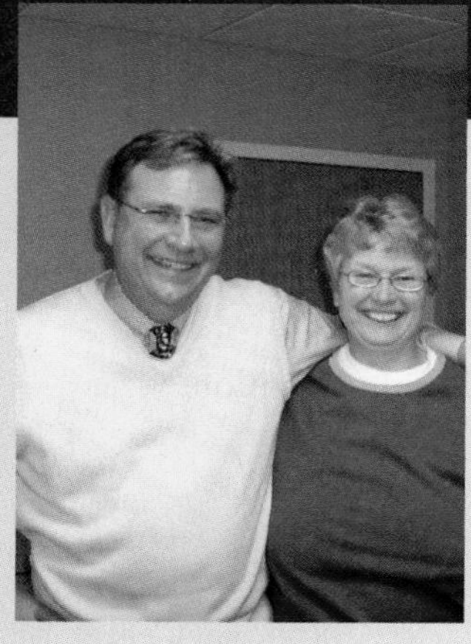

UNIT FOUR REFERENCES

Baumgartner WA: What's new in cardiac surgery, *J Am College Surg* March:345-355, 2001.

Berlin JA, Colditz G: A meta-analysis of physical activity in the prevention of coronary heart disease, *Am J Epidemiol* 132:612-628, 1990.

Certification and registration as a massage practitioner in Maryland. Accessed November 5, 2002, at www.mdmassage.org/certnreg.htm

Chaitow L: *Fibromyalgia syndrome: a practitioner's guide to treatment,* London, 2000, Churchill Livingstone.

Chaitow L, Bradley D, Gilbert C: *Multidisciplinary approaches to breathing pattern disorder,* London, 2002, Churchill Livingstone.

Medical school admission requirements, 2001-2002: United States and Canada. (51st ed). Washington, D.C.: Association of American Medical Colleges, c2000.

Corbin L: Safety and efficacy of massage therapy for patients with cancer, Cancer Control 12:158-164, 2005.

D'Avanzo CE, Geissler EM: *Mosby's pocket guide series: cultural health assessment,* ed 3, St Louis, 2003, Mosby.

Kao GD, Devine P: Use of complementary health practices by prostate carcinoma patients undergoing radiation therapy, Cancer 88:615-619, 2000.

Mack MJ: Minimally invasive and robotic surgery, *JAMA* February:568-572, 2001.

Millbank Memorial Fund: *Enhancing the accountability of alternative medicine,* New York, 1998, The Fund 1-8877748-18-0.

Monahan L: *A practical guide to health assessment,* ed 2, Philadelphia, 2002, WB Saunders.

Moore CM: *Mosby's pocket guide series: nutritional care,* ed 4, St Louis, 2001, Mosby.

Peters D, Chaitow L, Harris G, Morrison S: *Integrating complementary therapies in primary care,* Philadelphia, 2002, Churchill Livingstone.

Rattray F, Ludwig L: *Clinical massage therapy: understanding, assessing and treating over 70 conditions,* Ontario, 2000, Talus.

Redwood D, Cleveland C: *Fundamentals of chiropractic,* St Louis, 2003, Mosby.

Rich GJ, editor: *Massage therapy: the evidence for practice,* St Louis, 2002, Mosby.

Salvo SG, Anderson SK: *Mosby's pathology for massage therapists,* St Louis, 2004, Mosby.

Seidel H, Ball J, Dains J, Benedict W: *Mosby's physical examination handbook,* ed 3, St Louis, 2003, Mosby.

Skidmore-Roth L: *Mosby's nursing drug reference,* St Louis, 2002, Mosby.

Studdert DM, Eisenberg DM, Miller FH et al: (1998). Medical malpractice implications of alternative medicine, *JAMA* 280:1610-1615, 1998.

Young A, Kennedy D: *Kinn's the medical assistant; an applied learning approach,* ed 9, St. Louis, 2003, Elsevier.

Additional Resources

AHCPR
www.ahcpr.gov/consumer

American Botanical Council
www.herbalgram.org/

American Heart Association Biostatistical Fact Sheets
americanheart.org/statistics/biostats/index.html
americanheart.org/Heart_and_Stroke_A_Z_Guide/

ASPET Herbal and Medicinal Plant Interest Group
www.faseb.org/aspet/H&MIG3.htm#top

Children's Health Information Network
www.tchin.org/

Columbia University Fact Sheets on Alternative Medicine http://cpmcnet.columbia.edu/dept/rosenthal/factsheets.html

CPR You can do it!
weber.u.washington.edu/~gingy/cpr.html#choice

Heart Failure Online
www.heartfailure.org

Herb Research Foundation
http://www.herbs.org
Phytochemical Database
www.orst.edu/dept/lpi/

Life and Health Insurance Foundation for Education
www.health-line.org

Mended Hearts
www.mendedhearts.org/

National Center for Complementary and Alternative Medicine (NCCAM)
http://nccam.nih.gov/health/practitioner

National Center for Health Statistics
www.cdc.gov/nchs/

National Institutes of Health, National Center for Complementary and Alternative Medicine
http://altmed.od.nih.gov/nccam/

Open the Door to a Healthy Heart
www.healthyfridge.org

Pediatric Cardiology Almanac
www.neosoft.com/~r/pierce/pc.htm

Phytochemical Database
www.orst.edu/dept/lpi/

The Heart: Online Exploration
http://sln.fi.edu/biosci/heart.html

University of Texas Center for Alternative Medicine Research
www.sph.uth.tmc.edu:8052/utcam/

University of Washington Medicinal Herb Garden
www.nnlm.nlm.nih.gov/pnr/uwmhg/

You've had a heart attack—what now?
weber.u.washington.edu/~bmperra/heart_help.html

Minimally Invasive Heart Surgery. American Heart Association Web site, 2000.

Coronary Artery Disease Treatment—Surgery. Cleveland Clinic Heart Center Web site, April 2001.

Minimally Invasive Direct Coronary Artery Bypass, MIDCAB. Brown University Division of Biology and Medicine Web site.

Mayo Clinic Health Letter, May 1994.

Dr. David Allie, M.D., Cardiovascular Institute of the South

HealthAnswers (Orbis-AHCN); Ask the Doctor, Infinity Heart Institute

Virtual Hospital, Iowa CHAMPS

Dean Santerre, Anatomy of the Human Heart

Dr. Joseph Galichia, Heart Homepage

www.medicineNet.com

APPENDIX

MASSAGE PROTOCOLS

General Protocol, 759

Seated Massage Protocol, 782

Palliative Protocol, 783

Low Back Massage Protocol, 786

Protocol to Address Breathing Function, 791

GENERAL PROTOCOL

This series of photographs can be used as a visual slide show. It provides an example of how the general protocol can be implemented. The general protocol is also demonstrated in the DVD that accompanies this text.

The general protocol and variations demonstrate massage application on patients in the prone, supine, and side-lying positions. Examples of the seated protocol are provided after the general protocol.

The sequence can be used in conjunction with the written protocol in Chapter 11 (also supported by anatomic drawings) by matching up the photographs with the corresponding description. The written protocol is presented within an extensive and detailed discussion, and the illustrations here provide a series of visual "snapshots" that capture an entire concept. Truly a picture is worth a thousand words.

The photographic sequence that follows tells a visual story, just as the DVD tells a visual and auditory story, and the written protocol obviously tells the written story. The written protocol is also available on the Evolve Web site; it can be printed and used with both the photographs and the DVD.

These examples illustrate an effective and logical massage application, incorporating assessment and intervention based on outcomes. However, you probably will not implement it precisely as presented, because massage applications must be personalized to meet the needs of each individual patient. Nevertheless, for learning purposes, you should practice the protocol as shown, especially applications that are new to you, so that you can expand your skills as a massage practitioner. The models used throughout this text, including these protocols, represent the expansive diversity of cultures, gender, age, lifestyle, and more. When working in healthcare, the massage professional will serve many different people. Nonjudgmental massage application is necessary even when personal belief systems are challenged. We hope that you will appreciate the diversity as much as we did when creating this text.

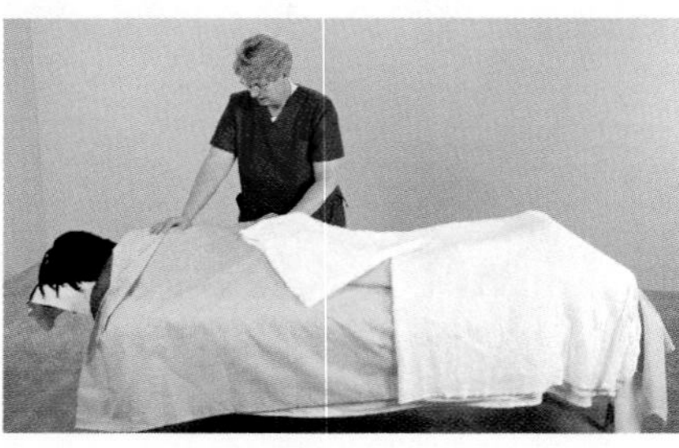

A-1 ■ Massage application begins with the massage practitioner using focused intention, the patient in the prone position, and full draping in place. (Subsequent illustrations use minimal draping to improve visual clarity.)

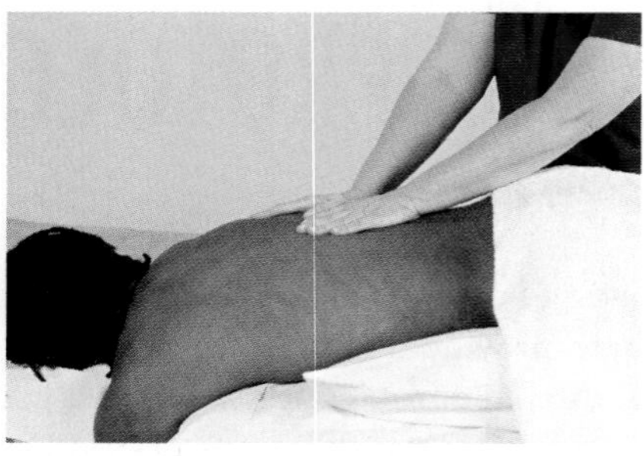

A-3 ■ Hand placement for lymphatic drainage. Primary focus: fluid drainage.

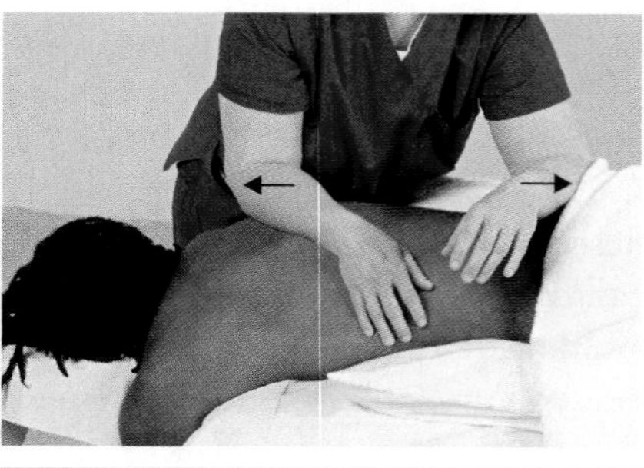

A-5 ■ Tension force applied to the skin and superficial fascia. Primary focus: connective tissue pliability.

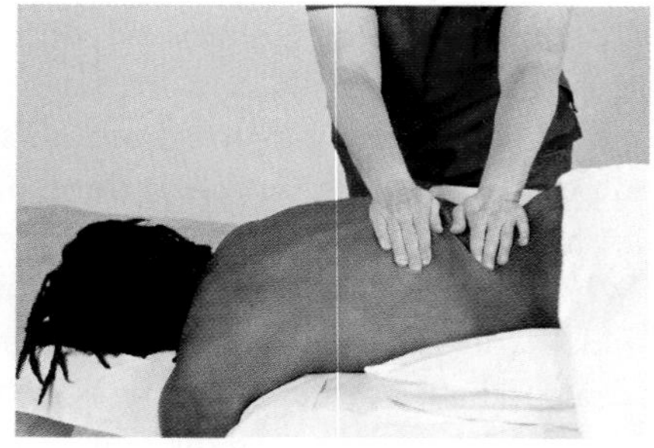

A-7 ■ Kneading to introduce torsion forces to assess tissue texture, increase tissue pliability, and influence fluid movement.

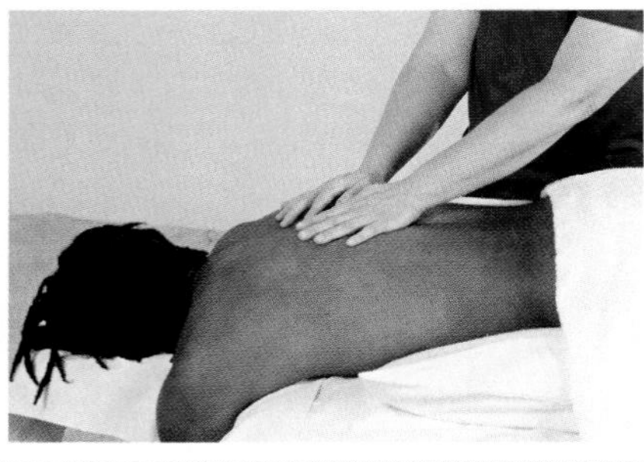

A-2 ■ Palpation and assessment of the skin.

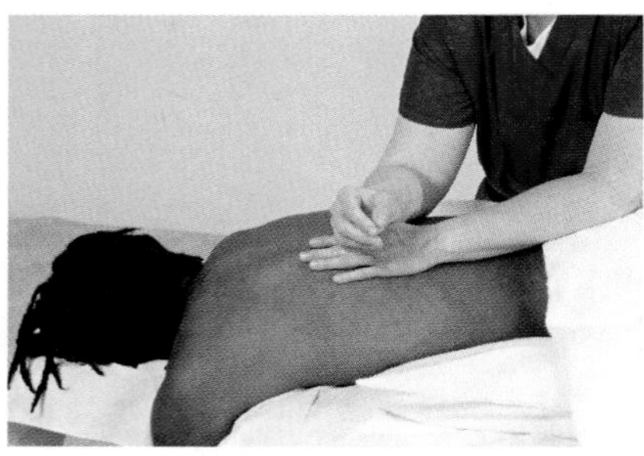

A-4 ■ Forearm gliding—light, medium, or deep pressure to address different tissue layers. Light to moderate drag, slow speed. Primary focus: assessment of tissue texture.

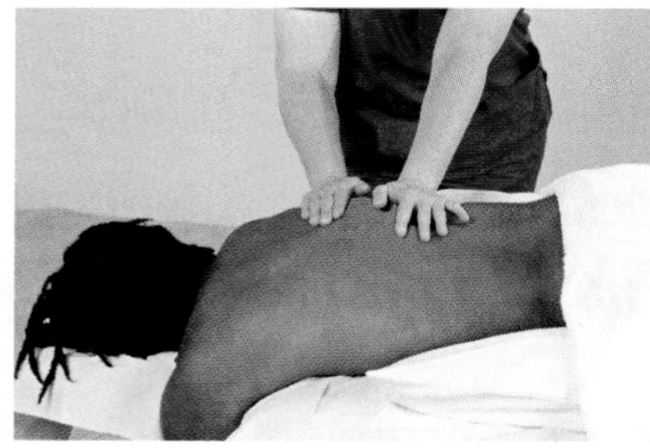

A-6 ■ Palm gliding—light, medium, or deep pressure. Light to moderate drag, slow speed. Primary focus: assessment of tissue texture and movement of tissue layers.

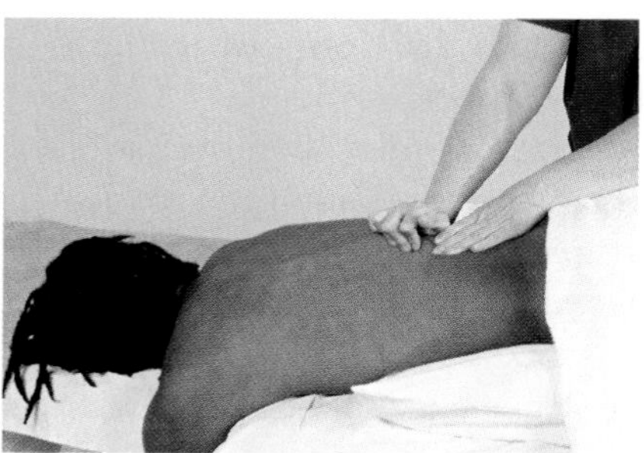

A-8 ■ Palm compression—to produce bending and compressive force. Slow to static speed, maximum drag. Primary focus: introduction of mechanical forces into tissue.

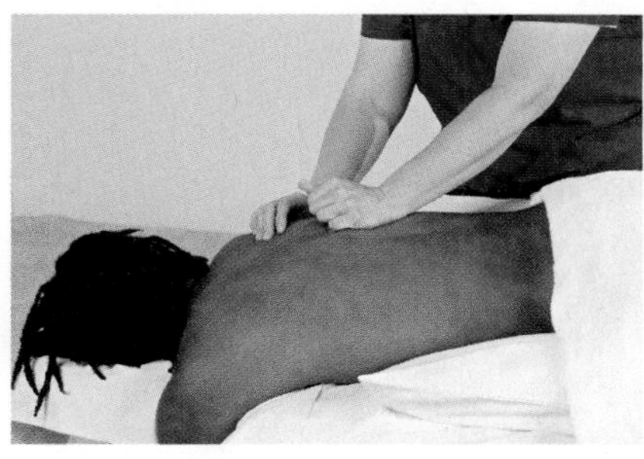

A-9 ■ Kneading and skin rolling. Primary focus: assessment of skin and superficial fascia.

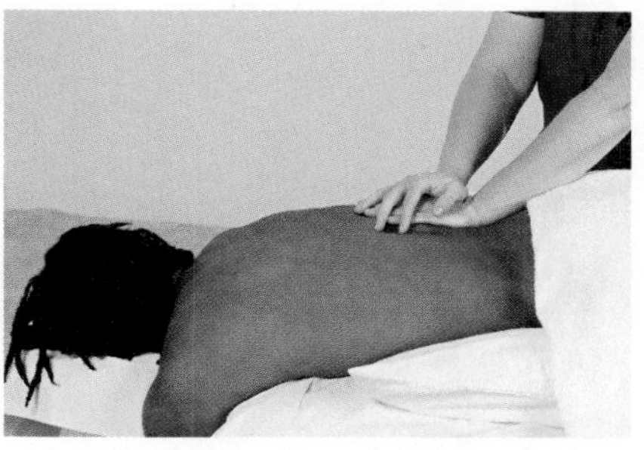

A-10 ■ Rhythmic compression to assess mobility of the ribs and vertebrae, increase fluid movement, and improve respiratory function.

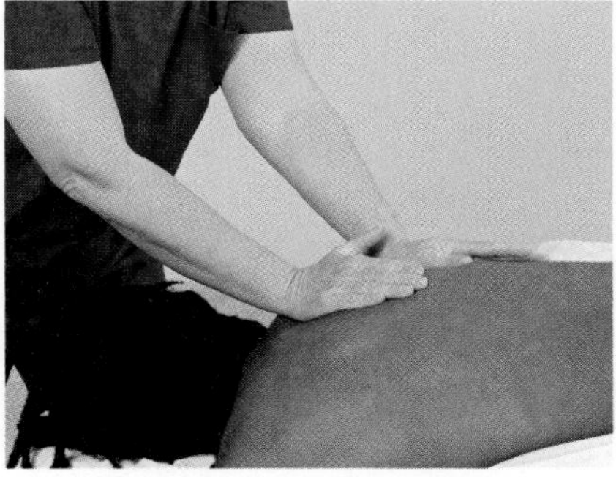

A-11 ■ Palm gliding for assessment and lymphatic drainage.

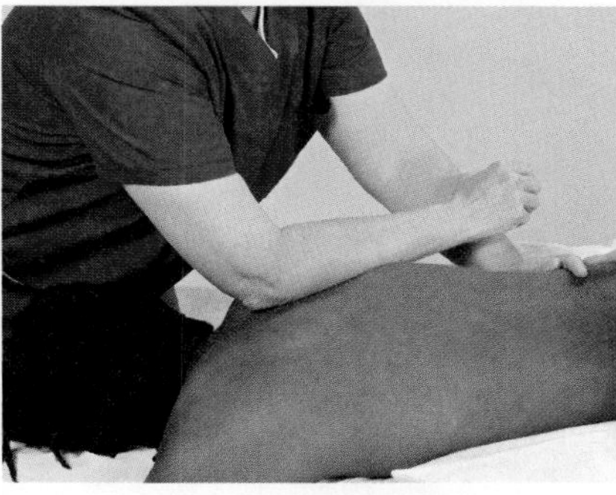

A-12 ■ Forearm gliding and compression: various pressure depths, speeds, and drag.

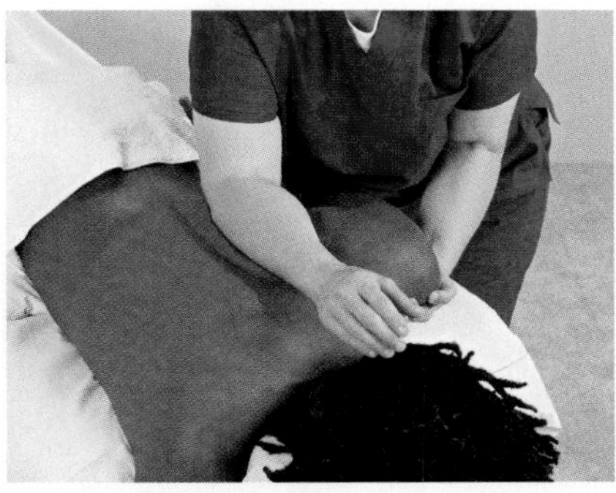

A-13 ■ Position for combined loading: compression and movement of the scapular region.

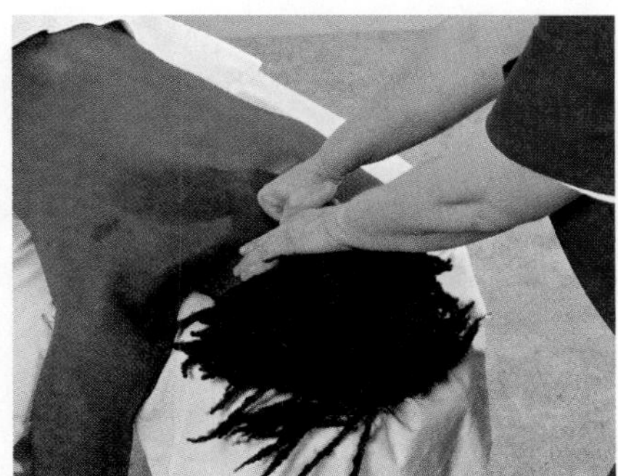

A-14 ■ Fist gliding or compression of the upper shoulder and neck region. Primary focus: assessment and treatment.

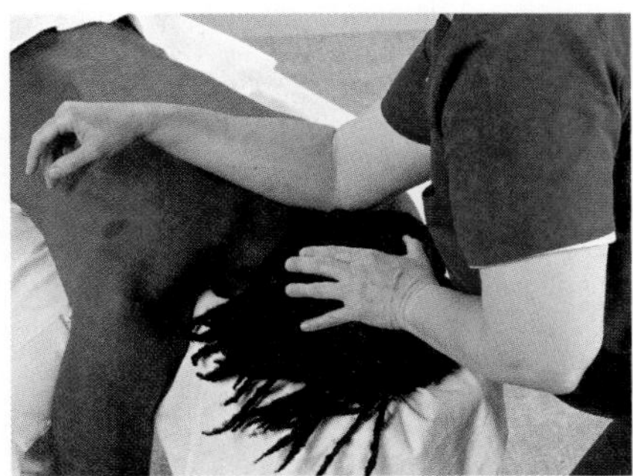

A-15 ■ Forearm gliding or compression of the upper shoulder and neck region. Primary focus: assessment and treatment.

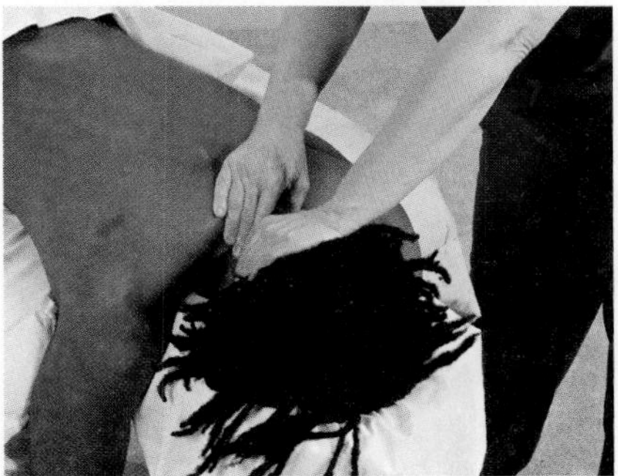

A-16 ■ Kneading to introduce torsion forces to assess tissue texture and to address muscle motor tone, fascial tone, and fluid movement.

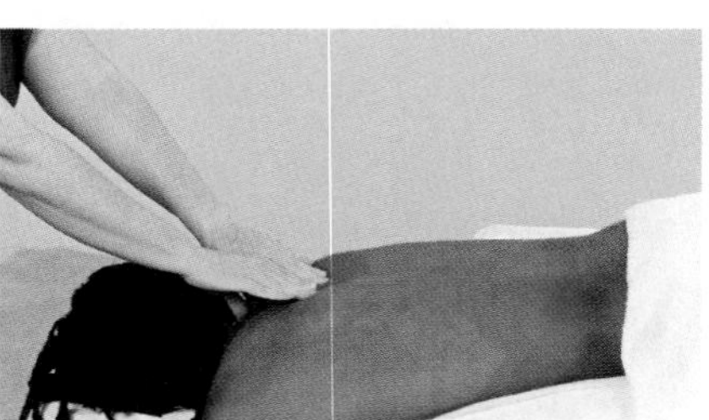

A-17 ■ Inhibitory pressure using the stable hand.

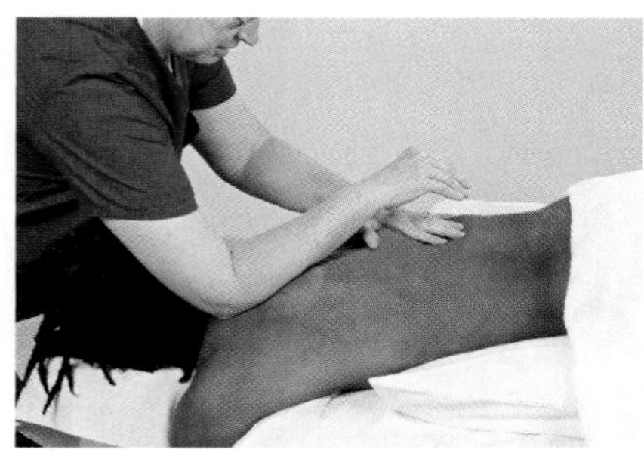

A-18 ■ Inhibitory pressure using the forearm.

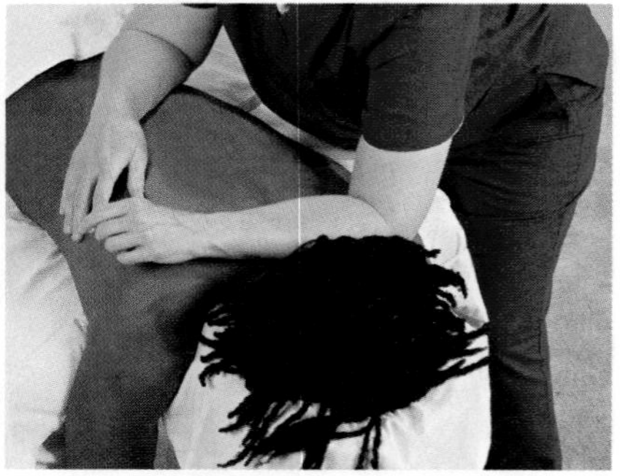

A-19 ■ Forearm inhibitory pressure against the occipital region.

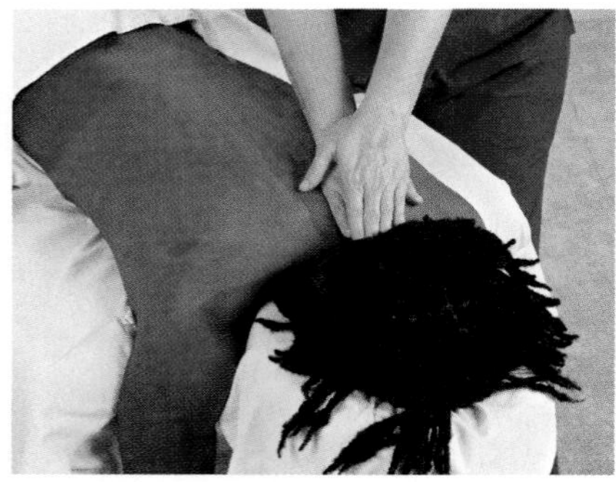

A-20 ■ Inhibitory pressure using the stable hand in the cervical and occipital regions.

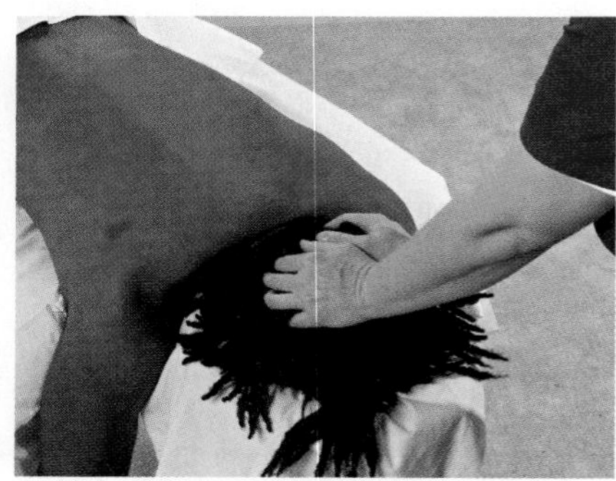

A-21 ■ Massage of the occipital region.

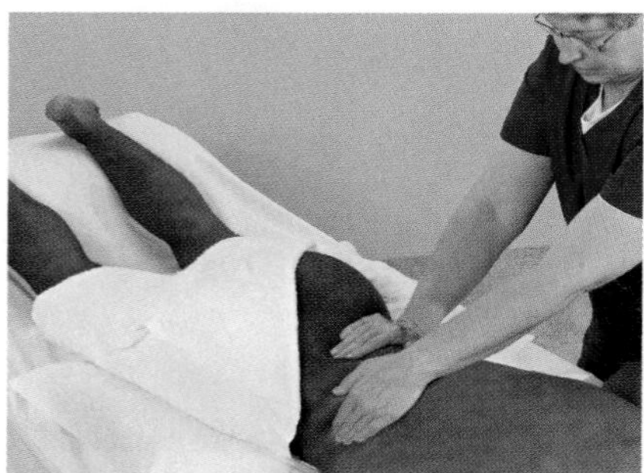

A-22 ■ Kneading of lumbar tissue.

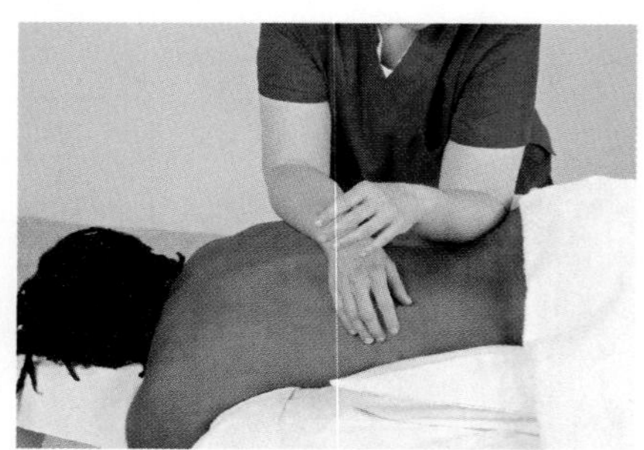

A-23 ■ Inhibitory pressure to a lumbar trigger point.

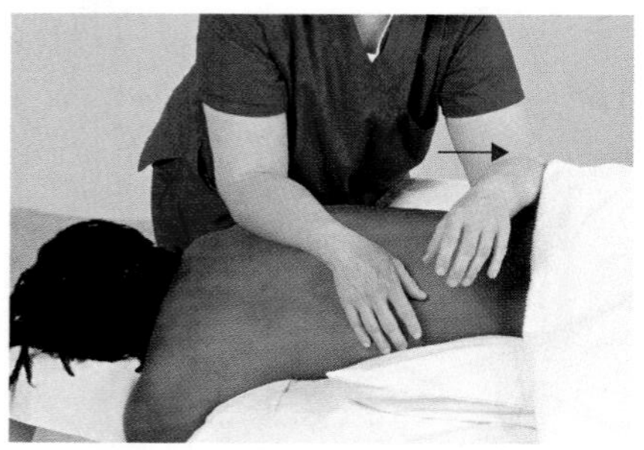

A-24 ■ Direct tissue lengthening of a trigger point area using tension force.

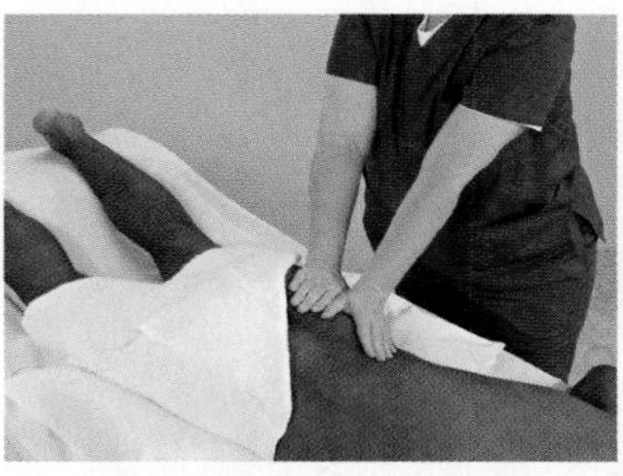

A-25 ■ Palpation assessment of the skin and superficial fascia of the gluteal area; also the position for lymphatic drainage.

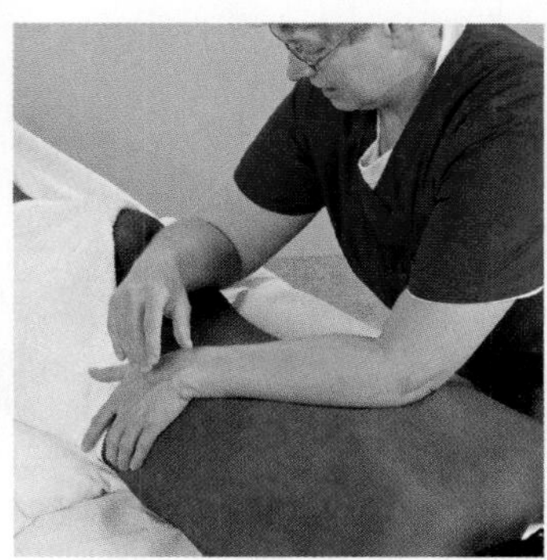

A-26 ■ Forearm gliding using various pressure depths, directions, and speeds to assess the gluteal area.

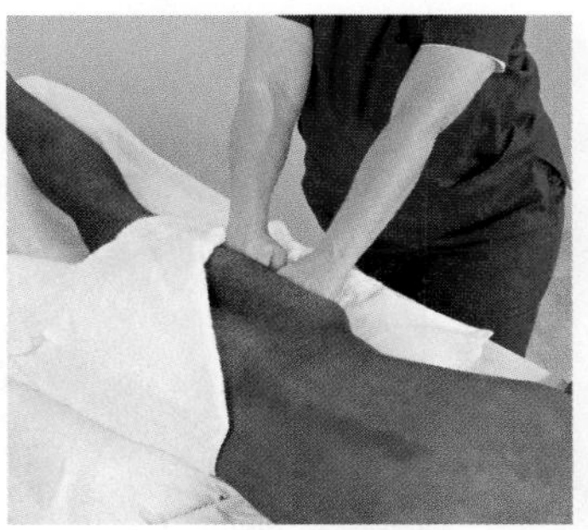

A-27 ■ Fist compression to the gluteal area.

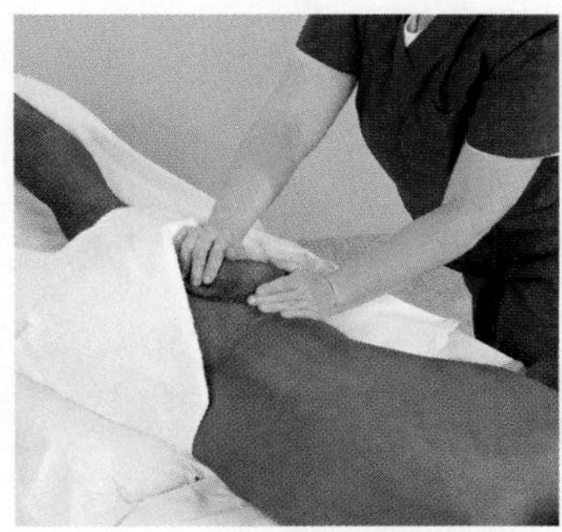

A-28 ■ Kneading of the gluteal area.

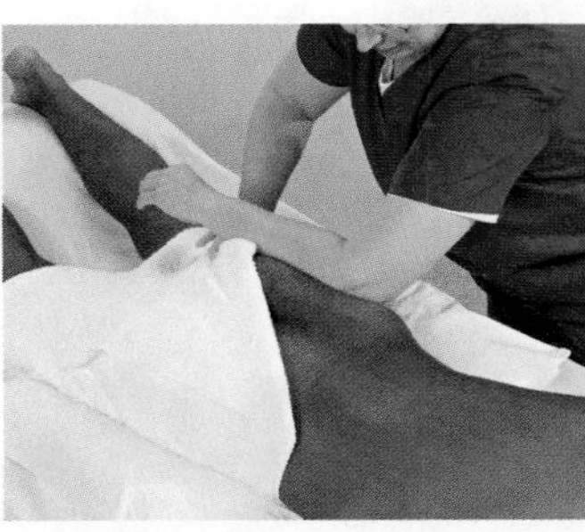

A-29 ■ Inhibitory pressure to the gluteal area.

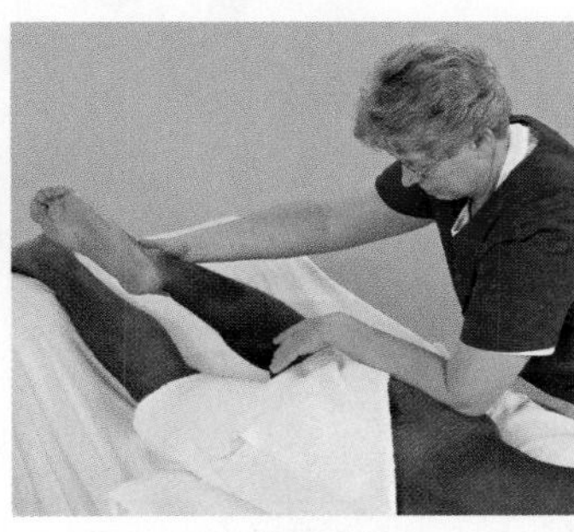

A-30 ■ Inhibitory pressure with movement combined loading. Movement can be passive to introduce mechanical force or active to introduce muscle energy methods.

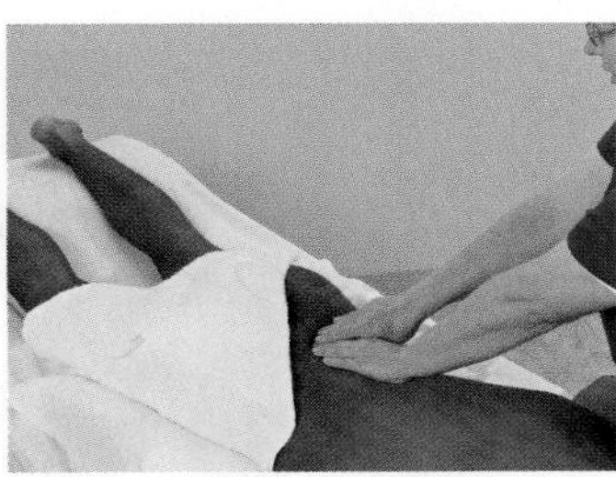

A-31 ■ Inhibitory pressure in the sacroiliac (SI) joint area.

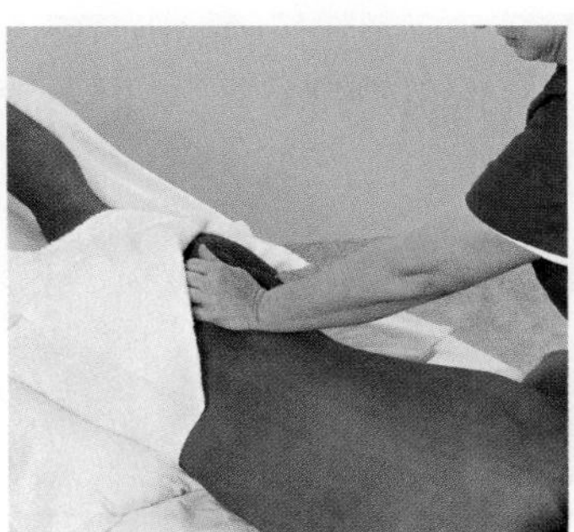

A-32 ■ Compression against the sacrum.

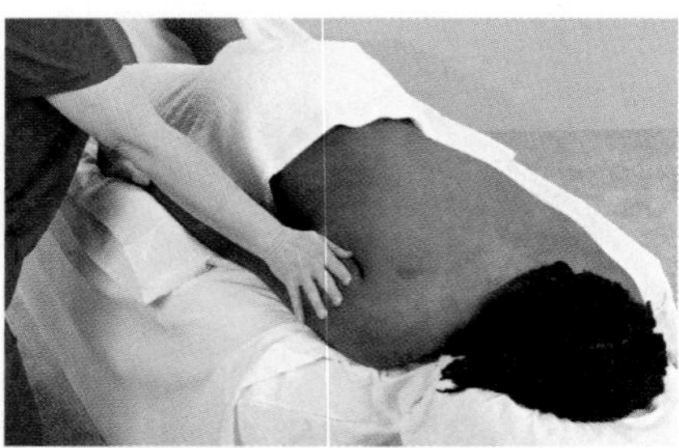

A-33 ■ Palm gliding using various pressure depths, speeds, and directions to assess tissue and to address fluid movement, muscle motor tone, and fascial tone.

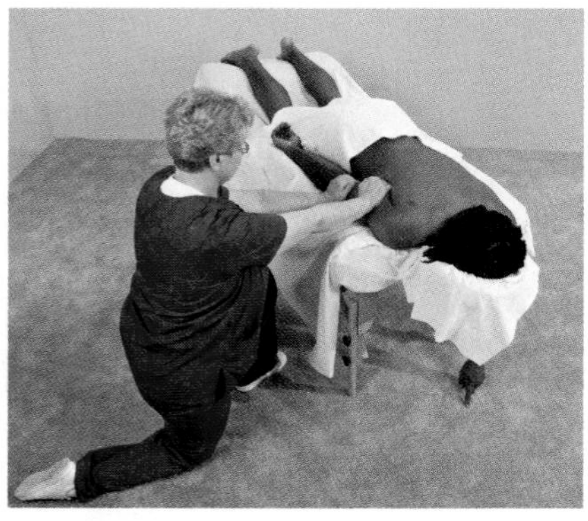

A-34 ■ Effective body mechanics for kneading the arm (patient prone).

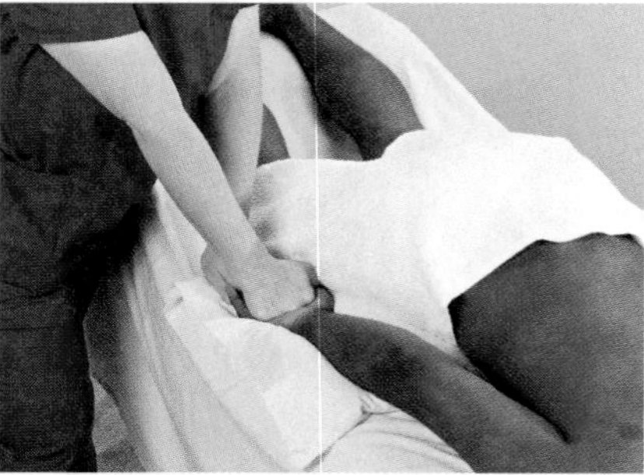

A-35 ■ Fist compression of the palm.

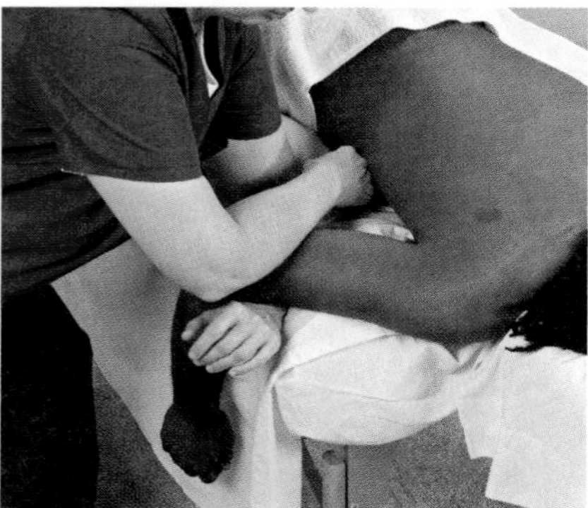

A-36 ■ Forearm compressive gliding of the triceps area.

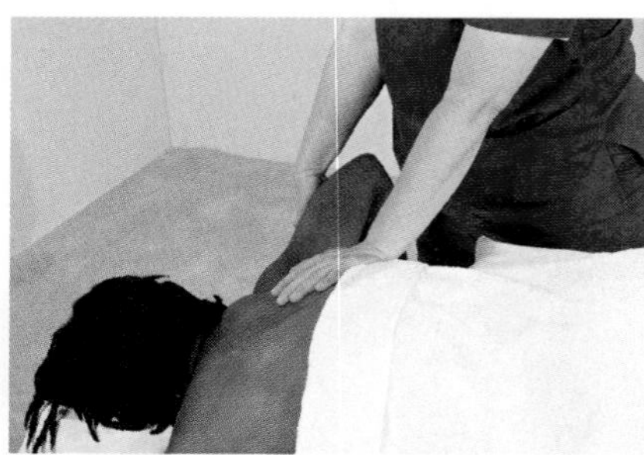

A-37 ■ Shoulder area: position for active and passive range of motion, muscle testing, and muscle energy methods for lengthening and stretching.

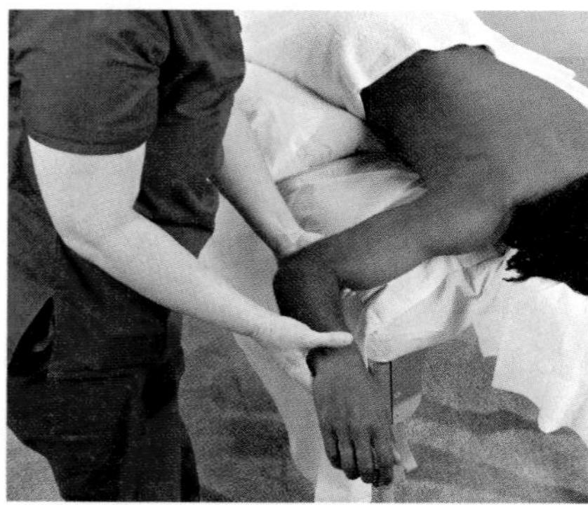

A-38 ■ Shoulder and arm: position for active and passive range of motion, muscle testing, muscle energy methods, and oscillation for lengthening and stretching.

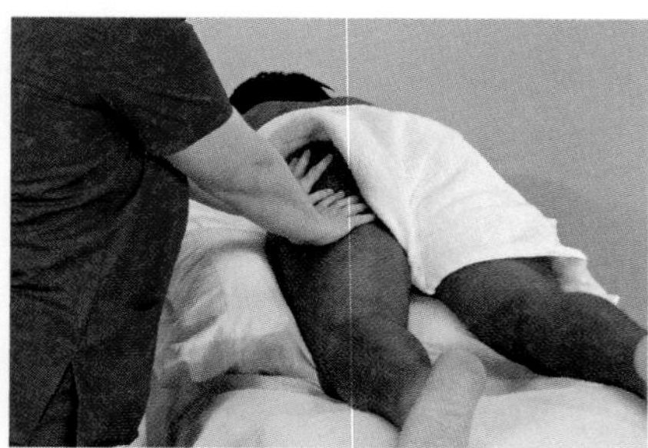

A-39 ■ Palpation of the skin of the lower limb—assessment using skin drag, tissue bind, hot and cold.

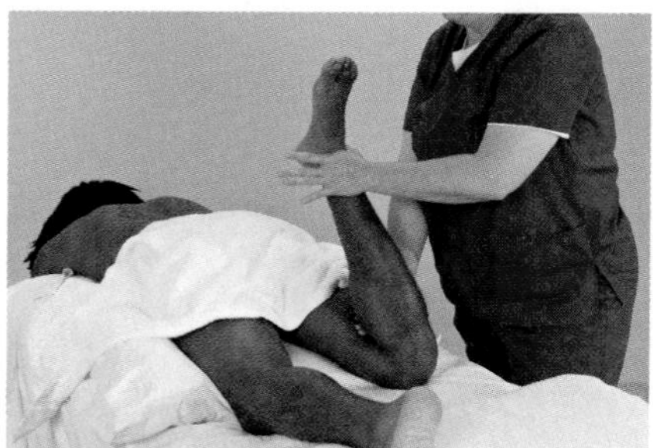

A-40 ■ Position for various assessment and intervention procedures incorporating movement: active and passive range of motion.

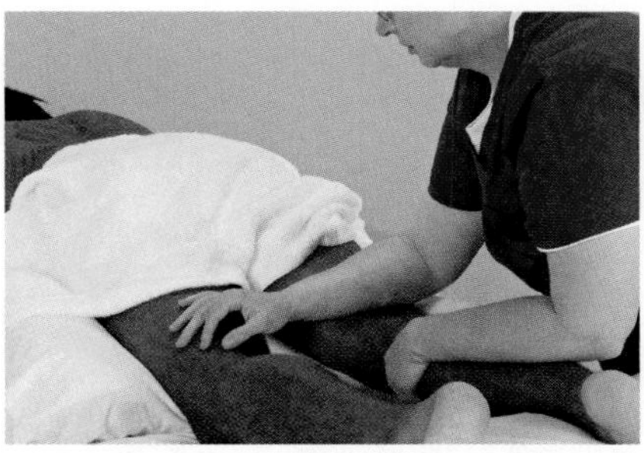

A-41 ■ Gliding in the thigh region (patient prone). Various pressure depths, speeds, directions, as well as drag assessment, to address fluid movement, muscle and motor tone, and fascial tone to increase pliability.

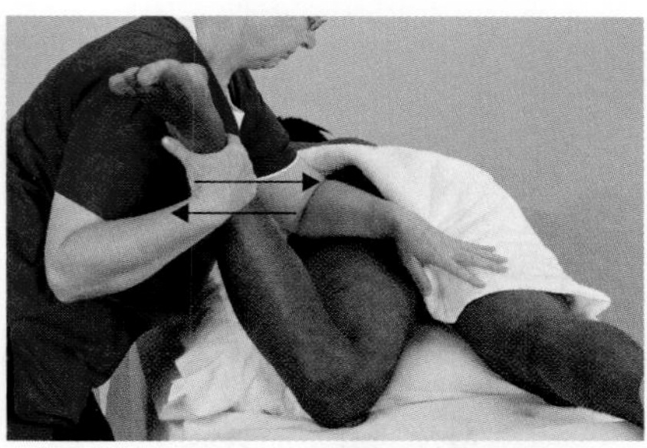

A-42 ■ Combined loading: compression and movement.

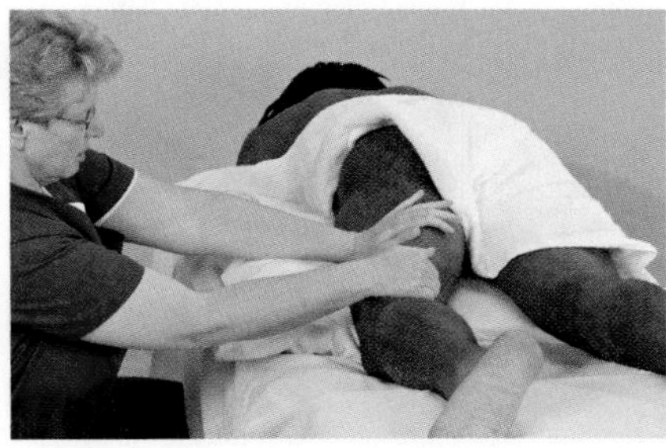

A-43 ■ Kneading of the thigh (patient prone)—therapist kneeling.

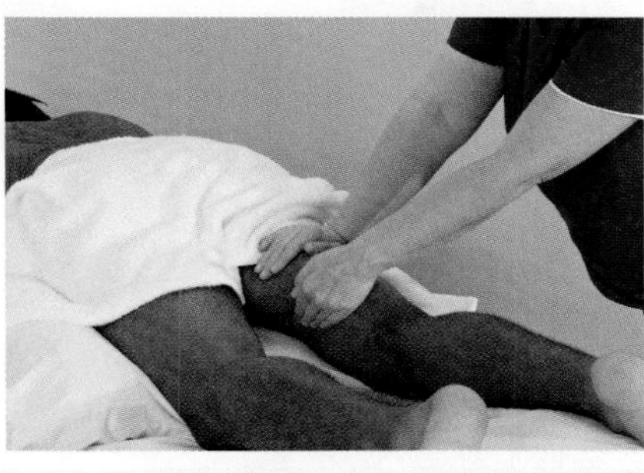

A-44 ■ Kneading of the thigh (patient prone)—therapist standing.

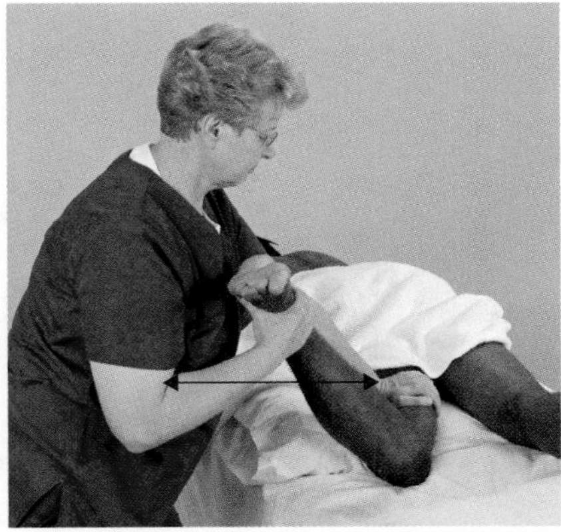

A-45 ■ Combined loading: compression, bend force, and movement.

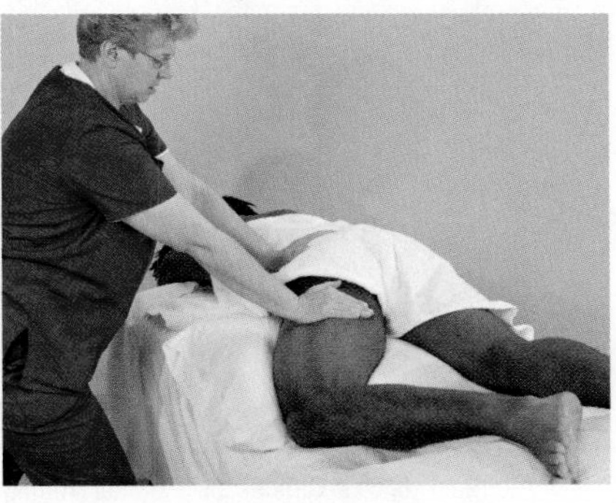

A-46 ■ Position for accessing the lateral thigh (patient prone).

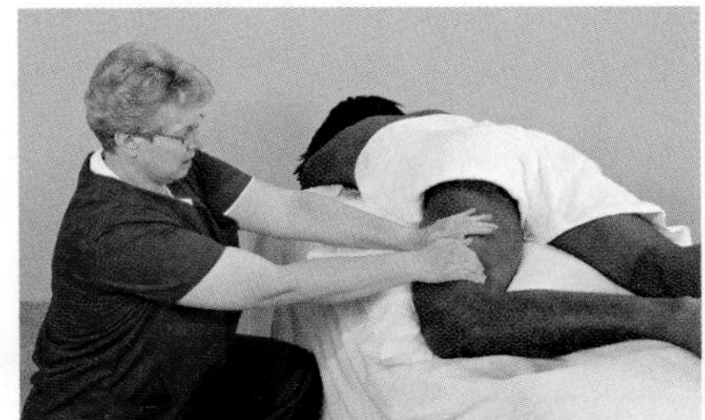

A-47 ■ Shear force to the iliotibial (IT) band—therapist kneeling.

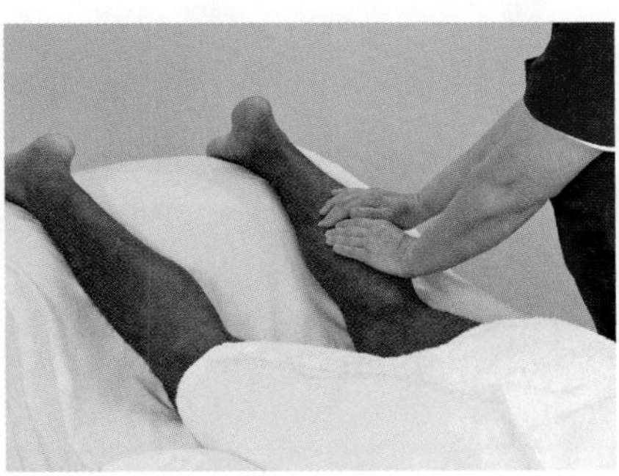

A-48 ■ Assessment of the skin and superficial fascia of the calf.

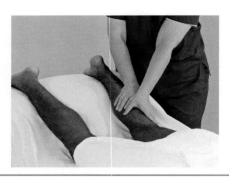

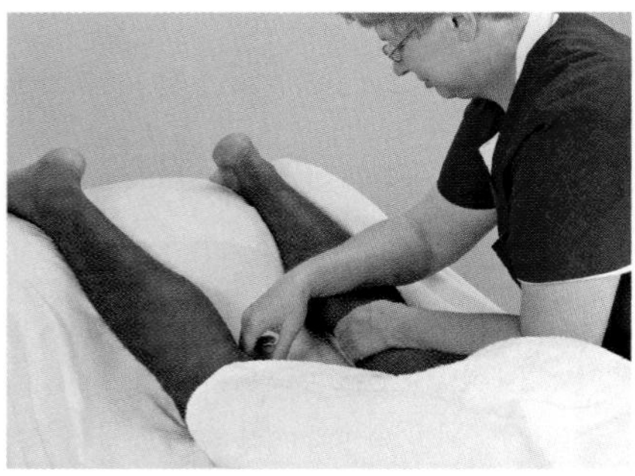

A-49 ■ Lymphatic drainage.

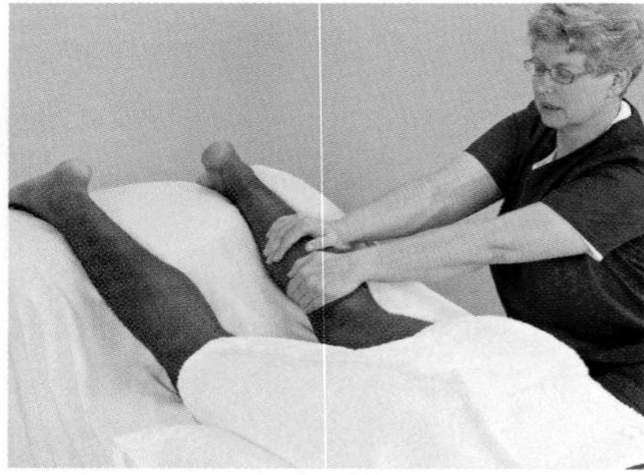

A-50 ■ Gliding to apply tension and compression force for assessment and treatment.

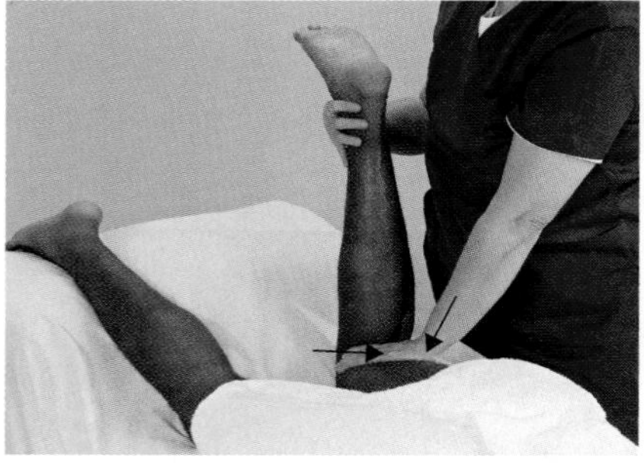

A-51 ■ Kneading of the calf—therapist kneeling.

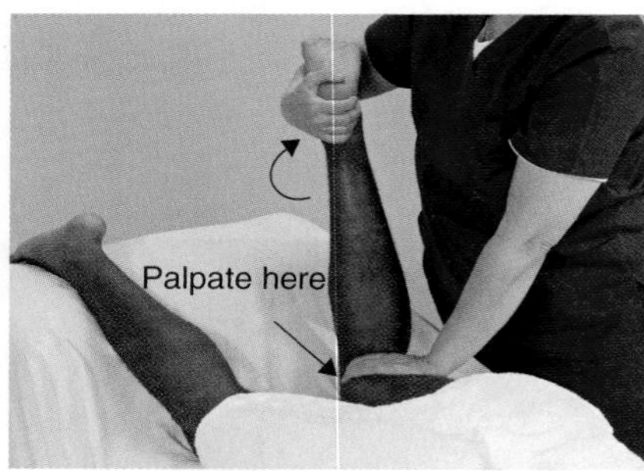

A-52 ■ Inhibitory pressure to the gastrocnemius and hamstring attachments.

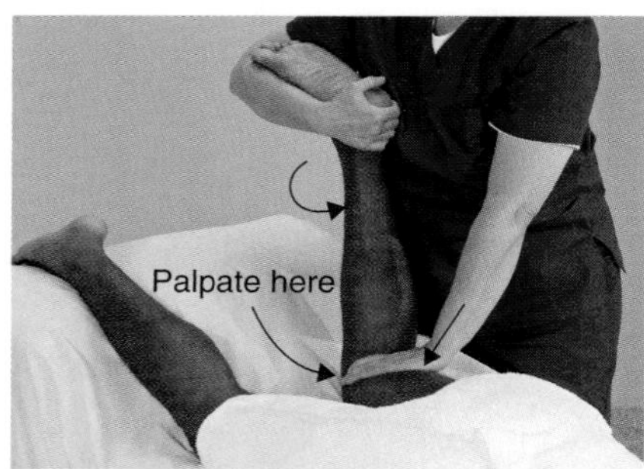

A-53 ■ Assessment and treatment of external rotation of the knee.

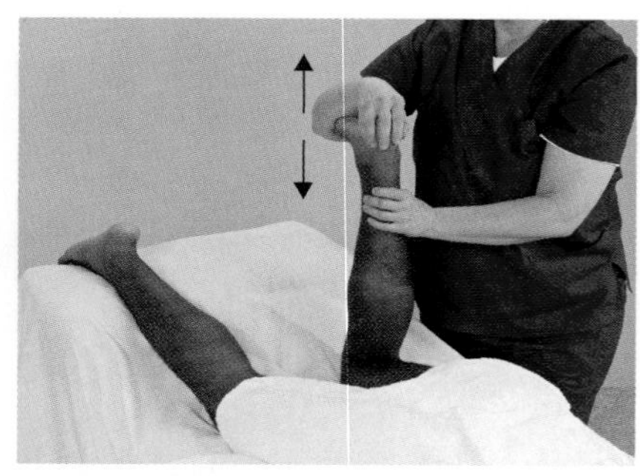

A-54 ■ Assessment and treatment of internal rotation of the knee.

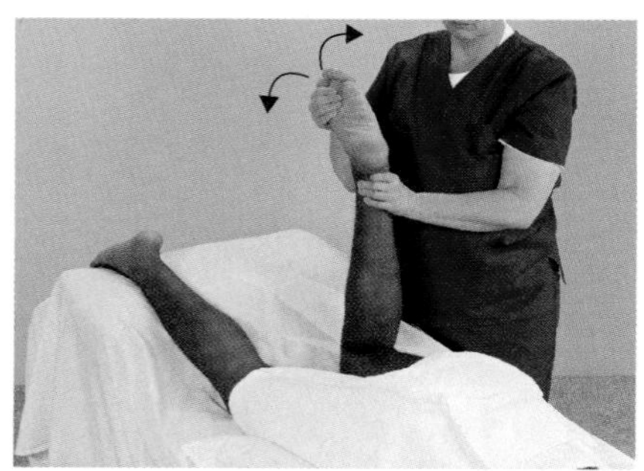

A-55 ■ Assessment and treatment of ankle movement: dorsiflexion–plantar flexion.

A-56 ■ Assessment and treatment of the ankle: inversion (supination), eversion (pronation).

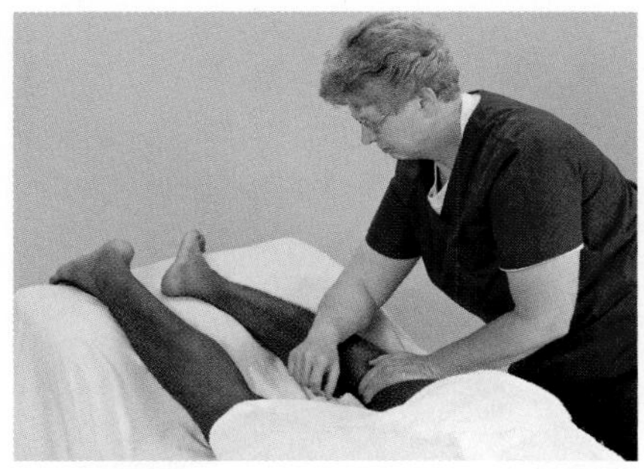

A-57 ■ Position for addressing lateral leg with patient prone.

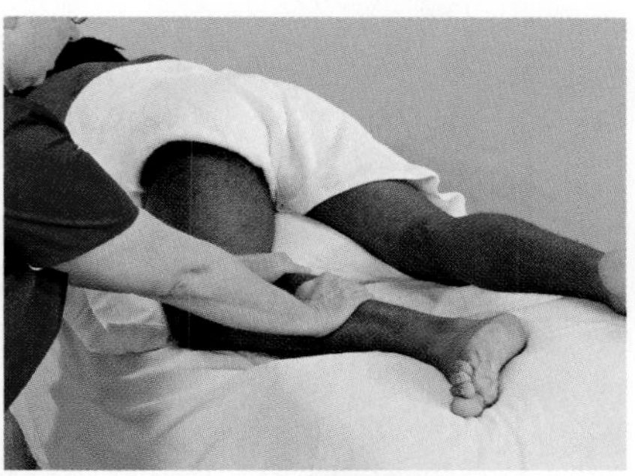

A-58 ■ Kneading of the lateral leg: patient prone.

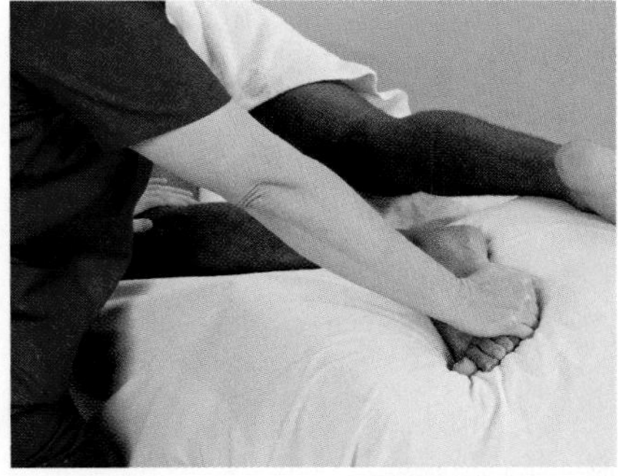

A-59 ■ Compression and joint movement of foot: patient prone.

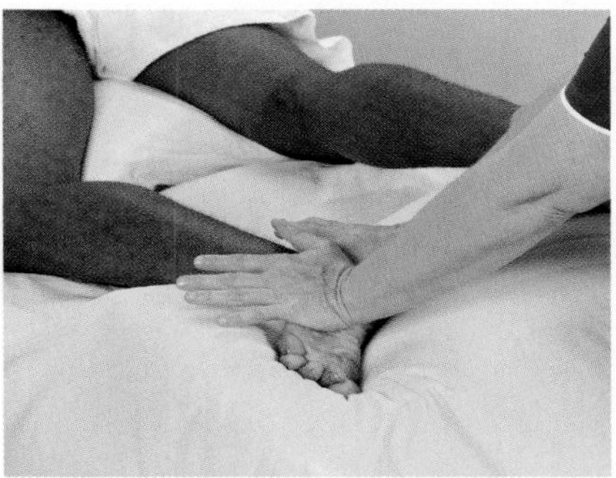

A-60 ■ Compression and joint movement—foot: patient prone.

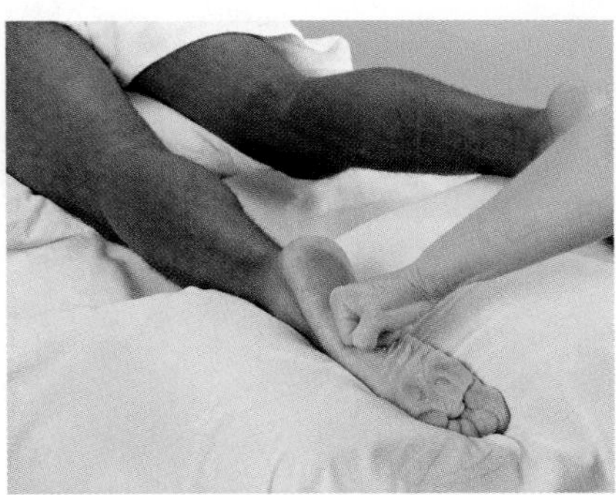

A-61 ■ Compression of the sole of the foot with a loose fist.

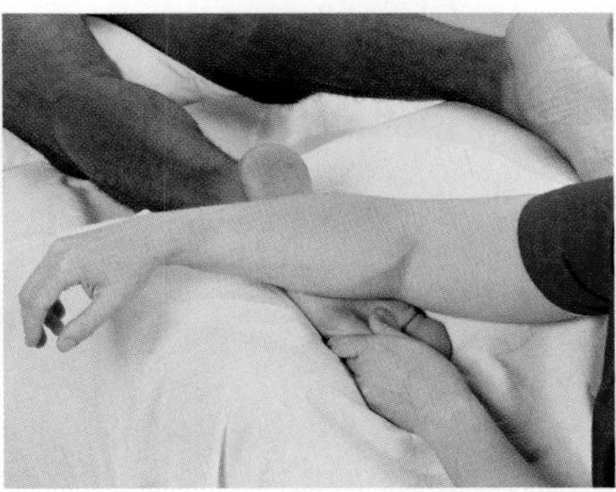

A-62 ■ Compression of the sole of the foot with the forearm.

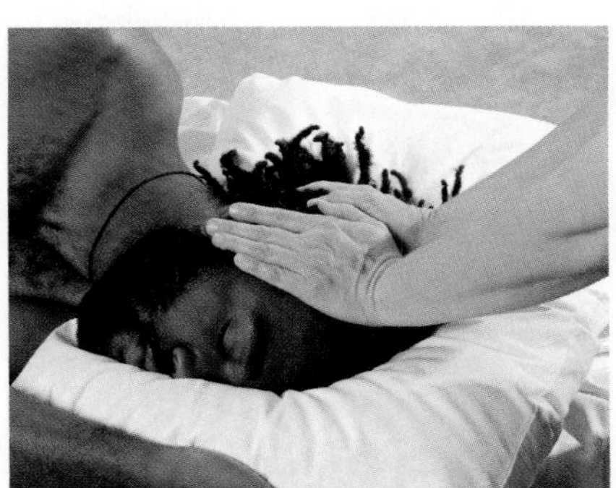

A-63 ■ Head, face, and neck in side-lying position.

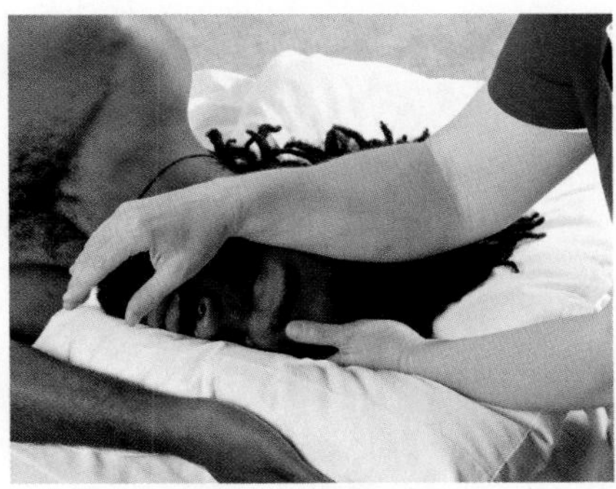

A-64 ■ Compression of the temporalis muscle.

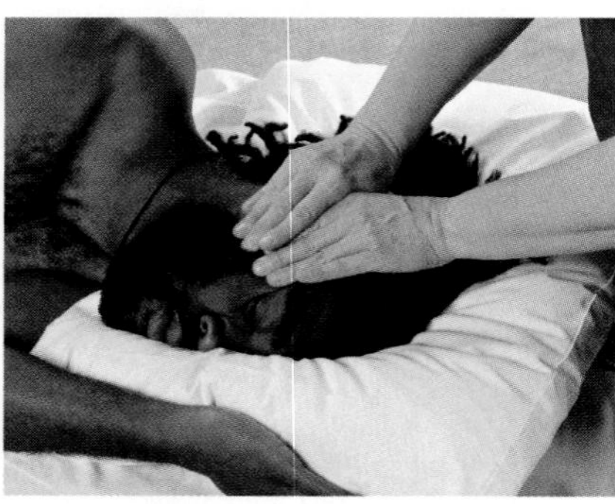

A-65 ■ Inhibitory pressure of soft tissue in the temporomandibular joint (TMJ) area.

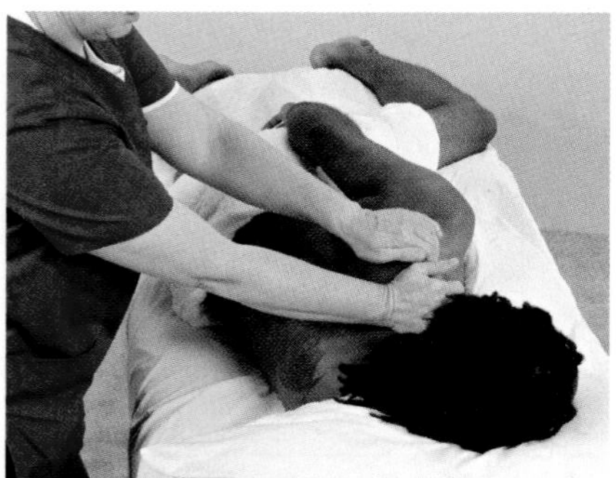

A-66 ■ Kneading of shoulder areas (patient side-lying).

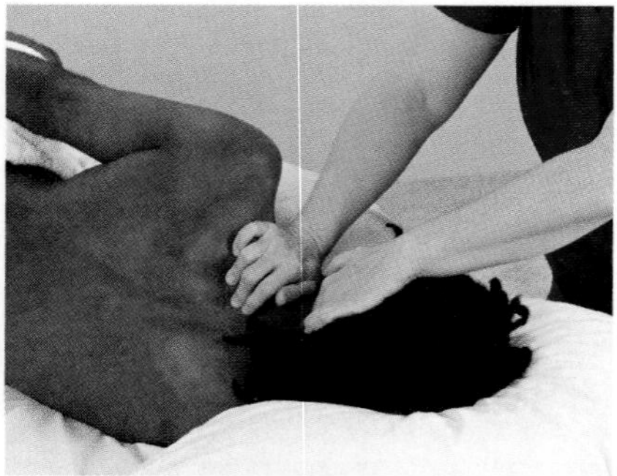

A-67 ■ Kneading of the neck and upper shoulder (patient side-lying).

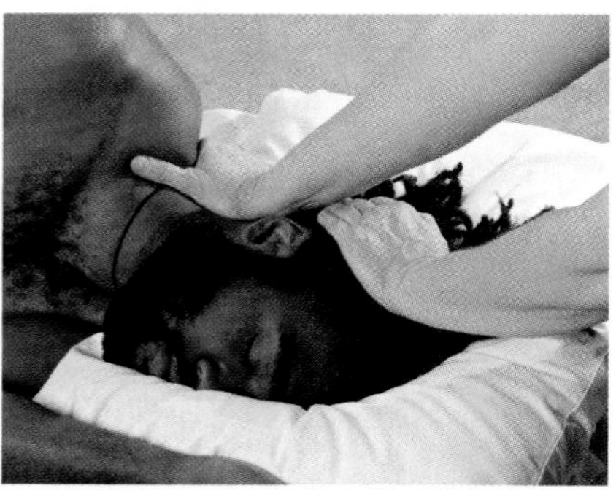

A-68 ■ Palm compression to the neck.

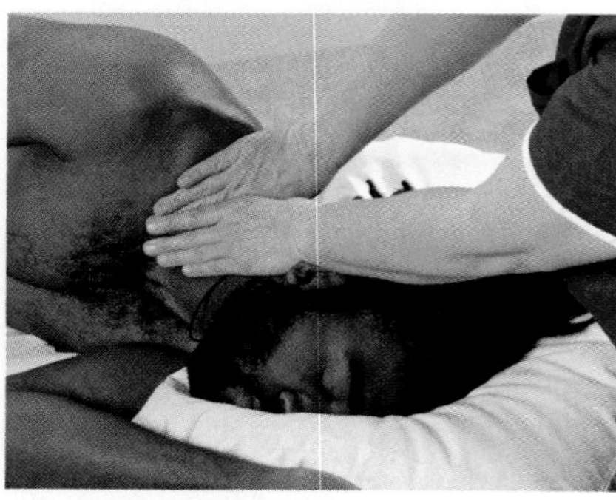

A-69 ■ Lymphatic drainage.

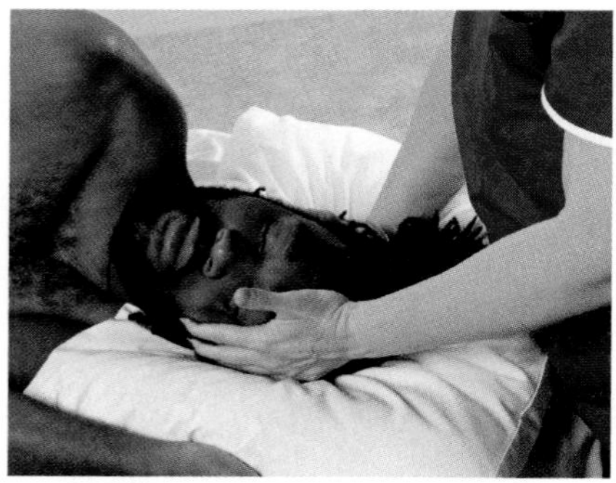

A-70 ■ Position for movement methods for the cervical area.

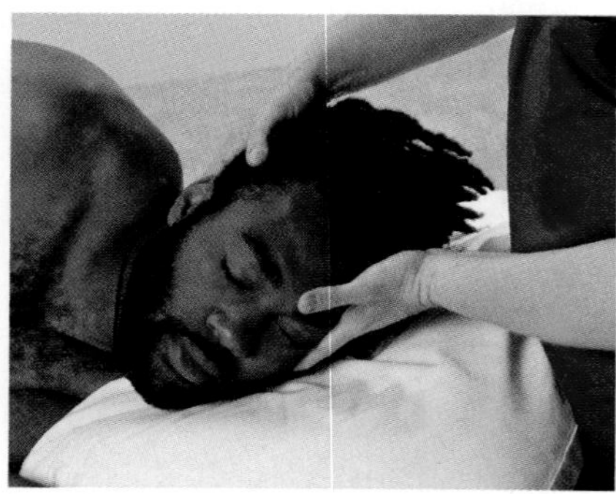

A-71 ■ Range of motion of the cervical area.

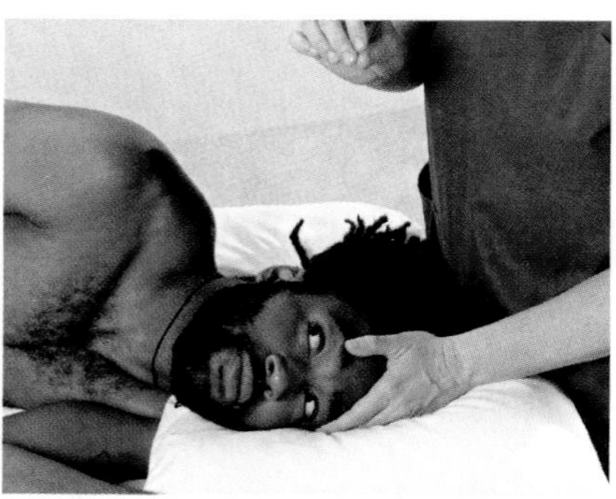

A-72 ■ Muscle energy methods for the cervical area using eye positions.

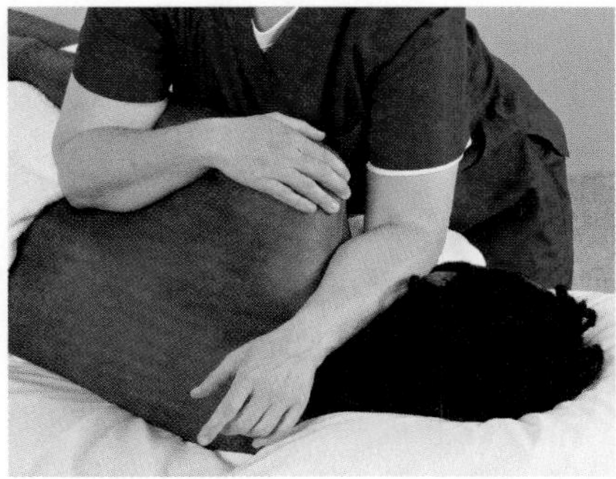

A-73 ■ Compression to the upper cervical and occipital areas; the patient moves the head and/or eyes in a circle to achieve combined loading.

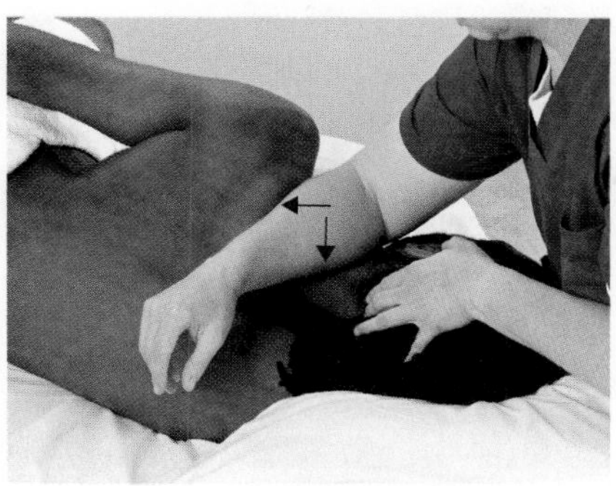

A-74 ■ Compression to the lower cervical area and upper shoulder; the patient moves the shoulder to achieve combined loading.

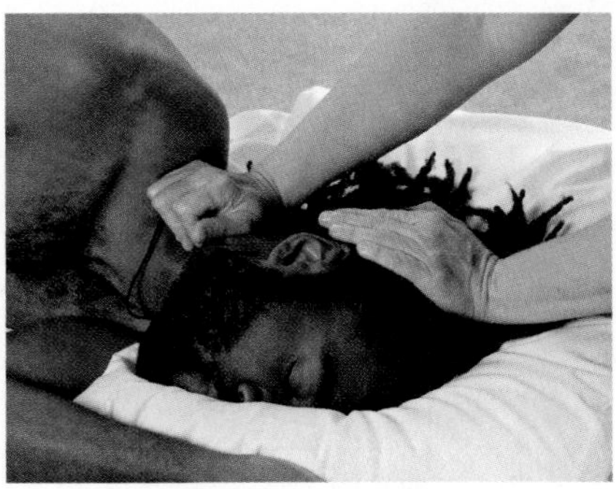

A-75 ■ Position for inhibition and stretching of the sternocleidomastoid muscle (patient side-lying).

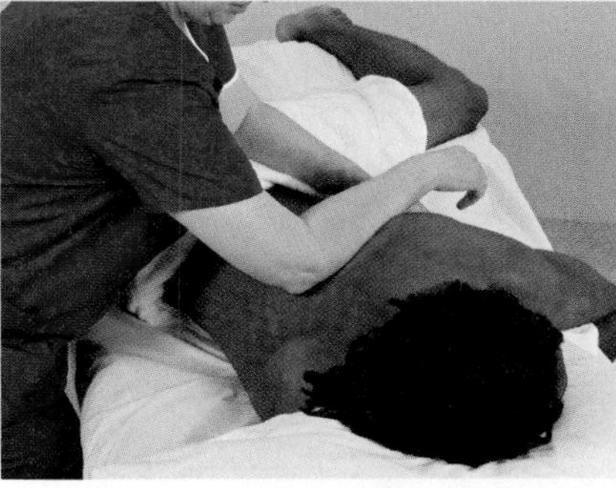

A-76 ■ Position for assessing and treating the back (patient side-lying): gliding at various pressure depths, speeds, durations, and drag, depending on the desired outcome.

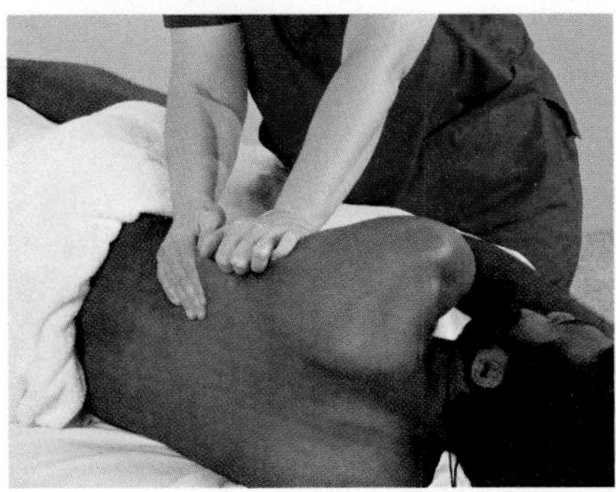

A-77 ■ Kneading with patient in the side-lying position.

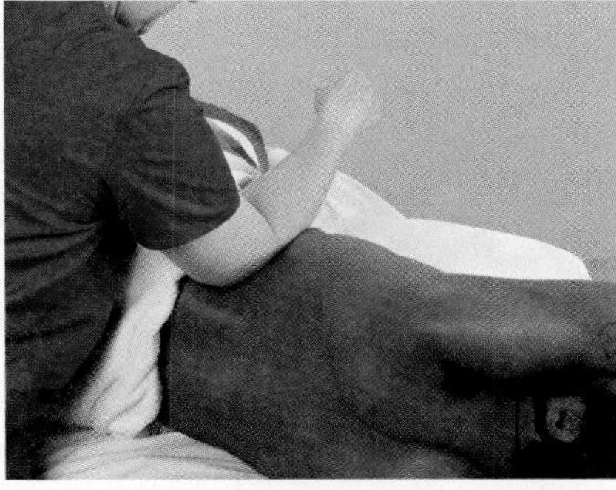

A-78 ■ Inhibitory pressure in the lumbar region (patient side-lying).

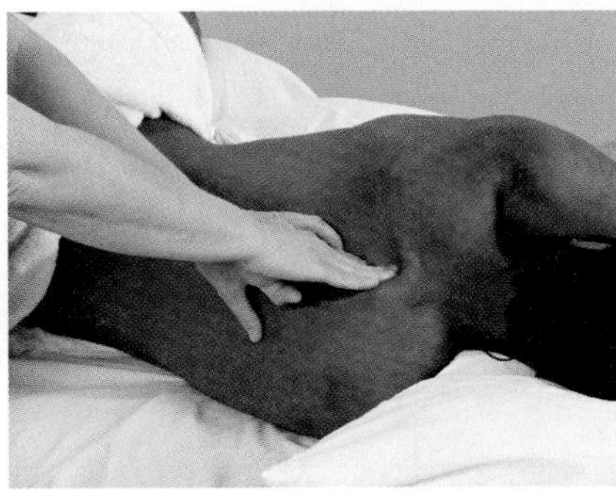

A-79 ■ Massage of the deep muscles along the vertebral column.

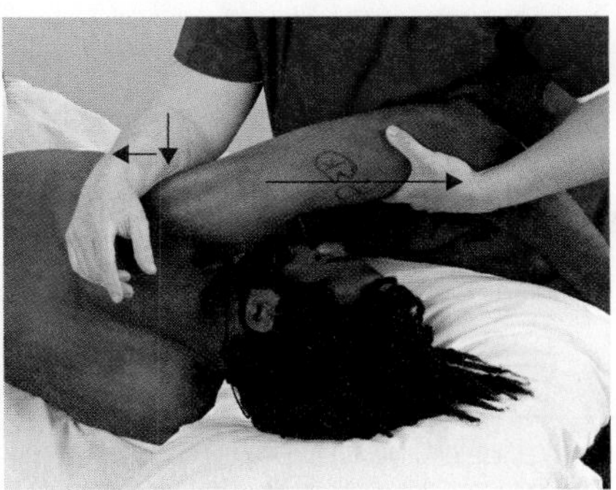

A-80 ■ Side-lying position for addressing the shoulder adductor: compression, gliding, and movement.

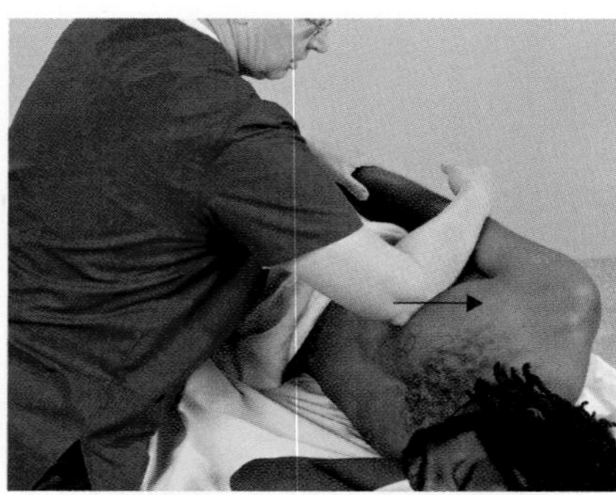

A-81 ■ Position for addressing the anterior thorax (patient side-lying).

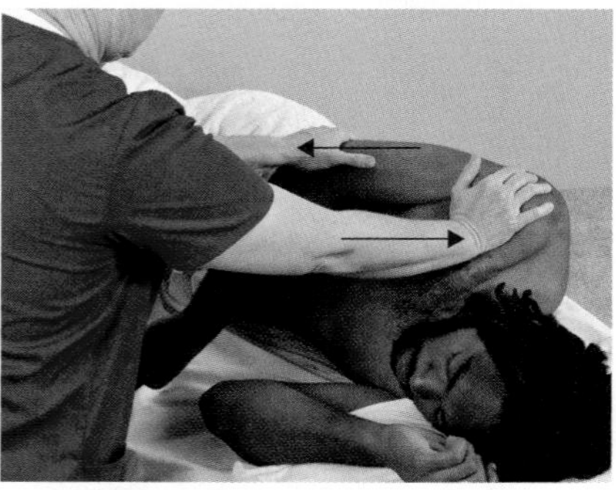

A-82 ■ Kneading and compression using counterpressure.

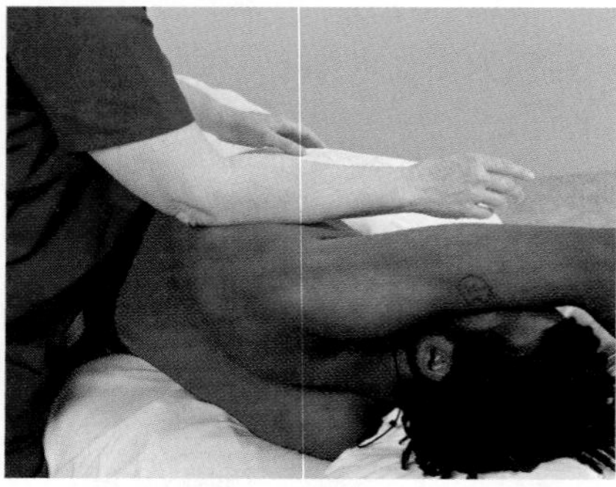

A-83 ■ Position for addressing rib movement (especially effective for the anterior serratus).

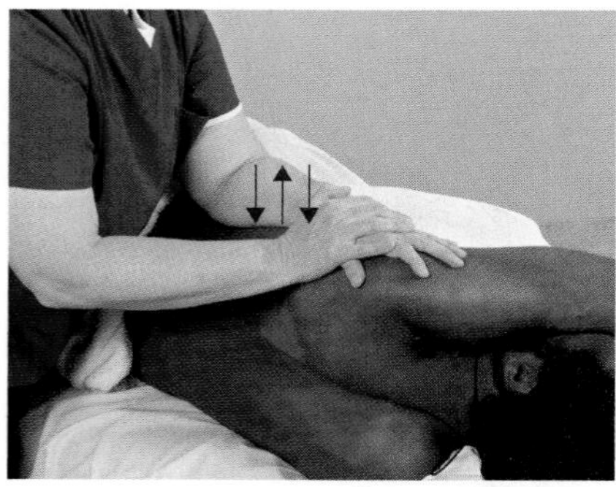

A-84 ■ Position for rib movement.

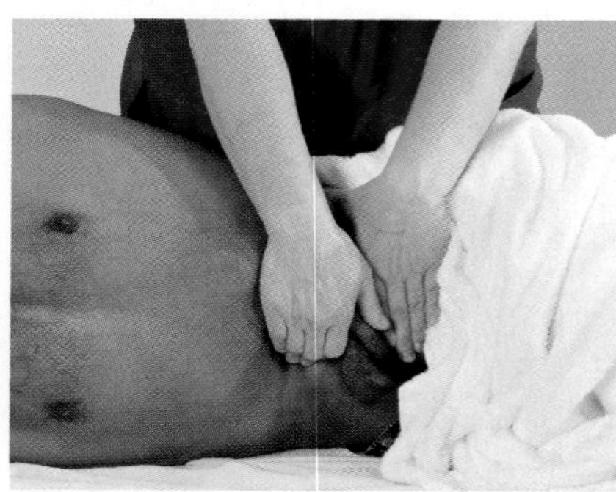

A-85 ■ Position for massage of the abdomen (patient side-lying).

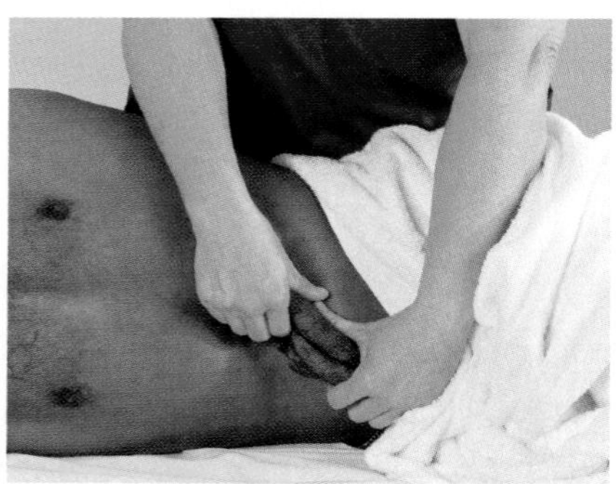

A-86 ■ Combined loading to the rectus abdominis: bend and shear forces.

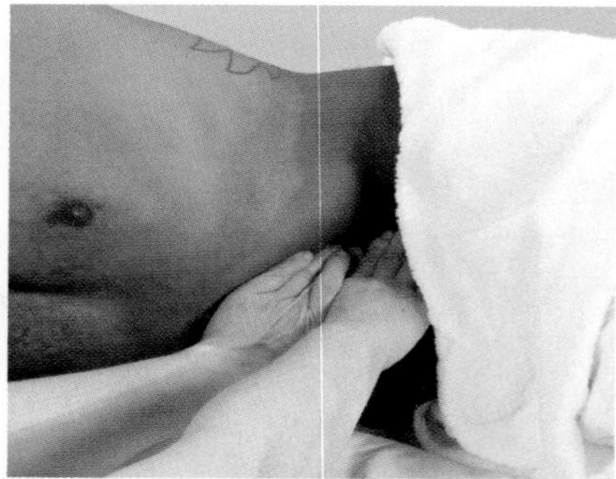

A-87 ■ Position for deeper massage of the abdomen and for psoas release (patient side-lying)—therapist kneeling.

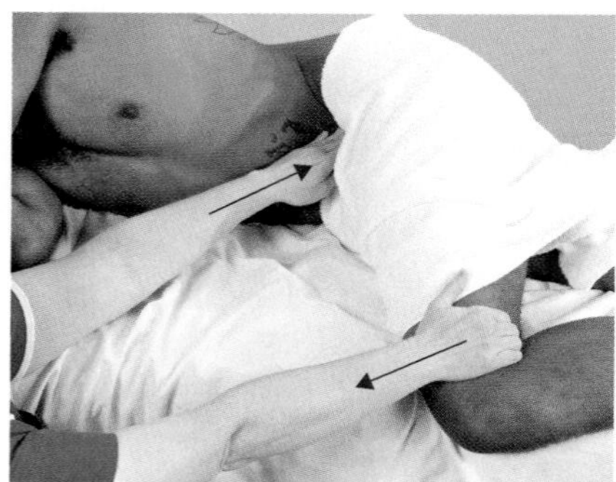

A-88 ■ Combined loading to the psoas: compression and bend forces—therapist kneeling.

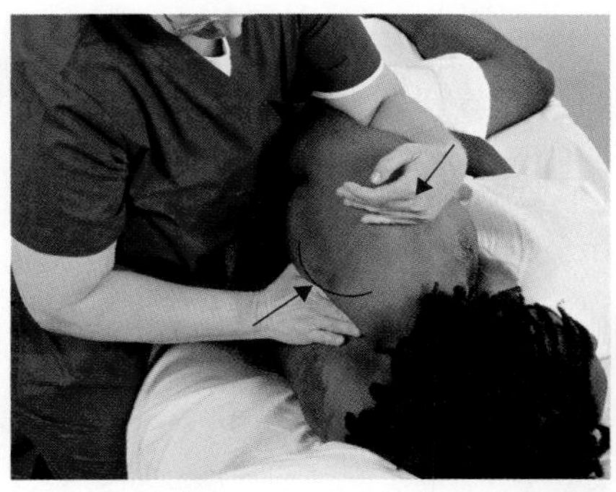

A-89 ■ Position for addressing the scapular border and for providing movement to the scapula with the patient in the side-lying position.

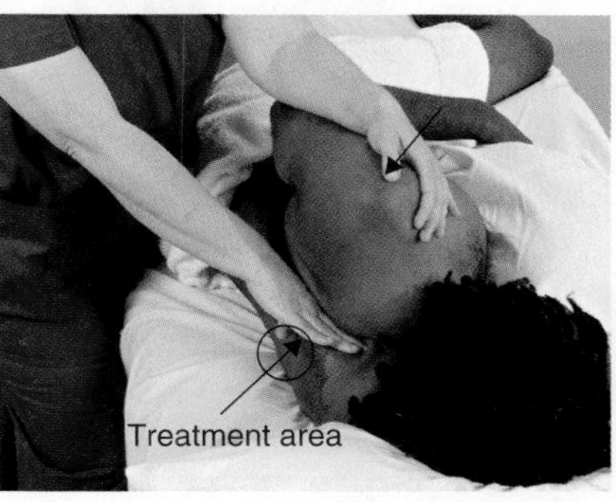

A-90 ■ Position for addressing the scapular border (this position is most effective for the target area in the circle).

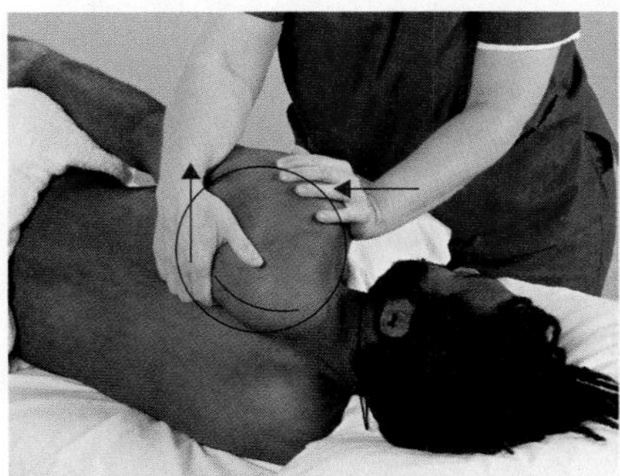

A-91 ■ Alternate position for addressing the scapula (the target area is circled).

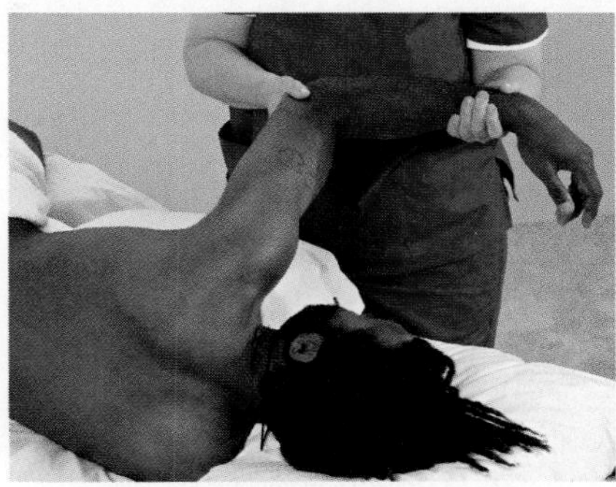

A-92 ■ Position for upper limb movement methods.

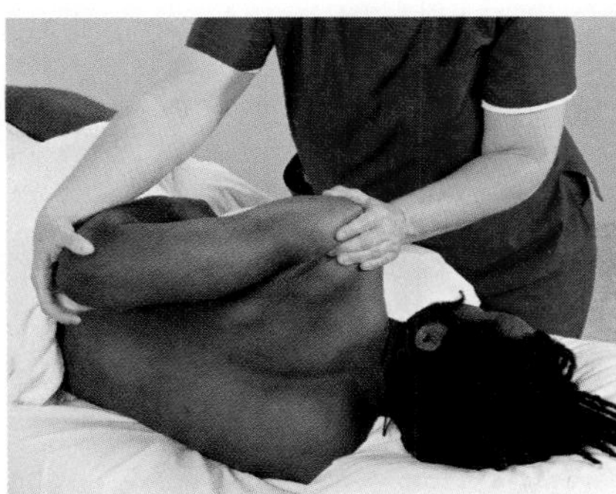

A-93 ■ Position for upper limb movement methods.

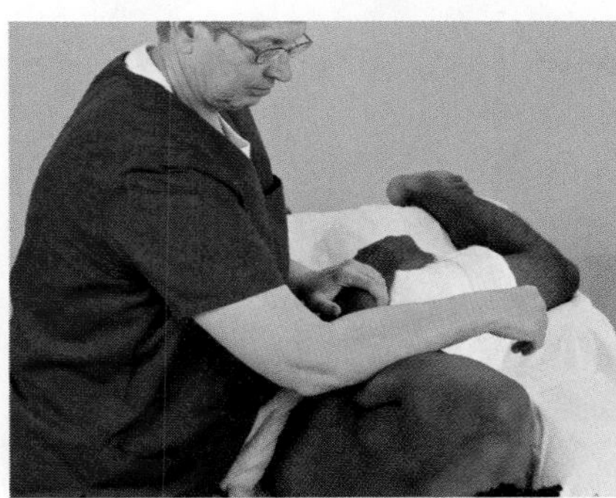

A-94 ■ Gliding of the arm (patient side-lying).

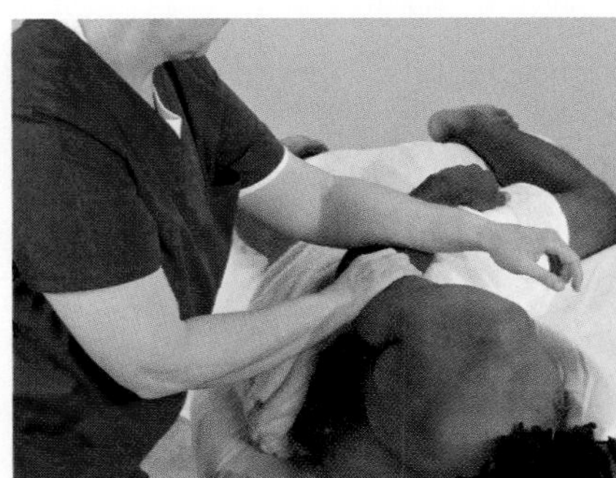

A-95 ■ Inhibitory pressure on the wrist extensors.

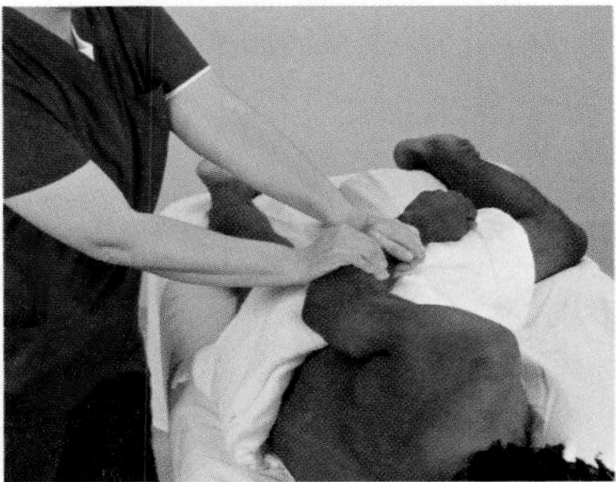

A-96 ■ Kneading of the arm (patient side-lying).

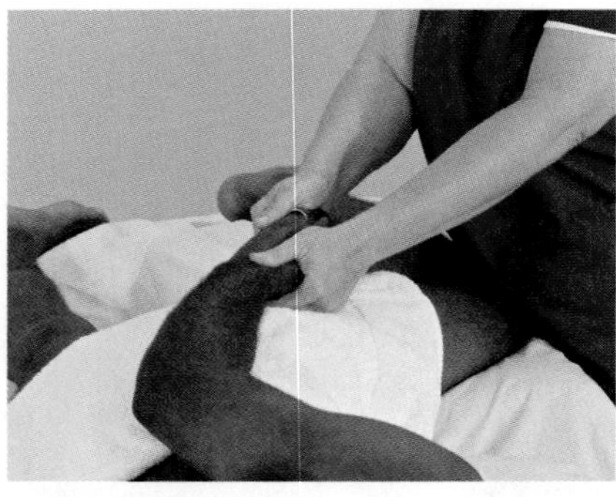

A-97 ■ Massage of the hand (patient side-lying).

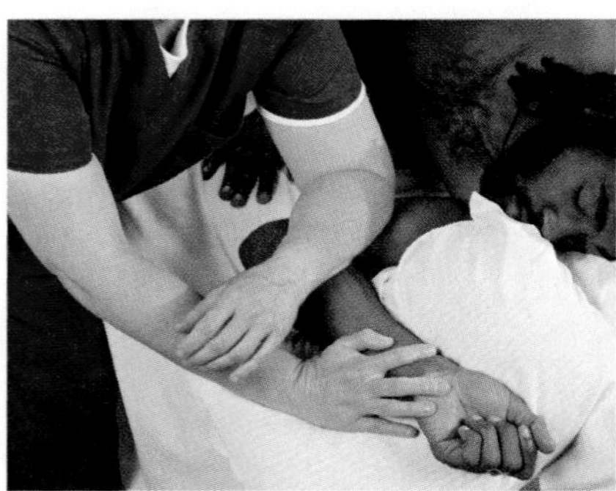

A-98 ■ Position for the arm: compression and gliding.

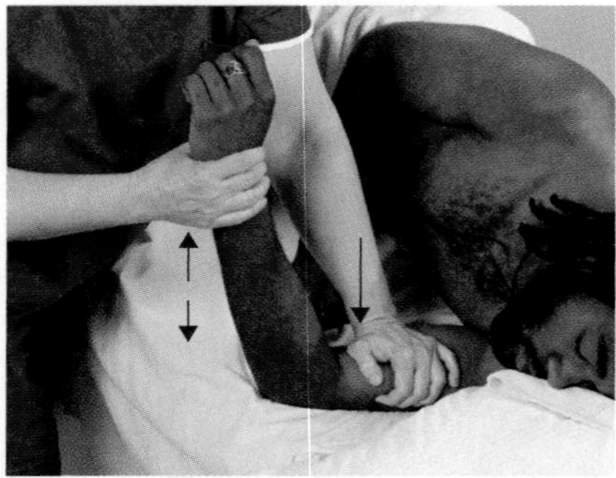

A-99 ■ Combined loading: compression and movement. Internal and external rotation, effective alternative for kneading methods.

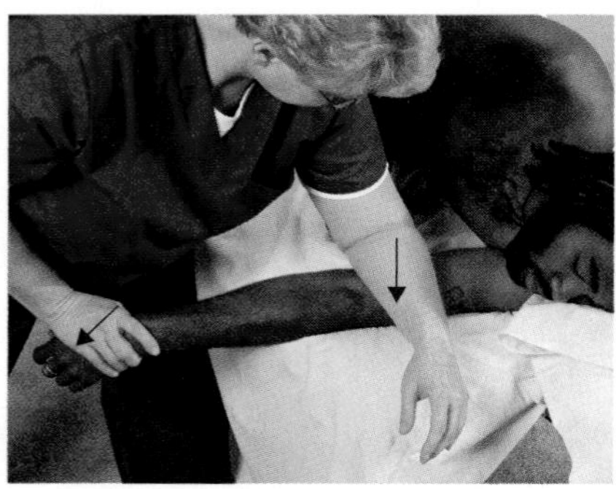

A-100 ■ Position for combined loading. Compression and lengthening (tension force) can be considered active release and stretch.

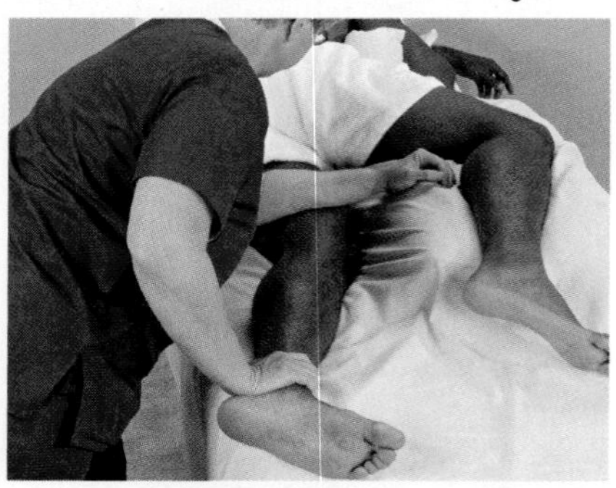

A-101 ■ Thigh position (patient side-lying): gliding used at various pressure depths, speeds, directions, and durations for assessment and treatment.

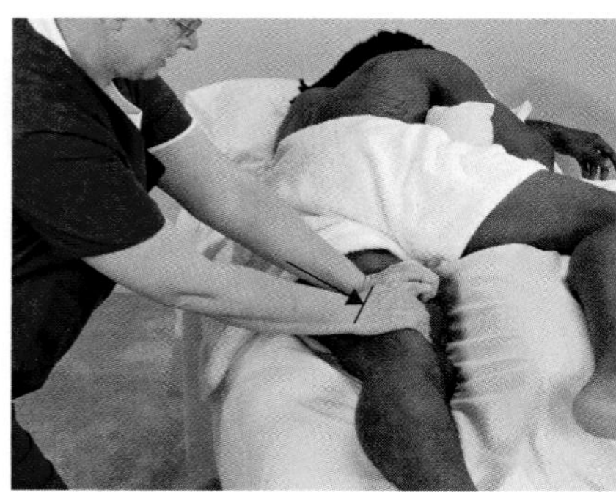

A-102 ■ Kneading of the thigh (patient side-lying): direction of mechanical force is 90° against soft tissue.

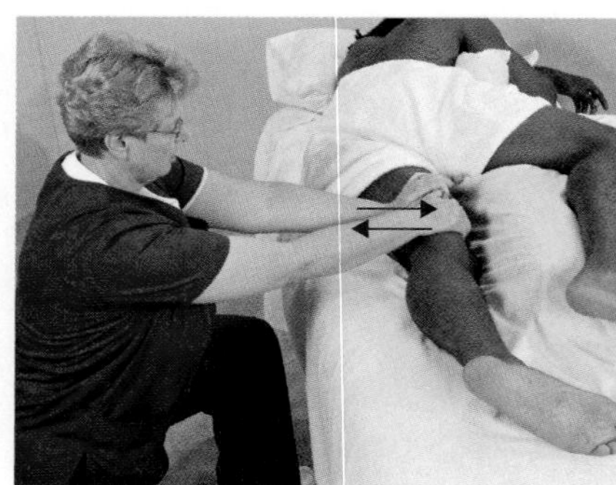

A-103 ■ Kneading while kneeling directs mechanical force horizontally. This position is effective for application of bend, shear, and torsion forces.

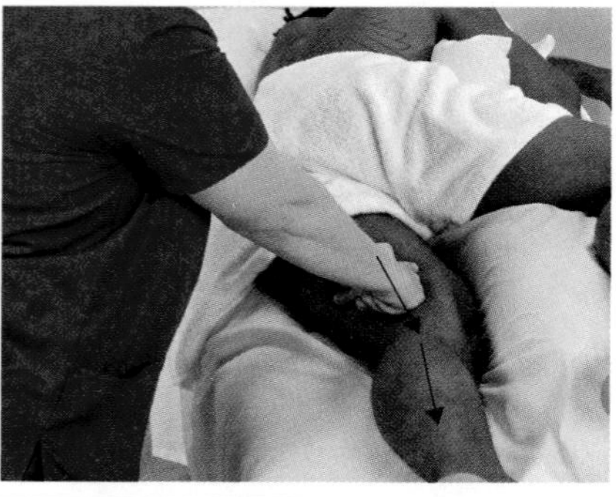

A-104 ■ Loose fist compression to address arterial blood flow, motor tone, and fascial tone.

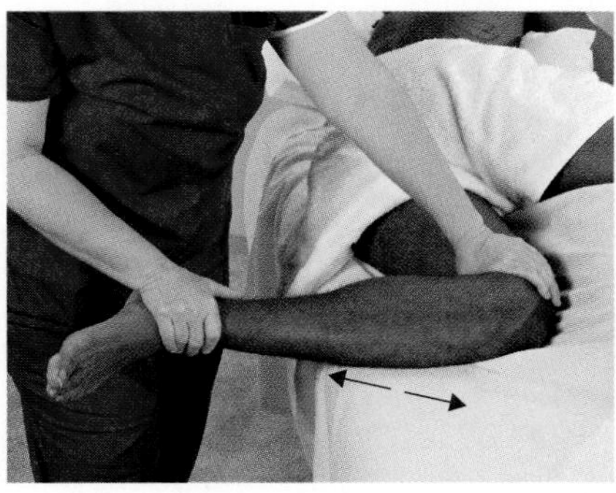

A-105 ■ Position for all movement assessment and intervention methods for the knee, side-lying position.

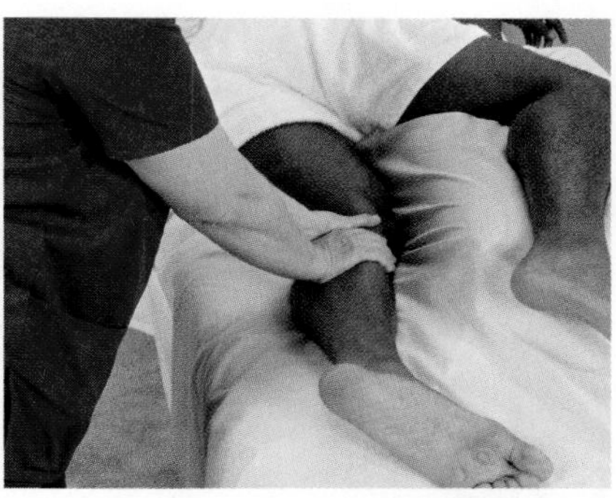

A-106 ■ Lymphatic drainage of the lower limb (patient side-lying).

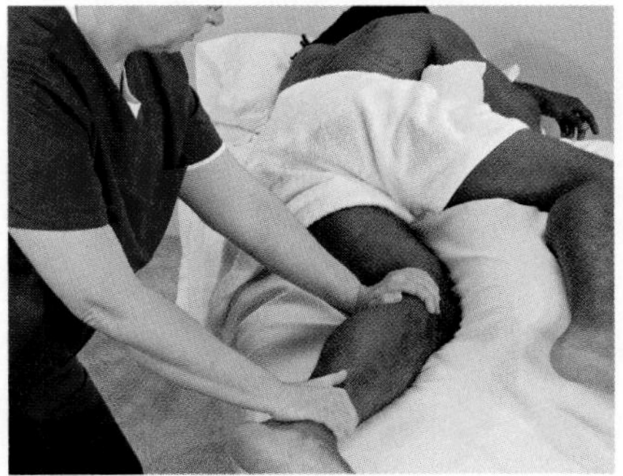

A-107 ■ Lymphatic drainage of the knee joint: rhythmic pumping.

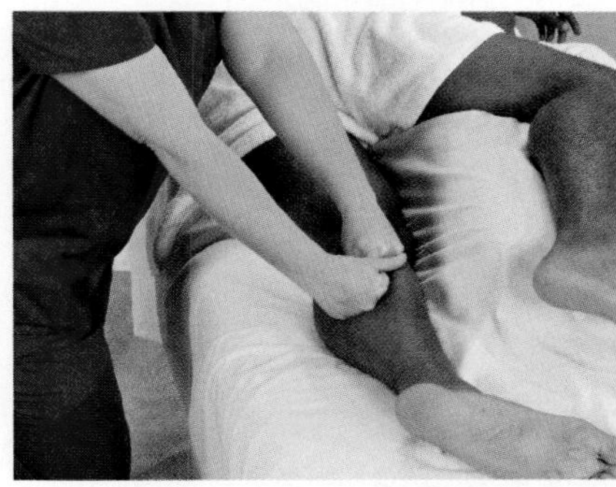

A-108 ■ Loose fist gliding and compression of the calf to address fluid movement, primary arterial flow, muscle and motor tone, and fascial tone.

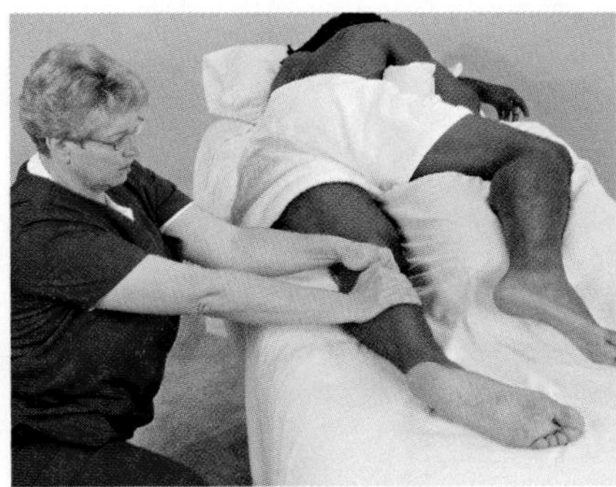

A-109 ■ Kneading of the calf to assess and influence muscle movement, fascial tone, and movement of fluid, especially in the microvascular structures.

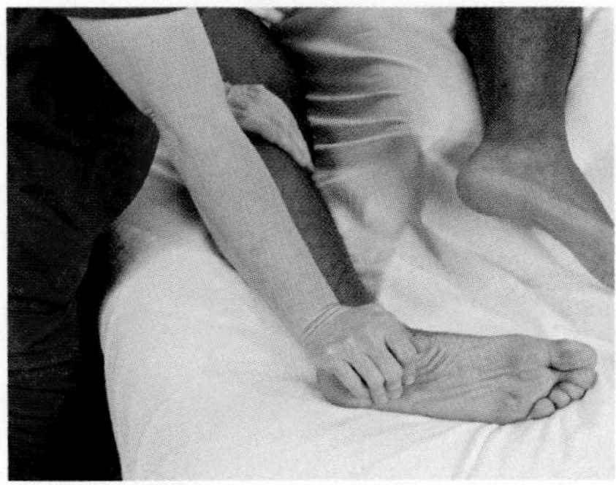

A-110 ■ Compression of the heel.

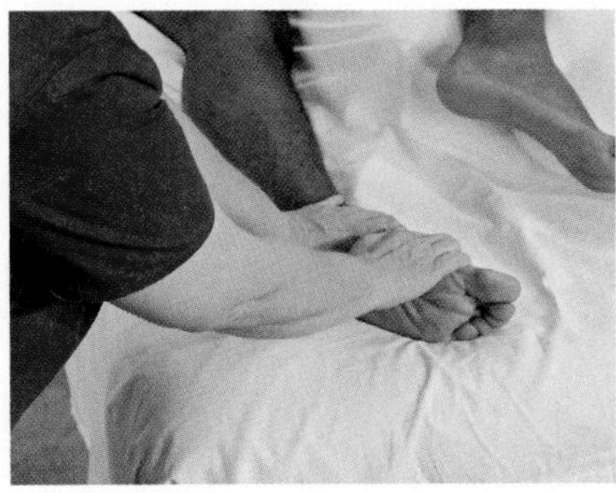

A-111 ■ Applying shear, bend, and torsion forcers to the medial foot, side-lying position.

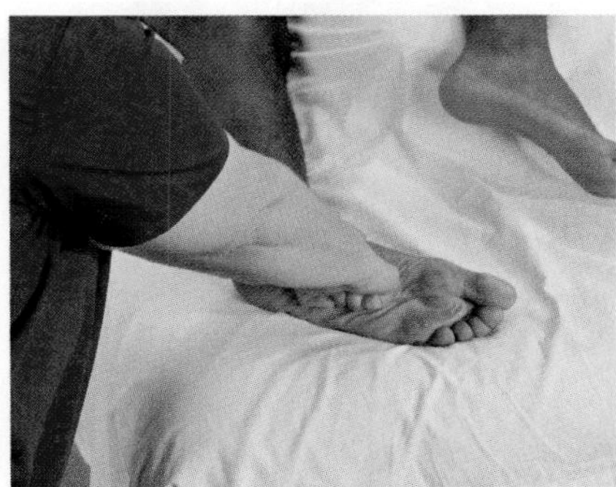

A-112 ■ Loose fist compression of the sole of the foot. Rhythmic compression stimulates the lymphatic plexus.

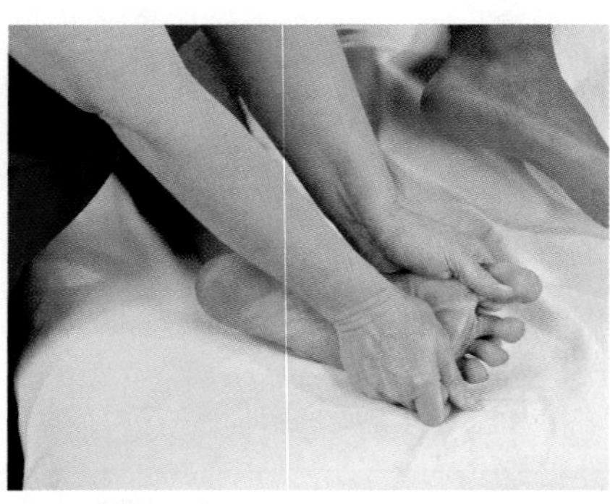

A-113 ■ Spreading the toes to lengthen the intrinsic muscles of the foot.

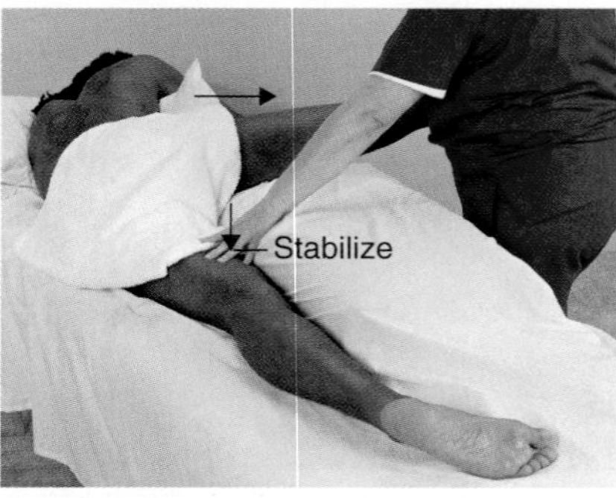

A-115 ■ Position for lengthening the hamstring muscle (patient side-lying).

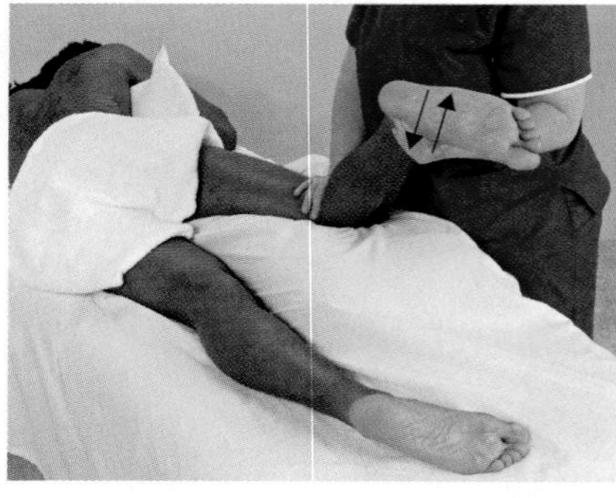

A-117 ■ Position for assessing and treating hip structures: flexion and internal rotation.

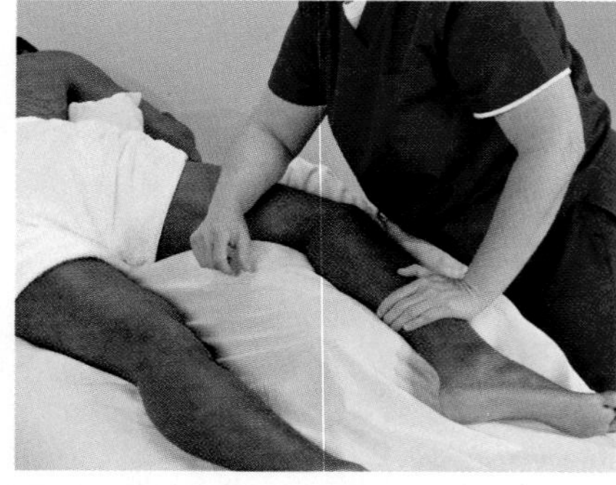

A-119 ■ Gliding lateral leg (patient side-lying).

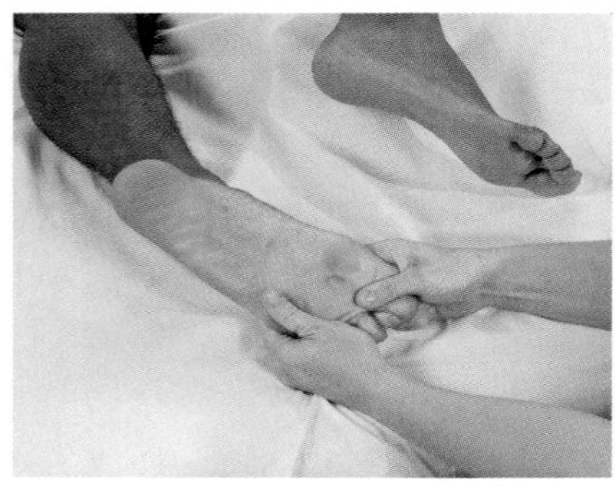

A-114 ■ Incorporating reflexology (patient side-lying).

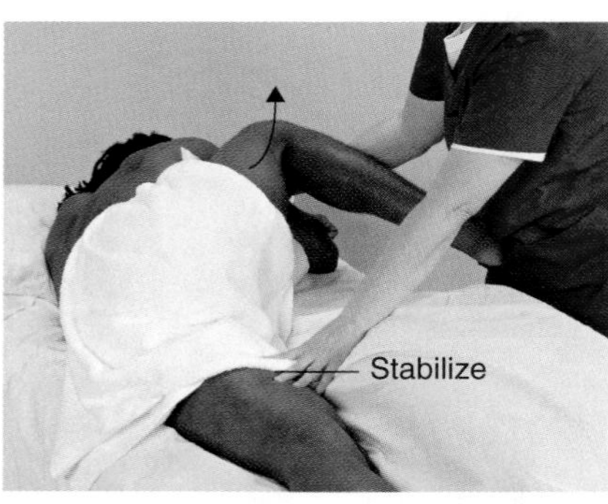

A-116 ■ Position for movement methods for hip (patient side-lying): flexion and external rotation.

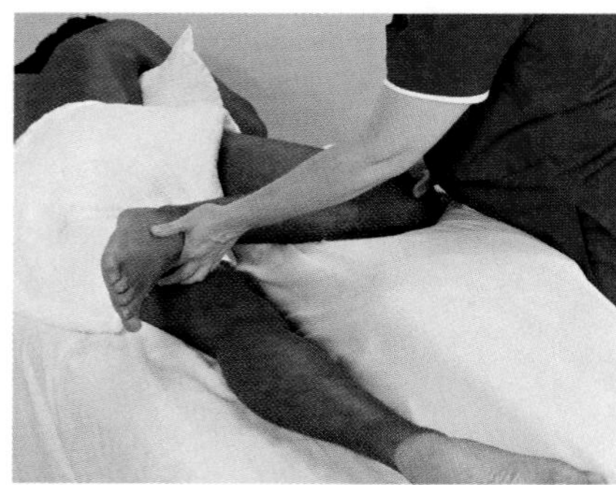

A-118 ■ Position for all movement assessment and treatment of lower limb (patient side-lying).

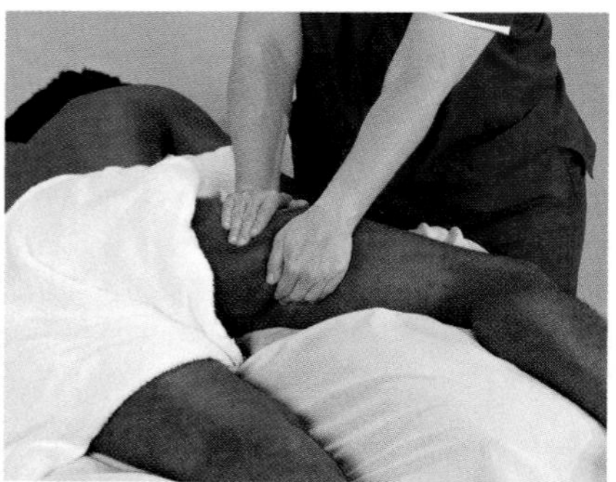

A-120 ■ Kneading of the lateral and posterior thigh (patient side-lying).

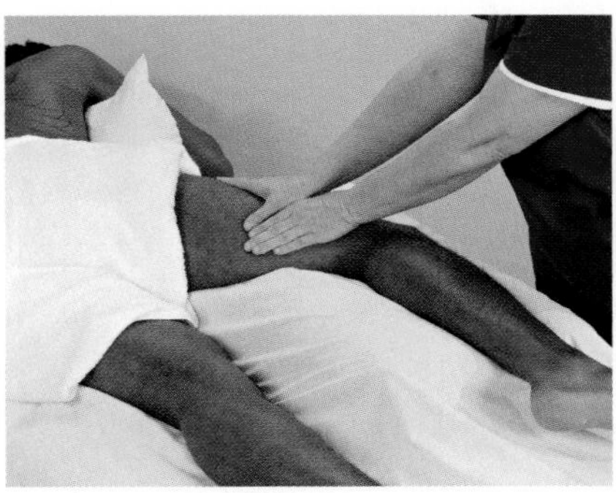

A-121 ■ Lymphatic drainage.

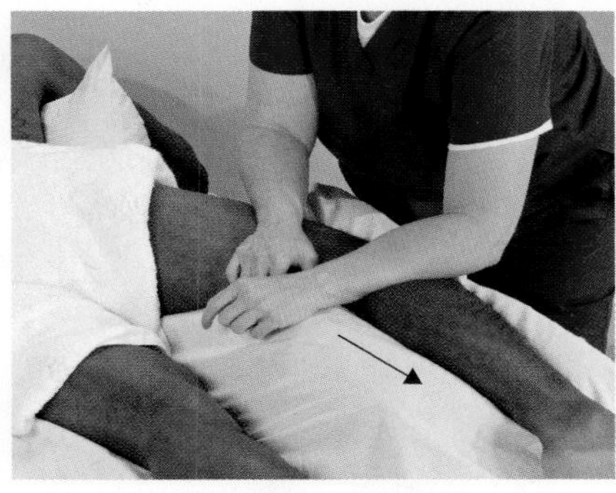

A-122 ■ Gliding of the lateral lower limb (patient side-lying).

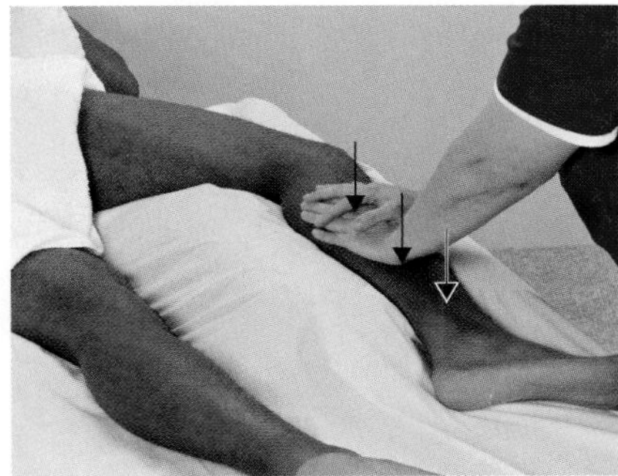

A-123 ■ Compression with the palms to address fluid movement, particularly arterial blood flow.

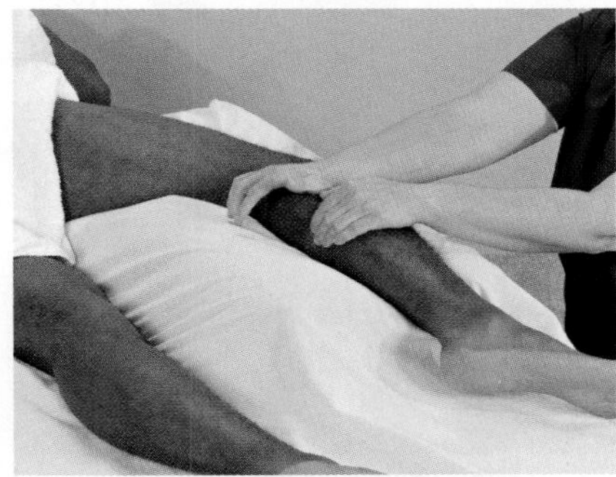

A-124 ■ Kneading of the lateral lower limb (therapist kneeling).

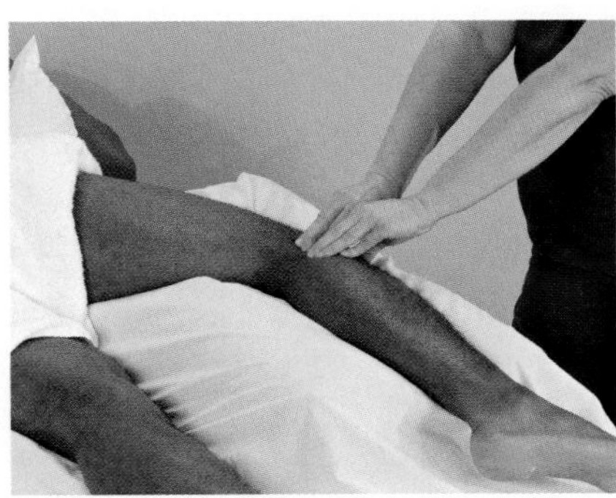

A-125 ■ Side-lying position for frictioning of lateral knee structures.

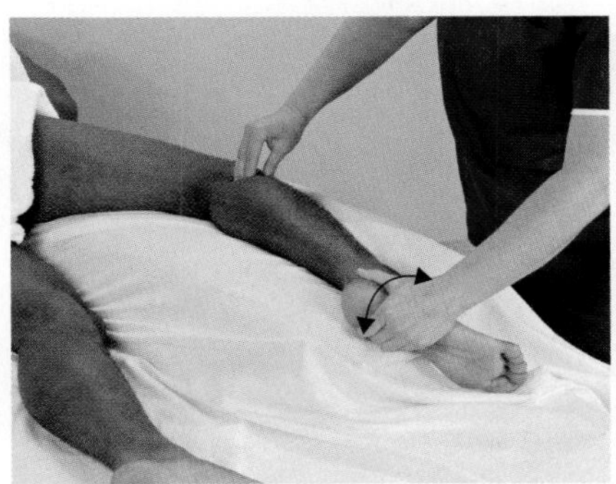

A-126 ■ Position for assessing and treating fibular head joint movement.

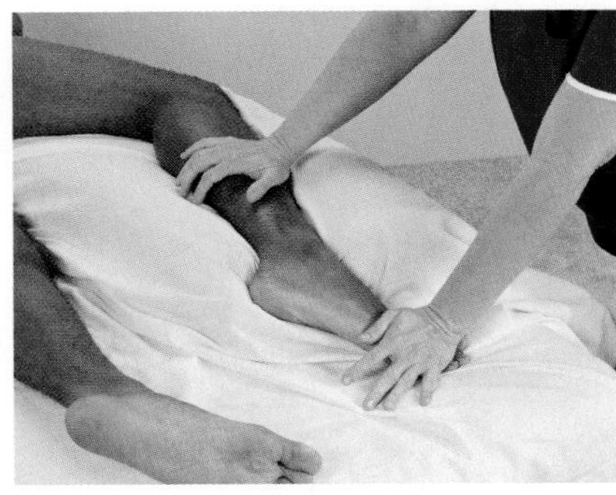

A-127 ■ Position for assessing and treating the lateral leg, pin and stretch (patient side-lying).

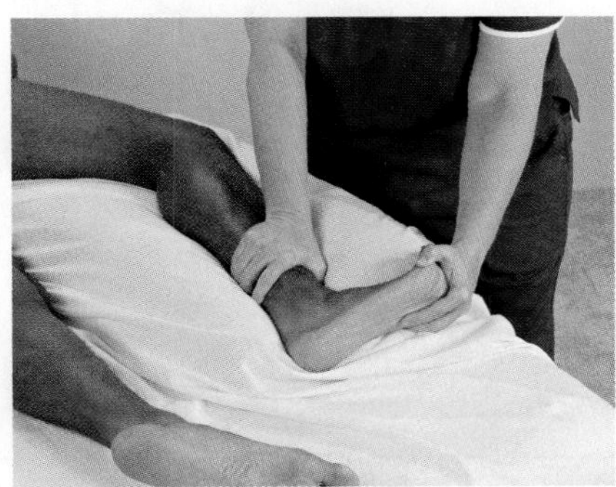

A-128 ■ Position for assessing and treating the foot using movement (patient side-lying).

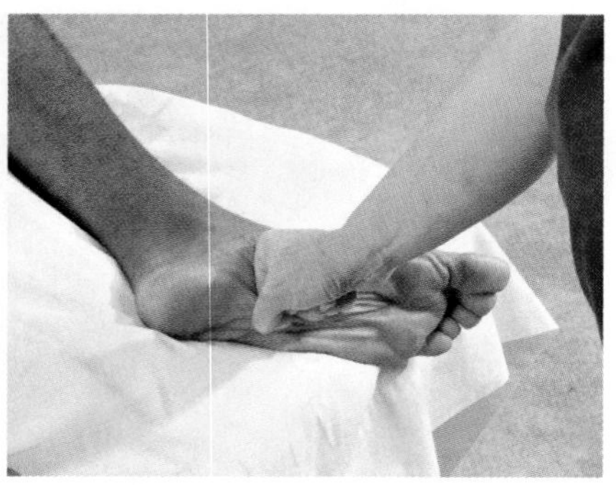

A-129 ■ Position for massage of the foot (patient supine).

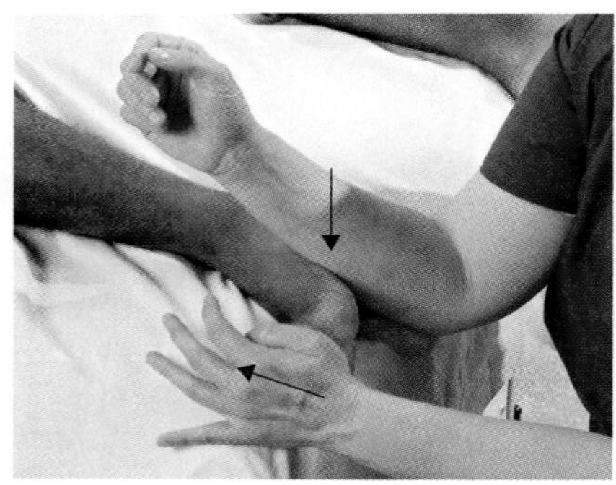

A-130 ■ Compression and tension forces, combined loading.

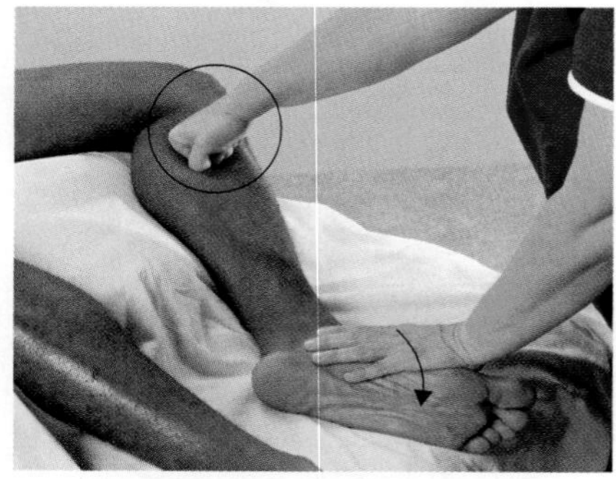

A-131 ■ Compression and movement at knee attachment structures. Notice the position of the leg.

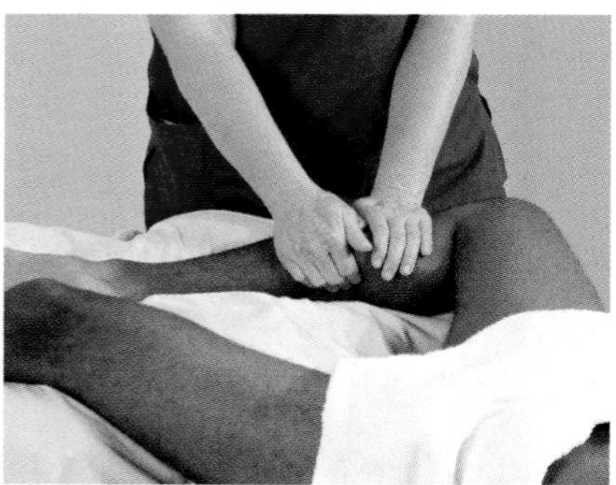

A-132 ■ Kneading of the medial and posterior calf (patient supine).

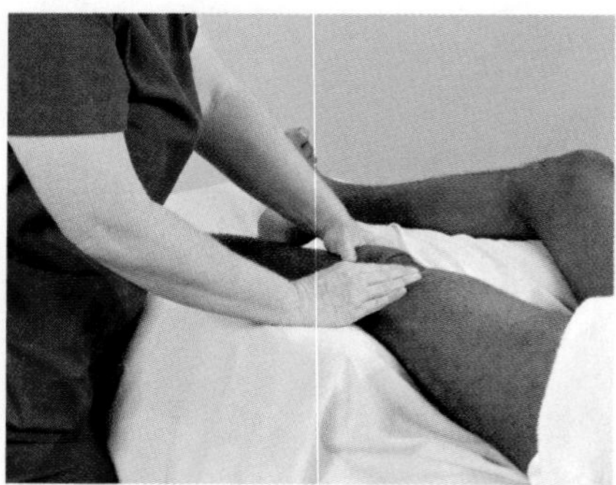

A-133 ■ Palpation assessment of patellar mobility.

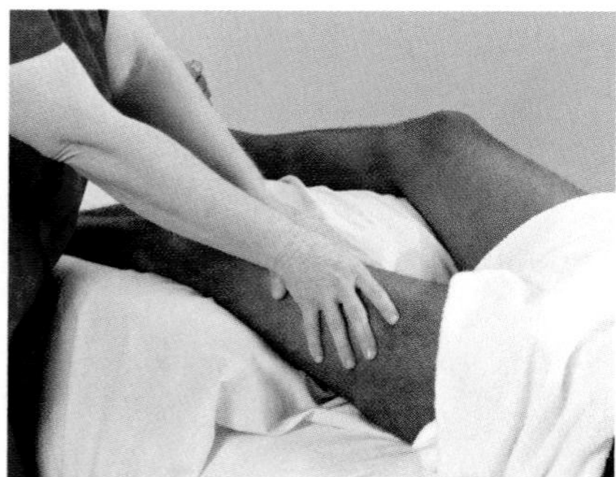

A-134 ■ Palpation assessment using the hand to identify edema, tissue bind, and areas that are moist, warm, or cool.

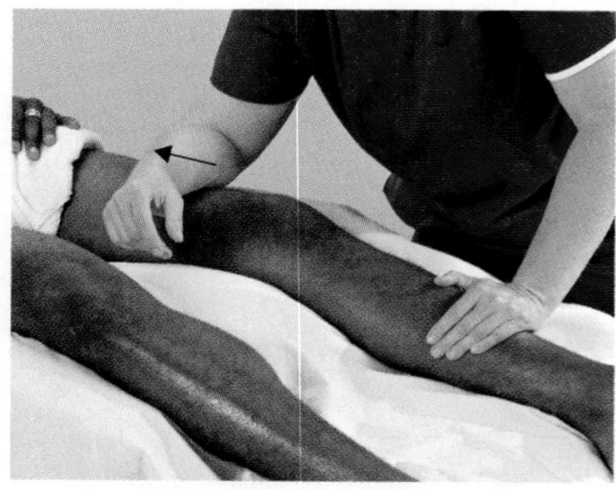

A-135 ■ Forearm gliding to influence fluid movement: primarily venous blood or reduce motor tone.

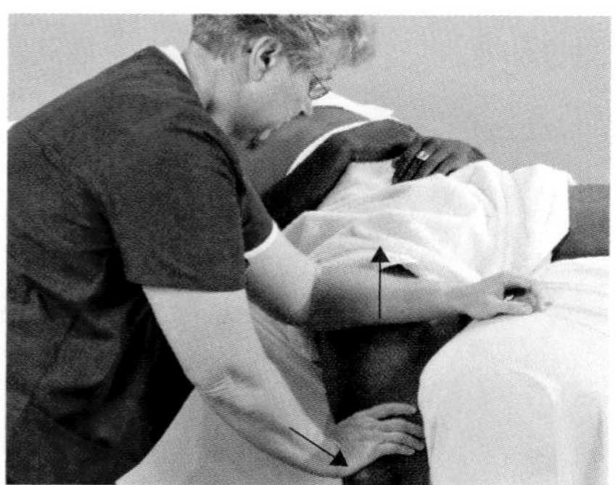

A-136 ■ Thigh extension at hip and knee with gliding.

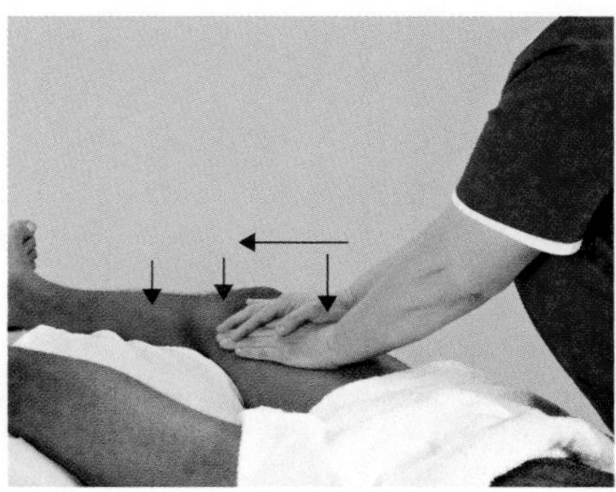

A-137 ■ Rhythmic compression to encourage arterial blood flow.

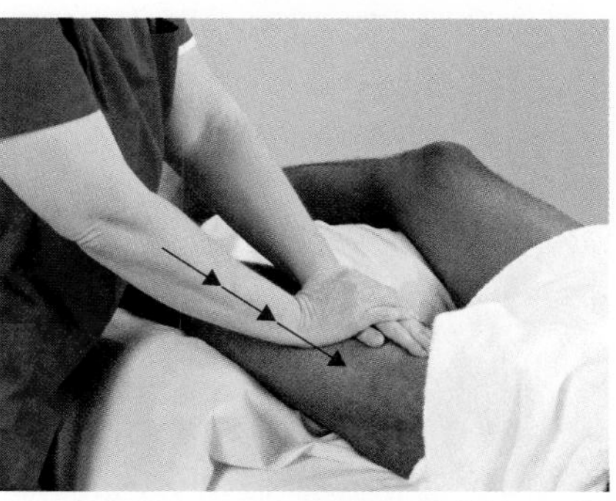

A-138 ■ Beginning position for gliding to support venous return blood flow.

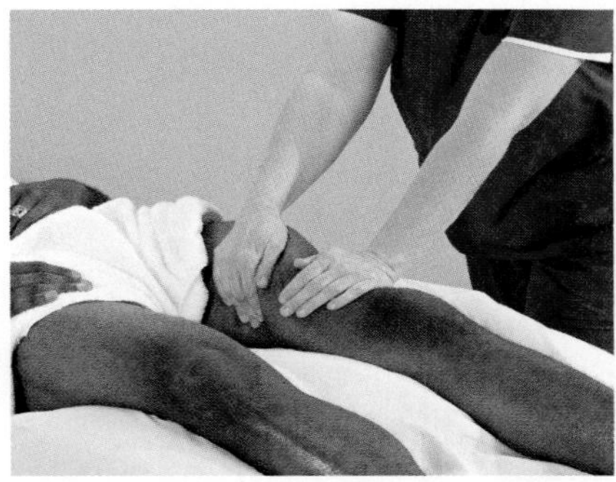

A-139 ■ Kneading of the thigh (patient supine and therapist standing) influences fluid movement and muscle, motor, and fascial tone.

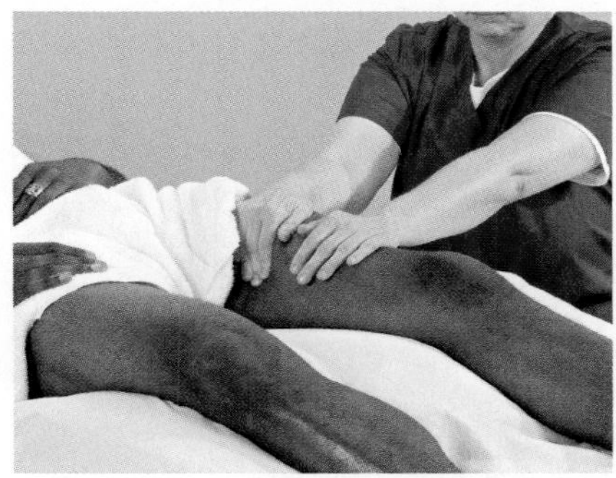

A-140 ■ Kneading of the thigh (patient supine and therapist kneeling).

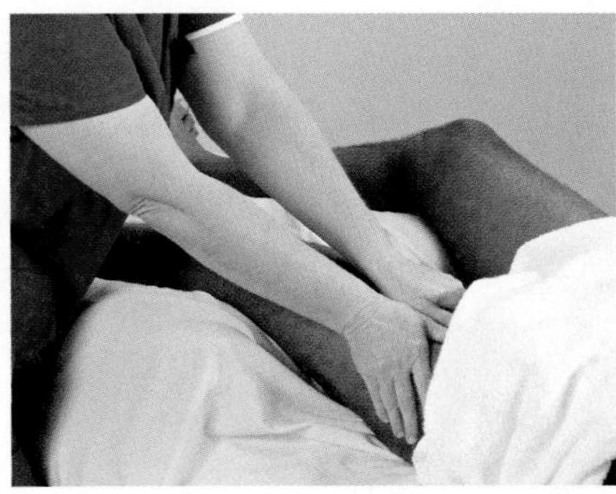

A-141 ■ Lymphatic drainage (patient supine).

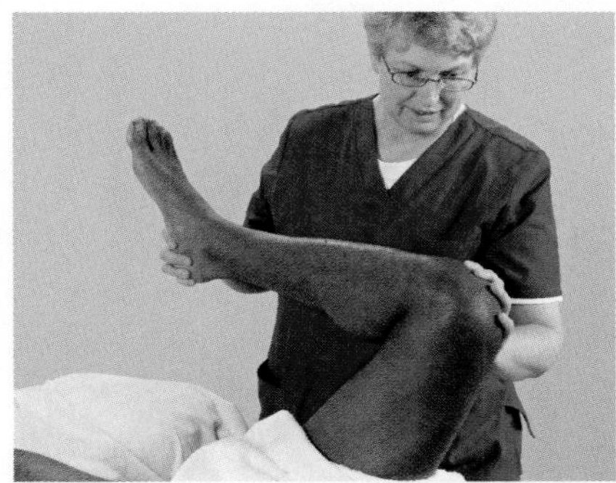

A-142 ■ Passive and active range of motion during lymphatic drainage—patient supine.

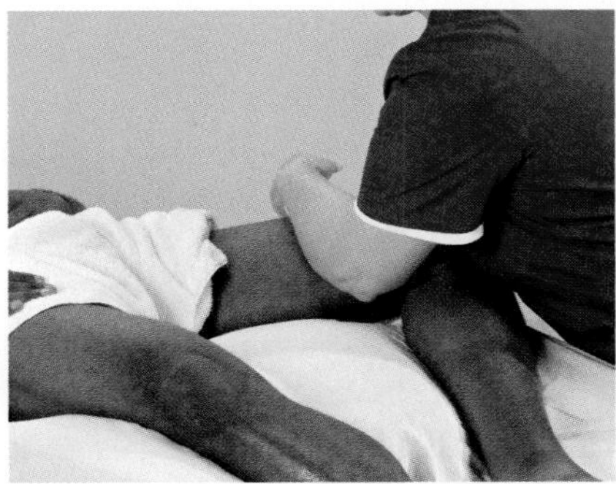

A-143 ■ Position to access the medial thigh—patient supine.

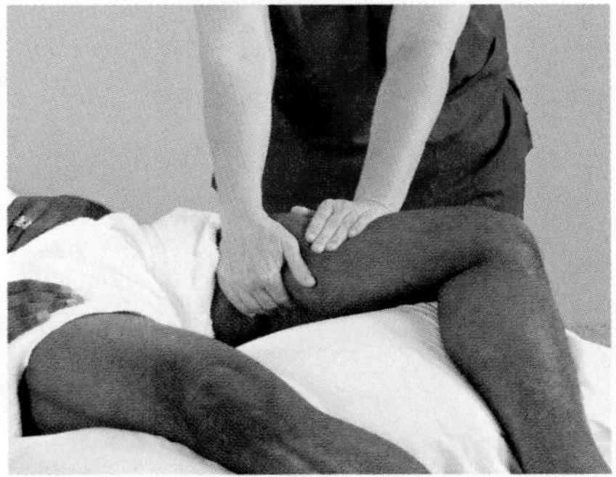

A-144 ■ Kneading of the medial thigh (patient supine).

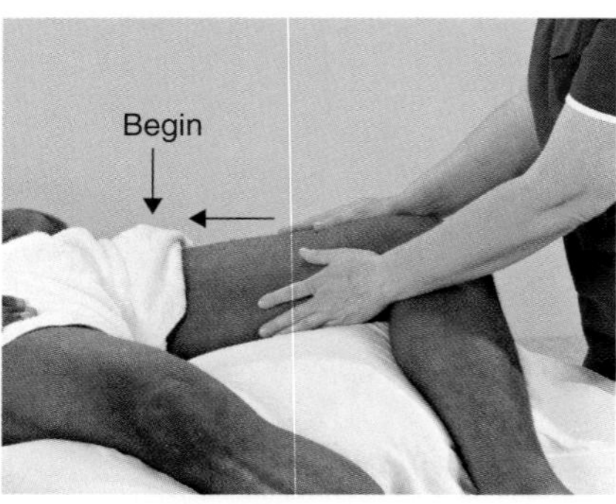

A-145 ■ Lymphatic drainage—skin drag method.

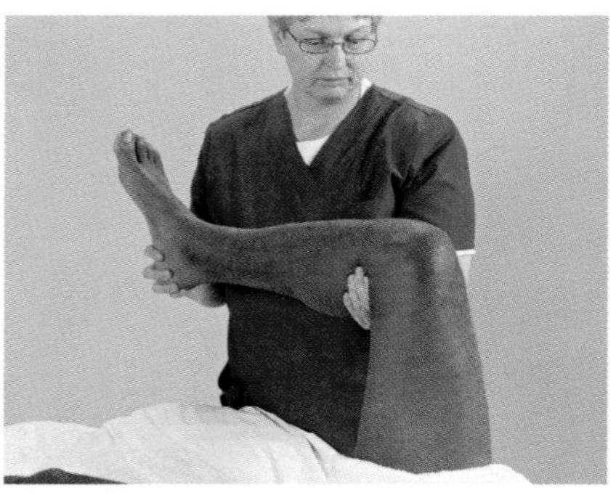

A-146 ■ Positioning for movement methods, such as joint movement and muscle energy methods.

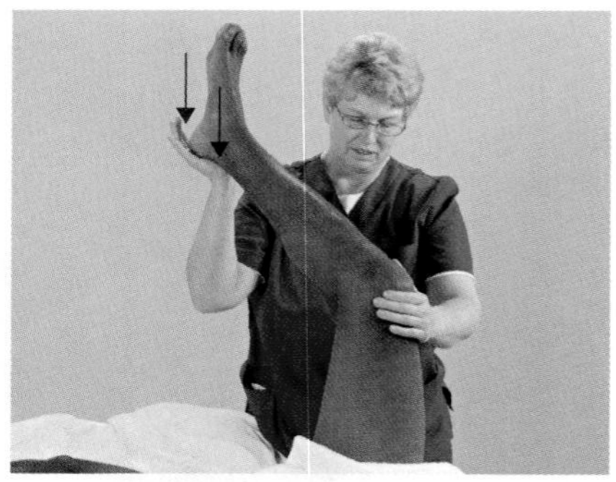

A-147 ■ Application of muscle energy methods.

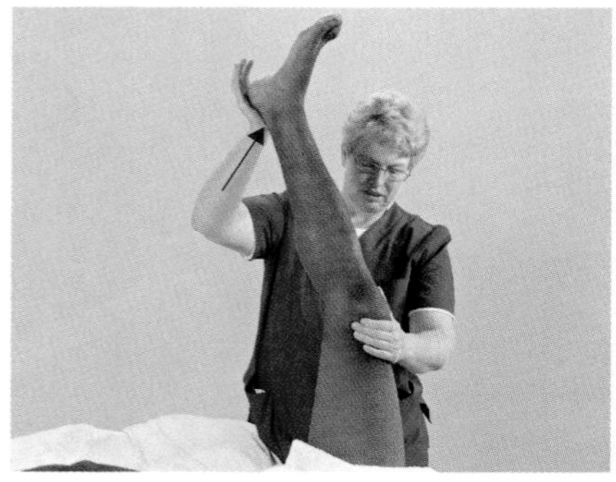

A-148 ■ Lengthening and stretching of the hamstrings (patient supine).

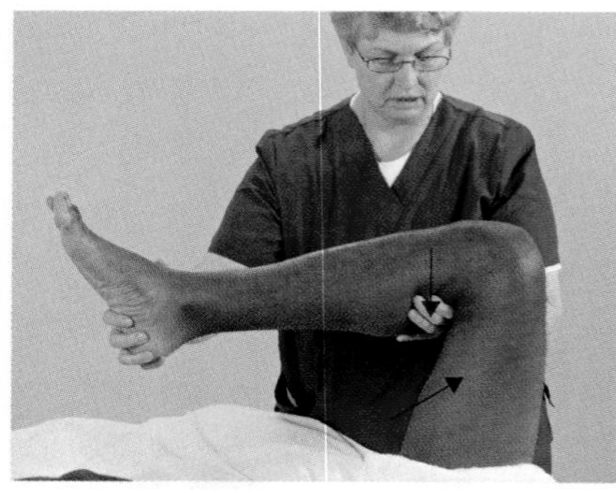

A-149 ■ External rotation assessment and treatment of the hip.

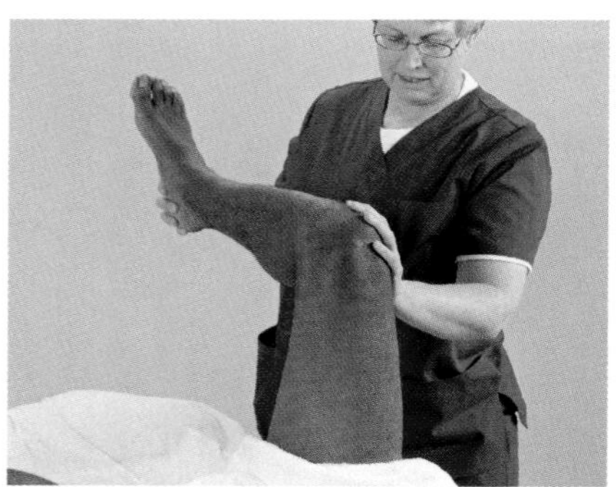

A-150 ■ Internal rotation assessment and treatment of the hip.

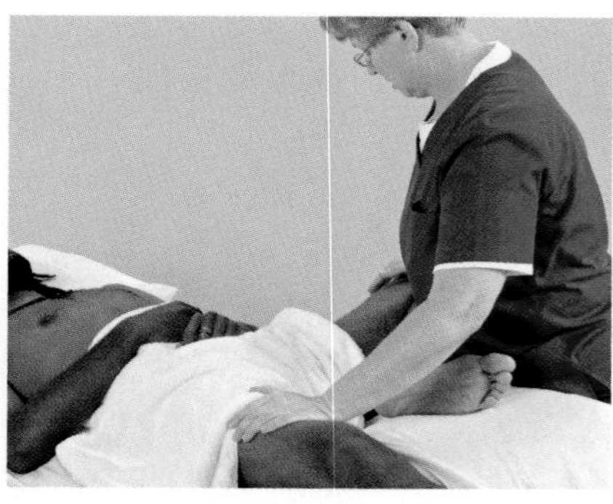

A-151 ■ Position of the medial thigh for movement methods.

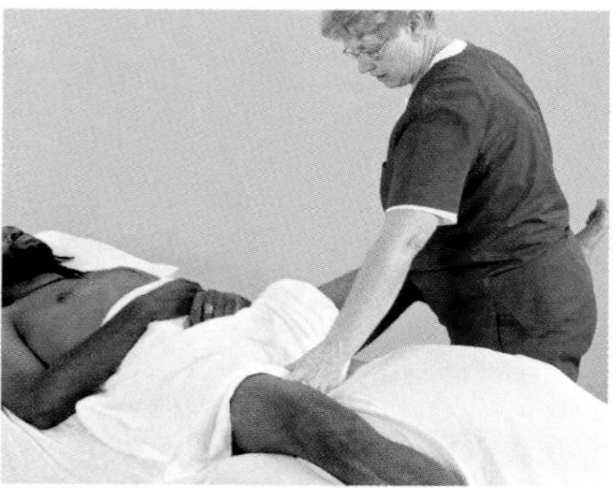

A-152 ■ Muscle energy methods for lengthening of the adductors.

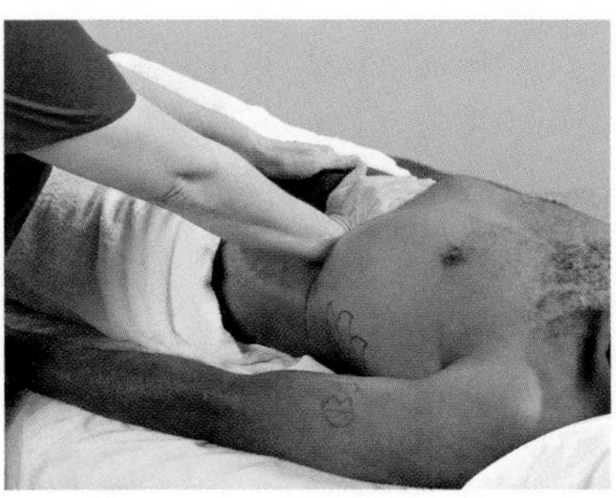

A-153 ■ Position for abdominal massage. Note that the knees are bent to soften the abdominal muscles.

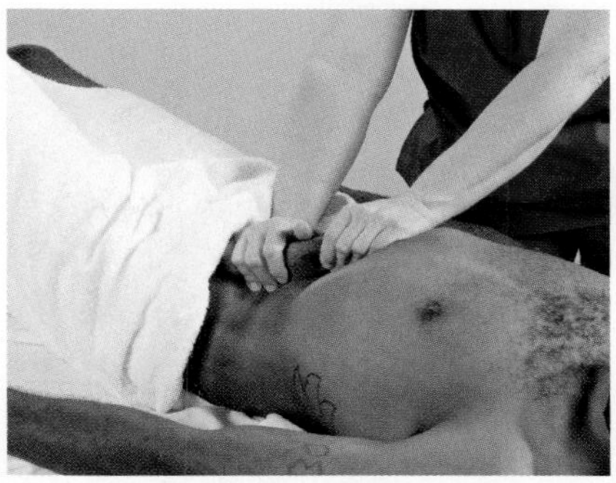

A-154 ■ Kneading of the rectus abdominis to reduce motor tone and increase tissue pliability.

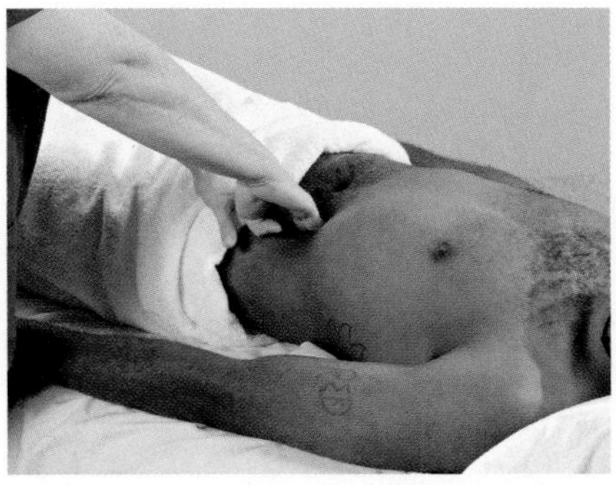

A-155 ■ Position for psoas release (inhibition) (patient supine).

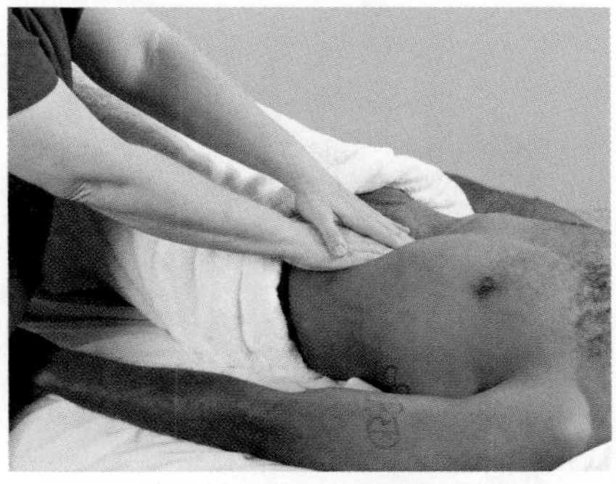

A-156 ■ Position for diaphragm release.

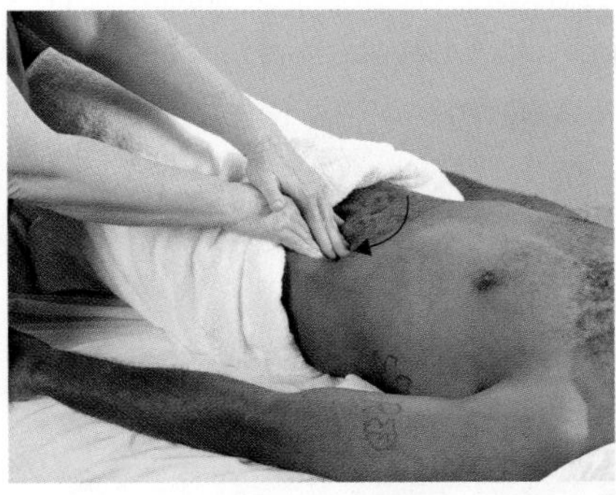

A-157 ■ Position for massage of the large intestine.

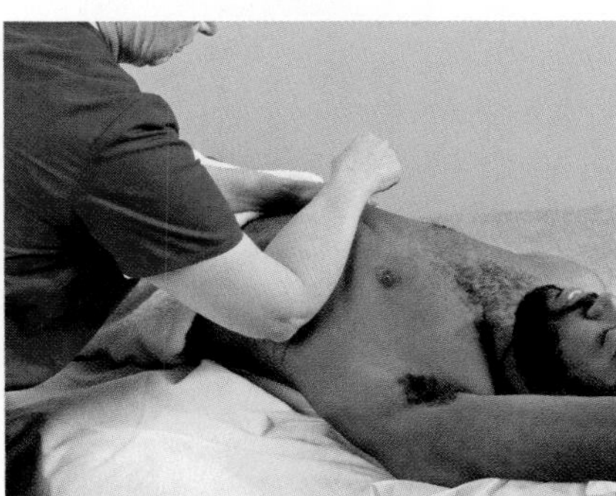

A-158 ■ Forearm compression and gliding to the anterior thorax. Primary focus: assessment and intervention for breathing function.

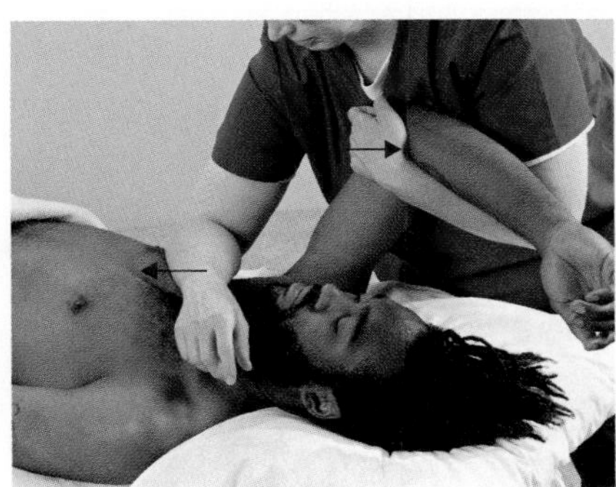

A-159 ■ Compression and gliding of the upper anterior thorax.

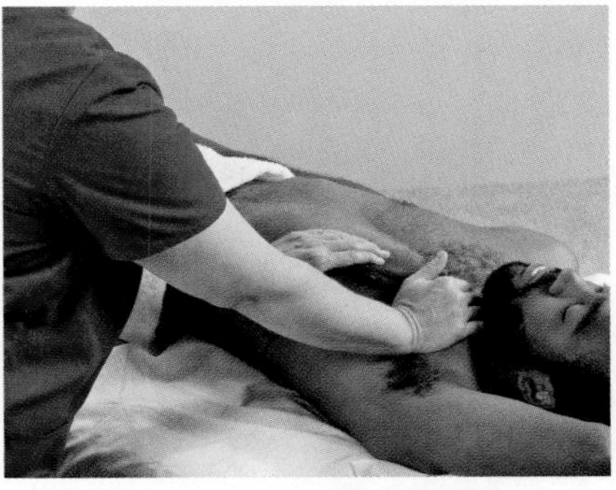

A-160 ■ Kneading of the pectoralis major.

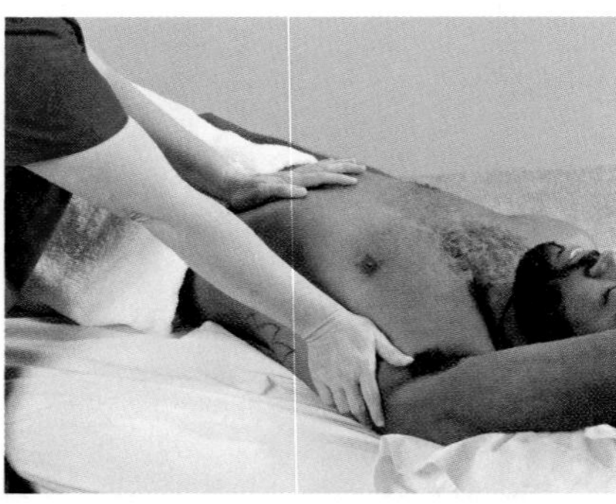

A-161 ■ Lymphatic drainage.

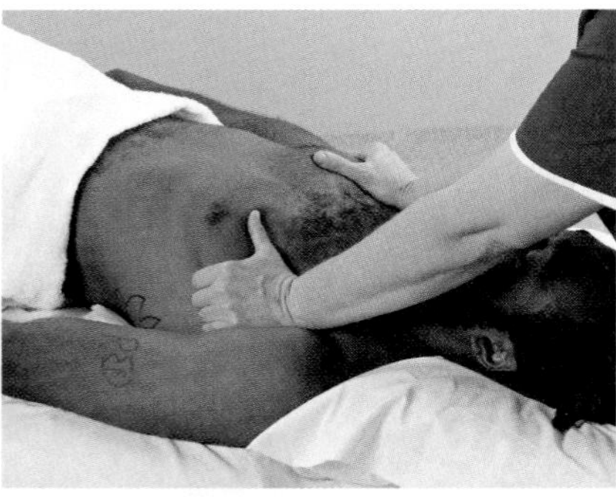

A-162 ■ Bilateral use of the hands to apply various mechanical forces (primarily compression, bend, and shear forces); also applicable for rhythmic pumping of the thorax.

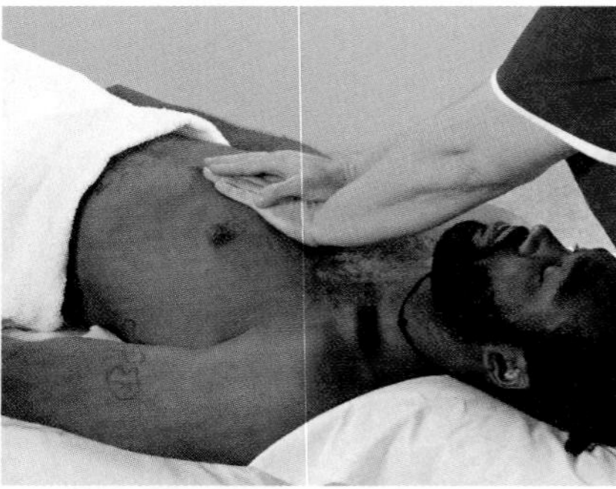

A-163 ■ Rhythmic compression at the sternum to assess rib mobility and breathing function and to pump the lymphatics.

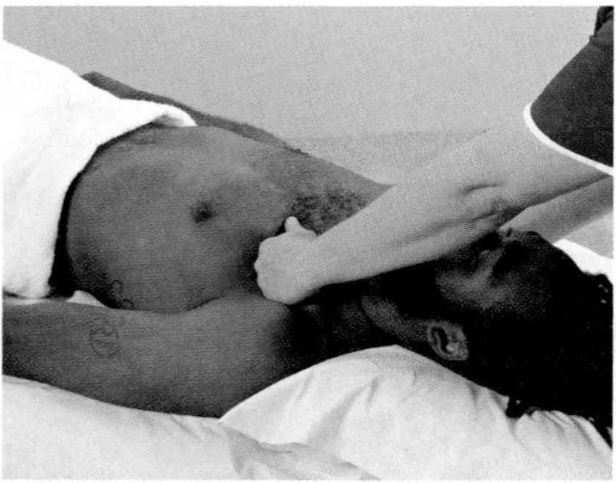

A-164 ■ Loose fist compression. Primary focus: pumping of the lymphatics and support of breathing function; reduction of motor tone in the pectoralis major and pectoralis minor.

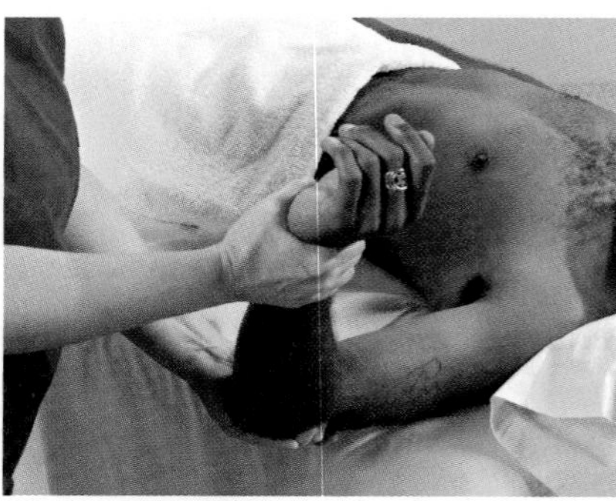

A-165 ■ Position for all movement-based assessment and treatment of upper limb (patient supine).

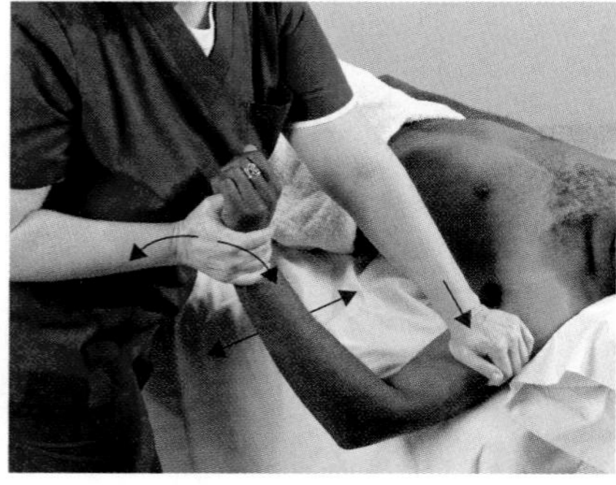

A-166 ■ Combined loading of the arm: compression and movement.

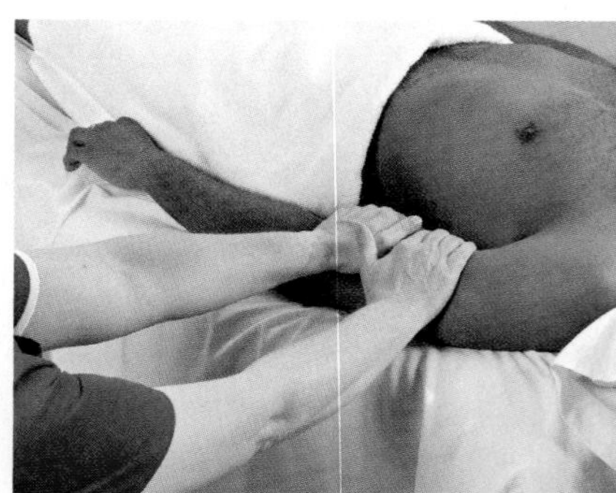

A-167 ■ Kneading of the arm (patient supine and therapist kneeling).

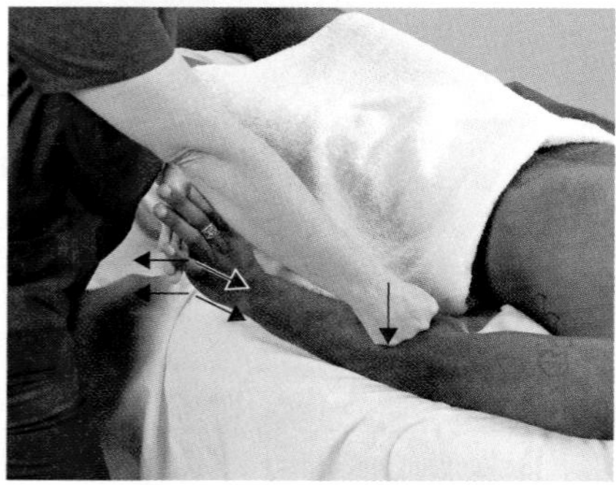

A-168 ■ Loose fist compression of the wrist extensors with active movement.

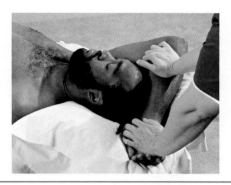

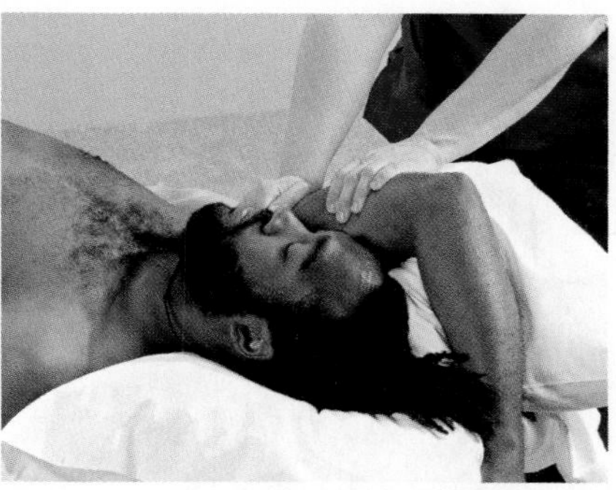

A-169 ■ Position for massage of the arm (patient supine).

A-170 ■ Kneading of the arm (patient supine).

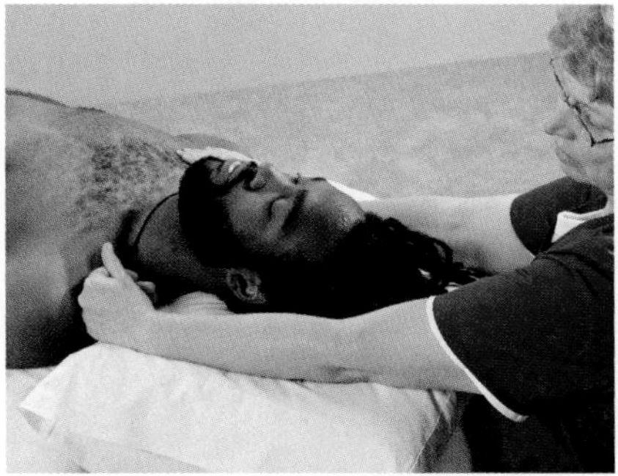

A-171 ■ Loose fist compression and gliding of the upper shoulder and neck (therapist kneeling).

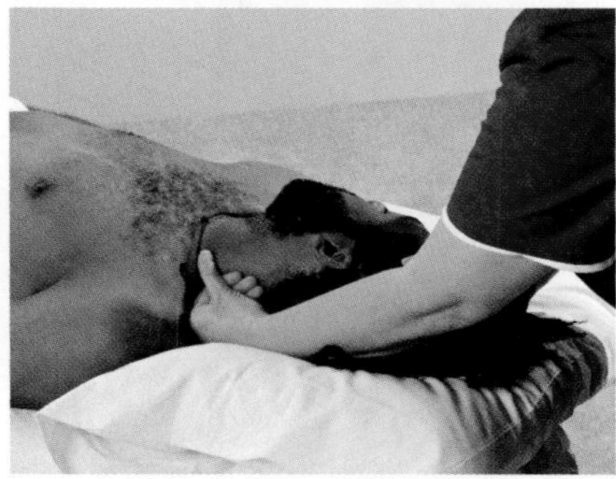

A-172 ■ Lymphatic drainage.

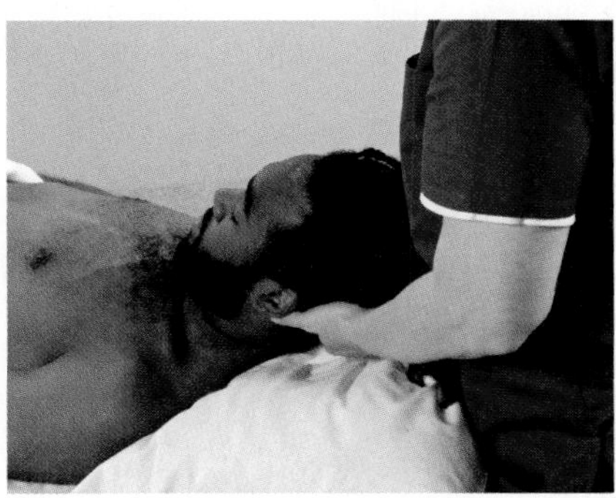

A-173 ■ Position for all movement methods, including assessment of the cervical area (patient supine).

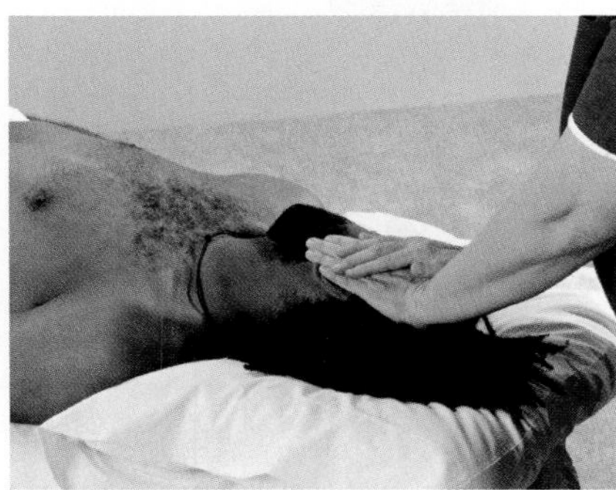

A-174 ■ Head turned to the side to allow access to the muscles of mastication.

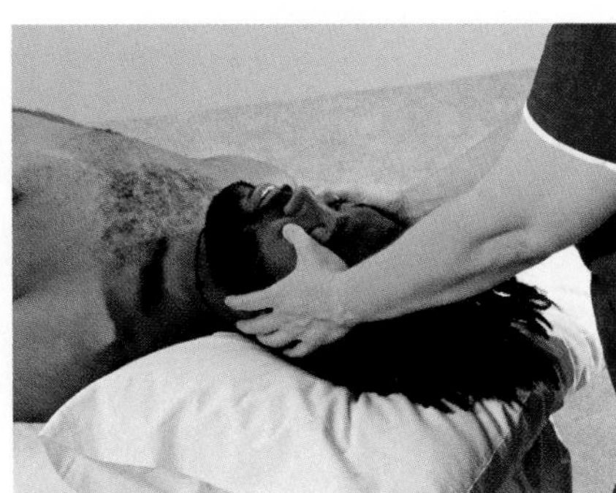

A-175 ■ Massage of the sinuses.

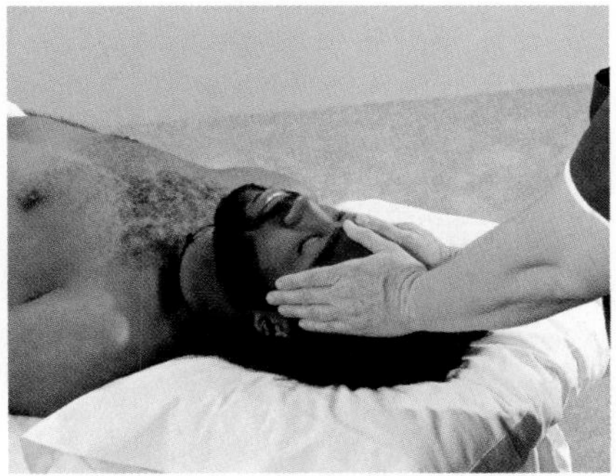

A-176 ■ Focused intention.

SEATED MASSAGE PROTOCOL

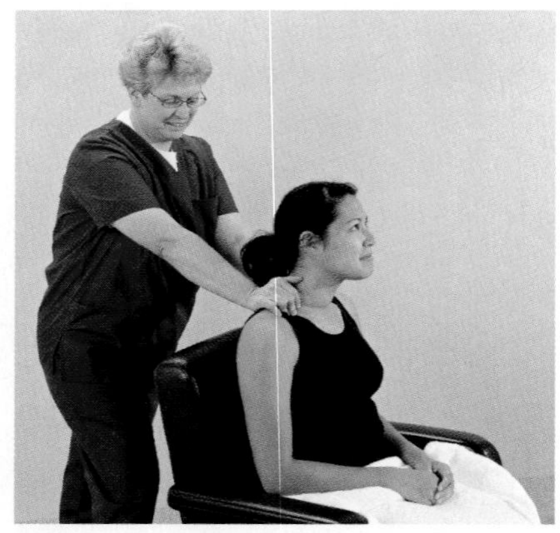

B-1 ■ Examples of massage application with the patient in the seated position: kneading of the neck and shoulders.

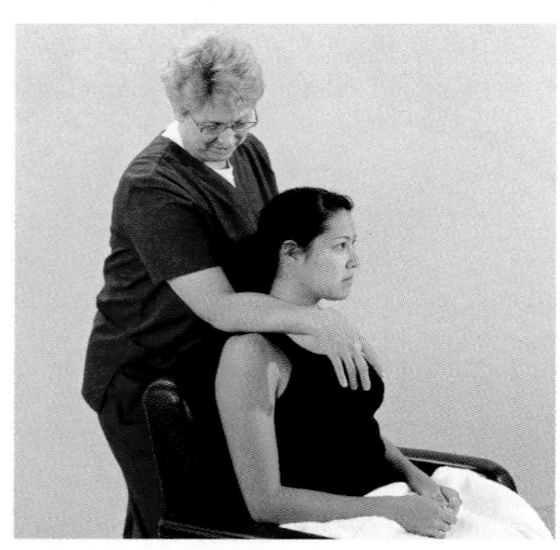

B-2 ■ Compression of the shoulder.

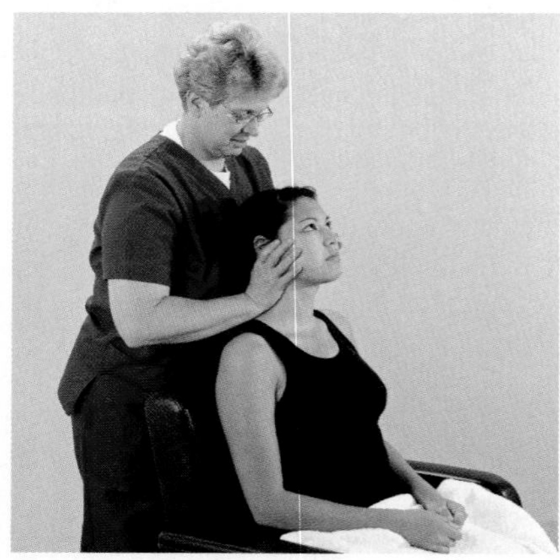

B-3 ■ Position for oscillation and stretching of cervical area.

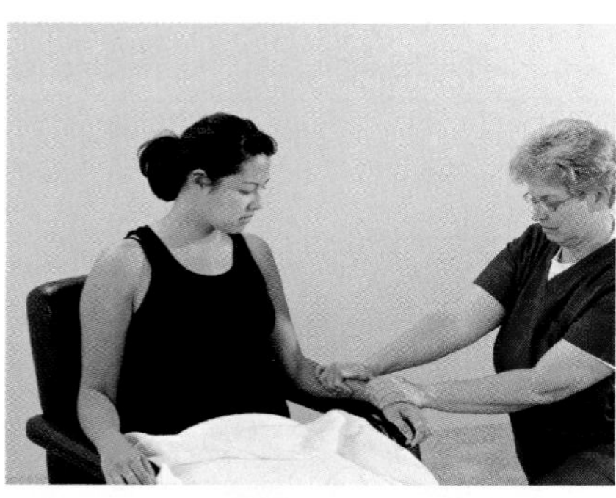

B-4 ■ Massage of the arm—therapist kneeling.

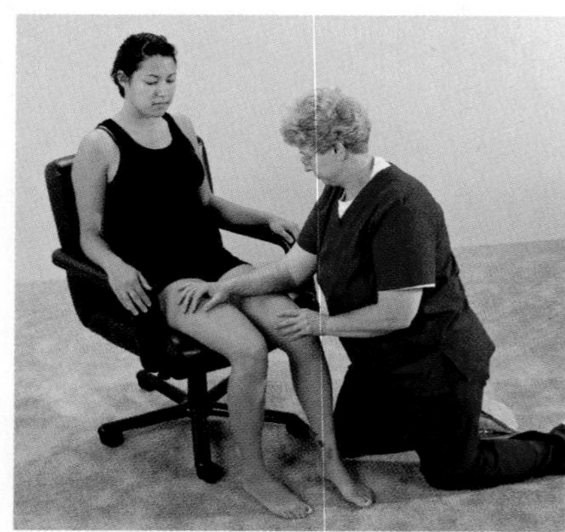

B-5 ■ Gliding of the leg.

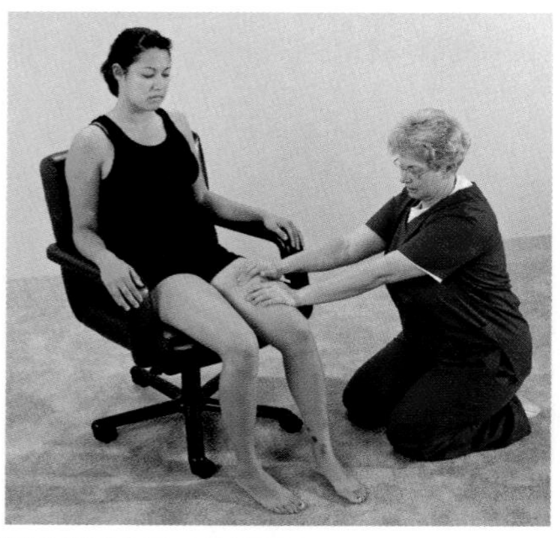

B-6 ■ Kneading of the leg.

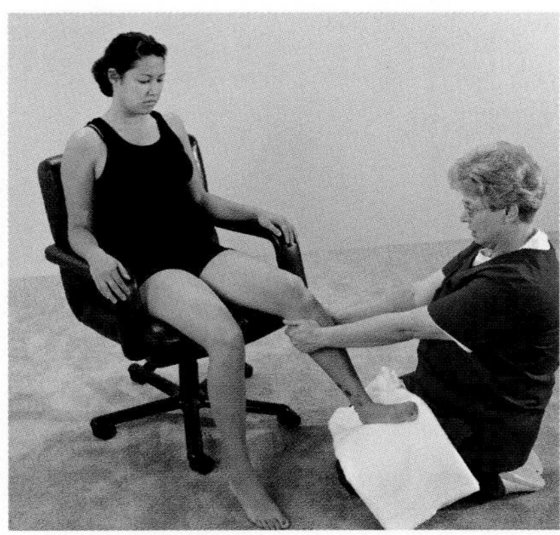

B-7 ■ Massage of the calf.

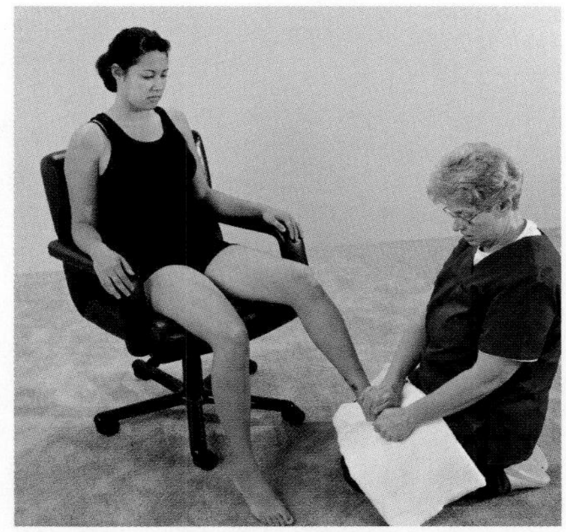

B-8 ■ Massage of the foot.

PALLIATIVE PROTOCOL

Typically, palliative care is less specific in focus, less intense for assessment, and targets pain and mood management. Pressure levels vary based on the particular situation and what the patient finds pleasurable. Occasional use of inhibitory pressure (if the sensation is one of a "good hurt") is appropriate, as is incorporating fluid movement methods, with appropriate caution. As a general rule, if the application will improve the patient's well-being and not increase adaptive load, then it is appropriate.

The written description of the palliative protocol is presented in Chapter 11.

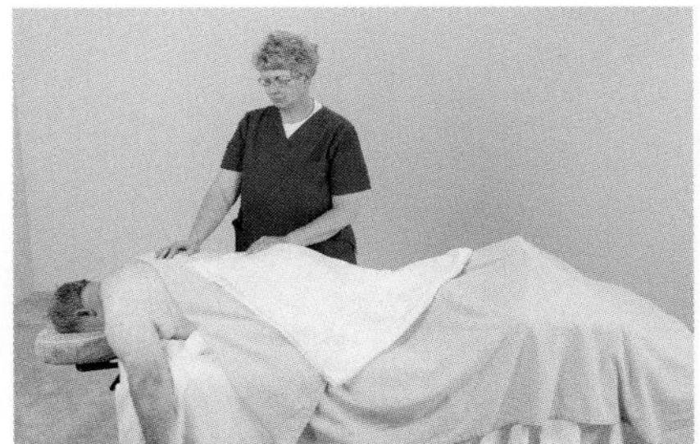

C-1 ■ Focus and intention are always important.

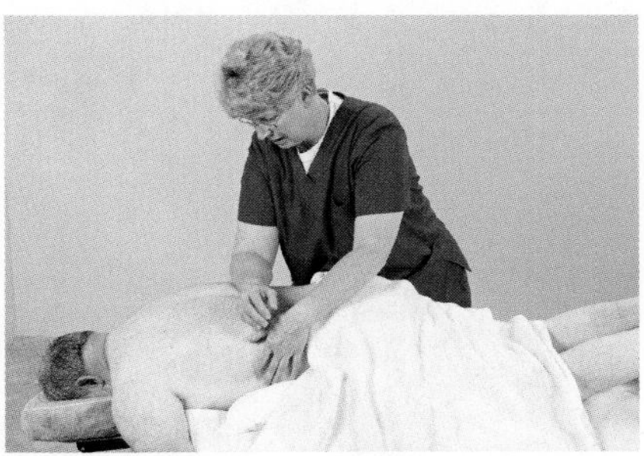

C-2 ■ Use broad-based compression with moderate pressure (less if indicated), little or no drag, and a rhythmic application.

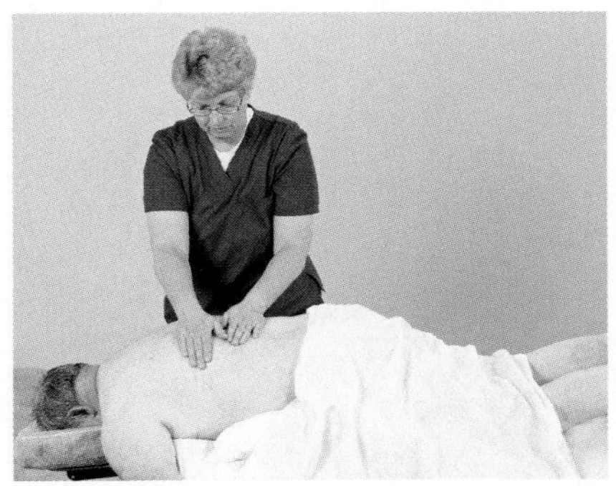

C-3 ■ Kneading should be pleasurable.

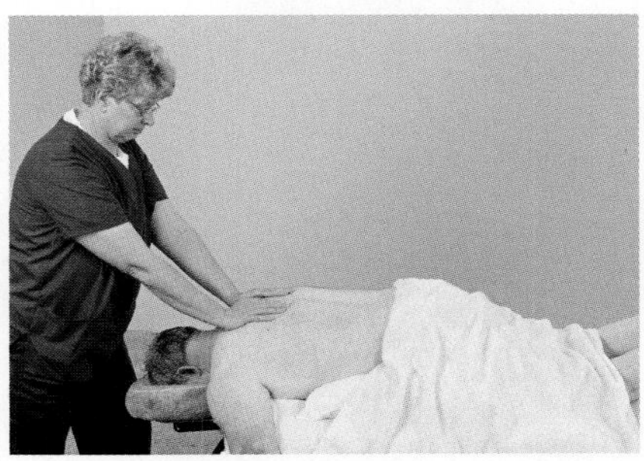

C-4 ■ When using the palms, maintain good body mechanics to avoid "poking" the patient.

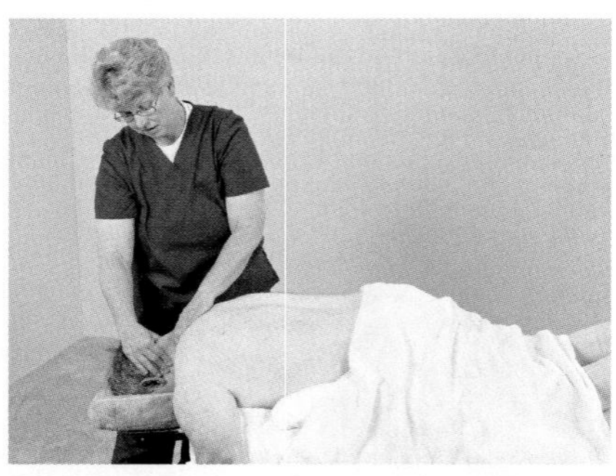

C-5 ■ Kneading of the neck tissues (patient prone).

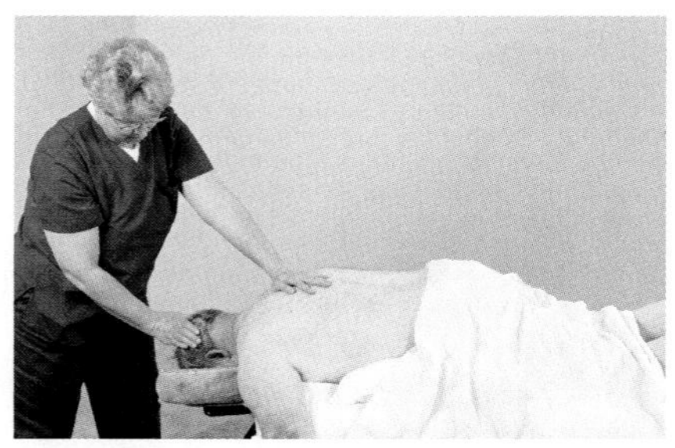

C-6 ■ Massage of the scalp (patient prone).

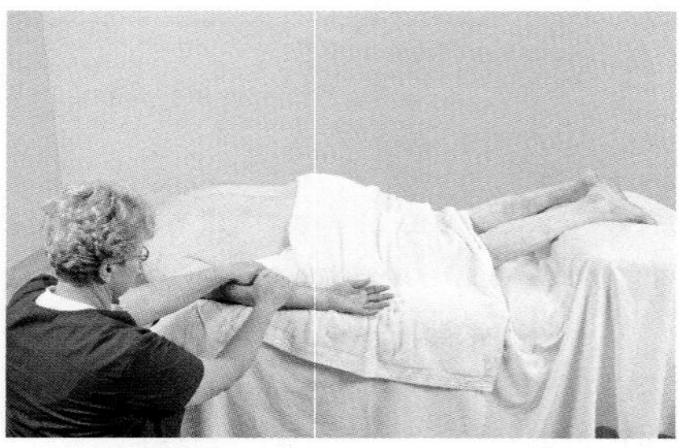

C-7 ■ Kneeling while providing massage modulates the depth of pressure will support efficient body mechanics.

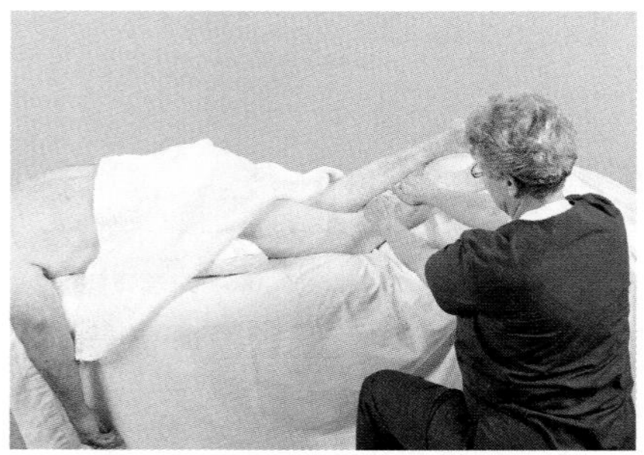

C-8 ■ Kneading of the calf—patient prone.

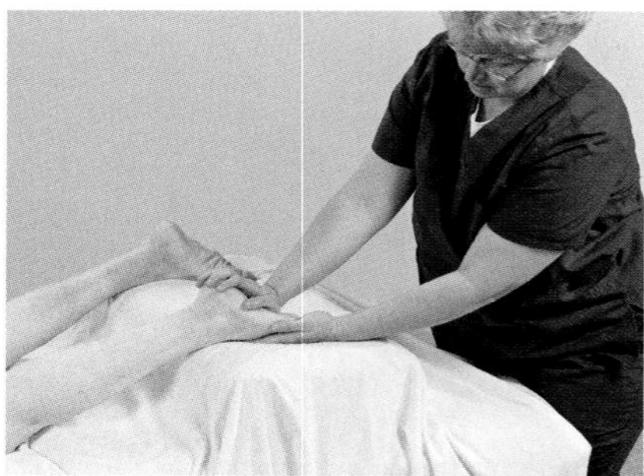

C-9 ■ Massage of the foot typically is pleasurable; maintain broad-based contact to modulate pressure and prevent tissue damage.

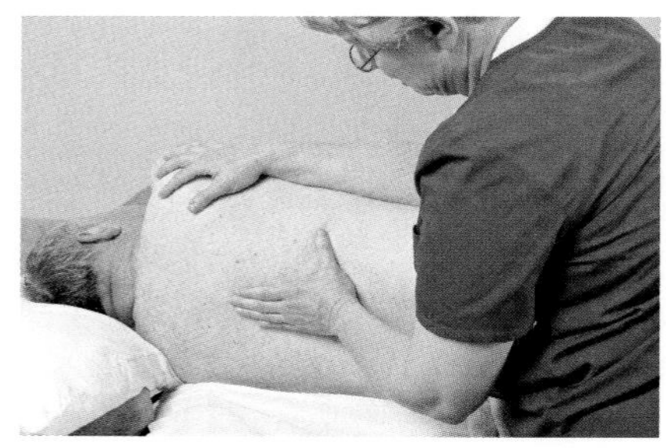

C-10 ■ The side-lying (lateral recumbent) position with bolstering often is most comfortable for the patient.

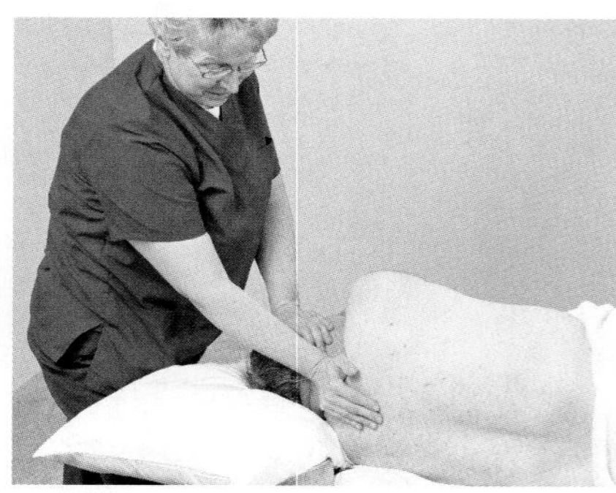

C-11 ■ Access to the head, neck, and shoulders (patient side-lying).

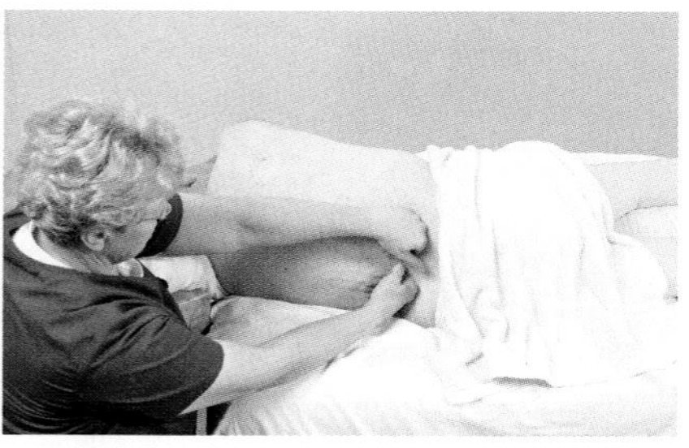

C-12 ■ Loose fist massage of the back—therapist kneeling.

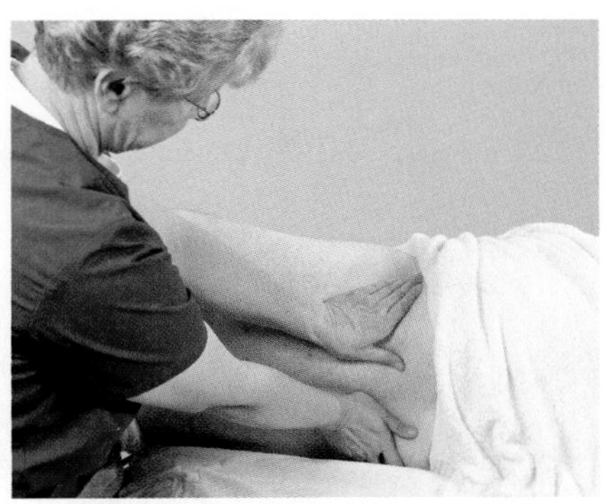

C-13 ■ Rhythmic compression with rocking in the lumbar region.

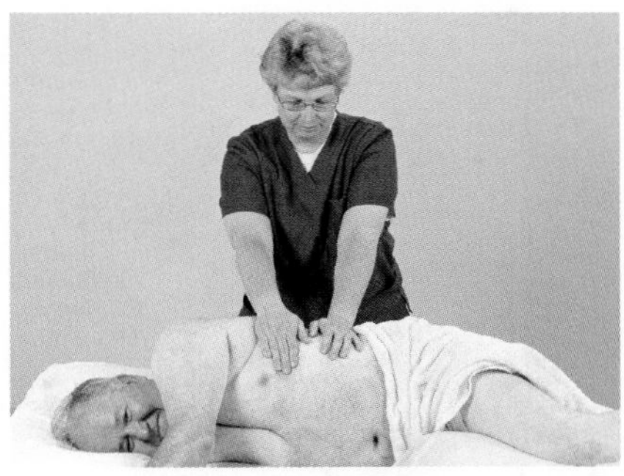

C-14 ■ Kneading of the lateral torso.

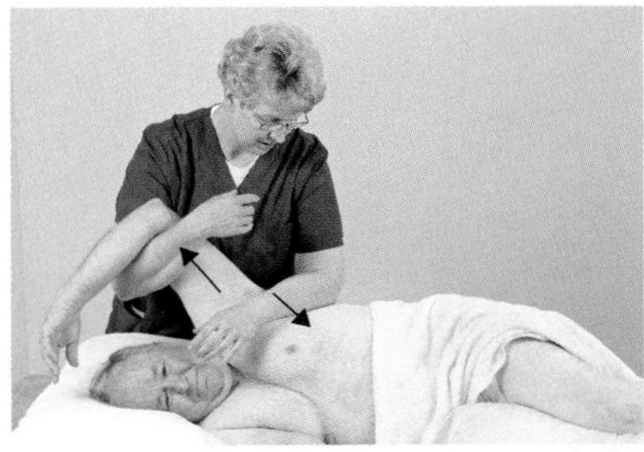

C-15 ■ Gentle combined loading. Primary focus: influence breathing function.

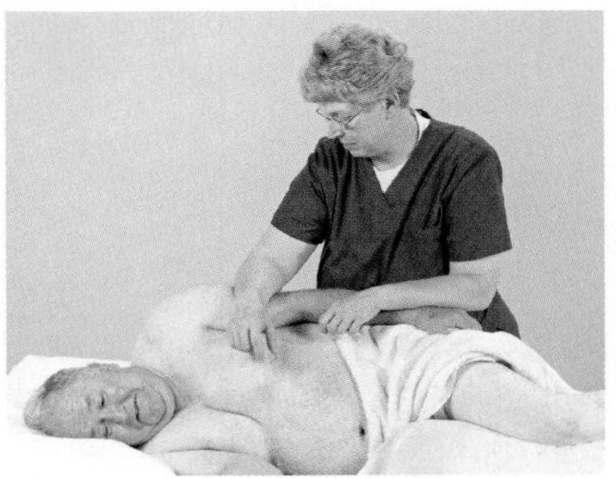

C-16 ■ Gliding of the arm—patient side-lying.

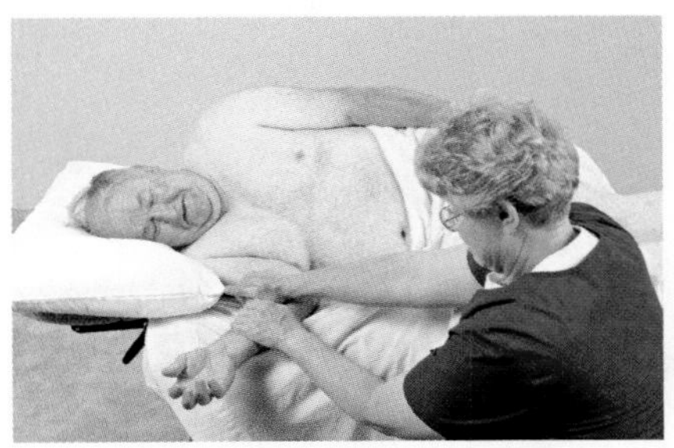

C-17 ■ Kneading of the arm—therapist kneeling.

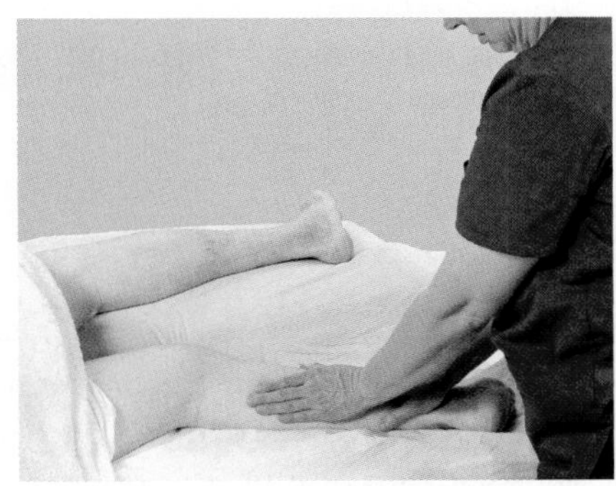

C-18 ■ Palm gliding of the lower limbs to address motor tone and fluid movement.

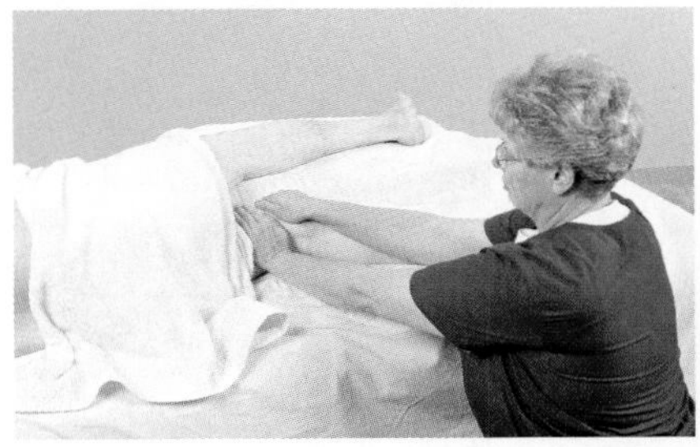

C-19 ■ Application of massage with the therapist kneeling; kneeling helps modulate the depth of pressure—patient side-lying.

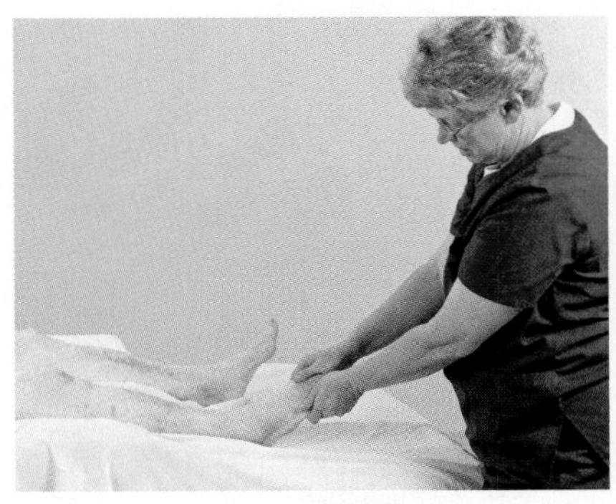

C-20 ■ Massage of the foot (patient supine).

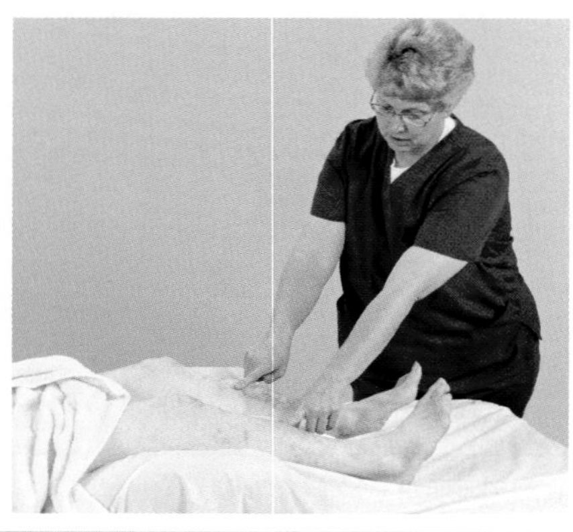

C-21 ■ Assess for areas of caution and regional contraindications.

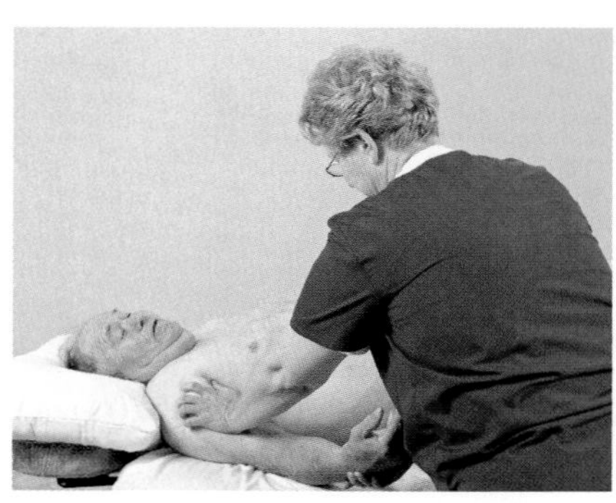

C-23 ■ Massage of the arm and hand (patient supine).

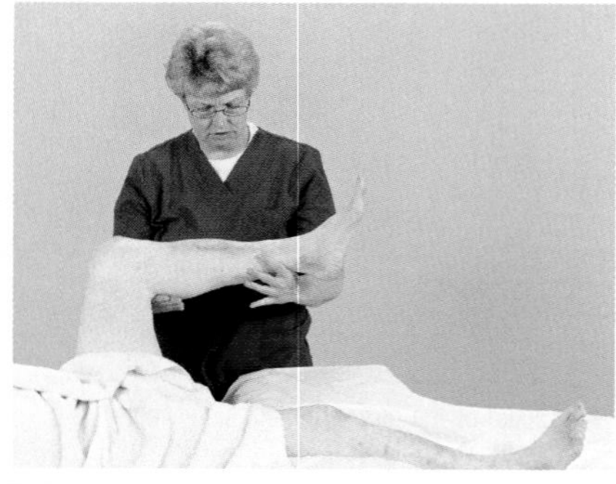

C-22 ■ Rhythmic joint movement and oscillation can be used over areas where direct massage is contraindicated.

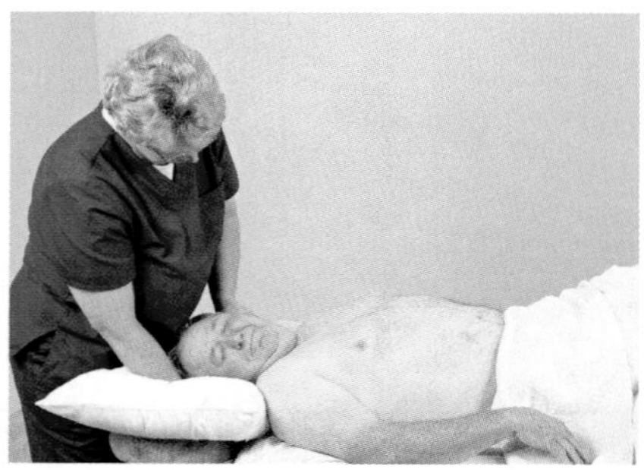

C-24 ■ Gentle pressure and oscillation at the neck combined with massage of the face are soothing.

LOW BACK MASSAGE PROTOCOL

The following photographs present an example of how massage methods can be combined to address nonspecific back pain of muscular origin.

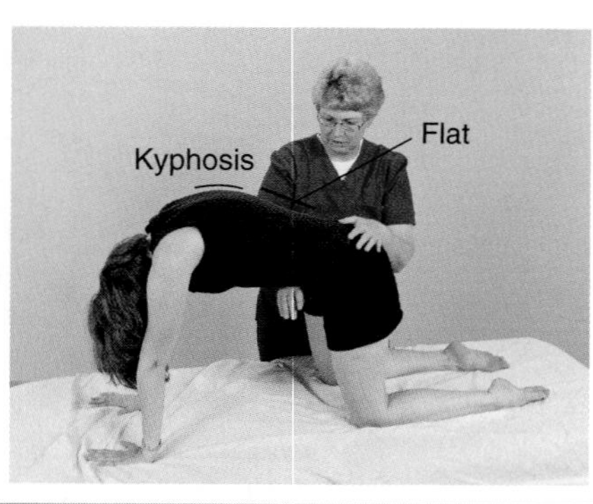

D-1 ■ Assess the spinal curvature.

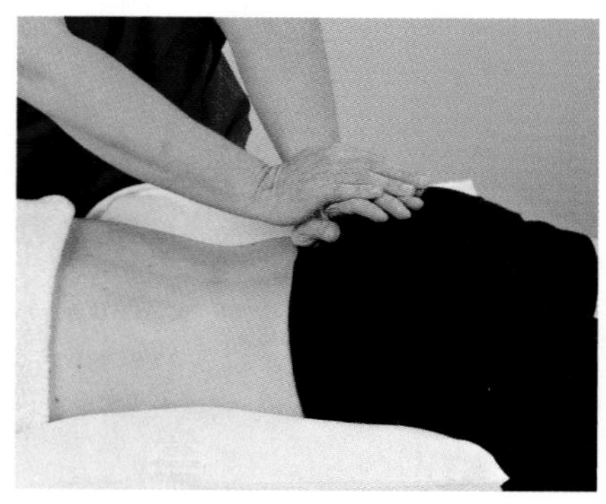

D-2 ■ Compress the sacroiliac (SI) joint area to identify symptoms.

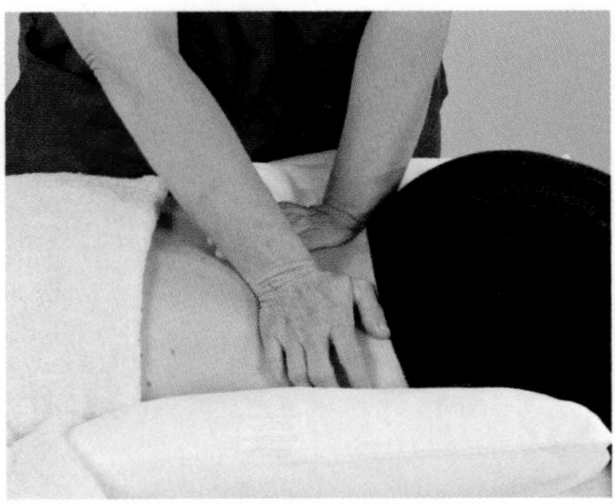

D-3 ■ Assess for psoas involvement by applying bilateral pressure in the lumbar area.

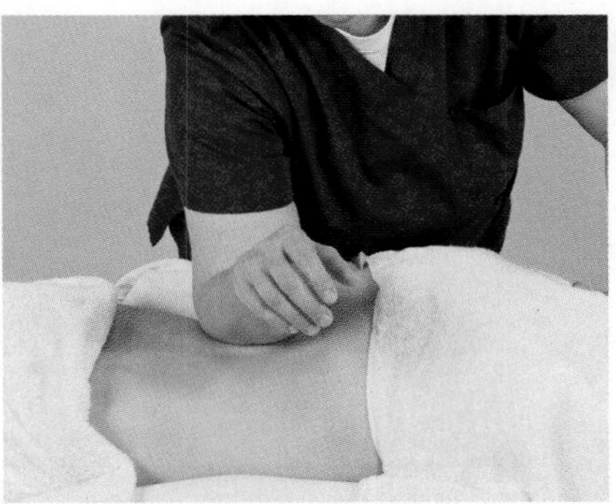

D-4 ■ Apply compression to one side of the lumbar region to assess for quadratus lumborum involvement.

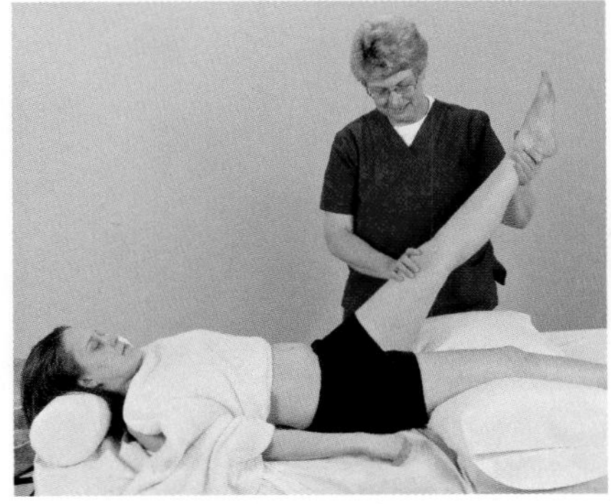

D-5 ■ Assess the length of the hamstring.

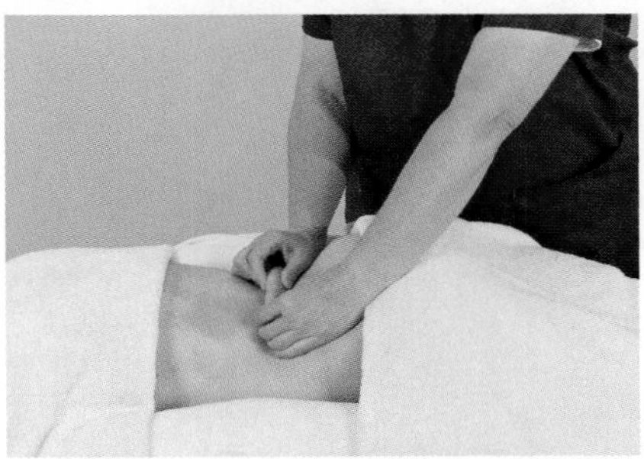

D-6 ■ Assess for tissue bind with skin rolling.

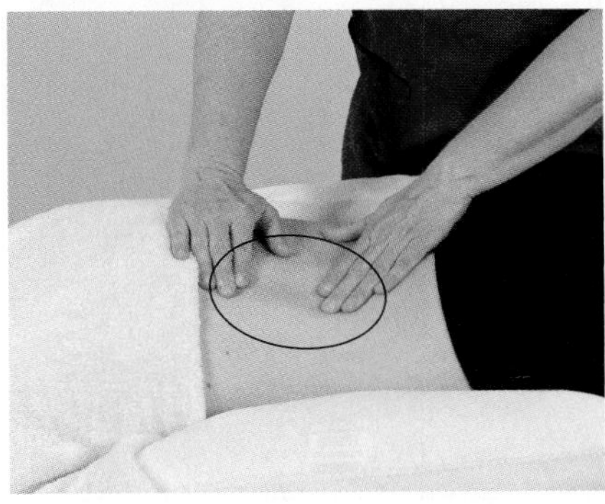

D-7 ■ Assess tissue pliability and also for histamine response.

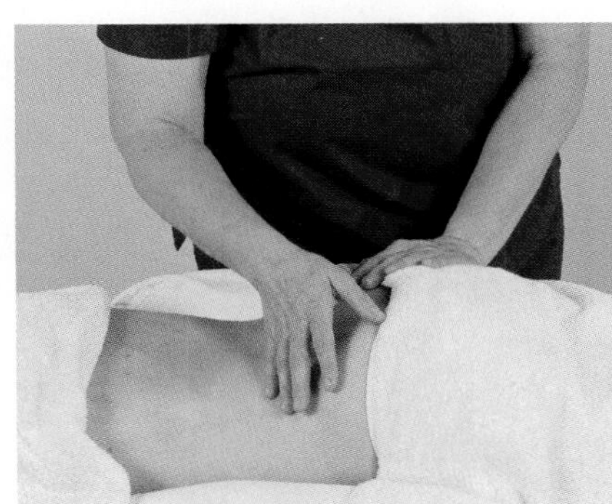

D-8 ■ Massage the area to prepare for specific work.

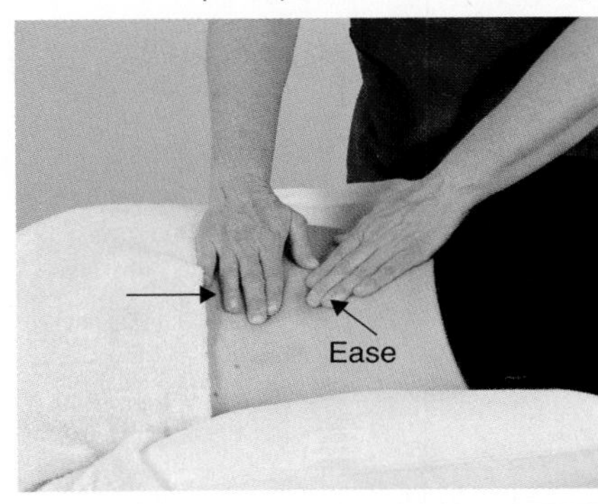

D-9 ■ Use indirect function methods on binding tissue.

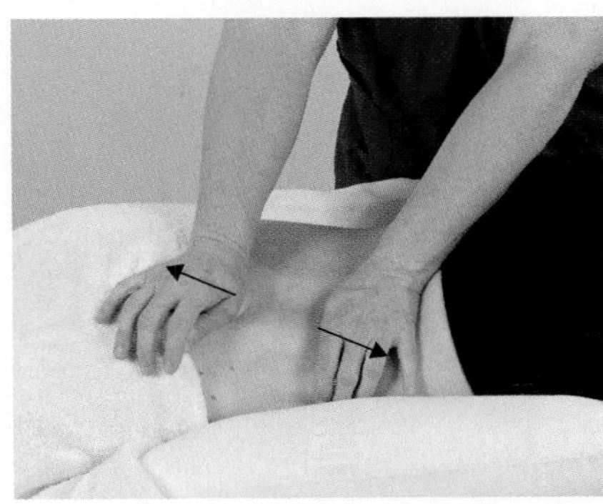

D-10 ■ Next, apply tension force to stretch (move the tissues to bind).

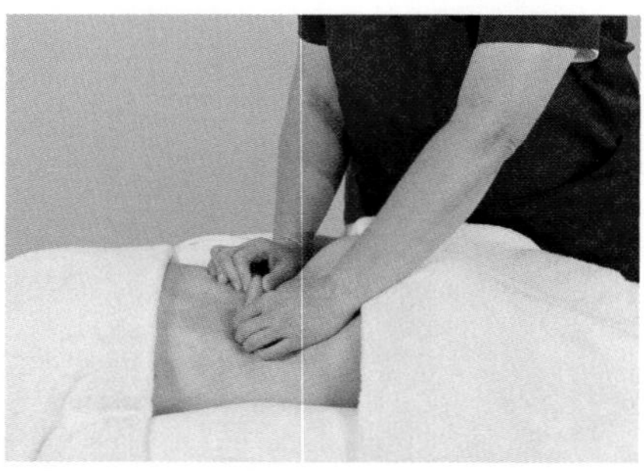

D-11 ■ Address binding tissue with bend and shear forces applied during skin rolling.

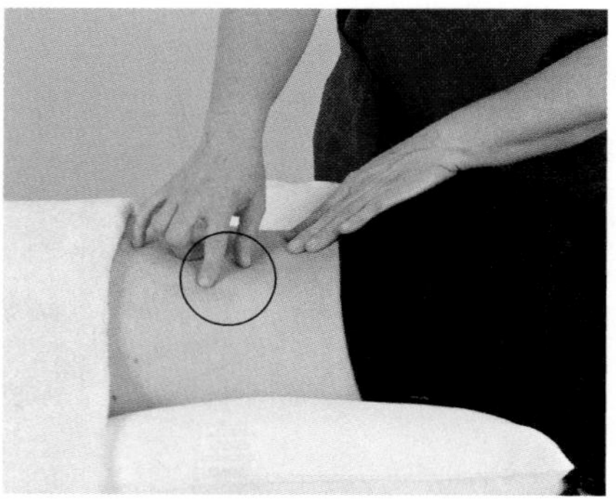

D-12 ■ Identify potential trigger points with drag palpation of the skin.

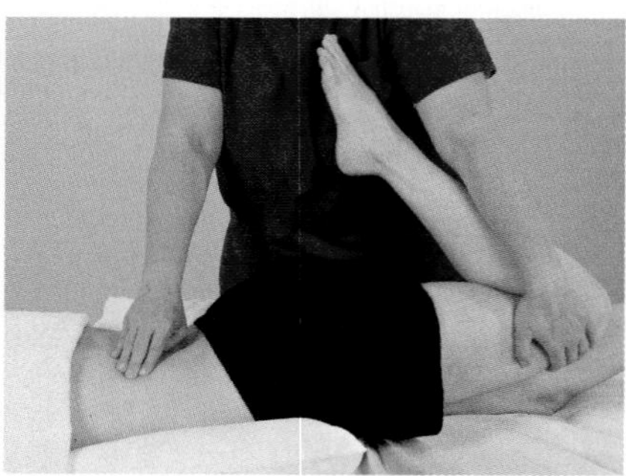

D-13 ■ Address trigger points with positional release.

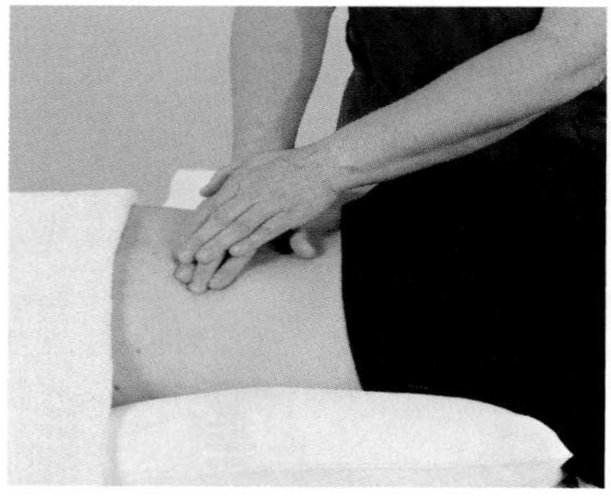

D-14 ■ Address trigger points with inhibitory pressure.

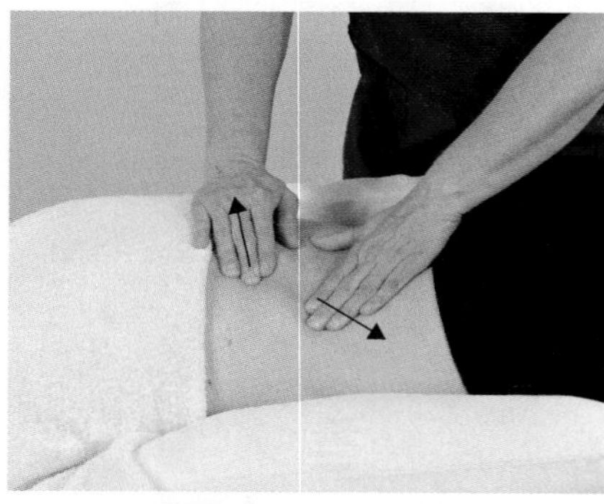

D-15 ■ Stretch the area with direct tissue stretching.

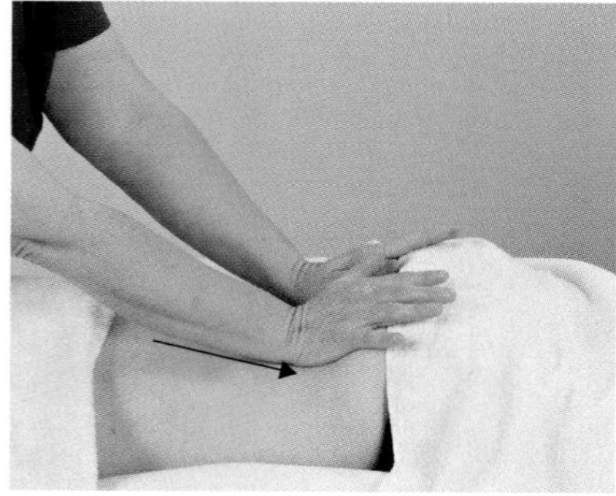

D-16 ■ Apply connective tissue stretching using gliding with drag.

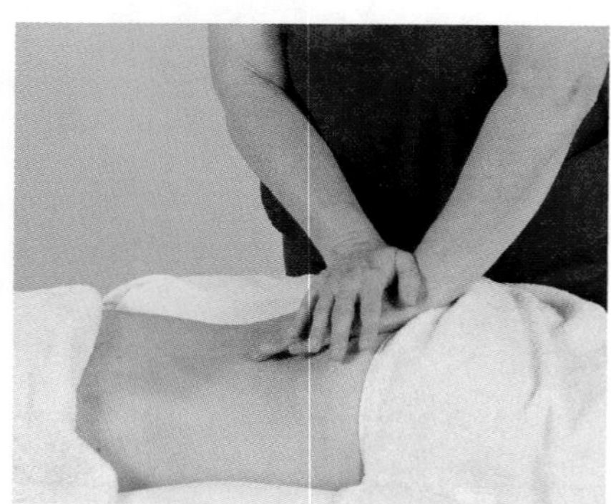

D-17 ■ Rhythmically compress the sacrum.

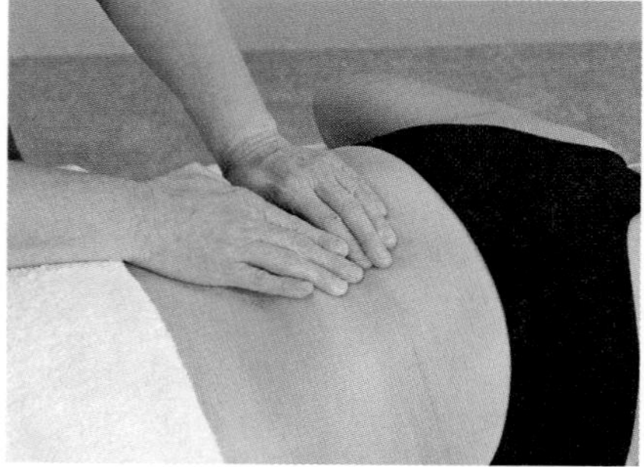

D-18 ■ Provide deep massage in flat areas of spinal column, especially the paraspinals (multifidus rotator release).

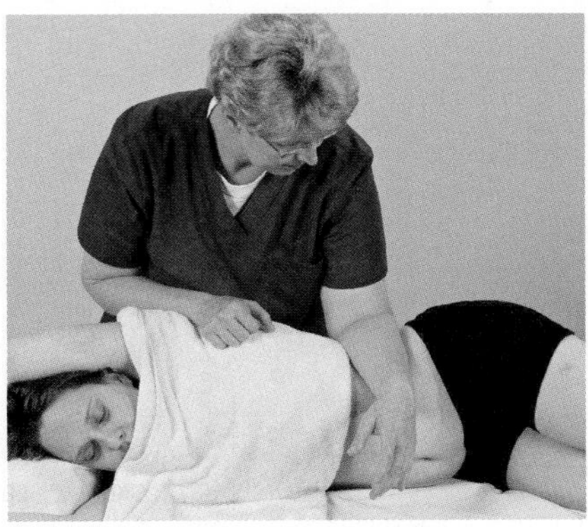

D-19 ■ Perform quadratus lumborum release.

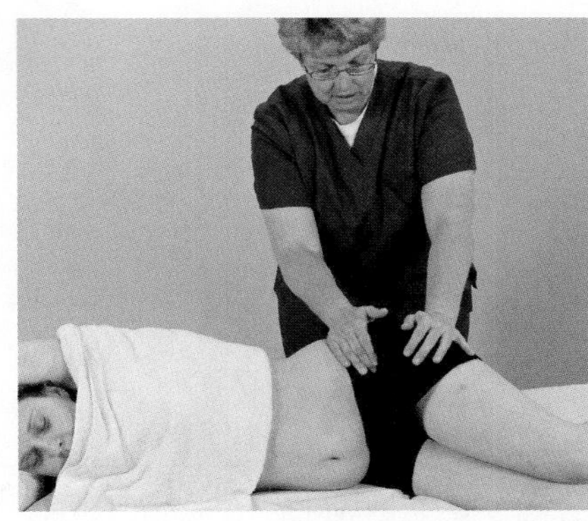

D-20 ■ Mobilize the SI joint in multiple directions.

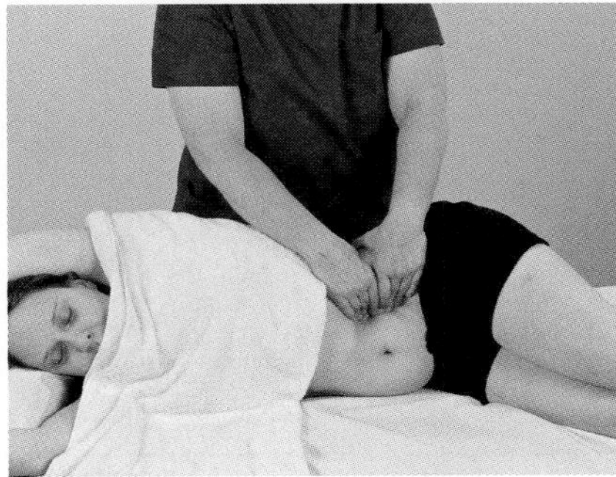

D-21 ■ Perform psoas release (all positions are appropriate).

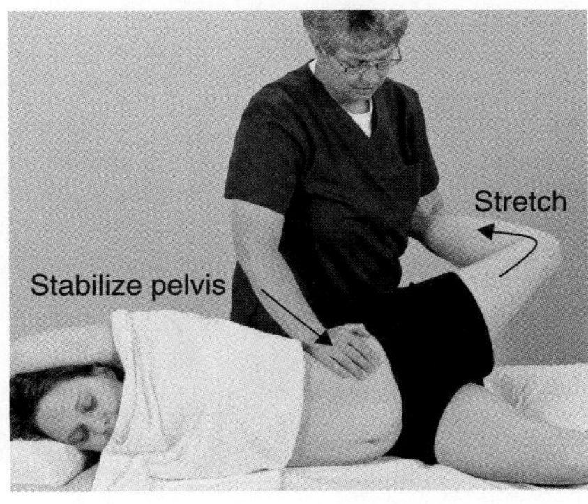

D-22 ■ Stretch the psoas.

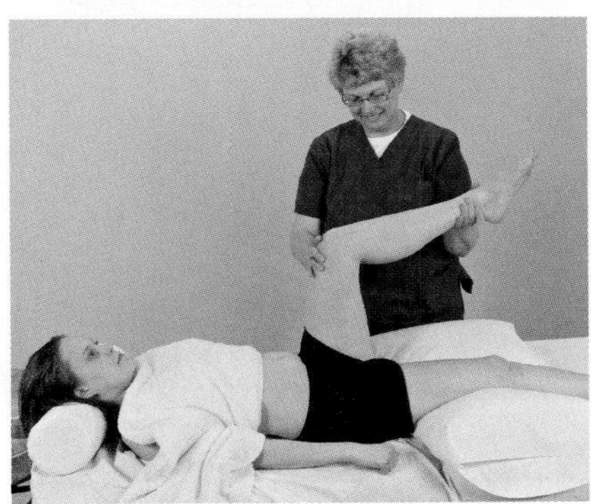

D-23 ■ Use various muscle energy methods to increase tolerance to stretching of the hamstrings.

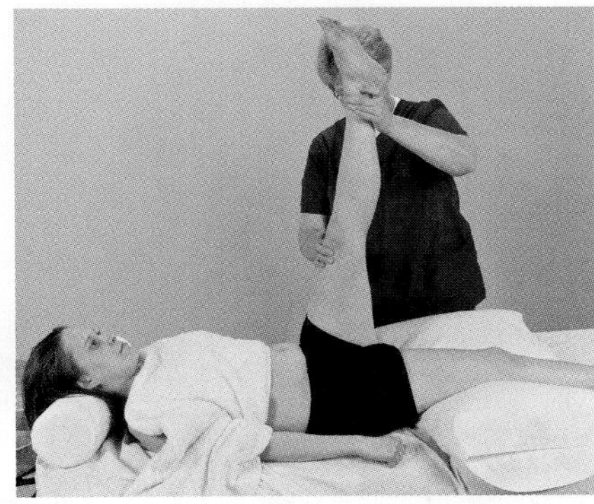

D-24 ■ Stretch (lengthen) the hamstrings.

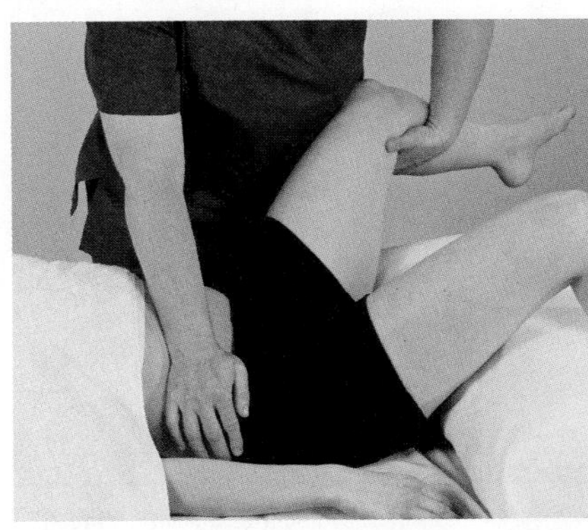

D-25 ■ Assess for and correct rotation/tilting inflares and outflares of the pelvis.

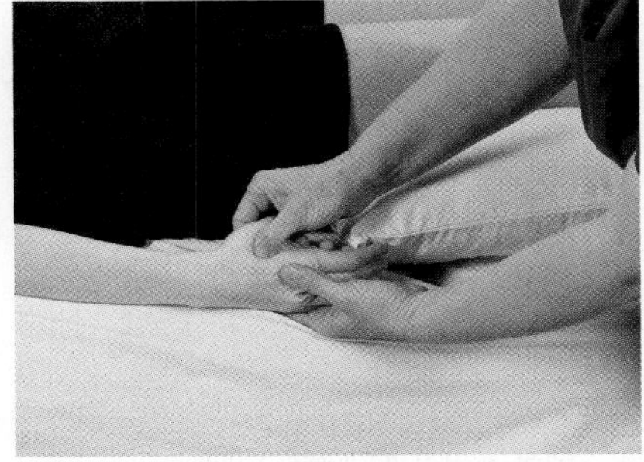

D-26 ■ Apply pressure to acupuncture points known to modulate pain.

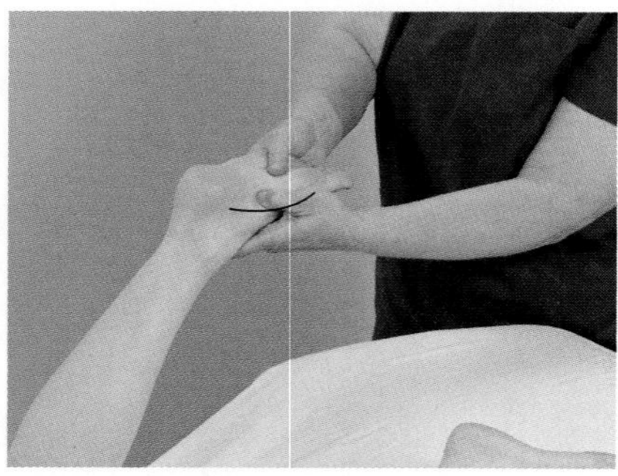

D-27 ■ Massage reflexology points related to the low back.

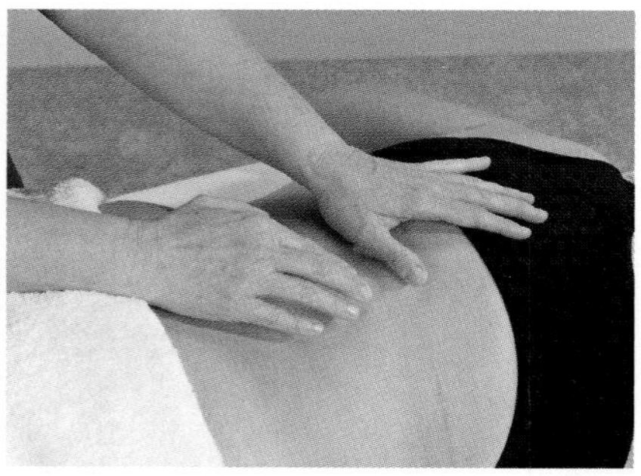

D-28 ■ Incorporate near-touch energy-based methods when appropriate.

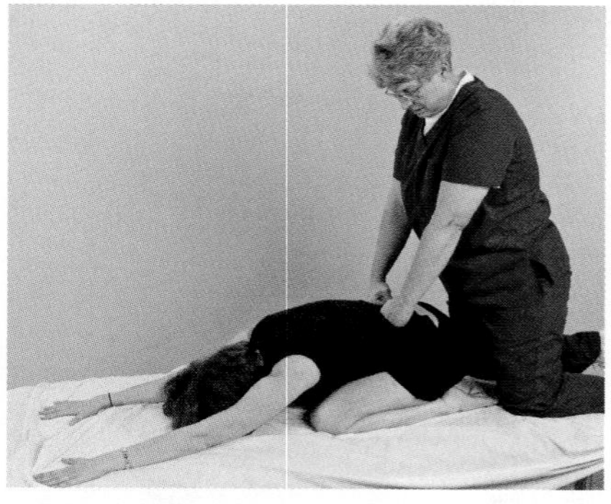

D-29 ■ Compression of the lumbar area (caution for knee flexibility).

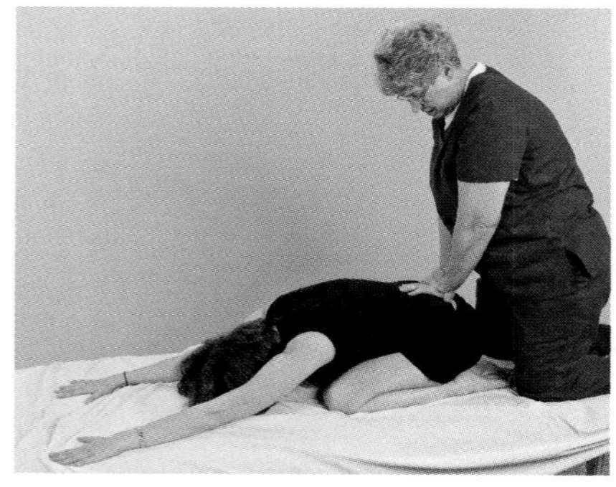

D-30 ■ Stretching of the lumbar area (caution for knee flexibility).

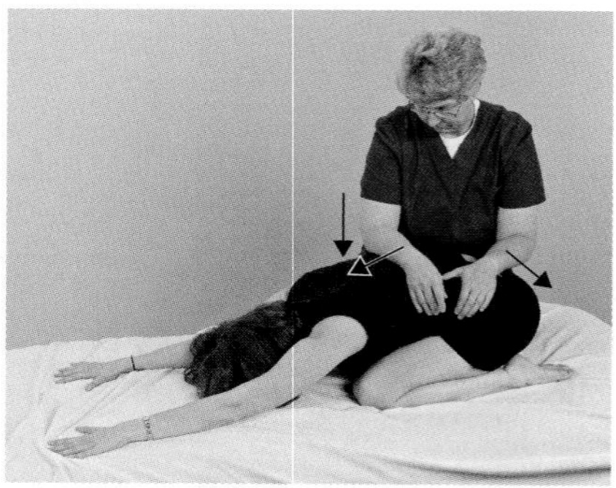

D-31 ■ Modified stretch position (caution for knee and shoulder mobility).

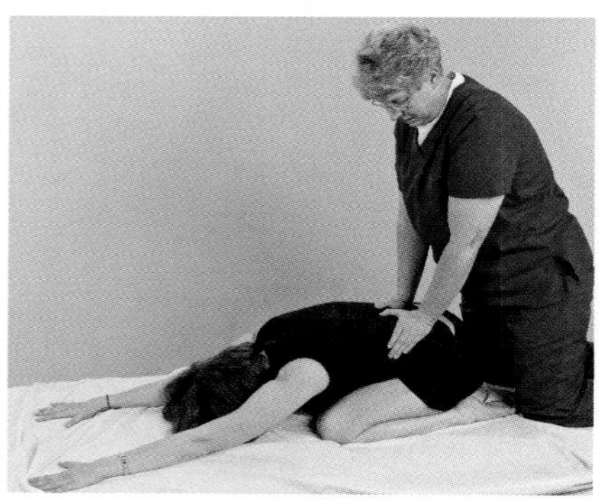

D-32 ■ Use oscillation to relax the back. Sway back and forth, rhythmically alternating compression with hands (caution for knee mobility).

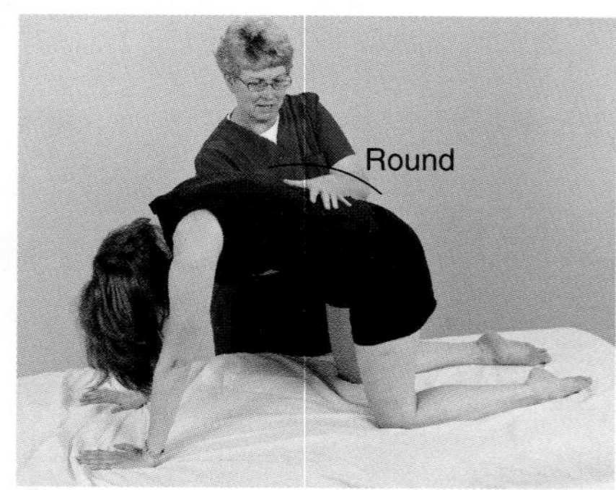

D-33 ■ Active assisted movement to mobilize an area.

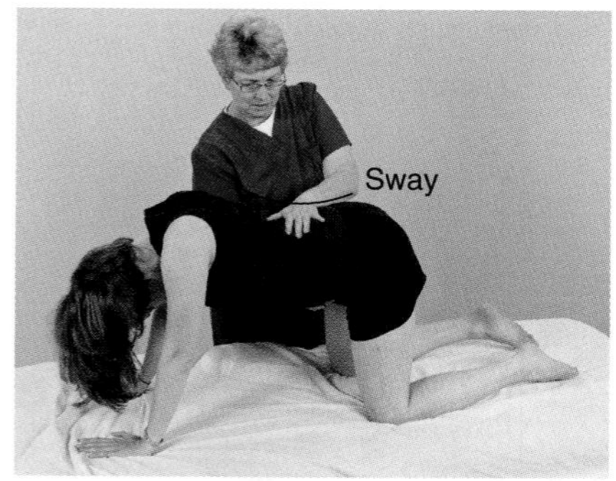

D-34 ■ Active assisted movement to mobilize an area.

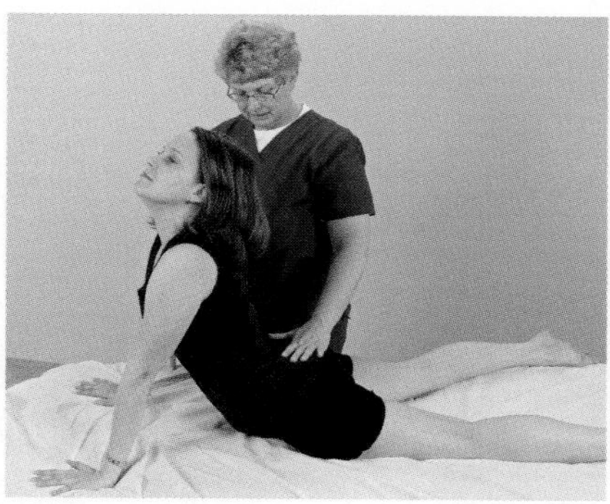

D-35 ■ Monitor active movement to lengthen anterior muscles and connective tissue—use caution with disk involvement.

PROTOCOL TO ADDRESS BREATHING FUNCTION

The following photographs show how various massage applications can be used together to influence breathing function. As always, the specific methods chosen and their application vary, depending on the individual patient, and cautions that need to be observed.

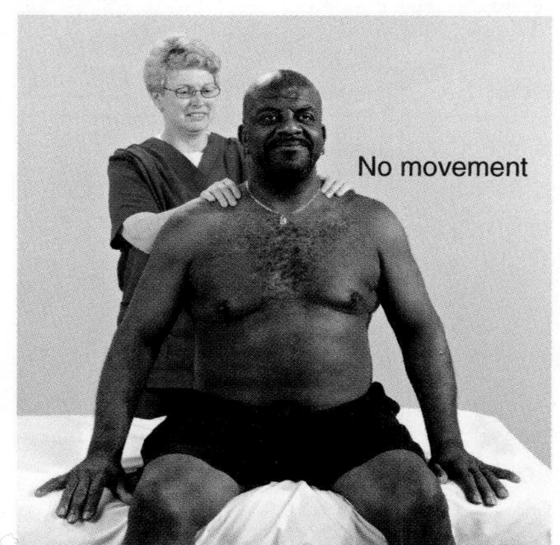

E-1 ■ Assess for shoulder movement during inspiration; the shoulders should not move during quiet inspiration.

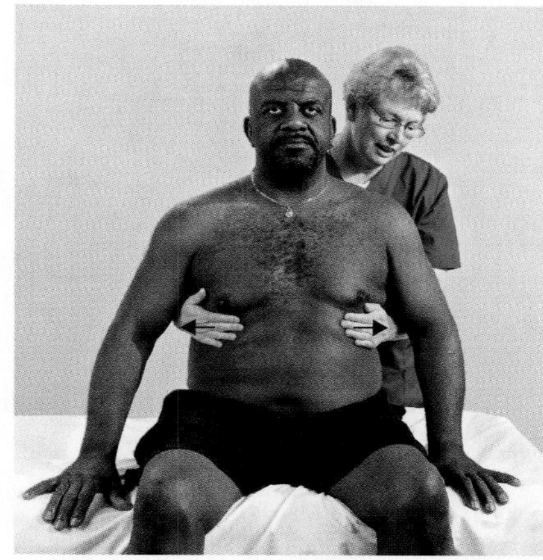

E-2 ■ Assess for rib movement during inspiration; the ribs should move outward during inhalation.

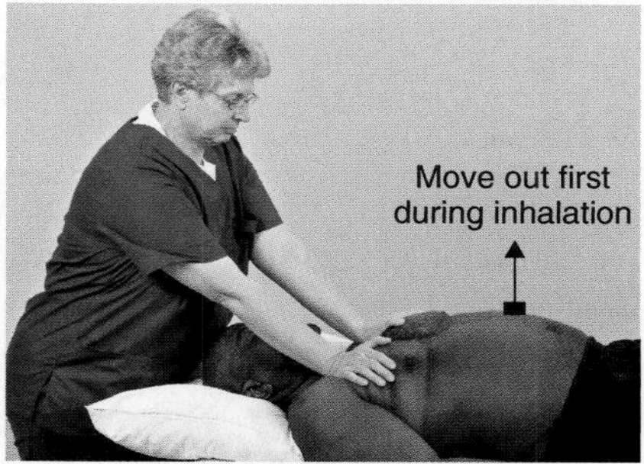

E-3 ■ Assess for movement in the upper chest during inspiration; the chest should not move before the abdomen.

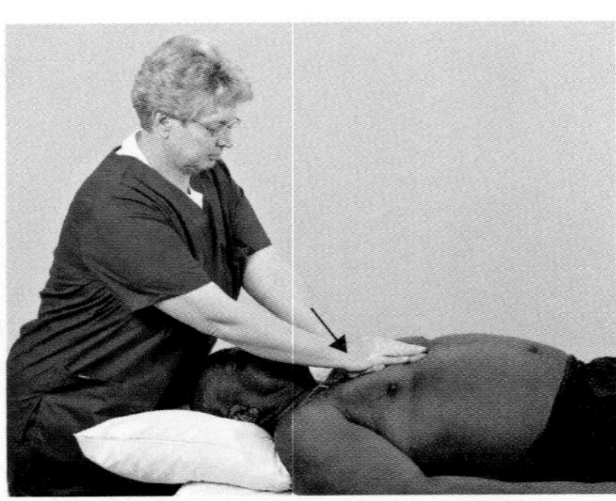

E-4 ■ Assess for rib and sternum springing by applying compression over the sternum and feeling for a tiny amount of give, followed by recoil to the original position.

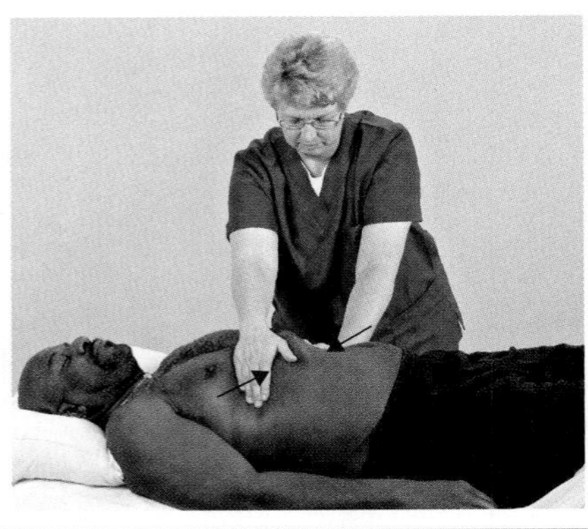

E-5 ■ Assess for lower rib movement using compression; the ribs should move slightly and then recoil to the original position.

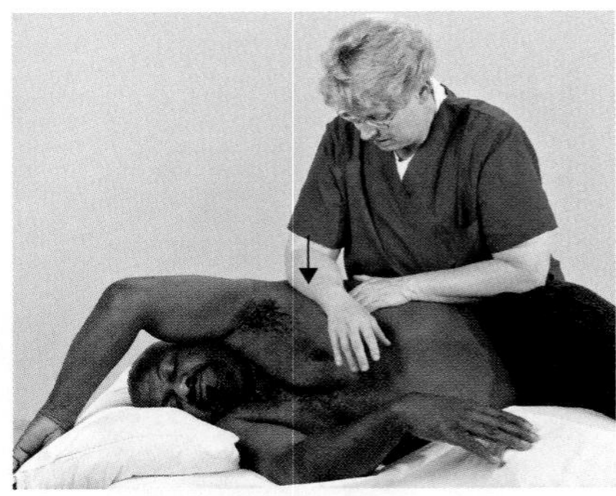

E-6 ■ Assess for rib movement using compression; the ribs should move slightly.

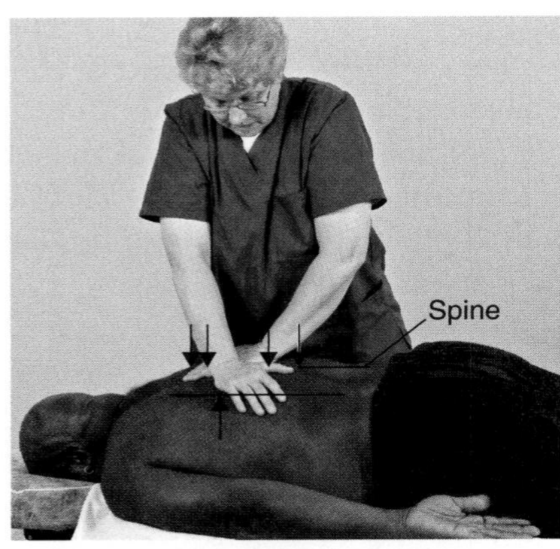

E-7 ■ Assess for rib movement (posterior) by applying compression to the ribs from T1 to T12; apply compression on either side of the vertebral column, not over the spine.

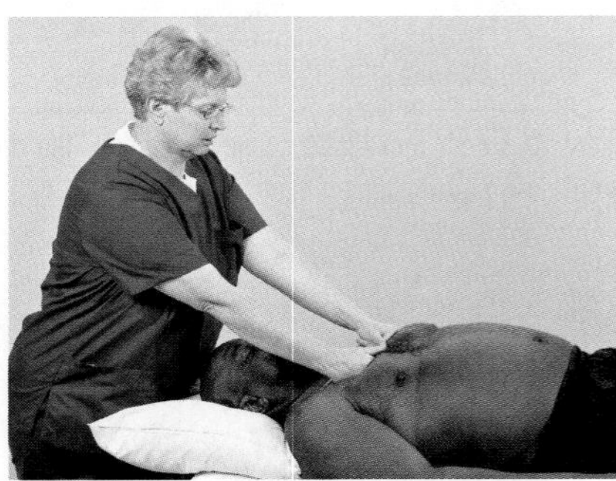

E-8 ■ Massage application to increase the pliability of the thorax soft tissue and to reduce motor tone, especially in the pectoralis minor.

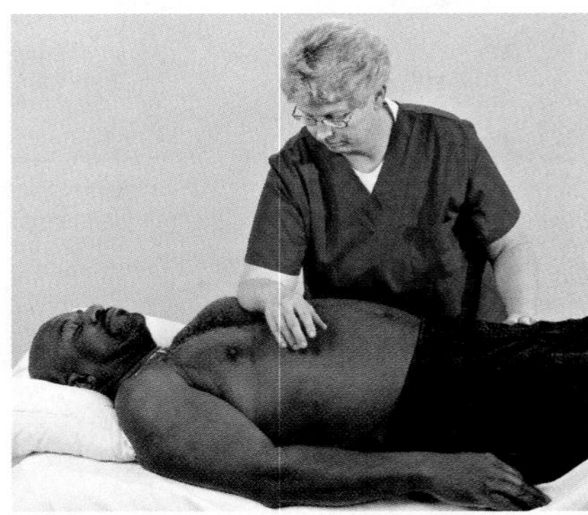

E-9 ■ Massage the area to increase the mobility of the thorax, supine.

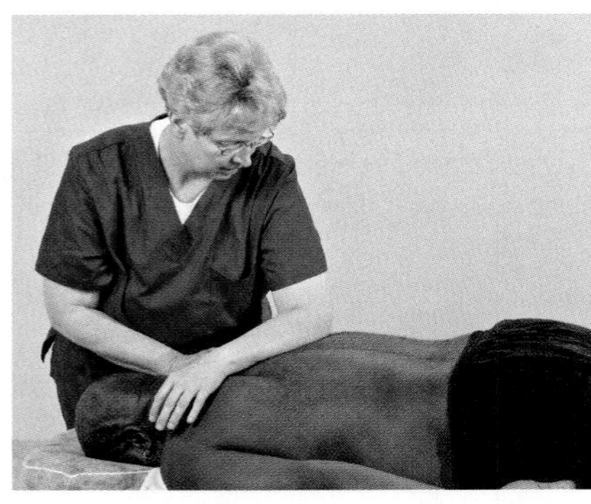

E-10 ■ Massage the area to increase the mobility the thorax, prone.

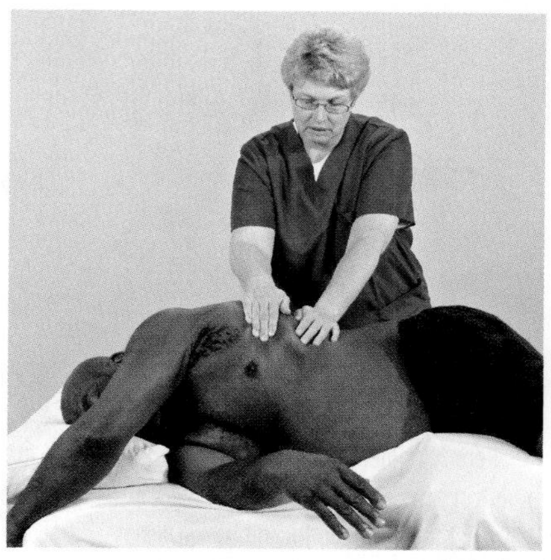

E-11 ■ Massage the area to increase the mobility of the thorax, side-lying.

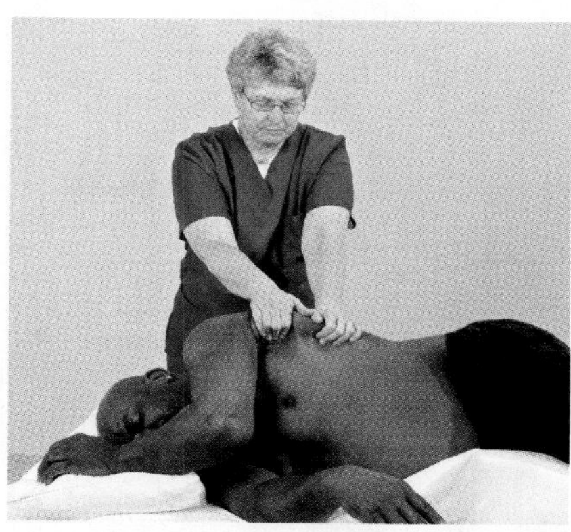

E-12 ■ Introduce torsion force to increase the pliability of binding tissue.

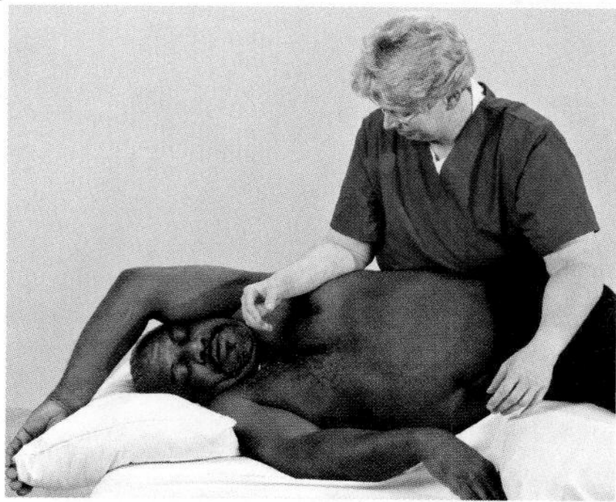

E-13 ■ Reduce motor tone in the latissimus dorsi, teres major, teres minor, and triceps, especially at the attachment to the scapula.

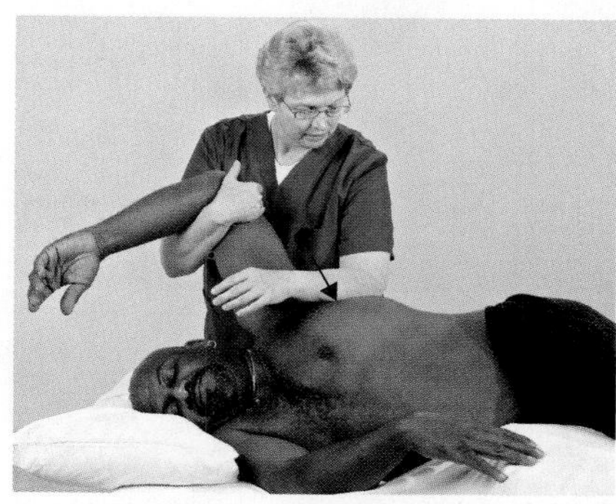

E-14 ■ Reduce motor tone in the anterior serratus.

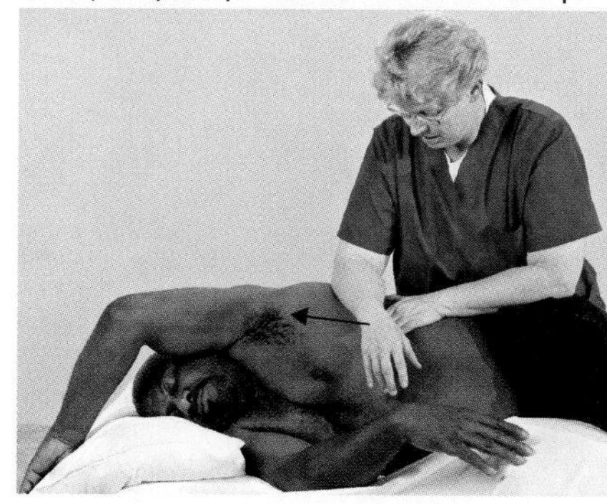

E-15 ■ Apply tension force to lengthen the anterior serratus.

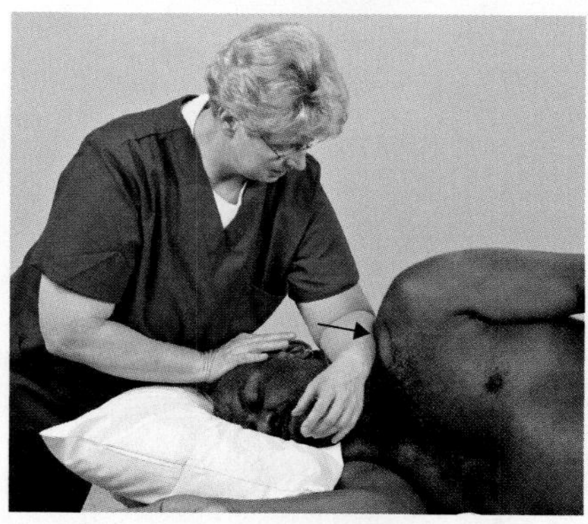

E-16 ■ Reduce motor tone in the upper trapezius, broad-based compression.

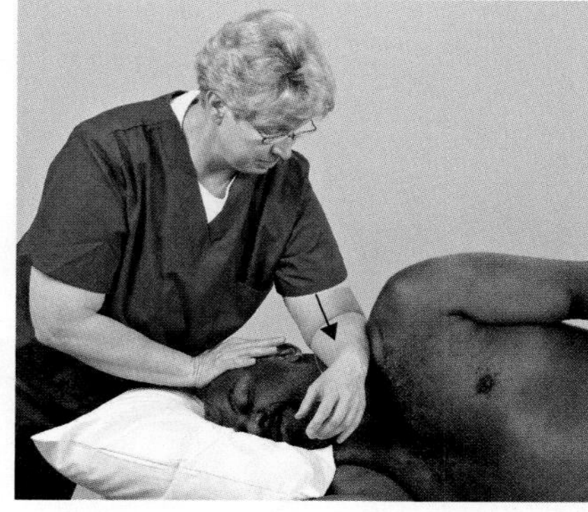

E-17 ■ Reduce motor tone in the scalenes.

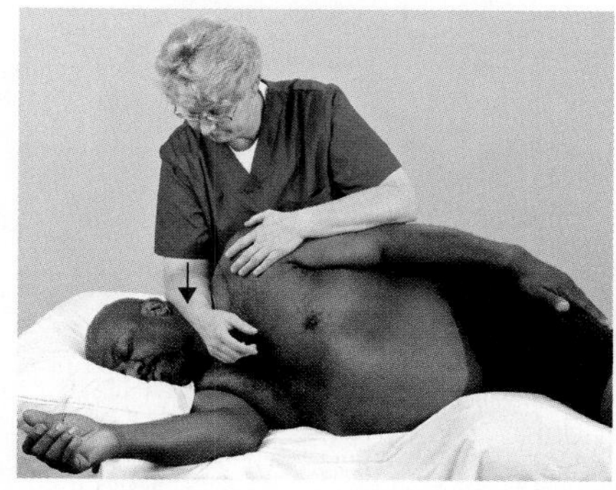

E-18 ■ Reduce motor tone in the occipital base area and the sternocleidomastoid.

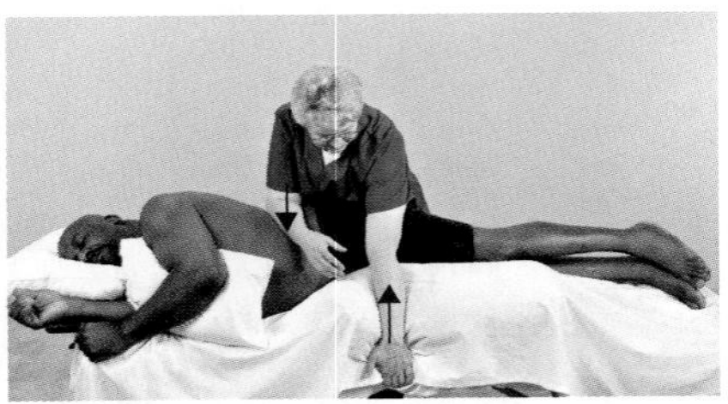

E-19 ■ Reduce motor tone in the lumbar area and the quadratus lumborum, using counterpressure if necessary.

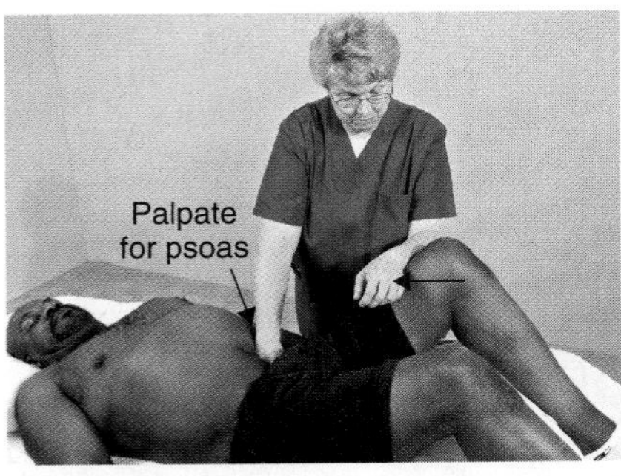

E-20 ■ Reduce motor tone in the psoas. Make sure the psoas is accessed by having the patient push the leg against the therapist's arm while the therapist feels for contraction of the psoas.

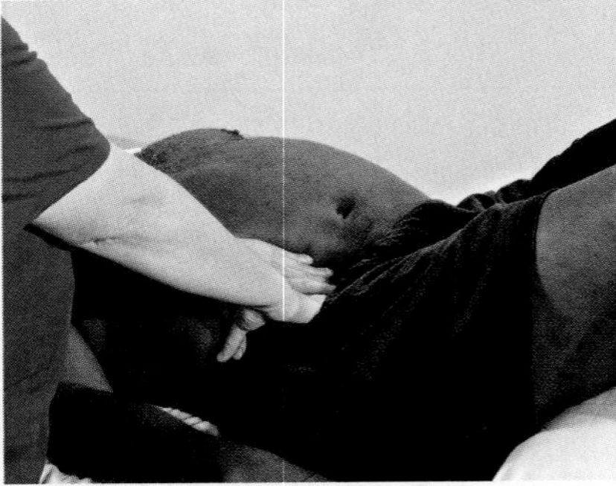

E-21 ■ Applying inhibitory pressure to the psoas (be sure to stabilize the fingers).

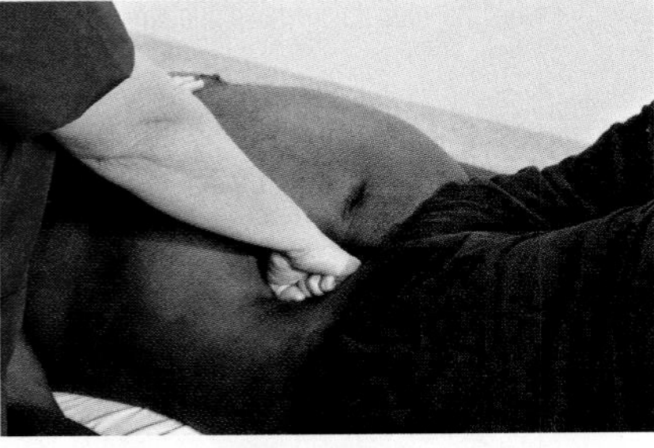

E-22 ■ The fist can be used if stabilized fingers would feel too "pokey" to the patient.

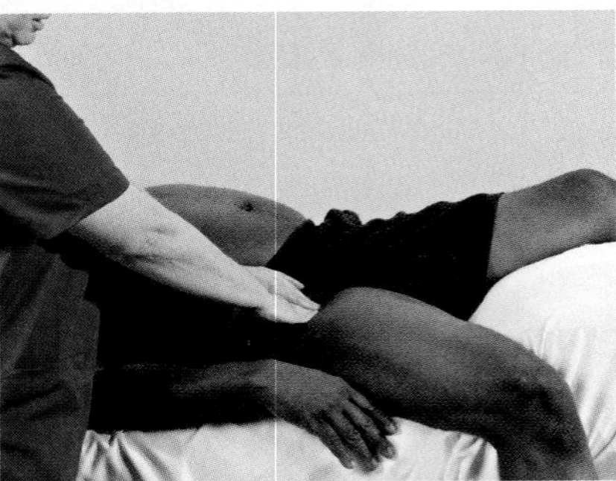

E-23 ■ The psoas also can be inhibited near the distal attachment.

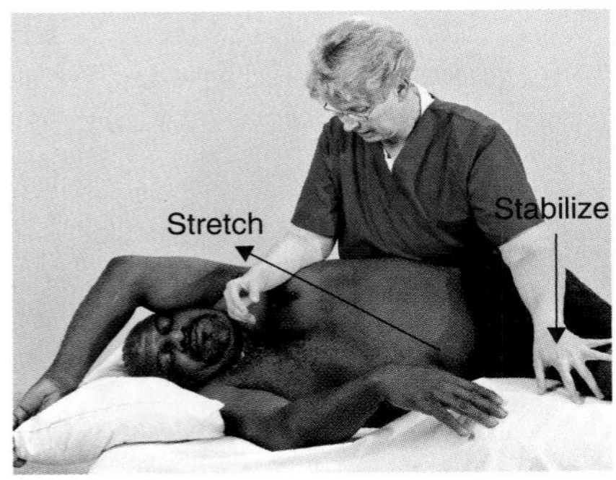

E-24 ■ Lengthen and stretch the anterior thorax.

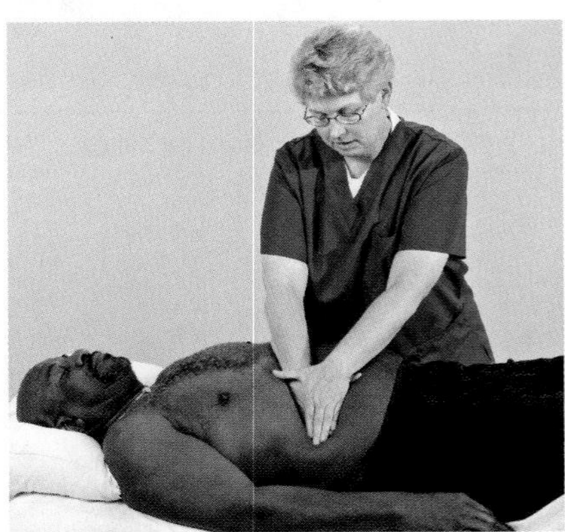

E-25 ■ Massage the area around the lower ribs to prepare for diaphragm release.

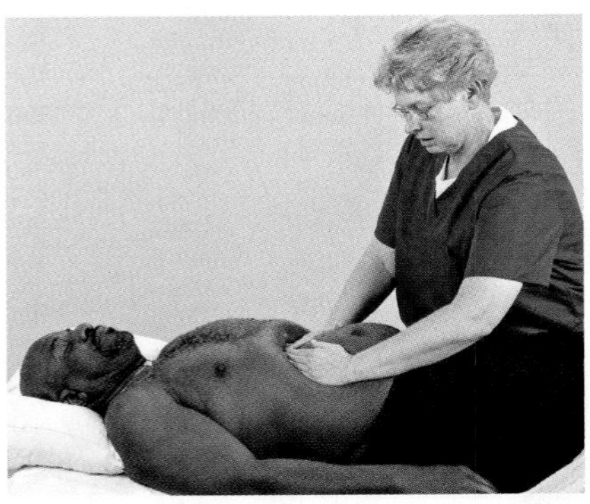

E-26 ■ Diaphragm release.

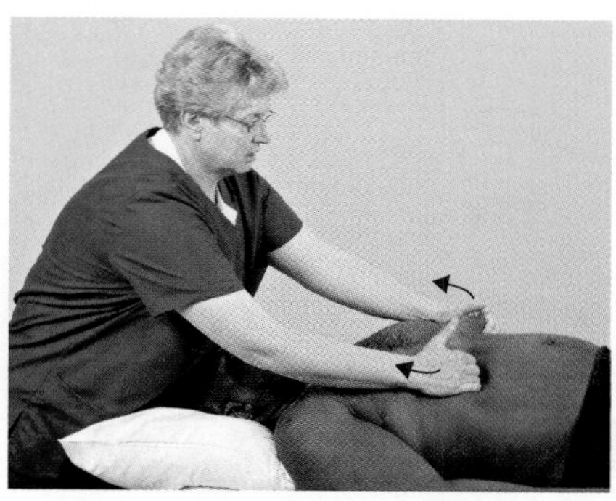

E-27 ■ Gently stretch the tissue around the lower ribs.

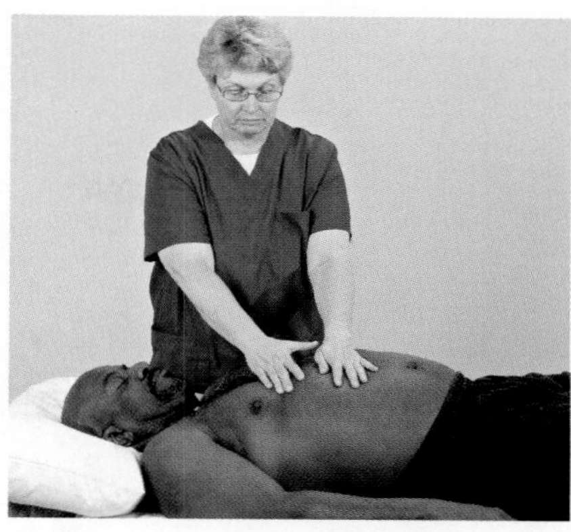

E-28 ■ Use drag palpation to identify tender points. Typically, no more than five or six areas are addressed during a session.

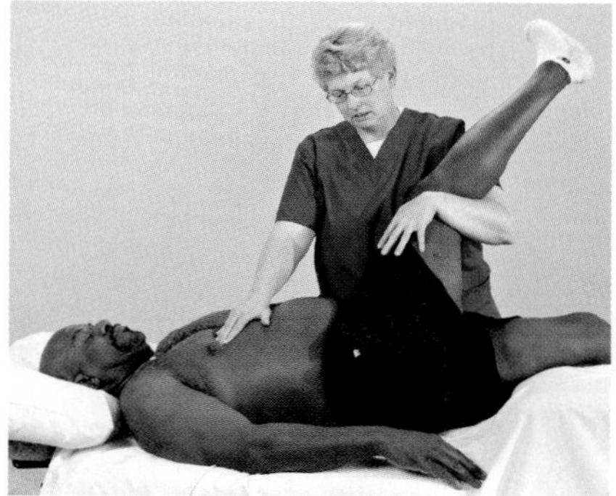

E-29 ■ Use positional release to address tender points.

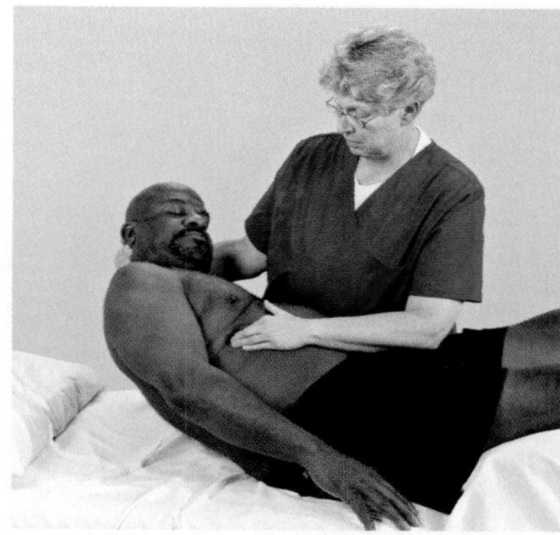

E-30 ■ Use multiple positions for positional release if required.

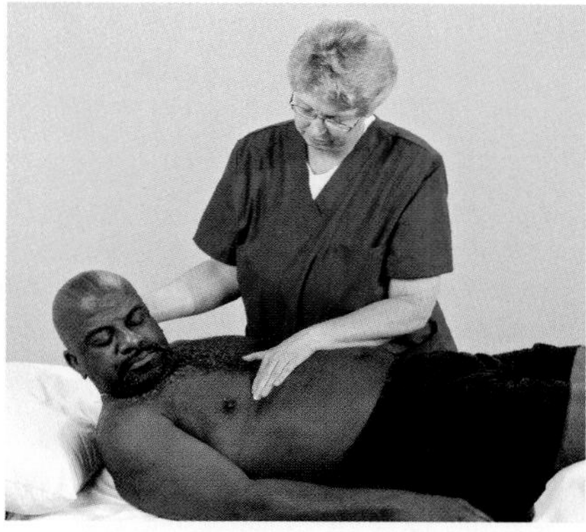

E-31 ■ Use multiple positions for positional release.

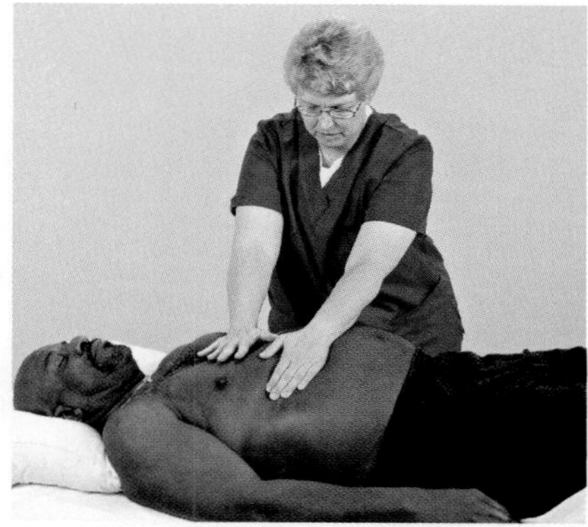

E-32 ■ Massage the area and continue with the general massage. Repeat the assessment to identify improvement.

INDEX

A

Abdomen
  general massage protocols, 387f, 396, 397f, 398-400
  massage illustration, 305f
  muscles
    shortening with breathing pattern disorders, 478-479
  observation and palpation of, 272, 273f-274f
  physical examination of, 256
Abdominal viscera, 304
Abrasions, 655f
Absence seizures, 638
Abstracts
  definition of research article, 45, 49b
Acceptance
  during grieving process, 588-590
  stage of death and dying, 584-585
Accessible populations, 32
Acetylcholine, 547-548
Achilles tendon
  shortening of, 267f, 268
Aching pain, 488
Acid-base balance, 161-162
Acidosis, 161-162
Acquired immunity, 495-496
Acquired immunodeficiency syndrome (AIDS), 9
Action potential, 146
Active assisted movements, 222
Active assistive range-of-motion (AAROM), 223, 530-531
Active joint movements, 222
Active range-of-motion (AROM)
  defining, 272
  exercise, 528
Active release technique, 343-344
Active resistive movements, 222
Active resistive range-of-motion, 223-224
Acupressure, 355, 356f, 357b, 358, 359f
Acupuncture
  for back pain, 602
  description of, 355, 356f, 357b, 358-359, 490-491
  occupational definition
    and scope of practice of, 13b
  for pain, 490-491
Acute care
  illustration of, 14f
Acute illnesses, 468
Acute infections, 198
Acute inflammation, 494-495, 501
Acute injuries, 468
Acute pain
  versus chronic, 485-486
  triggers of, 485
Acute reinjury
  of chronic condition, 461
Acute renal failure; *See also* kidneys
  description of, 631
Adaptation
  to fitness programs, 99
Adaptive capacity
  definition of, 88
Adaptive mechanisms, 6
Addictions
  benefits of massage for, 556
  types of, 104-105
Adhesions, 177-178
Adipose tissue
  percentage of water in, 160t
Adjunct therapies
  unique circumstances and
    essential oils, 435, 437, 438t, 439
    hydrotherapy, 435, 436b
    magnets, 440-442
    probiotics, 440
    the sleeping patient, 434-435
    vibrational methods, 439-440
Adjustment disorders, 557b
Adjustments
  for back pain, 602
  in chiropractic, 59
  definition of, 67
Adjuvant drugs, 490
Admitting diagnosis
  body system review, 255
  history of, 254-255
  during massage assessment process, 254-256
  physical examination, 255-256
Adolescents
  benefits of massage for, 573
  illustration of massage for, 569f-570f

Adult Hodgkin's lymphoma
  case study on, 681-687
Adverse reactions, 523
Aerobic exercise training, 99, 100, 531
Aerobic system, 99
Agility
  assessing during examination, 265
Aging
  and back pain, 596-607
  collagen reduction with, 177-178
  as factor for illness and injury, 455
  and geriatric massage, 537-555 (*See* older adults)
  nervous system conditions with, 546-549
  and vision, 549-550
Aging process
  and geriatric massage, 537-555
Agitation-quality mechanical force, 494
Agnosia, 567
Agonists
  definition of, 185
  muscles functioning as, 269
Agoraphobia, 558-559
Alcohol
  addiction to, 104-105, 556
  and aging, 537-538
  and depression, 560-561
  and liver disease, 632-634
  and pain tolerance, 483
Alkalosis, 161-162
Allergies
  related to chronic inflammation, 125t
Allostasis, 459b
Allowable charges, 80
Alpha levels, 36
Alpha nerves, 185-186
Alternative health systems
  types of, 9
Alternative hypotheses, 35
Alternative medicine
  definition of, 6
Alzheimer's disease
  benefits of massage for, 549, 566-567
  description and stages of, 547-548
  medical treatment of, 548-549
  related to chronic inflammation, 125t
Ambulatory surgery, 517b
Americans with Disabilities Act, 574
Amputation
  case study on, 714-720
  and gait, 290, 293
Amygdala, 145
Amyloid plaques, 547
Anaerobic system, 99
Anatomic barriers
  restricting ROM, 275-276
Anatomy;*See also* anatomy and physiology
  definition of, 143
Anatomy and physiology
  cardiovascular system, 162-169
    blood, 168
    blood pressure and pulse, 165-168
    pathologic conditions of, 168-169
  fluid dynamics, 159-162
  importance of learning, 295
  joints
    degeneration, 183-184
    stability, 182-183
    structure and function, 181-182
  muscles
    functional movement of, 184-185, 188-191, 191f-192f, 193-194
    kinetic chain, 186-187, 188f
    types of actions, 185-186
  myofascial form and function, 175-181
    fascia, 179-180
    periosteum, 179
  neuroendocrine structure and function, 144-147
    autonomic nervous system, 152-153, 154t, 155-159
    chemoreceptors, 150-152
    emotional states, 153, 155-156
Anatomy and physiology *(Continued)*
    energy systems, 157-159
    entrainment, 156
    epithelial tissue, 148-150
    gate control theory, 156-157
    parasympathetic nervous system, 153
    peripheral nervous system, 147-148
    somatic nervous system, 148-150
    the spinal cord, 147
    sympathetic nervous system, 153
  respiratory system
    breathing mechanics, 169-170, 171f-173f
    respiratory rate, 174-175
  summary of massage and, 194b
Anemia
  as chemotherapy side effect, 629-630
  related to chronic inflammation, 125t
Anger
  stage of death and dying, 584
Ankles
  general massage protocols, 426, 427f, 428
  important structures of, 427f
  observation and palpation of, 272, 273f-274f
  overuse problems with, 269, 272
  reflexology, 352-354
  sprain
    case study on, 682, 692
Antagonists
  definition of, 185
  muscles functioning as, 269
Anterior rotation, 375, 377f, 378
Anterior serratus muscles
  specific release techniques, 367-368, 368f
Anterior torso
  general massage protocols, 387f, 396, 398-400
  illustration of important structures of, 397f
  palliative protocol for, 429
Antibodies, 495-496
Anticipatory anxiety, 558
Antiemetics, 629
Antigen-presenting cells, 496-497
Antiinflammatory diet
  elements of, 463b
Antioxidants, 523
Antiphospholipid syndrome, 510b
Anxiety
  benefits of massage for, 121-122, 556-557
  definition of, 122, 556
  disorders
    description of, 557b
Aortic valve stenosis
  related to chronic inflammation, 125t
Aphasia, 566
Apnea
  breathing, 169
  sleep, 651
Approximation, 230, 276
Apraxia, 566-567
Arms
  general massage protocols, 409, 410f, 411-414
  important structures of, 410f
  observation and palpation of, 272, 273f-274f
  palliative protocol for, 429
Arnica montana, 440
Aromatherapy
  description of, 435, 437
  examples of uses, 438t
  for respiratory disorders, 175
Arterial blood flow, 164
Arterial circulation
  illustration of massage for, 328f
  methods of increasing, 327-329
Arteries
  circulation, 324-327, 328f
  compression over, 321f
  of face and head, 384f
Arteriole tone, 166
Arterioles, 162
Arteriosclerosis, 607, 749-753

Arthritis
and back pain, 596
case study on, 720-729
chronic pain with, 486
massage for, 183, 184f
related to chronic inflammation, 125t
Arthrokinematic inhibition, 190
Arthrokinematic reflexes, 181, 186
Arthroscopic surgery, 517-518
Arthrosis, 183, 184f
Asian massage
concepts of
acupuncture and acupressure, 355, 356f, 357b, 358
focused massage applications for, 355-356, 357b, 358-359
meridians, 355-356, 357b
Yin and Yang theory, 355
Assessment process
admitting diagnosis, 254-256
analysis of, 311-312
clinical reasoning during, 251-252
confidentiality, 260-261
of gait, 283, 290, 291f-293f, 293
introduction to, 250-251
kinetic chain analysis, 272-273, 280-282, 294-295, 296b-297b
massage treatment orders, 252-253
massage-specific, 261-306
medical records, 256-260
muscle firing patterns, 282-283, 284b-289b
muscle-strength testing, 278-280
musculoskeletal conditions, 261
outcome goals, 252
palpation, 295-306
physician's treatment orders, 252-253
resourceful compensation, 308
sacroiliac joint function, 293-294
short-term and long-term goals, 253-254
summary of, 310-312
treatment plan development, 309-312
understanding findings of, 306, 308
Assessments;*See also* assessment process
of breathing pattern disorders, 477-478
in case studies, 680
definition of, 250
of pain, 492t
Assistive devices
caution when massaging clients with, 132-133, 134f, 135
Assistive therapies
for independence, 528-529
Asthma
causes of, 499-500
related to chronic inflammation, 125t
Ataxic cerebral palsy, 639
Atherosclerosis
and inflammation, 500
Athetoid cerebral palsy, 639
Athletes
defining, 536
massage strategies for, 536-537
Athletic training
occupational definition
and scope of practice of, 13b
Atrophy
assessment of, 265-266
with cerebral palsy, 639-640
Attention deficit disorder (ADD), 559
Audits
by complementary medicine practitioners
in professional practice model, 12b
Autism, 559
Autoimmune diseases
causes of, 498-499, 504-505
and inflammatory response, 463
list of, 510b
massage strategies for, 510-511
medical treatment of, 505-506
types of, 506-510
diabetes mellitus type 1, 506-507, 510b
Graves disease, 509-510, 510b
Guillain-Barre syndrome, 507, 510b
Autoimmune diseases *(Continued)*
hematologic disorders, 507, 510b
inflammatory bowel disease, 506, 510b
lupus, 509, 510b
multiple sclerosis, 507-508, 510b, 640
myasthenia gravis, 508, 510b
psoriasis, 508, 510b
rheumatoid arthritis, 508, 510b
scleroderma, 508-509
Sjögren's syndrome, 509, 510b
thyroid diseases, 509-510
vasculitis syndromes, 510
Autonomic nervous system (ANS)
anatomy, physiology and massage, 152-153, 154t, 155-159
description and function of, 152-153
disruption and breathing disorders, 474
Avulsions, 655f
Axons, 145, 500

B
Babies;*See* infants
Bacilli, 199
Back pain
clinical reasoning process
assessment of, 597, 598f, 599f
disks, 597, 598f
major muscles involved in, 599f-601f
prevention of, 603
specific massage strategies for, 603-607
symptoms and diagnosis of, 597
treatment of, 597, 601-603, 603-607
description of, 485-486, 596-607
massage strategies for, 603-607
muscles involved in, 596-607, 599f-601f
Backs
keeping therapist's straight, 240, 241f-244f
Backward-tilting pelvis
description of, 456-457
Bacterial infections
and fibromyalgia, 610
inflammation with, 625
massage contraindicated for, 129
morphology and transmission of, 199
Balance
assessment of, 271f-272f
lack of body
landmarks to identify, 268b
Bargaining
stage of death and dying, 584
Baroreceptors
and medulla, 168
Basal ganglia, 145
Basilar artery migraine, 621
B-cells, 496-498
Behavior modification
and additions, 104-105
and fibromyalgia, 610
for pain relief, 491
Behavioral patterns
changing, 88
Behaviors
component of wellness, 104
defining in wellness terms, 104-105
and pain, 642b
Behcet's disease, 510b
Bending forces
definition of, 214
illustration of, 215f-216f
stretching with, 239f
Bereavement
process of, 588-589
Best practice
description of, 56, 58
future of, 73-74
and patient's bill of rights, 57b
Between-subjects independent variables, 43-44
Billing
and coding guidelines, 79b
Bind, 316, 341f-342f

Biochemistry
  influences on health, 460f
  the mind and neurosomatic disorders, 458b-459b
Biofeedback
  for pain relief, 491
Biologic therapy, 630
Biologically based therapies, 9
Biomechanics
  importance of understanding, 269, 272, 273f, 274
  influences on health, 460f
Biomedical model, 6-7
Biopsychosocial model, 6
Bipolar disorder, 559, 560
Bladder
  meridians relating to, 356f, 357b
Blast cells, 168
Bleeding disorders
  massage contraindicated for, 131
Blinded and open studies, 45
Blinded (masked) studies, 45
Blood
  clotting, 168, 635-636
  components of, 168
  disorders and contraindications, 131
  hydrostatic pressure, 160
  percentage of water in, 160t
  poisoning, 123
  as target for autoimmune diseases, 510b
Blood clots
  and stroke, 635-636
Blood flow
  massage to stimulate, 324-326
Blood pressure
  definition of, 165-166
Blood vessels
  definition of, 165-166
  microcirculation, 328-329
  palpation of, 300
Blood-brain barrier, 500, 524
Body;*See also* full body massage
  areas in general maintenance protocol, 283f
  areas of symmetry, 519f, 520b
  movements of, 225f
  natural protective mechanisms for, 626f
  quadrants of, 280-282
  rhythmic function, 306, 307f
  signaling homeostatic balance, 117
  wellness components
    behaviors, 104
    breathing, 96-97, 98f
    demands, 94-95
    loss, 95
    mind/body relationship, 103-106
    nutrition, 95-96
    physical fitness, 97, 99-101
    relaxation, 101-102
    sleep, 102-103
Body fluids
  description of, 159-162
  and edema, 320-321
  focused massage applications for, 317-318
  and hydrostatic pressure, 317
  and inflammation, 318
  intra *versus* extracellular, 317
  lymphatic drainage, 322-323, 324f
  and the lymphatic system, 318-320
  targeting massage to move, 326-327
Body mechanics
  and back pain, 596
  concepts of
    and massage application techniques, 237, 239-240, 241f-244f
  counterpressure, 240, 241f-242f
  fundamentals of, 241f-244f
  of massage therapist, 237, 239-240, 241f-244f
  on mats, 240, 243f-244f, 245
Body rhythms
  palpation of, 304
Body systems
  classifying massage application by, 451
  review of, 255
Boggy end-feel, 276
Bones;*See also* fractures
  and back pain, 596-607
  palpation of, 303-304
  percentage of water in, 160t
Bony end-feel, 276
Botanical medicine, 69
Botulinum toxin, 528
Brachial plexus
  description and illustration of, 152
Bradycardia, 166
Bradypnea, 174
Brain
  anatomy and physiology of, 144-147, 634-640
  attack (*See* stroke)
  chemical imbalances in, 559
  complexity of, 145, 634-635
  medulla and baroreceptors, 168
  neurological diseases of, 634-639
  and pain, 484-485
  percentage of water in, 160t
  sensitization, 153
  traumatic injuries to, 636-637
Brain attack, 635-636
Brain infarction, 635
Brainstem
  functions of, 635
  stimulation of, 151
Breasts
  physical examination of, 256
Breathing;*See also* breathing pattern disorders
  component of wellness, 96-97, 98f
  control of, 170, 171f
  deep, 91, 467
  definition of, 169
  and eye movement
    massage application techniques, 226-227, 228f
  function
    photographs illustrating massage protocols, 791-795
  mechanics of, 169-170, 171f-173f, 174-175
  and palpation, 304-305
  pattern disorder
    description of, 174, 476-480
    illustration of negative effects of, 475f
  phases of, 97, 98f
  as primary benefit of massage, 15
  problems with, 96-97
  qi gong exercises, 358
  reflexes that affect, 174
  retraining, 480-481, 482f
  signs and symptoms of problems, 476-477, 477b
Breathing pattern disorders
  assessment of, 477-478
  breathing retraining, 480-481, 482f
  definition of, 174, 474
  health conditions related to, 483b
  interventions, 477b, 478-480
  physical changes with, 476, 477b
  signs and symptoms of, 476
  specific massage strategies, 478-480
Bright pain, 488
Bruises
  assessing during examination, 265
  clinical reasoning process, 656-657, 659-660
  fluid drainage around, 326
Burning pain, 488
Burnout
  Sandy Fritz on professional, 16
Burns
  accommodating, 577
  exercise regimens benefiting, 529t
  and inflammation, 499
  types of, 499
Bursae
  description of, 143

Business structures
in healthcare, 69-70

C

Calf muscles, 368, 478-479, 649f
Cancer
chronic pain with, 486
clinical reasoning process
characteristics and statistics, 626-627
diagnosis of, 627-628
massage strategies for, 630
treatment, 628-630
diagnosis of, 627-628
and hospice care, 585-586
and inflammation, 500-501
location and types of, 627b
related to chronic inflammation, 125t
treatment of, 628-630
Capillaries
definition of, 160
Capsular stretch end-feel, 276
Carbon dioxide
transport of
and oxygen, 170
Cardiac arrest
causes of, 168-169
Cardiac disease
massage contraindicated for, 131
Cardiovascular diseases
description and treatment of, 607-608
and inflammation, 500
massage strategies for, 608, 609f
Cardiovascular system, 162-169
assessment of, 255
benefits of massage on, 163-165, 169
blood, 168
blood pressure and pulse, 165-168
breathing pattern disorder signs in, 476
changes with exercises, 100
clinical reasoning process
description and treatment of, 607-608
massage strategies for, 608, 609f
and entrainment, 163
and geriatric massage, 542-543
harmful unrelieved pain effects, 493t
pathologic conditions of, 168-169
surgery, 517b
sympathetic and parasympathetic response, 154t
therapeutic exercise benefiting, 529t
Career development
for massage therapists, 82-84
Carotidynia migraine, 621
Carpal tunnel syndrome, 644-645, 645f
Cartilage
description of, 143
Case studies
Case 1
on adult Hodgkin's lymphoma, 681-687
on ankle sprain, 682, 692
on stuttering, 681-682, 687-693
Case 2
on lupus and pregnancy, 693-705
Case 3
on diabetes mellitus and depression, 705-713
Case 4
on amputation, 714-720
on hepatitis C, 713-714
Case 5
on arthritis, 720-729
on drug addiction, 722-723
on knee replacement, 720, 723-729
on pain, 720-729
on restless leg syndrome, 720-721
Case 6
on migraines, 729, 731-732
on peptic ulcers, 730-731
on premenstrual syndrome, 732-737
Case studies *(Continued)*
Case 7
on Parkinson's disease, 737-742
Case 8
on coronary heart diseases, 742-753
methods, 48, 50
overview of
documentation methods, 680-681
problem-oriented medical records (POMR), 680-681
SOAP format, 680-681
SOAPIE format, 681
standard format for each, 679-680
Case-report methods, 48, 50
Cataracts
description of, 550
Causes
versus symptoms, 455
Cautions
concerning lymphatic drainage, 322, 335
conditions requiring massage, 128
definition of, 126
Cell-mediated immunity, 200
Cells
and aging process, 538
cancer, 500-501
illustration of twisting reaction, 175, 176f
types of immune, 496-498
Centers for Disease Control and Prevention (CDC)
on Standard Precautions, 200-206
Central pain syndrome, 486
Cerebellum
stimulation of, 151
Cerebral cortex, 635
Cerebral palsy (CP)
categories of, 639-640
Cerebrospinal fluid (CSF), 635
Cerebrovascular accident (CVA)
causes and types of, 635-636
Cervical lordosis
description of, 456-457
Cervical plexus
illustration of, 152f
impingement of, 151, 152f
Cervical spine
and posture and gravity, 267f, 268
Charting;*See* documentation
Chemical addictions, 556
Chemokines, 497, 500-501
Chemoreceptors
anatomy, physiology and massage, 150-152
definition of, 148
and massage, 150-151
Chemotaxis
definition of, 123
Chemotherapy, 629-630
Chest
physical examination of, 256
Chief complaint, 254
Child abuse, 260-261
Childbirth
research on massage and pain of, 30-39, 40f
Children
benefits of massage for, 569f-570f, 573
Chiropractic
diagnoses and treatment in, 67-68
education and license requirements, 66-67
history of, 66
methods of treatment, 68, 602
occupational definition
and scope of practice of, 13b
Chiropractors
educational requirements, 58-59, 66-67
employing massage therapists, 59
focus of, 58
spinal manipulation by, 602
Chondrocytes, 182
Chronic fatigue syndromes, 609, 612-613

Chronic illnesses
benefits of massage for, 119-121
definition of, 467-468
Chronic infections, 198
Chronic inflammation, 495
Chronic local inflammation, 502
Chronic pain
versus acute, 485-486
definition of, 485
syndromes, 609-613
Chronic pain syndromes;*See also* fibromyalgia
massage for, 612
risk factors and symptoms of, 610-611
treatment of, 611-612
Chronic renal failure, 632, 661-664
Chronic stress
signs of, 90-91
Chronic trauma, 461
Circulation
changes with inflammation, 124f
general massage protocols for
abdomen, 387f, 396, 398-400
anterior torso, 387f, 396, 398-400
approach and sequence, 382, 383f
arms, 409, 410f, 411-414
face and head, 382-388
forearms, wrists and hands, 414-416
hips, 416, 417f, 418-421
legs, ankles and feet, 426, 427f, 428
neck, 392, 393f, 394-396
occipital base, 388-392
posterior torso, 400-405
shoulders, 405-409
thighs, 421, 422f, 423-426
increasing arterial, 327-329
of lymph, 318-320
massage
description of, 324
illustration of, 325f
methods of, 324-326
meridians relating to, 356f, 357b
as primary benefit of massage, 15
Circulatory system;*See also* circulation
focused massage applications for, 318-323, 324f
methods of increasing arterial, 327-329
Cirrhosis, 633, 634f
Clavicles
observation and palpation of, 272, 273f-274f
Clients
characteristics of, 56, 58
defining in massage, 4-5
versus patients, 56
and patient's bill of rights, 57b
populations of
classifying massage application by, 451
positioning of, 241f-244f
Clinical reasoning
definition of, 251
and massage client medications, 525
process (*See* clinical reasoning process)
Clinical reasoning process
approach to massage, 596
for back pain
assessment of, 597, 598f, 599f
disks, 597, 598f
major muscles involved in, 599f-601f
prevention of, 603
specific massage strategies for, 603-607, Appendix
symptoms and diagnosis of, 597
treatment of, 597, 601-603, 603-607
for cancer
characteristics and statistics, 626-627
diagnosis of, 627-628
massage strategies for, 630
treatment, 628-630
for cardiovascular/ respiratory diseases
description and treatment of, 607-608
massage strategies for, 608, 609f
Clinical reasoning process *(Continued)*
in case studies, 680
for chronic fatigue syndromes, 612-613
for chronic pain syndromes, 609-613
for chronic renal failure, 661-664
for contusions, 656-657, 659-660
definition of, 251
for headaches, 613-614
migraines, 613, 620-621
tension, 622-624
vascular, 613-614, 620-622
for infections
bacterial, 624-625
massage for, 626
parasitic, 625-626
viral, 625
for kidney disease, 630-632, 661-664
for liver disease, 632-634
during massage assessment process, 251-252
for neurologic diseases, 634-646
brain, 634-639
complex regional pain syndrome, 640-642
disk herniation, 645-646
multiple sclerosis, 639-640
nerve and spinal cord, 642-645
nerve impingement, 642-646
peripheral neuropathy, 640
for orthopedics, 647-648, 649f-650f
for sleep disorders, 647, 650-652
for treatment plan development, 660-661
for wounds, 652-656, 657f-658f
Clotting
blood, 168
Clotting factors, 168, 498
Cluster headaches, 620
Cocci, 199
Co-contraction
of muscles, 185
Coding
and billing guidelines, 79b
Cognition
definition of, 546-547
and dementia, 547-548
problems with fibromyalgia, 610
Cognitive behavioral therapy, 89
Cognitive system
disorders
dementia and delirium, 546-547
description of, 557b
and fibromyalgia, 610-612
harmful unrelieved pain effects, 493t
Cold therapy
hydrotherapy using, 435, 436b
for pain, 490
Collagen
definition of, 177
fibers and massage, 184
and massage, 177-178
Colon
general protocol for, 400
massage illustration, 305f
meridians relating to, 356f, 357b
Combined loading
definition of, 214
illustration of, 215f-216f
Comfort
as primary benefit of massage, 15
Communication
in immune system, 497
Communication skills
barriers to effective, 79
and conflict resolution, 74-79
importance of good, 74-75
and listening, 74-75
Comparison treatment control groups, 44
Complement system
of molecules, 496-498
Complementary
definition of, 6

Complementary and alternative medicine (CAM)
definition of, 6
history of, 8-9
pain treatments, 490-492
Complementary medicine
conditions aided by, 10-11
energy systems
description and illustration of, 157-159, 158f
practitioners
in professional practice model, 12b
professional practice model for
key constituents of, 12b
Complex regional pain syndrome
chronic pain with, 486
definition of, 126
description and massage for, 641
Compression
application methods, 217f, 219
definition of, 214
illustrations of, 215f-216f
over arteries and veins, 324-326
spinal cord, 634
Compression loading
description of, 213-214
illustration of, 215f
Compressive forces
and depth of pressure, 210
illustration of different, 136f
and seven tissue levels, 135-138
Computerized documentation, 82
Computerized patient records (CPRs), 82, 258-259
Concentric actions
of muscles, 185
Conception vessel meridians, 356f, 357b
Concluding sections
of research articles, 31b, 47, 49b
Concussions
symptoms of, 637
Confidence interval (CI), 37
Confidentiality
importance of, 73
during massage assessment process, 260-261
in massage therapy, 82
Conflict
causes of, 75-76, 79
climate, 78
common skills during, 78-79
dealing with, 77-78
mediating, 75-76
types of, 76-77
Confounding variables, 33
Confusion
with Alzheimer's disease, 548
Congestive heart failure
illustration of signs of, 131f
related to chronic inflammation, 125t
symptoms of, 132
Connective tissue
and aging process, 538
focused massage applications for, 340, 341f, 342-344
general massage protocols for
abdomen, 387f, 396, 398-400
anterior torso, 387f, 396, 398-400
approach and sequence, 382, 383f
arms, 409, 410f, 411-414
face and head, 382-388
forearms, wrists and hands, 414-416
hips, 416, 417f, 418-421
legs, ankles and feet, 426, 427f, 428
neck, 392, 393f, 394-396
occipital base, 388-392
posterior torso, 400-405
shoulders, 405-409
thighs, 421, 422f, 423-426
methods of massage, 316-317
properties of, 180f
types and descriptions of, 179-181
Contact relax, 227, 229f
Contact-relax-antagonist-contract method
massage application technique, 228, 230f
Contractures
with cerebral palsy (CP), 639-640
Contraindications
definition of, 126
for lymphatic drainage, 322, 335
massage
acute local soft tissue inflammation, 128
avoidance or alteration, 128
bleeding disorders, 131
bone and joint injuries, 128
cardiac disease, 131-132
deep vein thrombosis (DVT), 128-129
defining *versus* cautions, 126-128
diabetes, 129, 130f
endangerment sites, 132
infections, 129
kidney disease, 131, 630-631, 661-664
medical devices, 132-133, 134f, 135
myositis ossificans, 129-130
open wounds, 130
pressure and intensity levels, 135-138
tumors, 130-131
varicose veins, 131
regional *versus* general, 1216-127
Control, 105
Control groups, 42-43
Contusions
assessing during examination, 265
brain, 636-637
clinical reasoning process, 656-657, 659-660
fluid drainage around, 326
Conventional healthcare, 7
Coping
with aging process, 538
and commitment, control and challenge, 105
with illness or injury, 92-94
with stress, 89-90
Cordotomy, 489
Core
of body, 187
stabilization, 241f-244f
Coronary artery bypass graft (CABG) surgery, 742-749
Coronary heart diseases
case study on, 742-753
Corporation, 71
Corticosteroids, 528
Cortisol
and stress, 155
Council on Chiropractic Education (CCE), 66
Counseling, 69
Counterirritants
for pain relief, 491-492
Counterirritation, 157, 484, 491, 624
Counterpressure, 226
technique of, 240, 241f-242f
Cranial nerves
anatomy and physiology of, 147-148
Crawford, Cindy C., 157-159
Crisis intervention, 564-565
Critical incident
with trauma, 563-564
Critical stress levels, 89
Crohn's disease, 510b
Cross-directional tissue stretching, 236-237, 238f
Cryosurgery, 517b
Cultures
CAM approaches based on, 7-8
Curettage, 517b
Cytokines, 497

D

Dao yin, 358
Data
conflicts, 776
quality, 81

Death; *See also* end-of-life care
 and dignity, 6
 and hospice care, 585-586
 process of, 583-584
 signs of approaching, 588
 stages of, 584-585
Debridement, 517b
Decision-making
 ethical, 6
Deconditioning, 99
Deductive approach, 25, 26f
Deep breathing, 91
Deep fascia
 palpation of, 302
Deep heat therapies, 529
Deep lateral hip rotators
 specific release techniques, 373-374
Deep pain, 488
Deep second-degree burns, 499
Deep somatic tissues, 180
Deep tissue massage
 confusion concerning term, 344
Deep transverse friction, 218f, 221-222
Deep vein thrombosis, 299
Defensive measures, 89
Deformation
 defining, 461
Degenerative diseases
 chronic pain with, 486
Degenerative joint disease
 description of, 183
 illustration of, 184f
Dehydration
 causes of, 161, 162
 and headaches, 623
 in older adults, 555
 physical effects of, 162, 163f
Delayed onset muscle soreness (DOMS), 326
Delirium
 definition of, 546-547
 and dementia
  benefits of massage for, 549, 566-567
Demands
 component of wellness, 94-95
Dementia
 definition of, 546-547
 and delirium
  benefits of massage for, 549, 566-567
Dendrites, 500
Denial
 during grieving process, 588-590
 with illness or injury, 92-94
 stage of death and dying, 584
 and stress, 89
Dentistry
 occupational definition
  and scope of practice of, 13b
Dentists, 59
Dependency anxiety, 558
Dependent variables, 32
Depression
 with Alzheimer's disease, 548-549
 benefits of massage for, 121-122
 and brain chemistry, 559
 definition of, 122
 and diabetes mellitus
  case study on, 705-713
 major, 561
 in older adults
  benefits of massage for, 449, 554
 postpartum, 582-583
 stage of death and dying, 584-585
 statistics and symptoms of, 560
Depth of pressure
 illustration of, 212f
 massage guidelines for, 210
Dermatitis herpetiformis, 510b
Developmental system
 harmful unrelieved pain effects, 493t
Diabetes mellitus
 complications of, 130f
 and depression
  case study on, 705-713
 insulin injection sites, 130f
 and kidney disease, 630-631
 type 1
  as autoimmune disorder, 504
  massage strategies for, 506-507
Diagnosis
 admitting
  body system review, 255
  history of, 254-255
  during massage assessment process, 254-256
  physical examination, 255-256
 cancer, 627-628
 in case studies, 680
 of kidney disease, 630-632
 and pain, 486
Diagnostic and Statistical Manual of Mental Disorders (DSM-IV), 555
Diaphragm
 and breathing mechanics, 169-170, 171f-173f, 174-175
 general protocol for, 400
 illustration of, 369f
 specific release techniques, 368-369
Diastolic pressure
 definition of, 165-166
Diencephalon, 635
Diet
 and aging, 537-538
 basics of balanced, 95-96
 massage complementing, 531
Diffusion
 and oxygen/ carbon dioxide transport, 170
 principle of, 435
 water loss from, 160t
Digestive system
 and geriatric massage, 543
 surgery, 517b
 sympathetic and parasympathetic response, 154t
Direct manipulation
 massage application technique, 229-231, 232f
Direct techniques, 316-317
Direct trauma, 461
Direction
 illustration of, 212f-213f
 massage guidelines for, 210
Disabilities
 versus handicaps, 454
 physical
  definitions concerning, 574-575
  visual, hearing and speech, 575-576
Discharge summary
 documentation for, 257
Discussion sections
 of research articles, 47, 49b
Diseases; *See also* illnesses
 chronic, 467-468
 classifying massage application by, 451
 definition of, 198
 and geriatric massage, 538
 long-term debilitating, 468
 and posture, 266-267
 related to chronic inflammation, 125t
 and sanitation, 198
 treated by physical medicine, 529
Disks
 herniated, 597, 598f
  description and illustration of, 645, 646f
Disposable gloves; *See* gloves
Dissociative disorders, 557b
Distraction
 for pain relief, 491-492
Diversity
 in clinical settings, 7, 8f
Doctors of chiropractic (DCs)
 description of, 58
 history of, 8-9

Doctors of naturopathy (NDs)
description of, 59
history and philosophies of, 8-9, 65-66
Doctors of osteopathy (DOs)
description of, 58
history of, 8-9
Doctors of physical therapy (DPTs), 60-61
Documentation
case studies illustrating, 680-681
common styles of, 257-259
by complementary medicine practitioners
in professional practice model, 12b
computerized, 82
definition of, 256
discharge summary, 257
flow charts, 257
importance of, 80-82, 256
problem-oriented, 257-258
progress notes, 258
rules for completing, 256-259
technologic advances, 258-259
Dopamine, 146, 523
Double-blind research procedures, 45
Drag
definition of massage, 135
illustration of, 212f-213f
massage guidelines for, 137t, 210
and pain management, 494
scales for, 137
Dreaming, 102
Drug abuse
and addiction, 104-105, 521, 722-723
massage for withdrawal, 556
Drug addiction
case study on, 722-723
Drug therapy
and massage
interaction of, 526b-527b
Drugs
addiction to, 104-105, 521, 722-723
allergies, 523-524
information for massage therapists, 524-525
and massage, 526b-527b
versus medications, 520
routes of administration, 524
Duration
of exercise, 99-100
guidelines for massage, 137t, 211
of inflammation, 494-495
of massage, 135, 137t
Dying;*See also* end-of-life care
and hospice care, 585-586
process of, 583-584
stages of, 584-585

E

Earlier trauma, 461
Ears
assessment of, 255
infections
chronic pain with, 486
observation and palpation of, 272, 273f-274f
Eating disorders, 557b, 561-562
Eccentric actions
of muscles, 185
Edema
assessment of pitting, 300f
causes of, 320-321
and fibromyalgia, 610
and fluid dynamics, 320-321
and interstitial fluid, 162, 164f
reduction
for pain relief, 493
relief as primary benefit of massage, 15, 338, 339f, 340
Education
by complementary medicine practitioners
in professional practice model, 12b
for massage therapists, 11, 13b, 14
Effect size, 37
Elasticity
of soft tissue, 177
Elbows
observation and palpation of, 272, 273f-274f
Elderly;*See* geriatric population; older adults
Elective surgery, 517b
Electrocorticography, 638
Electrolytes
description of, 160
Electromagnetic currents
travel pattern of, 158f
Electronic health records (EHRs), 82, 258-259
Electronic patient records (EPRs), 258-259
Electronic record-keeping systems, 82, 258-259
Electrosurgery, 517b
Emotional health
defining, 103-104
with injuries and illness, 457-458, 458b-459b
and psychogenic pain, 485
trauma, 460-461
Emotional states
anatomy, physiology and massage, 153, 155-156
benefits of massage for, 153, 155-156
Emotions
defining, 103-104
Empty end-feel, 276
End stage renal failure
contraindications of massage for, 126, 661-664
description and causes of, 630-631
Endangerment sites
diagram illustrating nervous system, 133f
for massage, 132
End-feel
types of, 276
Endocrine system
and fibromyalgia, 610
harmful unrelieved pain effects, 493t
massage effect on, 144-145
surgery, 517b
as target for autoimmune diseases, 510b
therapeutic exercise benefiting, 529t
End-of-life care
anorexia, 587
challenge of massage with, 583
elimination/ constipation, 587
massage during, 590
mouth care, 587
pain management, 586-587
psychiatric health, 587-588
Endorphins
and pain relief, 492-493
Endotoxin, 498
Endurance, 99, 528
Energy medicine
electromagnetic currents, 158f
summary of, 158-159
Energy systems
anatomy, physiology and massage, 157-159
description and illustration of, 157-159, 158f
therapies, 9
Enkephalins, 156
Entrainment
anatomy, physiology and massage, 156
and cardiovascular system, 163
definition of, 156
Entrapment
spinal cord, 634
Environmental protection
OSHA on safety and, 203, 205
Epidural steroid injections, 528
Epilepsy, 637-639
Epinephrine, 147
Epithelial tissue
anatomy, physiology and massage, 148-150
Essential oils
examples and uses of, 438t, 624
principles and benefits of, 435, 437, 438t, 439
Ethical considerations
in research, 39-41

Ethical dilemma, 72-73
Ethical distress, 72-73
Ethics
  definition of, 72
  and massage therapy, 6
Etiquette, 72-73
Evaluations
  in case studies, 680
  of pain, 486, 488
  in research, 24-25
Evidence-based research
  of massage effectiveness, 12b
Exercise
  and aging, 537-538
  for back pain, 602
  and cardiovascular health, 608
  component of wellness, 97, 99-101
  developing a program, 101
  diseases benefiting from, 529t
  injuries, 455
  lack of
    and edema, 320-321
  regimens, 529t, 530
  for strengthening back, 601
  therapeutic, 528, 529t, 530
Experimental validity, 37-38
Expiration
  and breathing retraining, 480-481
  description and phases of, 97
  illustration of, 171f, 173f
  mechanism of, 98f
Expiratory reserve volume, 170
External control, 105
External respiration
  definition of, 169
External validity, 38
Extracellular fluids
  versus intracellular
    and fluid dynamics, 317
Extracorporeal circulation, 517b
Extraneous variables, 32-33
Extremities
  physical examination of, 256
Eyes
  assessment of, 255
  movement during muscle energy massage, 226, 228f
  observation and palpation of, 272, 273f-274f
  sympathetic and parasympathetic response, 154t
  vision changes in older adults, 549-550

F
Face
  general massage protocols, 382-388
  important structures of, 384f
  palliative protocol for, 428
Factitious disorders, 557b
Factors
  definition and example of, 24-25
Faith, 106
Family history
  assessment of, 254-255
Fascia
  description and illustration of, 179-180
  general massage protocols for
    abdomen, 387f, 396, 398-400
    anterior torso, 387f, 396, 398-400
    approach and sequence, 382, 383f
    arms, 409, 410f, 411-414
    face and head, 382-388
    forearms, wrists and hands, 414-416
    hips, 416, 417f, 418-421
    legs, ankles and feet, 426, 427f, 428
    neck, 392, 393f, 394-396
    occipital base, 388-392
    posterior torso, 400-405
    shoulders, 405-409
    thighs, 421, 422f, 423-426
Fascial sheaths
  palpation of, 302
Fascicles
  of muscles, 184
Fatigue
  as chemotherapy side effect, 629-630
  chronic syndrome, 612-613
  with depression or anxiety, 561
  injuries due to, 455
  reduction
    as primary benefit of massage, 15
Fatigue syndromes
  benefits of massage for, 126, 612-613
Feelings
  defining in wellness terms, 104
Feet
  general massage protocols, 426, 427f, 428
  important structures of, 427f
  methods of massage for, 354-355
  observation and palpation of, 272, 273f-274f
  palliative protocol for, 430
  reflexology, 352-354, 354f
  symmetry and posture, 267f, 268-269
Femoral joints, 416, 417f, 418-421
Fetus
  in utero, 580f
Fibrin, 168
Fibromyalgia
  chronic pain with, 486
  massage for, 612
  and myofascial pain, 487b
  related to chronic inflammation, 125t
  risk factors and symptoms of, 610-611
  treatment of, 611-612
Fibrosis
  definition of, 178
  of joint capsule, 181
  process of, 503
  related to chronic inflammation, 125t
Fibrous joint capsule, 181
Fight-or-flight, 474, 476
Fingers
  observation and palpation of, 272, 273f-274f
Firing patterns
  assessing during examination, 265
Fitness
  definition of, 97
  maintaining, 100
Flat back posture, 267f
Flexibility
  and aging process, 538
  massage to improve, 97, 530-532
Flexor muscles
  and postural dysfunction, 269, 270f-271f
Flora, 199
Flow charts
  documentation using, 257
Fluid dynamics
  and edema, 320-321
  focused massage applications for, 317-318
  and hydrostatic pressure, 317
  and inflammation, 318
  intra *versus* extracellular, 317
  and joint swelling, 338, 339f, 340
  lymphatic drainage, 322-323, 324f
  and the lymphatic system, 318-320
  principles of, 159-162
Fluids
  balance of, 161
  body, 159-162
    and edema, 320-321
    focused massage applications for, 317-318
    and hydrostatic pressure, 317
    and inflammation, 318
    intra *versus* extracellular, 317
    lymphatic drainage, 322-323, 324f
    and the lymphatic system, 318-320
  general massage protocols for
    abdomen, 387f, 396, 398-400
    anterior torso, 387f, 396, 398-400
    approach and sequence, 382, 383f

Fluids *(Continued)*
arms, 409, 410f, 411-414
face and head, 382-388
forearms, wrists and hands, 414-416
hips, 416, 417f, 418-421
legs, ankles and feet, 426, 427f, 428
neck, 392, 393f, 394-396
occipital base, 388-392
posterior torso, 400-405
shoulders, 405-409
thighs, 421, 422f, 423-426
hydrostatic pressure of
and flow, 166-167
imbalance benefited by massage, 15
targeting massage to move body, 326-327
viscosity, 167
Focused massage applications
and fluid dynamics, 317-318
Fomites, 199-200
Force couples
definition of, 187
illustration of, 189f
Force stability
definition of, 182-183
Forces
couples, 187
defining, 461
mechanical, 211-214
bending, shear, and rotational loading, 214
compression loading, 213-214
definition of massage, 209-210
illustration of different, 215f-218f
massage application techniques, 211, 213-214
structural effects, 211
tension loading, 211, 213
types of, 211, 213-214
Forearms
general massage protocols, 414-416
illustration of, 415f
Form stability
definition of, 182-183
Forward-tilting pelvis
description of, 456-457
Fractures
and osteoporosis, 545f
stress, 597
types of, 648f-650f
Fragile
awareness of older adults being, 541f
definition of, 6
Free radicals, 498, 523
Frequency
of exercise, 100
massage guidelines for, 211
Friction
deep transverse, 218f, 221-222
description and techniques, 221-222
illustration of, 218f
Frontal plane movement, 187, 188f, 225f, 270f
Full body massage
and breathing, 479
and pain management, 494
protocols for general maintenance
abdomen, 387f, 396, 398-400
anterior torso, 387f, 396, 398-400
approach and sequence, 382, 383f
arms, 409, 410f, 411-414
face and head, 382-388
forearms, wrists and hands, 414-416
hips, 416, 417f, 418-421
legs, ankles and feet, 426, 427f, 428
neck, 392, 393f, 394-396
occipital base, 388-392
posterior torso, 400-405
shoulders, 405-409
thighs, 421, 422f, 423-426
sequence and body areas, 382, 383f
Full body pronation, 188-189
Functional assessment
definition of, 250
of movement, 274-275
Functional movement patterns
biomechanics of, 188-193
and muscles, 187, 188f
Functional strength, 189
Functional techniques
focused massage applications for, 316-317
Fungal infections
massage contraindicated for, 129
Fungi
transmission of, 199

G

Gait
assessing
during massage assessment process, 283, 290, 291f-293f, 293
during physical examination, 265
biomechanics of, 189
and kinetic chain, 282
muscle testing as intervention tool, 297b
optimum, 290
and thigh massage, 421
Galea aponeurotica, 387
Gallbladder
meridians relating to, 356f, 357b
Gastrointestinal system
assessment of, 255
breathing pattern disorder signs in, 476
and fibromyalgia, 610
and geriatric massage, 543
harmful unrelieved pain effects, 493t
as target for autoimmune diseases, 510b
Gastrointestinal tract
water loss from, 160t
Gate control theory
anatomy, physiology and massage, 156-157
and pain management, 494
Gender, 557b
General adaptation syndrome, 89
General constitutional application, 118
General protocols
photographs illustrating massage protocols, 759-781
Generalized anxiety disorder, 557-558
Genetics
and autoimmune disorders, 504-505
and fibromyalgia, 610
Genitals
physical examination of, 256
Genitourinary system
harmful unrelieved pain effects, 493t
Geriatric population
and aging process, 537-539
cardiovascular conditions, 542-543
digestive/ gastrointestinal conditions, 543
and disease risks, 538
examples of interaction with, 539f-541f
exercise regimens benefiting, 529t
goals of massage for, 538-539
hearing conditions, 542t, 550-551
illness and injury in, 455
integumentary system, 543-544
interactions with, 539f-541f
massage therapist understanding of, 537-538
and mental health, 555
musculoskeletal system, 542t, 544
nervous system, 542t, 546-549
and nutrition, 551
osteoporosis, 545, 546b
physical changes with aging, 542t
pulmonary conditions, 542t, 549
reproductive conditions, 542t, 552-553
similarities in, 537-538, 539f-541f, 542-555
sleep disorders, 553
specific massage techniques for, 554-555
support systems for, 553
urinary conditions, 542f, 551-552
vision conditions, 542t, 549-550

Glaucoma
  description of, 550
Gliding
  definition of massage, 135
  fundamentals of, 241f-242f
  strokes
    description and illustration of, 216, 217f
Global muscles
  definition of, 187
Gloves
  CDC guidelines for, 203
  proper removal of disposable, 203, 204f
Gluteus maximus
  general protocol for, 416, 417f, 418-421
Glycemic demand, 96
Goals
  short and long-term, 253-254
Golgi tendon organs, 148, 150, 216, 217f, 230-231
Governor vessel meridians, 356f, 357b
Grand mal seizures, 638
Graves disease, 509-510, 510b
Gravity
  and body balance, 280-282
  center of massage therapist's, 240, 241f-244f
  increasing venous flow, 165, 169
  and posture, 268-269
Gray matter, 145
Grief
  physical symptoms of, 589, 590b
  process of, 588-590
Groin muscles
  specific release techniques, 373-374
Group-specific research
  or single-case focus, 44
Growth hormones, 147
Guarding
  contractions, 186
  definition of, 181
Guided imagery, 91
Guillain-Barre syndrome
  massage strategies for, 507
Guilt
  during grieving process, 588-590
Gynecology
  exercise regimens benefiting, 529t

H

Habits
  and posture, 266-267
  types of, 266
Hair
  assessment of, 299
  and head massage, 386-388
  loss
    as chemotherapy side effect, 629-630
Hamstrings
  specific release techniques, 363, 364f-365f
  symmetry and posture, 267f, 268
Hand washing
  importance of, 201
  technique for, 202f, 203
Handicaps
  versus disabilities, 454
Hands
  general massage protocols, 414-416
  illustration of, 415f
  palliative protocol for, 429
Hardiness
  definition of, 468
Harm
  versus hurt, 454
Hashimoto's thyroiditis, 509-510, 510b
Head
  assessment of, 255
  general massage protocols, 382-388
  important structures of, 384f
  observation and palpation of, 272, 273f-274f
Head *(Continued)*
  occipital base, 388-392
  palliative protocol for, 428
Headache-free migraines, 621
Headaches
  clinical reasoning process, 613
    migraines, 613, 620-621
    tension, 613, 622-624
    vascular, 613, 620-623
  and fibromyalgia, 610
  illustration of massage for, 614f-617f
  massage strategies for, 623-624
  possible causes of, 621-623
  self-help for, 624
Healing
  and complementary medicine, 7
  definition of, 6
  goals of massage in phases of, 505b
  and intention, 157-159
  massage approaches during, 462b
  massage during surgical stages of, 518-520
  regeneration and remodeling, 501
  and rehabilitation process
    three phases of, 93
  stages of, 504t
    and massage interventions, 119t
  stages of pain during, 276-277
  straining restorative mechanism, 118
  time, 463-464
Healing process
  following trauma, 461
  and inflammation, 505b
Health
  influences on, 460f
Health and safety
  by complementary medicine practitioners
    in professional practice model, 12b
Health insurance
  billing and coding guidelines, 79b
  covering massage, 83
  reimbursement of massage therapy, 5
Health Insurance Portability and Accountability Act (HIPAA)
  components of, 73b
  and confidentiality, 260-261
Healthcare
  assessment of
    admitting diagnosis, 254-256
    body system review, 255
    physical examination, 255-256
  hierarchy, 50
  illustration of work in, 5f
  and massage, 3-17
  population similarities in
    athletes, 536-537
    geriatrics, 537-538, 539f-541f, 542-555
    hearing impairment, 575-576
    mental health, 555-567
    mobility impairment, 576
    pediatrics, 567, 568f-570f, 571-574
    physical disabilities, 574-577
    pregnancy, 577, 578f-579f, 580-583
    terminal illness/ end-of-life care, 583-591
    visual impairment, 575
Healthcare environments
  business structures in, 69-70
  integrating massage into, 56, 61-72
  licensed or certified professionals, 60-61
  massage therapists getting jobs in, 82-84
  settings for massage therapists, 69-70
  types of professions in, 56, 58-61
Healthcare professionals
  appearance and attitude
    when greeting a client, 74f
  licensing and certification, 60-61
  occupational definitions
    and scope of practice for, 13b-14b
  types of doctorates in, 58-60
Healthy behavior
  example of, 15f

Hearing impairment
and geriatric massage, 550-551
interacting with patients with, 575
population similarities in, 575-576
Heart
meridians relating to, 356f, 357b
percentage of water in, 160t
physical examination of, 256
sympathetic and parasympathetic response, 154t
Heart attack
causes of, 168-169
early warning signs of, 609f
and inflammation, 500
related to chronic inflammation, 125t
Heart disease
and edema, 321
and inflammation, 500
Heart failure
massage contraindicated for, 131
Heart rate
definition of, 166
Heat therapy
hydrotherapy using, 435, 436b
for pain, 490
Heels
symmetry and posture, 267f, 268-269
HEENT
assessment of, 255-256
Hematologic disorders
massage strategies for, 507
Hematopoiesis, 168
Hemiparesis, 636
Hemorrhagic stroke, 635-636
Hepatitis C
case study on, 713-714
Herbs, 96, 175, 520, 521, 523
Heredity
and aging process, 538
and osteoporosis, 545f
and posture, 266-267
Herniated disks, 597, 598f
description and illustration of, 645, 646f
High velocity, low amplitude (HVLA) thrusts, 67
Hip abduction, 286b
Hip extension, 285b
Hippocampus, 145
Hips
general massage protocols, 416, 417f, 418-421
illustration of, 377f, 417f
observation and palpation of, 272, 273f-274f
overuse problems with, 269, 272
palliative protocol for, 429-430
specific release techniques, 374-375, 376f, 377f, 378
symmetry and posture, 267f, 268
Homeopathic medicine, 68, 439-440
Homeostasis
definition of, 64, 117
supported by nervous system, 153
Homeostatic balance
body signals, 117
Hope, 106
Hormonal therapy
for cancer, 630
Hormones
and osteoporosis, 545f
and pain, 492-493
and stress, 89
Hospice care
and comfort of massage, 585-586
massage during, 590
Host
infection transmission from, 199-200
Human body; *See* body
Human immunodeficiency virus (HIV), 9
Humoral immunity, 200
Hurt
versus harm, 454
Hydrokinetics, 317-318
Hydrostatic pressure
definition of, 160, 166, 317
and fluid dynamics, 317
and fluid flow, 166-167
illustration of effect of, 167f, 317f
Hydrotherapy
principles and benefits of, 435, 436b
Hymel, Glenn M.
on research, 22-51
Hyperactivity, 559
Hyperkalemia, 632
Hypermobility
and gait, 290
of joints, 272, 274
Hyperpnea, 174
Hyperstimulation analgesia, 157, 484
Hypertension
definition of, 166
Hypnosis
for pain relief, 491-492
Hypomobility
and gait, 290
of joints, 272, 274
Hypothalamus, 144
Hypotheses, 34-35

I

Ice
hydrotherapy using, 435, 436b, 490
Ideal posture, 267f
Iliac crest
observation and palpation of, 272, 273f-274f
Illnesses; *See also* clinical reasoning process
assessing pain of, 262-263
causes of, 462-463
definition of, 454
as homeostatic imbalance, 117-118
overview of
causes *versus* symptoms, 455
chronic, 467
common causes, 455-459, 460f
defining *versus* injuries, 454
the healing process, 461
healing time, 463-464
hurt *versus* harm, 454
massage's role in recovery, 467
prevention of, 455
PRICE therapy, 465
recovery expectations, 463-464
recovery process, 465-467
terminology of, 454
treatment of, 464-465
types of, 461-462
and stress, 92-94
stress warning signs, 93
treatment
drug therapy and massage interaction, 526b-527b
flexibility techniques, 531
massage therapy supporting, 515, 518-520, 531
nutrition, mental health and lifestyle, 531
pharmacology for massage, 520-521, 523-525, 526b-527b
physical medicine, 525, 528-532
surgery, 516-520
and therapeutic exercise, 528, 529t, 530
Imagery
for pain relief, 491
Immune cells
types of, 496-498
Immune complex
description of, 497
Immune response
cellular action during, 496
Immune system
communication, 497
defending against infections, 200
and fibromyalgia, 610
function of, 495
harmful unrelieved pain effects, 493t

Immune system *(Continued)*
and homeostatic balance, 117-118
and inflammation, 495-498
influences on, 460f
natural protective mechanisms, 626f
and stress, 105
Immunizations
Hepatitis B, 205
for infection control, 200
Impingement
of nerves, 151
Impingement syndromes
and soft tissue dysfunction, 125-126
Impulse control disorders, 557b
Incontinence
with Alzheimer's disease, 548
in older adults, 551-552
Independent variables (IVs)
between and within, 43-44
definition and example of, 32
groups or levels, 41-42
Indirect functional techniques
for trigger points, 348
Indirect techniques
of massage, 316
Indirect trauma, 461
Infants
developmental sequence, 572b
illustration of massage for, 568f
and toddlers
massage for, 571-573
Infections
as chemotherapy side effect, 629-630
classification of, 198
clinical reasoning process
bacterial, 625
massage for, 626
parasitic, 625-626
viral, 625
control by complementary medicine practitioners
in professional practice model, 12b
and fibromyalgia, 610
and inflammation, 499
massage contraindicated for, 129, 626
massage for subacute, 626
transmission of
bacteria, 199
fungi, 199
host, 199-200
portals of entry, 200
protozoa, 199
rickettsiae, 199
viruses, 198-199
Inflammation
burns, 499
and cancer, 500-501
and cardiovascular disease, 500
cellular reactions during, 498-499
chronic local, 502
disorders related to, 125t
causing edema, 321
and fluid dynamics, 318
healing process, 505b
the immune system, 495-498
and infections, trauma, burns, 499
inflammatory response, 498-499
massage strategies for, 503-504
nerve disorders, 500
and pain management, 494-495
pathology of, 498-499
phases of, 500-501, 504t
process of, 123, 504t
respiratory disorders, 499-500
trauma, 499
types of, 494-495
Inflammatory bowel disease
massage strategies for, 506
Inflammatory diseases
chronic pain with, 486
Inflammatory mediators
definition of, 498
Inflammatory process
defending against infections, 200
description of, 123, 125
diagram illustrating, 124f
phases of, 123, 504t
Inflammatory reaction, 119t
Inflammatory response
cellular reactions during, 498-499
description and illustration of, 498-499
flow chart illustrating, 124f, 625f
Inflare, 378
Information
guidelines for release of, 260-261
in patient history, 261-262
resources for research, 23-24
Informed consent, 73
Inhibition-prone mover muscles, 190b
Injections
for back pain, 602
for peripheral neuropathy, 640-641
Injuries;*See also* clinical reasoning process
assessing pain of, 262-263
definition of, 454
joint, tendon and ligament, 177-178
overview of
causes *versus* symptoms, 455
chronic, 467
common causes, 455-459, 460f
defining *versus* illnesses, 454
the healing process, 461
healing time, 463-464
hurt *versus* harm, 454
massage's role in recovery, 467
prevention of, 455
PRICE therapy, 465
recovery expectations, 463-464
recovery process, 465-467
terminology of, 454
treatment of, 464-465
types of, 461-462
present, 254
schematic of cycle, 456f
severity and massage, 6
and stress, 92-94
stress warning signs, 93
treated by physical medicine, 529
treatment
drug therapy and massage interaction, 526b-527b
flexibility techniques, 531
massage therapy supporting, 515, 518-520, 531
nutrition, mental health and lifestyle, 531
pharmacology for massage, 520-521, 523-525, 526b-527b
physical medicine, 525, 528-532
surgery, 516-520
and therapeutic exercise, 528, 529t, 530
Injury cycle, 456f
Innate immunity, 495-496
Insomnia
and aging, 537-538, 553
and back pain, 596
benefits of massage for, 15, 123
common causes of, 651b
with fibromyalgia, 610
and stress, 91
treatment of, 650-651
and wellness, 102-103
Inspiration
description and phases of, 97
illustration of, 171f, 173f
mechanism of, 98f
Inspiratory reserve volume, 170
Insurance
of complementary medicine practitioners
in professional practice model, 12b
Intact groups, 41
Integrated medicine
definition of, 9-10

Integrated muscle energy approach
massage application technique, 232-234
Integumentary system
assessment of, 255
and geriatric massage, 543-544
as target for autoimmune diseases, 510b
Intensity
of exercise, 99
seven pressure levels of, 135-138
Intensity levels
using caution with, 135-138
Intention
definitions of, 157-158
Interdisciplinary teams
characteristics of, 72
massage therapists joining, 74
Interest conflicts, 76
Interferon, 198-199, 498
Interleukins, 498
Internal control, 105
Internal derangement end-feel, 276
Internal respiration, 169
Internal response
defining, 461
Internal validity, 37-38
Interspinales muscles, 363, 364, 366f
Interstitial fluid
assessing volume of, 335-336
and edema, 162, 164f
increase with edema, 320-321
Intertransversarii muscles, 363, 364, 366f
Intervening variables, 33-34
Intestines
percentage of water in, 160t
Intracellular fluids
versus extracellular
and fluid dynamics, 317
Intrafusal fibers, 149-150
Intraoperative period, 517b
Introductory sections
of research articles, 45, 49b
Involuntary muscle contractions, 186
Irritation, 157
Ischemic stroke, 635-636
Isolation
stage of death and dying, 584
Isometric actions
of muscles, 185
Isometric contractions
description of, 226
Isometric exercises, 528
Isotonic contractions
description of, 226
Isotonic exercises, 528
Isotonic movements
description of, 226

J

Joint arthrokinematics, 189
Joint capsule
definition of, 181
and injuries, 178
Joint movements
benefits and methods of, 222-225
massage application techniques, 222-225
and pain relief, 485
Joint play
definition of, 350
focused massage applications for, 222-225, 350, 352
illustration of, 353f
and joint arthrokinetics, 189
Joint receptors
four types of, 181
Joints
assessment, 275-276
and back pain, 596-607
close-packed positions of, 184t
and collagen, 177-178
degeneration, 183-184
Joints *(Continued)*
edema at, 338, 339f, 340
end-feel, 276
flexibility, 97, 530-532
general massage protocols for
abdomen, 387f, 396, 398-400
anterior torso, 387f, 396, 398-400
approach and sequence, 382, 383f
arms, 409, 410f, 411-414
face and head, 382-388
forearms, wrists and hands, 414-416
hips, 416, 417f, 418-421
legs, ankles and feet, 426, 427f, 428
neck, 392, 393f, 394-396
occipital base, 388-392
posterior torso, 400-405
shoulders, 405-409
thighs, 421, 422f, 423-426
hypermobility and hypomobility, 272, 274, 290
least-packed positions of, 183t, 353t
massage application techniques on, 182
mobilization goals, 183-184
mobilization with movement (MWM), 350, 353f
movement
guidelines for, 224-225
patterns, 272, 274-276
in pronation and supination, 189b
types of, 222-225
overuse problems with, 269, 272
palpation of, 303
stability, 182-183, 238f
stacking of, 239-240, 241f-244f
structure and function, 181-182
Jonas, Wayne B., 157-159
Justification
definition of, 251

K

Ketogenic diet, 638-639
Kidney disease
chronic renal failure, 632, 661-664
clinical reasoning process, 630-632, 661-664
diagnosis, symptoms and treatment, 630-632
and edema, 321
massage contraindicated for, 131, 632, 663-664
treatment of, 632-633
Kidney failure
related to chronic inflammation, 125t
Kidneys
changes in older adults, 551-552
chronic renal failure, 632, 661-664
end stage renal failure
contraindications of massage for, 126, 630-631, 661-664
as endangerment site for massage, 132, 133f
meridians relating to, 356f, 357b
percentage of water in, 160t
sympathetic and parasympathetic response, 154t
water loss from, 160t
Kinetic chain
analysis
during massage assessment process, 272-273, 294-295, 296b-297b
components of, 186f
defining, 272, 274
dysfunction, 190-191, 192f
functions of, 186-187
and gait, 282
protocol testing, 296b-297b
serial distortion pattern, 191, 191f-192f, 193
Kneading
body mechanics of, 242f-243f
description and illustration of, 217f, 218
Knee extension, 288b
Knee flexion, 287b
Knee joints
arthroscopic surgery, 517-518
Knee replacement
case study on, 720, 723-729
Kneeling, 242f

Knees
  illustration of, 422f
  location of injuries to, 650f
  observation and palpation of, 272, 273f-274f
  overuse problems with, 269, 272
  symmetry and posture, 267f, 268
Kübler-Ross, Elisabeth, 584
Kypholordotic posture, 267f

L
Lacerations, 655-656
Laparoscope, 516
Laparoscopic surgery, 516
Large intestine
  meridians relating to, 356f, 357b
Laser surgery, 517b
Latent infections, 198
Latissimus dorsi
  shortening with breathing pattern disorders, 478-479
Laughter, 91
Learning disorders, 559
Leathery end-feel, 276
Legs
  general massage protocols, 426, 427f, 428
  important structures of, 427f
  observation and palpation of, 272, 273f-274f
  palliative protocol for, 430
Length-tension relationship
  definition of, 186
Leukotriene inhibitors, 500
Levator scapulae
  shortening with breathing pattern disorders, 478-479
Levels of significance, 36-37
License
  of complementary medicine practitioners
    in professional practice model, 12b
Licensed practical nurses (LPNs), 60
Lifestyle
  adjustments for stress, 91
  and aging, 537-538
  and back pain, 596
  and fibromyalgia, 610
  increasing injury/illness risks, 457
  massage complementing, 531
  and osteoporosis, 545f
Ligaments
  and back pain, 596-607
  description of, 143
  injuries to, 177-178
Ligand-gated channel
  definition of, 146
Limbic system, 144
Lipopolysaccharide (LPS), 498
Literature reviews, 45-46
Liver
  cirrhosis of, 633, 634f
  meridians relating to, 356f, 357b
  percentage of water in, 160t
  sympathetic and parasympathetic response, 154t
Liver disease
  clinical reasoning process, 632-634
  description and causes of, 632-633
  massage for, 633-634
  types of, 633
Load
  definition of, 461
Local muscles
  definition of, 187
Localized pain, 486
Long-term care facilities
  massage therapy in, 70
Long-term goals
  for massage therapists, 253-254
Loss
  component of wellness, 95
Love, 106
Low back
  causes of pain in, 485-486
  photographs illustrating massage protocols, 786-791
Lower crossed syndrome
  flowchart of, 192f
Lumbar lordosis
  description of, 456-457
Lumbar plexus
  description and illustration of, 152
Lumbar spine
  and back pain, 604-605
  and posture and gravity, 267f, 268
Lung volumes, 170
Lungs
  meridians relating to, 356f, 357b
  percentage of water in, 160t
  water loss from, 160t
Lupus
  as autoimmune disorder, 504, 509, 510b
  and pregnancy
    case study on, 693-705
  related to chronic inflammation, 125t
Lyme disease, 199
Lymph
  circulation of, 318-320
  facilitating flow of, 319f
Lymph nodes
  definition of, 318, 319f
  palpation of, 300-301
Lymphadenopathy
  definition of, 123
Lymphangitis
  massage contraindicated for, 129
Lymphatic drainage
  contraindications and cautions concerning, 322, 335
  and fluid dynamics, 322-323, 324f
  focused massage applications for, 329-330, 331f-334f, 335-338, 339f, 340
  general massage protocols for
    abdomen, 387f, 396, 398-400
    anterior torso, 387f, 396, 398-400
    approach and sequence, 382, 383f
    arms, 409, 410f, 411-414
    face and head, 382-388
    forearms, wrists and hands, 414-416
    hips, 416, 417f, 418-421
    legs, ankles and feet, 426, 427f, 428
    neck, 392, 393f, 394-396
    occipital base, 388-392
    posterior torso, 400-405
    shoulders, 405-409
    thighs, 421, 422f, 423-426
  at joints, 338, 339f
  massage
    benefits of, 322
    principles and indications for, 322-323
  for pain relief, 493
  procedure for, 331f-334f, 336-338
Lymphatic system
  diagrams illustrating, 318f-320f
  and fluid dynamics, 318-320
  focused massage applications for, 318-323, 324f
  organs of
    illustration of, 318f
Lymphedema, 321
  illustration of, 164f

M
Macrophages, 200, 496-498
Macular degeneration
  description of, 550
Magnetic therapy
  north and south poles in, 441b
  principles and benefits of, 440-442
Major histocompatibility complex (MHC), 496
Major surgery, 516
Manipulated independent variables, 32
Manipulation
  and body-based methods, 9
  in chiropractic, 59
  definition of, 67

Massage; *See also* massage applications; massage protocols
anatomy and physiology role in, 142-144
application movements, 143-144
application on cardiovascular system, 165, 169
assessment process
admitting diagnosis, 254-256
analysis of, 311-312
clinical reasoning process, 251-252
confidentiality, 260-261
of gait, 283, 290, 291f-293f, 293
introduction to, 250-251
kinetic chain analysis, 272-273, 280-282, 294-295, 296b-297b
massage-specific, 261-306
medical records, 256-260
muscle firing patterns, 282-283, 284b-289b
muscle-strength testing, 278-280
musculoskeletal conditions, 261
outcome goals, 252
palpation, 295-306
physician's treatment orders, 252-253
resourceful compensation, 308
sacroiliac joint function, 293-294
short-term and long-term goals, 253-254
summary of, 310-312
treatment orders, 252-253
treatment plan development, 309-312
understanding findings of, 306, 308
and autoimmune diseases
causes of, 504-505
medical treatment of, 505-506
strategies for, 510-511
types of, 506-510
for behavior modification, 104-105
benefits of
for addictions, 556
for adolescents, 573
for Alzheimer's disease, 549, 566-567
for anxiety, 121-122, 556-557
for cardiovascular system, 163-165, 169
for children, 569f-570f, 573
chronic illnesses, 119-121
for condition management, 120
for delirium and dementia, 549, 566-567
for dementia and delirium, 549, 566-567
for depression, 121-122, 560-561
for depression in older adults, 449, 554
for emotional conditions, 153, 155-156
for fatigue syndromes, 126, 612-613
for insomnia, 15, 123
for joint movements, 222-225
for lymphatic drainage, 322
for mental health, 122, 555-556
for mood management, 121-122
for pain, 126
for palliative care, 120-121
for pleasure and relaxation, 121
posttraumatic stress disorder, 562-565
for psychiatric disorders, 556-560
for relaxation, 121
for sleep, 123
for stages of tissue healing, 119t
for stress, 121-122
for treatment goals, 118-121
for venous system, 164-165
for breathing pattern disorders
assessment of, 477-478
breathing retraining, 480-481, 482f
definition of, 474
health conditions related to, 483b
interventions, 477b, 478-480
physical changes with, 476, 477b
signs and symptoms of, 476
specific massage strategies, 478-480
and client best practice, 56-57
contraindications
acute local soft tissue inflammation, 128
avoidance or alteration, 128
bleeding disorders, 131
bone and joint injuries, 128

Massage *(Continued)*
cardiac disease, 131-132
deep vein thrombosis (DVT), 128-129
defining *versus* cautions, 126-128
diabetes, 129, 130f
end stage renal failure, 126, 630-631, 661-664
endangerment sites, 132
infections, 129
kidney disease, 131
medical devices, 132-133, 134f, 135
myositis ossificans, 129-130
open wounds, 130
pressure and intensity levels, 135-138
tumors, 130-131
varicose veins, 131
definition of, 3-5
effectiveness of, 11, 12b
focused application of
Asian massage concepts, 355-356, 357b, 358-359
circulatory system, 318-323, 324f
connective tissue, 340, 341f, 342-344
fluid dynamics, 317-318
functional techniques, 316-317
increasing arterial circulation, 327-329
joint play, 350, 352
lymphatic drainage, 329-330, 331f-334f, 335-338, 339f, 340
lymphatic system, 318-323, 324f
motor tone inhibition techniques, 360-363, 364f, 365-375, 376f-377f, 378
pin and stretch, 343-344
reflexology, 352-355
specific release methods, 360-363, 364f, 365-375, 376f-377f, 378
targeting fluid movement, 326-327
tissue movement methods, 343-350, 351f-352f
trigger points, 344-350, 351f-352f
venous return, 329
in hospice setting, 590
illustration of strokes and compression, 215f-218f
indications for
anxiety, depression and mood, 121-122
impingement disorders, 125-126
inflammation management, 122, 124f, 125
mental health disorders, 122
pain and fatigue syndrome, 126
posttraumatic stress disorder, 121-122
relaxation and pleasure, 121
soft tissue dysfunction, 125-126
stress-related disorders, 121-123
and inflammation
and cancer, 500-501
and cardiovascular disease, 500
chronic local, 502
healing process, 505b
the immune system, 495-498
and infections, trauma, burns, 499
inflammatory response, 498-499
massage strategies for, 503-504
nerve disorders, 500
phases of, 500-501, 504t
respiratory disorders, 499-500
types of, 494-495
insurance coverage of, 5
integration into conventional healthcare, 11, 14
methods of
and forces, 214, 215f, 216, 217f, 218-222
model of practice, 11, 12b
outcomes and goals of, 118-121
and pain
acute *versus* chronic, 485-486
assessment factors, 492t
definitions associated with, 481, 483
diagnosis of, 486
evaluation of, 486, 488
medical treatment for, 488-492
medications, 488-492
messages, 483-485
sensations of, 485
strategies for, 492-494

Massage *(Continued)*
three major components of, 484-485
unrelieved effects, 493t
for pain management, 93-94
palpation techniques (*See* palpation)
physiological benefits of, 154t, 155-156
primary benefits of, 15
and relaxation therapy, 91-92
research literature example, 30-39, 40f
role in recovery process, 467
sanitation in
and blood-borne pathogen standards, 200-206
and diseases, 198
and environmental protection guidelines, 203, 205
hand washing, 201, 202f, 203
hepatitis B vaccinations, 205
housekeeping controls, 205
importance in massage therapy, 197
and infection transmission, 198-200
OSHA mission, 200
postexposure follow-up, 205-206
on short tight muscles, 282f
stages of healing associated with, 119t
strategies
for dementia and AD patients, 549
for surgical patients, 518-520
techniques and movements
components of, 210-211, 212f
treatment goal patterns, 118-121, 253-254
Massage applications
affecting vestibular apparatus, 151
body mechanics
concepts of, 237, 239-240, 241f-244f
counterpressure, 240, 241f-242f
on mats, 240, 243f-244f, 245
focused therapy
Asian massage concepts, 355-356, 357b, 358-359
circulatory system, 318-323, 324f
connective tissue, 340, 341f, 342-344
fluid dynamics, 317-318
functional techniques, 316-317
increasing arterial circulation, 327-329
joint play, 350, 352
lymphatic drainage, 329-330, 331f-334f, 335-338, 339f, 340
lymphatic system, 318-323, 324f
motor tone inhibition techniques, 360-363, 364f, 365-375, 376f-377f, 378
pin and stretch, 343-344
reflexology, 352-355
specific release methods, 360-363, 364f, 365-375, 376f-377f, 378
targeting fluid movement, 326-327
tissue movement methods, 343-350, 351f-352f
trigger points, 344-350, 351f-352f
venous return, 329
on joints, 182
on muscle dysfunction conditions, 193, 194b
muscle energy techniques, 225-234
breathing and eye movement, 226-227, 228f
contact-relax-antagonist-contract method, 228, 230f
direct manipulation, 229-231, 232f
focus of, 225-226
the integrated approach, 232-234
muscle contraction types, 226
positional release techniques, 231-232, 233f
postisometric relaxation (PIR), 227, 229f
pulsed muscle energy, 229, 231f
reciprocal inhibition (RI), 227-228, 229f
on muscles, 184-185
for myofascial form and function, 180-181, 183-184
for respiratory system, 174-175
review of, 209-245
components of, 210-211, 212f
joint movement methods, 222-225
mechanical forces, 211, 213-214
methods of, 214, 215f, 216, 217f, 218-222
qualities of touch, 210-211, 212f-213f
stretching, 234-237, 238f-239f
Massage protocols
for athletes, 536-537
for general maintenance
abdomen, 387f, 396, 398-400
anterior torso, 387f, 396, 398-400
approach and sequence, 382, 383f
arms, 409, 410f, 411-414
face and head, 382-388
forearms, wrists and hands, 414-416
hips, 416, 417f, 418-421
legs, ankles and feet, 426, 427f, 428
neck, 392, 393f, 394-396
occipital base, 388-392
posterior torso, 400-405
shoulders, 405-409
thighs, 421, 422f, 423-426
for joint edema, 338, 339f, 340
for lymphatic drainage, 331f-334f, 336-338
palliative massage considerations, 428-430
photographs illustrating
breathing function protocols, 791-795
general protocols, 759-781
low back protocols, 786-791
seated protocols, 782-786
Massage therapists
basic pharmacology for, 520-521, 523-524
body mechanics, 237, 239-240
in case studies, 680
choosing career as, 5-6
diversity of, 4f
dress and attitude of, 74
educational requirements, 11, 13b, 14, 61-62
getting jobs in healthcare settings, 82-84
pay scale comparison, 62-63
as team players, 5
Massage therapy;*See* massage
Massage Therapy Foundation
on guidelines for case reports, 50
Mats
used in massage, 240, 243f-244f, 245
Maturation
in tissue healing, 119t
Means testing, 71
Measurements
in research, 24-25
Mechanical forces
agitation-quality, 494
bending, shear, and rotational loading, 214
compression loading, 213-214
definition of massage, 209-210
illustration of different, 215f-218f
massage application techniques, 211, 213-214
structural effects, 211
tension loading, 211, 213
types of, 211, 213-214
Mechanical stress
defining, 461
Mechanoreceptors
definition of, 148
and pain relief, 485
responding to, 148
Mediation, 75-76
Medicaid
benefits of, 80
origins of, 71
Medical/ clinical massage; *See* massage
Medical devices
caution when massaging clients with, 132-133, 134f, 135
Medical doctors (MDs)
description of, 58
Medical history, 254
Medical practices
business structures in, 69-70
Medical records;*See also* documentation
during massage assessment process, 256-260
rules for completing, 259-260
Medical responsibility
of complementary medicine practitioners
in professional practice model, 12b

Medical treatment
of autoimmune diseases, 505-506
for illnesses and injuries
drug therapy and massage interaction, 526b-527b
flexibility techniques, 531
massage therapy supporting, 515, 518-520, 531
nutrition, mental health and lifestyle, 531
pharmacology for massage, 520-521, 523-525, 526b-527b
physical medicine, 525, 528-532
surgery, 516-520
and therapeutic exercise, 528, 529t, 530
for pain, 488-492
Medically fragile
definition of, 6
Medicare
benefits of, 80
origins of, 71
Medications
Alzheimer's disease, 548
anatomic distribution of, 524
for back pain, 602
versus drugs, 520
information for massage therapists, 524-525
and massage
interaction of, 526b-527b
metabolism, 524-525
modes of action, 523
for pain, 488-492
routes of administration, 524
side effects of, 520, 548
Medicine
occupational definition
and scope of practice of, 13b
Meditation, 92, 175, 491
Medulla
and baroreceptors, 168
Melanoma, 501
Memory
loss
with Alzheimer's disease, 548
with concussions and stroke, 635-637
with fibromyalgia, 610
Menopause, 552
Menstrual cycles
and edema, 321
Mental health
and addictions, 556
Alzheimer's disease, 547-549, 566-567
assessing during examination, 256
benefits of massage for, 122, 555-556
delirium and dementia, 546-547, 566-567
disorder classification and categories, 555, 557b
drugs and massage, 526b-527b
with the dying, 587-588
eating disorders, 561-562
and geriatric massage, 555
massage complementing, 531
in older adults
Alzheimer's disease, 547-549, 566-567
delirium and dementia, 546-547, 566-567
pain/ fatigue syndromes, 561
population similarities in, 555-567
posttraumatic stress disorder, 562-565
psychiatric disorders
anxiety, 556-559
brain chemical imbalances, 559-560
depression, 560-561
and psychogenic pain, 485
psychotic disorders, 565-566
trauma, 460-461
Meridians
and Asian massage, 355-356, 357b
definition of, 355
example of massage, 359f
illustration of, 356f
twelve main, 357b
Metabolic system
changes with exercises, 100-101
harmful unrelieved pain effects, 493t
Metabolism
of medications, 524-525
Methods sections
in Chang example, 31b
of research articles, 31b, 46-47, 49b
Microcirculation, 165
blood vessel, 328-329
illustration of, 329f
Microsurgery, 517b
Microtrauma
in muscles, 269, 272
Migraine with aura, 621
Migraine without aura, 621
Migraines
case study on, 729, 731-732
chronic pain with, 486
description of, 613-614, 620-622
and sternocleidomastoid release, 362
triggers and symptoms, 621
Military, 71-72, 562-563
Mind
biochemistry and neurosomatic disorders, 458b-459b
and matter, 157-159
Mind and spirit
aspect of treatment, 6
Mind-body
interventions, 9
relationship between
component of wellness, 103-106
and recovery process, 469
Mindfulness
concept of, 102
Minor surgery, 517b
Mixed cerebral palsy, 639
Mobility
assessing during examination, 265
and movement, 350, 352, 353f
Mobility impairments
interacting with patients with, 576
population similarities in, 576
Mobilization with movement (MWM), 350, 352, 353f
Monoplegia, 636, 643-644
Mood disorders
description of, 557b
Mood management
benefits of massage for, 121-122
on treatment plan, 250
Morning sickness, 580
Morphology
of bacteria, 199
Motor nerves, 185-186
Motor tone
definition of, 149
Motor tone inhibition techniques
focused massage applications for, 360-363, 364f, 365-375, 376f-377f, 378
Movements
active, 272, 273f, 274
assessment of, 269, 270f
biomechanics of, 188-193
joint
methods of, 222-225
of massage therapists
and tension forces, 214, 215f, 216, 217f, 218-222
and muscle energy techniques, 225-234
patterns, 187, 188f, 275
phasic/ mover muscles role in, 190
and posture, 269, 270f-271f
quadrants, 280f
Mover muscles, 279
Multifidi muscles, 363, 364, 366f
Multiple isotonic contractions, 226
Multiple sclerosis (MS)
as autoimmune disease, 510b
description and statistics of, 640
and inflammation, 500
massage strategies for, 507-508, 640
Muscle contractions
increasing venous flow, 165, 169
types of, 226

Muscle energy
  definition of, 226
Muscle energy techniques
  massage application techniques on, 225-234
    breathing and eye movement, 226-227, 228f
    contact-relax-antagonist-contract method, 228, 230f
    direct manipulation, 229-231, 232f
    focus of, 225-226
    the integrated approach, 232-234
    muscle contraction types, 226
    positional release techniques, 231-232, 233f
    postisometric relaxation (PIR), 227, 229f
    pulsed muscle energy, 229, 231f
    reciprocal inhibition (RI), 227-228, 229f
  and pain management, 494
Muscle firing patterns
  during massage assessment process, 282-283, 284b-289b
Muscle inhibition, 601f
Muscle movements
  and pain relief, 485
Muscle pain, 488-489
Muscle pump
  increasing venous flow, 165, 169
Muscle relaxants, 489-490
Muscle spasm end-feel, 276
Muscle spindle cells
  description and illustration of, 149-150
  direct manipulation of, 230-231
  gliding strokes on, 216, 217f
Muscle strength
  and movement, 269, 270f-271f
  testing and findings, 278-279
Muscle tone
  definition of, 149
  general massage protocols for
    abdomen, 387f, 396, 398-400
    anterior torso, 387f, 396, 398-400
    approach and sequence, 382, 383f
    arms, 409, 410f, 411-414
    face and head, 382-388
    forearms, wrists and hands, 414-416
    hips, 416, 417f, 418-421
    legs, ankles and feet, 426, 427f, 428
    neck, 392, 393f, 394-396
    occipital base, 388-392
    posterior torso, 400-405
    shoulders, 405-409
    thighs, 421, 422f, 423-426
Muscles; *See also* muscle energy techniques
  activation sequence, 283
  and back pain, 596-607, 599f-601f
  and collagen, 177-178
  contraction types, 226
  dysfunction conditions
    massage application techniques on, 184-185, 193, 194b
  of face and head, 384f
  functional movement, 184-185, 187-193, 191f-192f, 193-194, 269, 270f-271f
  general massage protocols for
    abdomen, 387f, 396, 398-400
    anterior torso, 387f, 396, 398-400
    approach and sequence, 382, 383f
    arms, 409, 410f, 411-414
    face and head, 382-388
    forearms, wrists and hands, 414-416
    hips, 416, 417f, 418-421
    legs, ankles and feet, 426, 427f, 428
    neck, 392, 393f, 394-396
    occipital base, 388-392
    posterior torso, 400-405
    shoulders, 405-409
    thighs, 421, 422f, 423-426
  groups and functions, 190-191
  imbalances in, 190-191, 192f
  inhibition, 601f
  kinetic chain, 186-187, 188f
  lengthening, 230-231
  massage to lengthen, 282f
  movers and stabilizers, 190b
Muscles *(Continued)*
  palpation of, 300-304
  percentage of water in, 160t
  and posture, 269, 270f-271f
  roles of, 185f
  sensory nerve receptors of, 149-150
  short and tight, 193
  shortening
    with breathing pattern disorders, 478-479
    and lengthening, 279-281, 283f
  soreness and overuse, 269, 272
  strength testing, 278-280
  sympathetic and parasympathetic response, 154t
  tension, 175-177
  tonic/ postural stabilizing, 190
  trigger points
    active and latent, 346b
    assessment of, 347
    definition of, 344-345
    diagram illustrating common, 348f
    focused massage applications for, 344-350, 351f-352f
    myofascial, 345f
    palpation of, 300-304, 347b
    perpetuating factors, 346-347
    theory of formation, 346b
    treatment methods, 345-350
  types of actions, 185-186
  weakness
    causing illness or injury, 4457
Muscular end-feel, 276
Musculoskeletal system
  and back pain, 597
  breathing pattern disorder signs in, 476
  conditions
    assessment of, 261
  and geriatric massage, 544
  harmful unrelieved pain effects, 493t
  massage-specific assessment of, 261
  as target for autoimmune diseases, 510b
Musculotendinous junctions, 148, 150, 300-302
Myasthenia gravis, 508, 510b
Mycotic infections, 199
Myocardial infarction
  causes of, 168-169
  early warning signs of, 609f
  related to chronic inflammation, 125t
Myoclonic seizures, 638
Myofascia, 184
Myofascial form and function, 175-181
  fascia, 179-180
  massage application techniques on, 180-181, 183-184
  periosteum, 179
  trigger points, 345f
Myofascial pain
  and fibromyalgia, 487b
Myositis ossificans, 129-130

N
Nails
  assessment of, 299
Narcolepsy, 652
National Center for Complementary and Alternative Medicine (NCCAM), 7, 8
Naturopathic medicine
  focus and training in, 65-66
  history of, 64-65
  occupational definition
    and scope of practice of, 13b
  principles of, 65
Naturopathy;*See* naturopathic medicine
Nausea
  as chemotherapy side effect, 629-630
Near-touch palpation, 298
Neck
  general massage protocols, 392, 393f, 394-396
  important structures of, 393f
  massage techniques for, 361, 392, 394-396
  palliative protocol for, 428-429
  physical examination of, 255-256

Negotiation, 75-76
Nephrologists, 631
Nerve disorders
  and inflammation, 500
Nerve fibers, 484
Nerve impingement
  definition of, 643
  massage for, 645, 646
Nerve root compression, 645
Nerves
  and back pain, 596-607
  impingement of, 151
  injuries, 642-650
Nervous system
  anatomy and physiology of
    massage influence on, 144-147
  endangerment sites, 133f
  and geriatric massage, 546-549
  as target for autoimmune diseases, 510b
Neuroendocrine structure, 144-147
  autonomic nervous system, 152-153, 154t, 155-159
  chemoreceptors, 150-152
  emotional states, 153, 155-156
  energy systems, 157-159
  entrainment, 156
  epithelial tissue, 148-150
  gate control theory, 156-157
  parasympathetic nervous system, 153
  peripheral nervous system, 147-148
  somatic nervous system, 148-150
  the spinal cord, 147
  sympathetic nervous system, 153
Neurofibrillary tangles (NFTs), 547
Neurogenic pain, 150, 486
Neurologic diseases
  clinical reasoning process, 634-646
    brain, 634-639
    complex regional pain syndrome, 640-642
    disk herniation, 645-646
    multiple sclerosis, 639-640
    nerve and spinal cord, 642-645
    nerve impingement, 642-646
    peripheral neuropathy, 640
Neurological system
  assessment of, 255
  breathing pattern disorder signs in, 476
  physical examination of, 256
Neurology
  exercise regimens benefiting, 529t
Neuromuscular reflex patterns
  in neck, 395-396
Neurons, 145
Neurosomatic disorders, 458b-459b
Neurotic disorders
  description of, 557b
Neurotransmitters, 146
Neutrophils
  and immune response, 496-498
Nitric oxide, 498
No treatment control groups, 42
Nociceptors
  definition of, 148
  and pain, 484
  role of, 147
Nodal points, 494
Nonmanipulated independent variables, 41
Nonprofit hospitals, 69
Nonsteroidal antiinflammatory drugs (NSAIDs), 465, 483, 489-490, 613
Norepinephrine, 146
Nose
  assessment of, 255
Null (statistical) hypotheses, 35
Nurse anesthetists, 60
Nursing
  occupational definition
    and scope of practice of, 13b
Nutrition
  basics of, 95-96
  component of wellness, 95-96
Nutrition *(Continued)*
  and geriatric massage, 551
  and herbs, 520-521, 523
  massage complementing, 531
  in naturopathic medicine, 68
  and stress, 91
Nutritional supplements, 96, 520, 531

O

Objective assessment
  physical, 265-266
Observation and palpation
  to assess body areas, 272, 273f-274f
Obsessive compulsive disorder (OCD), 559-560
Obstetrics
  exercise regimens benefiting, 529t
  surgery, 517b
Occipital base
  general massage protocols, 388-392
  illustration of important structures, 389f
  specific release techniques, 361
Occulopelvic reflexes, 186
Occupational definitions
  and scopes of practice
    for various medical professionals, 13b-14b
Older adults
  and aging process, 537-539
  benefits of exercise for, 529t, 530
  cardiovascular conditions, 542-543
  digestive/ gastrointestinal conditions, 543
  and disease risks, 538
  examples of interaction with, 539f-541f
  goals of massage for, 538-539
  hearing conditions in, 550-551
  illness and injury in, 455
  integumentary system, 543-544
  massage therapist understanding of, 537-538
  and mental health, 555
  musculoskeletal system, 544
  nervous system conditions in, 546-549
  and nutrition, 551
  osteoporosis, 545, 546b
  physical changes with aging, 542t
  pulmonary conditions, 549
  reproductive conditions, 552-553
  sleep disorders, 553
  specific massage techniques for, 554-555
  support systems for, 553
  urinary conditions in, 551-552
  vision conditions in, 549-550
Open procedure surgery, 516
Open study, 45
Open wounds
  as massage contraindication, 130
Ophthalmologic surgery, 517b
Ophthalmoplegic migraine, 621
Opioids, 489-490
Optometrists, 59
Oral surgery, 517b
Organs
  affected by sympathetic and parasympathetic divisions, 154t
  percentage of water and loss, 160t
Orthopedics
  clinical reasoning process, 647-648, 649f-650f
  exercise regimens benefiting, 529t
Oscillation
  description and illustration of, 217f, 219-220
Osmotic pressure, 160
Osteoarthritis
  chronic pain with, 486
  and joint degeneration, 183, 184f
  and joint edema, 338, 339f, 340
Osteoblasts, 179
Osteopathic manipulative therapy (OMT), 63
Osteopathic medicine
  history of, 63
  occupational definition
    and scope of practice of, 13b
  philosophy and characteristics of, 63-64

Osteoporosis
causes and consequences of, 545f
chronic pain with, 486
and geriatric massage, 545, 546b
risk factors for, 546b
Ostomy, 517b
Otorhinolaryngologic surgery, 517b
Outcome goals
definition of, 252
during massage assessment process, 252
Outcome-based process
massage as, 3-4, 6
Outcomes
classifying massage application by, 451
intentions, 157-159
or benefits of massage, 121
and pressure level guidelines, 137t
for stress management with massage, 122-123
three goal patterns of, 118-119
Outflare, 378
Overpressure
definition of, 276
Overuse syndrome, 269, 272
Overuse trauma, 461
Oxygen
transport of
and carbon dioxide, 170
Oxytocin, 147

P

P values, 36-37
Pain; *See also* acute pain; chronic pain
acute *versus* chronic, 485-486
causing altered gait, 290
assessment factors, 492t
behaviors, 642b
benefits of massage for, 126
case study on, 720-729
as chemotherapy side effect, 629-630
chronic syndrome, 610-612
complexity of, 126
components of, 484-485
control mechanisms for, 606-607
counteracted by massage pleasure, 155
decreasing range of motion, 276-277
definitions associated with, 481, 483
with depression or anxiety, 561
descriptive words, 263-264
diagnosis of, 486
evaluation of, 486, 488
and fatigue syndromes
benefits of massage for, 561
with healing, 276-277
of integrated muscle energy approach, 232-234
management (*See* pain management)
medical treatment for, 488-492
medications, 488-492
messages, 483-485
muscle, 488
neurogenic, 150
with palpation, 295
rating scales, 262f
referred, 127f
research on massage and, 30-39, 40f
sensations of, 485
strategies for, 492-494
three major components of, 484-485
treatment and medications, 488-493
two types of, 483
unrelieved effects, 493t
Pain management
with massage, 474
massage applications for, 494
massage therapy's role in, 94
as primary benefit of massage, 15
spinal cord, brain, and peripheral nerves, 484-485
on treatment plan, 250
Pain scales
for children, 262f
description and illustration of, 488, 489f
Pain threshold, 483
Pain tolerance, 483
Pain-spasm-pain cycle, 488
Paired functional areas
and range of motion, 519f, 520b
Palliative care
benefits of massage for, 120-121
definition of, 585-586
protocol for athletes, 536
Palliative massage
for posttraumatic stress, 564
Palliative protocol
for ill, fragile, pre or postoperative patients, 428-430
Palpation
of body rhythms and respiration, 304-305
of bones, 303-304
during examination, 265
illustration of, 301f
of joints and ligaments, 303-304
levels and types of, 298-304
during massage assessment process, 295-306
of muscles, 295
near-touch, 298
pressure used during, 297-298
of skin surface, 298-299
of superficial fascia, 299-300
of tendons, 302
of trigger points, 347b
Pancreas
sympathetic and parasympathetic response, 154t
Pancreatitis
related to chronic inflammation, 125t
Panic attack, 558
Parameters, 36
Paraplegia, 636, 643-644
Parasitic infections
description and inflammation with, 626
Parasympathetic dominance
enhanced
as primary benefit of massage, 15
and pain management, 494
Parasympathetic nervous system
anatomy, physiology and massage, 153
organs affected by, 154t
Parkinson's disease
case study on, 737-742
Partnerships, 71
PARTS acronym, 67
Passive range-of-motion (PROM), 272, 274, 530-531
Patella
observation and palpation of, 272, 273f-274f
Pathogens, 499
blood-borne, 201, 202f, 203, 204f, 205-206
Pathologic barriers
restricting ROM, 275-276
Pathologic conditions
classifying massage application by, 451
Pathomechanics, 456
Patient history
information in, 261-262
Patient records
guidelines for creating, 81-82
Patients
versus clients, 56
in massage, 5
sleeping, 434-435
Patient's bill of rights, 57b
Pay scales, 62-63
Pectoralis major and minor muscles
shortening with breathing pattern disorders, 478-479
specific release techniques, 367-368, 368f
Pediatric population
adolescents, 573
age range and characteristics of, 567, 569
children, 569f-570f, 573
illustration of massage techniques for, 568f-570f

Pediatric population *(Continued)*
infants and toddlers, 571-573
pain, 262f
population similarities in, 567, 568f-570f, 571-574
special medical issues in, 573-574
Pelvis
forward-tilting, 456-457
illustration of, 377f
sacrum moving within
and back pain, 605f, 606
specific release techniques, 375, 377f, 378
Pemphigus vulgaris, 510b
Peptic ulcers
case study on, 730-731
Perceptual dominance, 483
Percussion
description of, 220-221
illustration of, 218f
slapping, 218f
Periodic limb movement disorder, 651-652
Periosteum
description and illustration of, 179
Peripheral nervous system (PNS)
anatomy, physiology and massage, 147-148
and pain, 484
Peripheral neuropathy
chronic pain with, 486
description and massage for, 640-641
Peripheral resistance, 167
Permeability
definition of, 327
Pernicious anemia, 510b
Perpendicularity
of massage therapist, 239, 241f-244f
Personal history
assessment of, 254
Personality conflicts, 76
Personality disorders, 557b
Petit mall seizures, 638
PH balance, 161-162
Phagocytosis
definition of, 123
Pharmacology
basic massage therapist, 520-521, 523-524
Phasic muscles, 190, 279-280
Phlebitis, 608
Phobias, 559
Physiatrists, 528
Physical disabilities
definitions concerning, 574-575
population similarities in, 574-577
Physical examination
format of, 255-256
procedures for, 272, 273f-274f
Physical fitness;*See also* exercise
component of wellness, 97, 99-101
definition of, 97
mechanical aids for, 531
Physical medicine, 69, 525, 528
Physical therapists (PTs), 61
Physical therapy
for back pain, 602
for fibromyalgia, 611
occupational definition
and scope of practice of, 13b-14b
Physical trauma, 460-461
Physician assistants (PAs), 61
Physicians
referrals and preauthorization, 5
treatment orders, 252-253
Physiologic barriers
restricting ROM, 275-276
Physiology;*See also* anatomy and physiology
importance in massage therapy, 142-143
Piezoelectricity, 178
Pin and stretch
focused massage applications for, 343-344
technique of, 235, 343-344, 344f
Pitting edema, 162, 300f
Placebo-attention control groups, 42
Placebos
power of, 491b
Placebo-sham treatment control groups, 42-43
Plasma, 168
Plasticity
of soft tissue, 177
Platelets, 498
Pleasure
benefits of massage for, 15, 121
counteracting pain, 155
versus pain during massage, 381-382
Podiatrists, 59
Podiatry
occupational definition
and scope of practice of, 14b
Populations
definition and example of, 31-32
Portals of entry
infection transmission through, 200
Positional release techniques
of massage application, 231-232, 233f
Posterior rotation, 375, 377f, 378
Posterior torso
general massage protocols, 400-405
illustration of important structures, 401f
palliative protocol for, 429
Postisometric relaxation (PIR), 227, 229f
Postsurgical massage, 5f
Post-test, 44
Posttraumatic stress disorder
benefits of massage for, 562-565
definition of, 121-122, 562
description of, 557b
types of, 562-563
Postural deviations
and injuries/ illnesses, 455-457
Postural imbalances, 267f
Postural muscles, 279
Posture
and back pain, 596
balance and imbalance diagram, 280-281, 281f
causes of dysfunction, 269
deviations causing injury, 455-457
distortions
and integrated muscle energy approach, 232-234
effects of imbalances, 267f
of massage therapist, 240, 241f-244f
and muscle function, 269, 270f-271f
muscles involved in, 279-280
physical assessment of, 266, 267f, 268
and symmetry, 268b
three major factors influencing, 266
tonic/ postural stabilizing muscles, 190
Prayer, 92
Preeclampsia, 582
Preexisting conditions, 73b
Prefrontal cortex, 145
Pregnancy
disorders with, 582-583
first trimester, 580-581
labor, 582
and lupus
case study on, 693-705
population similarities in, 577, 578f-579f, 580-583
prenatal massage, 577, 578f-579f
second trimester, 581-582
third trimester, 582
Preliminary sections
of research articles, 45, 49b
Premenstrual syndrome
case study on, 732-737
Presbyopia, 549
Prescriptions
massage, 5
Present illnesses
defining, 254

Pressure
definition of massage, 135
guidelines for, 137t
levels
of compressive force, 135
depth and pain relief, 494
illustration of different, 136f
intensity awareness and caution, 135
on trigger points, 344-349
and weight transfer, 239, 241f-244f
Presurgery plan
based on relaxation, 250
Pretest, 44
Prevention
of back pain, 603
of illness or injury, 455, 4546f
in naturopathic medicine, 65
PRICE therapy
components of, 465b
description of, 465
and fluid movements, 326
during healing stage 1, 119t
Pricking pain, 488
Primary biliary cirrhosis, 510b
Privacy standards
by HIPAA, 260-261
Probability
and P values, 36-37
of type 1 error, 36
Probiotics
principles and benefits of, 440
Problem-oriented medical records (POMR), 680-681
documentation of, 257-258
Prodromal period, 198
Professional boundaries
in massage therapy, 6
Professional literature review
research question, 31
Professional practice model
for complementary medicine
key constituents of, 12b
Professionals
appearance and attitude
when greeting a client, 74f
occupational definitions
and scope of practice for, 13b-14b
Progress notes
documentation, 258
Progressive muscle relaxation, 91, 466-467
Projected pain, 486
Pronation, 188-189
Pronation distortion syndrome
flowchart of, 192f
Proprioceptive neuromuscular facilitation (PNF), 530
Proprioceptors
definition of, 148
function of, 147
Prostaglandins, 498
Prosthesis implantation, 517b
Protozoa
transmission of, 199
Psoas
general protocol for, 400, 416, 417f, 418-421
low back pain, 605-606
shortening with breathing pattern disorders, 478-479
specific release techniques, 365-367, 370-371, 372f
Psoriasis
as autoimmune condition, 510b
massage strategies for, 508
related to chronic inflammation, 125t
Psychiatric disorders
benefits of massage for
anxiety, 556-559
brain chemical imbalances, 559-560
dementia and AD, 549
depression, 560-561
exercise regimens benefiting, 529t
Psychiatrists
definition of, 555
Psychogenic pain, 485
Psychological system
breathing pattern disorder signs in, 476
stages
and emotional factors, 457-458, 458b-459b
and healing, 467
Psychologists
definition of, 555
Psychology
occupational definition
and scope of practice of, 14b
Psychosocial
history
assessment of, 254
influences on health, 460f
Psychotic disorders, 565-566
PubMed, 50
Pulmonary system
and geriatric massage, 549
therapeutic exercise benefiting, 529t
Pulse
definition of, 166
Pulsed muscle energy, 229, 231f
Pus, 123

Q
Qi, 7
Qi gong, 358
Quadrants
of body movements, 280f
Quadratus lumborum
and back pain, 605
shortening with breathing pattern disorders, 478-479
specific release techniques, 373
Quadriplegia, 636, 643-644
Qualifiable goals, 252
Qualifications
of complementary medicine practitioners
in professional practice model, 12b
Qualitative research
categories and strategies of, 28-29
Qualities of touch
techniques and movements, 210-211, 212f-213f
Quality health data, 81
Quality of life
harmful unrelieved pain effects, 493t
Quality standards
by complementary medicine practitioners
in professional practice model, 12b
Quantifiable goals, 252
Quantitative research
categories and strategies of, 28
Questions
before massage therapy, 264-265
when taking patient histories, 262

R
Radiating pain, 488
Radiation therapy, 629
Radiculopathy, 597
Random assignment, 32, 41
Random selection, 32
Randomization
definition and example of, 32
Randomized clinical trials, 44
Randomized controlled trial (RCT) research method; *See* true experimental (RCT) research method
Range of motion (ROM)
active, 223-224
assessment of, 265, 275-276
degrees of, 277f
interpreting, 277-278
joint movement method, 222-225
measurement of, 274, 276-277
shoulders, 405f, 406-409
Rapid eye movement (REM), 650
Reactive oxygen intermediate molecules, 496-498
Reciprocal inhibition (RI), 193, 227-228, 229f
Reconstructive surgery, 517b

Record keeping
common styles of, 257-259
by complementary medicine practitioners
in professional practice model, 12b
computerized, 82
definition of, 256
discharge summary, 257
flow charts, 257
importance of, 80-82, 256
problem-oriented, 257-258
progress notes, 258
rules for completing, 256-259
technologic advances, 258-259
Recovery
process of, 465-467
realistic expectations for, 463
Rectus abdominis
specific release techniques, 362-363
Red blood cells, 168
Referrals
by physicians, 5
Referred pain
definition of, 488
diagram illustrating locations of, 127f
Reflex sympathetic dystrophy, 126, 486, 641
Reflexes
arthrokinematic, 181
muscle, 186
that affect breathing, 174
Reflexology
focused massage applications for, 352-355
generalized chart, 354f
and pain management, 494
Regeneration
definition of, 503
and repair, 501
Registered nurses (RNs), 60
Registration
of complementary medicine practitioners
in professional practice model, 12b
Rehabilitation process
for athletes, 536-537
exercise regimens benefiting, 529t
and healing
three phases of, 93
for stroke, 635-636
Relaxation
benefits of massage for, 121
component of wellness, 101-102
for pain relief, 491
progressive, 466-467
for stress reduction, 91-92
types of, 101
Remodeling phase
definition of, 501
following surgery, 520
Renal dialysis, 133
Repetitive injuries, 461-462
Repetitive motion activities, 455-457
Replacement, 503
Reproductive system
assessment of, 255
and geriatric massage, 552-553
sympathetic and parasympathetic response, 154t
Rescue Remedy, 439
Research
blinded and open studies, 45
in case studies, 680
categories, 25, 26f, 27-28, 27f
by complementary medicine practitioners, 12b
continuum, 26, 27f
control groups, 42-43
criteria for critiquing, 48, 49b
the deductive approach, 25, 26f
definition and origins of, 24
derived evidence of massage effectiveness, 12b
design notation, 38-39, 39, 40f
designs and procedures, 29-30
ethics, 39-41
Research *(Continued)*
experimental validity, 37-38
framework of research articles, 45-47, 49b
group-specific or single-case focus, 44
hypotheses, 34-35
independent variable groups or levels, 41-42
informational resources, 23-24
integrative, 29, 30f
introduction to, 23-24
between and within IVs, 43-44
matrix, 50
measurement, statistics and evaluation, 24-25
methods, 28-29
on naturopathic medicine, 69
nonmanipulated independent variables, 41
objectives for students, 22-23
parameters and statistics, 36
pretest and post-test, 44
process
example of, 30-39, 40f
five levels of, 25, 26f
and professional literature review, 31
qualitative, quantitative and integrative, 28-29
questions, 24, 31
random assignment or intact groups, 41
randomized controlled or clinical trials, 44-45
the research continuum, 26, 27f
single-subject/ single-case, 48, 50
statistical analysis, 36-37
strategies, 28
true experimental (RCT) research method
and case example, 30-39, 40f
Research articles
framework of, 45-47, 49b
Research studies
criteria for critiquing, 49b
Research universe
three subsets of, 25f
Reserve volume, 170
Reservoir host, 199-200
Resistance
defining, 461
in fluid dynamics, 167
testing
procedure for, 275
Resistive strength training (RST), 530
Resourceful compensation
patterns of, 308
Resources
for anatomy and physiology, 143b
for research information, 23-24
Respect
importance of maintaining, 6
Respiration
accessory muscles of, 476-477, 477b
definition of, 169
muscles of, 172f
and palpation, 304-305
Respiratory pump
increasing venous flow, 165, 169
Respiratory rate
definition of, 174
Respiratory system
assessment of, 255
breathing mechanics, 169-170, 171f-173f
breathing pattern disorder signs in, 476
changes with exercises, 100
clinical reasoning process
description and treatment of, 607-608
discussion of, 169-170, 171f-173f, 174-175
disorders
and inflammation, 499-500
harmful unrelieved pain effects, 493t
massage application techniques on, 174-175
pathologic conditions of, 174
respiratory rate, 174
sympathetic and parasympathetic response, 154t
Response to stress
common physiologic, 345b

Resting position
description and illustration of, 214, 216, 217f
Restless leg syndrome, 610, 651-652
case study on, 720-721
Results section
in Chang example, 31b
of research articles, 31b, 47, 49b
Rheumatoid arthritis
as autoimmune disorder, 510b
chronic pain with, 486, 496
exercise regimens benefiting, 529t
and joint edema, 338, 339f, 340
massage strategies for, 508
Rhomboid muscles
shortening with breathing pattern disorders, 478-479
specific release techniques, 367-368, 368f
Rhythm
massage guidelines, 211
Ribs
observation and palpation of, 272, 273f-274f
Rickettsiae
transmission of, 199
Righting reflexes, 186
Rights
definition of, 72-73
Rocking
technique of, 217f, 219-220
Rocky Mountain spotted fever, 199
Rolf, Ida, 7
Rotator muscles, 363, 364, 366f
Routine orders, 253

S

Sacral plexus
description and illustration of, 152
Sacral spine
and back pain, 605, 605f
illustration of, 401f
and posture and gravity, 267f, 268
Sacroiliac joint
assessing, 294f-295f
and back pain, 604-605
function of, 293-294
general massage of, 416, 417f, 418-421
specific release techniques, 374-375, 376f
Sadness
during grieving process, 588-590
Sagittal plane movement, 187, 188f, 225f, 270f-271f
Salaries, 62-63
Samples
definition and example of, 31-32
Sanitation
and diseases, 198
goal of, 198
importance in massage therapy, 197
and infection transmission
bacteria, 199
fungi, 199
host, 199-200
portals of entry, 200
protozoa, 199
rickettsiae, 199
viruses, 198-199
Occupational Safety and Health Administration (OSHA)
on blood-borne pathogen standards, 200-206
environmental protection guidelines, 203, 205
hand washing, 201, 202f, 203
hepatitis B vaccinations, 205
housekeeping controls, 205
mission of, 200
postexposure follow-up, 205-206
Scalenes
shortening with breathing pattern disorders, 478-479
specific release techniques, 360-361
Scalp, 383-384, 384f, 387, 624
Scapula
observation and palpation of, 272, 273f-274f
Scar tissue
management of, 250, 521f-522f
massage strategies for, 656, 658f
Schizophrenia
and brain chemistry, 559
Sciatic nerve
and back pain, 597
illustration of, 417f
Sciatica, 597
Scleroderma, 508-509, 510b
Seasonal affective disorder (SAD), 559
Seated protocols
photographs illustrating massage protocols, 782-786
Secondary gain, 458, 468
Second-degree burns, 499
Sedentary lifestyle
and back pain, 596
Seizures, 637-639
Self-concept
importance of good, 105
Self-interpretation, 265
Selye, Hans
on stress, 89, 563
Sensations
of pain, 485
Sensitization
of brain, 153
definition and causes of, 153
and pain, 481-482
Sensory losses
with stroke, 636
Sensory nerve receptors
five types of muscle, 149
four categories of, 148
of muscle, 149-150
supplying each muscle, 185-186
Sensory nerves
and aging, 542t
four categories of, 148
Separation anxiety, 558
Sepsis, 499
Septicemia, 123
Serial distortion pattern
of kinetic chain, 191, 191f-192f, 193
Serotonin, 146, 493, 494
Serratus anterior
shortening with breathing pattern disorders, 478-479
Sexual disorders, 557b
Shaking, 217f, 219-220
Shear forces
definition of, 214
illustration of, 215f-216f
illustration of stretching with, 239f
Shock
during grieving process, 588-590
Short tight muscles, 279-281, 282f
Short-term goals
for massage therapists, 253-254
Shoulder flexion, 289b
Shoulders
assessing movement of, 270f-271f
general massage protocols, 405-409
illustration of important structures of, 405f
observation and palpation of, 272, 273f-274f
palliative protocol for, 429
specific release techniques, 365-367
Side effects
versus adverse reactions, 523
of chemotherapy, 629-630
of medications
and massage, 527b
Single-blind research procedures, 45
Single-case experimental methods, 48, 50
Single-case quantitative analysis methods, 48, 50
Single-subject/ single-case research methods, 48, 50
Sinus headaches, 617f-618f
Size
accommodating body, 576-577
Sjögren's syndrome, 509, 510b

Skeletal muscles
palpation of, 300
Skeleton
percentage of water in, 160t
Skin
assessing during examination, 265
as extension of nervous system, 148
general massage protocols for
abdomen, 387f, 396, 398-400
anterior torso, 387f, 396, 398-400
approach and sequence, 382, 383f
arms, 409, 410f, 411-414
face and head, 382-388
forearms, wrists and hands, 414-416
hips, 416, 417f, 418-421
legs, ankles and feet, 426, 427f, 428
neck, 392, 393f, 394-396
occipital base, 388-392
posterior torso, 400-405
shoulders, 405-409
thighs, 421, 422f, 423-426
hot areas and cold areas, 298-299
observation and palpation of, 272, 273f-274f
percentage of water in, 160t
physical examination of, 255-256
sympathetic and parasympathetic response, 154t
water loss from, 160t
Skin rolling
description and illustration of, 217f, 218-219
Skull
bones of, 382
Sleep
and aging, 537-538, 553
and back pain, 596
benefits of massage for, 15, 123
component of wellness, 102-103
disorders
clinical reasoning process, 647, 650-652
common causes of insomnia, 651b
with fibromyalgia, 610
and geriatric massage, 553
massage strategies for, 652
treatment of, 650-651
five stages of, 650
hygiene, 651b
and stress, 91
for wellness, 102-103
Sleep apnea, 651
Sleeping patient, 434-435
Slow infections, 198
Small intestine
meridians relating to, 356f, 357b
Smoking
and aging, 537-538
SOAP charting
in case studies, 680
format for, 680-681
method of, 258f
SOAPIE format, 681
Soft tissue
changes and breathing disorders, 477b
dysfunction and impingement syndromes, 125-126
elasticity and plasticity, 177
normalization
as primary benefit of massage, 15
Soft tissue approximation end-feel, 276
Sole proprietorship, 70-71
Somatic motor nerves
definition of, 148
Somatic nervous system
anatomy, physiology and massage, 148-150
Somatic pain, 483
Somatic sensory nerves, 148
Somatoform disorders, 557b
Spastic cerebral palsy, 639
Specific release techniques
anterior serratus muscles, 367-368, 368f
deep lateral hip rotators, 373-374
diaphragm, 368-369
Specific release techniques *(Continued)*
focused massage applications for, 360-363, 364f, 365-375, 376f-377f, 378
groin muscles, 373-374
hamstrings, 363, 364f-365f
hips, 374-375, 376f, 377f, 378
multifidi, rotators, intertransversarii, and interspinales, 363, 364, 366f
the occipital base, 361
pelvic alignment, 375, 377f, 378
the psoas, 370-371, 372f
quadratus lumborum, 373
rectus abdominis, 362-363
sacroiliac joint, 374-375, 376f
the scalenes, 360-361
the sternocleidomastoid muscles, 362
subscapularis, 365-367
Speech impairments
interacting with patients with, 575
with stroke, 635-636
Speed
guidelines for massage, 137t
of joint movement, 222
of manipulation
massage guidelines for, 210-211
Spinal cord
anatomy, physiology and massage, 147
curvatures of, 267f, 269, 270f
diagram illustrating, 643f
injuries, 642-643
levels of possible injury to, 643f
neurological diseases of, 634-639
and pain, 484
Spinal cord injuries
description and massage strategies, 642-644
and fibromyalgia, 610
Spinal manipulation
for back pain, 602
Spinal meningitis
and back pain, 596
Spinal nerves
anatomy and physiology of, 147-148, 642-650
diagram illustrating, 644f
Spinal stenosis, 597
Spine
anatomy, physiology and massage, 147
curvatures of, 267f, 269, 270f
observation and palpation of, 272, 273f-274f
and osteoporosis, 545f
Spiral form, 175, 176f
Spirilla, 199
Spiritual health
and healing, 105-106
Spleen
meridians relating to, 356f, 357b
percentage of water in, 160t
Splinting contractions, 186
Spondyloarthropathies, 510b
Spores, 199
Sports
and back pain, 596
Sprains
chronic pain with, 486
pain associated with, 262-263
Springy block end-feel, 276
Spurs, 179
Squat assessment, 272
Stability
assessment of, 265, 271f-272f
procedure for testing, 275
Stabilizers
muscles functioning as, 269
Stacking of joints, 239-240, 241f-244f
Stamina
assessing during examination, 265
Stance phase
components of gait, 291f
Standard Precautions
Centers for Disease Control and Prevention (CDC) on, 200-206

Standard treatment control groups, 42
Standing orders, 253
Statistical analysis, 36-37
Statistical power, 37
Statistics
  and parameters, 36
  in research, 24-25
Status migraine, 621
Stem cells, 168
Sternocleidomastoid muscles
  shortening with breathing pattern disorders, 478-479
  specific release techniques, 362
Stomach
  meridians relating to, 356f, 357b
Strains
  microtrauma, 269, 272
  muscle, 176-177
  pain associated with, 262-263
Stranger anxiety, 558
Strength testing
  assessing during examination, 265
  muscles, 278-280
  procedure for, 274-275, 278-280
Stress
  benefits of massage for, 121-122
  common responses to, 90b
  definition of, 88
  external factors related to, 89-90
  and fibromyalgia, 610
  management outcomes for massage, 122-123
  mechanical and repetitive, 177-178
  and movement, 269
  physiology of, 90
  and posture, 266, 267f, 268-269
Stress fractures
  definition of, 597
  illustration of, 598f
Stress responses
  list of common, 90b, 345b
Stressors, 88
Stretching
  definition of, 234
  before exercise, 97-98
  and gait improvement, 293
  illustration of, 238f-239f
  longitudinal, 236-237
  massage application technique, 234-237
  and pain management, 494
  before sleep, 103
  techniques and movements, 234-237, 238f-239f
Stroke
  description of, 634-635
  and inflammation, 500
  massage strategies for, 636
  rehabilitation for, 635-636
  related to chronic inflammation, 125t
  warning signs of, 636
Stroking techniques
  increasing venous flow, 165, 169
  for lymph flow, 319f
  for lymphatic drainage, 324f
Stuttering
  case study on, 681-682, 687-693
Subluxations
  description of, 67-68
  and nerve root compression, 645
Subscapularis
  specific release techniques, 365-367
Superficial second-degree burns, 499
Supination, 188-189
Support systems
  and geriatric massage, 553-554
Surgery
  for back pain, 602-603
  cancer, 628-629
  common procedures and terminology, 517b
  definition of, 516
  exercise regimens benefiting, 529t
Surgery *(Continued)*
  general categories of
    arthroscopic, 517-518
    laparoscopic, 516
    open procedure, 516
  massage following, 518-519
  for pain, 489
  types of, 516, 517b
Surgical complications
  related to chronic inflammation, 125t
Surgical decompression, 517b
Susceptible host, 200
Swayback posture, 267f
Sweat
  water loss from, 160t
Swing phase
  components of gait, 292f-293f
Symmetry
  diagram of areas of, 310f
  landmarks that identify lack of, 268b
Sympathetic dominance
  reduced
    as primary benefit of massage, 15
Sympathetic nervous system
  anatomy, physiology and massage, 153
  organs affected by, 154t
Symptoms
  descriptive words for assessing, 263-264
Synapses, 144
Synergist muscle, 185
Synergistic dominance, 193, 283
Synovial joints, 182, 350, 352, 353f
Synovial membrane, 181-182
Systemic lupus erythematosus
  as autoimmune disorder, 504, 509, 510b
  and pregnancy, 693-705
  related to chronic inflammation, 125t
Systolic pressure
  definition of, 165-166

T

Tachycardia, 166
Tachypnea, 174
Tai ji quan, 358
Targeting fluid movement
  focused massage applications for, 326-327
T-cells, 496-498
Temporal arteritis, 510b
Tendonitis, 302, 486
Tendons
  and back pain, 596-607
  description of, 143
  general massage protocols for
    abdomen, 387f, 396, 398-400
    anterior torso, 387f, 396, 398-400
    approach and sequence, 382, 383f
    arms, 409, 410f, 411-414
    face and head, 382-388
    forearms, wrists and hands, 414-416
    hips, 416, 417f, 418-421
    legs, ankles and feet, 426, 427f, 428
    neck, 392, 393f, 394-396
    occipital base, 388-392
    posterior torso, 400-405
    shoulders, 405-409
    thighs, 421, 422f, 423-426
  injuries to, 177-178
  palpation of, 302
Tenoperiosteal junction
  description and illustration of, 179
Tense and relax, 227, 229f
Tensegrity, 175
Tensile forces, 211, 213
Tension
  breathing pattern disorder causing, 476
  forces
    definition of, 213, 214
    illustration of, 215f-216f

Tension *(Continued)*
muscle
and posture, 279
and soft tissue, 175-177
Tension headaches
massage strategies for, 614f-617f, 623-624
Terminal illnesses
anorexia, 587
cancer, 630
challenge of massage with, 583
elimination/ constipation issues, 587
massage during, 590
mouth care, 587
pain management, 586-587
population similarities in, 583-591
Terminology
surgical, 517b
Testing
kinetic chain protocol, 296b-297b
means, 71
muscle-strength, 278-280
range of motion (ROM)
active, 223-224
assessment of, 265, 275-276
degrees of, 277f
interpreting, 277-278
joint movement method, 222-225
measurement of, 274, 276-277
shoulders, 405f, 406-409
resistance, 275
stability, 275
two-joint muscle, 278b
Therapeutic massage;*See* massage
Thighs
general massage protocols, 421, 422f, 423-426
illustration of important structures, 422f
palliative protocol for, 430
Third-party payers, 80
Thoracic kyphosis
description of, 456-457
Thoracic spine
illustration of, 366f
and posture and gravity, 267f, 268
Thoracic surgery, 517b
Throat
assessment of, 255
Thrombocytopenia
as chemotherapy side effect, 629-630
Thrombophlebitis, 608
Thyroid diseases
massage strategies for, 509-510
Tidal volume, 170
Tightness-prone stabilizer muscles, 190b
Tinea, 199
Tissue movement methods
focused massage applications for, 343-350, 351f-352f
Tissue stretch end-feel, 276
Tissues
and aging process, 538
general massage protocols for connective
abdomen, 387f, 396, 398-400
anterior torso, 387f, 396, 398-400
approach and sequence, 382, 383f
arms, 409, 410f, 411-414
face and head, 382-388
forearms, wrists and hands, 414-416
hips, 416, 417f, 418-421
legs, ankles and feet, 426, 427f, 428
neck, 392, 393f, 394-396
occipital base, 388-392
posterior torso, 400-405
shoulders, 405-409
thighs, 421, 422f, 423-426
movement techniques, 343-350, 351f-352f
percentage of water in, 160t
pliability
assessing during examination, 265
seven layers of, 135, 136f
stages of healing associated with massage, 119t, 498
Toddlers
illustration of massage for, 569f
and infants
massage for, 571-573
Tonic/ postural stabilizing muscles, 190
Tonic-clonic seizures, 638
Touch
importance for older adults, 555
and pain relief, 485
qualities of
photographs illustrating, 212f-213f
techniques and movements, 210-211, 212f-213f
and sensory nerves, 148-149
and wellness, 104
Toxic effects, 523
Traditional Chinese medicine (TCM)
Asian massage
acupuncture and acupressure, 355, 356f, 357b, 358
focused massage applications for, 355-356, 357b, 358-359
meridians, 355-356, 357b
Yin and Yang theory, 355
and complementary and alternative medicine, 7
Traditional medicine
integration with complementary, 11, 12b
Trager, Milton, 7
Training
by complementary medicine practitioners
in professional practice model, 12b
Training stimulus threshold, 99
Transcutaneous electrical nerve stimulation (TENS), 488-489
Transient ischemic attack (TIAs), 635-636
Transplantation, 517b
Transverse plane
movement, 225f, 271f
rotational movement, 187, 188f
Trauma
brain, 461-462, 636-637
causes of, 460-461
definition of, 121
and inflammation, 499
Traumatic brain injuries
description of, 461-462
symptoms and treatment of, 636-637
Traumatic injuries, 461-462, 499, 636-637
Traumatic stress
definition of, 562-563
Treatment; *See also* massage; treatment plans
in case studies, 680
focused massage applications
Asian massage concepts, 355-356, 357b, 358-359
circulatory system, 318-323, 324f
connective tissue, 340, 341f, 342-344
fluid dynamics, 317-318
functional techniques, 316-317
increasing arterial circulation, 327-329
joint play, 350, 352
lymphatic drainage, 329-330, 331f-334f, 335-338, 339f, 340
lymphatic system, 318-323, 324f
motor tone inhibition techniques, 360-363, 364f, 365-375, 376f-377f, 378
pin and stretch, 343-344
reflexology, 352-355
specific release methods, 360-363, 364f, 365-375, 376f-377f, 378
targeting fluid movement, 326-327
tissue movement methods, 343-350, 351f-352f
trigger points, 344-350, 351f-352f
venous return, 329
goal patterns for massage, 118-121, 250
of illnesses and injuries
cancer, 628-629
drug therapy and massage interaction, 526b-527b
flexibility techniques, 531
massage strategies, 464-465
massage therapy supporting, 515, 518-520, 531
nutrition, mental health and lifestyle, 531
pharmacology for massage, 520-521, 523-525, 526b-527b
physical medicine, 525, 528-532
surgery, 516-520
and therapeutic exercise, 528, 529t, 530

Treatment *(Continued)*
methods for trigger points, 345-350
mind and spirit aspect of, 6-7
Treatment goals
importance of defining, 250
Treatment orders
during massage assessment process, 252-253
Treatment plans
algorithm for developing, 309f
in case studies, 680
description of, 252
development
and clinical reasoning process, 660-661
during massage assessment process, 309-312
Trigeminal neuralgia, 486
Trigger points
active and latent, 346b
assessment of, 347
definition of, 344-345
diagram illustrating common, 348f, 351f-352f
in fibromyalgia, 487b
focused massage applications for, 344-350, 351f-352f
general massage protocols for, 387f, 396, 398-400
myofascial, 345f
and pain management, 494
palpation of, 300-304, 347b
perpetuating factors, 346-347
in shoulder, 408
theory of formation, 346b
treatment methods, 345-350
Triple-heater (TH)
meridians relating to, 356f, 357b
True experimental (RCT) research method
case example, 30-39, 40f
example of, 30-39, 40f
randomized controlled trials, 44-45
schematic illustration of, 39, 40f
Trunk
flexion, 284b
observation and palpation of, 272, 273f-274f
Tumor necrosis factor (TNF), 498
Tumors
cancer, 627
as massage contraindication, 130-131
Two-joint muscle testing, 278b
Type 1 error, 36

U
Ulcerative colitis, 510b
Unrelieved pain, 493t
Upper crossed syndrome
flowchart of, 191f
Upper trapezius
shortening with breathing pattern disorders, 478-479
Urinary incontinence
in older adults, 551-552
Urinary system
assessment of, 255
and geriatric massage, 551-552
sympathetic and parasympathetic response, 154t
Urination
and fibromyalgia, 610
Urine
and kidney disease, 631-632
water loss from, 160t
Urogenital surgery, 517b

V
Vagus nerve stimulator, 638
Values conflicts, 76
Variables
definition and example of, 24-25, 32
Varicose veins
massage contraindicated for, 131
Vascular cell adhesion molecule-1 (VCAM-1), 500
Vascular dementia, 567
Vascular headaches, 613-614, 619f-620f, 620-623
Vascular resistance, 167
Vascular system
and entrainment, 156
phase of inflammation, 501
Vasculitis, 510b
Vasculitis syndromes, 510
Veins
circulation, 164-165, 324-326
of face and head, 384f
sympathetic and parasympathetic response, 154t
Venous circulation, 164-165, 324-326
Venous return
examples of massage for, 330f
focused massage applications for, 329
maintaining, 164
supporting, 329
Venous system
benefits of massage for, 164-165
Ventilation, 474
Ventricles
definition of, 165-166
Venules, 165
Vertebrae
stress fractures, 598f
Vestibular apparatus, 151
Veterans, 71-72, 562-563
Vibration
methods of
principles and benefits of, 439-440
and pain relief, 485
technique of, 217f, 220
Viral infections
description and inflammation with, 625-626
and fibromyalgia, 610
massage contraindicated for, 129
transmission of, 198-199
Viruses;*See* viral infections
Visceral pain, 483
Visceral sensory nerves, 148
Viscosity
definition of fluid, 167
Vision
and aging, 549-550
assessing during examination, 265
Vision impairment
and geriatric massage, 549-550
interacting with patients with, 575
population similarities in, 575
Visualization, 91, 467
Vital capacity, 170
Vital signs
physical examination of, 255-256
Vitamins, 521, 523
Vitiligo, 510b

W
Waist
observation and palpation of, 272, 273f-274f
Waiting-list control groups, 42
Water; *See also* fluid dynamics
content in body, 159, 160t
function in human body, 159b
importance of drinking, 96
loss from organs, 160t
Weight transfer
of massage therapist, 239, 241f-244f
Wellness
components of
behaviors, 104
breathing, 96-97, 98f
demands, 94-95
loss, 95
mind/body relationship, 103-106
nutrition, 95-96
physical fitness, 97, 99-101
relaxation, 101-102
sleep, 102-103
defining in whole person, 88, 94
questions regarding, 262

Wellness programs
  growing popularity of, 6
White blood cells, 168, 496-498
White matter, 145
Whole person
  defining wellness in, 88
  emphasis on, 8
  philosophy in naturopathic medicine, 65
Withdrawal reflexes, 186
Within-subjects independent variables, 43-44
Wong-Baker FACES pain rating scale, 262f
Word repetition, 91
Wounds
  and clinical reasoning process, 652-656, 657f-658f
Wrists
  general massage protocols, 414-416
  illustration of, 415f

Y

Yield point, 461
Yin and Yang theory
  Asian massage, 355
  illustration of meridian locations, 356f, 357b
Yoga, 381